Fibromyalgia & Other Central Pain Syndromes

Fibromyalgia & Other Central Pain Syndromes

Editors

Daniel J. Wallace, MD
Clinical Professor of Medicine
David Geffen School of Medicine
University of California—Los Angeles
Attending Physician
Cedars-Sinai Medical Center
Los Angeles, California

Daniel J. Clauw, MD
Professor of Medicine
Division of Rheumatology
Assistant Dean
Clinical and Translational Research
Director
Chronic Pain and Fatigue Research Center
University of Michigan Medical School
Ann Arbor, Michigan

LIPPINCOTT WILLIAMS & WILKINS
A **Wolters Kluwer** Company
Philadelphia • Baltimore • New York • London
Buenos Aires • Hong Kong • Sydney • Tokyo

Acquisitions Editor: Sonya Seigafuse
Developmental Editor: Julia Seto
Project Manager: Nicole Walz
Senior Manufacturing Manager: Ben Rivera
Senior Marketing Manager: Kathy Neely
Creative Director: Doug Smock
Cover Designer: Karen Kappe
Production Services: Laserwords Private Limited
Printer: Edwards Brothers

Library of Congress Cataloging-in-Publication Data

Fibromyalgia and other central pain syndromes / editors, Daniel J. Wallace, Daniel J. Clauw.–1st ed.
   p. ; cm.
  Includes bibliographical references and index.
  ISBN 0-7817-5261-2
   1. Fibromyalgia. 2. Myofascial pain syndromes. 3. Chronic pain.
I. Wallace, Daniel J. (Daniel Jeffrey), 1949- II. Clauw, Daniel J. [DNLM:
1. Fibromyalgia--physiopathology. 2. Central Nervous System--physiopathology.
3. Chronic Disease. 4. Pain--physiopathology. WE 544 F4414 2005]
RC927.3.F518 2005
616.7'42--dc22

2005002006

Care has been taken to confirm the accuracy of the information presented and to describe generally accepted practices. However, the authors, editors, and publisher are not responsible for errors or omissions or for any consequences from application of the information in this book and make no warranty, expressed or implied, with respect to the currency, completeness, or accuracy of the contents of the publication. Application of this information in a particular situation remains the professional responsibility of the practitioner.

The authors, editors, and publisher have exerted every effort to ensure that drug selection and dosage set forth in this text are in accordance with current recommendations and practice at the time of publication. However, in view of ongoing research, changes in government regulations, and the constant flow of information relating to drug therapy and drug reactions, the reader is urged to check the package insert for each drug for any change in indications and dosage and for added warnings and precautions. This is particularly important when the recommended agent is a new or infrequently employed drug.

Some drugs and medical devices presented in this publication have Food and Drug Administration (FDA) clearance for limited use in restricted research settings. It is the responsibility of health care providers to ascertain the FDA status of each drug or device planned for use in their clinical practice.

The publishers have made every effort to trace copyright holders for borrowed material. If they have inadvertently overlooked any, they will be pleased to make the necessary arrangements at the first opportunity.

To purchase additional copies of this book, call our customer service department at (800) 638-3030 or fax orders to (301) 824-7390. Lippincott Williams & Wilkins customer service representatives are available from 8:30 am to 6:30 pm, EST, Monday through Friday, for telephone access. Visit Lippincott Williams & Wilkins on the Internet: http://www.lww.com.

10 9 8 7 6 5 4 3 2 1

PREFACE

As practitioners of rheumatology, a craft that encompasses 150 disorders of the musculoskeletal and immune systems, our denizens have been responsible for many classic textbooks that embody increased understanding of the discipline. These encompass *Arthritis and Allied Conditions, Dubois' Lupus Erythematosus,* and *Kelley's Textbook of Rheumatology,* among others. In the last decade seminal works pertaining to rheumatoid arthritis, osteoporosis, scleroderma, and the spondyloarthropathies have appeared. Up to now, however, no textbook on fibromyalgia has been published. It is now time to correct this oversight. Fibromyalgia is the second or third most common reason for referral to a rheumatologist, and it ranks high in new patient visits to other musculoskeletal specialists. Fifteen billion dollars are spent annually in the United States diagnosing and treating fibromyalgia. We now have a statistically validated definition for the syndrome, epidemiologic surveys have been published, its etiopathogenesis is being elucidated, and in the last decade a body of work has been published relating to fibromyalgia that is firmly evidence-based. We realize that fibromyalgia is a syndrome and not a disease, that some of our colleagues believe that labeling patients as such stigmatizes them, and that there is a significant overlay with other pain and behavioral conditions. This effort serves to be a compendium of the rapidly growing knowledge base relating to fibromyalgia and centrally mediated pain syndromes and is meant to serve rheumatology, other musculoskeletal specialties, allied health professionals, and basic science investigators in their quest to understand and improve the management of this often mysterious syndrome.

The authors would like to thank Julia Seto and Danette Sommers at Lippincott Williams & Wilkins for their encouragement and assistance. Dr. Wallace wishes to acknowledge Janice, Phil, Sarah, and Naomi Wallace and Jody Stanley for their support. Dr. Clauw would like to thank his family, his numerous colleagues at the Chronic Pain and Fatigue Research Center, and patients with fibromyalgia and related conditions, who have and continue to provide tremendous inspiration for research into these conditions.

Daniel J. Wallace
Daniel J. Clauw
Los Angeles, California
Ann Arbor, Michigan

October, 2004

CONTRIBUTING AUTHORS

Graciela S. Alarcón, MD, MPH
Professor of Medicine
Jane Knight Lowe Chair of Medicine in Rheumatology
Department of Medicine-Clinical Immunology and
    Rheumatology
University of Alabama at Birmingham
Birmingham, Alabama

Lesley M. Arnold, MD
Associate Professor
Department of Psychiatry
University of Cincinnati College of Medicine
Cincinnati, Ohio

Robert Bennett MD, FRCP
Professor of Medicine
Department of Medicine
Oregon Health & Science University
Portland, Oregon

Rafael Benoliel, BDS(Hons), LDS RCS Eng
Senior Lecturer
Department of Oral Medicine
The Hebrew University
Jerusalem, Israel

Chairman
Department of Oral Medicine
Hadassah
Jerusalem, Israel

Stephanie A. Bolling, MS, PT, OCS
Physical Therapy Specialist
Cedars–Sinai Medical Center
Los Angeles, California

Laurence A. Bradley, PhD
Professor of Medicine
Jane Knight Lowe Chair of Medicine in Rheumatology
Department of Medicine-Clinical
Immunology and Rheumatology
University of Alabama at Birmingham
Birmingham, Alabama

Lin Chang, MD
Associate Professor of Medicine
David Geffen School of Medicine
University of California—Los Angeles
Los Angeles, California

Co-Director
Center for Neurovisceral Science and Women's Health
David Geffen School of Medicine
University of California—Los Angeles
Los Angeles, California

Lan Chen MD, PhD
Clinical Assistant Professor
University of Pennsylvania School of Medicine
Philadelphia, Pennsylvania

Attending Physician
University of Pennsylvania Medical
    Center-Presbyterian
Philadelphia, Pennsylvania

Daniel J. Clauw, MD
Professor of Medicine
Division of Rheumatology
Assistant Dean
Clinical and Translational Research
Director
Chronic Pain and Fatigue Research Center
University of Michigan Medical School
Ann Arbor, Michigan

Leslie J. Crofford, MD
Professor
Department of Internal Medicine
University of Kentucky
Lexington, Kentucky

Chief
Division of Rheumatology
Gloria W. Singletary Chair and Director
Women's Health Program
University of Kentucky
Lexington, Kentucky

Atul Deodhar, MD, MRCP
Associate Professor of Medicine
Division of Arthritis & Rheumatic Diseases
Oregon Health & Science University
Portland, Oregon

Medical Director
Rheumatology Clinic
Oregon Health & Science University
Portland, Oregon

Eli Eliav, DMD, MSc, PhD
Associate Professor
Carmel Endowed Chair in Algesiology
Department of Diagnostic Sciences
New Jersey Dental School
University of Medicine and Dentistry of New Jersey
Newark, New Jersey

Edzard Ernst, MD, PhD, FRCP, FRCPEd
Professor
Director and Laing Chair in Complementary Medicine
Department of Complementary Medicine
Peninsula Medical School
Universities of Exeter & Plymouth
Exeter, United Kingdom

Michael E. Geisser, PhD
Associate Professor
Department of Physical Medicine and
    Rehabilitation
University of Michigan Medical School
Ann Arbor, Michigan

Thorsten Giesecke, MD
Junior Faculty
Faculty of Medicine
University of Cologne
Cologne, Germany

Assistant Medical Director
Pain Clinic
Department of Anesthesiology
University Hospital of Cologne
Cologne, Germany

Jodi Goldman-Knaub PT
Physical Therapy Specialist
Department of Rehabilitation Medicine
The Veterans Administration Medical Center
Philadelphia, Pennsylvania

Owner/Director
Breakthru Physical Therapy
Medford, New Jersey

Richard H. Gracely, PhD
Professor
Department of Rheumatology and Neurology
University of Michigan Medical School
Ann Arbor, Michigan

Ann Arbor Veteran's Administration
    Medical Center
Ann Arbor, Michigan

David S. Hallegua, MD
Assistant Professor
Division of Rheumatology
David Geffen School of Medicine
University of California—Los Angeles
Los Angeles, California

Consultant
Division of Rheumatology
Cedars-Sinai Medical Center
Los Angeles, California

Lucinda A. Harris, MS, MD
Senior Associate Consultant
Division of Gastroenterology and Hepatology
Mayo Clinic—Scottsdale
Scottsdale, Arizona

Arash A. Horizon, MD, FACR
Clinical Instructor
David Geffen School of Medicine
University of California—Los Angeles
Los Angeles, California

Attending Staff
Division of Rheumatology
Cedars-Sinai Medical Center
Los Angeles, California

Maura Daly Iversen, MPH, DPT, SD
Professor
Associate Director
Graduate Programs in Physical Therapy
Massachusetts General Hospital Institute of Health
    Professions
Charlestown, Massachusetts

Instructor in Medicine
Brigham & Women's Hospital
Division of Rheumatology, Immunology & Allergy
Boston, Massachusetts

Franklin Kozin, MD
Staff Physician
Department of Rheumatology
Scripps Clinic Medical Group
La Jolla, California

James G. MacFarlane PhD, Dip ABSM
Assistant Professor of Psychiatry
Department of Psychiatry
University of Toronto
Toronto, Canada

Lab Director
Sleep Disorders Clinic
Centre for Sleep & Chronobiology
Toronto, Canada

Kaisa Mannerkorpi PhD, PT
Research Associate
Department of Rheumatology
Göteborg University
Göteborg, Sweden

Physical Therapist
Department of Physiotherapy
Sahlgrenska University Hospital
Göteborg, Sweden

Susan A. Martin, MSPH
Director
Outcomes Research
Pfizer Inc.
Ann Arbor, Michigan

Manuel Martinez-Lavin
Full Professor
Department of Rheumatology
National Autonomous University of Mexico
Mexico City, Mexico

Head
Department of Rheumatology
National Institute of Cardiology
Mexico City, Mexico

John McBeth, MA, PhD
Lecturer
ARC Epidemiology Unit
University of Manchester
Manchester, United Kingdom

Samuel A. McLean, MD, MPH
Department of Emergency Medicine
University of Michigan Medical School
Ann Arbor, Michigan

Harvey Moldofsky MD, Dip Psych, FRCP(C), FAPA
Professor Emeritus
Faculty of Medicine
University of Toronto
Toronto, Canada

Sleep Disorders Clinic
Centre for Sleep & Chronobiology
Toronto, Canada

Sally Pullman-Mooar MD, FACP, FACR
Clinical Associate Professor
Division of Rheumatology
University of Pennsylvania School
    of Medicine
Philadelphia, Pennsylvania

Staff Rheumatologist
Department of Medicine
Philadelphia Veterans Administration
    Medical Center
Philadelphia, Pennsylvania

I. Jon Russell, MD, PhD
Associate Professor of Medicine
Department of Medicine—Division Clinical
    Immunology and Rheumatology
Director
University Clinical Research Center
University of Texas Health Science Centerat
    San Antonio
San Antonio, Texas

Medical Staff
Department of Rheumatology
University Hospital Medical Center
San Antonio, Texas

Medical Attending Physician
Consultant Rheumatologist
Audie Murphy South Texas Veterans
    Medical Center
San Antonio, Texas

David D. Sherry, MD
Professor
Department of Pediatrics
University of Pennsylvania School of Medicine
Philadelphia, Pennsylvania

Director
Clinical Rheumatology
Attending Physician
Chronic Pain Clinic
Department of Pediatrics
The Children's Hospital of Philadelphia
Philadelphia, Pennsylvania

Stuart L. Silverman, MD
Clinical Professor of Medicine
Division of Rheumatology
David Geffen School of Medicine
University of California—Los Angeles

Division of Rheumatology
Cedars-Sinai Medical Center
Los Angeles, California

Hugh A. Smythe, MD, FRCPC
Professor
Department of Medicine
University of Toronto
Toronto, Canada

Consultant
Department of Medicine
Toronto Western Hospital
Toronto, Canada

Haiko Sprott, MD
Privatdozent
Medical Faculty
University of Zurich
Zurich, Switzerland

Senior Physician
Department of Rheumatology
Institute of Physical Medicine
University Hospital Zurich
Zurich, Switzerland

Roland Staud, MD
Professor of Medicine
Department of Medicine
University of Florida
Gainesville, Florida

Department of Medicine
Shands Hospital
Gainesville, Florida

Thomas M. Susko, MD
Assistant Clinical Professor of Medicine
Department of Rheumatology
Cedars-Sinai Medical Center
Los Angeles, California

Medical Staff
Department of Medicine
Saint John's Health Center
Santa Monica, California

Swamy Venuturupalli, MD, FACR
Attending Rheumatologist
Clinical Instructor of Medicine
Division of Rheumatology
David Geffen School of Medicine
University of California—Los Angeles
Los Angeles, California

Attending Physician
Division of Rheumatology
Cedars-Sinai Medical Center
Los Angeles, California

Daniel J. Wallace, MD, FACP, FACR
Clinical Professor of Medicine
David Geffen School of Medicine
University of California—Los Angeles
Los Angeles, California

Attending Physician
Division of Rheumatology
Cedars-Sinai Medical Center
Los Angeles, California

Michael H. Weisman, MD
Professor of Medicine
David Geffen School of Medicine
University of California—Los Angeles
Los Angeles, California

Director
Division of Rheumatology
Cedars-Sinai Medical Center
Los Angeles, California

Kevin P. White, MD, PhD
President and CEO
Clinical Trials Design, Inc.
London, Canada

Rheumatologist
London, Canada

David A. Williams, PhD
Associate Professor
Department of Internal Medicine-Rheumatology
University of Michigan Medical School
Ann Arbor, Michigan

Muhammad B. Yunus, MD, FACP, FACR, FRCP Edin
Professor of Medicine
Section of Rheumatology
University of Illinois College of Medicine at Peoria
Peoria, Illinois

CONTENTS

INTRODUCTION TO FIBROMYALGIA AND RELATED PROBLEMS

Hugh A. Smythe

Each generation believes that it has invented sex; similarly, each generation of rheumatologists has to rediscover the burden of fibromyalgia and related syndromes. The understanding of the nature of fibromyalgia has developed in a stuttering fashion, with contributions from many generations of medical scientists. Some of this understanding may even be lost before the next surge. The pace of advances has quickened since the publication of the 1990 *Criteria for the Classification of Fibromyalgia*. What has been learned has filled a book—this book—but we have not yet achieved consensus on causes and treatment strategies. Meanwhile, certain historic insights have been lost over the Internet horizon. My role is not only to celebrate the achievements of my colleagues but also to fill in some gaps.

There are many problems, but I will begin with two. The first is that many rheumatologists are not doing tender point counts. They are not only missing fibromyalgia but are also missing concomitant fibromyalgia. This is of special concern at this time because powerful, new biologic therapies are becoming available, and aggressive therapies are being advocated in early stages of disease. The patients being entered in large-scale trials are those who are still symptomatic after conventional therapies. This selection process will enrich such studies with patients with both rheumatoid arthritis and fibromyalgia (RA/FM). Dr. Wolfe estimated that 17.1% of the 11,886 patients referred by rheumatologists to The National Data Bank for Rheumatic Diseases for participation in therapeutic trials had (previously unrecognized) fibromyalgia-like features. The diagnosis was based on a questionnaire, and Dr. Wolfe argued that tender point counts were unnecessary. In "unresponsive" patients with RA, referred by rheumatologists to tertiary care centers, this diagnosis may be an underestimate of the selection bias favoring the referral of patients with RA/FM. My colleagues had earlier performed extensive studies of tenderness in several patient groups. Using dolorimetry as well as standard tender point counts, we found that 25 of the 51 referred subjects with RA met the American College of Rheumatology (ACR) criteria for fibromyalgia, as compared to 10 subjects in each of the groups with psoriatic arthritis ($n = 50$) and acquired immunodeficiency syndrome ($n = 51$). A similarly high prevalence of concomitant fibromyalgia was found in patients with lupus and were reported in many other diseases.

Patients with RA/FM should not be denied entry into controlled trials, but the disease should be recognized before the patient's entry by using appropriate and standard criteria, and their response to treatment should be followed and appropriate outcome measures should be similarly predefined. There is evidence that cytokines that are active in the inflammatory response are also active as pain messengers in the central nervous system, but we may hesitate to use powerful immunosuppressive therapies in patients with only mild RA but with severe pain and fatigue of other origin. These concerns have been expressed by others. It should also be noted that many questionnaires designed to measure the activity of RA are seriously misleading in the presence of fibromyalgia, so that joint tenderness and reported "swelling" do not reliably predict the presence of synovial inflammation or effusions.

The second major problem is that many rheumatologists do not understand the significance of the tender sites. It is assumed that reported tenderness equates with reported pain. The most valuable sites are those that are remote from the areas of perceived pain. It can also be helpful when the regions of perceived pain are *not* tender, particularly as a clinical change in patients beginning to respond to therapy. These situations need not have anything to do with fibromyalgia and is more often relevant to regional pain problems.

What is FM? It seems that many rheumatologists do not know the answer! Yet it is so simple in all its fundamental aspects—FM is referred pain and the amplifying factors. The pain is of deep, somatic origin. The areas where the referred pain is perceived are innocent, and the source of the pain is unknown to the patient and to many health professionals too. There are many referred pain syndromes, and the subgroup labeled FM is at the more severe end of the pain spectrum and is complicated further by fatigue, physical deconditioning, and other symptoms. If you understand referred pain, you know 90% of fibromyalgia pathogenesis, assessment, and treatment. If you understand the amplifying factors, you know 50% of fibromyalgia pathogenesis, but only 20% of that needed for effective treatment. Referred pain interacts with amplification factors.

The remarkable evolution of human brain function occurred very recently, perhaps 50,000 years ago. We developed the ability to think in abstract terms and to use language and symbols to understand and transmit new concepts to our friends and offspring. It is fascinating that the earliest evidences of high-level use of symbols by modern humans are artistic; the cave paintings in southern France and Spain, about 30,000 years old, show color, shading, perspective, and motion…not just things. Agriculture, architecture, alphabets, and algebra came much later.

But we still cannot feel the deep structures of our body, and specifically the bones deep in the low neck and low back. These structures were not included in the famous map of the sensory cortex constructed by Penfield. They are not included in Kellgren's "body image." My consultation letters must begin: "It may be helpful to preview the findings at today's examination. There are major mechanical problems in the lowest part of the lower cervical and lumbar spine, problems which have not been specifically identified and dealt with in the treatment program to date." The details of the findings are then reviewed, and the treatment program follows. I often do not need the label "fibromyalgia," but do need tender point counts.

Kellgren's experimental work on referred pain must be rediscovered. He later suggested that "this false localization over muscles has been responsible for old concepts such as 'fibrositis,'" but he left us with no clinical strategy to test this hypothesis. He did, however, describe the "The deep tender spot, frequently lies outside the distribution of the pain, …the patient is not aware of its existence until it is discovered by the physician." This is clearly distinguished from the more diffuse tenderness to be found in regions to which pain is referred. Let me now jump to the very specific set of 24 tender sites (and 6 control sites) studied, 18 of which were incorporated in the *American College of Rheumatology 1990 Criteria for the Classification of Fibromyalgia.* Many of these sites, such as midtrapezius, suboccipital, scapular, and buttock sites, lie in regions to which pain is commonly referred, and are of use only when they are not tender. By contrast, low anterior cervical and medial knee tenderness (and other sites) are located in regions where there is no local pain, so that "the patient is not aware of its existence until it is discovered by the physician." This finding, and interactions among sleep disturbance, pain, and tenderness described by Moldofsky, were all objective findings available in the 1970s and reproduced by all who cared to look for these findings.

The patients often state that they have "pain all over." This is not correct. The symptom patterns are characteristic. In the upper body, referred symptoms (pain or pain equivalents such as numbness, tingling, tightness, stiffness, and swelling) may affect the forehead, eyes, jaw (the distribution of the first division of the trigeminal nerve), the back of neck, anterior chest (cervical nerves), the trapezius (spinal accessory nerves), other muscles that control the shoulders, as well as the arm, forearm, hand and fingers (not the tongue, nor the nipples, both of which are sensitive and are well represented in the cortex). The distribution of symptoms clearly cannot be explained by the anatomy of a single nerve or segment. The organizing principle is the neurology of eye–hand coordination, which has evolved spectacularly over 4 million years. Even the symptom of "dizziness" is consistent; it is a momentary unsteadiness rather than a spinning sensation.

Our bony structure has changed, along with the controlling neurology. Some of us can throw or hit a baseball or play a musical instrument; but we cannot sleep in the fetal position without, at some time, developing symptoms mentioned in the preceding text. We have long clavicles and broad shoulders. When we lie on our side, the lower shoulder tends to rise toward our cheek, so that the delivery of reliable support to the low neck is blocked.

We need to revisit the C6-7 syndrome. With a variety of neck support strategies during sleep, 151 subjects (91 with prior FM) had lost all of the previously marked tenderness in the upper body sites listed in the 1990 criteria set, but they remained symptomatic. They had a new pattern of tenderness. Now, there was a striking referred tenderness at the medial rather than the lateral elbow, and at the origin and insertion of pectoralis minor, from the fifth rib behind the outer breast to the tip and to the medial aspect of the coracoid process. (Clinical advice: ask a female patient to move the breast centrally before examining the lateral pectoral site.) This pattern was linked with marked tenderness in the bones and attached structures adjacent to the C6–7 disk but not at the C5–6 level. The distribution was commonly asymmetric, with strong correlations among the sites on the affected side. To recover, the patients had to learn precisely where the pain arose, and precisely how it had to be treated, none of which was intuitively apparent.

Apart from the coracoid tip, all of these sites were included among the 24 defined sites in the studies leading to the ACR criteria definition. These sites were dropped as redundant, or in the interests of delicacy. None of the sites are central to the areas of perceived pain. The symptoms related to the lateral pectoral site were 8 to 10 cm lower, near the rib margin or the "hypochondrium." Concerns about heart attacks were common, and at least seven of my patients had normal gallbladders removed.

Note also that the tender sites were a much more helpful guide to the specific site of origin of the symptoms than were the pain patterns. This is also their role in the study of regional pain patterns. Many athletes would be spared unnecessary and unhelpful surgical procedures if the examination of tender sites were understood to be essential in any patient with a pain problem.

In the lower body, analogous patterns of symptoms in patients are found. Diskography in the lumbar spine had earlier demonstrated the pain patterns referred from the lower spine. The most common areas of reference were to the low lumbar and trochanteric regions, but the spread of pain to the lower extremity, even as far as the foot, occurred following injection of any of the three lower spaces but was twice as common at L5 as it was at L3. A less common but important area of reference was the lower abdominal and inguinal regions, common sites of pain in patients with fibromyalgia. The pelvic floor is represented in the form of the irritable bowel and irritable bladder. The neuroanatomy of this pattern is not simple, but, functionally, the symptoms are all linked to the special demands of the upright posture.

Why did we begin to walk upright 4 million years ago with (often locked) lumbar hyperextension? We could not run faster or walk further. But it gave us the freedom to use our hands, and major changes in our thumbs, shoulders, and rib cage appeared rapidly. There were huge gains in function, at the cost of vulnerable low backs and low necks.

None of this is obvious. Without the discovery of the characteristic pattern of tender sites, the correct diagnosis is literally inconceivable; this is a clear example of "medically unexplained symptoms" (MUS). The psychosocial factors cannot play a role either, except as aggravating factors.

However, these factors would not account for the absence of previously discovered tenderness at midtrapezius, second rib, and outer elbow. (In the references to MUS , the authors comment on measures of anxiety, depression, somatization, hypochondriasis, and a tendency to seek alternative therapies. Is this not normal, given the failure of the health professionals to define and treat the origin of their symptoms?)

The 1990 criteria were designed to identify groups of patients suitable for research studies. They were not designed to assess relative severity nor to detect conscious or unconscious exaggeration of symptoms and associated disability. The ACR point count is a censored scale; it cannot be less than zero or greater than 18. When applied to patients with fibromyalgia, it cannot be less than 11 or greater than 18, so that discrimination among such patients, or among others with many pain complaints, is unsatisfactory. However, by combining an expanded list of tender sites, with emphasis on those remote from areas of pain; using dolorimetry on these sites and on control sites; and ascribing scores to a predefined list of pain behaviors, deliberate exaggeration was identified in approximately 90% of 45 subjects in blinded, randomized trials.

It should be argued that all rheumatologists should possess a dolorimeter, not only for patient assessments but also for teaching and to calibrate their own palpation technique. In a study of variation among observers, the mean initial value was 4.05 kg, but it varied from 1.78 to 8.92 kg. Training reduced observer variation by 65%, with reduction of mean absolute error from 1.25 kg to 0.44 kg. Naïve participants performed as well as experts, and there were no gender differences.

Many studies of pharmacotherapy have been performed, and we learn a great deal from those therapies that do *not* work. Nonsteroidal anti-inflammatory drugs (NSAIDs) give minimal relief; therefore cyclooxygenases 1, 2, and 3 are not important. Serotonin reuptake inhibitors give minimal, time-limited relief. Similarly, opioids give only modest relief. The use of small doses of tricyclics and opioids is not wicked, but is merely ineffective. In a randomized, double blind, placebo-controlled study of effects of epidural placebo, an opioid, and lidocaine in subjects with lower body pain and referred tenderness, there was no response to placebo, reduced pain with opioid, but total relief of both pain and tenderness with lidocaine. Perhaps fortunately, steroids make pain and tenderness worse. Early studies identifying elevated levels of substance P in the spinal fluid of patients with fibromyalgia have now been replicated. It seems likely the pain transmission in fibromyalgia is complex and redundant. Recent studies have implicated other cytokines that participate in inflammatory or immune responses but are often widely distributed in the nervous system (among others) where they act as intercellular messengers, performing a great variety of functions. Tumor necrosis factor (TNF) is one of these cytokines. It has been extensively studied in a model of chronic back pain. Many thousands of patients with RA have been treated with inhibitors of TNF, with great relief from pain, but we have not determined whether they act on neural pain transmission because neither the referring rheumatologists nor the principal investigators have ensured that tender point counts were part of the protocol! This concern has been expressed by others.

These comments return us to the introductory section. Fibromyalgia and regional pain syndromes are extremely common in the practices of all rheumatologists and, indeed, of all health practitioners. For most, they remain as MUS. The possibility of referred pain should be considered for any patient in pain, especially if the problem is confounded by the presence of other diagnoses. We should rediscover our history and the value of characteristic sites of referred tenderness as objective markers of the presence and severity of noninflammatory problems. Most often (but not always), the site of origin of the referred pain is in the low cervical or low lumbar spine, the anatomy of which is unique to humans. A variety of amplifying factors have been identified, and progress in identifying the anatomic, cellular, and neurochemical pathways involved has been dramatic.

In this review, I have not detailed the precise assessment and treatment techniques that follow from these insights. The principles can only be summarized in this review. The ultimate objective is to restore the patient to a high level of fitness and function. This cannot be achieved in the face of high-level pain and fatigue; therefore, the first phase must deal with the mechanical problems in the low neck and low back. The low-neck problems are due to stresses in the unsupported (or overrotated) low neck during sleep and are therefore closely related to the sleep disturbance and fatigue. Essentially, a list of alternative strategies is available to ensure reliable delivery of support to the low neck throughout the night.

The two lowest levels of the lumbar spine are vulnerable when loaded in locked hyperextension. Recurring back problems are commonly associated with weak lower abdominal muscles. This weakness must be identified and corrected by tough-but-safe, graded, sit-up exercises. For a patient with chronic back pain, the first technically correct, painless sit-up in the examiner's office is a huge victory as well as a reinforcement about the postural strategies needed to avoid hyperextension.

Progress is often slow. The therapist can only be a coach and a friend, and active commitment by the patient is essential to success. The patients need reinforcement and encouragement for further victories. Measured gains in strength and the loss of once marked tenderness at characteristic sites can be very reassuring and often occurs before symptom relief. This may take 2 years, and quicker relief should not be promised. The patient will forgive the physician if they attain relief in 6 months. In any case, the victory is theirs. It is only achieved through their efforts, and a search for passive therapies is understandable but is a mistake.

1

The History of Fibromyalgia

Daniel J. Wallace

Depictions of chronic widespread pain have appeared in literature since the dawn of literary embellished recorded time. For example, such references to the protagonist's symptoms and appearance appeared in the Babylonian epic of Gilgamesh (ca. 2800 B.C.) (1).

The Bible also includes references to chronic neuromuscular pain. Note the following passages from the Old Testament:

> ...and wearisome nights are appointed to me. When I lie down, I say, When shall I arise, and the night be gone? And I am full of tossings to and fro unto the dawning of the day. (Job 7:3–4)
>   ...the days of affliction have taken hold upon me. My bones are pierced in me in the night season: and my sinews take no rest. (Job 30:16–17)
>   Have mercy on me, O Lord; for I am weak: O Lord, heal me; for my bones are vexed. My soul is also sore vexed: but thou, O Lord, how long?...I am weary with my groaning; all the night make I my bed to swim; I water my couch with tears. (Psalm 6:2–6)
>   It is nothing to you, all that pass by? Behold ye and see if there be any pain like unto my pain, which is done unto me, wherewith the Lord hath afflicted me in the day of his fierce anger. From above hath he sent fire into my bones...and I am weary and faint all the day. (Jeremiah, in Lamentations 1:12–13)

Changes in weather and their association with symptoms were recorded by Shakespeare in *A Midsummer Night's Dream*: Therefore the moon, the governess of floods. Pale in her anger; washes all the air. That rheumatic diseases do abound. (Act 2, scene 34, I, 105).

CHRONIC WIDESPREAD PAIN OR FATIGUE AFTER SHAKESPEARE TO 1800

The word "rheumatism" was first used to denote a specific musculoskeletal syndrome by Guillaume de Bailou around 1592 and, more particularly, to be diagnostic of nonarticular musculoskeletal disorders by F.B. de Sauvages de la Croix in 1763 in the first modern classification of rheumatic diseases (2,3).

Robert Burton's treatise on "The Anatomy of Melancholy," published in 1621, noted that "the Minde most effectually works on the Body, producing by his passions and perturbations, miraculous alterations as Melancholy, Despaire, cruelle disease..." (4). Some people with melancholic depression were noted to have pain and fatigue as well. In 1750, Sir Richard Manningham described "febricula," or little fever, among mostly upper-class women who were afflicted with "listlessness, with great lassitude and weariness all over the body ... little flying pains ... the patient is a little ... forgetful." People with febricula were sedentary and studious, and their symptoms were brought on by grief, intense thoughts, or taking cold (5). Robert Whytt (1714–1766) was the physician to King George III of Great Britain whenever the monarch visited Scotland. He blamed the female nervous system and reproductive system for women's proneness to hysteria. Nerves were "embued with feeling and there is a general sympathy which prevails through the whole system; so that there is a particular and very remarkable consent between various parts of the body" (6). He posited that nerves integrate bodily function and mediate emotion and mental shock, which he termed "sensibility." Whytt concluded that "all diseases may, in some sense, be called afflictions of the nervous system." William Cullen (1712–1790) was influenced by these writings and stated that "all diseases, in some sense, be called affections of the nervous system" (7).

A CONVERGENCE OF CONCEPTS

Several separate threads of evidence eventually converged into the concept of chronic widespread pain, chronic neuromuscular pain, and modern fibromyalgia. These include the development of the concept of myofascial tender points (TePs), neurasthenia, postinfectious fatigue, myasthenic syndrome, myalgic encephalomyelitis, posttraumatic fibromyalgia, and wartime/occupational continuous exposure musculoskeletal syndromes. Since they were not connected as a single concept until the work of this author, Smythe, Yunus, and Hench between 1975 and 1985, they will be discussed individually.

THE EVOLUTION OF TRIGGER POINTS AND "FIBROSITIS"

In 1821 the British physician R.P. Player observed that patients reported pain when certain vertebrae were pressed and "in many instances patients are surprised at the discovery of tenderness in a part, of whose implication in disease they had not the least suspicion" (8). This was duly noted again in the early 19th century by William Balfour of Edinburgh, who argued that chronic rheumatism included disorders of the "cellular membrane which abounds in the human body and connects every part" (9,10). The term "spinal irritation" entered our lexicon in 1828 largely due to the efforts of Thomas Brown of Glasgow, who noted that young women had painful tender spots in their spine on pinching. This pain was "in the majority of cases more severe than in those of real vertebral diseases" (8). In 1832, I. Parrish noted that irritation of the spinal marrow accounts for a "peculiar neurologic affection of females" (11). F. Velleix's 1841 treatise on neuralgia described points ("points douloureaux") painful to pressure without spontaneous pain that had a tendency to radiate and was associated with somatic symptoms (12). In 1843 the German physician Robert Froreip described a rheumatic state in which tender areas in the muscles were accompanied by pain, stiffness, and, occasionally, fever. This was deduced in the course of his studies with electricity and magnetic therapies (13). In the 1850s, Thomas Inman postulated that contraction or spasm of muscles caused rheumatic nodules. The Swedish massagist Unna Helleday described neuralgic pain spreading from nodules in rheumatic muscles in 1876 (14,15). A Boston physician, D. Graham, wrote in 1893 that pathologic basis of muscular rheumatism was "probably coagulation of the semi-fluid contractile muscular substance and adhesion of muscular fibrils" (16).

These observations set the stage for the English neurologist Sir William R. Gowers (1845–1915) to coin the term "fibrositis" in his 1904 treatise on lumbago (17). It was thought to be an inflammatory change in the fibrous tissues of the back muscles, which produced "muscular rheumatism" with or without the presence of trauma. Gowers did not describe diffuse body pain, only asymmetric regional pain. His discussion included considerations of pain amplification, lack of firm evidence for inflammation, improvement with gentle manipulation, counterirritation, and even cocaine injections, fatigue, and sleep disturbances. The same year, in the first of several publications, Ralph Stockman of the University of Glasgow embraced the term fibrositis and purported histologically that these tissues consisted of "inflammatory hyperplasia of the connective tissue in patches ... confined to white fibrous tissue" (18). Although numerous other investigators failed to confirm these findings (discussed in detail in Reynolds's review article), Stockman's work and reputation was so influential and pervasive that it went unchallenged by orthodox medicine for over 30 years (19).

Sir Thomas Lewis and Jonas Kellgren published seminal studies in the 1930s documenting that injecting hypertonic saline into deep structures of blindfolded volunteers produced discomfort ("referred pain") in patterns demarcated chiefly by the segmental nerve supply (20). In 1937, Arthur Steindler followed up on earlier work relating to painful and tender areas and is credited with popularizing the term "trigger points" and injecting them with procaine (21). The 1930s and 1940s also saw the publication of studies from Michael Good in Great Britain, who exhaustively mapped out "myalgia spots," and Michael Kelly of Australia, who connected "visceral" pain syndromes with fibrositis (22,23). Janet Travell (1901–1997) was clearly influenced by the above-mentioned writings, beginning her own amazingly prolific career in 1942 (from 1961 to 1965 she was the chief White House physician to John F. Kennedy and then Lyndon B. Johnson). With David Simons, Travell is the de facto founder of the modern day discipline of physical medicine. She hypothesized etiologies for self-perpetuating pain–spasm–pain sequences (introducing the term "myofascial pain syndromes") and noted the chronicity of such complaints (24,25). We must be fair and credit European investigators who made similar, important observations during the early 20th century but are not widely cited because their work was not published in English. These include Folke Lindstedt from Sweden, A. Reichart from Czechoslovakia, and Alfons Cornelius from Germany (26–28).

NEURASTHENIA

In the early 19th century, Austin Flint (for whom a murmur is named) used the term "nervous exhaustion" to describe chronic fatigue (29). These concepts were popularized by the American neurologist George Beard (1839–1883), who, along with E. Van Drusen, coined the term "neurasthenia" in 1869 to describe the lack of strength of nerves. People with neurasthenia had deficient nerve tone, general debility, and were "living on a plane lower than normal" (30,31). Neurasthenia was popularized in American and Victorian literature and characterized by Miss Marchmont in Charlotte Bronte's *Villette* and Mrs. Snow in *Polyanna*, among many others (32). Beard was an enthusiast of all things electric and needed little prodding to apply "faradic current ... from head to toe." When nonorganic explanations were associated with some of the symptoms, the nascent discipline of psychiatry was assisted in its development. Silas Weir Mitchell (1829–1914) was a prominent Philadelphia society physician who initially worked with Civil War veterans who had difficulty adjusting to civilian life. He described neurasthenics as broken down and exhausted women who were "weak, pallid, flabby ... poor eaters, digesting ill, incapable of exercise" (33). Sir William Osler (1849–1919) wrote extensively about neurasthenia, with the longest section appearing in the 1899 edition of his medical textbook. He discussed concepts of referred hyperaesthesia and described "weariness on the least exertion, weakness, pain in the back, and aching in the legs" (34).

Social prejudice in the form of Victorian proprieties influenced attitudes and medical thinking (35–38). Neurasthenia became a middle-class phenomenon that assumed almost epidemic proportions, and treating it became very profitable. Practitioners extensively used rest cures, overfeeding, enemas, massage, and some electricity. Mitchell was said to make as much as $70,000 a year. Some condescending male physicians treated patients with electronic stimulation of pelvic areas (a form of masturbation) and female genital mutilating surgery such as removing the clitoris, while others proposed useless and meddlesome surgery for diagnoses such as "chronic appendicitis" (38).

After World War I the term neurasthenia disappeared, and it had no prominence in a landmark 1934 Mayo Clinic review of patients with "chronic nervous exhaustion" (39).

POSTINFECTIOUS FATIGUE SYNDROMES

The association between established infections and psychological or fatigue states was postulated in the neurasthenia literature. Van Deusen attributed it to malaria infestation in the 1860s, and Beard attributed it to "wasting fevers." The neurologist Francis X. Dercum (1856–1931) wrote that "Nervous exhaustion is also apt to follow certain acute illnesses such as typhoid fever, malaria and especially influenza" (40). In 1903, Gowers noted that "Neurasthenia may follow the infection disease, particularly influenza, typhoid fever and syphilis" (41). Osler referred to posttyphoidal neuromuscular symptoms as a variety of "Railway Spine." Other reports appeared connecting chronic fatigue with alimentary bacteria, streptococcus, and the effects of vaccination (42).

Chronic infection with brucellosis was a source of chronic fatigue, according to the American physician Alice Evans (43). Although serologic evidence was present in some, she stepped in more dangerous territory by stating in 1934 that she could make the diagnosis in those without bacteriologic evidence on the basis of clinical impression alone. In 1951, Spink related that no organic cause for persistent fatigue could be found in 13 of 65 infected patients in Minnesota who had symptoms lasting at least a year. Interestingly, "some of the individuals had clear cut emotional problems prior to the onset of brucellosis" (44). The importance of "pre-illness personality structure" was confirmed in a more rigorous analysis of "chronic brucellosis" patients at Johns Hopkins with chronic fatigue in 1959 (45).

By the 1970s chronic fatigue was attributed to a host of other noninfectious conditions such as hypoglycemia, "total allergy" syndrome, mercury amalgam fillings, and multiple chemical sensitivities (38; see Chapter 23). However, new organisms were associated with chronic fatigue syndromes. A best-selling book by a Tennessee family practitioner pronounced "chronic candidiasis" to be an "immunotoxin" whose uncontrolled growth led to depression, chronic fatigue, and abdominal distension (46). Even though double-blind, placebo-controlled studies showed that antifungal therapies did not have any effect on the condition, legions of patients still pursue this "idée fixe," which is difficult to dislodge from their minds and lifestyles. On the other hand, the Epstein-Barr virus (EBV) story led to a productive outcome for organized medicine. Since mononucleosis is caused by EBV (confirmed in 1968) and is a notorious fatigue inducer,

several studies conducted in the early 1980s concluded that the virus was the source of postinfectious chronic fatigue syndromes (47,48). This enthusiasm was tempered by reports demonstrating the ubiquity of elevated IgG EBV viral serologies, its lack of specificity, and failure to respond to antiviral therapy. Although true EBV infections with elevated IgM viral serologies are associated with chronic fatigue, these occurrences were relatively rare. EBV investigators (especially Gary Holmes) were responsible for working together to propose that "chronic fatigue syndrome" is an entity caused by EBV and other infections and developing the Centers for Disease Control 1988 classification for defining cases (49).

CHRONIC WIDESPREAD PAIN IN WARTIME

Complaints of chronic fatigue in military situations were reported among Captain Cook's crew on the *Resolution* in 1772 (50). Jones and Wessely surveyed the first 4,000 pension files of the Royal Hospital in Chelsea (United Kingdom) and found 11 examples of "functional debility" among veterans of the Crimean War, Boer War, and 19th-century campaigns in Afghanistan, Egypt, and the Sudan (51). Jacob Mendez da Costa was a Union surgeon in the U.S. Civil War (1861–1865). Trained in Paris, Prague, and Vienna, the future chairman of medicine at Jefferson Medical College described "effort syndrome" or "irritable heart" (52,53). Soldiers said to have "irritable heart" complained of shortness of breath, dizziness, palpitations, headache, digestive disturbances, chest pains, difficulty sleeping, and inexplicable chronic fatigue, which required their removal from the battlefield. No structural abnormalities were found, even at autopsy (when they died for other reasons). Da Costa posited that there was a "connection between functional derangement and organic change."

During the First World War (1914–1918), 600,000 cases of "Da Costa's syndrome" were diagnosed among the British forces, 44,000 of whom received medical pensions. In 1941, Wood suggested that patients with "Da Costa's syndrome" should be "informed of the nature of their illness and treated as psychoneurotics" (54). By that time World War II had broken out and the term "fibrositis" was now used. In 1942, Hutchison noted that 69% of all rheumatology referrals at his army hospital were for fibrositis (55):

> I met with instances where men have spent many weeks off duty "enjoying" physical therapy for fibrositis which was not longer existent and at which stage it had become wellnigh impossible to convince them that they were organically sound and fit for duty. Some cases have been referred to the psychiatrist.

On the other hand, also in 1942, Savage attributed most of his 141 fibrositis referrals to exacerbations induced by heavy equipment or drill, noting marked relief after procaine injections (56). Ellman's 1942 definition of fibrositis in the *Annals of the Rheumatic Diseases* encompassed strains, bursitis, psychogenic rheumatism, disc disease, and what we now know as fibromyalgia (57). In the U.S. military, Beeson (future editor of the Cecil medical textbook) described a syndrome of neck and shoulder pain for which no infectious or anatomic etiology could be found (58). At the American Red Cross-Harvard Field Hospital it affected mostly white women and was noted in 13% of the clerks, 6% of the soldiers, and 23% of the paramilitary staff. Ed Boland (who became the first practicing rheumatologist in Los Angeles and was an American Rheumatism Association president) wrote in 1943 that 24% of his 450 military referrals were for fibrositis (59). Their psychological profiles included several common features: concern over loss of security and separation from loved ones, concern over the loss of ability to control one's destiny, resentment of authority—especially when invested in persons felt to be inferior, fear of bodily harm, confusion in strange surroundings, crowding, regimentation, and competition, and concern for the safety and financial well-being of dependents. Further understandings of our concepts of fibromyalgia in wartime were advanced during the Vietnam conflict (1961–1975) when posttraumatic stress disorder (PTSD) was described and its features delineated. PTSD is a well-known feature of 10% to 20% of those with fibromyalgia, especially in those with a personal or family history of abuse, addiction, and violence (60).

MASS HYSTERIA AND MYALGIC ENCEPHALOMYELITIS/EPIDEMIC NEUROMYASTHENIA

Hysteria, fits, and demonic passions were described during the Renaissance in the context of religious experiences. Mass frenzies of St Vitus's dance in the Middle Ages and the actions of nuns in 17th-century France were popularized by Aldous Huxley's *Devils of Loudon* (61). In his discussion of magnetism theories, Eberhard Gmelin described a young woman in 1793 who was "able to remain out of bed only for a short time, sitting on a chair, nor is she able, without being supported by someone, to go from one chair to the next" (62). This resolved temporarily after she drank "magnetized" water. Jean-Baptiste Charcot described and codified "motor hysteria" (also called "Charcot's hysteria") in the late 19th century (63).

An offshoot of postinfectious fatigue syndromes known as *myalgic encephalomyelitis* or *epidemic neuromyasthenia* constituted several well-described "outbreaks" between 1934 and 1987 (64). These episodes differ from classic postinfectious fatigue syndromes in that there was a component of mass hysteria and panic associated with a confirmed infectious outbreak as precipitating factors. In 1934, Los Angeles was struck by a frightful epidemic of polio. Among those cared for at Los Angeles County General Hospital, 210 women began developing muscle tenderness, insomnia, emotional upset, sensory disturbances, localized muscle weakness, and neck and back stiffness. No fevers above 100 degrees were noted. Sixteen percent of the student nurses, 8% of the graduate nurses, and 2% of the hospital orderlies were afflicted. Although none tested positive for polio or any other organism, many were hospitalized or left their jobs for months. None died (65). In

1965 a 30-year follow-up of these patients showed that the initial symptoms were persistent in a large number of them and continued to affect their quality of life (66). Similar well-documented occurrences were noted in Iceland (1948), Adelaide, Australia (1949), New York (1950 and 1961), Copenhagen (1952), Middlesex and Coventry, England (1952 and 1953), Maryland (1953), Durban, South Africa (1955), London (1955 and 1970), Punta Gorda, Florida (1956), and, more recently, in New Zealand in 1982–1983 and the Lake Tahoe region of California/Nevada from 1984 to 1987 (67–73). Polio, Epstein-Barr, and influenza-like illnesses were usually part of the milieu. In 1994, Briggs and Levine examined 12 of the outbreaks (out of 46 published) in detail (64). They concluded that excessive fatigue, myalgias, headache, sleep disturbances, complaints of low-grade fever, and other constitutional symptoms were seen in most patients. Neurologic features were heterogeneous and inconsistent and usually more serious in reports prior to 1960. Most of the patients recovered, but a significant minority had a chronic relapsing course consistent with fibromyalgia.

MYASTHENIC SYNDROME

A small group of interested persons founded what became the Arthritis Foundation and the American College of Rheumatology in 1934. However, for all practical purposes, rheumatology did not exist as a discipline until after the Second World War. People with symptoms and signs of what we now term fibromyalgia presented to neurologists in large numbers beginning in the 1930s. In a fascinating story, some were thought to have a myasthenia gravis-like condition. Antibody testing to the anticholinesterase receptor was not yet available and tensilon testing had a subjective component. Further confusion was created when many of these people had dramatic responses to pyridostigmine, with flaring of symptoms when the drug was withdrawn (61).

J.E. Tether ran the myasthenia gravis clinic at Indiana University Medical Center for over 20 years. In 1961 he published the results of 2,327 patients referred to him, and 775 were said to have a "mild myasthenic state." They primarily consisted of women aged between 20 and 40 at diagnosis whose symptoms were either of gradual onset or followed a traumatic event. They complained of fatigue, tightness, stiffness and aching in the back of the neck, chest heaviness, intrascapular and lumbar area aching, and "sad, tired expressions" (74). These findings were replicated at Johns Hopkins by Johns and McQuillen, who commented on the ability of some women to tolerate near-lethal doses of pyridostigmine without untoward effects, dependency, or withdrawal syndromes (75). The same clinical picture was reported by Schwab and Perlo among 120 patients treated at the Myasthenia Gravis clinic at the Massachusetts General Hospital between 1954 and 1964; 37.6% had "chronic fatigue syndrome" and were described as asthenic individuals who had a "surprising tolerance to anticholinesterase medication" (76). At University of California Los Angeles (UCLA), Fullerton and Munsat, mentored by the world authority Christian Hermann, studied seven patients with "pseudo myasthenia gravis" in detail. All were women aged between 22 and 60. They had an average of 15 complaints each, including fatigue, dysmenorrhea, chest pain, and back pain, had undergone a surprisingly large number of pelvic operations, and were "doctor shoppers" until they were given a diagnosis of myasthenia gravis. At that point they became devotedly attached to the diagnosing physician. Psychiatric profiles revealed strict and repressive upbringings, hysteria, and marital problems (77).

The "myasthenic syndrome" has now come full circle. Evidence that pyridostigmine increases growth hormone secretion has led to studies evaluating its use in fibromyalgia (78).

RAILWAY SPINE, WHIPLASH, AND POSTTRAUMATIC MYOFASCIAL PAIN

In 1866, London surgeon John Eric Erichsen (1818–1896) described "Railway Spine" as a form of posttraumatic back pain that was more severe and of longer duration than expected from the attributed injury (79). In 1894, Osler wrote

> ...the condition follows an accident, often in a railway train...body shock or concussion is not necessary.... A slight blow, or a fall from a carriage or in the stairs may suffice.... Within a few weeks of the accident...the patient complains of headache and tired feelings, which may or may not have been associated with an actual trauma. He is sleepless and finds himself unable to concentrate...nervous irritability may develop, which may have a host of trivial manifestations.... He dwells constantly upon his condition, gets very despondent and low spirited...he may complain of numbness and tingling in the extremities, and in some cases of much pain in the back.... A condition of fright and excitement following an accident may persist for days or even weeks, and then gradually pass away.... The symptoms of neurasthenia...subsequently develop.... A majority of patients with traumatic hysteria recover. In railway cases, so long as litigation is pending, and the patient is in the hands of lawyers the symptoms usually persist... (80).

By 1910 references to "Railway Spine" in the literature and court cases related to it more or less disappeared.

The second wave of trauma-related litigation took place after Harold D. Crowe coined the term "whiplash" to describe eight cases of automobile-derived neck injuries in a lecture to San Francisco orthopedists in 1928 (81), followed by the first appearance of the term "trigger points" by Arthur Steindler in 1937 (21). The cause of such injuries has never been well established, but theories abounded. In 1957, Brendstrup et al. followed 32 posttraumatic patients with "interstitial myofascitis" who purportedly had increased mucopolysaccharides on muscle biopsy (82). In 1973, Awad "confirmed" these findings and hypothesized that trauma provoked platelet extravasation, which led to serotonin release and mast cell degranulation (83), and a year later his group suggested that this could be quantitated by a peculiar pattern of the five lactate dehydrogenase (LDH) isoenzymes (84). It would be another 25 years before serious work relating to posttraumatic fibromyalgia was published.

"CONTINUOUS" TRAUMA AND FIBROMYALGIA

Aside from military reports, the first suggestion that continuous trauma in the workplace could produce myofascial pain stems from reports commissioned by the Labor government in the United Kingdom relating to Welsh coal miners in the 1920s. These attributions quickly became consumed in issues relating to worker's compensation, which was first put into place by Otto von Bismarck in the late 19th century in Germany and adopted in the United States as part of Woodrow Wilson's progressive agenda between 1910 and 1920 (85,86). This is discussed in more detail in Chapter 33. The ongoing debate is clouded by the mid-1980s "epidemic" of "repetitive strain syndrome" in Australia, which resolved after changing the definitions for it, frequent resolution of complaints after receiving a monetary settlement (87), the addition of emotional stress to the "continuous trauma" definition, preemployment psychological personality profiles, which can predict who is at risk for filing "continuous trauma" complaints, and the length and character of exacerbations of minor preemployment complaints.

THE COMPLETION OF THE CYCLE

The Canadian rheumatologist Wallace Graham was the first North American to use the term fibrositis (in 1940), and he edited chapters on fibrositis for the first few editions of the Comroe/Hollander (later McCarty/Koopman) rheumatology textbook (88). He proposed the concept of "tension rheumatism" along with Ed Boland, which was challenged by Walter Bauer at Harvard and ultimately shown not to be the case by electrical silence in fibrositis muscles at electromyography (89). When Hugh Smythe at the University of Toronto was asked to take over writing the chapter after Graham's death, he initiated a series of remarkable studies. Between 1975 and 1977, Smythe and his colleague Harvey Modolfsky were the first investigators to connect TePs with systemic symptoms and a specific laboratory abnormality (90). This connection was an elaboration upon suggestions articulated by Traut in lectures given in the 1960s, some of which were attended by Smythe (91). They demonstrated reproducible TePs and showed that α-wave intrusion into δ-wave sleep was a pivotal feature of fibrosis, which they renamed "fibrositis syndrome." In the mid-1970s a rheumatologist at the Scripps Clinic, Kahler Hench (son of Phillip Hench, the only rheumatologist to win the Nobel Prize in Medicine for his work on the team that discovered cortisone), lectured that fibrositis was an inappropriate term because no inflammation was present. His suggestion that it be renamed "fibromyalgia" was adopted by Muhammad Yunus and his colleagues at the University of Illinois College of Medicine at Peoria whose 1981 seminal publication documented that numerous nonmusculoskeletal systemic complaints were statistically associated with the syndrome (92). In the mid-1980s this writer and Don Goldenberg related chronic fatigue syndrome, myasthenic syndrome, and epidemic neurasthenia as being conditions associated with chronic widespread pain and supported Yunus's suggestions that they all had "central sensitization" features of pain amplification in common (93). Yunus further documented the similarity, association, and connectivity of central sensitization syndromes (94). This culminated in an article and editorial in the *Journal of the American Medical Association* endorsing the concept of fibromyalgia (from Goldenberg and Robert Bennett) and led to the formation of an *ad hoc* committee that ultimately resulted in the American College of Rheumatology's criteria for the classification of fibromyalgia (95–97). The World Health Organization validated the concept of fibromyalgia with the Copenhagen declaration in 1992 (98). Papers in the last decade have reexamined famous personages in the context of how purported fibromyalgia affected their careers. These include Clara Schumann, Alfred Nobel, Charles Darwin, Florence Nightingale, Henry James's sister Alice, and Frida Kahlo (89,99–102).

THE DISSENTING VIEW: MEDICALLY UNEXPLAINED SYNDROMES

In 1965, C.K. Meador posited that when a specific disease is suspected but not found, the patient has a particular nondisease (103). A small but distinguished minority of academicians, some of whom are rheumatologists, have published numerous opinion pieces and editorials expressing the viewpoint that fibromyalgia is a nondisease or "medically unexplained syndrome" and does not in fact exist. None have undertaken an epidemiologic or evidence-based study supporting their hypothesis, which is why only a single paragraph is devoted to discussing this argument as a historical footnote. A few examples of this viewpoint are cited here (104–108). This writer shares the concerns that some of these thought leaders have expressed relating to medicalization, stigmatization, and the legal consequences of labeling some people as having fibromyalgia, but this does not nullify the validity of fibromyalgia existing as a syndrome (109).

SUMMARY POINTS

- Although the term "fibromyalgia" is relatively new, descriptions of the symptom complex we now label as fibromyalgia have occurred for millennia.
- The terms used to describe this syndrome have attempted to connote the current notion of what caused these symptoms; the current term fibromyalgia acknowledges that this is an idiopathic pain syndrome that affects the tissues.
- Although there are valid criticisms of the many legal and societal implications of the fibromyalgia construct, this does not diminish the legitimacy of those who are suffering from chronic widespread pain.

REFERENCES

1. Tablet X. *At the edge of the world, The Epic of Gilgamesh.* London: Penguin Classics, 1999.
2. Barnard CC. The famous Parisian physician Guilelmus Balloniu's book on rheumatism. *Br J Rheumatol* 1940;2:141–162.
3. De Sauvages de la Croix FM. *Nosologia methodica sistens morborum classes, genera et species juxt Sndenhami mentem et botanicum ordinem.* Amsterdam, 1763.
4. Burton R. *The anatomy of melancholy* (1621, Da Capo Press). Amsterdam: Theatrum Orbus Terrarum, 1971.
5. Manningham R. *The symptoms, nature, causes and cure of the febricula or little fever: commonly called the nervous or hysteric fever, the fever on the spritis; vapours, hypo, or spleen,* 2nd ed. London: J Robinson, 1750:52–53.
6. Weiner H. Was Robert Whytt (1714–1766) right? *Psychother Psychosom* 1986;45:5–13.
7. Cullen W. *Synopsis nosologiae methodicae,* 4th ed.. Edinburgh: W. Creech, 1785.
8. Weissman G. If leeches were a luxury. *MD Mag* 1992;8, 20.
9. Balfour W. Observations with cases illustrative of a new, simple, and expeditious mode of curing rheumatism and sprains. *London Med Phys J* 1824;51:446–462.
10. Balfour W. Observations on the pathology and cure of rheumatism. *Edinb Med Surg J* 1815;11:168–187.
11. Parrish I. Remarks on spinal irritation as connected with nervous diseases. *Am J Ment Sci* 1832;10:293–314.
12. Velleix F. *Traite des neuralgias au affections douloureuses des nerfes.* Paris: JP Balliere, 1841:654.
13. Froriep R. On the therapeutic application of electro-magnetism in the treatment of rheumatic and paralytic affections. Translated by RM Lawrence. London: Henry Renshaw, 1850.
14. Inman T. *On myalgia: its nature, causes and treatment,* 2nd ed. London: John Churchill, 1860.
15. Helleday U. Om myitis chronica (rheumatica). *Ark* 1876;8.
16. Graham D. Massage in muscular rheumatism, and its possible value in the diagnosis of muscular rheumatism from neuritis. *N Y St Med J* 1948;48:2050–2059.
17. Gowers WR. Lumbago: Its lesson and analogues. *Br Med J* 1904;1:117–121.
18. Stockman R. *Rheumatism and arthritis.* Edinburgh: W Green and Son Ltd, 1920:132.
19. Reynolds MD. The development of the concept of fibrositis. *J Hist Med Allied Sci* 1983;38:5–35.
20. Kellgren JH. Observations on referred pain arising from muscle. *Clin Sci* 1938;3:175–190.
21. Steindler A, Luck JV. Differential diagnosis of pain in the low back: allocation of the source of pain by the procaine hydrochloride method. *JAMA* 1938;110:106–113.
22. Kelly M. The nature of fibrositis. *Ann Rheum Dis* 1946;5:69–77.
23. Good MD. Objective diagnosis and curability of nonarticular rheumatism. *Br J Phys Med Ind Hyg* 1951;14:1–7.
24. Travell J. Referred pain from skeletal muscle. *N Y State Med J* 1952;55:331–339.
25. Travell JG, Simons DG. *Myofascial pain and dysfunction.* Baltimore, MD: Williams &Wilkins, 1983.
26. Lindstedt F. Zur kennetis der aetiologic und pathogenese der lumbago und ahnlicher ruckenschmerzen. *Act Med Scand* 1921;55:248–280.
27. Reichart A. Reflexschmerzen auf grund von myogelosen. *Deutsche Med Wschr* 1938;64:823–824.
28. Cornelius A. Narben und nerven. *Dtsch Militarztl Z* 1903;32:657–673.
29. Straus SE. History of chronic fatigue syndrome. *Rev Infect Dis* 1991;13 (Suppl. 1):S2–S7.
30. Beard G. Neurasthenia. *Boston Med Surg J* 1869;80:217–221.

31. Van Deusen E. Observations on a form of nervous prostration (Neurasthenia) culminating in insanity. *Am J Insanity* 1869;25:445–461.

32. Wallace DJ. How our understanding of fibromyalgia evolved. In: Wallace DJ, Wallace JB, eds. *All about fibromyalgia*. New York: Oxford University Press, 2002:3–6.

33. Mitchell SW. The treatment by rest, seclusion, etc. in relation to psychotherapy. *JAMA* 1908;25:2033–2037.

34. Osler W. *The principles and practice of medicine*. New York: D Appleton & Co, 1899.

35. Wessely S, Hotopf M. Is fibromyalgia a distinct clinical entity? Historical and epidemiological evidence. *Balliere's Clin Rheumatol* 1999;13:427–436.

36. Wessely S. History of postviral fatigue syndrome. *Br Med Bull* 1991;47:919–941.

37. Leitch AG. Neurasthenia, myalgic encephalomyelitis or cryptogenic chronic fatigue syndrome? *Q J Med* 1995;88:447–450.

38. Black J. Female genital mutilation: a contemporary issue, and a Victorian obsession. *J R Soc Med* 1997;90:402–405.

39. Macy JW, Allen EV. A justification for the diagnosis of chronic nervous exhaustion. *Ann Int Med* 1934;7:861–867.

40. Dercum C. The nervous disorders in women simulating pelvic disease: analysis of 591 cases. *JAMA* 1909;52:848–851.

41. Gowers WR. *A manual of diseases of the nervous system*, 2nd ed. Philadelphia, PA: Blaikston's Son & Co, 1903:1045–1050.

42. Benedek TG. Typhoid spine: somatic versus psychosomatic diagnosis in Osler's time. *Semin Arthritis Rheum* 1998;28:114–123.

43. Evans AC. Brucellosis in the United States. *Am J Public Health* 1947;37:139–151.

44. Spink WW. What is chronic brucellosis? *Ann Intern Med* 1951;35:358–374.

45. Imboden JB, Canter A, Cluff LE, et al. Psychologic aspects of delayed convalescence. *Arch Intern Med* 1959;103:406–414.

46. Crook WG. *The yeast connection: a medical breakthrough*, 3rd ed. Jackson, TN: Professional Books, 1983.

47. Jones JF, Ray CG, Minnich LL, et al. Evidence for active Epstein-Barr virus infection in patients with persistent, unexplained illness: elevated anti-early antigen antibodies. *Ann Intern Med* 1985;102:1–7.

48. Schooley R. Epstein-Barr virus. *Curr Opin Infect Dis* 1989;2:267–271.

49. Holmes GP, Kaplan JE, Gantz NM, et al. Chronic fatigue syndrome: a working case definition. *Ann Intern Med* 1988;108:387–389.

50. St George I. Did Cook's sailors have Tapanui flu?—chronic fatigue syndrome on the *Resolution*. *N Z J Med* 1998;109:15–17.

51. Jones E, Wessely S. Case of chronic fatigue syndrome after Crimean war and Indian mutiny. *Br Med J* 1999;319:18–25.

52. Wooley CF. *The irritable heart of soldiers and the origins of Anglo-American cardiology: the US Civil War (1861) to World War I*. Aldershot, Hampshire, UK: Ashgate, 2002.

53. Da Costa JM. Irritable heart: a clinical study of a form of functional cardiac disorder and its consequence. *Am J Med Sci* 1871;121:17–52.

54. Wood P. Da Costa's syndrome (or effort syndrome). *Br Med J* 1941;767–772, 805–811, 845–851.

55. Hutchison R. Nonarticular rheumatism in the army: symptomatology, aetiology, treatment. *Glasgow Med J* 1942;137:33–42.

56. Savage O. Management of rheumatic diseases in the armed forces. *Br Med J* 1942;2:336–338.

57. Ellman P, Savage OA, Wittkower E, et al. A biographical study of fifty civilian and military cases from the Rheumatic unit, St Stephen's Hospital (London County Council), and a military hospital. *Ann Rheum Dis* 1942;3:56–76.

58. Beeson P, Scott T. Clinical epidemiological and experimental observations in an acute myalgia of the neck and shoulders: its possible relation to certain cases of generalized fibrositis. *Proc R Soc Med* 1942;35:733–740.

59. Boland E, Corr W. Psychogenic rheumatism. *JAMA* 1943;123:805–809.

60. Sherman JJ, Turk CC, Okifuji A. Prevalence and impact of post-traumatic stress disorder-like symptoms on patients with fibromyalgia syndrome. *Clin J Pain* 2000;16:127–134.

61. Wallace DJ. Fibromyalgia: Unusual historical aspects and new pathologic insights. *Mt Sinai J Med* 1984;51:124–131.

62. Gmelin E. *Materialien fur die anthropologie: v. 2 untersuchungen uber den thierischen magnetismus*. Heilbronn: Johann Daniel Class, 1793:25.

63. Lagier R. Nosology versus pathology, two approaches to rheumatic diseases illustrated by Alfred Baring Garrod and Jean-Martin Charcot. *Rheumatology* 2001;40:367–471.

64. Briggs NC, Levine PH. A comparative review of systemic and neurologic symptomatology in 12 outbreaks collectively described as chronic fatigue syndrome, epidemic neuromyasthenia and myalgic encephalomyelitis. *Clin Infect Dis* 1994;18 (Suppl. 1):S32–S42.

65. Gilliam AG. *Epidemiological study of an epidemic, diagnosed as poliomyelitis, occurring among the personnel of the Los Angeles County General Hospital during the summer of 1934*. Washington, DC: U.S. Public Health Service Division of Infectious Diseases, National Institutes of Health, 1938:1–90.

66. Marinacci A, Von Hagen K. The value of the electromyolgram in the diagnosis of Iceland disease. *Electromyography* 1965;5:241–251.

67. Shekelov A, Habel K, Veeder E, et al. Epidemic neuromyasthenia: an outbreak of poliomyelitis illness in student nurses. *N Engl J Med* 1957;257:345–355.

68. Poskanzer DC, Henderson DA, Kunkle EC, et al. Epidemic neuromyasthenia: an outbreak in Punta Gorda, Florida. *N Engl J Med* 1957;257:356–363.

69. Dillon MJ. Epidemic neuromyasthenia at the hospital for sick children, Great Ormond Street, London. *Postgrad Med J* 1978;54:725–730.

70. Acheson ED. Benign myalgic encephalomyelitis (Iceland) disease. *Am J Med* 1959;26:569–575.

71. McEvedy CP, Beard AW. The Royal free epidemic of 1955: a reconsideration. *Br Med J* 1970;1:7–11.

72. Parish JG. Early outbreaks of 'epidemic neuromyasthenia.' *Postgrad Med J* 1978;54:711–717.

73. Shorter E. *Chronic fatigue in historical perspective, chronic fatigue syndrome*. Chichester: Wiley, 1993:6–22; Ciba Foundation Symposium 173,

74. Tether JE. Mild myasthenic state. In: Viets JR, ed. *Myasthenia gravis: the second international symposium proceedings*. Springfield, IL: Charles C Thomas Publisher, 1961:444–463.

75. Johns RJ, McQuillen MP. Syndromes simulating myasthenia gravis: asthenia with anticholinesterase tolerance. *Ann N Y Acad Sci* 1966;135:385–397.

76. Schwab RS, Perlo VP. Syndromes simulating myasthenia gravis. *Ann N Y Acad Sci* 1966;135:350–366.

77. Fullerton DT, Munsat TL. Pseudo-myasthenia gravis: a conversion reaction. *J Nerv Ment Dis* 1966;142:78–86.

78. Pavia ES, Deodhar A, Jones KD, et al. Impaired growth hormone secretion in fibromyalgia patients: evidence for augmented hypothalamic somatostatin tone. *Arthritis Rheum* 2002;46:1344–1350.

79. Erichsen JE. *On concussion of the spine, nervous shock, and other obscure injuries of the nervous system*. New York: W Wood & Co, 1875:7–8.

80. Osler W. The traumatic neuroses: railway brain and railway spine; traumatic hysteria. In: Osler W, ed. *The principles and practice of medicine*. New York: D Appleton & Co, 1894:981–985.

81. Crowe HD. A new diagnostic sign in neck injuries. *Calif Med* 1964;100:12–13.

82. Brendstrup P, Jesperson K, Asboe-Hansen G. Morphological and clinical connective tissue changes in fibrositic muscles. *Ann Rheum Dis* 1957;16:438–440.

83. Awad EA. Interstitial myofibrositis. *Arch Phys Med Rehabil* 1973;54:449–453.

84. Ibrahim GA, Awad EA, Kottke FJ. Interstitial myofasciitis: serum and muscle enzymes and lactate dehydrogenase isoenzymes. *Arch Phys Med Rehabil* 1973;55:23–28.

85. Hadler NM. *Occupational musculoskeletal disorders*. New York: Raven Press, 1993.

86. Wallace DJ, Hallegua DS. Quality-of-life, legal-financial and disability issues in fibromyalgia. *Curr Pain Headache Rep* 2001;5:313–319.

87. Littlejohn GO. Fibromyalgia syndrome and disability: the neurogenic model. *Med J Aust* 1998;168:398–401.

88. Graham W. Fibrositis. In: Comroe B, ed. *Arthritis and allied conditions*. Philadelphia, PA: Lea & Febiger, 1949:633.

89. Smythe H. Fibrositis syndrome: a historical perspective. *J Rheumatol* 1989;16(Suppl. 19):2–6.

90. Smythe HA, Moldofsky H. Two contributions to understanding of the "fibrositis" syndrome. *Bull Rheum Dis* 1977–1978; 28:928–931.

91. Traut EF. Fibrositis. *J Am Ger Assn* 1968;16:531–538.

92. Yunus M, Masi AT, Calabro JJ, et al. Primary fibromyalgia (fibrositis): clinical study of 50 patients with matched normal controls. *Semin Arthritis Rheum* 1981;11:151–170.

93. Buchwald D, Goldenberg DL, Sullivan JL, et al. The 'chronic Epstein-Barr virus infection' syndrome and primary fibromyalgia. *Arthritis Rheum* 1987;30:1132–1136.

94. Yunus MB. Primary fibromyalgia syndrome: current concepts. *Compr Ther* 1984;10:21–28.

95. Goldenberg DL. Fibromyalgia syndrome: An emerging but controversial condition. *JAMA* 1987;257:2782–2787.

96. Bennett RM. Fibromyalgia. *JAMA* 257:2802–2803.

97. Wolfe F, Smythe HA, Yunus MB, et al. The American College of Rheumatology 1990 criteria for the classification of fibromyalgia. Report of the Multicenter Criteria Committee. *Arthritis Rheum* 1990;33:160–172.

98. Csillage C. Fibromyalgia: the Copenhagen declaration. *Lancet* 1992;340:663–664.

99. Martinez-Lavin M, Amigo M-C, Coindreau J, et al. Fibromyalgia in Frida Kahlo's life and art. *Arthritis Rheum* 2000; 43:708–709.

100. Holmin LR. Alfred Nobel: Could he have had fibromyalgia? *J Clin Rheumatol* 1996;2:251–256.

101. Hingsten CM. The painful perils of a pair of pianists: the chronic pain of Clara Schumann and Sergei Rachmaninov. *Semin Neurology* 1999;19 (Suppl. 1):29–34.

102. Brown J. *Charles Darwin: the power of place*. New York: Knopf, 2002.

103. Meador CK. The art and science of nondisease. *N Engl J Med* 1965;272:92–95.

104. Bohr T. Problems with myofascial pain syndrome and fibromyalgia syndrome. *Neurology* 1996;46:593–597.

105. Butler CC, Evans M, Greaves D, et al. Medically unexplained symptoms: the biopsychosocial model found wanting. *J R Soc Med* 2004;97:219–221.

106. Ehrlich GE. Pain is real; fibromyalgia isn't. *J Rheumatol* 2003;30:1666–1667.

107. Hadler NM. "Fibromyalgia" and the medicalization of misery. *J Rheumatol* 2003;30:1668–1670.

108. Wessely S. Chronic fatigue: symptoms and syndrome. *Ann Intern Med* 2001;134:838–843.

109. Wallace DJ. To fibromyalgia nihilists: stop pontificating and test your hypothesis [Editorial]. *J Rheumatol* 2004; 31:632.

2

The Taxonomy of Chronic Pain: Moving Toward More Mechanistic Classifications

Daniel J. Clauw

POPULATION-BASED STUDIES OF CHRONIC PAIN

Population-based studies indicate that approximately 10% of the population suffers from chronic widespread pain, which is usually defined as pain above and below the waist and on both sides of the body (1,2). Nearly twice as many people suffer from chronic regional pain. Just as with other chronic somatic symptoms, chronic pain is more common in women than in men (see Figure 2-1).

Population-based studies usually obtain such information from surveys. Unfortunately, no detailed clinical evaluations have been performed on people identified through surveys as suffering from chronic pain to ascertain the precise cause. Thus we can only infer what might be *causing* pain in this large portion of the population with this symptom.

CAUSES OF CHRONIC PAIN

Table 2-1 represents one historical system used to broadly characterize the causes of chronic pain. The first category of disorders would be systemic autoimmune or inflammatory conditions. The second category would be disorders characterized by damage of peripheral tissues, as occurs in osteoarthritis or neuropathy. The final category would be a group of idiopathic conditions of which we do not know the precise cause.

Figure 2-2 represents an attempt to reconcile the known frequency of chronic regional and widespread pain and the known causes of pain in order to estimate the relative mechanistic contributions to the chronic pain seen in the population. Although systemic autoimmune and inflammatory disorders

are always a concern when a patient presents with pain, these conditions are relatively uncommon. The most common systemic inflammatory rheumatic disorder is rheumatoid arthritis, which affects approximately 1% of the population (3). Ankylosing spondylitis and polyarticular gout each affect approximately 0.5% of the population, and other inflammatory disorders, such as systemic lupus erythematosus (SLE), scleroderma, and so on, are considerably less common. In aggregate, then, systemic inflammatory conditions likely affect approximately 2% to 3% of the population. Most of these conditions lead to widespread rather than regional pain. Thus, approximately 20% to 30% of the widespread pain seen in the population—and an even smaller percentage of regional pain—is likely due to a systemic inflammatory disease.

The next group of conditions, where there is mechanical damage to tissues, is considerably more difficult to characterize. Because of the nature of these entities, they are more likely to lead to regional than widespread pain. Osteoarthritis (degenerative joint disease) is the most common condition in this category. Osteoarthritis is very uncommon in the young, and the prevalence increases with age. For example, radiographic evidence of osteoarthritis of the knee occurs in 27% of those under age 70, and 44% of those over age 80 (3,4). Other chronic pain conditions due to damage of tissues would include neuropathic pain, pain due to neural entrapment or vascular compromise, and an assortment of endocrine and other conditions, all of which are relatively uncommon.

Conditions acknowledged to be "idiopathic" make up by far the largest category of pain conditions. As the prevalence figures in Figure 2-1 indicate, a substantial proportion of the population suffers from one or more of these conditions.

Many disorders are difficult to place into one of these categories because the clinical term used to describe the

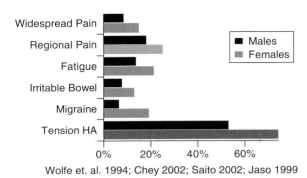

Figure 2-1. Prevalence of somatic symptoms/syndromes in the United States.

TABLE 2-1	Causes of Pain

- Inflammation
  - Rheumatoid arthritis
  - SLE
  - Inflammatory bowel disease
- Damage
  - Osteoarthritis
  - Tendinitis/bursitis
  - Neurological and endocrine disorders
- Idiopathic disorders

SLE, systemic lupus erythematosus.

condition is a "location" rather than a "disease." In fact, many pain conditions are labeled largely by the location where they occur, some of which are depicted in Figure 2-3.

Chronic low back pain (CLBP) gives an excellent illustration of the problems with labeling a chronic pain syndrome by its location. This is an extremely common problem, especially in industrialized countries. Although acute low back pain affects 70% to 85% of all people at some time in their life, 90% of affected individuals recover, typically within 12 weeks (5). Recovery after 12 weeks is slow and uncertain, and this subset of patients who develop CLBP is the group responsible for major expenses in the health-care and disability systems (5,6). CLBP affects approximately 5% of the population, with the prevalence varying depending on exactly on how it is defined.

Despite the problem's magnitude, little is known about the precise cause of CLBP. There is often a mismatch between objective findings and symptoms. Despite advances in imaging, in most patients it is impossible to determine whether identifiable structural or mechanical abnormalities are responsible for symptoms (7). Moreover, even when anatomic abnormalities are detected, the significance is unclear, since bulging disks or annular tears are found in high percentages of asymptomatic patients (8,9).

Because of this mismatch between objective findings and pain, investigators have assumed that psychosocial factors must be responsible for much of CLBP. These studies suggest that increasing age, female gender, lower levels of formal education, depression, stress, job dissatisfaction,

and disability/compensation issues may play some role in expression of symptoms and in chronicity (10–14). Nonetheless, all the known anatomic, demographic, and psychosocial factors that might cause CLBP do not explain the symptoms in a significant number of subjects (15). These patients are referred to as having "idiopathic" or "nonspecific" CLBP, and this may comprise 60% to 70% of CLBP patients.

This brief overview suggests that our current classification systems for chronic pain are unsatisfactory because the overwhelming majority of people with chronic pain have conditions that (1) are merely labeled by the anatomic location of the pain or (2) are acknowledged to be "idiopathic." The obvious corollary of not understanding the underlying mechanism of pain is that treatments are likely to be less effective.

To amplify the problem with our current taxonomy systems, even when someone has a "disease," we may not necessarily know what is causing the pain. Two prototypical "diseases" are presented to illustrate this point, an inflammatory disease (SLE) and a mechanical disorder (osteoarthritis).

SYSTEMIC LUPUS ERYTHEMATOSUS

In many ways SLE is the prototypical autoimmune disease, in which hyperactivity of the immune system leads to immune complex formation and deposition in various end-organs. These immune changes can theoretically lead to pain either

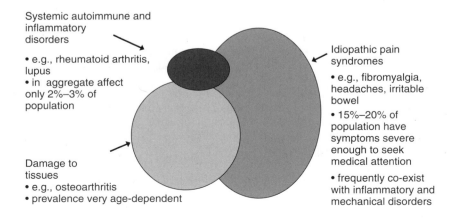

Systemic autoimmune and inflammatory disorders

- e.g., rheumatoid arthritis, lupus
- in aggregate affect only 2%–3% of population

Damage to tissues
- e.g., osteoarthritis
- prevalence very age-dependent

Idiopathic pain syndromes

- e.g., fibromyalgia, headaches, irritable bowel
- 15%–20% of population have symptoms severe enough to seek medical attention
- frequently co-exist with inflammatory and mechanical disorders

Figure 2-2. What's causing the pain?

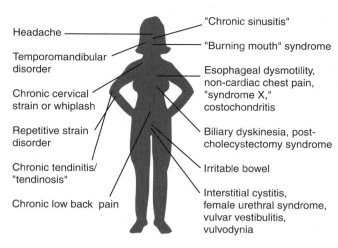

Headache

Temporomandibular disorder

Chronic cervical strain or whiplash

Repetitive strain disorder

Chronic tendinitis/ "tendinosis"

Chronic low back pain

"Chronic sinusitis"

"Burning mouth" syndrome

Esophageal dysmotility, non-cardiac chest pain, "syndrome X," costochondritis

Biliary dyskinesia, post-cholecystectomy syndrome

Irritable bowel

Interstitial cystitis, female urethral syndrome, vulvar vestibulitis, vulvodynia

Figure 2-3. Pain syndromes by location.

directly (because of inflammation) or indirectly (by causing tissue damage). To aid in the study of SLE, composite indices have been developed and validated that summarize either the disease's immune activity (e.g., the SLE Disease Activity Index—SLEDAI), or the amount of tissue damage the disease has caused (e.g., the Systemic Lupus International Coordinating Committee/American College of Rheumatology Damage Index). If the "disease" SLE is responsible for the pain and the other symptoms people with this condition are experiencing, then some combination of the degree of inflammation and the amount of damage from the SLE should predict the amount of pain and other symptoms. In fact, this is not the case. Neither of these indices correlates well with pain, fatigue, function, or other symptoms of SLE (16–18). Instead, the presence or absence of comorbid fibromyalgia (which occurs in approximately 20% of patients with SLE as well as other autoimmune disorders) is the biggest predictor of pain, fatigue, and function in SLE patients (19,20).

OSTEOARTHRITIS

If SLE is the classic inflammatory rheumatic disease, osteoarthritis is the classic mechanical or "wear-and-tear" condition. In this condition cartilage damage and new bone formation (osteophytes) occur in the joints. Again, if damage to the cartilage and bone is the "disease," the magnitude of one or both of these pathologic changes should predict symptoms. However, population-based studies suggest that there is a significant disparity between the degree of peripheral damage noted on radiographs and the pain and functional limitations that patients with this condition experience. The most dramatic evidence of this is that in all the population databases that have examined osteoarthritis, between 30% and 60% of patients with moderate to severe radiographic changes of osteoarthritis are *totally asymptomatic,* and approximately 10% of patients with moderate to severe knee pain have normal radiographs (21,22).

Just as with CLBP, this disparity between radiographic features and symptoms has caused investigators to explore the notion that psychological factors may be responsible for this discordance. Again, these studies have suggested that

psychological factors such as anxiety and depression do account for some of this variance in pain and other symptoms, but only a small degree (23,24).

Another recurring "trap" we fall into in clinical medicine is that when there is discordance between objective abnormalities identified in diagnostic testing and the symptoms an individual is experiencing, we erroneously conclude that our diagnostic tests are not sensitive enough. In osteoarthritis, investigators have hypothesized that the reason that plain radiographs only partly explain pain and other symptoms is that this technique does not permit visualization of cartilage defects, bone marrow edema, and other lesions that may be causing pain. Although early studies of these hypotheses suggested this may be the case, more recent studies suggest that although these types of magnetic resonance imaging (MRI) abnormalities are important, they likewise do not consistently cause pain (25,26).

NOCICEPTION AND PAIN

Any new system for characterizing chronic pain by the underlying cause must be based on a contemporary understanding of pain mechanisms. Until relatively recently, most pain had been thought to be due to activation of peripheral nociceptive nerves. These afferent neurons located in the skin, muscles, joints, and other tissues become depolarized in response to thermal, mechanical, or chemical stimuli. Once a nociceptor is activated, the depolarization is carried to the spinal cord, primarily by lightly myelinated A-delta or unmyelinated C fibers, or both. The A-delta fibers are considered to transduce the first pain that is felt as a sharp, pricking quality, whereas the "second pain" is conducted via the C fibers and leads to a more prolonged, deep quality of pain (27).

This nociceptive information first undergoes integration and modification at the levels of the dorsal horn/column through interaction with interneurons and descending supraspinal pathways. Interneurons receive and modulate signals from many sensory levels (i.e., wide dynamic range neurons) and thus are thought to be responsible for phenomena such as referred pain. Descending supraspinal information originates in various subcortical regions and travels caudally to the spinal cord. Under normal conditions these descending influences are inhibitory and thus are capable of attenuating or even eliminating the conduction of nociceptive information from the periphery to central structures (28). This mechanism is likely responsible for the fact that much nociceptive information that is transmitted to the spinal cord via nociceptive neurons and serves no adaptive role (i.e., is not damaging tissues) is "filtered out" by descending pathways that are tonically active. (An example would be that although with prolonged sitting pressure nociceptors in the back and buttocks are constantly activated, these sensations are not typically felt and certainly are not judged as painful.) These descending antinociceptive pathways can be more active during stress or in response to repeated painful stimuli, and neuromodulators such as opioids, serotonin, and norepinephrine play roles in transmitting this inhibitory information (28,29).

If interneurons or antinociceptive processes occurring in the dorsal horn do not filter or modulate nociceptive information, most of this information projects contralaterally and continues upward through a variety of ascending pathways. These various ascending pathways and circuits are responsible for the localization, attention, movement, and emotion associated with "pain" (27,30).

NONNOCICEPTIVE PAIN

Recent research into several "idiopathic" conditions suggests that the pain in these conditions is not occurring because of inflammation or damage in peripheral tissues and thus is not truly "nociceptive" pain. The best example of this would be fibromyalgia, the second most common rheumatic disease (1). Although people with fibromyalgia have the most severe pain and disability of any rheumatic disease, there is virtual unanimity that there is no inflammation (thus the abandonment of the term fibrositis) or damage in tissues. Instead, fibromyalgia pain is likely due to a central nervous system disturbance in pain processing in the absence of appropriate nociceptive input (31). Other similar nonnociceptive "central" pain syndromes include irritable bowel syndrome (IBS), temporomandibular disorders, and a variety of other regional pain syndromes that are discussed in this text (32–35).

In reviewing potential mechanisms by which pain could occur in the absence of nociceptive input, even lay persons are aware that psychological and cognitive processes are capable of leading to pain. But a plethora of neurobiological mechanisms have been identified in animal models that can lead to pain in the absence of normal nociceptive input. Some of these processes are listed in Table 2-2. In general terms, an "increased gain" in pain processing can occur either because of increased sensitivity of peripheral nociceptive neurons or because of increased sensitivity (or lack of antinociceptive activity) of central nervous system function. The clinical correlates of this increased gain in pain processing systems include hyperalgesia (increased pain in response to normally painful stimuli) or allodynia (pain in response to normally nonpainful stimuli), or both.

Some of the conditions in which peripheral or visceral hyperalgesia has been identified are noted in Table 2-3 (36–42). Although skeptics sometimes question the veracity

TABLE 2-2 Neurobiological Mechanisms That Can Cause Pain in the Absence of Appropriate Nociceptive Input

Peripheral
- Sensitization of C- or A-delta neurons
- Recruitment of silent nociceptors (e.g., A-beta fibers in inflammation)
- Alteration in phenotype
- Hyperinnervation
Central
- Deafferentation (i.e., as in phantom limb)
- Central sensitization (e.g., wind-up)
- Decreased descending antinociceptive activity

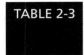

TABLE 2-3 Conditions Characterized by Widespread Peripheral or Visceral Hyperalgesia/Allodynia

Fibromyalgia
Irritable bowel syndrome
Temporomandibular disorder
Tension headache
"Trapezius myalgia"
Atypical facial pain
Vulvodynia/vulvar vestibulitis

of these findings because they rely on patient self-report of pain and thus could be due to psychological factors, more sophisticated pain testing paradigms have suggested that these findings are not likely to be due to psychological factors (43,44). Instead, these findings implicate central neurobiological mechanisms that exacerbate pain (e.g., "wind-up") or the absence of processes that normally inhibit the ascending transmission of pain-related activity (39,45,46).

To further strengthen the veracity and meaning of these findings of hyperalgesia/allodynia assessed by patient self-report, functional imaging techniques can allow the objective visualization of pain processing. These methods can use infusion of radioactive tracers (30,47) or, in the case of functional magnetic resonance imaging (fMRI), use the magnetic character of the level of oxygen in the blood as an indirect, intrinsic tracer (see Chapter 8) (48). Functional imaging studies have shown that painful stimulation produces increased neural activity in structures involved in the processing of sensation, movement, cognition, and emotion (30,49,50). Functional imaging studies in chronic pain states characterized by hyperalgesia/allodynia, such as IBS and fibromyalgia syndrome (FMS), have corroborated patients' self-reports of mechanical hyperalgesia, identifying objective evidence of augmented neural responses to pressure stimuli in the viscera and periphery, and are reviewed in detail in Chapter 8 (51–54).

EXAMINING THE ROLE OF NONNOCICEPTIVE PAIN IN CHRONIC LOW BACK PAIN

As noted earlier, CLBP is an example of a condition labeled on the basis of location rather than underlying "disease," and the role of mechanical and psychological factors have been examined in detail. However, in a recent cross-sectional study of CLBP, a simple laboratory measure of pressure pain sensitivity performed at the thumb (i.e., a "neutral" site) was a better correlate of pain and functional status than any other demographic, psychological, or radiographic variable (55). Subsequent studies have also detected lowered pain thresholds at neutral sites in low back pain patients (36) and lowered thresholds in patients with regional or widespread pain that do not have the 11 tender points (TePs) required for the diagnosis of fibromyalgia (56). In a subsequent study, people with idiopathic CLBP were studied using more sophisticated measures of pressure pain sensitivity that are not influenced by psychological status, and again these patients were found to be much more tender than normal controls and in fact had overall tenderness comparable to fibromyalgia patients (57). Moreover, these patients had the same types of objective abnormalities of augmented central pain processing on functional MRI that were seen in a group of fibromyalgia patients. Taken together, these data suggest that a subset of people with CLBP have nonnociceptive pain as a major underlying mechanism for their pain.

THE ROLE OF PSYCHOLOGICAL, COGNITIVE, AND BEHAVIORAL FACTORS IN CHRONIC PAIN

To emphasize the point that purely neurobiological mechanisms can cause nonnociceptive pain, up to this point in this chapter the role of psychological, cognitive, and behavioral factors in chronic pain has been minimized. However, these factors play extremely important roles in some groups of chronic pain patients (e.g., those in tertiary care centers or with high levels of disability) and in some people with chronic pain (58,59). These factors are examined in detail in Chapter 14 and Chapter 29 and are noted in Table 2-4.

A recent study in fibromyalgia illustrates how in an entirely nonnociceptive pain condition psychological and cognitive factors can interact with neurobiological factors to lead to the same expression of symptoms (57). In this study 97 patients who all met the American College of Rheumatology (ACR) criteria for fibromyalgia (i.e., chronic widespread pain and more than 11/18 TePs) were studied for the relative contributions of psychological, cognitive, and neurobiological factors in contributing to their symptoms. These patients all finished the same battery of self-report questionnaires and experimental pain testing. Analyzed variables were taken from several domains including (1) mood (depression, anxiety), (2) negative cognitions (catastrophizing and external locus of control), and (3) degree of hyperalgesia/allodynia (pressure pain sensitivity measured by sophisticated measures not influenced by psychological status). Cluster analytic procedures were used to identify subgroups on the basis of these domains. Three clusters best fit these data (see Figure 2-4). One subgroup (Group 1; $n = 50$) was characterized by normal mood ratings, low levels

| TABLE 2-4 | The Role of Psychological, Cognitive, and Behavioral Factors in Chronic Pain |

- Psychological (e.g., depression, anxiety, fear)
- Cognitions/beliefs (e.g., locus of control, helplessness, catastrophizing)
- Social (e.g., family, job, medicolegal)
- Behaviors (decreased activity/deconditioning, insomnia, substance abuse)

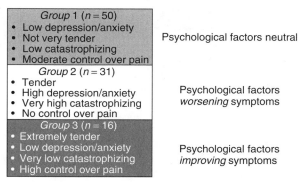

Figure 2-4. Subgroups of fibromyalgia patients.

of catastrophizing, moderate levels of personal control of pain, and low levels of tenderness (they were tender enough to meet ACR TeP criteria, but the least tender of the three groups when using the more sophisticated measures of pain sensitivity). It appeared as though psychological factors were "neutral" in this group and were neither worsening nor improving their pain. A second subgroup (Group 2; $n = 31$) displayed significant depression or anxiety, or both, the highest values on catastrophizing, the lowest values of locus of control, and intermediate tenderness. In this group psychological and cognitive factors were likely causing, perpetuating, or maintaining their pain. The third group (Group 3; $n = 16$) also had normal mood ratings but had very low levels of catastrophizing and the highest level of perceived control over pain. Despite this, they had the most pronounced tenderness. In these individuals, neurobiological factors (i.e., extreme levels of hyperalgesia/allodynia) were clearly causing pain, and if anything, these individuals' psychological and cognitive states were *improving,* not worsening, their pain (i.e., they were *above normal* psychologically).

A MECHANISTIC CHARACTERIZATION OF CHRONIC PAIN PATIENTS

Table 2-5 gives a suggested mechanistic characterization scheme for chronic pain. In this simplistic scheme pain is considered to be nociceptive (because there is an appropriate inflammatory or mechanical stimulus in the periphery) or nonnociceptive (i.e., "central pain"). In general, conditions such as osteoarthritis, rheumatoid arthritis, and cancer pain are considered prototypical nociceptive pain syndromes. However, certain people with these conditions may have elements of nonnociceptive pain, thus accounting for the fact that there is sometimes a mismatch between the degree of joint space damage, inflammation, extent of metastatic disease, and the amount of pain an individual is experiencing.

The differential diagnosis of individuals along such lines is outlined in Chapters 24 and 25, but nonnociceptive pain should not be considered only when no peripheral abnormalities are noted or when there is a disparity between objective peripheral findings and symptoms. Table 2-6 lists other clinical clues to the presence of central, nonnociceptive pain.

TABLE 2-5	Mechanistic Characterization of Chronic Pain

Peripheral (nociceptive)	Central (nonnociceptive)
– Primarily due to *inflammation* or mechanical damage in periphery	– Primarily due to a central disturbance in pain processing
– NSAID, opioid responsive	– Tricyclic, neuroactive compounds most effective
– Responds to procedures	– Psychological, behavioral factors more prominent
– Behavioral factors minor	– Examples
– Examples	• Fibromyalgia
• Osteoarthritis	• Irritable bowel syndrome
• Rheumatoid arthritis	• Tension and migraine headache
• Cancer pain	• Interstitial cystitis/vulvodynia, noncardiac chest pain, and so on

NSAID, nonsteroidal anti-inflammatory drugs.

In some cases a peripheral nociceptive abnormality can be identified in an individual, but the distribution of the pain exceeds that noted (e.g., the individual with a single herniated disk who has diffuse back pain and paresthesias). As noted, the presence of tenderness (allodynia/hyperalgesia) is a mechanistic clue that an individual has a globally heightened state of pain processing. In some cases the presence of nonnociceptive pain is not suspected until the individual is found to be unresponsive to nonsteroidal anti-inflammatory drugs (NSAIDs), opioids, nerve blocks, or other therapies that typically ameliorate nociceptive pain. Finally, nonnociceptive pain is sometimes identifiable by the "company it keeps." Patients with nonnociceptive pain syndromes not only have pain in several locations (and it is important to consider headache, frequent sore throat, tender nodes, and visceral pain as "pain") but also frequently experience fatigue, insomnia, sleep disturbances, memory problems, and so on.

This most important reason to move to this type of classification system is because nociceptive and nonnociceptive pain respond differently to therapeutic interventions. NSAIDs and opioids are more effective for nociceptive than nonnociceptive pain. People with nociceptive pain are also much more likely to benefit from procedures aimed at correcting peripheral abnormalities, such as joint replacement, nerve blocks, and so on. In contrast, different classes of drugs that primarily work on central nervous system function, such as tricyclic compounds, are more effective for nonnociceptive pain. Although psychological, cognitive, and behavioral factors are more common in nonnociceptive than nociceptive pain conditions, these should be identified and addressed in all chronic pain patients. Finally, although this chapter has emphasized

identifying and treating nonnociceptive pain in people with conditions heretofore suspected to be nociceptive, the converse is also true. For example, although we consider conditions such as fibromyalgia to be primarily nonnociceptive, if these patients have comorbid arthritis or other mechanical or inflammatory conditions, these should be identified and treated. This is especially important because we know that continuous peripheral nociceptive input can lead to phenomena such as wind-up and central sensitization. Thus, if nociceptive stimuli are present in an individual with nonnociceptive pain and are not appropriately addressed, this is doubly important; the nociceptive pain will continue unabated, and this can worsen the nonnociceptive component of that individual's pain.

SUMMARY POINTS

- Most chronic pain states are acknowledged to be idiopathic or are simply labeled by the location of the pain (e.g., chronic low back pain).
- Even when chronic pain occurs in the setting of diseases in which the underlying pathophysiology is understood, there is often a significant disparity between the degree of inflammation or damage in peripheral structures (i.e., nociceptive input) and the pain and other symptoms that the individual is experiencing.
- When pain is not occurring because of peripheral nociceptive input, this does not mean that psychological or behavioral factors are responsible.
- Many neurobiological mechanisms can cause an increase in the "gain" or "volume control" on pain processing systems, and these seem to be the primary underlying abnormality in nonnociceptive pain syndromes such as fibromyalgia, irritable bowel syndrome, tension headache, and so on.
- Characterizing an individual's pain as nociceptive or nonnociceptive (acknowledging that in many cases both are present) is more useful than our present classification schemes and logically leads to the most effective treatments for a given individual.

TABLE 2-6	Recognizing Central Pain Clinically

- Peripheral factors inadequate to account for symptoms
- Pain outside distribution affected by the suspected peripheral disorder
- Hyperalgesia/allodynia present
- Unresponsiveness to "peripheral therapies"
- Accompanying symptoms (fatigue, cognitive dysfunction, distress)

■ IMPLICATIONS FOR PRACTICE

- Nociceptive pain is primarily due to damage or inflammation of peripheral structures and typically is responsive to NSAIDs, opioids, and other classic classes of analgesics.
- Nonnociceptive pain is either unresponsive or much less responsive to these classic analgesics, whereas tricyclic compounds and other neuroactive drugs are the most effective pharmacologic therapies.
- It is common for a given individual to have elements of both nociceptive and nonnociceptive pain. Both these elements must be addressed and aggressively managed.
- Psychological, behavioral, and cognitive factors can play a role in any chronic pain patient, and these factors likewise should be assessed and managed independent of the nociceptive or nonnociceptive pain.

REFERENCES

1. Wolfe F, Ross K, Anderson J, et al. The prevalence and characteristics of fibromyalgia in the general population. *Arthritis Rheum* 1995;38(1):19–28.
2. Croft P, Rigby AS, Boswell R, et al. The prevalence of chronic widespread pain in the general population. *J Rheumatol* 1993;20(4):710–713.
3. Lawrence RC, Helmick CG, Arnett FC, et al. Estimates of the prevalence of arthritis and selected musculoskeletal disorders in the United States. *Arthritis Rheum* 1998;41(5):778–799.
4. Felson DT, Naimark A, Anderson J, et al. The prevalence of knee osteoarthritis in the elderly. The Framingham Osteoarthritis Study. *Arthritis Rheum* 1987;30(8):914–918.
5. Shekelle PG, Markovich M, Louie R. An epidemiologic study of episodes of back pain care. *Spine* 1995;20(15):1668–1673.
6. Andersson GB. Epidemiological features of chronic low-back pain. *Lancet* 1999;354(9178):581–585.
7. Nachemson AL. Low back pain in the year 2000—"back" to the future. *Bull Hosp Jt Dis* 1996;55(3):119–121.
8. Jensen MC, Brant-Zawadzki MN, Obuchowski N, et al. Magnetic resonance imaging of the lumbar spine in people without back pain. *N Engl J Med* 1994;331(2):69–73.
9. Boden SD, McCowin PR, Davis DO, et al. Abnormal magnetic-resonance scans of the cervical spine in asymptomatic subjects. A prospective investigation. *J Bone Jt Surg Am* 1990;72(8):1178–1184.
10. Bigos SJ, Battie MC, Spengler DM, et al. A prospective study of work perceptions and psychosocial factors affecting the report of back injury. *Spine* 1991;16(1):1–6.
11. Burton AK, Tillotson KM, Main CJ, et al. Psychosocial predictors of outcome in acute and subchronic low back trouble. *Spine* 1995;20(6):722–728.
12. Croft PR, Papageorgiou AC, Ferry S, et al. Psychologic distress and low back pain. Evidence from a prospective study in the general population. *Spine* 1995;20(24):2731–2737.
13. Frymoyer JW, Rosen JC, Clements J, et al. Psychologic factors in low-back-pain disability. *Clin Orthop* 1985;195:178–184.
14. Greenough CG, Fraser RD. Comparison of eight psychometric instruments in unselected patients with back pain. *Spine* 1991;16(9):1068–1074.
15. Linton SJ. A review of psychological risk factors in back and neck pain. *Spine* 2000;25(9):1148–1156.
16. Urowitz MB, Gladman DD. Measures of disease activity and damage in SLE. *Baillieres Clin Rheumatol* 1998;12(3):405–413.
17. Wang B, Gladman DD, Urowitz MB. Fatigue in lupus is not correlated with disease activity. *J Rheumatol* 1998;25(5):892–895.
18. Neville C, Clarke AE, Joseph L, et al. Learning from discordance in patient and physician global assessments of systemic lupus erythematosus disease activity. *J Rheumatol* 2000;27(3):675–679.
19. Gladman DD, Urowitz MB, Gough J, et al. Fibromyalgia is a major contributor to quality of life in lupus. *J Rheumatol* 1997;24(11):2145–2148.
20. Clauw DJ, Katz P. The overlap between fibromyalgia and inflammatory rheumatic diseases: when and why does it occur? *J Clin Rheumatol* 1995;1:335–341.
21. Creamer P, Keen M, Zananiri F, et al. Quantitative magnetic resonance imaging of the knee: a method of measuring response to intra-articular treatments. *Ann Rheum Dis* 1997;56(6):378–381.
22. Hannan MT, Felson DT, Pincus T. Analysis of the discordance between radiographic changes and knee pain in osteoarthritis of the knee. *J Rheumatol* 2000;27(6):1513–1517.
23. Creamer P, Hochberg MC. The relationship between psychosocial variables and pain reporting in osteoarthritis of the knee. *Arthritis Care Res* 1998;11(1):60–65.
24. Creamer P, Lethbridge-Cejku M, Costa P, et al. The relationship of anxiety and depression with self-reported knee pain in the community: data from the Baltimore Longitudinal Study of Aging. *Arthritis Care Res* 1999;12(1):3–7.
25. Felson DT, Chaisson CE, Hill CL, et al. The association of bone marrow lesions with pain in knee osteoarthritis. *Ann Intern Med* 2001;134(7):541–549.
26. Hill CL, Gale DR, Chaisson CE, et al. Periarticular lesions detected on magnetic resonance imaging: prevalence in knees with and without symptoms. *Arthritis Rheum* 2003;48(10):2836–2844.
27. Willis WD, Westlund KN. Neuroanatomy of the pain system and of the pathways that modulate pain. *J Clin Neurophysiol* 1997;14(1):2–31.
28. Millan MJ. Descending control of pain. *Prog Neurobiol* 2002;66(6):355–474.
29. Crofford LJ, Casey KL. Central modulation of pain perception. *Rheum Dis Clin North Am* 1999;25(1):1–13.
30. Casey KL. Match and mismatch: identifying the neuronal determinants of pain. *Ann Intern Med* 1996;124(11):995–998.
31. Yunus MB. Towards a model of pathophysiology of fibromyalgia: aberrant central pain mechanisms with peripheral modulation. *J Rheumatol* 1992;19(6):846–850.
32. Clauw DJ, Crofford LJ. Chronic widespread pain and fibromyalgia: what we know, and what we need to know. *Best Pract Res Clin Rheumatol* 2003;17(4):685–701.
33. Clauw DJ, Chrousos GP. Chronic pain and fatigue syndromes: overlapping clinical and neuroendocrine features and potential pathogenic mechanisms. *Neuroimmunomodulation* 1997;4(3):134–153.
34. Schwetz I, Bradesi S, Mayer EA. Current insights into the pathophysiology of irritable bowel syndrome. *Curr Gastroenterol Rep* 2003;5(4):331–336.
35. Bragdon EE, Light KC, Costello NL, et al. Group differences in pain modulation: pain-free women compared to pain-free men and to women with TMD. *Pain* 2002;96(3):227–237.
36. Wilder-Smith OH, Tassonyi E, Arendt-Nielsen L. Preoperative back pain is associated with diverse manifestations of central neuroplasticity. *Pain* 2002;97(3):189–194.
37. Kashima K, Rahman OI, Sakoda S, et al. Increased pain sensitivity of the upper extremities of TMD patients with myalgia to experimentally-evoked noxious stimulation: possibility of worsened endogenous opioid systems. *Cranio* 1999;17(4):241–246.

38. Maixner W, Fillingim R, Booker D, et al. Sensitivity of patients with painful temporomandibular disorders to experimentally evoked pain. *Pain* 1995;63(3):341–351.

39. Leffler AS, Hansson P, Kosek E. Somatosensory perception in a remote pain-free area and function of diffuse noxious inhibitory controls (DNIC) in patients suffering from long-term trapezius myalgia. *Eur J Pain* 2002;6(2):149–159.

40. Whitehead WE, Holtkotter B, Enck P, et al. Tolerance for rectosigmoid distention in irritable bowel syndrome. *Gastroenterology* 1990;98(5 Pt 1):1187–1192.

41. Gibson SJ, Littlejohn GO, Gorman MM, et al. Altered heat pain thresholds and cerebral event-related potentials following painful CO_2 laser stimulation in subjects with fibromyalgia syndrome. *Pain* 1994;58(2):185–193.

42. Kosek E, Ekholm J, Hansson P. Increased pressure pain sensibility in fibromyalgia patients is located deep to the skin but not restricted to muscle tissue. *Pain* 1995;63(3):335–339 [published erratum appears in *Pain* 1996 Mar;64(3):605].

43. Petzke F, Gracely RH, Park KM, et al. What do tender points measure? Influence of distress on 4 measures of tenderness. *J Rheumatol* 2003;30(3):567–574.

44. Petzke F, Clauw DJ, Ambrose K, et al. Increased pain sensitivity in fibromyalgia: effects of stimulus type and mode of presentation. *Pain* 2003;105(3):403–413.

45. Staud R, Vierck CJ, Cannon RL, et al. Abnormal sensitization and temporal summation of second pain (wind-up) in patients with fibromyalgia syndrome. *Pain* 2001;91(1–2):165–175.

46. Kosek E, Hansson P. Modulatory influence on somatosensory perception from vibration and heterotopic noxious conditioning stimulation (HNCS) in fibromyalgia patients and healthy subjects. *Pain* 1997;70(1):41–51.

47. Casey KL, Minoshima S, Morrow TJ, et al. Comparison of human cerebral activation pattern during cutaneous warmth, heat pain, and deep cold pain. *J Neurophysiol* 1996;76(1):571–581.

48. Gelnar PA, Krauss BR, Sheehe PR, et al. A comparative fMRI study of cortical representations for thermal painful, vibrotactile, and motor performance tasks. *Neuroimage* 1999;10(4):460–482.

49. Derbyshire SW. Imaging the brain in pain. *APS Bull* 1999;9(3):7–8.

50. Peyron R, Garcia-Larrea L, Gregoire MC, et al. Haemodynamic brain responses to acute pain in humans: sensory and attentional networks. *Brain* 1999;122(Pt 9):1765–1780.

51. Mountz JM, Bradley LA, Modell JG, et al. Fibromyalgia in women. Abnormalities of regional cerebral blood flow in the thalamus and the caudate nucleus are associated with low pain threshold levels. *Arthritis Rheum* 1995;38(7):926–938.

52. Gracely RH, Petzke F, Wolf JM, et al. Functional magnetic resonance imaging evidence of augmented pain processing in fibromyalgia. *Arthritis Rheum* 2002;46(5):1333–1343.

53. Silverman DH, Munakata JA, Ennes H, et al. Regional cerebral activity in normal and pathological perception of visceral pain. *Gastroenterology* 1997;112(1):64–72.

54. Derbyshire SW, Jones AK, Devani P, et al. Cerebral responses to pain in patients with atypical facial pain measured by positron emission tomography. *J Neurol Neurosurg Psychiatry* 1994;57(10):1166–1172.

55. Clauw DJ, Williams D, Lauerman W, et al. Pain sensitivity as a correlate of clinical status in individuals with chronic low back pain. *Spine* 1999;24(19):2035–2041.

56. Carli G, Suman AL, Biasi G, et al. Reactivity to superficial and deep stimuli in patients with chronic musculoskeletal pain. *Pain* 2002;100(3):259–269.

57. Giesecke T, Williams DA, Harris RE, et al. Subgroupings of fibromyalgia patients on the basis of pressure pain thresholds and psychological factors. *Arthritis Rheum* 2003;48(10):2916–2922.

58. Drossman DA, McKee DC, Sandler RS, et al. Psychosocial factors in the irritable bowel syndrome. A multivariate study of patients and nonpatients with irritable bowel syndrome. *Gastroenterology* 1988;95(3):701–708.

59. Aaron LA, Bradley LA, Alarcon GS, et al. Psychiatric diagnoses in patients with fibromyalgia are related to health care-seeking behavior rather than to illness. *Arthritis Rheum* 1996;39(3):436–445.

3

The Epidemiology of Chronic Widespread Pain and Fibromyalgia

John McBeth

Chronic generalized body pain, classified as fibromyalgia when in the presence of widespread tenderness or other somatic symptoms, has been described for centuries (see Chapter 1) (1). The past 20 years have seen an increase in the number of studies examining the prevalence, characteristic features, etiology, natural history, and individual and societal impact of symptoms. The aim of this chapter is to collate that information and highlight the salient findings. However, before doing so it is useful to briefly discuss the issues surrounding the classification of chronic widespread pain and fibromyalgia.

DEFINING CHRONIC WIDESPREAD PAIN AND FIBROMYALGIA

Throughout the literature, "diagnostic criteria" and "classification criteria" are used interchangeably when discussing case definition, and this can often lead to confusion. In epidemiological studies it is more appropriate to discuss syndromes such as fibromyalgia in terms of classification criteria, since this term implies the identification of a homogenous group of persons with regard to symptoms. Epidemiological studies that investigate disease prevalence or etiological risk factors using the same classification criteria can then be compared and contrasted. In this chapter the term "classification criteria" will be used when discussing case definition.

In describing the clinical presentation of fibrositis, Smythe (2) identified what is generally accepted as the defining characteristics of the fibromyalgia syndrome. Widespread pain was described occurring in "deep tissues" such as muscles and tendon insertions. Notable was the presence of local points of tenderness that on palpation elicited pain. These descriptive criteria were further refined when Smythe and Moldofsky (3) proposed the first generally accepted criteria for the classification of fibromyalgia. Widespread aching, disturbed sleep, and normal laboratory studies were proposed as inclusion criteria. Tender points (TePs) were identified as central to diagnosis with a total of 12 of 14 "active" sites required. In recent years the development of fibromyalgia classification criteria has followed two clear lines (4,5): Some researchers have retained the broad scope of Smythe and Moldofsky (3) (including primary/secondary distinctions and other diagnostic variables unrelated to pain but which may act to modulate pain, such as disturbed sleep) (6), while others have restricted the description and focused almost exclusively on the syndrome's musculoskeletal aspects (4).

Noting the impact of the fibromyalgia syndrome and the lack of a commonly agreed classification criteria, Yunus et al. (6) studied a group of 63 fibromyalgia patients. Patients were classified as having fibromyalgia when generalized musculoskeletal aching or stiffness, or both, present for at least 3 months at three or more anatomic sites in the absence of an underlying condition were identified. All subjects had TePs but no predefined number was required for entry into the study. As controls, two groups were identified. "Pain controls" consisted of 32 mild rheumatoid patients and 31 patients with trauma-associated localized musculoskeletal pain. Thirty normal controls without significant pain were also included. Fibromyalgia patients could be discriminated from both control groups by a combination of six diverse historical features, ranging from pain at seven or more sites to poor sleep, and seven pairs of TePs. On the basis of these results, classification criteria for fibromyalgia were proposed, which had a sensitivity (the proportion of subjects correctly classified as having fibromyalgia) of 92% and specificity (the proportion of subjects correctly classified as not having fibromyalgia) of 94%.

Focusing on the symptom of widespread pain, Wolfe et al. (4), in a 16-center study, proposed criteria for the classification of fibromyalgia [the American College of Rheumatology (ACR) criteria]. Four specific objectives were stated: (1) to provide a consensus definition of fibromyalgia, (2) to establish new classification criteria, (3) to study the relationship of primary fibromyalgia to secondary/concomitant fibromyalgia, and (4) to examine the relationship between previous criteria sets with the new definition. Trained blinded assessors interviewed and examined 293 fibromyalgia patients and 265 control patients. The fibromyalgia patients were considered to have the disorder by the clinical diagnosis normally used by the investigator at the various centers. Age-matched and sex-matched patients with a variety of pain disorders, including low back pain syndromes and trauma-related pain syndromes, were used as controls. The presence of 11 of 18 TePs in the presence of widespread pain (see Figure 3-1) enabled fibromyalgia patients to be distinguished from controls with a sensitivity of 88% and a specificity of 81%. The primary and secondary distinction at the diagnostic level was abandoned as none of the criteria distinguished between the two. In this way these two defining features could diagnose fibromyalgia.

Subsequent studies have demonstrated that although chronic widespread pain and widespread tenderness are associated, the relationship is by no means linear (7). Persons with no pain may have a high TeP count and others with chronic widespread pain may have a low count (7). It appears that both TePs and pain exist as continua in the general population with fibromyalgia representing a subset of persons with chronic widespread pain who additionally have a high TeP count. The strength of the classification criteria lies in enabling researchers to identify and investigate a homogenous group of subjects with the fibromyalgia syndrome, with the ACR criteria coming to be the most widely used in studies.

However, it has been noted that patterns of pain distribution involving only a few local areas would qualify as widespread under the ACR definition (8), while cases of clinically meaningful widespread pain may be excluded. Macfarlane et al. (9) have proposed a more stringent (the "Manchester") definition that identifies a group of subjects whose pain is more likely to be widespread (Figure 3-1). This definition requires more diffuse limb pain, present in two or more sections of contralateral limbs, and axial pain, present for at least 3 months. When compared to persons classified using the ACR criteria, an increased severity of symptoms associated with fibromyalgia, such as fatigue, TePs, and sleep disruption, have been demonstrated in persons with chronic widespread pain identified using the Manchester criteria (9). Although any distinction between persons with regional pain and those with chronic widespread pain is arbitrary, the Manchester definition does have construct validity, identifying a group of persons with more severe disability and higher levels of associated symptoms (10).

THE PREVALENCE OF CHRONIC WIDESPREAD PAIN AND FIBROMYALGIA

PREVALENCE OR INCIDENCE RATES?

In epidemiological studies estimates of the frequency of chronic widespread pain and fibromyalgia are often reported as prevalence (the proportion of persons in a population with symptoms at a particular time or during a particular period) or incidence rates (the proportion of new cases or first-ever episodes). However, identifying a true incident rate is problematic because many cases may resolve and recur over a period of time. In addition, many individuals may experience their first-ever onset in childhood. For these reasons it is most appropriate to discuss these symptoms in terms of prevalence rates.

PREVALENCE ESTIMATES IN THE GENERAL POPULATION

Although there are no studies of the cumulative lifetime prevalence of chronic widespread pain, it is clear that a significant proportion of cases persist (11,12) and that symptoms do not generally respond well to contemporary treatments (13). A limited number of studies have specifically examined the prevalence of chronic widespread pain in the adult population (see Table 3-1). Of those available, one was conducted in the United States (14), two in the United Kingdom (10,15), one in Canada (16), and one in Sweden (17). In a random sample of community-based subjects, Wolfe et al. (14) reported a prevalence rate of chronic widespread pain using the ACR definition of 10.6%. The prevalence of chronic widespread pain was observed to increase with age in both men and women, and women were more likely to report symptoms when compared to men at all ages. This rate was similar to that reported in a survey of community subjects in the United Kingdom (15). In that study, of the 1,340 subjects who responded to a postal questionnaire, 13% (the crude prevalence rate) reported having experienced pain symptoms that satisfied the ACR criteria for chronic widespread pain. When these rates were standardized to the population of England and Wales, the adjusted prevalence rate was 11.2%. Rates were 7% higher in women when compared to men (16% vs. 9% respectively) with an overall tendency to increase with age in both sexes. Hunt and colleagues (10) examined the prevalence of chronic widespread pain, defined using both the ACR criteria and the more stringent "Manchester" criteria. The prevalence of ACR-defined chronic widespread pain of 12.9% was similar to that reported previously, while the prevalence using the Manchester definition was, as expected, lower at 4.7%. Lower rates of ACR-defined chronic widespread pain have been reported. In a telephone survey conducted in Ontario, White et al. (16) reported a prevalence of chronic widespread pain of 7.3% while an even lower rate of 4.2% has been reported in a Swedish population (17).

A number of studies have assessed the prevalence of fibromyalgia in the general population (Table 3-1), with rates ranging from approximately 1% to 11%. Overall, the population prevalence is estimated to be 2% (32). Two of the earliest studies (18,19) reported rates of around 1% using the definition of fibromyalgia described by Yunus et al. (6). Wolfe et al. (14) reported an overall prevalence of 2% with higher rates in women and an increase with age. Standardizing these data to the population of the United States, the prevalence of fibromyalgia has been estimated to be 34 per 1,000 women and 5 per 1,000 men across all age groups (32). A slightly higher rate was reported in a population study of adults in Canada (16). Of the 3,395 subjects who responded, 248 (7.3%) reported widespread pain and 176 (78%) participated in a physical examination. The adjusted (for nonparticipation in

ACR coding

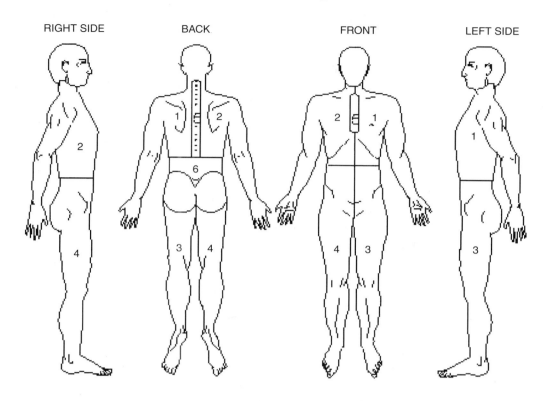

Manchester coding

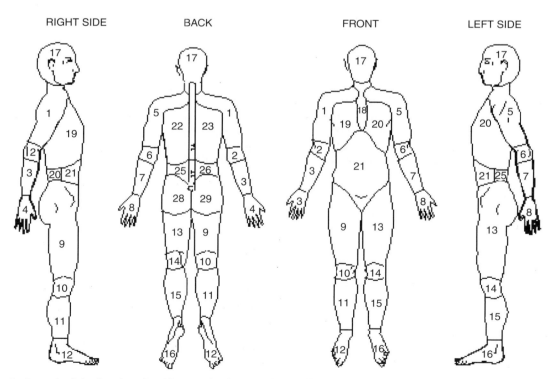

Figure 3-1.   Coding schedules for chronic widespread pain: American College of Rheumatology (ACR) and Manchester definitions.

TABLE 3-1	Prevalence of Fibromyalgia and Chronic Widespread Pain				
REFERENCE	STUDY SETTING	AGE GROUP (YEARS)	STUDY POPULATION	FM/CWP CLASSIFICATION	PREVALENCE (%)
Fibromyalgia					
Jacobsson et al., 1989 (18)	Sweden	50–70	876	Yunus	1.0
Makela & Heliovaara, 1991 (19)	Finland	≥30	7,217	Yunus	0.75
Prescott et al., 1993 (20)	Denmark	18–79	1,219	ACR	0.66
Wolfe et al., 1995 (14)	US		3,006	ACR	2.0
Jacobsson et al., 1996 (21)	Pima Indians, US	35–70	105	ACR	0
Forseth et al., 1997 (22)	Norway	20–49	2,498 (women)	ACR	10.5
Farooqi & Gibson, 1998 (16,23,24)	Punjabi, Pakistan	≥14	700	Unclear	2.1
White KP et al., 1999 (25)	Ontario		3,395	ACR	3.3
Carmona et al., 2001 (26)	Spain	≥20	2,998	ACR	2.4
White & Thompson, 2003 (27)	Amish community, Canada	≥18	179	ACR	7.3
Chronic Widespread Pain					
Croft et al., 1993 (15)	UK	18–65	1,340	ACR	11.2
Wolfe et al., 1995 (14)	US		3,006	ACR	10.6
Andersson et al., 1996 (28)	Sweden	25–74	1,609	Chronic pain, multiple locations	10.7
Hunt et al., 1999 (10)	UK	18–65	1,953	i) Manchester definition	4.7
				ii) ACR	12.9
White et al., 1999 (16,23,24)	Ontario		3,395	ACR	7.3
Buskila et al., 2000 (29)	Israel	≥18	4,643	ACR	9.9
Bergman et al., 2001 (30)	Sweden	≥18	2,425	ACR	11.4
White & Thompson, 2003 (27)	Amish community, Canada	≥18	179	ACR	14.5
Schochat & Raspe, 2003 (31)	Germany	35–74	3,174 (women)	ACR	13.5

FM, fibromyalgia; CWP, chronic widespread pain; ACR, American College of Rheumatology.

examination and weighted by the number of adults in each household) rate of fibromyalgia was reported to be 3.3%, with a higher rate in women (4.9%) compared to men (1.6%). One study has examined the prevalence of fibromyalgia in the northern region of Pakistan (25), although the classification criteria used was unclear. Overall, the prevalence rate was found to be 2.1% with a male-to-female ratio of 1:13. Interestingly, there was a significant discrepancy in the prevalence rate between those persons who lived in an urban area and were poor (3.2%) and those who lived in the same area but were classified as affluent (1.1%). A higher rate of 7.3% has also been reported in a rural Amish community, suggesting that this is not a symptom localized to industrialized or urban populations (27).

PREVALENCE ESTIMATES IN PRIMARY CARE

There are no prevalence estimates of chronic widespread pain and only one available of the prevalence of fibromyalgia in primary care (33). Of 692 patients examined, 2.1% satisfied the investigators' classification criteria for fibromyalgia defined as unexplained diffuse musculoskeletal aching present for 3 months or more and having four or more TePs. Other investigators have examined the prevalence of fibromyalgia in a diverse range of specialist clinics, including rheumatology, spine, and systemic lupus erythematosus clinics. These studies have reported rates of fibromyalgia ranging from 2% to 22%. However, they most certainly will not reflect the true prevalence in primary care since these rates are likely to be elevated because of differences in referral procedures and other factors associated with consultation at specialist clinics.

PREVALENCE IN OCCUPATIONAL SETTINGS

To date no studies have been conducted to specifically determine the prevalence rate of chronic widespread pain or fibromyalgia in an occupational setting. A population-based study in Finland (19) reported that the prevalence of fibromyalgia was lowest among professional workers (0%), rising to 0.5% in those employed in industry, 0.8% in service workers, and 1.5% in agricultural workers. The highest prevalence rate of 1.9% was among those who had never been employed (19).

TRENDS IN CHRONIC WIDESPREAD PAIN AND FIBROMYALGIA

Whether chronic widespread pain and fibromyalgia are increasing in prevalence is unknown. General population estimates do seem to be stable at around 10% to 13% between populations. Whether these rates are increasing within populations remains to be examined. Two studies conducted 7 years apart in different regions of South Manchester in the United Kingdom used the same definition for chronic widespread pain (10,15). Unadjusted prevalence estimates were similar in both studies, being 13.1% and 12.9% for the earlier and later studies respectively (10,15). Population-based studies that have followed up the same populations have found that although a large proportion of subjects change pain status after 1 (12), 2 (11), and 7 years (34), movement of subjects in and out of pain state results in the prevalence of chronic widespread pain remaining stable.

Nevertheless, it has been reported that claims for fibromyalgia "have reached near epidemic proportions" in those seeking some form of compensation through the legal system (35,36). A survey conducted among 100 Canadian rheumatologists found that fibromyalgia was the only condition that most of the respondents felt was increasing in incidence, with almost 70% observing an increase in the prevalence in their clinic over the past 5 years (37). Similarly, between 1987 and 1996, Andersson et al. (38) reported an increase in the prevalence of primary care consultations as a result of pain and that this increased consultation rate was primarily due to fibromyalgia. However, increases in the prevalence of fibromyalgia in the rheumatology clinic and primary care setting will be partly explained by the increased awareness of the fibromyalgia syndrome, in particular, with the development of the ACR criteria in 1990.

HIGH RISK GROUPS

With few exceptions (39–41), those persons at high risk of the onset of new widespread pain and fibromyalgia have been identified through cross-sectional studies. Such studies cannot distinguish the temporal relationship between risk factors and symptom onset and cannot identify true etiological risk factors. Nevertheless, they do give us an insight into factors that are commonly associated with symptoms (see Table 3-2) and that may usefully be investigated as potential risk factors.

INDIVIDUAL RISK FACTORS

In persons with chronic widespread pain and fibromyalgia, the influence of age and gender is clear. Women are consistently more likely to report chronic widespread pain, to satisfy criteria for fibromyalgia on examination (14,15), and to have more associated symptoms, including fatigue and irritable bowel syndrome (IBS) (51). For both women and men, self-reported widespread pain symptoms tended to increase with age. As previously noted, a study conducted in the United States, Wolfe et al. (14), found similar patterns for both age and gender-specific rates of ACR-defined chronic widespread pain in community subjects as those found in a U.K. population (15). The only difference was that in the latter study the prevalence started to decrease in

those aged 70 and over, although the small number of subjects in the upper age ranges in both studies may account for this discrepancy (52).

Why are these differences observed? Aging is associated with degenerative processes, and these may explain the observed increased likelihood of symptom reporting in older persons. Alternatively, following symptom onset it is likely that symptoms become chronic and the increase with age is the result of an accumulation of cases that have persisted over time. In older age groups we tend to observe a falloff in symptoms, and that may be attributed to either a change in those risk factors associated with further symptom onset or persistence (for example, a change in workplace mechanical factors after retirement from the workforce) or that chronic widespread pain may be associated with an increased risk of mortality (52).

A number of hypotheses may explain the excess symptom reporting among women (53). These include an increased sensitivity to pain or lower pain thresholds (54), a tendency to appraise and label stimuli as being more noxious (55), and the role of socialization in encouraging gender differences in the expression of symptoms (56) and willingness to seek health care (57). One appealing hypothesis is the role of hormonal factors. In a small clinic-based study of 16 patients, women with fibromyalgia reported significant changes in pain symptoms throughout the menstrual cycle (58). Fibromyalgia patients are also more likely to retrospectively recall a worsening of pain and associated symptoms during pregnancy and the postpartum period (59), to have a later menarche, or to have never been pregnant (60). However, a recent population-based study has found that hormonal factors, as measured by length of menstrual cycle, length of a period, and current oral contraceptive pill use and duration of use, among premenopausal or perimenopausal women was not associated with having chronic widespread pain (61). Among postmenopausal women, neither age at menopause nor hormone replacement therapy use was associated. Although the authors concluded that hormonal factors were unlikely to explain the observed gender differences in chronic widespread pain, the relationship between hormonal factors and symptom *severity* in persons with chronic widespread pain is still largely unknown.

There is a wealth of data examining risk factors for regional chronic pain syndromes such as low back pain, with associations reported with socioeconomic factors, individual factors such as body mass index (BMI), and health behaviors, including smoking and diet (62). Cross-sectional studies have shown similar associations with persons with chronic widespread pain and fibromyalgia, reporting lower levels of education and higher rates of unemployment and divorce (23). Others have demonstrated that among a group of fibromyalgia patients, factors such as smoking (43) and a high BMI (44) were associated with symptom severity. Although there is a paucity of prospective data, one recent study has examined these factors in relation to symptom onset. In a population-based survey of Swedish residents, Bergman and colleagues (46) followed up subjects who had responded to an original questionnaire that gathered details on pain status and a range of individual risk factors 3 years previously. At follow-up those persons who reported chronic widespread pain were identified. Compared to those without new chronic widespread pain at follow-up, those with new symptoms were

TABLE 3-2 Risk Factors for Chronic Widespread Pain and Fibromyalgia

REFERENCE	STUDY DESIGN	RISK FACTOR	STRENGTH AND DESCRIPTION OF ASSOCIATION
Vaeroy et al., 1988 (42)	Cross sectional	Smoking	Associated with higher substance P levels, possibly symptom severity
Croft et al., 1993 (15)	Cross sectional	Age	Positive linear relationship
		Gender	F (16%) > M (9%)
		Sleep disturbance	OR = 2.1 (1.4, 3.1)
Wolfe et al., 1995 (14)	Cross sectional	Age	Positive linear relationship
		Gender	F > M
Buskila et al., 1997 (49)	Prospective case-control	Traumatic injury	Higher rate of new onset fibromyalgia in subjects with neck injury (21.6%) compared to those with leg fractures (1.7%)
Forseth et al., 1999 (39,40)	Prospective	Previous pain ≥6 years	OR = 3.5 (1.0, 10.4)
		Altered bowel habit	OR = 3.0 (1.1, 8.0)
		Depression	OR = 6.3 (1.4, 24.8)
Hunt et al., 1999[a] (10)	Cross sectional	Age	Positive linear relationship
		Gender	F > M
		Fatigue	OR = 3.6 (2.2, 5.9)
McBeth et al., 2001 (12,41,45)	Prospective	Other (nonpain) somatic symptoms	OR = 3.3 (1.5, 7.4)
		Illness behavior	OR = 9.0 (3.7, 22.2)
Al-Allaf et al., 2002 (50)	Case-control	Traumatic physical events	Compared with controls, increased rates of surgery (38.2% v 26.2%) and occupational injury (14.7%, 4.8%)
Bergman et al., 2002 (46)	Prospective	Socioeconomic group	Inverse linear relationship
		Immigrant status	OR = 1.84 (0.96, 3.5)
		Smoking	OR = 1.65 (0.95, 2.9)
		Family history of chronic pain	OR = 1.87 (1.1, 3.1)
Yunus et al., 2002a (43)	Cross sectional	Smoking	Associated with symptom severity
Yunus et al., 2002b (44)	Cross sectional	BMI	Associated with symptom severity
Harkness et al., 2003 (48)	Prospective	Occupational exposures:	
		Lifting heavy weights	OR = 1.9 (1.1, 3.3)
		Prolonged squatting	OR = 2.9 (1.8, 4.9)
		Low job satisfaction	OR = 2.1 (0.9, 4.6)
		Monotonous work	OR = 2.4 (1.5, 3.9)
Imbierowicz & Egle, 2003 (47)	Retrospective case-control	Adverse childhood events	Compared with controls, increased rates of self-reported sexual (10.5% v 0%) and physical (31.6% v 11.4%) abuse

OR, odds ratio; BMI, body mass index.
[a]Manchester defined chronic widespread pain.

significantly older and more likely to have reported some pain at the time of the original study. Other factors, including low socioeconomic status, being an immigrant to Sweden, and being a current smoker, predicted new symptom onset although, statistically, these associations were not significant.

PSYCHOLOGICAL DISTRESS

Community subjects with chronic widespread pain (in comparison to those without such symptoms) more commonly report other somatic symptoms, negative life events (63), psychological distress (11), and an increased focus on bodily symptoms (10). Both community and clinic patients are also more likely to have a diagnosis of a psychiatric disorder, particularly depression and anxiety (15,64). Nonetheless,

the precise nature of the relationship between distress and pain symptoms is unclear, as studies are unable to distinguish whether depressive illness is a consequence of chronic pain, whether it precedes the onset of pain symptoms, or whether both depression and chronic pain share a common pathway but are unrelated. One prospective study has examined the role of several factors, including self-reported depression, in the onset of fibromyalgia (39). Among a group of 175 women, 43 (25%) satisfied criteria for fibromyalgia after 5.5 years of follow-up. Self-reported depression at baseline was associated with a more than sixfold increased likelihood of reporting fibromyalgia at follow-up and was found to be the strongest independent predictor. A subsequent study has lent support to this hypothesis. In the first population-based prospective study to examine predictors of new onset chronic widespread pain in a general population sample, indicators of somatization (the tendency to report distress as physical symptoms, for which health care is sought) measured at baseline (41) and aspects of illness behavior (65,66) predicted the development of new chronic widespread pain in the following 12-month period.

It has been hypothesized that the relationship between psychological distress and widespread pain in adulthood may be explained by exposure to adverse early life events. Indeed, clinic and community subjects with chronic widespread pain are more likely to report exposure to childhood events such as parental divorce or abuse (67,68), events that have historically (69) and more recently (70,71) been related to the presence of chronic localized pain. It has been argued that these reports are associated with consultation behavior and medication usage rather than symptoms *per se* (72), although in a comparison with other chronic pain patients, persons with fibromyalgia were found to report significantly increased rates of, among other factors, sexual abuse, physical abuse, and parental drug and alcohol addiction (47). Similar associations have been found in persons with high TeP counts (73), although these may be overestimated because of differential recall of adverse childhood events between persons according to their health status in adulthood (45). A study that identified a group of young adults on whom documented evidence of early adverse events was available found that, prospectively, factors such as sexual and physical abuse did not predict who would have pain. When asked to recall their early childhoods, those with pain were more likely to recall an adverse childhood event than those currently pain free (74). However, as a "gold standard," the study relied on evidence of abuse as documented by a criminal court, although it is unclear how complete such records are. Etiological hypotheses have suggested the role of biochemical "abnormalities," such as altered hypothalamic-pituitary-adrenal stress axis function (75), which are also associated with adverse early life events, in symptom onset. Although consistent evidence is lacking, this may provide one plausible mechanism through which such adverse events may lead to future chronic widespread pain (76).

Although high levels of occupational-related psychological distress have been linked to regional pain syndromes (77), few data examine the association with widespread pain syndromes. One study examined the relationship between work-related "physical stress" (although how the exposure was defined is unclear) and fibromyalgia (19), reporting that symptom prevalence increased as the level of work-related stress increased. Others have examined the relationship between work-related psychological distress and chronic widespread pain and fibromyalgia (19,78,79). Makela and Heliovaara (80) examined "mental stress" and found that there was no association with the prevalence of fibromyalgia. An examination of the work-related psychosocial environment as based on the Demand-Control-Support model proposed by Karasek and Theorell (81) found that reports of high job demands and low levels of social support were associated with a twofold increased likelihood of new symptom onset when compared to those not reporting these exposures.

DISTURBED SLEEP

Fibromyalgia patients report disturbed sleeping patterns, including light sleep that is often interrupted and unrefreshing.

Such patterns are thought to disrupt the restorative nature of sleep and may lead to the increased stiffness and pain upon wakening and daytime fatigue (82) commonly reported by patients. Indeed, self-reported nonrestorative sleep has been identified as being one of the most common symptoms among a group of fibromyalgia patients, second only to muscle and joint pain (14,83). In a study of factors associated with chronic unexplained musculoskeletal aching, subjects with severe symptoms could be distinguished from those with moderate symptoms by their reports of difficulty in sleeping and of fatigue upon wakening (84). Poor sleep is also significantly associated with an increased number of TePs (85).

The Alpha-delta (α-δ) Sleep Anomaly

Such evidence of disturbed sleep architecture has been taken to indicate an involvement of nonrestorative sleep in the development and persistence of fibromyalgia symptoms. Specifically, the α-δ sleep anomaly, an intrusive electroencephalogram (EEG) defined sleep pattern (86), has been postulated as a possible causal mechanism. Normal human sleep is usually classified into four nonrapid eye movement (NREM) sleep stages and one rapid eye movement (REM) stage. The α-δ sleep anomaly describes α-like waves, thought to be a waking rhythm, superimposing upon the more normal δ waves during deep NREM sleep. In this way normal restorative deep sleep is interrupted by periods of miniarousal or temporary wakening.

Evidence appears to support the contention that sleep is associated with a refreshing restorative process. An increase in time spent in δ sleep results in a decrease in reported pain and altered mood symptoms (87). Conversely, an increase in α sleep results in an increase in reported pain. In this sense, α-δ sleep could be regarded as a biologic indicator of nonrestorative sleep. In an uncontrolled study, Moldofsky et al. (88) investigated the sleep patterns and musculoskeletal symptoms in a group of fibromyalgia patients. On examining the EEG sleep patterns of a group of ten patients who had satisfied their criteria for "fibrositis syndrome," they found that 70% displayed α-δ sleep patterns. This anomaly was identified as occurring more frequently during fibromyalgia patients' sleep patterns than controls and chronic insomniacs (89).

In a persuasive study, an attempt to answer the question of whether this relationship was causal, α-δ sleep has been induced in healthy controls by exposing them to brief auditory stimulation during periods of NREM sleep (90). Periods of δ sleep deprivation resulted in reports of temporary musculoskeletal symptoms, including muscular fatigue and tenderness at identified TeP sites and mood disorders. The authors hypothesized that the external stimulation used to induce α-δ sleep patterns in controls was a plausible model for some form of internal arousal mechanism in fibromyalgia patients, which acted to intrude on restorative δ sleep, thus producing fibromyalgia-like symptoms. It was further suggested that the fibromyalgia syndrome be considered a "nonrestorative sleep complex" based on an internal mechanism, which might be associated with a disorder of serotonin metabolism. Others have hypothesized that such disturbed sleep patterns disrupt growth hormone levels in fibromyalgia patients, leading to impaired muscle repair and thereby predisposing some individuals to develop widespread pain (91).

Identifying the etiology of fibromyalgia in such a way is problematic. NREM α-δ sleep is not specific to fibromyalgia. It was initially noted occurring in a heterogeneous psychiatric population (86) and has been identified in osteoarthritis (OA) patients (92), rheumatoid arthritis patients (93), and control subjects with no pain (94). Sometimes such intrusive sleep patterns are absent in fibromyalgia patients altogether. Doherty and Smith (95) studied a group of fibromyalgia and OA patients. All complained of pain and interrupted sleep, yet no period of α-δ sleep was identified in any patient. Rains and Penzien (96) found that of 1,076 patients attending a sleep disorders center, 5% ($n = 54$) displayed the α-δ anomaly. Of those, 21 persons had a previous diagnosis of fibromyalgia, 15 had a psychiatric disorder, and 18 had other, nonpainful or sleep, conditions. A comparison between these three groups found no difference in sleep architecture.

It would appear that disturbed sleep, and more specifically the α-δ sleep anomaly, is a common feature in both a variety of "pain" disorders and in pain-free persons. Chronic widespread pain can be present in the absence of identifiable sleep disruption, while intrusive α sleep patterns may not necessarily lead to the development of pain. Although nonrestorative sleep, as identified by this pattern, is not necessary for the development of symptoms specific to fibromyalgia, it is likely that sleep disturbances may function to exacerbate pain symptoms.

"TRAUMA-RELATED" FIBROMYALGIA

Intense debate has surrounded the theory of trauma-related fibromyalgia, and this topic is reviewed in detail in Chapter 22. It has been hypothesized that "trauma," whether occurring because of a high-impact traumatic physical event, in the workplace as a result of low-level mechanical trauma, or because of a major psychological trauma in adulthood, may be a precipitating factor for the development of symptoms (97).

Based upon patient self-reports, Greenfield et al. (97) reported that of 127 consecutive patients presenting to rheumatology clinics, 23% could be classified as having "reactive fibromyalgia"—that is, the onset of fibromyalgia occurred after an identifiable traumatic event. About half of those persons with "reactive fibromyalgia" reported a fracture, traffic accident, or back or shoulder injury prior to symptom onset. Although such reports are subject to recall bias, these observations were subsequently confirmed in a retrospective case–control study (50). In a survey of 136 patients with fibromyalgia and a group of age-matched and sex-matched controls attending the same hospital for non-rheumatological diseases, subjects completed a questionnaire that inquired about any trauma they had experienced in the 6-month period before the first symptoms of their disorder. Trauma was defined as a fracture, surgery, childbirth or miscarriage, or traffic or other accident, for which the subject had attended an emergency room, a general practitioner, or other health care specialty. Overall, fibromyalgia patients reported a greater number of traumatic events, with significantly increased rates of surgery and workplace injuries. Importantly, the authors were able to validate the accuracy of

subjects' reports by examining their health care records held by their general practitioner and found no differences in the recall of events between cases and controls. Interestingly, there were no differences in the rate of reported road traffic accidents, an event associated with whiplash injuries and commonly thought to be associated with widespread pain symptom onset. Indeed, a prospective study found that fibromyalgia was 13 times more common in persons who had sustained a cervical spine injury when compared to those with leg fractures (49). However, this finding was perhaps unsurprising, considering that 10 of the 18 TeP sites used in the classification of fibromyalgia are located in the region around the cervical spine (98). A reevaluation of those persons who had originally developed fibromyalgia ($n = 20:9$ male, 11 female) 3 years later found that 60% ($n = 12:1$ male, 11 female) still reported symptoms (99).

Although the relationship between workplace low-level trauma arising from activities involving repetitive movements, poor posture, or working with heavy loads has been established in relation to regional pain symptoms (100), little is known of their role in widespread pain. Two prospective studies have been conducted (78) and have found limited supporting evidence. Workplace activities, including lifting, carrying, pushing or pulling heavy weights, prolonged periods of kneeling, and repetitive wrist movements significantly predicted the onset of widespread pain in those persons initially symptom free. Other factors associated with the working environment, such as low levels of job satisfaction and social support and high levels of monotonous work, were equally important.

Concurrent with the hypothesis linking traumatic childhood events and chronic widespread pain and fibromyalgia is the hypothesis that major psychological trauma as an adult precipitates symptom onset. This is evidenced by the reported relationship of high rates of posttraumatic stress disorder-type symptoms in patients with fibromyalgia (101) and high rates of fibromyalgia-type symptoms in Gulf War veterans (102). Evidence documenting the impact of the World Trade Center terrorist attacks of September 11, 2001 lent support to this hypothesis, noting that chronic pain patients were reporting increased pain severity (103). However, a community-based survey has elegantly challenged those findings (103). A cohort of women in the New York/New Jersey metropolitan area, who had completed a survey of psychiatric symptoms and pain prior to the terrorist attacks of September 11, were asked about their current pain status 6 months following the attacks. The data indicated that a prior report of depression was associated, albeit nonsignificantly, with postattack fibromyalgia-type symptoms. However, being exposed to one or more specific events related to the attacks (including being in the direct vicinity of the attack, the death of a close relative or friend, and subsequent unemployment) was not associated with symptoms.

NATURAL HISTORY

PROGNOSIS

Despite the high prevalence of chronic widespread pain and fibromyalgia in clinics and in the general population, little work has been done to address the issue of prognosis. Hospital and specialist clinic series suggest it is a difficult condition to treat, and currently used pharmacological (analgesics, anti-inflammatory drugs, antidepressants) and nonpharmacological (physical activity, educational programs) therapies appear rarely to result in rapid or complete recovery (104). However, such series are dominated by persons with a long history of symptoms and many associated features of chronic fibromyalgia. One study has reported that most of the patients (47%) had improved or no longer satisfied the criteria for fibromyalgia after 2 years and minimal intervention (105). In a population-based study of persons with chronic widespread pain, only 35% still had the condition after a follow-up period of between 1 and 3 years (11). The authors concluded that in the community, chronic widespread pain has a generally good prognosis. However, this and other studies (12,34,106) indicate that persons with additional symptoms that are often associated with fibromyalgia, such as high levels of psychological distress, fatigue, and high levels of consultation to primary care, are more likely to have pain symptoms that persist over time.

IMPACT ON HEALTH CARE SYSTEMS AND SOCIETY

The impact of chronic widespread pain and fibromyalgia is far reaching, affecting society as a whole in terms of economics and lost productivity and on the individuals themselves, having implications in terms of physical functioning and perhaps even mortality.

HEALTH CARE SYSTEM COSTS

Fibromyalgia has been shown to be associated with high medical service utilization costs in Canada (24,107) and the United States (108,109). White et al. (24) reported that the annual costs of fibromyalgia patients were twice that of persons with chronic widespread pain and pain-free controls. Wolfe et al. (108) estimated that annual health service costs per patient were $2,274, and this was mainly attributed to hospitalizations, prescription drugs, and outpatient service costs. In the first stage of a multicenter clinic-based study of 538 fibromyalgia patients selected from a total of 1,604, Wolfe et al. (108) found that patients averaged almost ten outpatient medical visits a year. When nontraditional treatments such as acupuncture were included, these patients averaged almost one visit per month. In each 6-month period patients used an average of three fibromyalgia-related drugs. In addition, when compared to patients with other rheumatic disorders, fibromyalgia patients were more likely to have increased lifetime rates of surgical procedures. In the second stage of that study, work disability was assessed for the total sample population (110). Although most patients (64%) reported being able to work, more than 16% reported receiving disability payments, compared to only 2.2% of the population of the United States. A further study in the United States measured the total economic costs of fibromyalgia, through the use of insurance claims data, in an employed population (109). The total cost to the employer, which included direct (medical) and indirect (disability claims and

partial absenteeism) costs, was $7,776 per employee. These costs were categorized into health care, disability, and absenteeism payments, which comprised approximately one-half, one-third, and one-fifth of the total costs, respectively. The total cost per employee increased to over $14,000 for those who had disability claims for any reason, although only 1% of those persons with fibromyalgia made a claim directly related to their fibromyalgia symptoms, with other disorders (back pain and musculoskeletal and connective tissue disorders) being the main reasons for disability claims.

INDIVIDUAL COSTS

The impact of chronic widespread pain and fibromyalgia on individuals is high, with a significant proportion reporting lost days at work and many persons reporting some form of disability (110,111). In a follow-up study of fibromyalgia patients who had visited a rheumatology clinic, almost a third of patients regarded themselves as being "heavily dependent" (13). Fibromyalgia patients are likely to attribute their symptoms to a specific traumatic event (50) and are consequently more likely to experience higher levels of disability (112). Of a series of clinic patients seen at a rheumatology clinic, those with fibromyalgia had a similar number of functional limitations as patients with rheumatoid arthritis and higher rates than those patients in five other groups of rheumatic disorders, including osteoarthritis of the hands and knees, low back and neck pain, and degenerative overlap syndromes (113). However, there is discordance between physician-assessed and patient-assessed levels of disability (114), with patients perceiving more physical limitations. Not surprisingly, fibromyalgia patients also report limitations in their ability to work (115,116), and employment status among patients has been found to be associated with better functional status, lower levels of fatigue, and less pain (117).

LONG-TERM CONSEQUENCES OF MUSCULOSKELETAL PAIN

The long-term consequences of chronic widespread musculoskeletal pain are unknown. Previous studies have demonstrated associations between regional pain symptoms and higher rates of mortality (118), although these findings are not consistent (119). In a 25-year follow-up study, Wolfe et al. (120) reported a significant increased mortality among a group of 80 fibromyalgia patients, with rates from infections, pneumonia, and accidental deaths increased (120). A subsequent population-based study reported an excess mortality among subjects with widespread pain after 8 years of follow-up, with the excess almost entirely due to deaths from cancer (121). On further investigation, widespread pain was found to be significantly associated with a subsequent increased risk of cancer incidence and reduced survival (122). Among a cohort of 214 individuals on whom detailed pain information was available at baseline, persons with widespread pain, when compared to those pain-free at baseline, had an increased rate of mortality after 12 years. The cause of death was not available for this group of subjects, and the investigators were unable to determine the cause-specific increase. Although these reports are suggestive, they are preliminary and must await confirmation by large, well-conducted studies that follow subjects over long periods of time.

SUMMARY POINTS

- Chronic widespread pain affects roughly 10% of the population.
- Approximately 20% of these individuals, primarily women, will meet the ACR classification criteria for fibromyalgia.
- In the few studies that have examined the issue, chronic widespread pain is at least as common (or more common) in rural and nonindustrialized populations as in urban or industrialized regions.
- There are no data examining longitudinal trends in the prevalence of chronic widespread pain.
- Risk factors for the development or persistence of chronic widespread pain include female gender, increasing age, distress, the presence of other somatic symptoms, smoking, and higher BMI.
- Chronic widespread pain is associated with high health care costs and considerable disability.

REFERENCES

1. Gran JT. The epidemiology of chronic generalized musculoskeletal pain. *Best Pract Res Clin Rheumatol* 2003;17: 547–561.
2. Smythe HA. Non-articular rheumatism and the fibrositis syndrome. In: Hollender JL, McCarthy DJ, eds. *Arthritis and allied conditions.* Philadelphia, PA: Lea & Febiger, 1972.
3. Smythe HA, Moldofsky H. Two contributions to understanding of the "fibrositis" syndrome. *Bull Rheum Dis* 1977;28: 928–931.
4. Wolfe F, Smythe HA, Yunus MB, et al. The American College of Rheumatology 1990 criteria for the classification of fibromyalgia. *Arthritis Rheum* 1990;33:160–172.
5. Raspe H, Croft P. Fibromyalgia. *Baillieres Clin Rheumatol* 1995;9:599–614.
6. Yunus MB, Masi AT, Aldag JC. Preliminary criteria for primary fibromyalgia syndrome (PFS): multivariate analysis of a consecutive series of PFS, other pain patients, and normal subjects. *Clin Exp Rheumatol* 1989;7:63–69.
7. Croft P, Schollum J, Silman A. Population study of tender point counts and pain as evidence of fibromyalgia. *Br Med J* 1994;309:696–699.
8. Schochat T, Croft P, Raspe H. The epidemiology of fibromyalgia. Workshop of the standing committee on epidemiology, European League Against Rheumatism (EULAR), Bad Sackingen, 19-21 November 1992. *Br J Rheumatol* 1994;33: 783–786.
9. Macfarlane GJ, Croft PR, Schollum J, et al. Widespread pain: is an improved classification possible? *J Rheumatol* 1996;23:1628–1632.
10. Hunt IM, Silman AJ, Benjamin S, et al. The prevalence and associated features of chronic widespread pain in the community using the 'Manchester' definition of chronic widespread pain. *Rheumatology (Oxford)* 1999;38:275–279.
11. Macfarlane GJ, Thomas E, Papageorgiou AC, et al. The natural history of chronic pain in the community: a better prognosis than in the clinic? *J Rheumatol* 1996;23:1617–1620.
12. McBeth J, Macfarlane GJ, Hunt IM, et al. Risk factors for persistent chronic widespread pain: a community-based study. *Rheumatology (Oxford)* 2001;40:95–101.
13. Ledingham J, Doherty S, Doherty M. Primary fibromyalgia syndromes—an outcome study. *Rheumatology (Oxford)* 1993;32:139–142.
14. Wolfe F, Ross K, Anderson J, et al. The prevalence and characteristics of fibromyalgia in the general population. *Arthritis Rheum* 1995;38:19–28.
15. Croft P, Rigby AS, Boswell R, et al. The prevalence of chronic widespread pain in the general population. *J Rheumatol* 1993;20:710–713.
16. White KP, Speechley M, Harth M, et al. The London fibromyalgia epidemiology study: the prevalence of fibromyalgia syndrome in London, Ontario. *J Rheumatol* 1999;26:1570–1576.
17. Lindell L, Bergman S, Petersson IF, et al. Prevalence of fibromyalgia and chronic widespread pain. *Scand J Prim Health Care* 2000;18:149–153.
18. Jacobsson L, Lindgarde F, Manthorpe R. The commonest rheumatic complaints of over six weeks' duration in a twelve-month period in a defined Swedish population. Prevalences and relationships. *Scand J Rheumatol* 1989;18:353–360.
19. Makela M, Heliovaara M. Prevalence of primary fibromyalgia in the Finnish population. *Br Med J* 1991;303:216–219.
20. Prescott E, Jacobsen S, Kjoller M, et al. Fibromyalgia in the adult Danish population: I. A prevalence study. *Scand J Rheumatol* 1993;22(5):233–237.
21. Jacobsson LT, Nagi DK, Pillemer SR, et al. Low prevalences of chronic widespread pain and shoulder disorders among the Pima Indians. *J Rheumatol* 1996;23(5):907–909.
22. Forseth KO, Gran JT, Husby G. A population study of the incidence of fibromylagia among women aged 16–55 yr. *Br J Rheumatol* 1997;36(12):1318–1323.
23. White KP, Speechley M, Harth M, et al. The London fibromyalgia epidemiology study: comparing the demographic and clinical characteristics in 100 random community cases of fibromyalgia versus controls. *J Rheumatol* 1999;26:1577–1585.
24. White KP, Speechley M, Harth M, et al. The London fibromyalgia epidemiology study: direct health care costs of fibromyalgia syndromes in London, Ontario. *J Rheumatol* 1999;26:885–889.
25. Farooqi A, Gibson T. Prevalence of the major rheumatic disorders in the adult population of north Pakistan. *Br J Rheumatol* 1998;37:491–495.
26. Carmona L, Ballina J, Gabriel R, et al. The burden of musculoskeletal diseases in the general population of Spain: results from a national survey. *Ann Rheum Dis* 2001;60(11): 1040–1045.
27. White KP, Thompson J. Fibromyalgia syndrome in an Amish community: a controlled study to determine disease and symptom prevalence. *J Rheumatol* 2003;30:1835–1840.
28. Andersson HI, Ejlertsson G, Leden I. Characersitics of subjects with chronic pain, in relation to local and widespread pain report. A prospective study of symptoms, clinical findings and blood tests in subgroups of a geographically defined population. *Scand J Rheumatol* 1996;25(3):146–154.
29. Buskila D, Abramov G, Biton A, et al. The prevalence of pain complaints in a general population in Israel and its implications for utilization of health services. *J Rheumatol* 2000;27(6):1521–1525.
30. Bergman S, Herrstrom P, Hogstrom K, et al. Chronic musculoskeletal pain, prevalence rates, and sociodemographic associations in a Swedish population study. *J Rheumatol* 2001;28(6):1369–1377.
31. Schochat T, Raspe H. Elements of fibromyalgia in an open population. *Rheumatology (Oxford)* 2003;42(7):829–835.
32. Lawrence RC, Helmick CG, Arnett FC, et al. Estimates of the prevalence of arthritis and selected musculoskeletal disorders in the United States. *Arthritis Rheum* 1998;41:778–799.
33. Hartz A, Kirchdoerfer E. Undetected fibrositis in primary care practice. *J Fam Pract* 1987;25:365–369.
34. Papageorgiou AC, Silman AJ, Macfarlane GJ. Chronic widespread pain in the population: a seven year follow up study. *Ann Rheum Dis* 2002;61:1071–1074.
35. Wolfe F. The fibromyalgia problem. *J Rheumatol* 1997;24: 1247–1249.
36. Littlejohn G. Medicolegal aspects of fibrositis syndrome. *J Rheumatol Suppl* 1989;19:169–173.

37. White KP, Speechley M, Harth M, et al. Fibromyalgia in rheumatology practice: a survey of Canadian rheumatologists. *J Rheumatol* 1995;22:722–726.
38. Andersson HI, Ejlertsson G, Leden I, et al. Musculoskeletal chronic pain in general practice. Studies of health care utilisation in comparison with pain prevalence. *Scand J Prim Health Care* 1999;17:87–92.
39. Forseth KO, Husby G, Gran JT, et al. Prognostic factors for the development of fibromyalgia in women with self-reported musculoskeletal pain. A prospective study. *J Rheumatol* 1999;26:2458–2467.
40. Forseth KO, Forre O, Gran JT. A 5.5 year prospective study of self-reported musculoskeletal pain and of fibromyalgia in a female population: significance and natural history. *Clin Rheumatol* 1999;18:114–121.
41. McBeth J, Macfarlane GJ, Benjamin S, et al. Features of somatization predict the onset of chronic widespread pain: results of a large population-based study. *Arthritis Rheum* 2001;44:940–946.
42. Vaeroy H, Helle R, Forre O, et al. Elevated CSF levels of substance P and high incidence of Raynaud phenomenon in patients with fibromyalgia: new features for diagnosis. *Pain* 1988;32(1):21–26.
43. Yunus MB, Arslan S, Aldag JC. Relationship between fibromyalgia features and smoking. *Scand J Rheumatol* 2002;31:301–305.
44. Yunus MB, Arslan S, Aldag JC. Relationship between body mass index and fibromyalgia features. *Scand J Rheumatol* 2002;31:27–31.
45. McBeth J, Morris S, Benjamin S, et al. Associations between adverse events in childhood and chronic widespread pain in adulthood: are they explained by differential recall? *J Rheumatol* 2001;28:2305–2309.
46. Bergman S, Herrstrom P, Jacobsson LT, et al. Chronic widespread pain: a three year followup of pain distribution and risk factors. *J Rheumatol* 2002;29:818–825.
47. Imbierowicz K, Egle UT. Childhood adversities in patients with fibromyalgia and somatoform pain disorder. *Eur J Pain* 2003;7:113–119.
48. Harkness EF, Macfarlane GJ, Nahit ES, et al. Risk factors for new-onset low back pain amongst cohorts of newly employed workers. *Rheumatology (Oxford)* 2003;42(8):959–968.
49. Buskila D, Neumann L, Vaisberg G, et al. Increased rates of fibromyalgia following cervical spine injury. A controlled study of 161 cases of traumatic injury. *Arthritis Rheum* 1997;40:446–452.
50. Al Allaf AW, Dunbar KL, Hallum NS, et al. A case-control study examining the role of physical trauma in the onset of fibromyalgia syndrome. *Rheumatology (Oxford)* 2002;41:450–453.
51. Yunus MB, Inanici F, Aldag JC, et al. Fibromyalgia in men: comparison of clinical features with women. *J Rheumatol* 2000;27:485–490.
52. LeResche L. Gender considerations in the epidemiology of chronic pain. In: Crombie IK, Croft PR Linton SJ et al., eds. *Epidemiology of pain: a report of the task force on epidemiology of the International Association for the Study of Pain.* Seattle, WA: IASP Press, 1999:43–52.
53. Barsky AJ, Peekna HM, Borus JF. Somatic symptom reporting in women and men. *J Gen Intern Med* 2001;16:266–275.
54. Chesterton LS, Barlas P, Foster NE, et al. Gender differences in pressure pain threshold in healthy humans. *Pain* 2003;101:259–266.
55. Unruh AM, Ritchie J, Merskey H. Does gender affect appraisal of pain and pain coping strategies? *Clin J Pain* 1999;15:31–40.
56. Dao TT, LeResche L. Gender differences in pain. *J Orofac Pain* 2000;14:169–184.
57. Adamson J, Ben Shlomo Y, Chaturvedi N, et al. Ethnicity, socio-economic position and gender—do they affect reported health-care seeking behaviour? *Soc Sci Med* 2003;57:895–904.
58. Anderberg UM. Comment on: Johns and Littlejohn, the role of sex hormones in pain response. *Pain* 2000;87:109–111.
59. Ostensen M, Rugelsjoen A, Wigers SH. The effect of reproductive events and alterations of sex hormone levels on the symptoms of fibromyalgia. *Scand J Rheumatol* 1997;26:355–360.
60. Schochat T, Beckmann C. Sociodemographic characteristics, risk factors and reproductive history in subjects with fibromyalgia—results of a population-based case–control study. *Z Rheumatol* 2003;62:46–59.
61. Macfarlane TV, Blinkhorn A, Worthington HV, et al. Sex hormonal factors and chronic widespread pain: a population study among women. *Rheumatology (Oxford)* 2002;41:454–457.
62. Dionne CE. Low back pain. In: Crombie IK, Croft PR, Linton SJ et al., eds. *Epidemiology of pain: a report of the task force on epidemiology of the International Association for the Study of Pain.* Seattle, WA: IASP Press, 1999:283–297.
63. Wigers SH. Fibromyalgia outcome: the predictive values of symptom duration, physical activity, disability pension, and critical life events—a 4.5 year prospective study. *J Psychosom Res* 1996;41:235–243.
64. Benjamin S, Morris S, McBeth J, et al. The association between chronic widespread pain and mental disorder: a population-based study. *Arthritis Rheum* 2000;43:561–567.
65. Speckens AE, Van Hemert AM, Spinhoven P, et al. The diagnostic and prognostic significance of the Whitely index, the illness attitude scales and the somatosensory amplification scale. *Psychol Med* 1996;26:1085–1090.
66. Speckens AE, Spinhoven P, Sloekers PP, et al. A validation study of the Whitely index, the illness attitude scales, and the somatosensory amplification scale in general medical and general practice patients. *J Psychosom Res* 1996;40:95–104.
67. Taylor ML, Trotter DR, Csuka ME. The prevalence of sexual abuse in women with fibromyalgia. *Arthritis Rheum* 1995;38:229–234.
68. Boisset-Pioro MH, Esdaile JM, Fitzcharles MA. Sexual and physical abuse in women with fibromyalgia syndrome. *Arthritis Rheum* 1995;38:235–241.
69. Engel GL. Psychogenic pain and pain-prone patient. *Am J Med* 1959;26:899–918.
70. Linton SJ. A population-based study of the relationship between sexual abuse and back pain: establishing a link. *Pain* 1997;73:47–53.
71. Goldberg RT, Pachas WN, Keith D. Relationship between traumatic events in childhood and chronic pain. *Disabil Rehabil* 1999;21:23–30.
72. Alexander RW, Bradley LA, Alarcon GS, et al. Sexual and physical abuse in women with fibromyalgia: association with outpatient health care utilization and pain medication usage. *Arthritis Care Res* 1998;11:102–115.
73. McBeth J, Macfarlane GJ, Benjamin S, et al. The association between tender points, psychological distress, and adverse childhood experiences: a community-based study. *Arthritis Rheum* 1999;42:1397–1404.
74. Raphael KG, Widom CS, Lange G. Childhood victimization and pain in adulthood: a prospective investigation. *Pain* 2001;92:283–293.
75. Torpy DJ, Papanicolaou DA, Lotsikas AJ, et al. Responses of the sympathetic nervous system and the hypothalamic-pituitary-adrenal axis to interleukin-6: a pilot study in fibromyalgia. *Arthritis Rheum* 2000;43:872–880.
76. Winfield JB. Pain in fibromyalgia. *Rheum Dis Clin North Am* 1999;25:55–79.
77. Leclerc A, Chastang JF, Niedhammer I, et al. Incidence of shoulder pain in repetitive work. *Occup Environ Med* 2004;61:39–44.
78. McBeth J, Harkness EF, Silman AJ, et al. The role of workplace low-level mechanical trauma, posture and environment in the onset of chronic widespread pain. *Rheumatology (Oxford)* 2003;42:1486–1494.

79. Elaine FH, Macfarlane GJ, Nahit, E, et al. Mechanical injury and psychosocial factors in the workplace predict the onset of widespread body pain: a 2-year prospective study among cohorts of newly-employed workers. *Arthritis Rheum* 2004; 50(5):1655–1664.

80. Altman DG. *Practical statistics for medical research.* London: Chapman & Hall, 1991.

81. Karasek RA, Theorell T. *Healthy work: stress, productivity and reconstruction of working life.* New York: Basic Books, 1990.

82. Campbell SM, Clark S, Tindall EA, et al. Clinical characteristics of fibrositis. I. A "blinded," controlled study of symptoms and tender points. *Arthritis Rheum* 1983;26:817–824.

83. Wolfe F, Hawley DJ, Cathey MA, et al. Fibrositis: symptom frequency and criteria for diagnosis. An evaluation of 291 rheumatic disease patients and 58 normal individuals. *J Rheumatol* 1985;12:1159–1163.

84. Kolar E, Hartz A, Roumm A, et al. Factors associated with severity of symptoms in patients with chronic unexplained muscular aching. *Ann Rheum Dis* 1989;48:317–321.

85. Jacobsen S, Danneskiold-Samsoe B. Inter-relations between clinical parameters and muscle function in patients with primary fibromyalgia. *Clin Exp Rheumatol* 1989;7:493–498.

86. Hauri P, Hawkins DR. Alpha-delta sleep. *Electroencephalogr Clin Neurophysiol* 1973;34:233–237.

87. Moldofsky H, Lue FA. The relationship of alpha and delta EEG frequencies to pain and mood in 'fibrositis' patients treated with chlorpromazine and L-tryptophan. *Electroencephalogr Clin Neurophysiol* 1980;50:71–80.

88. Moldofsky H, Scarisbrick P, England R, et al. Musculoskeletal symptoms and non-REM sleep disturbance in patients with "fibrositis syndrome" and healthy subjects. *Psychosom Med* 1975;37:341–351.

89. Gupta MA, Moldofsky H. Dysthymic disorder and rheumatic pain modulation disorder (fibrositis syndrome): a comparison of symptoms and sleep physiology. *Can J Psychiatry* 1986;31:608–616.

90. Moldofsky H, Scarisbrick P. Induction of neurasthenic musculoskeletal pain syndrome by selective sleep stage deprivation. *Psychosom Med* 1976;38:35–44.

91. Bennett RM, Clark SR, Campbell SM, et al. Low levels of somatomedin C in patients with the fibromyalgia syndrome. A possible link between sleep and muscle pain. *Arthritis Rheum* 1992;35:1113–1116.

92. Moldofsky H. Sleep influences on regional and diffuse pain syndromes associated with osteoarthritis. *Semin Arthritis Rheum* 1989;18:18–21.

93. Mahowald MW, Mahowald ML, Bundlie SR, et al. Sleep fragmentation in rheumatoid arthritis. *Arthritis Rheum* 1989; 32:974–983.

94. Dumermuth G, Walz W, Scollo-Lavizzari G, et al. Spectral analysis of EEG activity in different sleep stages in normal adults. *Eur Neurol* 1972;7:265–296.

95. Doherty M, Smith J. Elusive 'alpha-delta' sleep in fibromyalgia and osteoarthritis. *Ann Rheum Dis* 1993;52:245.

96. Rains JC, Penzien DB. Sleep and chronic pain: challenges to the alpha-EEG sleep pattern as a pain specific sleep anomaly. *J Psychosom Res* 2003;54:77–83.

97. Greenfield S, Fitzcharles MA, Esdaile JM. Reactive fibromyalgia syndrome. *Arthritis Rheum* 1992;35:678–681.

98. Smith MD. Relationship of fibromyalgia to site and type of trauma: comment on the articles by Buskila et al. and Aaron et al. *Arthritis Rheum* 1998;41:378–379.

99. Neumann L, Zeldets V, Bolotin A, et al. Outcome of posttraumatic fibromyalgia: a 3-year follow-up of 78 cases of cervical spine injuries. *Semin Arthritis Rheum* 2003;32:320–325.

100. Latza U, Karmaus W, Sturmer T, et al. Cohort study of occupational risk factors of low back pain in construction workers. *Occup Environ Med* 2000;57:28–34.

101. Sherman JJ, Turk DC, Okifuji A. Prevalence and impact of posttraumatic stress disorder-like symptoms on patients with fibromyalgia syndrome. *Clin J Pain* 2000;16: 127–134.

102. Bourdette DN, McCauley LA, Barkhuizen A, et al. Symptom factor analysis, clinical findings, and functional status in a population-based case control study of Gulf War unexplained illness. *J Occup Environ Med* 2001;43:1026–1040.

103. Raphael KG, Natelson BH, Janal MN, et al. A community-based survey of fibromyalgia-like pain complaints following the World Trade Center terrorist attacks. *Pain* 2002;100:131–139.

104. Carette S, Oakson G, Guimont C, et al. Sleep electroencephalography and the clinical response to amitriptyline in patients with fibromyalgia. *Arthritis Rheum* 1995;38: 1211–1217.

105. Granges G, Zilko P, Littlejohn GO. Fibromyalgia syndrome: assessment of the severity of the condition 2 years after diagnosis. *J Rheumatol* 1994;21:523–529.

106. Andersson HI. The course of non-malignant chronic pain: a 12-year follow-up of a cohort from the general population. *Eur J Pain* 2004;8:47–53.

107. Cameron RS. The cost of long term disability due to fibromyalgia, chronic fatigue syndrome and repetitive strain injury. *J Musc Pain* 1995;3:169–172.

108. Wolfe F, Anderson J, Harkness D, et al. A prospective, longitudinal, multicenter study of service utilization and costs in fibromyalgia. *Arthritis Rheum* 1997;40:1560–1570.

109. Robinson RL, Birnbarm HG, Morley MA, et al. Economic cost and epidemiological characteristics of patients with fibromyalgia claims. *J Rheum* 2003;30:1318–1325.

110. Wolfe F, Anderson J, Harkness D, et al. Work and disability status of persons with fibromyalgia. *J Rheumatol* 1997;24: 1171–1178.

111. Katz J, Heft M. The epidemiology of self-reported TMJ sounds and pain in young adults in Israel. *J Public Health Dent* 2002;62:177–179.

112. Geisser ME, Roth RS, Bachman JE, et al. The relationship between symptoms of post-traumatic stress disorder and pain, affective disturbance and disability among patients with accident and non-accident related pain. *Pain* 1996;66:207–214.

113. Hawley DJ, Wolfe F. Pain, disability, and pain/disability relationships in seven rheumatic disorders: a study of 1,522 patients. *J Rheumatol* 1991;18:1552–1557.

114. Dobkin PL, De Civita M, Abrahamowicz M, et al. Patient-physician discordance in fibromyalgia. *J Rheumatol* 2003; 30:1326–1334.

115. Wolfe F, Anderson J, Harkness D, et al. Work and disability status of persons with fibromyalgia. *J Rheumatol* 1997;24: 1171–1178.

116. Henriksson C, Liedberg G. Factors of importance for work disability in women with fibromyalgia. *J Rheumatol* 2000; 27:1271–1276.

117. Reisine S, Fifield J, Walsh SJ, et al. Do employment and family work affect the health status of women with fibromyalgia? *J Rheumatol* 2003;30:2045–2053.

118. Penttinen J. Back pain and risk of fatal ischaemic heart disease: 13 year follow up of Finnish farmers. *Br Med J* 1994; 309:1267–1268.

119. Heliovaara M, Makela M, Aromaa A, et al. Low back pain and subsequent cardiovascular mortality. *Spine* 1995;20: 2109–2111.

120. Wolfe F, Hawley DJ, Anderson J. The long term outcomes of fibromyalgia: rates and predictions of mortality in fibromyalgia after 25 years of follow-up. *Arthritis Rheum* 1999;42:S135.

121. Macfarlane GJ, McBeth J, Silman AJ. Widespread body pain and mortality: prospective population based study. *Br Med J* 2001;323:662–665.

122. McBeth J, Silman AJ, Macfarlane GJ. Association of widespread body pain with an increased risk of cancer and reduced cancer survival: a prospective, population-based study. *Arthritis Rheum* 2003;48:1686–1692.

4

The Concept of Central Sensitivity Syndromes

Muhammad B. Yunus

HISTORY OF CENTRAL SENSITIVITY SYNDROMES

Central sensitivity syndromes (CSS) comprise a similar and overlapping group of syndromes without demonstrable structural pathology and are bound by a common pathophysiologic mechanism of central sensitization (CS). Currently, members of this group include fibromyalgia syndromes (FMS), chronic headaches, irritable bowel syndromes (IBS), chronic fatigue syndromes (CFS), myofascial pain syndromes (MPS), restless legs syndromes (RLS), periodic limb movement disorder (PLMD), temporomandibular disorder (TMD), multiple chemical sensitivity (MCS), female urethral syndromes (FUS), interstitial cystitis (IC), primary dysmenorrhea (PD)/"functional" chronic pelvic pain, posttraumatic stress disorder (PTSD), and depression. Evidence of CS is lacking in some of these syndromes at this time, but it is reasonable to include them on clinical grounds.

Many of the above listed nonpsychiatric "functional" syndromes were fairly well described as discrete conditions at least in the earlier part of the last century (1,2). Comorbidity among several psychiatric conditions—anxiety and depression, for example—has been known since the early 20th century (3). However, knowledge of an association between the nonpsychiatric CSS conditions is recent. Although the overlapping nature and concurrence of the above-mentioned nonpsychiatric "functional" conditions (FMS, IBS, headaches, etc.) are now taken for granted (4), the birth of such a concept occurred only 21 to 24 years ago (5,6). Such a concept was not accepted or acceptable in the 1980s, particularly in the earlier part of the decade. Virtually all residents and attending physicians were resistant to such an idea. The connection between the musculoskeletal pain of FMS and the colonic pain of IBS was intriguing and not obvious. The first clue that these conditions are associated came in the publication of a paper in 1981 that for the first time showed an association of IBS, tension-type headaches (TTH), and migraine

with FMS in a controlled study (5). Subsequently, in 1984, Yunus described the overlapping clinical similarities of FMS, IBS, TTH, and PD, and clearly depicted their interconnectedness by a Venn diagram (see Figure 4-1) (6). It was also noted that many of the overlapping conditions were present in the same patient. Interestingly, the common binder of these syndromes was suggested to be muscle spasm (6), since there was pain and tenderness in the respective muscles of these conditions and patients often described muscle spasm as part of their complaints. At that time CS as a probable pathophysiologic mechanism of these conditions was not generally appreciated. Muscle tension was a popular postulated mechanism of chronic muscle pain; the term "tension myalgia" had been used in the Mayo Clinic since 1950 (7). However, later studies failed to demonstrate objective muscle spasm in FMS by electromyography (8,9). In an uncontrolled study, electromyographic hyperactivity was demonstrated, but there was no correlation between this finding and perceived muscle tension (10). The association of IBS, headaches, and PD with FMS was further confirmed in controlled studies when they were found to be more common in FMS as compared with another chronic pain disease of "organic" etiology—for example, rheumatoid arthritis (RA) as well as normal controls (11).

In 1989, Hudson and Pope used the term "affective spectrum disorder" for some of the conditions mentioned above, as well as several psychiatric disorders, including depression and obsessive–compulsive disorder (12). The term "affective" implied that somehow all these conditions were related to depression, contrary to the authors' intention. In 1994, the term "dysfunctional spectrum syndromes" was suggested because the common pathophysiology that binds these overlapping related syndromes (and others subsequently added) was postulated to be a dysfunction of the neuroendocrine system (13). However, the word "dysfunction" was too broad. As evidence accumulated, it became known that the major neuroendocrine aberration in FMS is CS (14). In 2000, Yunus reviewed the evidence for CS among other fibromyalgia-related syndromes, besides FMS, and coined the term "central sensitivity syndromes" (15), a

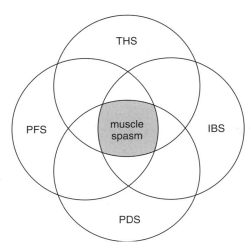

Figure 4-1. The original Venn diagram of 1984 first depicting the interrelationships between several members of the central sensitivity syndromes family. THS, tension headache syndromes; IBS, irritable bowel syndromes; PDS, primary dysmenorrhea syndromes; PFS, primary fibromyalgia syndromes. Muscle spasm was thought to be the common mechanism. (From Yunus MB. Primary fibromyalgia syndromes: current concepts. *Compr Ther* 1984;10:21–28, with permission.)

group terminology for FMS and other overlapping syndromes, as explained above. The term, implying both clinical and pathophysiologic features of these syndromes, seems appropriate, and we have continued to use it (16,17).

NOMENCLATURES USED IN THE LITERATURE

The terms "functional," "functional somatic syndromes," "somatoform disorders," and "medically unexplained symptoms" have all been used in the literature to describe a group of illnesses/diseases that show no structural pathology and demonstrate psychological distress among the sufferers (18–20). However, these terms are largely irrelevant to the currently proposed terminology and concept of CSS since they do not state that these syndromes are mutually associated and share many overlapping features as a group. Recently, Barsky and Borus stated that "each individual somatic syndrome is seen in a heterogeneous group of patients," missing the common link of CS (20). In fact, some authors wrongly emphasize that there is "absence of proven pathophysiology" (19) and "uncertainty ... about the presence of demonstrable pathophysiology" (20). These authors incorrectly state or imply that these "functional" conditions are predominantly, if not exclusively, based on psychopathology. The term "functional" is intriguing, considering that the problem in these conditions is a *dys*function of the neuroendocrine system (13). In this regard, such terms as "medically unexplained symptoms" (21,22), "somatoform disorders" (19), and "unexplained clinical conditions" (4) are particularly troubling, since they imply an absence of physiological mechanism that might explain the symptoms of these illnesses or diseases, despite the evidence to the contrary. The authors ignore the currently demonstrated pathophysiology of CS and involved neurotransmitters that explain symptoms (16,17,23). Only three terminologies used in the literature (besides CSS) indicate a common binding thread between the members of CSS—"stress-related syndromes" (24), "affective spectrum disorder" (12), and "dysfunctional spectrum syndromes" (13). The history of CSS is shown in Table 4-1.

In the nosology of CSS, we prefer "sensitivity" to "sensitization," since sensitivity is a common clinical manifestation of CS with hypersensitivity to various noxious and nonnoxious stimuli at the periphery (mechanical, electrical, heat, cold, ischemic, touch) as well as sensitivity to environmental stimuli—for example, temperature, smell, noise, and chemicals. Moreover, the term "sensitization" implies an active response to some peripheral or environmental stimuli. We

TABLE 4-1	History of Central Sensitivity Syndromes (CSS)
Yunus, 1981	First data based demonstration of an association between FMS with headaches and irritable bowel syndromes in FMS (5).
Yunus, 1984	First conceptual depiction (by a Venn diagram) of an interrelationship between several CSS members with similar and overlapping features; muscle spasm is suggested to be the common pathologic mechanism of these syndromes (6).
Yunus, 1985	Use of the term "stress-related syndromes" (24).
Hudson, 1989	"Affective" mechanism is suggested for FMS and other overlapping syndromes (psychiatric as well as medical functional conditions) described as "affective spectrum disorder" (12).
Yunus, 1994	The collective term "dysfunctional spectrum syndromes" is suggested, implying the dysfunction of the neurohormonal system as the common mechanism between the CSS members (13).
Bennett, 1999	A review of the literature showing the evidence for central sensitization in FMS (14).
Yunus, 2000	The new term "central sensitivity syndromes" is coined based on the evidence that FMS and several members of the CSS family demonstrate central sensitization to multiple stimuli (15). CSS is both a clinical and pathogenetic term.

FMS, fibromyalgia syndromes.

had suggested that some persons may be genetically or otherwise intrinsically predisposed to hypersensitivity without such stimulus (15). Thus, the nomenclature "central sensitivity syndromes" paints both a clinical and pathophysiologic picture.

THE CONCEPT OF CENTRAL SENSITIVITY SYNDROMES

CSS is a unifying concept for FMS and other related syndromes mentioned above based on their clinical similarities and overlaps, mutual associations, and presence of CS. Common clinical similarities include predominantly or exclusively female gender; a common age distribution of 30 to 60 years; pain or discomfort; fatigue; poor sleep; hyperalgesia/sensitivity to physical, psychological, environmental, and chemical stimuli; paresthesia in a number of CSS conditions; and an absence of structural pathology.

CENTRAL SENSITIZATION

The physiology of CS has been well described elsewhere in this book (Chapters 5,6). The clinical manifestations of CS in humans are amplified pain, hyperalgesia, spread of pain, unpleasant sensations after a physical stimulus (e.g., mechanical, heat, and others), and chronicity. Basically, in animal models and experimental human laboratories, CS is defined as hyperexcitability of the central nervous system (CNS) following a peripheral stimulus, giving rise to the above clinical manifestations resulting from an altered sensory processing. The neurochemistry of CS involves release of substance P (SP) presynaptically in the dorsal horn and removal of magnesium block of N-methyl-D-aspartate (NMDA) receptor channel allowing excitatory amino acids (EAAs) (glutamate, aspartate) to activate the postsynaptic NMDA receptor with remarkable chemical and even some morphologic changes in the CNS postsynaptic cells and their membranes—for example, influx of calcium, activation of second messengers, expression of *c-fos*—and alteration of cell membrane permeability. Besides SP and EAA, other c-fiber peptides may also be involved—for example, calcitonin gene-related peptide (CGRP), neurokinin A, galanin, cholecystokinin, vaso-active intestinal peptide, nerve growth factor (NGF), and somatostatin (25,26). Also important are the neurotransmitters that dampen excessive sensitization—for example, serotonin, norepinephrine, and enkephalins (26)—since their decreased availability will accentuate CS.

MUTUAL ASSOCIATIONS

In an excellent review, Aaron and Buchwald have documented the mutual associations between different members of the CSS family (4). These have been updated in this chapter by additional references; important studies are shown in Table 4-2.

An association between FMS (or an increased prevalence by comparison with known population control) and several members of the CSS have been well demonstrated by using normal controls as well as other chronic pain controls, several with structural pathology. FMS is associated with IBS (5,11,27,30,31,34,36,39,40,47,48,51,61–65), TTH (5,11,31, 56,62), migraine (5,37,56), CFS (29,36,37,52,65), RLS (41), PLMD (53), TMD (42,47,48,65), MCS (54,55,65), regional soft tissue pain (49), PD (11,31), FUS (32,38), IC (44,65), and PTSD (60,66). Bidirectional associations/increased prevalence by known population occurrence have also been documented—for example, increased frequency of FMS in IBS (50,63,64), CFS (55,65), migraine (57), TMD (65), RSTP (49), and IC (67). Selected studies of other mutual associations are shown in Table 4-2. However, references have been provided for all of them (5,11,27–68).

EVIDENCE OF CENTRAL SENSITIZATION AMONG CENTRAL SENSITIVITY SYNDROMES MEMBERS

Until recently, local or peripheral factors were emphasized in the pathogenesis of CSS conditions. For example, for a long time there was focus on muscles in FMS (69) and gut motility in IBS (70–72). Previous muscle biopsies in FMS prior to 1989 were either uncontrolled or otherwise poorly designed. Later, a blinded controlled study of muscle histology in FMS showed negative results (73). This was helpful in focusing on CNS dysfunction with aberrant pain mechanism in this condition (74). Only recently has there been a deemphasis of the role of gut motility in IBS, with greater focus on the CNS dysfunction, including CS (75).

In recent years, strong evidence for CS has been presented in a number of CSS disorders—for example, FMS (76–100), headaches (101–110), IBS (111–121), CFS (33,122), RLS (123), and TMD (124–127). Selected studies from among the above references are shown in Table 4-3. As compared with controls, FMS patients showed significantly decreased pain threshold and tolerance along with other features of CS—for example, spread of pain, prolonged duration of pain, and unpleasant dysesthesia to multimodal stimuli—for example, mechanical pressure (107,111–114,123,127), heat (107, 108,112,118,119,121,122,126,127), cold (80,84,91,93,95), cutaneous electric (78,80), deep muscle electric (86), deep muscle hypertonic saline (86), and vibration (85). Allodynia was also observed (84,93,95,98). Cortical dysfunction was shown by several methodologies—for example, single-photon-emission computed tomography (SPECT) (82,89), positron-emission tomography (PET) using [^{15}O] butanol (94), functional Magnetic Resonance Imaging (fMRI) (92), single and double magnetic stimulation (88), and cerebral evoked potential (79). Temporal summation was demonstrated for deep (muscle), mechanical pressure (98), deep electrical (86,87), and cutaneous heat (90). Significantly, CS has been objectively established in FMS (as opposed to subjective pain response) by decreased spinal nociceptive flexion reflex (NFR) threshold by two independent studies (95,100).

Similar evidence has been published in other CSS members besides FMS—for example, TTH (100–102,104–106), migraine headaches (102,104,107–110), IBS (111–121), and TMD (124). Limited studies have been carried out in CFS (33,122) and RLS (123) showing evidence of CS.

TABLE 4-2 Selected Studies Showing Mutual Associations of Fibromyalgia and Other Central Sensitivity Syndromes (CSS) Conditions[a,b]

CONDITIONS STUDIED (CRITERIA USED)	CONDITIONS EXAMINED FOR ASSOCIATION (CRITERIA USED)	FIRST AUTHOR (REF); YEAR	STUDY SUBJECTS	RESULTS AND COMMENTS
FMS (modified Smythe)	IBS (Almy), TH (Adams), migraine (Plum)	Yunus (5); 1981	50 FMS, 50 HC	FMS—32% had IBS, HC—8% (p<0.01); FMS—44% had HA (combined tension and migraine), HC—16% (p<0.01)
FMS (Yunus)	HA (ND), IBS (ND)	Bengtsson (27); 1986	50 FMS, 30 RA	FMS—44% had IBS, RA—43% (NS); FMS—56% had HA, RA—20% (p<0.01)
IBS (author)	HA (ND), PD (ND)	Whorwell (28); 1986	100 IBS; 100 HC	IBS—68% had PD, HC—72 (NS); IBS—increased frequency of urination
FMS (Yunus)	CFS symptoms	Buchwald (29); 1987	50 FMS	FMS patients had symptoms of CFS, e.g., sore throat (54%), adenopathy (33%), low grade fever 28%. *No control group.*
FMS (author)	IBS (Kruis)	Romano (30); 1988	100 FMS (primary), 100 arthritic patients	FMS—49% had IBS; Arthritic control—9% (p<0.001)
FMS (Yunus)	IBS (Whitehead), TTH (Adams), PD (Weingold)	Yunus (11); 1989	113 FMS, 77 RA, 67 HC	FMS—41% had IBS, RA—1%, HC—6%; FMS 56% had TTH, RA—14%, HC—10%; FMS—45% had PD, RA—12%, HC—17% (p<0.005 for IBS, TTH, and PD)
FMS (participants of the study)	IBS, HA, primary dysmenorrhea (PD)	Wolfe (31); 1990	293 FMS, 265 rheumatic diseases control	FMS—36% had IBS, controls—9%; FMS—54% had HA, control—35.5% (p<0.001 for both IBS and HA); FMS—41% had PD, controls—32% (p<0.037)
FMS (Wolfe 1989)	FUS (Gallagher)	Wallace (32); 1990	50 FMS, 50 rheum. dis. cont.	FMS—12% had FUS. *Retrospective chart review may have underestimated frequency of FUS.*
Chronic fatigue (CF)/CFS (CDC 1988)	FMS (Yunus—slight modification)	Goldenberg (33); 1990	27 CF (16 had CFS) 20 FMS	CF—70% had diffuse pain; mean TePs—19.9 FMS, 11.6 CF, 2.1 HC. *Separate data on CFS not shown. Small n.*
FMS (Smythe)	IBS (Drossman)	Triadafilopoulos (34); 1991	123 FMS, 54 DJD, 46 HC	FMS—60% had IBS symptoms vs. 13% in DJD (p<0.001)
FMS (Yunus)	CFS (1988 CDC)	Wysenbeek (35); 1991	33 FMS	21% of FMS had CFS. *No control group.*
FMS (ACR)	IBS (Thompson), migraine (IHS), CFS (Holmes), depression (DSM III)	Hudson (36); 1992	33 FMS (family study)	FMS—current IBS had 39%, migraine in 45%, CFS in 42%, major depression in 18%, panic disorder 15%. *No control group.*
FMS (ACR), CFS (CDC), MCS (Cullen)	CFS, MCS	Buchwald (37); 1994	30 FMS, 30 CFS, 30 MCS	FMS—70% had CFS, 40% itching skin, 27% hoarseness of voice (2 MCS symptoms). MCS—30% had CFS. *No controls.*
FMS (ACR)	FUS (Gallagher)	Paira (38); 1994	212 FMS, 212 rheum. dis. cont.	FMS—18% FUS. *Retrospective chart review.*
FMS (ACR)	IBS	Wolfe (39); 1995	Population study of FMS (n = 60)	Odds ratio of having IBS in FMS was 2.49 compared with those without FMS.

(continued)

Condition (criteria)	Associated condition (criteria)	Reference; year	Sample	Results
FMS (ACR)	IBS	Sivri (40); 1996	75 FMS, 50 HC	FMS—42% had IBS, HC—16% ($p<0.05$)
FMS (ACR)	RLS (published features from the literature)	Yunus (41); 1996	115 FMS, 54 RA, 88 HC	FMS—31% had RLS, RA—15%, HC—2% ($p<0.02$ FMS vs. RA, <0.001 for FMS vs. HC)
FMS (ACR)	M-TMD (RDC)	Plesh (42); 1996	60 FMS	FMS—75% had M-TMD. *No controls.*
IBS (Thompson)	Chronic pelvic pain	Walker (43);1996	60 IBS, 26 IBD	IBS—35% chronic pelvic pain, IBD—14% ($p<0.05$)
FMS (ACR), IC (NIH)	FMS (ACR), IC (NIH)	Clauw (44); 1997	60 FMS, 30 IC, 30 HC	FMS and IC shared several genitourinary and musculoskeletal symptoms (significantly higher than HC)
TMD (RDC)	FMS (ACR)	Wright (45); 1997	104 TMD	13% of TMD patients had FMS. *No controls.*
PTSD (DSM-IV)	FMS (ACR)	Amir (46)	29 PTSD and 37 HC	21% of MCS had FMS vs. none among HC
FMS (ND)	M-TMD (based on multiple literature)	Cimino (47); 1998	23 FMS, 23 M-TMD	Similar features of TMD in FMS and TMD (no significant difference)
FMS (ACR), CFS (CDC-1988)	IBS, M-TMD, PMS (physician diagnosed)	Korszun (48); 1998	92 FMS /CFS (FMS-36, CFS 34, both 22), 39 had TMD	FMS/CFS—39 (42%) had TMD; those with TMD—46% IBS, 42% PMS, 19% ICS
RSTP/modified MPS (regional pain and TePs)	FMS (ACR)	Inanici (49); 1999	630 FMS, 91 RSTP, 166 HC	High prevalence of FMS symptoms (fatigue, poor sleep, IBS, TTH, paresthesia, etc.) in RSTP, all of which are significantly higher than HC ($p<0.001$)
IBS (Rome), FMS (ACR)	FMS, IBS	Sperber (36); 1999	79 IBS, 100 FMS, 72 HC	IBS—31.6% had FMS, HC—4.2% ($p<0.001$); FMS—32% had IBS, HC—no data
IBS (Rome)	FMS (ACR)	Barton (50); 1999	46 IBS, 46 HC	IBS—28% had FMS, HC—11% ($p<0.064$)
FMS (ACR)	IBS, TTH (ND, but same as ref.11)	Yunus (51); 2000	536 female FMS	FMS—40% had IBS, 54.7% TTH. *No female control group.*
FMS (ACR)	IBS (Alamy), TH (Adams)	Yunus (51); 2000	67 male FMS; 36 male HC	Male FMS—14% had IBS, HC—0% ($p<0.005$); FMS—51% had TTH, HC—11% ($p<0.001$)
FMS (ACR)	CFS (CDC)	White (52); 2000	69 FMS, 26 with widespread pain (WSP) only, 16 localized pain (LP)	FMS—58% CFS by CDC criteria, WSP—26% CSF, LP—2.5% CFS 1 ($p<0.0006$). *A population study.*
Juvenile FMS (Yunus and Masi)	PLMD (evaluated by polysomnography)	Tayag-Kier (53); 2000	16 juvenile FMS (mean age 15), 14 HC	PLMD score 9 times higher in FMS than controls.

TABLE 4-2 Continued

CONDITIONS STUDIED (CRITERIA USED)	CONDITIONS EXAMINED FOR ASSOCIATION (CRITERIA USED)	FIRST AUTHOR (REF); YEAR	STUDY SUBJECTS	RESULTS AND COMMENTS
CFS (1988 CDC)	MCS (authors' symptom evaluation)	Nawab (54); 2000	73 CFS, 39 HC	CFS patients had higher MCS symptom score than HC ($p<0.001$)
CFS (1994 CDC)	MCS (Bartha), FMS (ACR)	Jason (55); 2000	166 CFS, 47 HC	CFS—41% had MCS, HC—17%; CFS—16% had FMS, HC—0% ($p<0.01$ for both). *Population study.*
FMS (ACR)	TTH, migraine (IHS) IBS (Manning)	Choudhury (56); 2001	30 FMS, 30 RA, 30 HC	FMS—60% had TTH, RA—7%, HC—10% ($p<0.001$); FMS—13% migraine, RA—0%, HC—3% (NS); FMS—30% had IBS, RA—3%, HC—7% ($p<0.02$ for both)
T-migraine (Silberstein and Lipton)	FMS (ACR)	Peres (57); 2001	101 T-migraine	T-migraine—35.6% had FMS. *No controls.*
IBS (Rome)	FMS (ACR)	Lubrano (58); 2001	130 IBS	20% of IBS had FMS. *No control group.*
Chronic migraine	CFS (CDC)	Peres (59); 2002	63 chronic migraine	FMS—51% had CFS (CDC—excluding headache item)
WSP	PTSD (PTSD checklist)	Raphael (60); 2004	1,312 women from the community	Odds of having PTSD among those having WSP was 3 times those without WSP.

ACR, American College of Rheumatology; CDC, Centers for Disease Control; CFS, chronic fatigue syndrome; DJD, degenerative joint disease; FMS, Fibromyalgia; FUS, female urethral syndromes; HA, headaches; HC, healthy control; IA, inflammatory arthritis; IBD, inflammatory bowel disease; IBS, irritable bowel syndromes; IC, interstitial cystitis; IHS, International Headache Society; MCS, multiple chemical sensitivity; M-TMD, myofascial temporomandibular disorder; ND, not defined; NIH, National Institutes of Health; NS, not significant; PD, primary dysmenorrhea; PLMD, periodic limb movement disorder; PMS, premenstrual syndromes; PTSD, posttraumatic stress disorder; RA, rheumatoid arthritis; RDC, Research Diagnostic Criteria (for TMD); RLS, restless legs syndromes; RSTP, regional soft tissue pain; T-migraine, transformed migraine; TMD, temporomandibular disorder; TePs, tender points; TTH, tension-type headache; WSP, widespread pain; LP, localized pain.

[a]Studies in this table were selected, in general, on the basis of sample size, design (e.g., control group), and importance based on other judgmental criteria. However, all published studies are referenced.

[b]For references of various disease criteria used, please check the original articles cited.

TABLE 4-3	Evidence for Central Sensitization among Central Sensitivity Syndromes (CSS) Conditions[a,b]		
CONDITIONS STUDIED (CRITERIA)	**FIRST AUTHOR (REF); YEAR**	**STUDY METHODOLOGY**	**RESULTS AND COMMENTS**
FMS (various)	Multiple (5,11,57, 60,66,106)	Clinical evaluation with history and TePs examination/algometry.	Diffuse pain, TePs (hyperalgesia), and ↓ pain threshold and tolerance; correlation between sites of TePs and control points; dysesthesia following TePs palpation. These findings suggest central sensitization.
FMS (ACR)	Lautenbacher (80); 1994	26 FMS and 26 HC tested for PPT and response to heat and electrocutaneous stimuli (ECS).	FMS patients had significantly ↓ detection threshold for pressure (both at TePs and control site), heat, and ECS; among nonpainful stimuli, only cold threshold in FMS was significantly lower in FMS than the HC group.
FMS (ACR)	Sorensen (81); 1995	31 FMS; pain intensity, threshold and tolerance was measured before, during, and after randomized and blinded (RB) I.V. infusion of morphine, lidocaine, and ketamine.	Morphine had no effect; lidocaine and ketamine decreased pain intensity both during and after I.V. infusion; TePs, pain threshold and tolerance also decreased significantly in response to ketamine, an NMDA receptor antagonist, suggesting central sensitization.
FMS (ACR)	Mountz (82); 1995	10 FMS, 7 HC; rCBF by SPECT and PPT by dolorimeter.	Significantly ↓ rCBF in thalami, caudate nucleus, and cortices, as well as ↓ PPT in both TePs and control sites.
FMS (ACR)	Bendtsen (83); 1996	25 FMS, 25 HC; blinded evaluation of 7 pressure intensities in muscles measured by a palpometer.	Hyperalgesia and qualitatively different stimulus-response function in FMS, compared with HC.
FMS (ACR)	Kosek (84); 1996	10 FMS, 10 HC studied for perception sensitivity to pressure (algometry), heat (Thermotest), and low-threshold mechanoreceptor (Von Frey) at both painful (as symptom) and nonpainful sites.	FMS patients showed significant hypersensitivity to pressure, heat and cold pain at all sites, and nonnoxious heat and cold as well as light touch at painful sites (by symptom). Thus, FMS patients had generalized multimodal hypersensitivity, even to nonnoxious stimuli, and even at nonpainful sites.
FMS (ACR)	Kosek (85); 1997	10 FMS, 10 HC; effects of vibration, pressure pain, and HNCS (tourniquet test) on somatosensory input (QST).	Effect of vibratory stimulus in FMS was similar to HC; ↓ PPT by algometry, and no modulation of PPT by HNCS in FMS, suggesting an abnormal HNCS in FMS.
FMS (ACR)	Sorensen (86); 1998	12 FMS, 12 HC; a RB study of single and repeated I.M. electrical stimulus vs. hypertonic saline (HS) injection in anterior tibial muscle (AT); PPT (by algometry).	In FMS, there was significantly ↓ PPT and evidence of summation from repeated I.M. electrical stimulus and increased pain from injection of saline, with longer duration and spread of pain. Electrical stimulation of the skin provided similar results between patients and controls.
FMS (ACR)	Graven-Nielsen (87); 2000	15 FMS to study effect of ketamine vs. placebo on PPT, I.M. HS induced pain intensity, referral pain, and summation following I.M. electrical stimulation.	Ketamine significantly increased PPT, decreased pain intensity and area of referred pain, as well as temporal summation from repeated I.M. electrical stimulation in FMS, as compared with placebo controls.
FMS (ACR)	Salerno (88); 2000	13 FMS, 13 HC; investigation of the motor cortex by single and double magnetic stimulation.	FMS patients showed significant cortical dysfunction with a ↓ in both excitatory and inhibitory circuitry, as compared to controls.
FMS (ACR)	Kwiatek (89); 2000	17 FMS, 22 HC; assessment of rCBF by SPECT and advanced analytic technique.	Significant reduction of rCBF in right thalamus and pontine tegmentum (confirming previous finding of decreased rCBF in thalamus).
FMS (ACR)	Staud (90); 2001	59 FMS, 65 HC; a study to determine temporal summation (TS) in FMS by repetitive thermal stimuli.	Significantly greater sensory magnitude with greater after-sensations of pain that lasted longer in FMS, suggesting TS. *Larger n in this study provides greater reliability.*

(continued)

TABLE 4-3	Continued		

CONDITIONS STUDIED (CRITERIA)	FIRST AUTHOR (REF); YEAR	STUDY METHODOLOGY	RESULTS AND COMMENTS
FMS (ACR)	Price (91); 2002	16 FMS, 14 HC; similar design as (119), plus assessment of repeated cold pain stimuli on TS, and pharmacologic study (placebo vs. fentanyl with naloxone reversibility) to determine if central modulation played a role in TS in FMS.	Previous observation of heat-induced TS was confirmed, with an additional finding that cold stimuli also produce TS, with attenuation of TS by both saline placebo and fentanyl; effect of naloxone was similar between placebo and fentanyl group suggesting that central pain modulatory system may be involved in TS, but the effect in FMS is similar to that in HC.
FMS (ACR)	Gracely (92); 2002	16 (nondepressed) FMS, 16 HC; an fMRI study of rCBF under 2 conditions: (a) HC received similar pressure to thumbnail as FMS (b) adequate pressure to cause similar pain in both FMS and HC groups.	PPT was lower in FMS. Similar pressure paradigm caused no common regions of activation between FMS and HC, whereas stimuli causing similar pain produced activation patterns in many areas that were similar in patients and controls, suggesting augmented pain processing in FMS.
FMS (ACR)	Berglund (93); 2002	20 FMS, 20 HC; Thermotest was used for temperature and Frey nylon for tactile stimulation. Thenar eminence and 2 areas of spontaneous pain were sites of experiment.	FMS patients had significantly ↓ perception threshold and tolerance for heat and cold pain with increased intensity of tactile sensation; cold pain was qualitatively different than HC with dysesthesia. Tactile threshold was also low. Such multimodal hyperalgesia may be integrated at the insular cortex level in FMS.
FMS (ACR)	Desmeules (95); 2003	85 FMS and 40 HC were studied by thermal, mechanical, and electric stimuli using QST; pain was assessed by subjective reporting and NFR, a specific and objective test for central nociceptive pathways.	Significantly ↓ pressure, cold and heat pain threshold, and much ↓ cold pressor pain threshold in FMS; a significantly ↓ NFR threshold suggesting central allodynia. The results strongly suggest central sensitization (CS) in FMS. *This study remarkably shows an objective evidence of CS that does not rely upon self-reported pain.*
FMS (ACR)	Staud (96); 2003	12 FMS and 20 HC; force-controlled mechanical stimulation was applied to forearm flexor digitorum muscle in brief, repeated (at interval of 3 or 5s) to study TS.	Deep muscular pain produced significant TS in FMS as compared with HC. *Previous studies showed TS from stimulation of cutaneous nociceptors; this study adds that CS may occur from stimulation of deep tissues, i.e., muscle nociceptors.*
FMS (ACR)	Staud (97); 2003	11 female (F) FMS, 22 F HC, 11 male HC; effect of DNIC (induced by immersion in hot water bath) on TS (induced by repeated heat stimuli) was studied.	DNIC, a central inhibitory mechanism, attenuated thermal TS in male HC, not in female HC. DNIC + distraction, but not DNIC alone, caused inhibition of TS in F-FMS patients. Inhibition of DNIC in F-FMS may be related to F-gender.
FMS (ACR)	Geisser (98); 2003	20 FMS and 20 HC subjected to both noxious and innocuous heat plus pressure stimuli.	FMS—significantly ↓ PPT to pressure, and to both heat stimuli. Catastrophizing correlated with increased pain perception.
FMS (ACR)	Petzke (99); 2003	43 FMS, 28 HC assessed for pressure and heat sensitivity by both ascending and random stimuli.	Pain sensitivity to both pressure and heat at both threshold and suprathreshold stimuli was significantly greater in FMS than HC. Higher rating of pain by random (vs. ascending) stimuli was similar in two groups. *This study establishes that there is no reporting bias in FMS.*
FMS (ACR)	Banic (100); 2004	22 FMS, 27 whiplash patients, and 29 HC; nociceptive withdrawal reflex evaluated by transcutaneous electrical stimulus, both single and repeated, and EMG.	Reflex thresholds were significantly ↓ both in FMS and whiplash patients after both stimuli, compared with HC, suggesting spinal cord hyperexcitability in both groups of patients. *These results suggest that whiplash injury is based on CS also.*

(continued)

TABLE 4-3 Continued

CONDITIONS STUDIED (CRITERIA)	FIRST AUTHOR (REF); YEAR	STUDY METHODOLOGY	RESULTS AND COMMENTS
TTH (IHS)	Langemark (101); 1989	50 TTH for PPT; 32 TTH and 24 HC tested at temporal and occipital regions for heat thresholds and nonpainful temperature changes.	TTH patients had significantly ↓ threshold for heat as compared with HC, with no difference in nonpainful temperature change between TTH and HC.
TTH/migraine (without aura) (IHS)	Schoenen (102); 1991	32 TTH, 20 HC, 10 migraine without aura were tested for PPT (algometer) at suboccipital, temple, forehead, and Achilles tendon sites.	PPT in TTH was significantly ↓ at cranial as well as Achilles tendon sites, compared with HC; TTH was significantly lower than HC only at forehead.
TTH (international diagnostic criteria)	Langemark (103); 1993	40 TTH and 23 HC tested for NFR (by sural nerve stimulation; muscular response obtained from biceps femoris muscle).	Compared with HC, TTH patients had significantly ↓ threshold in pain tolerance and in NFR (a spinal reflex with supraspinal influence that is not under a subject's voluntary control). The results suggest CS.
Migraine (without aura) (IHS)	Nicolodi (104); 1993	61 migraine patients (MP) (intercritical period) and 60 HC were subjected to HAVD causing local pain, followed by HS injection into antecubital vein during a 1 minute circulatory blockage.	93% of MP vs. none in the HC group complained of pain following HAVD test. Mean ± SEM concentration (%) of NaCl needed to cause pain among MP and HC were 2.82 ± 0.16 and 13.2 ± 0.6, respectively. Thus pain threshold of visceral pain away from the head was greatly ↓ in migraine patients compared with HC, suggesting CS.
TTH (IHS)	Bendtsen (105); 1996	Pericranial muscles in 40 TTH (chronic myofascial pain) and 40 HC were subjected to 7 different pressure intensities using a palpometer.	Pericranial tenderness was ↑ in patients than HC ($p<0.00001$); in a highly tender muscle, the stimulus-response function was linear (i.e., qualitatively different from normal muscle), suggesting sensitized CNS.
TTH (IHS)	Bendtsen (106); 1996	Pericranial PPT and pain detection (manual and an electronic algometer) as well as relative electrical pain threshold (REPT) (by constant current stimulator) in pericranial muscles and finger were tested in 40 TTH and 40 HC subjects.	TTH patients were significantly more tender than HC at all sites; PPT and detection were significantly ↓ in fingers in TTH; REPT in labial commissure was also significantly decreased in TTH compared with HC—all suggesting generalized pain sensitivity among TTH patients.
TTH (IHS); FMS (ACR)	Okifuji (107); 1999	70 HA without a history of widespread pain (63% migraine, 8% TTH, 11% mixed) were tested for manual TePs using 0–10 scale for pain.	40% of HA patients had 11 or more TePs at widespread locations, suggesting a state of generalized hyperalgesia in HA, as well as an overlap with FMS.
Migraine (without aura) (IHS)	Burstein (108); 2000	42 migraine patients were tested for heat, cold, and mechanical pain thresholds in periorbital and forearm skin during or outside of a migraine attack.	79% of migraine patients consistently exhibited allodynia, i.e., pain to normally innocuous stimulus (as defined by pain threshold values from an earlier study by the authors) during an attack, compared with attack-free period, suggesting CS.
Migraine (IHS)	Weissman-Fogel (110); 2003	34 migraine patients during attack-free period and 28 HC were tested for mechanical, thermal, and electric pain threshold; TS measured by repeated stimulation.	Patients showed significantly ↓ threshold to mechanical stimuli as well as TS. ↑ summation suggests ↑ membrane excitability of central trigeminovascular neurons, even in the absence of a migraine attack.
IBS (author)	Whitehead (111); 1990	16 IBS and 18 HC investigated for pain tolerance and the influence of anxiety, depression, and neuroticism on the pain tolerance.	Patients demonstrated significantly decreased pain tolerance to rectal balloon distension compared with HC, and the results were not affected by any of the psychometric tests.

(continued)

TABLE 4-3	Continued		
CONDITIONS STUDIED (CRITERIA)	**FIRST AUTHOR (REF); YEAR**	**STUDY METHODOLOGY**	**RESULTS AND COMMENTS**
IBS (Rome)	Trimble (112); 1995	12 IBS, 10 functional dyspepsia (FD), 32 HC; pain perception threshold tested by rectal and esophageal balloon distension.	IBS patients had significantly ↓ threshold for pain as well as discomfort both in the rectum and the esophagus, suggesting that there is generalized gut hypersensitivity in IBS.
IBS (Rome)	Mertz (113); 1995	100 IBS and 15 HC; rectal balloon distension and manometer used to study threshold for aversive reaction (TAR).	IBS patients had significantly ↓ TAR (94%), as well as ↑ intensity of pain, associated with altered viscerosomatic referral (perineal and lower abdomen areas).
IBS (Rome); FMS (ACR)	Chun (115); 1999	15 IBS, 10 FMS, 12 HC, and 10 with sphincter of Oddi (III) dysfunction (SOD); pain threshold assessed by rectal distension and psychological factors by SCL-90-R and MPI.	IBS patients showed significantly decreased rectal pain threshold compared with HC; FMS and SOD patients were not significantly different from HC. Pain threshold was not related to psychological distress.
IBS (Rome)	Schmulson (116); 2000	42 IBS, 19 HC; nonbiased tracking protocol for phasic rectal distension before and after repetitive sigmoid distension.	IBS patients had significantly lower threshold for discomfort both at baseline and after sigmoid distension compared with HC.
IBS (Rome)	Chan (118); 2001	22 IBS, 22 HC; CEP recorded before and after a meal in response to rhythmic rectal distension.	IBS patients showed significantly higher occurrence of CEP early peaks as well as shorter CEP both before and after a meal.
IBS (Rome)	Naliboff (119); 2001	12 IBS (nonconstipated), 12 HC; rCBF assessed by $H_2^{15}O$-water PET following moderate (45 mm Hg) rectal distension, both actual and anticipated, before and after a series of repetitive noxious sigmoid distension.	Brain area activation was similar between actual and anticipated stimuli in both groups. Compared with HC, IBS patients showed ↑ activation in certain areas, e.g., rostral anterior and posterior ACC, right PFC, and ↓ in others, e.g., perigenual cortex and temporal lobe, suggesting aberrant perceptual responses of central origin.
IBS (Rome II)	Verne (120); 2001	12 IBS (mostly diarrhea predominant), 17 HC rated unpleasantness to both sigmoid distension and cutaneous thermal stimuli in hand and foot.	Compared with HC, IBS patients demonstrated significant allodynia/hyperalgesia and increased pain intensity mostly in rectum and foot, but also to a smaller extent in the hand. Thus hyperalgesia in IBS is widespread, suggesting CS.
IBS (Rome II)	Verne (121); 2003	9 IBS, 9 HC; fMRI used to assess brain activities to both rectal (distension) and cutaneous stimuli (heat).	IBS patients rated significantly ↑ intensity and unpleasantness in both visceral and cutaneous stimuli, and ↑ brain activation in somatosensory cortex and thalamus (somatosensory processing), as well as insular, PFC, and cingulated (affective processing).
CFS (CDC)	Vecchiet (122); 1996	21 CFS, 30 HC; pain threshold to electric stimulation was assessed in deltoid, trapezius and quadriceps muscles, and the overlying skin and subcutis.	Pain threshold in CFS was significantly ↓ in muscles. Diffuse hyperalgesia in muscles suggest CS. *Muscle biopsy in 9 CFS and 9 HC showed degenerative changes in CFS. However, non-blindedness and small n make these changes unreliable.*
RLS (International RLS Study Group)	Stiasny-Kolster (123); 2004	11 RLS, 11 HC; effect of pricking pain obtained with 7 calibrated punctate mechanical stimulators (activating A-delta mechano-receptors) was studied in legs and hands.	Compared with HC, RLS patients had significantly higher pin-prick rating pain both in hands and feet (more pronounced in feet), suggesting generalized hyperalgesia (CS).
TMD (RDC)	Maixner (124); 1995	52 TMD, 23 HC; thermal and ischemic pain threshold and tolerance assessed on the forearm.	TMD patients had significantly ↓ thermal threshold, and ↓ ischemic threshold and tolerance, suggesting generalized CNS sensitization.

(continued)

TABLE 4-3	Continued		

CONDITIONS STUDIED (CRITERIA)	FIRST AUTHOR (REF); YEAR	STUDY METHODOLOGY	RESULTS AND COMMENTS
TMD (RDC)	Maixner (125); 1998	23 TMD, 24 HC; temporal summation of noxious thermal pain assessed in face and forearm (sustained noxious heat) and the ventral palm (C-fiber mediated repetitive brief trains of noxious heat).	TMD patients showed significantly greater C-fiber mediated TS, and a greater magnitude of sustained heat pain. Discrimination and detection of small increments of heat (noxious-adapting temperature) were similar between the 2 groups. TS at distant sites support CS.
TMD (authors)	Kashima (126); 1999	20 TMD, 20 HC; ischemic stimulus at a distant site, i.e., hand, was used to assess pain qualities. PPT (algometer) was measured before, during, and after ischemic pain.	TMD patients had significantly greater pain intensity, unpleasant scores, and lower pain threshold than HC. PPT and tolerance before ischemic pain were also significantly lower among patients.
TMD- (specified as myofascial) (RDC)	Svensson (127); 2001	22 TMD (TMD clinic) and 21 controls from general dentistry clinic without TMD were assessed for deep tonic pain (masseter and anterior tibial muscles), PPT in the muscles, and heat pain threshold over the skin of the muscles.	Deep pain from hypertonic saline was significantly more painful in masseter (with greater area of pain), but not in anterior tibial muscle in TMD vs. controls; PPT was significantly ↓ at both muscle sites, but there was no significant difference in the heat pain threshold between TMD and controls.

For abbreviations, also see footnote in Table 4-2. ACC, anterior cingulate cortex; CNS, central nervous system; DNIC, diffuse noxious inhibitory control; ECS, electrocutaneous stimulation; EMG, electromyography; fMRI, functional magnetic resonance imaging; HAVD, hand arm vein distension test; HNCS, heterotropic noxious conditioning stimulation; HS, hypertonic saline; IM, intramuscular; MPI, multidimensional pain inventory; NFR, nociceptive flexion reflex; PET, positron-emission tomography; PFC, prefrontal cortex; PPT, pressure pain threshold; QST, quantitative sensory testing; rCBF, regional cerebral blood flow; RDC, research diagnostic criteria for TMD; RB, randomized and blinded; SPECT, single-photon-emission computed tomography; TS, temporal summation; CEP, cerebral evoked potential; TMD, temporomandibular disorder; ↑, increase(d); ↓, decrease(d).
[a]Studies in this table were selected, in general, on the basis of sample size, design (e.g., control group), and importance based on other judgmental criteria. However, all published studies are referenced in the text.
[b]For references of various disease criteria used, please check the original articles cited.

Limitations of several mutual associations as well as human experimental studies described above should be noted—for example, small sample size, an absence of uniform criteria used, lack of adjustment for gender effect, and a lack of subgrouping—for example, constipation versus diarrhea-dominated symptoms in IBS. Interestingly, however, almost all studies converge on the same, consistent results—for example, significantly decreased pain threshold and tolerance to various stimuli as compared with healthy controls, with demonstration in many studies of characteristic central pain components—for example, dysesthesia and unpleasant nature as well as spread of pain among the CSS patients.

Although direct proof is lacking for CS in MCS and PTSD, there is indirect and hypothetical evidence that CS may indeed occur in these syndromes as well. MCS is associated with FMS (65,54,55), and 30% of MCS patients have CFS (37). Sorg (128) and Bell (129) have proposed a time-dependent sensitization (TDS) model for MCS. TDS was described in rodents that develop increased behavioral and neurochemical responses on repeat exposure to psychostimulant drugs (130). Both Bell and Sorg have stated several similarities between TDS and MCS: (a) initiation by a single or repeated exposure (requiring lower doses) to a chemical stimulus; (b) lasting changes in subsequent reactivity to low levels of chemically unrelated substances; (c) occurrence of further sensitization to other types of stimuli, including psychological stress (cross-sensitization), after exposure to one stimulus; (d) female vulnerability; (e) both conditioned and unconditioned amplification of responses; (f) sensitization following withdrawal from a stimulus and its reappearance with repeat exposure; and (g) no changes in baseline animal activity or human clinical symptoms if exposure to a chemical is avoided. It has been argued that the limbic system is involved in MCS (128,129).

PTSD is associated with FMS (88,96), and FMS is associated with PTSD (46), demonstrating increased sensitivity to mechanical pressure in this disorder. PTSD can be explained on the same TDS model as MCS. In this model, a single stressor of large magnitude (or multiple exposures of lower intensity) can cause sensitization leading to PTSD with greater vulnerability upon subsequent stressful events (131). Aberrations in sympathetic and HPA-axis functions, as well as abnormal cortical functions by neuroimaging (including symptom provocative tests by visual reexposure to the vivid initial traumatic exposure) in PTSD, have been reviewed (132).

DEPRESSION AND OTHER PSYCHIATRIC DISORDERS

A large number of studies have long established comorbidity of depression and other psychiatric disorders with members of the CSS family. These have been reviewed (13,19,20,22,133,134). On the basis of a lack of excessive depression in comparison with controls in our center (13), including a blinded study by DSM-III criteria (135), as well as several other studies showing the same results (13), I was reluctant to include depression as part of the CSS spectrum, arguing that depression and FMS are different diseases (13), in opposition to the views of others (12,19,20,133,134). More important, a convincing binding factor to link depression with other CSS diseases was lacking. Now a wide body of literature from other centers supports the view that depression, indeed, is more significantly common in FMS and other related CSS syndromes than in various control groups. Additionally, it is more than likely that there is CS in depression (to be described below). Hence depression is now added to my previously published Venn diagram (13) (see Figure 4-2). However, many of the authors of "psychiatric/psychological doctrine," as mentioned above, have put the psychological status and psychosocial factors at the center stage of pathogenesis of these diseases, with which I disagree. Only a minority of patients, about one-third, have significant psychological distress (136), and there are important biological bases of CSS conditions, as has been shown earlier.

Although there is currently a lack of direct evidence of CS with regard to sensory functions in depression, Robert Post of the National Institutes of Health (NIH) has presented strong theoretical arguments that depression is also based on CS (137). Essentially, the theory is based on kindling and TDS models. It is now recognized that most cases of depression follow stressful events, mostly of a psychosocial nature, that initiate various biological processes, including gene transcription and other neurochemical-hormonal aberrations in animal models. These lead to intracellular changes and subsequent CS (137). With multiple exposure to stress, even of less severity, there is progressive sensitization of the CNS. Neuronal hyperexcitability now becomes self-sustained, so that even without discernable stress, depression becomes chronic (137). A similar paradigm has been suggested for other psychiatric diseases—anxiety disorders, for example (138).

AN INTEGRATIVE MODEL FOR CENTRAL SENSITIVITY SYNDROMES

Although this chapter has emphasized nociceptive-biologic components of disease pathogenesis, it must be remembered that CS itself is modulated by several factors—for example, genetic, environmental, and psychological. Neuroendocrine factors and the autonomic nervous system likely modulate CS (139–141). Although there is no psychological bias in pain reporting (i.e., response bias due to hypervigilence or expectancies) (99), psychology does play a role in pain processing through nociceptive neurons. Placebo, for example, works through the expectation of pain relief that is mediated by the endogenous opioid system (142). Trauma, poor sleep, and psychosocial distress, including depression and mental stress, all play a role (13,16,17,143). Adverse childhood experiences may also be a factor (144–146). Many of these factors may be bidirectionally related to CS.

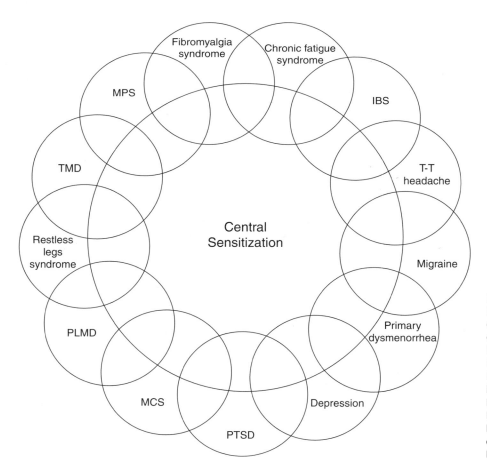

Figure 4-2. Currently proposed members of the central sensitivity syndromes (CSS) group, incorporating depression. The common pathophysiologic binding glue for these interrelated syndromes is central sensitization. IBS, irritable bowel syndromes; T-T headache, tension-type headache; PTSD, posttraumatic stress disorder; MCS, multiple chemical sensitivity; PLMD, periodic limb movement disorder; TMD, temporomandibilar disorder; MPS, myofascial pain syndromes.

SIGNIFICANCE OF CENTRAL SENSITIVITY SYNDROMES AS A NEW PARADIGM IN DISEASE/ILLNESS

CSS is a new paradigm. It arose from the concept that FMS, IBS, TTH, migraine, and similar members of the CSS family are interrelated with a common pathogenetic factor, first proposed in 1984 (6). However, that common factor remained conjectural and elusive for some time. The initial speculation was muscle spasm (6); subsequently depression was implied in the term "affective spectrum disorder" (12). We now know that neither is true. Depression is not at the top of the "command chain," since depression itself may be the result of CS. A review of the evidence for the presence of CS among CSS members other than FMS (justifying the nomenclature "CSS") was first proposed in 2000 (15). Since then the evidence has grown stronger among diseases that were already known to show CS, and new data are now available for other members of the family—for example, RLS (123).

So we ask, what does this mean in practical as well as hypothetical terms? A majority of our patients who seek health care most likely belongs to the CSS as a group, with enormous cost to the system. Other implications are that we need to put greater emphasis on physician training for recognition and proper treatment of these common and distressing disorders and make a national commitment for further research with greater availability of funds. Since these disorders are related, a pathogenetic factor that has been elucidated in one member may also apply to the other (being cognizant that some aspects of pathogenesis—for example, genetics and neurohormonal dysfunctions—may be dissimilar among the individual syndromes), and one treatment that has been found to be effective in one may also be shown to work in other members by appropriate clinical trials. In clinical terms, the knowledge of mutual associations helps early and easier diagnosis, avoiding unnecessary and expensive investigations, and one treatment that is effective (by clinical trials) in one may also be tried in others, even in the absence of proper studies on the basis of a common pathophysiology of CS. Perhaps most exciting is that new drugs can be tested in a human experimental laboratory, showing their effect or lack of it on CS, that can now be measured quantitatively. Such findings will help to conduct randomized and blinded clinical trials.

SUMMARY POINTS

- The notion that conditions such as fibromyalgia, IBS, tension headache, and a number of other conditions may all be related and share common pathophysiologic mechanisms is relatively new and is generally acknowledged to have been first suggested by Yunus.
- The term "central sensitivity syndromes" is currently preferred by Yunus to describe these conditions; other terms currently being used include functional somatic syndromes, chronic multisymptom illnesses, somatoform disorders, and medically unexplained symptoms.

- Persons with any one of the illnesses in this spectrum are more likely to have another, and there is a strong familial predisposition for the same.
- Pathogenesis and treatment in one may be shared by the others.

ACKNOWLEDGMENT

I wish to thank Dr. Fatma Inanici for critiquing the manuscript and offering invaluable suggestions.

REFERENCES

1. Osler W. Mucous colitis. In: Osler W, ed. *The principles and practice of medicine*. New York: D. Appleton and Company, 1906:530–531.
2. Osler W. Migraine. In: Osler W, ed. *The principles and practice of medicine*. New York: D. Appleton and Company, 1906:1066–1068.
3. Lewis A. Melancholia: a clinical survey of depressive states. *J Ment Sci* 1934;80:277–378.
4. Aaron LA, Buchwald D. A review of the evidence for overlap among unexplained clinical conditions. *Ann Intern Med* 2001;134:868–881.
5. Yunus MB, Masi AT, Calabro JJ, et al. Primary fibromyalgia (fibrositis): clinical study of 50 patients with matched normal controls. *Semin Arthritis Rheum* 1981;11:151–171.
6. Yunus MB. Primary fibromyalgia syndrome: current concepts. *Compr Ther* 1984;10:21–28.
7. Thompson JM. Tension myalgia as a diagnosis at the Mayo Clinic and its relationship to fibrositis, fibromyalgia, and myofascial pain syndrome. *Mayo Clin Proc* 1990;65:1237–1248.
8. Zidar J, Backman E, Bengtsson A, et al. Quantitative EMG and muscle tension in painful muscles in fibromyalgia. *Pain* 1990;40:249–254.
9. Durette MR, Rodriquez AA, Agre JC, et al. Needle electromyographic evaluation of patients with myofascial or fibromyalgic pain. *Am J Phys Med Rehabil* 1991;70:154–156.
10. Kendall SA, Elert J, Ekselius L, et al. Are perceived muscle tension, electromyographic hyperactivity and personality traits correlated in the fibromyalgia syndrome? *J Rehabil Med* 2002;34:73–79.
11. Yunus MB, Masi AT, Aldag JC. A controlled study of primary fibromyalgia syndrome: clinical features and association with other functional syndromes. *J Rheumatol* 1989;19:62–71.
12. Hudson JI, Pope HG, Jr. Fibromyalgia and psychopathology: is fibromyalgia a form of "affective spectrum disorder"? *J Rheumatol* 1989;19(Suppl.):15–22.
13. Yunus MB. Psychological aspects of fibromyalgia syndrome: a component of the dysfunctional spectrum syndrome. *Baillieres Clin Rheumatol* 1994;8:811–837.
14. Bennett RM. Emerging concepts in the neurobiology of chrome pain: evidence of abnormal sensory processing in fibromyalgia. *Mayo Clin Proc* 1999;74:385–398.
15. Yunus MB. Central sensitivity syndromes: a unified concept for fibromyalgia and other similar maladies. *J Indian Rheum Assoc* 2000;8:27–33.
16. Yunus MB, Inanici F. Clinical characteristics and biopathophysiological mechanisms of fibromyalgia syndrome. In: Baldry P, ed. *Myofascial pain and fibromyalgia syndromes: a clinical guide to diagnosis and management*. Edinburgh: Churchill Livingstone, 2001:351–377.
17. Yunus MB, Inanici F. Fibromyalgia syndrome: clinical features, diagnosis and biophysiological mechanisms. In:

Rachlin ES, ed. *Myofascial pain and fibromyalgia: trigger point management*. Philadelphia, PA: Mosby, 2002:3–31.

18. Lipkin M. Functional or organic? A pointless question. *Ann Intern Med* 1969;71:1013–1017.

19. Manu P, ed. *Functional somatic syndromes: etiology, diagnosis and treatment*. Cambridge, MA: Cambridge University Press, 1998.

20. Barsky AJ, Borus JF. Functional somatic syndromes. *Ann Intern Med* 1999;130:910–921.

21. Richardson RD, Engel CC Jr. Evaluation and management of medically unexplained physical symptoms. *Neurologist* 2004;10(1):18–30.

22. Sharpe M. Medically unexplained symptoms and syndromes. *Clin Med* 2002;2(6):501–514.

23. Yunus MB. Suffering, science and sabotage. *J Musculoskelet Pain* 2004;12(2):3–18.

24. Yunus MB, Masi AT. Association of primary fibromyalgia syndrome with stress-related syndromes [Abstr.]. *Clin Res* 1985;33(4):923A.

25. Coderre TJ, Katz J, Vaccarino AL, et al. Contribution of central neuroplasticity to pathological pain: review of clinical and experimental evidence. *Pain* 1993;52:259–285.

26. Besson JM. The neurobiology of pain. *Lancet* 1999;353: 1610–1615.

27. Bengtsson A, Henriksson KG, Jorfeldt L, et al. Primary fibromyalgia. A clinical and laboratory study of 55 patients. *Scand J Rheumatol* 1986;15:340–347.

28. Whorwell PJ, McCallum M, Creed FH, et al. Non-colonic features of irritable bowel syndrome. *Gut* 1986;27:37–40.

29. Buchwald D, Goldenberg DL, Sullivan JL, et al. The "chronic, active Epstein-Barr virus infection" syndrome and primary fibromyalgia. *Arthritis Rheum* 1987;30: 1132–1136.

30. Romano TJ. Coexistence of irritable bowel syndrome and fibromyalgia. *W V Med J* 1988;84:16–18.

31. Wolfe F, Smythe HA, Yunus MB et al., The American College of Rheumatology 1990 criteria for the classification of fibromyalgia. Report of the Multicenter Criteria Committee. *Arthritis Rheum* 1990;33: 160–172.

32. Wallace DJ. Genitourinary manifestations of fibrositis: an increased association with the female urethral syndrome. *J Rheumatol* 1990;17:238–239.

33. Goldenberg DL, Simms RW, Geiger A, et al. High frequency of fibromyalgia in patients with chronic fatigue seen in a primary care service. *Arthritis Rheum* 1990;33: 381–387.

34. Triadafilopoulos G, Simms RW, Goldenberg DL. Bowel dysfunction in fibromyalgia syndrome. *Dig Dis Sci* 1991;36(1): 59–64.

35. Wysenbeek AJ, Shapira Y, Leibovici L. Primary fibromyalgia and the chronic fatigue syndrome. *Rheumatol Int* 1991; 10(6):227–229.

36. Hudson JI, Goldenberg DL, Pope HG Jr, et al. Comorbidity of fibromyalgia with medical and psychiatric disorders. *Am J Med* 1992;92:363–367.

37. Buchwald D, Garrity D. Comparison of patients with chronic fatigue syndrome, fibromyalgia, and multiple chemical sensitivities. *Arch Intern Med* 1994;154:2049–2053.

38. Paira SO. Fibromyalgia associated with female urethral syndrome. *Clin Rheumatol* 1994;13:88–89.

39. Wolfe F, Ross K, Anderson J, et al. The prevalence and characteristics of fibromyalgia in the general population. *Arthritis Rheum* 1995;38:19–28.

40. Sivri A, Cindas A, Dincer F, et al. Bowel dysfunction and irritable bowel syndrome in fibromyalgia patients. *Clin Rheumatol* 1996;15:283–286.

41. Yunus MB, Aldag JC. Restless legs syndrome and leg cramps in fibromyalgia syndrome: a controlled study. *Br Med J* 1996;312:1339.

42. Plesh O, Wolfe F, Lane N. The relationship between fibromyalgia and temporomandibular disorders: prevalence and symptom severity. *J Rheumatol* 1996;23:1948–1952.

43. Walker EA, Gelfand AN, Gelfand MD, et al. Chronic pelvic pain and gynecological symptoms in women with irritable bowel syndrome. *J Psychosom Obstet Gynaecol* 1996;17: 39–46.

44. Clauw DJ, Schmidt M, Radulovic D, et al. The relationship between fibromyalgia and interstitial cystitis. *J Psychiatr Res* 1997;31:125–131.

45. Wright EF, Des Rosier KF, Clark MK, et al. Identifying undiagnosed rheumatic disorders among patients with TMD. *J Am Dent Assoc* 1997;128:738–744.

46. Amir M, Kaplan Z, Neuman L, et al. Posttraumatic stress disorder, tenderness and fibromyalgia. *J Psychosom Res* 1997;42:607–613.

47. Cimino R, Michelotti A, Stradi R, et al. Comparison of clinical and psychologic features of fibromyalgia and masticatory myofascial pain. *J Orofac Pain* 1998;12:35–41.

48. Korszun A, Papadopoulos E, Demitrack M, et al. The relationship between temporomandibular disorders and stress-associated syndromes. *Oral Surg Oral Med Oral Pathol Oral Radiol Endod* 1998;86:416–420.

49. Inanici F, Yunus MB, Aldag JC. Clinical features and psychological factors in soft tissue pain: comparison with fibromyalgia syndrome. *J Musculoskelet Pain* 1999;7(1/2): 293–301.

50. Barton A, Pal B, Whorwell PJ, et al. Increased prevalence of sicca complex and fibromyalgia in patients with irritable bowel syndrome. *Am J Gastroenterol* 1999;94:1898–1901.

51. Yunus MB, Inanici F, Aldag JC, et al. Fibromyalgia in men: comparison of features with women. *J Rheumatol* 2000;27: 485–490.

52. White KP, Speechley M, Harth M, et al. Co-existence of chronic fatigue syndrome with fibromyalgia syndrome in the general population. A controlled study. *Scand J Rheumatol* 2000;29:44–51.

53. Tayag-Kier CE, Keenan GF, Scalzi LV, et al. Sleep and periodic limb movement in sleep in juvenile fibromyalgia. *Pediatrics* 2000;106:E70.

54. Nawab SS, Miller CS, Dale JK, et al. Self-reported sensitivity to chemical exposures in five clinical populations and healthy controls. *Psychiatry Res* 2000;95:67–74.

55. Jason LA, Taylor RR, Kennedy CL. Chronic fatigue syndrome, fibromyalgia, and multiple chemical sensitivities in a community-based sample of persons with chronic fatigue syndrome-like symptoms. *Psychosom Med* 2000;62:655–663.

56. Choudhury AK, Yunus MB, Haq SA, et al. Clinical features of fibromyalgia in a Bangladeshi population. *J Musculoskelet Pain* 2001;9:25–33.

57. Peres MF, Young WB, Kaup AO, et al. Fibromyalgia is common in patients with transformed migraine. *Neurology* 2001; 57:1326–1328.

58. Lubrano E, Iovino P, Tremolaterra F, et al. Fibromyalgia in patients with irritable bowel syndrome. An association with the severity of the intestinal disorder. *Int J Colorectal Dis* 2001;16:211–215.

59. Peres MFP, Zukerman E, Young WB, et al. Fatigue in chronic migraine patients. *Cephalalgia* 2002;22:720–724.

60. Raphael KG, Janal MN, Nayak S. Comorbidity of fibromyalgia and posttraumatic stress disorder symptoms in a community sample of women. *Pain Med* 2004;5:33–41.

61. Campbell SM, Clark S, Tindall EA, et al. Clinical characteristics of fibrositis: I. A "blinded" controlled study of symptoms and tender points. *Arthritis Rheum* 1983;26:817–824.

62. Goldenberg DL. Fibromyalgia syndrome: an emerging but controversial condition. *JAMA* 1987;257:2782–2787.

63. Veale D, Kavanagh G, Fielding JF, et al. Primary fibromyalgia and the irritable bowel syndrome: different expressions

of a common pathogenetic process. *Br J Rheumatol* 1991;30: 220–222.

64. Sperber AD, Atzmon Y, Neumann L, et al. Fibromyalgia in the irritable bowel syndrome: studies of prevalence and clinical implications. *Am J Gastroenterol* 1999;94:3541–3546.

65. Aaron LA, Burke MM, Buchwald D. Overlapping conditions among patients with chronic fatigue syndrome, fibromyalgia, and temporomandibular disorder. *Arch Intern Med* 2000; 160:221–227.

66. Sherman JJ, Turk DC, Okifuji A. Prevalence and impact of posttraumatic stress disorder-like symptoms on patients with fibromyalgia syndrome. *Clin J Pain* 2000;16:127–134.

67. Alagiri M, Chottiner S, Ratner V, et al. Interstitial cystitis: unexplained associations with other chronic disease and pain syndromes. *Urology* 1997;49(5A Suppl):52–57.

68. Slotkoff AT, Radulovic DA, Clauw DJ. The relationship between fibromyalgia and the multiple chemical sensitivity syndrome. *Scand J Rheumatol* 1997;26:364–367.

69. Simms RW. Is there muscle pathology in fibromyalgia syndrome? *Rheum Dis Clin North Am* 1996;22:245–266.

70. Whitehead WF, Engel BT, Schuster MM. Irritable bowel syndrome. *Dig Dis Sci* 1980;25:404–413.

71. McKee DP, Quigley EMM. Intestinal motility in irritable bowel syndrome: is IBS a motility disorder? Part 2. *Dig Dis Sci* 1993;38:1773–1782.

72. McKee DP, Quigley EMM. Intestinal motility in irritable bowel syndrome: is IBS a motility disorder? Part 1. *Dig Dis Sci* 1993;38:1761–1772.

73. Yunus MB, Kalyan-Raman UP, Masi AT, et al. Electron microscopic studies of muscle biopsy in primary fibromyalgia: a controlled and blinded study. *J Rheumatol* 1989;16:97–101.

74. Yunus MB. Towards a model of pathophysiology of fibromyalgia: aberrant central pain mechanisms with peripheral modulation. *J Rheumatol* 1992;19:846–850.

75. Mayer EA. Emerging disease model for functional gastrointestinal disorders. *Am J Med* 1999;107:12S–19S.

76. Granges G, Littlejohn G. Pressure pain threshold in pain-free subjects, in patients with chronic regional pain syndromes, and in patients with fibromyalgia syndrome. *Arthritis Rheum* 1993;36:642–646.

77. McDermid AJ, Rollman GB, McCain GA. Generalized hypervigilance in fibromyalgia: evidence of perceptual amplification. *Pain* 1996;66:133–144.

78. Arroyo JF, Cohen ML. Abnormal responses to electrocutaneous stimulation in fibromyalgia. *J Rheumatol* 1993;20:1925–1931.

79. Gibson SJ, Littlejohn GO, Gorman MM, et al. Altered heat pain thresholds and cerebral event-related potentials following painful CO_2 laser stimulation in subjects with fibromyalgia syndrome. *Pain* 1994;58:185–193.

80. Lautenbacher S, Rollman GB, McCain GA. Multi-method assessment of experimental and clinical pain in patients with fibromyalgia. *Pain* 1994;59:45–53.

81. Sorensen J, Bengtsson A, Backman E, et al. Pain analysis in patients with fibromyalgia. Effects of intravenous morphine, lidocaine, and ketamine. *Scand J Rheumatol* 1995;24:360–365.

82. Mountz JM, Bradley LA, Modell JG, et al. Fibromyalgia in women. Abnormalities of regional cerebral blood flow in the thalamus and the caudate nucleus are associated with low pain threshold levels. *Arthritis Rheum* 1995;38: 926–938.

83. Bendtsen L, Jensen R, Olesen J. Qualitatively altered nociception in chronic myofascial pain. *Pain* 1996;65:259–264.

84. Kosek E, Ekholm J, Hansson P. Sensory dysfunction in fibromyalgia patients with implications for pathogenic mechanisms. *Pain* 1996;68:375–383.

85. Kosek E, Hansson P. Modulatory influence on somatosensory perception from vibration and heterotopic noxious conditioning stimulation (HNCS) in fibromyalgia patients and healthy subjects. *Pain* 1997;70:41–51.

86. Sorensen J, Graven-Nielsen T, Henriksson KG, et al. Hyperexcitability in fibromyalgia. *J Rheumatol* 1998;25:152–155.

87. Graven-Nielsen T, Aspegren Kendall S, Henriksson KG, et al. Ketamine reduces muscle pain, temporal summation, and referred pain in fibromyalgia patients. *Pain* 2000;85:483–491.

88. Salerno A, Thomas E, Olive P, et al. Motor cortical dysfunction disclosed by single and double magnetic stimulation in patients with fibromyalgia. *Clin Neurophysiol* 2000;111:994–1001.

89. Kwiatek R, Barnden L, Tedman R, et al. Regional cerebral blood flow in fibromyalgia: single-photon-emission computed tomography evidence of reduction in the pontine tegmentum and thalami. *Arthritis Rheum* 2000;43:2823–2833.

90. Staud R, Vierck CJ, Cannon RL, et al. Abnormal sensitization and temporal summation of second pain (wind-up) in patients with fibromyalgia syndrome. *Pain* 2001;91:165–175.

91. Price DD, Staud R, Robinson ME, et al. Enhanced temporal summation of second pain and its central modulation in fibromyalgia patients. *Pain* 2002;99:49–59.

92. Gracely RH, Petzke F, Wolf JM, et al. Functional magnetic resonance imaging evidence of augmented pain processing in fibromyalgia. *Arthritis Rheum* 2002;46:1333–1343.

93. Berglund B, Harju EL, Kosek E, et al. Quantitative and qualitative perceptual analysis of cold dysesthesia and hyperalgesia in fibromyalgia. *Pain* 2002;96:177–187.

94. Wik G, Fischer H, Bragee B, et al. Retrosplenial cortical activation in the fibromyalgia syndrome. *NeuroReport* 2003; 14:619–621.

95. Desmeules JA, Cedraschi C, Rapiti E, et al. Neurophysiologic evidence for a central sensitization in patients with fibromyalgia. *Arthritis Rheum* 2003;48:1420–1429.

96. Staud R, Cannon RC, Mauderli AP, et al. Temporal summation of pain from mechanical stimulation of muscle tissue in normal controls and subjects with fibromyalgia syndrome. *Pain* 2003;102:87–95.

97. Staud R, Robinson ME, Vierck CJ, et al. Diffuse noxious inhibitory controls (DNIC) attenuate temporal summation of second pain in normal males but not in normal females or fibromyalgia patients. *Pain* 2003;101:167–174.

98. Geisser ME, Casey KL, Brucksch CB, et al. Perception of noxious and innocuous heat stimulation among healthy women and women with fibromyalgia: association with mood, somatic focus, and catastrophizing. *Pain* 2003;102: 243–250.

99. Petzke F, Clauw DJ, Ambrose K, et al. Increased pain sensitivity in fibromyalgia: effects of stimulus type and mode of presentation. *Pain* 2003;105:403–413.

100. Banic B, Petersen-Felix S, Andersen OK, et al. Evidence for spinal cord hypersensitivity in chronic pain after whiplash injury and in fibromyalgia. *Pain* 2004;107:7–15.

101. Langemark M, Jensen K, Jensen TS, et al. Pressure pain thresholds and thermal nociceptive thresholds in chronic tension-type headache. *Pain* 1989;38:203–210.

102. Schoenen J, Bottin D, Hardy F, et al. Cephalic and extracephalic pressure pain thresholds in chronic tension-type headache. *Pain* 1991;47:145–149.

103. Langemark M, Bach FW, Jensen TS, et al. Decreased nociceptive flexion reflex threshold in chronic tension-type headache. *Arch Neurol* 1993;50:1061–1064.

104. Nicolodi M, Sicuteri R, Coppola G, et al. Visceral pain threshold is deeply lowered far from the head in migraine. *Headache* 1994;34:12–19.

105. Bendtsen L, Jensen R, Olsen J. Qualitatively altered nociception in chronic myofascial pain. *Pain* 1996;65:259–264.

106. Bendtsen L, Jensen R, Olesen J. Decreased pain detection and tolerance thresholds in chronic tension-type headache. *Arch Neurol* 1996;53:373–376.

107. Okifuji A, Turk DC, Marcus DA. Comparison of generalized and localized hyperalgesia in patients with recurrent headache and fibromyalgia. *Psychosom Med* 1999;61:771–780.

108. Burstein R, Yarnitsky D, Goor-Aryeh I, et al. An association between migraine and cutaneous allodynia. *Ann Neurol* 2000;47:614–624.

109. de Tommaso M, Guido M, Libro G, et al. Abnormal brain processing of cutaneous pain in migraine patients during the attack. *Neurosci Lett* 2002;333:29–32.

110. Weissman-Fogel I, Sprecher E, Granovsky Y, et al. Repeated noxious stimulation of the skin enhances cutaneous pain perception of migraine patients in between attacks: clinical evidence for continuous sub-threshold increase in membrane excitability of central trigeminovascular neurons. *Pain* 2003; 104:693–700.

111. Whitehead WE, Holtkotter B, Enck P, et al. Tolerance for rectosigmoid distention in irritable bowel syndrome. *Gastroenterology* 1990;98:1187–1192.

112. Trimble KC, Farouk R, Pryde A, et al. Heightened visceral sensation in functional gastrointestinal disease is not site-specific. Evidence for a generalized disorder of gut sensitivity. *Dig Dis Sci* 1995;40:1607–1613.

113. Mertz H, Naliboff B, Munakata J, et al. Altered rectal perception is a biological marker of patients with irritable bowel syndrome. *Gastroenterology* 1995;109:40–52.

114. Silverman DH, Munakata JA, Ennes H, et al. Regional cerebral activity in normal and pathological perception of visceral pain. *Gastroenterology* 1997;112:64–72.

115. Chun A, Desautels S, Slivka A, et al. Visceral algesia in irritable bowel syndrome, fibromyalgia, and sphincter of oddi dysfunction, type III. *Dig Dis Sci* 1999;44:631–636.

116. Schmulson M, Chang L, Naliboff B, et al. Correlation of symptom criteria with perception thresholds during rectosigmoid distension in irritable bowel syndrome patients. *Am J Gastroenterol* 2000;95:152–156.

117. Lembo T, Naliboff BD, Matin K, et al. Irritable bowel syndrome patients show altered sensitivity to exogenous opioids. *Pain* 2000;87:137–147.

118. Chan YK, Herkes GK, Badcock C, et al. Alterations in cerebral potentials evoked by rectal distension in irritable bowel syndrome. *Am J Gastroenterol* 2001;96:2413–2417.

119. Naliboff BD, Derbyshire SW, Munakata J, et al. Cerebral activation in patients with irritable bowel syndrome and control subjects during rectosigmoid stimulation. *Psychosom Med* 2001;63:365–375.

120. Verne GN, Robinson ME, Price DD. Hypersensitivity to visceral and cutaneous pain in the irritable bowel syndrome. *Pain* 2001;93:7–14.

121. Verne GN, Himes NC, Robinson ME, et al. Central representation of visceral and cutaneous hypersensitivity in the irritable bowel syndrome. *Pain* 2003;103:99–110.

122. Vecchiet L, Montanari G, Pizzigallo E, et al. Sensory characterization of somatic parietal tissues in humans with chronic fatigue syndrome. *Neurosci Lett* 1996;208:117–120.

123. Stiasny-Kolster K, Magerl W, Oertel WH, et al. Static mechanical hyperalgesia without dynamic tactile allodynia in patients with restless legs syndrome. *Brain* 2004;127:773–782.

124. Maixner W, Fillingim R, Booker D, et al. Sensitivity of patients with painful temporomandibular disorders to experimentally evoked pain. *Pain* 1995;63:341–351.

125. Maixner W, Fillingim R, Sigurdsson A, et al. Sensitivity of patients with painful temporomandibular disorders to experimentally evoked pain: evidence for altered temporal summation of pain. *Pain* 1998;76:71–81.

126. Kashima K, Rahman OI, Sakoda S, et al. Increased pain sensitivity of the upper extremities of TMD patients with myalgia to experimentally-evoked noxious stimulation: possibility of worsened endogenous opioid systems. *Cranio* 1999;17:241–246.

127. Svensson P, List T, Hector G. Analysis of stimulus-evoked pain in patients with myofascial temporomandibular pain disorders. *Pain* 2001;92:399–409.

128. Sorg BA, Hooks MS, Kalivas PW. Neuroanatomy and neurochemical mechanisms of time-dependent sensitization. *Toxicol Ind Health* 1994;10:369–386.

129. Bell IR. White paper: neuropsychiatric aspects of sensitivity to low-level chemicals: a neural sensitization model. *Toxicol Ind Health* 1994;10:277–312.

130. Antelman SM. Stressor-induced sensitization to subsequent stress: implications for the development and treatment of clinical disorders. In: Kalivas PW, Barnes CD, eds. *Sensitization in the nervous system.* New Jersey: Telford Press, 1988: 227–256.

131. Post RM, Weiss SRB, Li H, et al. Sensitization components of post-traumatic stress disorder: implications for therapeutics. *Semin Clin Neuropsychiatry* 1999;4:282–294.

132. van der Kolk B. The psychobiology of posttraumatic stress disorder. *J Clin Psychiatry* 1997;58(Suppl. 9):16–24.

133. Hudson JI, Pope HG. The concept of affective spectrum disorder: relationship to fibromyalgia and other syndromes of chronic fatigue and chronic muscle pain. *Baillieres Clin Rheumatol* 1994;8:839–856.

134. Gruber AJ, Hudson JI, Pope HG Jr. The management of treatment-resistant depression in disorders on the interface of psychiatry and medicine. Fibromyalgia, chronic fatigue syndrome, migraine, irritable bowel syndrome, atypical facial pain, and premenstrual dysphoric disorder. *Psychiatr Clin North Am* 1996;19:351–369.

135. Ahles TA, Khan SA, Yunus MB, et al. Psychiatric status of patients with primary fibromyalgia, patients with rheumatoid arthritis, and subjects without pain: a blinded comparison of DSM III diagnoses. *Am J Psychiatry* 1991;148: 1721–1726.

136. Giesecke T, Williams DA, Harris RE, et al. Subgrouping of fibromyalgia patients on the basis of pressure-pain thresholds and psychological factors. *Arthritis Rheum* 2003;48: 2916–2922.

137. Post RM. Transduction of psychosocial stress into the neurobiology of recurrent affective disorder. *Am J Psychiatry* 1992;149:999–1010.

138. Post RM, Weiss SRB. Sensitization and kindling phenomena in mood, anxiety, and obsessive-compulsive disorders: the role of serotonergic mechanism in illness progression. *Biol Psychiatry* 1998;44:193–206.

139. Cleare AJ. The neuroendocrinology of chronic fatigue syndrome. *Endocr Rev* 2003;24:236–252.

140. Crofford LJ, Demitrack MA. Evidence that abnormalities of central neurohormonal systems are key to understanding fibromyalgia and chronic fatigue syndrome. *Rheum Dis Clin North Am* 1996;22(2):267–284.

141. Natelson BH. Chronic fatigue syndrome. *JAMA* 2001;285(20): 2557–2559.

142. Benedetti F, Amanzio M. The neurobiology of placebo analgesia: from endogenous opioids to cholecystokinin. *Prog Neurobiol* 1997;52:109–125.

143. Bradley LA, Alarcon GS, Koopman WJ. Fibromyalgia. In: *Arthritis and allied conditions: a textbook of rheumatology.* Philadelphia, PA: Lippincott Williams & Wilkins, 2001: 1811–1844.

144. McBeth J, Macfarlane GJ, Benjamin S, et al. The association between tender points, psychological distress, and adverse childhood experiences: a community-based study. *Arthritis Rheum* 1999;42:1397–1404.

145. Salmon P, Skaife K, Rhodes J. Abuse, dissociation, and somatization in irritable bowel syndrome: towards an explanatory model. *J Behav Med* 2003;26:1–18.

146. Goodwin RD, Hoven CW, Murison R, et al. Association between childhood physical abuse and gastrointestinal disorders and migraine in adulthood. *Am J Public Health* 2003; 93:1065–1067.

5

The Neurobiology of Chronic Musculoskeletal Pain (Including Chronic Regional Pain)

Roland Staud

To understand the mechanisms of pain, one has to recognize the multiple dimensions of the pain experience. Over the last 30 years it has become increasingly evident that pain is a complex experience involving sensory, cognitive-evaluative, and affective-motivational dimensions. Pain cannot be explained by neurophysiologic, psychophysical, or psychological concepts alone, but it can be conceptualized as an adaptive sensation and early warning to protect the body from tissue injury. After injury has occurred, pain may aid in repair of tissue damage through multiple adaptive mechanisms, including hypersensitivity to normally innocuous stimuli.

Pain has been classified as acute and chronic pain. Chronic pain, however, is not just simply persistent "acute pain." Chronic pain differs from acute pain by being more diffuse and by often spreading to areas beyond the original site of injury (enlargement of receptive fields). Furthermore, chronic pain often starts as localized or regional pain, which then expands to adjacent areas over time. The relationship between the reported severity of chronic pain and tissue pathology is frequently poor or absent. Thus a frequent problem in the evaluation and treatment of chronic pain is the common belief of health care providers that these patients are exaggerating and embellishing a minor pain problem and that it is because of secondary motives that they do not improve. Questioning the veracity and ulterior motives of pain patients, however, is counterproductive. As a consequence of persistent chronic pain, most people experience negative emotions and behaviors that are often counterproductive in coping with their chronic pain problem.

Chronic pain patients almost always display findings related to central nervous system (CNS) pain-processing abnormalities, including secondary hyperalgesia, allodynia, and abnormal temporal summation of second pain (termed windup, or WU). Fibromyalgia syndrome (FMS) is a good example of this process, but other chronic pain syndromes—including chronic

low back pain, regional pain syndromes, irritable bowel syndrome, chronic fatigue syndrome, osteoarthritis, postherpetic neuralgia, and chronic headaches—demonstrate similar characteristics. This chapter will deal with the neurobiological abnormalities related to FMS and other chronic pain states.

PATHOPHYSIOLOGIC BASIS FOR PAIN

The International Association for the Study of Pain has defined pain as " ... an unpleasant sensory and emotional experience associated with actual or potential tissue damage, or described in terms of such damage" (1). Although this definition explicitly affirms that pain includes both a sensory and an affective-evaluative component and acknowledges that pain may occur in the absence of obvious peripheral or visceral pathologic features, it requires the threat of actual or potential tissue damage. This relationship, however, is not obvious for many patients with chronic pain syndromes, including FMS. Therefore, in 1999 a new definition of pain was proposed (2) that described pain as a "somatic perception containing: (a) a bodily sensation with qualities like those reported during tissue damaging stimulations, (b) an experimental threat associated with this sensation, and (c) a feeling of unpleasantness or other negative emotion based on this experienced threat."

NOCICEPTION AND PAIN

To comprehend chronic pain, one must integrate the sensory and affective evaluative elements of the pain experience. Focusing exclusively on the psychological aspects of pain or addressing only the sensory component and ignoring the affective dimensions are equally misguided approaches.

Pain is almost always related to impulse input that originates from nociceptors in somatic or visceral tissues. These impulses travel in myelinated (A-δ) and unmyelinated (C) peripheral nerves, which first project in the dorsal horn to nociceptor specific (NS) neurons and wide-dynamic range (WDR) neurons before they transmit to the thalamus, anterior cingulate cortex (ACC), anterior insular cortex, and somatosensory cortex, which include some of the most important CNS pain-processing regions. Some of these areas are related to somatotopic, affective, and cognitive evaluations of these impulses. The activation of these areas results in the pain experience and subsequent reflex and reflective behaviors. Whereas reflex and reflective behaviors are aimed at eliminating acute pain, similar mechanisms are not operative in chronic pain syndromes, including FMS. FMS patients, like most chronic pain sufferers, do not display the pain behaviors usually seen in acute pain, including increased perspiration and blood pressure, hyperthermia, and tachycardia. FMS patients have low pain thresholds (hyperalgesia) and report amplified pain with a variety of nociceptive stimuli, including pressure, heat, cold, and electrical current. Because no consistent tissue abnormalities have been detected in FMS, central pain processing abnormalities need to be considered as important contributors for the heightened pain sensitivity of these patients. As discussed in detail below, there is compelling evidence that the pain of FMS patients is related to central sensitization.

ROLE OF DIFFERENT NOCICEPTORS FOR PAIN

Pain signaling results from activation of a heterogeneous group of nociceptors which either express the neuropeptide substance P (SP) and calcitonin gene-related peptide (CGRP) or isolectin B_4 (IB_4) (3). Their sensory neurons terminate in the dorsal horn of the spinal cord, mainly in lamina I and II. These spinal cord regions also contain postsynaptic neurons that express pain-related receptors such as SP receptor, neurokinin-1 or protein kinase C-γ receptor, transient receptor potential channel, vanilloid subfamily member 1 (TRPV1), and its homolog TRPVL-1 (4). Several tissue nociceptors have been recently identified that can be activated by noxious heat (TRPV1 and TRPVL-1) (5) or mechanical stimuli (acid-sensing ion channels, ASICs) (6,7). Although IB_4 positive neurons can express several of these receptors, they are the only ones to display the purino-receptor P2X3 (8). This latter receptor is activated by purines like adenosine triphosphate (ATP), which are frequently released after tissue injury. Very little is known about the receptor expression of neurons that innervate different tissues of the body, but some tissues seem to contain special pain receptors. Much information has been obtained from animal models lacking specific pain receptors. Inbred mice without TRPV1 receptors show decreased response to noxious heat but normal mechanical nociception (9). Alternatively, mice without P2X3 receptors show no reduced nociceptive behavior. Because of the intricate interactions of many receptors involved in nociceptor excitation, neither genetic nor pharmacologic modification of a single receptor system has shown significant effects on pain perception.

NORMAL PAIN PROCESSING

Experimental pain stimuli can reliably evoke perceptions of pain when applied to somatic or intestinal tissues of human subjects (10–14). Pain that results from impulse conduction in peripheral C (unmyelinated) afferent axons increases in intensity when experimental pain stimuli are applied more often than once every 3 seconds (0.3 Hz). This progressive increase represents temporal summation (WU) and has been demonstrated to result from central rather than peripheral nervous system mechanisms. This form of sensitization is central, since in studies of this phenomenon the input from C nociceptors to WDR or NS neurons has been shown to decline or stay the same with stimulus repetition (10,11). Several ascending pain pathways, particularly the spinothalamic pathway, project from spinal neurons to brainstem and cortical regions (15). Although somatosensory input to the hypothalamus mostly ascends via an indirect, multisynaptic pathway, several other pathways connect the spinal cord dorsal horn directly to brainstem and limbic system areas. These pathways include a spinohypothalamic pathway (16) and a spinopontoamygdaloid pathway (17). In addition, individual spinal cord neurons often project in more than one of these pathways. Somatosensory nuclei of the thalamus [ventroposterior lateral nucleus (VPL) and ventroposterior inferior nucleus (VPI)] relay nociceptive information to somatosensory (S1 and S2) cortices (2,18). Importantly, however, all projections converge on the same limbic and subcortical structures that are directly accessed by ascending spinal pathways.

PAIN MODULATING SYSTEMS

Inhibition of pain is essential when safety is more important than attention to a source of pain. Yet pain represents an essential signal when something needs to be done about a damaged body area. Under the influence of cortico-reticular signals, the reticular formation of the brain stem is involved in either facilitation or inhibition of pain perception (19). At least five spinoreticular/reticulospinal loops on each side of the spinal cord are involved in pain processing that may be either inhibitory or facilitatory. They connect the spinal cord to the following areas of the brainstem.

ASCENDING PAIN MODULATING PATHWAYS

- the dorsolateral pontine tegmentum
- the rostral ventral medulla
- the dorsal medulla
- the caudal medulla
- the lateral hypothalamus

The effect of stimulating some of these centers can last from an hour to several days. In addition, several distinct pathways involved in pain processing descend from the brain to the spinal cord.

DESCENDING PAIN MODULATING PATHWAYS

These descending pathways originate from the brain or brainstem, specifically from the cerebral cortex and pass to the

- nucleus gracilis and cuneatus
- reticular formation
- thalamus
- periaqueductal gray matter

They can pass to the dorsal horn directly via the raphe nuclei of the medulla or via the locus ceruleus.

Pain can be down-regulated by an endogenous antinociceptive system that is activated by exercise, stress, and noxious stimuli (20). The neurons related to antinociception originate in the rostral ventromedial medulla (RVM) and the periaqueductal gray of the brain stem, including so-called "on" and "off" cells (20). Specific mechanisms that activate these neurons are only incompletely understood, but some of the neurotransmitters involved in antinociception include γ-aminobutyric acid, nitric oxide, adenosine, and met-enkephalin. The activity of spinal neurons is also modulated through afferent activity in descending antinociceptive spinal tracts (see above). Inhibition of this modulatory system may result in activation of otherwise silent intraspinal synapses, with a resultant expansion of receptive fields (21,22). Thus, decreased activation of the spinal descending inhibitory pathways can lead to simultaneous amplification of peripheral nociceptive afferent impulses and enlargement of receptive fields. At the spinal level, serotonin is the major neurotransmitter in this descending system.

PERIPHERAL SENSITIZATION

Peripheral sensitization is defined as a reduction in the threshold of nociceptive afferent receptors caused by a local change in the sensitivity of sensory fibers initiated by tissue damage (23). Peripheral sensitization almost always depends on local inflammation, which can lead to decreased nociceptor thresholds. Several mechanisms have been described that can account for peripheral sensitization. These include prostaglandins, kallidin, and bradykinin (BK), which are commonly released during tissue injury or inflammation. The activation of nociceptors by BK is mediated through the membrane-bound B_2 receptor, which is coupled to a G-protein. This G-protein in turn can activate phospholipase C and protein kinase C (PKC), which phosphorylate neuronal ion channels and thus modulate their excitability. Such B_2 receptor mediated activation of nociceptors has been described in skin, muscle, joints, and visceral organs (24–27). BK can also activate cyclooxygenase (COX), which transforms arachidonic acid to prostaglandins. Importantly, BK has been shown to sensitize sensory fibers to physical and chemical stimuli by synergistic interactions with other peripheral inflammatory mediators, such as prostaglandin E_2, I_2, serotonin, cytokines (IL-1, IL-6, TNF-α) (26,28) neuropeptides such as SP, neurokinin A, and calcitonin gene-related peptide (CGRP) (29) or through histamine release from mast cells (30). Conversely, the same chemical pain mediators can also sensitize nociceptors, which can then become activated by low concentrations of BK (31,32).

CENTRAL SENSITIZATION

Tissue sensitization after injury has long been recognized as an important contribution to pain, particularly after the pioneering studies of Lewis (33) and Hardy (34). These investigators distinguished two zones of increased pain sensitivity that include (a) the area of tissue injury (primary hyperalgesia) and (b) an area of uninjured tissue (secondary hyperalgesia) that is particularly sensitive to mechanical stimuli. Mechanical, electrical, and chemically induced painful sensations in these areas are signaled by nociceptive afferents, which encode the magnitude of the perceived pain by their discharge intensity (35). Primary hyperalgesia is related to changes of the properties of primary nociceptive afferents, whereas secondary hyperalgesia requires functional changes in the CNS (neuroplasticity). These changes are relevant for many forms of hyperalgesia that can present clinically as incident-related pain. Such CNS changes may result in central sensitization that manifests itself as (a) increased excitability of spinal cord neurons after an injury (36), (b) enlargement of these neurons' receptive fields, (c) reduction in pain threshold, and (d) recruitment of novel afferent inputs (37,38). Behaviorally, centrally sensitized patients report abnormal or heightened pain sensitivity with spreading of hypersensitivity to uninjured sites and the generation of pain by low threshold mechanoreceptors that are normally silent in pain processing (39). Thus, tissue injury may not only cause pain but also an expansion of dorsal horn receptive fields and central sensitization.

SPINAL MECHANISMS RELATED TO CENTRAL SENSITIZATION

Sensory input can originate from any body tissue, but activation of muscle nociceptors, in contrast to skin nociceptors, is substantially more powerful in causing central sensitization (40). The areas involved in spinal pain processing of pain are located in lamina I, II, V, VI, and X of the spinal cord. These regions are involved in pain processing and rostral transmission of nociceptive information (26–28,41). Within the spinal cord, excitatory as well as inhibitory neurons modulate nociceptive signals, resulting in both amplification as well as attenuation of pain signals. Several neurotransmitters, including glutamate, aspartate, vasoactive intestinal peptide (VIP), SP, cholecystokinin (CCK), and neurotensin, have been found to enhance neural transmission (42). Inhibitory dorsal horn interneurons that attenuate nociception often produce high concentrations of gamma-amino-butyric acid (GABA), an important inhibitor of nociceptive neurons

(43,44). In addition, cholinergic interneurons, acting via muscarinic and nicotinic receptors, also seem to play an important role in antinociception (20). After spinal cord processing, the nociceptive information is transmitted via projection neurons to supraspinal pain centers. Central sensitization, however, may not solely depend on neuronal mechanisms. As discussed below, activation of glial cells by cytokines, chemokines, or neurotransmitters may also contribute significantly to enhanced central pain mechanisms.

N-METHYL-D-ASPARTATE RECEPTOR SYSTEM

The amino acid glutamate is the main excitatory neurotransmitter in the human CNS. It can activate three types of ionotroptic receptors [α-amino-3-hydroxy-5-methyl-4-isoxazole propionate (AMPA), kainate, and N-methyl-D-aspartate (NMDA) receptors], all of which are important for pain signaling. NMDA receptors not only are abundant in the spinal cord but also are ubiquitously distributed throughout the brain. They are fundamental to excitatory neurotransmission and

critical for normal CNS function. The activation of NMDA receptors requires the presence of glutamate and glycine to open the ion channel and permit calcium entry into the cell. Under resting conditions, magnesium blocks the NMDA receptor's ion channel, but during depolarization this block is removed and calcium can enter the cell. NMDA receptors can trigger nociceptive signaling cascades, including calcium-dependent phosphorylation of PKC that results in immediate-early gene phosphorylation, activation of multiple genes, and long-term synaptic changes. Excessive activation of NMDA receptors, however, can lead to excitotoxicity (a mechanism relevant for various CNS disorders) (see Figure 5-1).

NMDA receptors are most commonly composed of one NR1 subunit in combination with one or more NR2 subunits (45) and, less commonly, one NR3 subunit (46). Not only are there four known NR2 subunits (A–D) but also several alternatively spliced NR1 variants that contribute to the diversity of the NMDA receptor system. In addition, there are important differences in NMDA subunit expression throughout the CNS. Whereas NR1 and NR2A are widely distributed in the CNS, NR2B appears to be restricted to the forebrain and NR2C to the cerebellum.

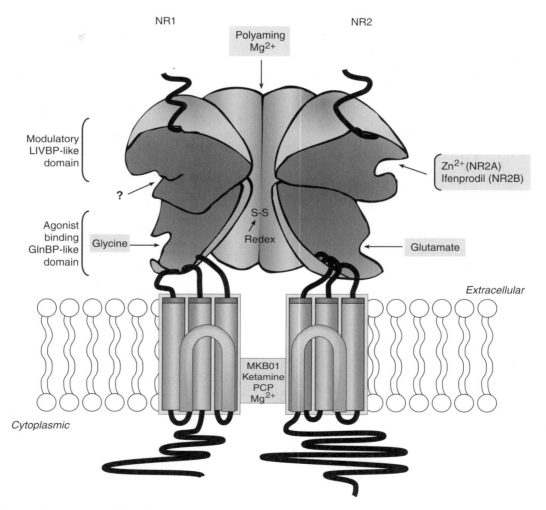

Figure 5-1. *N*-methyl-D-aspartate (NMDA) receptors most frequently consist of one NR1 and two NR2 subunits. The great variability of the NMDA receptor is attributable to the availability of four different NR2 subunits and several alternatively spliced NR1 variants. (From Kemp JA, McKernan RM. NMDA receptor pathways as drug targets. *Nat Neurosci* 2002;5:1039–1042, with permission.)

ROLE OF *N*-METHYL-D-ASPARTATE, NITRIC OXIDE, AND OPIOID RECEPTORS IN CENTRAL SENSITIZATION

NMDA and opioid receptor systems are considered central to nociception and antinociception. The relationship between these systems is not only functional but also spatial within multiple CNS regions (47). These receptor systems are found concentrated in presynaptic and postsynaptic sites of the dorsal horn (particularly lamina II), suggesting a close functional relationship (48). More recently, opioid and NMDA receptors have also been detected on peripheral processes of primary afferent neurons in animals (49–51) and in humans (52). These peripheral receptors show a strong similarity to those in the spinal cord and brain (53). Opioids can directly and indirectly modulate NMDA receptor activity (54–57) and affect the NMDA receptor mediated calcium influx into neurons similar to PKC (58,59), nitric oxide synthase (NOS), and phospholipase A$_2$ (60,61). NMDA receptor activation is also linked to nitric oxide (NO) production (62,63). Because NO is a gaseous molecule, it can diffuse into adjacent neurons and glia, resulting in their activation (64). It has a high affinity to guanyl cyclase, which may result in activation of Guanine-mono-phosphate (GMP) dependent protein kinase (PKG). This enzyme has been found to be involved in neurotransmitter release, learning, and memory (65). These receptor mechanisms have also been implicated in the maintenance of hyperalgesia in several animal models of persistent neuropathic pain (66). The neuropeptides SP and CGRP are both involved in pain signaling, which can lead not only to NMDA receptor but also to NOS activation (67,68). It has been hypothesized that NO release in lamina I and II after nociceptive activity can result in the release of SP and CGRP from C fibers, representing one mechanism of central sensitization (69), followed by spinal hyperexcitability, hyperalgesia, and allodynia. An important method to detect central sensitization is to measure temporal summation of second pain or WU (70) (see Figure 5-2).

Second pain is transmitted through unmyelinated C fibers to dorsal horn nociceptive neurons via synapses that use glutamate as a neurotransmitter. During volleys of C-fiber transmitted stimuli, NMDA receptors of second order neurons become activated, resulting in the removal of a magnesium block within the receptor (71–73). This event leads to calcium influx into the nerve cell and subsequent activation of protein kinase C, NOS, and COX. As a result, significantly increased firing rates of the nociceptive neurons can be observed, thus strongly amplifying peripheral input. WU can also be elicited in human subjects if identical nociceptive stimuli are applied to the skin or muscles more often than once every 3 seconds. This progressive increase represents WU and has been demonstrated to result from a central rather than a peripheral nervous system mechanism because the input from C nociceptors has been shown to decline or stay the same with stimulus repetition (10,74).

SUBSTANCE P, NERVE GROWTH FACTOR, AMINO ACIDS

Many studies have demonstrated the important role of excitatory amino acids, such as glutamate, and neuropeptides, such as SP, in the generation of chronic pain and central sensitization. SP is an important nociceptive neurotransmitter. It lowers the threshold of synaptic excitability, resulting in the unmasking of normally silent interspinal synapses and the sensitization of second order spinal neurons (75,76). Activation of NMDA receptors has a permissive effect on release of SP into the dorsal horn of the spinal cord (77). Furthermore, SP can extend long distances in the spinal cord and sensitize dorsal horn neurons at some distance from the initial input locus. This results in an expansion of receptive fields and the activation of wide-dynamic neurons by non-nociceptive afferent impulses. These alterations in the dorsal horn can result in increased internalization of SP receptors, increased expression of c-fos (a proto-oncogene induced by

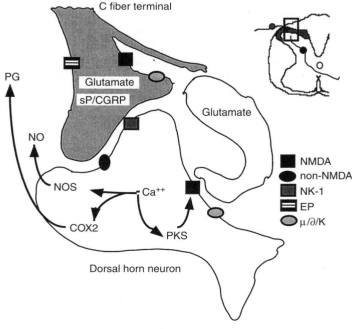

Figure 5-2. Processing of nociceptive information in the dorsal horn of the spinal cord. Primary afferent C-fibers release neuropeptides (e.g., substance P/CGRP, etc.) and glutamate. Peptides and excitatory amino acids result in excitation of second-order neurons—interneurons excited by afferent barrage induce excitation in second-order neuron via NMDA receptors, which lead to an increase in intracellular Ca^{2+}, activation of phospholipase A2, nitric oxide synthase (NOS), and phosphorylating enzymes. Prostaglandins and nitric oxide (NO) are formed and released. These agents diffuse extracellularly and facilitate transmitter release (retrograde transmission) from primary and nonprimary afferent terminals by either a direct cellular action (e.g., NO) or by an interaction with specific receptors. Phosphorylation of intracellular protein (e.g., enzymes and receptors such as NMDA) leads to additional enhanced sensitivity. [From Yaksh TL, Hua XY, Kalcheva I, et al. The spinal biology in humans and animals of pain states generated by persistent small afferent input. *PNAS* 1999;96(14):7680–7686, with permission.]

increased neuronal activity), and persistent structural changes (78). One study showed that activation of NMDA receptors in the spinal cord causes the release of SP and dramatic structural changes in the dendrites of neurons that display SP receptors (79). Increased production of SP within the spinal cord has been detected in the cerebrospinal fluid of pain patients (80). Several studies have shown a threefold increase of SP in the cerebrospinal fluid of patients with FMS in comparison with NC subjects (81,82). In addition, animal models of hyperalgesia have strongly supported the notion that SP is a major etiologic factor in central sensitization, thus highlighting the probable relevance of SP in human pain states (83). Finally, the increased levels of SP in the spinal fluid of patients with FMS may indicate a causal relationship with the observed central sensitization and therefore be relevant to the pathogenesis of FMS.

NERVE GROWTH FACTOR

Nerve growth factor (NGF) is expressed in nociceptive sensory C-fiber neurons and transported anterogradely to the dorsal horn of the spinal cord (84). Peripheral inflammation substantially up-regulates NGF in the dorsal root ganglion, resulting in increased sensitivity of the nociceptors (hyperalgesia). Both intradermal (85) and systemic application of NGF (86) have been found to result in pain reminiscent of FMS. The duration and severity of pain varied in a dose-dependent manner, and women appeared to be more susceptible than men. Increased concentrations of NGF in the spinal fluid of FMS patients have been described previously (87). Therefore, NGF may play an important role in FMS pain. NGF may also represent a promising therapeutic target for the treatment of FMS pain. In animal experiments the systemic administration of anti-NGF neutralizing antibodies prevented not only pain but also the up-regulation of neuropeptides and the inflammation-induced expression of the immediate-early gene c-fos in dorsal horn neurons (88).

CYTOKINES: ROLE OF ASTROCYTES AND MICROGLIA FOR CHRONIC PAIN

There has been recent recognition of neuroinflammation and neuroimmune activation in the pathogenesis of pain, particularly in patients with HIV, Alzheimer disease, Parkinson disease, spinal cord injury, and demyelinating diseases (89). Various events can result in a CNS immune response, including infections and trauma. Much of this response involves migration of cells to the site of injury, resulting in the activation of endothelial cells, microglia, and astrocytes. Activation of these cells can lead to subsequent production of cytokines, chemokines, and the expression of cell surface antigens (90). Because of neuroinflammatory activation following peripheral and central neurologic injury, similar events are conceivable in patients with FMS.

More than 70% of the cells in the brain and spinal cord are glial cells (microglia, astrocytes, and oligodendrocytes). Besides providing structural support for neurons, they have recently been found to play a key role in the neuromodulation and neuroimmunity of the CNS (91,92). Microglia are cells of monocytic origin that can function as antigen presenting cells

of the CNS. Although it is not yet well understood what signals lead to initial glial activation, the subsequent intracellular messengers include glutamate and calcium, leading to protein phosphorylation with subsequent nuclear factor-kappa B (NF-kB) activation and its downstream effects (93). NF-kB is an important transcription factor for many genes relevant for cell survival and functional integrity. Some of these genes control the synthesis of important mediators of inflammation and pain, including SP, COX, NOS, IL-6, IL-1β, and dynorphin. Cytokines and growth factors have been strongly implicated in the generation of chronic pain states at peripheral and central sites (94). It is well established that activated glial cells can also lead to the production of excitatory amino acids and subsequent eicosanoid secretion (95). Some of the most frequently used anti-inflammatory medications, like acetylsalicylic acid and glucocorticoids, inhibit NF-kB (96). Of possible future importance for the treatment of chronic pain is evidence of pain reduction in rodents with anti-inflammatory cytokines (97).

METHODS USED FOR PAIN TESTING

QUANTITATIVE SENSORY TESTING

Quantitative sensory or psychophysical testing is a well-established method for studying thermal, mechanical, electrical, and light touch sensitivity in human subjects (98,99). Different instruments permit measurement of pressure, warm, cold, and thermal pain thresholds, and the use of validated methods has enabled the application of controlled and quantifiable natural thermal or pressure stimuli to evoke specific threshold and suprathreshold sensations that are psychophysically measurable (see Figure 5-3).

Algometry

In 1949, Steinbrocker (100) provided the first documentation of utilizing a pressure gauge to measure palpation forces for the purposes of physical diagnosis. But it was not until 1954 that Keele coined the term "algometer" (101). Much of the early research on pressure pain testing was done by Andrew Fischer, who is generally recognized as the "father" of algometry (102). Algometers are sometimes referred to as dolorimeters, palpameters, algesiometers, or pressure threshold meters. They are designed to quantify and document levels of tenderness via pressure pain threshold measurement and pain sensitivity via pain tolerance measurements. Pressure threshold is defined as the minimum pressure (force) required for causing pain. The size of most algometers' footplates is 1 cm^2, and pressure is usually increased by 1 kg/sec during testing procedures. Pressure pain threshold measurements of FMS subjects and NC are typically performed over tender points (TePs) or areas of muscle tenderness (sometimes referred to as trigger points) (see below). Normal data for male and females have been determined for many muscles in which tender or trigger points are frequently found (102). Algometers are also frequently used for TeP determinations in FMS and are thus very useful for study purposes (103). It needs to be remembered, however, that TePs, as part of FMS, show little correlation with clinical pain intensity but are strongly associated

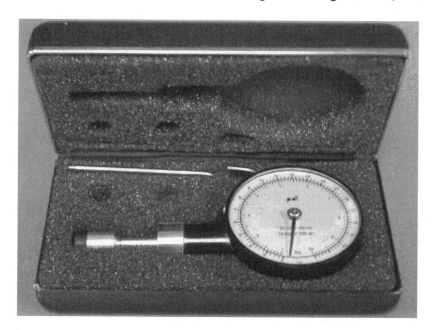

Figure 5-3. Mechanical pressure algometer used for pain threshold and tender point (TeP) testing. The size of the footplate is 1 cm².

with specific components of psychological distress, as well as characteristics of somatization (104).

Method of Limits

The simplest technique for measuring pain threshold is the method of limits. There are two forms of the method of limits: the ascending method of limits and the descending method of limits. To determine pain threshold using the method of limits, a subject is presented with a series of nociceptive (hot, cold, pressure, electric current) stimuli that change in intensity, and the subject is asked when he or she can or cannot perceive the stimulus.

Method of Constant Stimuli

The problem with the method of limits is that the descending method produces threshold values lower than the values obtained by the ascending method. This problem can be overcome with the method of "constant stimuli," which uses a train of nociceptive stimuli ranging from clearly perceivable and clearly not perceivable that is randomly presented to a study subject. Each time the stimulus is presented the subjects indicate whether or not they perceived the stimulus.

Staircase Method

This method represents a more efficient version of the "method of limits." Here the level of the stimulus is adjusted in steps until the observer either can or cannot feel the stimulus but does not start over with each trial.

NEURAL IMAGING OF PAIN

The most frequently used methods of measuring resting brain activity or the brain response to experimental stimuli

include positron-emission tomography (PET), single photon emission computed tomography (SPECT), and functional magnetic resonance imaging (fMRI). Brain activity after stimuli, as observed by PET and SPECT, is measured indirectly by measuring changes in regional cerebral blood flow (rCBF). fMRI detects brain activation in a different way. It provides images of pain-related alterations of neuronal activity by registering signal changes of blood deoxyhemoglobin concentration and blood volume (105).

Several clinical studies of brain imaging have shown that phasic noxious thermal stimuli result in increased rCBF of the contralateral thalamus, ACC, frontal cortex, and insula, as well as somatosensory cortices (SI and SII) (106–109).

Thalamic activation has been observed in acute pain states (110–112). In patients with chronic pain, however, measurement of rCBF showed a decrease of thalamic activity (106,113). A similarly decreased blood flow in the thalamus and caudate nuclei was also observed in FMS patients (114), sometimes only involving the right thalamus as well the inferior pontine tegmentum (115). These results strongly support the psychophysical data obtained in FMS patients, which indicate abnormalities of central pain processing. Several studies examined the pain experience and pain reporting to nociceptive mechanical stimuli in FMS patients compared to NC (116–118). fMRI of brain areas relevant to pain showed activation of the contralateral primary and secondary somatosensory cortex, ipsilateral cerebellum, contralateral insular cortex, basal ganglia, and superior temporal gyrus in all study subjects. Using identical stimuli, FMS patients showed more rCBF in all pain-related brain areas compared to NC (117). Although FMS patients required lower stimulus intensity to experience pain similar to NC, their patterns of brain activation were nearly identical to NC. These findings strongly support the role of cortical or subcortical amplification for the increased pain sensitivity in FMS.

NEUROPHYSIOLOGICAL ABNORMALITIES IN FIBROMYALGIA SYNDROME

FMS is a chronic pain syndrome characterized by generalized pain, TePs, disturbed sleep, and pronounced fatigue. Pain in FMS is consistently felt in the musculature and may be related to sensitization of CNS pain pathways. The pathogenesis of FMS is unknown, although abnormal concentration of CNS neuropeptides and alterations of the hypothalamic-pituitary-adrenal axis have been described (82,119–121). There is a large body of evidence for a generalized lowering of pressure pain thresholds in FMS patients (122–126). Importantly, mechanical allodynia of FMS patients is not limited to TePs, but appears to be widespread (126). In addition, almost all studies of FMS patients showed abnormalities of pain sensitivity while using different methods of psychophysical testing (see Table 5-1). Most investigations utilized thermal (heat and cold), mechanical, chemical, or electrical stimuli (single or repetitive) to the skin or muscles.

The noninvasive method of summation of second pain or WU can be used in FMS patients for evaluation of central sensitization (133). This technique reveals sensitivity to input from unmyelinated (C) afferents and the status of NMDA receptor systems that are implicated in a variety of chronic pain conditions. FMS patients showed excessive summation of second pain at a high rate of thermal stimulation [2s interstimulatory interval (ISI)] and abnormal WU at a slow rate (5s ISI) (see WU). Temporal summation depends on activation of NMDA transmitter systems by C nociceptors, and chronic central pain states can result from excessive temporal summation of pain (135,136).

TENDER POINTS

In 1990 the American College of Rheumatology identified 18 areas as TePs (103). In addition to chronic widespread pain, the presence of mechanical allodynia is required in at least 11 out of 18 TePs for the diagnosis of FMS. Abnormal tenderness, however, does not seem to be restricted to TeP sites in FMS,

but this abnormality is most frequently generalized (124,126). Most TePs are located at tendon insertion areas and have shown few detectable tissue abnormalities. Analysis of algesic substances at TeP sites by microdialysis showed no difference between FMS patients and NC (137), and magnetic resonance imaging of TePs was also unable to detect any specific abnormalities (138). Although there is evidence for local vasoconstriction of TeP areas in FMS (139), these findings may reflect physical deconditioning (140).

ROLE OF MUSCLES FOR CLINICAL PAIN IN FIBROMYALGIA SYNDROME

Since the predominant symptom in FMS is muscle pain and stiffness, many studies have focused on muscle tissue abnormalities in FMS (141,142). Light and electronmicroscopic evaluations identified moth-eaten and ragged-red fibers, indicating uneven and proliferating mitochondria. This finding suggests hypoperfusion of painful muscle tissues and has led to examinations of muscle microcirculation. Oxygen multipoint electrodes in trapezius muscles identified abnormal tissue oxygen pressures in FMS patients. Because microcirculation of muscle tissues is controlled by locally produced metabolites, humoral factors, and the sympathetic nervous system, several investigations focused on these possible mechanisms (141,143,144). Sympathetic ganglion blockade reversed the abnormal muscle findings. In addition, the amount of SP, a neurotransmitter stored within the afferent nociceptive fibers, was found to be increased in the trapezius muscles of FMS patients compared to NC (145).

Skeletal muscles have different fiber types, including type I, type IIA, and type IIB. Type I muscle fibers are associated with static muscle tone and posture. They are slow twitch, fatigue-resistant myocytes that contain a high number of mitochondria for oxidative phosphorylation. Type II fibers are fast twitch fibers and high contraction force over short periods. They fatigue easily, are rich in glycogen, and use anaerobic glycolysis for energy metabolism. Type I muscle fibers can transform into type II fibers depending on the demand placed on individual muscles. Therefore, inactivity and pain can be responsible in type II fiber loss/transformation.

TABLE 5-1	Psychophysical Studies of Patients with Fibromyalgia Syndrome (FMS)			
METHOD	**MODALITY**	**LOCALIZATION**	**YEAR**	**AUTHOR**
Electrical testing	Electrical	Upper limb	1993	(127)
Algometer	Mechanical	Hand	1994	(128)
Algometer	Mechanical	Muscle	1995	(126)
Heat testing	Thermal	Tender points	1994	(129)
Laser heat	Thermal	Hand	1996	(130)
Capsaicin	Chemical	Forearm	1998	(131)
Hypertonic saline	Chemical	Muscle	2000	(132)
Windup	Thermal	Skin	2001	(133)
Windup	Mechanical	Muscle	2003	(134)
Random staircase	Mechanical	Thumb	2003	(118)

Ionotropic and metabotropic pain receptors are found on peripheral unmyelinated sensory afferents in the skin and muscle (146). These polymodal muscle nociceptors are located along blood vessels, except capillaries (26), and comprise free nerve endings supplied by group III (thin myelinated) and group IV (nonmyelinated) afferents with conduction velocities of <30 m/s. The nerve endings have receptors for algesic substances like BK, serotonin, glutamate, and prostaglandin E2 (PGE-2) (147,148), which contribute to the sensitization of muscle nociceptors (149,150). This sensitization process by endogenous substances that are likely to be released during trauma or inflammatory injury is probably the best-established peripheral mechanism for muscle tenderness and hyperalgesia.

Although information on the receptor responses of muscle nociceptors is largely based on animal studies (151,152), similar findings have also been reported from human studies (153,154).

ABNORMAL MUSCLE HYPERSENSITIVITY IN FIBROMYALGIA SYNDROME

Powerful antinociceptive mechanisms become activated during muscle contraction in NC subjects (155). Specifically, during isometric muscle contraction of NC subjects, the mechanical pain threshold increases over the contracted muscles as well as over distal muscle areas (156). In FMS patients, however, the pain threshold decreased over all areas, more pronounced proximal to the muscle contraction compared to distal (157). This exercise-related hyperalgesia may be the result of either the sensitization of mechanoreceptors in FMS or the dysfunction of afferent pain inhibition activated by muscle contraction. These findings may explain some of the increased pain during exertion that is reported by FMS patients

MYOFASCIAL PAIN SYNDROME

Myofascial pain, or regional musculoskeletal pain, is one of the most common pain syndromes encountered in clinical practice. Myofascial pain represents the most common cause of chronic pain, including neck and shoulder pain, tension headaches, and lower back pain (158–161). Janet Travell introduced the term "myofascial pain" in the early 1950s. She also defined the term myofascial trigger point (TrP) and demonstrated with David Simons that individual muscles have specific nondermatomal patterns of TrP pain referral (162). In 1983 both authors first described the clinical picture and pathophysiology of a new syndrome that they named "myofascial pain syndrome" (MPS) (162,163).

MPS has been defined as a chronic pain syndrome accompanied by TrPs in one or more muscles or groups of muscles (164). Similar to FMS, it is found more frequently in women than in men. Besides the presence of TrPs and referred pain, MPS is frequently associated with limitation of movement, weakness, and autonomic dysfunction (163) similar to FMS.

TRIGGER POINTS

TrPs represent areas of local mechanical hyperalgesia that can be found in MPS and several chronic pain conditions, including FMS, osteoarthritis, and rheumatoid arthritis. They are defined as specific areas of hyperirritability in muscle, but they can also be detected in ligaments, tendons, periosteum, scar tissue, or skin (162,164). TrPs are located in palpable "taut bands" and produce local and referred pain, which is specific for the particular muscle. When TrPs are mechanically stimulated, so-called taut bands within a muscle, rather than the entire muscle, will contract (165). They are often associated with a local muscle "twitch response," which can easily be elicited by needling or palpation of the TrP (165,166). Latent TrPs are similar to active TrPs, but they are not associated with spontaneous pain and no referral of pain occurs. However, latent TrPs are painful when palpated.

RELATIONSHIP BETWEEN MYOFASCIAL PAIN AND FIBROMYALGIA SYNDROME

Approximately 70% of patients with FMS have TrPs (160). A TeP is considered to be different from a TrP because of the absence of referred pain, local twitch response, and a taut band in the muscle. The distinction between a TeP and a TrP requires careful physical examination. TrPs, however, are frequently located in areas of muscular TePs of patients with FMS (167,168), suggesting that some muscular TePs in patients with FMS may actually be TrPs (169).

The presence of TrPs in most, if not all, FMS patients represents strong evidence for local muscle abnormalities in this chronic musculoskeletal pain syndrome. Although it is unclear if TrPs are the cause or effect of muscle injury, they represent abnormally contracted muscle fibers. This muscle contraction can lead to accumulation of histamine, serotonin, tachykinins, and prostaglandins, which may result in the activation of local nociceptors. Prolonged muscle contractions may also result in local hypoxemia and energy depletion (162).

LACK OF EVIDENCE FOR PRIMARY HYPERALGESIA IN FIBROMYALGIA SYNDROME

Despite extensive investigation, no consistent inflammatory or other abnormal soft tissue changes have been detected in FMS patients (170). Nevertheless, several interesting new findings may be suggestive of peripheral sensitization in FMS patients. They include increased amounts of SP that have been detected in nerve fibers of FMS muscle tissue (145). SP is an important neurotransmitter of pain and usually not detectable in peripheral nerves. Therefore, this finding may indicate involvement of the afferent nervous system and may become relevant for the explanation of chronic FMS pain. It may also provide new and exciting avenues for research to see whether FMS pain may benefit from decreased peripheral nociceptive input and peripheral sensitization.

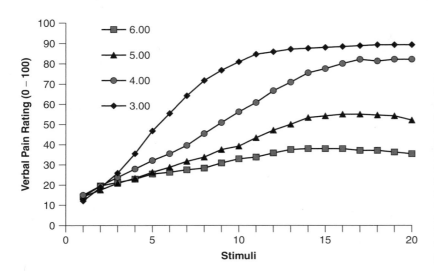

Figure 5-4. Windup (WU) of second pain in NC subjects. Twenty repetitive heat stimuli (52°C) were applied to the hand. Contact time was 0.7s; interstimulatory intervals (ISI) varied between 3s and 6s. Pain intensity of test stimuli was rated on a verbal rating scale from 0–100 (0 = no pain; 20 = min pain; 100 = unbearable pain). Only repetitive stimuli at short ISIs (3s) resulted in a significant increase of pain ratings, compared to long ISIs, which produced minimal pain sensations. (From Vierck CJ, Cannon RL, Fry G Jr, et al. Characteristics of temporal summation of second pain sensations elicited by brief contact of glabrous skin by a preheated thermode. *J Neurophysiol* 1997;78: 992–1002, with permission.)

PAIN AMPLIFICATION IN FIBROMYALGIA SYNDROME

TEMPORAL SUMMATION OF SECOND PAIN OR WINDUP

In 1965, Mendell and Wall reported for the first time that repetitive C-fiber stimulation can result in a progressive increase of electrical discharges from second order neurons in the spinal cord (171) (see Figure 5-4). This important mechanism of pain amplification in the dorsal horn neurons of the spinal cord is related to temporal summation of second pain or WU. First pain, which is conducted by myelinated A-δ pain fibers, is often described as sharp or lancinating, and most subjects can readily distinguish it from second pain. In contrast,

second pain (transmitted by unmyelinated C fibers), which is strongly related to chronic pain states, is most frequently reported as dull, aching, or burning (10,13,74,172,173). Second pain increases in intensity when painful stimuli are applied more often than once every 3 seconds. This progressive increase represents temporal summation (WU) and has been demonstrated to result from central rather than peripheral nervous system mechanisms, mostly because the input from C nociceptors has been shown to decline or stay the same with stimulus repetition (10,74). Animal studies have demonstrated similar WU of C afferent-mediated responses of dorsal horn nociceptive neurons, and this summation has been found to involve *N*-methyl-D-aspartate (NMDA) receptor mechanisms (71–73). Importantly, WU and second pain can be inhibited by application of NMDA receptor antagonists, including dextromethorphan (174) and ketamine (175) (see Figure 5-5).

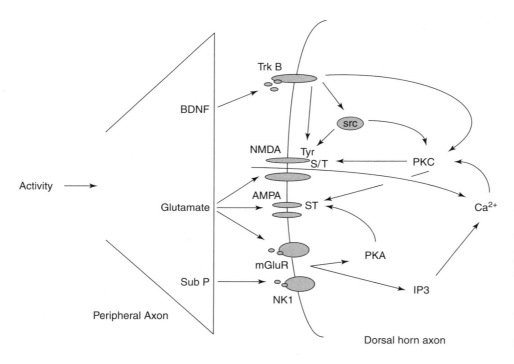

Figure 5-5. Posttranslational changes within dorsal horn neurons after release of transmitters from C-fiber central terminals. These transmitters/neuromodulators act on receptors and ion channels in the dorsal horn to activate protein kinases that phosphorylate membrane-bound *N*-methyl-D-aspartate (NMDA) and α-amino-3-hydroxy-5-methyl-4-isoxazole propionate (AMPA) receptors and alter their functional properties, increasing membrane excitability and thereby eliciting central sensitization. [From Woolf CJ, Costigan M. Transcriptional and posttranslational plasticity and the generation of inflammatory pain. *PNAS* 1999;96(14):7723–7730, with permission.]

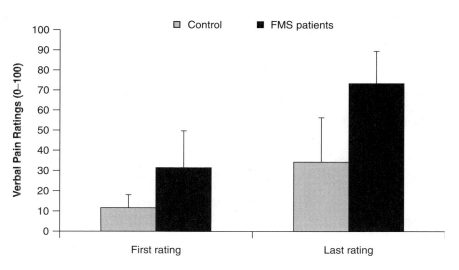

Figure 5-6. Windup (WU) of second pain in ten female fibromyalgia syndrome (FMS) patients and NCs, using 52°C repetitive heat stimuli to the hand. Contact time of each stimulus was 0.7s and ISI was 2s. Shown is only the rating of the first and last stimulus ($N = 20$) of each series. Pain intensity of test stimuli was rated on a verbal rating scale from 0–100 (same as in Figure 5-5). [From Staud R, Vierck CJ, Cannon RL, et al. Abnormal sensitization and temporal summation of second pain (wind-up) in patients with fibromyalgia syndrome. *Pain* 2001;91:165–175, with permission.]

ABNORMAL WINDUP OF FIBROMYALGIA SYNDROME PATIENTS

Abnormal WU and central sensitization may be relevant for FMS pain because this chronic pain syndrome is often associated with extensive secondary hyperalgesia and allodynia (176). Several recent studies have obtained psychophysical evidence that input to central nociceptive pathways is abnormally processed in patients with FMS (133,177–181).

Temporal summation of second pain was assessed, using a series of repetitive heat stimuli. Although WU pain was evoked in both NC and FMS patients, the perceived magnitude of the sensory response to the first stimulus within a series was greater for FMS patients compared to controls, as was the amount of temporal summation within a series (see Figure 5-6). Following the last stimulus in a series, after-sensations were greater in magnitude, lasted longer, and were more frequently painful in FMS subjects. These results indicate both augmentation and prolonged decay of nociceptive input in FMS patients and provide convincing evidence for the presence of central sensitization.

WINDUP MEASURES AS PREDICTORS OF CLINICAL PAIN INTENSITY IN FIBROMYALGIA SYNDROME PATIENTS

The important role of central pain mechanisms for clinical pain is also supported by their usefulness as predictors of pain intensity of FMS patients. Thermal WU ratings correlate well with clinical pain intensity (Pearson's r = 0.529), thus emphasizing the important role of these pain mechanisms for FMS. In addition, a statistical prediction model that includes TeP count, pain-related negative affect, and WU ratings has been shown to account for 50% of the variance in FMS clinical pain intensity (182) (see Figure 5-7).

EFFECT OF EXERCISE ON FIBROMYALGIA SYNDROME PAIN

Exercise has been shown to activate endogenous opioid and adrenergic systems, but attenuation of experimental pain has

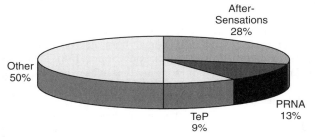

Figure 5-7. Predictors of clinical pain intensity of FMS patients. A statistical model consisting of WU after-sensations, pain-related negative affect (PRNA), and tender point (TeP) count, Accounts for 50% of FMS patients' variance in clinical pain intensity. (From Staud R, Robinson ME, Vierck CJ Jr, et al. Ratings of experimental pain and pain-related negative affect predict clinical pain in patients with fibromyalgia syndrome. *Pain* 2003;105:215–222, with permission.)

not been demonstrated consistently. In one study antinociceptive effects of exercise were assessed using a method of psychophysical testing that is especially sensitive to opioid modulation (179). Using a preheated thermode to the glabrous skin of the hand in a series of brief contacts, the perceived intensity of late thermal sensations increased following each successive contact. This temporal summation or WU depends upon input from unmyelinated (C) fiber afferents and provides information regarding the status of central NMDA receptor systems associated with pain. Using this method with a group of normal subjects, strenuous exercise substantially attenuated temporal summation of late pain sensations. In individuals diagnosed with FMS, however, second pain ratings increased significantly after exercise, an effect opposite to that obtained from age/sex matched control subjects (see Figure 5-8).

DIFFUSE NOXIOUS INHIBITORY CONTROLS IN FIBROMYALGIA SYNDROME

Diffuse noxious inhibitory controls (DNIC) is part of a central pain modulatory system that relies on spinal and supraspinal mechanisms (183,184). The activity of pain-signaling neurons in the spinal dorsal horn and in trigeminal nuclei can be inhibited

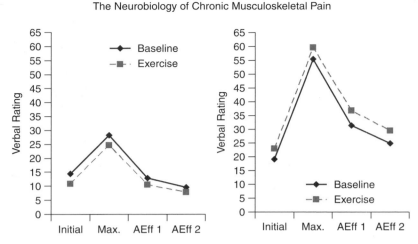

The Neurobiology of Chronic Musculoskeletal Pain

Figure 5-8. Ratings of late sensation magnitude in baseline testing sessions and 10 minutes after strenuous exercise, averaged across all series presented to control subjects (left panel) and fibromyalgia syndrome (FMS) subjects (right panel). Average ratings are shown for the initial stimulus in each series, the maximal sensation magnitude during series of contacts (max), and after-sensations at 15s (AEff1) and 120s (AEff2) following completion of the last series. Statistical tests revealing significant differences in exercise effects for control and FMS subjects utilized data from series presented at each ISI (not shown) and included all measures. [From Vierck CJ, Staud R, Price DD Jr, et al. The effect of maximal exercise on temporal summation of second pain (wind-up) in patients with fibromyalgia syndrome. *J Pain* 2001;2:334–344, with permission.]

by noxious stimuli applied to body areas far remote from the excitatory fields of these neurons (185–187). Down-regulation of pain threshold and pain can be demonstrated in NC during strong noxious stimulation (conditioning stimulus), thus effectively inhibiting dorsal horn neurons (including wide-dynamic neurons) to nociceptive input (188). This effect is known as DNIC. It appears that wide dynamic-range (WDR) neurons with nonnoxious and noxious input are especially sensitive to this inhibitory effect (185,189). Some controversy exists whether this antinociceptive mechanism is abnormal in FMS. Several investigators used tonic nociceptive stimuli in FMS patients and NC (190,191). The results indicated that the FMS patients showed significantly lower heat pain thresholds than did the NC. Thus conditioning tonic stimuli significantly increased the pain threshold in the NC but not in the FMS patients.

Several recent studies of FMS patients, however, did not confirm abnormal DNIC mechanisms in this chronic pain syndrome (192,193). It is well known that DNIC has a greater effect on second pain than on first pain. Therefore WU of second pain should be attenuated by a strong conditioning stimulus.

DNIC requires a strong conditioning stimulus for pain attenuation, which may be at least partly dependent on a distraction effect (194). To separately assess the contributions of distraction-related mechanisms to inhibition of second pain, the experiment was designed in such a way that directed the subjects' attention to either the test or conditioning stimulus. Noxious heat to the right hand was used as a test stimulus to generate WU of second pain. Immersion of the left hand into a hot water bath was the conditioning stimulus. However, when DNIC's effect on WU was compared in three groups of subjects, including NC males, NC females, and FMS female subjects (193), it significantly inhibited thermal WU pain in normal male subjects. Adding distraction to the DNIC effect did not increase the extent of this inhibition. In contrast, neither DNIC nor DNIC plus distraction attenuated thermal WU pain in NC females. DNIC plus distraction but not DNIC alone produced significant inhibition of thermal WU pain in female FMS patients. Theses results indicate that DNIC effects on experimental WU of second pain are gender specific, with women generally lacking this pain inhibitory mechanism (see Figures 5-9, 5-10).

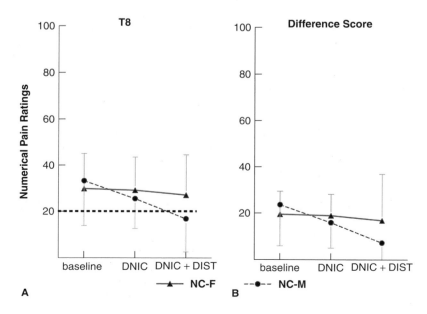

Figure 5-9. **A:** Windup (WU) ratings after the 8th tap (±SD) of NC-F and NC-M subjects at baseline, during DNIC and DNIC + DIST (plus distraction) conditions. The dashed line indicates pain threshold. **B:** Difference score (DS) (maximal windup minus baseline 1st tap ratings) of NC-F and NC-M during the same test conditions. Whereas pain ratings of NC-F remained unchanged during all conditions, NC-M subjects showed a significant reduction of windup (*p* = .042) during the conditioning stimulus. Ratings of DNIC + DIST were also statistically different from baseline, but not different from DNIC alone for NC-M subjects (*p* = .022). [From Staud R, Robinson ME, Vierck CJ, et al. Diffuse noxious inhibitory controls (DNIC) attenuate temporal summation of second pain in normal males but not in normal females or fibromyalgia patients. *Pain* 2003;101:167–174, with permission.]

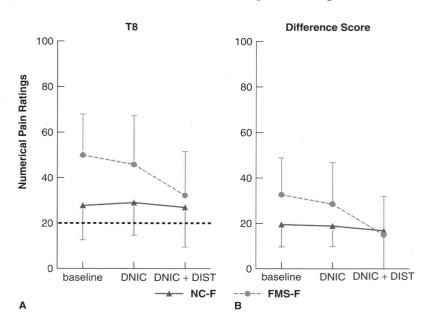

Figure 5-10. **A:** Windup (WU) ratings after the 8th tap (±SD) of NC-F and FMS-F patients at baseline, during DNIC and DNIC+DIST conditions. The dashed line indicates pain threshold. **B:** Difference score (DS) (maximal windup minus baseline 1st tap ratings) of NC-F and FMS-F during the same test conditions. Neither DNIC nor DNIC + DIST had an effect on windup in NC-F subjects. Although DNIC also had no effect on test stimuli in FMS-F patients, DNIC + DIST significantly reduced mean ratings of windup sensations in FMS-F patients [p = .043 (193)]. [From Staud R, Robinson ME, Vierck CJ, et al. Diffuse noxious inhibitory controls (DNIC) attenuate temporal summation of second pain in normal males but not in normal females or fibromyalgia patients. *Pain* 2003;101:167–174, with permission.]

GENETICS OF PAIN PROCESSING IN FIBROMYALGIA SYNDROME

Some preclinical and clinical studies suggest that individual responsiveness to painful stimuli is determined by genotype (193,195–197). Animal studies using 11 different mouse strains (198,199) showed significant influence of genotype on the response to painful stimulation. Consequently, the great variability in pain responses may be due to multiple factors, including quantitative differences in the representation of adapting and nonadapting nociceptors, inherited variation in numerous neurotransmitter systems (200), or other gene products, expressed in sensory neurons (201).

It has been suggested that the abnormally low plasma and CSF levels of serotonin of FMS patients may play an important role in the pathophysiology of this chronic pain disorder (202). Therefore the silent T102C polymorphism of the 5-HT2A-receptor gene was investigated in 168 FMS patients and 115 healthy controls (203). The results showed a significantly different genotype distribution in FMS patients with a decrease in T/T and an increase in both T/C and C/C genotypes as compared to the NC population (p = 0.008). A second study of this T102C polymorphism of the serotonin receptor gene, however, was unable to replicate these findings in FMS patients (204).

Interactions between multiple brain areas and neurochemical systems regulate responses to pain and other stressors. Catechol-O-methyltransferase (COMT) is a ubiquitous enzyme that inactivates catecholamines and catecholamine-containing drugs. Recent research on humans has focused on the influence of a common functional genetic polymorphism of the COMT gene that affects the metabolism of catecholamines, thus modulating subjects' responses to sustained pain (205). Individuals homozygous for the met^{158} allele of the COMT polymorphism ($val^{158}met$) showed diminished CNS μ-opioid responses to experimental pain stimuli compared to heterozygotes. In addition, homozygous individuals demonstrated higher sensory and affective pain ratings and more negative mood ratings. Opposite effects were observed in val^{158} homozygous patients. Thus the COMT $val^{158}met$ polymorphism may influence the human pain experience and may explain some of the interindividual differences in the adaptation and responses to pain and other stressful stimuli.

Importantly, the occurrence of COMT gene polymorphisms was also assessed in FMS patients (206). Three polymorphisms of the COMT gene could be detected in this population, including LL, LH, and HH. Although no significant differences were found between LL and LH separately, the LL and LH genotypes together were more frequently detected in FMS patients than in controls (p = 0.024). In addition, HH genotypes were significantly less often found in FMS patients than in NC (p = 0.04). Overall, these findings seem to indicate that genetic variants, including COMT polymorphism, may play an important role in chronic pain syndromes like FMS.

SUMMARY POINTS

- FMS patients show little evidence of peripheral tissue abnormalities and demonstrate convincing evidence of abnormal central pain processing, including central sensitization and WU.
- The precise cause for pain processing abnormalities in FMS is unknown, and future studies will be necessary to evaluate the role of genetic and environmental effects on these mechanisms.

■ IMPLICATIONS FOR PRACTICE

- When central sensitization has occurred in chronic pain patients, as has been noted in FMS, very little additional nociceptive input is required to maintain the sensitized state. Therefore, seemingly innocuous daily activities may contribute to the maintenance of chronic pain states.

- In addition, the decay of sensitization is very prolonged in FMS, and patients cannot expect drastic changes of their pain levels within short time intervals. Many analgesic medications do not seem to improve central sensitization, and some agents, like opioids, have been shown to maintain or even worsen this important central pain mechanism.
- Pharmacologic interventions that target glial activation hold great promise as future treatment options of central sensitization.

REFERENCES

1. Merskey H, Bogduk N. *Classification of chronic pain: description of chronic pain syndromes and definition of pain terms*, 2nd ed. Seattle, WA: IASP Press, 1994.
2. Price DD. *Psychological mechanisms of pain and analgesia: progress in pain research and management*, 15th ed. Seattle, WA: IASP Press, 1999.
3. Kitchener PD, Wilson P, Snow PJ. Selective labeling of primary sensory afferent terminals in lamina II of the dorsal horn by injection of Bandeiraea simplicifolia isolectin B4 into peripheral nerves. *Neuroscience* 1993;54:545–551.
4. Stucky CL, Gold MS, Zhang X. Mechanisms of pain. *Proc Natl Acad Sci* 2001;98:11845–11846.
5. Caterina MJ, Julius D. The vanilloid receptor: a molecular gateway to the pain pathway. *Annu Rev Neurosci* 2001;24:487–517.
6. Gunthorpe MJ, Smith GD, Davis JB, et al. Characterisation of a human acid-sensing ion channel (hASIC1a) endogenously expressed in HEK293 cells. *Pflugers Arch* 2001;442:668–674.
7. Krishtal O. The ASICs: signaling molecules? Modulators? *Trends Neurosci* 2003;26:477–483.
8. Burnstock G. P2 purinoceptors: historical perspective and classification. *Ciba Found Symp* 1996;198:1–28.
9. Caterina MJ, Leffler A, Malmberg AB, et al. Impaired nociception and pain sensation in mice lacking the capsaicin receptor. *Science* 2000;288:306–313.
10. Price DD. Characteristics of second pain and flexion reflexes indicative of prolonged central summation. *Exp Neurol* 1972;37:371–387.
11. Price DD, Dubner R. Mechanisms of first and second pain in the peripheral and central nervous systems. *J Invest Dermatol* 1977;69:167–171.
12. Yeomans DC, Proudfit HK. Nociceptive responses to high and low rates of noxious cutaneous heating are mediated by different nociceptors in the rat: electrophysiological evidence. *Pain* 1996;68:141–150.
13. Vierck CJ, Cannon RL, Fry G Jr, et al. Characteristics of temporal summation of second pain sensations elicited by brief contact of glabrous skin by a preheated thermode. *J Neurophysiol* 1997;78:992–1002.
14. Verne GN, Robinson ME, Price DD. Hypersensitivity to visceral and cutaneous pain in the irritable bowel syndrome. *Pain* 2001;93:7–14.
15. Price DD, Verne GN. Brain mechanisms of persistent pain states. *J Musculoskelet Pain* 2002;10:73–83.
16. Burstein R, Cliffer KD, Giesler GJ Jr. Direct somatosensory projections from the spinal cord to the hypothalamus and telencephalon. *J Neurosci* 1987;7:4159–4164.
17. Bernard JF, Besson JM. The spino(trigemino)pontoamygdaloid pathway: electrophysiological evidence for an involvement in pain processes. *J Neurophysiol* 1990;63:473–490.
18. Craig AD. *Forebrain areas involved in pain processing.* Paris: Eurotext, 1995:1325.
19. Millan MJ. Descending control of pain. *Prog Neurobiol* 2002;66:355–474.
20. Fields HL, Basbaum AI. Central nervous system mechanisms of pain modulation. In: Wall PD, Melzack R, eds. *Textbook of pain*, 4th ed. Edinburgh: Churchill Livingstone, 1999:309–329.
21. Hoheisel U, Mense S. Response behaviour of cat dorsal horn neurones receiving input from skeletal muscle and other deep somatic tissues. *J Physiol (London)* 1990;426:265–280.
22. Yu XM, Mense S. Response properties and descending control of rat dorsal horn neurons with deep receptive fields. *Neuroscience* 1990;39:823–831.
23. Treede RD, Meyer RA, Raja SN, et al. Peripheral and central mechanisms of cutaneous hyperalgesia. *Prog Neurobiol* 1992;38:397–421.
24. Fock S, Mense S. Excitatory effects of 5-hydroxytryptamine, histamine and potassium ions on muscular group IV afferent units: a comparison with bradykinin. *Brain Res* 1976;105:459–469.
25. Griesbacher T, Lembeck F. Effect of bradykinin antagonists on bradykinin-induced plasma extravasation, venoconstriction, prostaglandin E2 release, nociceptor stimulation and contraction of the iris sphincter muscle in the rabbit. *Br J Pharmacol* 1987;92:333–340.
26. Mense S. Nociception from skeletal muscle in relation to clinical muscle pain. *Pain* 1993;54:241–289.
27. Mense S. Nociceptors in skeletal muscle and their reaction to pathological tissue changes. In: Belmonte C, Cervero F, eds. *Neurobiology of nociceptors.* Oxford: Oxford University Press, 1996:184–201.
28. Schaible HG, Grubb BD. Afferent and spinal mechanisms of joint pain. *Pain* 1993;55:5–54.
29. Barber LA, Vasko MR. Activation of protein kinase C augments peptide release from rat sensory neurons. *J Neurochem* 1996;67:72–80.
30. Khasar SG, Ouseph AK, Chou B, et al. Is there more than one prostaglandin E receptor subtype mediating hyperalgesia in the rat hindpaw? *Neuroscience* 1995;64:1161–1165.
31. Abbott FV, Hong Y, Blier P. Persisting sensitization of the behavioural response to formalin-induced injury in the rat through activation of serotonin2A receptors. *Neuroscience* 1997;77:575–584.
32. Sann H, Pierau FK. Efferent functions of C-fiber nociceptors. *Z Rheumatol* 1998;57(Suppl. 2):8–13.
33. Lewis T. Experiments relating to cutaneous hyperalgesia and its spread through somatic fibres. *Clin Sci (Colch)* 1935;2:373–423.
34. Hardy JD, Wolff HG, Goodell H. Experimental evidence on the nature of cutaneous hyperalgesia. *J Clin Invest* 1950;29:115–140.
35. Koltzenburg M. Neural mechanisms of cutaneous nociceptive pain. *Clin J Pain* 2000;16:S131–S138.
36. Woolf CJ. Evidence for a central component of post-injury pain hypersensitivity. *Nature* 1983;306:686–688.
37. Cook AJ, Woolf CJ, Wall PD, et al. Dynamic receptive field plasticity in rat spinal cord dorsal horn following C-primary afferent input. *Nature* 1987;325:151–153.
38. Li J, Simone DA, Larson AA. Windup leads to characteristics of central sensitization. *Pain* 1999;79:75–82.
39. Torebjork HE, Lundberg LE, LaMotte RH. Central changes in processing of mechanoreceptive input in capsaicin-induced secondary hyperalgesia in humans. *J Physiol* 1992;448:765–780.
40. Wall PD, Woolf CJ. Muscle but not cutaneous C-afferent input produces prolonged increases in the excitability of the flexion reflex in the rat. *J Physiol Lond* 1984;356:443–458.

41. Schaible HG, Schmidt RF. Neurobiology of articular nociceptors. In: Belmonte C, Cervero. F, eds. *Neurobiology of nociceptors*. Oxford: Oxford University Press, 1996:202–219.

42. Coggeshall RE, Carlton SM. Receptor localization in the mammalian dorsal horn and primary afferent neurons. *Brain Res Rev* 1997;24:28–66.

43. Malcangio M, Bowery NG. GABA and its receptors in the spinal cord. *Trends Pharmacol Sci* 1996;17:457–462.

44. Schadrack J, Zieglgansberger W. Pharmacology of pain processing systems. *Z Rheumatol* 1998;57(Suppl. 2):1–4.

45. McBain CJ, Mayer ML. N-methyl-D-aspartic acid receptor structure and function. *Physiol Rev* 1994;74:723–760.

46. Chatterton JE, Awobuluyi M, Premkumar LS, et al. Excitatory glycine receptors containing the NR3 family of NMDA receptor subunits. *Nature* 2002;415:793–798.

47. Mao JR. NMDA and opioid receptors: their interactions in antinociception, tolerance and neuroplasticity. *Brain Res Rev* 1999;30:289–304.

48. Gracy KN, Svingos AL, Pickel VM. Dual ultrastructural localization of mu-opioid receptors and NMDA-type glutamate receptors in the shell of the rat nucleus accumbens. *J Neurosci* 1997;17:4839–4848.

49. Davidson EM, Coggeshall RE, Carlton SM. Peripheral NMDA and non-NMDA glutamate receptors contribute to nociceptive behaviors in the rat formalin test. *NeuroReport* 1997;8:941–946.

50. Coggeshall RE, Zhou S, Carlton SM. Opioid receptors on peripheral sensory axons. *Brain Res* 1997;764:126–132.

51. Kolesnikov Y, Pasternak GW. Topical opioids in mice: analgesia and reversal of tolerance by a topical N-methyl-D-aspartate antagonist. *J Pharmacol Exp Ther* 1999;290:247–252.

52. Stein C, Machelska H, Binder W, et al. Peripheral opioid analgesia. *Curr Opin Pharmacol* 2001;1:62–65.

53. Hassan AH, Ableitner A, Stein C, et al. Inflammation of the rat paw enhances axonal transport of opioid receptors in the sciatic nerve and increases their density in the inflamed tissue. *Neuroscience* 1993;55:185–195.

54. Chapman V, Haley JE, Dickenson AH. Electrophysiologic analysis of preemptive effects of spinal opioids on N-methyl-D-aspartate receptor-mediated events. *Anesthesiology* 1994; 81:1429–1435.

55. Sivilotti LG, Gerber G, Rawat B, et al. Morphine selectively depresses the slowest, NMDA-independent component of C-fibre-evoked synaptic activity in the rat spinal cord in vitro. *Eur J Neurosci* 1995;7:12–18.

56. Vaughan CW, Christie MJ. Presynaptic inhibitory action of opioids on synaptic transmission in the rat periaqueductal grey in vitro. *J Physiol* 1997;498(Pt 2):463–472.

57. Zhang KM, Wang XM, Mokha SS. Opioids modulate N-methyl-D-aspartic acid (NMDA)-evoked responses of neurons in the superficial and deeper dorsal horn of the medulla (trigeminal nucleus caudalis). *Brain Res* 1996;719: 229–233.

58. Basbaum AI. Spinal mechanisms of acute and persistent pain. *Reg Anesth Pain Med* 1999;24:59–67.

59. Mao J, Price DD, Mayer DJ. Mechanisms of hyperalgesia and morphine tolerance: a current view of their possible interactions. *Pain* 1995;62:259–274.

60. Coyle JT, Puttfarcken P. Oxidative stress, glutamate, and neurodegenerative disorders. *Science* 1993;262:689–695.

61. Bliss TV, Collingridge GL. A synaptic model of memory: long-term potentiation in the hippocampus. *Nature* 1993; 361:31–39.

62. Bredt DS, Snyder SH. Nitric oxide mediates glutamate-linked enhancement of cGMP levels in the cerebellum. *Proc Natl Acad Sci* 1989;86:9030–9033.

63. Brenman JE, Bredt DS. Synaptic signaling by nitric oxide. *Curr Opin Neurobiol* 1997;7:374–378.

64. Schuman EM, Madison DV. Nitric oxide and synaptic function. *Annu Rev Neurosci* 1994;17:153–183.

65. Wang X, Robinson PJ. Cyclic GMP-dependent protein kinase and cellular signaling in the nervous system. *J Neurochem* 1997;68:443–456.

66. Meller ST, Gebhart GF. Nitric oxide (NO) and nociceptive processing in the spinal cord. *Pain* 1993;52:127–136.

67. McMahon SB, Lewin GR, Wall PD. Central hyperexcitability triggered by noxious inputs. *Curr Opin Neurobiol* 1993;3: 602–610.

68. Radhakrishnan V, Yashpal K, Hui-Chan CW, et al. Implication of a nitric oxide synthase mechanism in the action of substance P: L-NAME blocks thermal hyperalgesia induced by endogenous and exogenous substance P in the rat. *Eur J Neurosci* 1995;7:1920–1925.

69. Aimar P, Pasti L, Carmignoto G, et al. Nitric oxide-producing islet cells modulate the release of sensory neuropeptides in the rat substantia gelatinosa. *J Neurosci* 1998;18:10375–10388.

70. Urban L, Thompson SW, Dray A. Modulation of spinal excitability: co-operation between neurokinin and excitatory amino acid neurotransmitters. *Trends Neurosci* 1994;17: 432–438.

71. Davies SN, Lodge D. Evidence for involvement of N-methyl-aspartate receptors in 'wind-up' of class 2 neurones in the dorsal horn of the rat. *Brain Res* 1987;424:402–406.

72. Dickenson AH, Sullivan AF. Evidence for a role of the NMDA receptor in the frequency dependent potentiation of deep rat dorsal horn nociceptive neurones following C fibre stimulation. *Neuropharmacology* 1987;26:1235–1238.

73. Dickenson AH. A cure for wind up: NMDA receptor antagonists as potential analgesics. *Trends Pharmacol Sci* 1990;11: 307–309.

74. Price DD, Hu JW, Dubner R, et al. Peripheral suppression of first pain and central summation of second pain evoked by noxious heat pulses. *Pain* 1977;3:57–68.

75. Liu H, Brown JL, Jasmin L, et al. Synaptic relationship between substance P and the substance P receptor: light and electron microscopic characterization of the mismatch between neuropeptides and their receptors. *Proc Natl Acad Sci* 1994;91: 1009–1013.

76. Liu H, Wang H, Sheng M, et al. Evidence for presynaptic N-methyl-D-aspartate autoreceptors in the spinal cord dorsal horn. *Proc Natl Acad Sci* 1994;91:8383–8387.

77. Liu H, Mantyh PW, Basbaum AI. NMDA-receptor regulation of substance P release from primary afferent nociceptors. *Nature* 1997;386:721–724.

78. Curran T, Morgan JI. Fos: an immediate-early transcription factor in neurons. *J Neurobiol* 1995;26:403–412.

79. Coderre TJ, Katz J, Vaccarino AL, et al. Contribution of central neuroplasticity to pathological pain: review of clinical and experimental evidence. *Pain* 1993;52:259–285.

80. Tsigos C, Diemel LT, White A, et al. Cerebrospinal fluid levels of substance P and calcitonin-gene-related peptide: correlation with sural nerve levels and neuropathic signs in sensory diabetic polyneuropathy. *Clin Sci (Colch)* 1993;84: 305–311.

81. Vaeroy H, Helle R, Forre O, et al. Elevated CSF levels of substance P and high incidence of Raynaud phenomenon in patients with fibromyalgia: new features for diagnosis. *Pain* 1988;32:21–26.

82. Russell IJ, Orr MD, Littman B, et al. Elevated cerebrospinal fluid levels of substance P in patients with the fibromyalgia syndrome. *Arthritis Rheum* 1994;37:1593–1601.

83. Watkins LR, Wiertelak EP, Furness LE, et al. Illness-induced hyperalgesia is mediated by spinal neuropeptides and excitatory amino acids. *Brain Res* 1994;664:17–24.

84. Mannion RJ, Costigan M, Decosterd I, et al. Neurotrophins: peripherally and centrally acting modulators of

tactile stimulus-induced inflammatory pain hypersensitivity. *Proc Natl Acad Sci* 1999;96:9385–9390.

85. Dyck PJ, Peroutka S, Rask C, et al. Intradermal recombinant human nerve growth factor induces pressure allodynia and lowered heat-pain threshold in humans. *Neurology* 1997;48: 501–505.

86. Petty BG, Cornblath DR, Adornato BT, et al. The effect of systemically administered recombinant human nerve growth factor in healthy human subjects. *Ann Neurol* 1994;36: 244–246.

87. Giovengo SL, Russell IJ, Larson AA. Increased concentrations of nerve growth factor in cerebrospinal fluid of patients with fibromyalgia. *J Rheumatol* 1999;26:1564–1569.

88. Woolf CJ, Safieh-Garabedian B, Ma QP, et al. Nerve growth factor contributes to the generation of inflammatory sensory hypersensitivity. *Neuroscience* 1994;62:327–331.

89. Ruffolo RR, Feuerstein GZ, Hunter AJ, et al. *Inflammatory cells and mediators in CNS diseases.* Amsterdam: Harwood Academic Press, 1999.

90. Watkins LR, Maier SF. *Cytokines and pain: progress in inflammation research.* Boston, MA: Birkhauser, 1999.

91. Kreutzberg GW. Microglia: a sensor for pathological events in the CNS. *Trends Neurosci* 1996;19:312–318.

92. Raivich G, Bluethmann H, Kreutzberg GW. Signaling molecules and neuroglial activation in the injured central nervous system. *Keio J Med* 1996;45:239–247.

93. Wooten MW. Function for NF-kB in neuronal survival: regulation by atypical protein kinase C. *J Neurosci Res* 1999;58: 607–611.

94. Woolf CJ, Allchorne A, Safieh-Garabedian B, et al. Cytokines, nerve growth factor and inflammatory hyperalgesia: the contribution of tumour necrosis factor alpha. *Br J Pharmacol* 1997; 121:417–424.

95. Wood PL. *Neuroinflammation: mechanism and management.* Totowa, NJ: Humana Press, 2000.

96. Crinelli R, Antonelli A, Bianchi M, et al. Selective inhibition of NF-kB activation and TNF-alpha production in macrophages by red blood cell-mediated delivery of dexamethasone. *Blood Cells Mol Dis* 2000;26:211–222.

97. Johansson A, Bennett GJ. Effect of local methylprednisolone on pain in a nerve injury model. A pilot study. *Reg Anesth* 1997;22:59–65.

98. Kosek E, Ekholm J, Hansson P. Sensory dysfunction in fibromyalgia patients with implications for pathogenic mechanisms. *Pain* 1996;68:375–383.

99. Sheps DS, McMahon RP, Light KC, et al. Low hot pain threshold predicts shorter time to exercise-induced angina: results from the psychophysiological investigations of myocardial ischemia (PIMI) study. *J Am Coll Cardiol* 1999;33:1855–1862.

100. Steinbrocker O. Simple pressure gauge for measured palpation in physical diagnosis and therapy. *Arch Phys Med* 1949;30:389–390.

101. Keele KD. Pain-sensitivity tests; the pressure algometer. *Lancet* 1954;1:636–639.

102. Fischer AA. Pressure algometry over normal muscles. Standard values, validity and reproducibility of pressure threshold. *Pain* 1987;30:115–126.

103. Wolfe F, Smythe HA, Yunus MB, et al. The American College of Rheumatology 1990 criteria for the classification of fibromyalgia. Report of the Multicenter Criteria Committee. *Arthritis Rheum* 1990;33:160–172.

104. McBeth J, Macfarlane GJ, Benjamin S, et al. The association between tender points, psychological distress, and adverse childhood experiences: a community-based study. *Arthritis Rheum* 1999;42:1397–1404.

105. Binder JR, Swanson SJ, Hammeke TA, et al. Determination of language dominance using functional MRI: a comparison with the Wada test. *Neurology* 1996;46:978–984.

106. Hui KKS, Liu J, Makris N, et al. Acupuncture modulates the limbic system and subcortical gray structures of the human brain: evidence from fMRI studies in normal subjects. *Hum Brain Mapp* 2000;9:13–25.

107. Coghill RC, Talbot JD, Evans AC, et al. Distributed processing of pain and vibration by the human brain. *J Neurosci* 1994;14:4095–4108.

108. Coghill RC, Sang CN, Berman KF, et al. Global cerebral blood flow decreases during pain. *J Cereb Blood Flow Metab* 1998;18:141–147.

109. Coghill RC, Gilron I, Iadarola MJ. Hemispheric lateralization of somatosensory processing. *J Neurophysiol* 2001;85: 2602–2612.

110. Xu X, Fukuyama H, Yazawa S, et al. Functional localization of pain perception in the human brain studied by PET. *NeuroReport* 1997;8:555–559.

111. Jones AK, Brown WD, Friston KJ, et al. Cortical and subcortical localization of response to pain in man using positron emission tomography. *Proc R Soc London B Biol Sci* 1991;244:39–44.

112. Sakiyama Y, Sato A, Senda M, et al. Positron emission tomography reveals changes in global and regional cerebral blood flow during noxious stimulation of normal and inflamed elbow joints in anesthetized cats. *Exp Brain Res* 1998;118:439–446.

113. Hsieh JC, Belfrage M, Stone-Elander S, et al. Central representation of chronic ongoing neuropathic pain studied by positron emission tomography. *Pain* 1995;63:225–236.

114. Mountz JM, Bradley LA, Modell JG, et al. Fibromyalgia in women. Abnormalities of regional cerebral blood flow in the thalamus and the caudate nucleus are associated with low pain threshold levels. *Arthritis Rheum* 1995;38:926–938.

115. Kwiatek R, Barnden L, Tedman R, et al. Regional cerebral blood flow in fibromyalgia: single-photon-emission computed tomography evidence of reduction in the pontine tegmentum and thalami. *Arthritis Rheum* 2000;43:2823–2833.

116. Petzke F, Clauw DJ, Wolf JM, et al. Pressure pain in fibromyalgia and healthy control: functional MRI of subjective pain experience versus objective stimulus intensity. *Arthritis Rheum* 2000;43:S400.

117. Gracely RH, Petzke F, Wolf JM, et al. Functional magnetic resonance imaging evidence of augmented pain processing in fibromyalgia. *Arthritis Rheum* 2002;46:1333–1343.

118. Petzke F, Clauw DJ, Ambrose K, et al. Increased pain sensitivity in fibromyalgia: effects of stimulus type and mode of presentation. *Pain* 2003;105:403–413.

119. Bradley LA, Alarcon GS, Sotolongo A, et al. Cerebrospinal fluid (CSF) levels of substance P (SP) are abnormal in patients with fibromyalgia (FM) regardless of traumatic or insidious pain onset. *Arthritis Rheum* 1998;41:S256.

120. Vaeroy H, Helle R, Forre O, et al. Elevated CSF levels of substance P and high incidence of Raynaud phenomenon in patients with fibromyalgia: new features for diagnosis. *Pain* 1988;32:21–26.

121. Neeck G, Crofford LJ. Neuroendocrine perturbations in fibromyalgia and chronic fatigue syndrome. *Rheum Dis Clin North Am* 2000;26:989–1002.

122. Lautenschlager J, Bruckle W, Schnorrenberger CC, et al. Measuring pressure pain of tendons and muscles in healthy probands and patients with generalized tendomyopathy (fibromyalgia syndrome). *Z Rheumatol* 1988;47:397–404.

123. Quimby LG, Block SR, Gratwick GM. Fibromyalgia: generalized pain intolerance and manifold symptom reporting. *J Rheumatol* 1988;15:1264–1270.

124. Tunks E, Crook J, Norman G, et al. Tender points in fibromyalgia. *Pain* 1988;34:11–19.

125. Mikkelsson M, Latikka P, Kautiainen H, et al. Muscle and bone pressure pain threshold and pain tolerance in fibromyalgia

patients and controls. *Arch Phys Med Rehabil* 1992;73: 814–818.

126. Kosek E, Ekholm J, Hansson P. Increased pressure pain sensibility in fibromyalgia patients is located deep to the skin but not restricted to muscle tissue. *Pain* 1995;63:335–339.

127. Arroyo JF, Cohen ML. Abnormal responses to electrocutaneous stimulation in fibromyalgia. *J Rheumatol* 1993;20:1925–1931.

128. Gibson SJ, Littlejohn GO, Gorman MM, et al. Altered heat pain thresholds and cerebral event-related potentials following painful CO_2 laser stimulation in subjects with fibromyalgia syndrome. *Pain* 1994;58:185–193.

129. Lautenbacher S, Rollman GB, McCain GA. Multi-method assessment of experimental and clinical pain in patients with fibromyalgia. *Pain* 1994;59:45–53.

130. Lorenz J, Grasedyck K, Bromm B. Middle and long latency somatosensory evoked potentials after painful laser stimulation in patients with fibromyalgia syndrome. *Electroencephalogr Clin Neurophysiol* 1996;100:165–168.

131. Morris V, Cruwys S, Kidd B. Increased capsaicin-induced secondary hyperalgesia as a marker of abnormal sensory activity in patients with fibromyalgia. *Neurosci Lett* 1998; 250:205–207.

132. Graven-Nielsen T, Aspegren-Kendall S, Henriksson KG, et al. Ketamine reduces muscle pain, temporal summation, and referred pain in fibromyalgia patients. *Pain* 2000;85:483–491.

133. Staud R, Vierck CJ, Cannon RL, et al. Abnormal sensitization and temporal summation of second pain (wind-up) in patients with fibromyalgia syndrome. *Pain* 2001;91:165–175.

134. Staud R, Cannon RC, Mauderli AP, et al. Temporal summation of pain from mechanical stimulation of muscle tissue in normal controls and subjects with fibromyalgia syndrome. *Pain* 2003;102:87–95.

135. Dickenson AH, Sullivan AF. NMDA receptors and central hyperalgesic states. *Pain* 1991;46:344–346.

136. Price DD, Mao J, Mayer DJ. Central neural mechanisms of normal and abnormal pain states. In: Fields HL, Liebeskind JC, eds. *Pharmacological approaches to the treatment of pain: new concepts and critical issues*. Seattle, WA: IASP Press, 1994:61–84.

137. Ashina M, Stallknecht B, Bendtsen L, et al. Tender points are not sites of ongoing inflammation—in vivo evidence in patients with chronic tension-type headache. *Cephalalgia* 2003;23:109–116.

138. Kravis MM, Munk PL, McCain GA, et al. MR imaging of muscle and tender points in fibromyalgia. *J Magn Reson Imaging* 1993;3:669–670.

139. Jeschonneck M, Grohmann G, Hein G, et al. Abnormal microcirculation and temperature in skin above tender points in patients with fibromyalgia. *Rheumatology* 2000;39:917–921.

140. Simms RW. Is there muscle pathology in fibromyalgia syndrome? *Rheum Dis Clin North Am* 1996;22:245–266.

141. Yunus MB, Kalyan-Raman UP. Muscle biopsy findings in primary fibromyalgia and other forms of nonarticular rheumatism. *Rheum Dis Clin North Am* 1989;15:115–134.

142. Bengtsson A. The muscle in fibromyalgia. *Rheumatology* 2002;41:721–724.

143. Kalyan-Raman UP, Kalyan-Raman K, Yunus MB, et al. Muscle pathology in primary fibromyalgia syndrome: a light microscopic, histochemical and ultrastructural study. *J Rheumatol* 1984;11:808–813.

144. Yunus MB, Kalyan-Raman UP, Masi AT, et al. Electron microscopic studies of muscle biopsy in primary fibromyalgia syndrome: a controlled and blinded study. *J Rheumatol* 1989;16:97–101.

145. De Stefano R, Selvi E, Villanova M, et al. Image analysis quantification of substance P immunoreactivity in the trapezius muscle of patients with fibromyalgia and myofascial pain syndrome. *J Rheumatol* 2000;27:2906–2910.

146. Cairns BE, Hu JW, Arendt-Nielsen L, et al. Sex-related differences in human pain and rat afferent discharge evoked by injection of glutamate into the masseter muscle. *J Neurophysiol* 2001;86:782–791.

147. Graven-Nielsen T, Mense S. The peripheral apparatus of muscle pain: evidence from animal and human studies. *Clin J Pain* 2001;17:2–10.

148. Svensson P, Cairns BE, Wang KL, et al. Glutamate-evoked pain and mechanical allodynia in the human masseter muscle. *Pain* 2003;101:221–227.

149. Marchettini P, Simone DA, Caputi G, et al. Pain from excitation of identified muscle nociceptors in humans. *Brain Res* 1996;740:109–116.

150. Simone DA, Marchettini P, Caputi G, et al. Identification of muscle afferents subserving sensation of deep pain in humans. *J Neurophysiol* 1994;72:883–889.

151. Kumazawa T, Mizumura K. The polymodal C-fiber receptor in the muscle of the dog. *Brain Res* 1976;101:589–593.

152. Mense S. Muscular nociceptors. *J Physiol (Paris)* 1977;73: 233–240.

153. Graven-Nielsen T, Mense S. The peripheral apparatus of muscle pain: evidence from animal and human studies. *Clin J Pain* 2001;17:2–10.

154. Sorensen J, Graven-Nielsen T, Henriksson KG, et al. Hyperexcitability in fibromyalgia. *J Rheumatol* 1998;25:152–155.

155. Mense S, Simons DG, Russell IJ. *Muscle pain: understanding its nature, diagnosis, and treatment*, Philadelphia, PA: Lippincott Williams & Wilkins, 2000.

156. Kosek E, Ekholm J. Modulation of pressure pain thresholds during and following isometric contraction. *Pain* 1995;61: 481–486.

157. Kosek E, Ekholm J, Hansson P. Modulation of pressure pain thresholds during and following isometric contraction in patients with fibromyalgia and in healthy controls. *Pain* 1996;64:415–423.

158. Borg-Stein J, Simons DG. Myofascial pain. *Arch Phys Med Rehabil* 2002;83:S40–S47.

159. Fricton JR. Myofascial pain. *Clin Rheumatol* 1994;8: 857–880.

160. Granges G, Littlejohn G. Prevalence of myofascial pain syndrome in fibromyalgia syndrome and regional pain syndrome: a comparative study. *J Musculoskelet Pain* 1993;1: 19–35.

161. Macfarlane GJ, Thomas E, Papageorgiou AC, et al. The natural history of chronic pain in the community: a better prognosis than in the clinic? *J Rheumatol* 1996;23: 1617–1620.

162. Travell JG, Simons LS, Simons DG. *Myofascial pain and dysfunction: the trigger point manual*, 2nd ed. New York: Lippincott, Williams & Wilkins, 1999.

163. Long SP, Kephart W. Myofascial pain syndrome. In: Ashburn MA, Rice LJ, eds. *The management of pain*. Philadelphia, PA: Churchill Livingstone, 1998:299–321.

164. Han SC, Harrison P. Myofascial pain syndrome and triggerpoint management. *Reg Anesth* 1997;22:89–101.

165. Chu J. Twitch response in myofascial trigger points. *J Musculoskelet Pain* 1998;6:99–116.

166. Chu J. Twitch-obtaining intramuscular stimulation: observations in the management of radiculopathic chronic low back pain. *J Musculoskelet Pain* 1999;7:131–146.

167. Wolfe F, Simons DG, Fricton JR, et al. The fibromyalgia and myofascial pain syndromes: a preliminary study of tender points and trigger points in persons with fibromyalgia, myofascial pain syndrome and no disease. *J Rheumatol* 1992; 19:944–951.

168. Borg-Stein J, Stein J. Trigger points and tender points: one and the same? Does injection treatment help? *Rheum Dis Clin North Am* 1996;22:305–322.

169. Inanici F, Yunus MB, Aldag JC. Clinical features and psychologic factors in regional soft tissue pain: comparison with fibromyalgia syndrome. *J Musculoskelet Pain* 1999;7:293–301.

170. Simms RW, Roy SH, Hrovat M, et al. Lack of association between fibromyalgia syndrome and abnormalities in muscle energy metabolism. *Arthritis Rheum* 1994;37:794–800.

171. Mendell LM, Wall PD. Responses of single dorsal cord cells to peripheral cutaneous unmyelinated fibres. *Nature* 1965; 206:97–99.

172. Price DD. *Psychologicial and neural mechanisms of pain.* New York: Raven Press, 1988.

173. Yeomans DC, Cooper BY, Vierck CJ Jr. Effects of systemic morphine on responses of primates to first or second pain sensations. *Pain* 1996;66:253–263.

174. Price DD, Mao J, Frenk H, et al. The N-methyl-D-aspartate receptor antagonist dextromethorphan selectively reduces temporal summation of second pain in man. *Pain* 1994;59: 165–174.

175. Arendt-Nielsen L, Petersen-Felix S, Fischer M, et al. The effect of N-methyl-D-aspartate antagonist (ketamine) on single and repeated nociceptive stimuli: a placebo-controlled experimental human study. *Anesth Analg* 1995;81:63–68.

176. Woolf CJ, Costigan M. Transcriptional and posttranslational plasticity and the generation of inflammatory pain. *Proc Natl Acad Sci* 1999;96:7723–7730.

177. Staud R, Domingo M. Evidence for abnormal pain processing in fibromyalgia syndrome. *Pain Med* 2001;2:208–215.

178. Staud R, Domingo M. New Insights into the pathogenesis of fibromyalgia syndrome. *Med Aspects Hum Sex* 2001;1: 51–57.

179. Vierck CJ, Staud R, Price DD Jr, et al. The effect of maximal exercise on temporal summation of second pain (wind-up) in patients with fibromyalgia syndrome. *J Pain* 2001;2:334–344.

180. Staud R. The evidence for involvement of central neural mechanisms in generating fibromyalgia pain. *Curr Rheumatol Rep* 2002;4:299–305.

181. Price DD, Staud R, Robinson ME, et al. Enhanced temporal summation of second pain and its central modulation in fibromyalgia patients. *Pain* 2002;99:49–59.

182. Staud R, Robinson ME, Vierck CJ Jr, et al. Ratings of experimental pain and pain-related negative affect predict clinical pain in patients with fibromyalgia syndrome. *Pain* 2003;105: 215–222.

183. Le Bars D, Villanueva L, Bouhassira D, et al. Diffuse noxious inhibitory controls (DNIC) in animals and in man. *Patol Fiziol Eksp Ter* 1992;4:55–65.

184. Bouhassira D, Bing Z, Le Bars D. Studies of brain structures involved in diffuse noxious inhibitory controls in the rat: the rostral ventromedial medulla. *J Physiol* 1993;463:667–687.

185. Le Bars D, Dickenson AH, Besson JM. Diffuse noxious inhibitory controls (DNIC). II. Lack of effect on non-convergent neurones, supraspinal involvement and theoretical implications. *Pain* 1979;6:305–327.

186. Dickenson AH, Le Bar D. Diffuse noxious inhibitory controls (DNIC) involve trigeminothalamic and spinothalamic neurones in the rat. *Exp Brain Res* 1983;49:174–180.

187. Morton CR, Du HJ, Xiao HM, et al. Inhibition of nociceptive responses of lumbar dorsal horn neurones by remote noxious afferent stimulation in the cat. *Pain* 1988;34:75–83.

188. Wall PD, Cronly-Dillon JR. Pain, itch, and vibration. *Arch Neurol* 1960;2:365–375.

189. Le Bars D, Dickenson AH, Besson JM. Diffuse noxious inhibitory controls (DNIC). I. Effects on dorsal horn convergent neurones in the rat. *Pain* 1979;6:283–304.

190. Lautenbacher S, Rollman GB. Possible deficiencies of pain modulation in fibromyalgia. *Clin J Pain* 1997;13:189–196.

191. Kosek E, Hansson P. Modulatory influence on somatosensory perception from vibration and heterotopic noxious conditioning stimulation (HNCS) in fibromyalgia patients and healthy subjects. *Pain* 1997;70:41–51.

192. Desmeules JA, Cedraschi C, Rapiti E, et al. Neurophysiologic evidence for a central sensitization in patients with fibromyalgia. *Arthritis Rheum* 2003;48:1420–1429.

193. Staud R, Robinson ME, Vierck CJ, et al. Diffuse noxious inhibitory controls (DNIC) attenuate temporal summation of second pain in normal males but not in normal females or fibromyalgia patients. *Pain* 2003;101:167–174.

194. Price DD, McHaffie JG. Effects of heterotopic conditioning stimuli on first and second pain: a psychophysical evaluation in humans. *Pain* 1988;34:245–252.

195. Lester N, Lefebvre JC, Keefe FJ. Pain in young adults: I. Relationship to gender and family pain history. *Clin J Pain* 1994;10:282–289.

196. Bachiocco V, Scesi M, Morselli AM, et al. Individual pain history and familial pain tolerance models: relationships to post-surgical pain. *Clin J Pain* 1993;9:266–271.

197. Honkasalo ML, Kaprio J, Winter T, et al. Migraine and concomitant symptoms among 8167 adult twin pairs. *Headache* 1995;35:70–78.

198. Mogil JS, Wilson SG, Bon K, et al. Heritability of nociception I: responses of 11 inbred mouse strains on 12 measures of nociception. *Pain* 1999;80:67–82.

199. Mogil JS, Wilson SG, Bon K, et al. Heritability of nociception II. 'Types' of nociception revealed by genetic correlation analysis. *Pain* 1999;80:83–93.

200. Fields HL, Heinricher MM, Mason P. Neurotransmitters in nociceptive modulatory circuits. *Annu Rev Neurosci* 1991; 14:219–245.

201. Akopian AN, Abson NC, Wood JN. Molecular genetic approaches to nociceptor development and function. *Trends Neurosci* 1996;19:240–246.

202. Russell IJ, Michalek JE, Vipraio GA, et al. Platelet 3H-imipramine uptake receptor density and serum serotonin levels in patients with fibromyalgia/fibrositis syndrome. *J Rheumatol* 1992;19:104–109.

203. Bondy B, Spaeth M, Offenbacher M, et al. The T102C polymorphism of the 5-HT2A-receptor gene in fibromyalgia. *Neurobiol Dis* 1999;6:433–439.

204. Gursoy S, Erdal E, Herken H, et al. Association of T102C polymorphism of the 5-HT2A receptor gene with pyschiatric status in fibromyalgia syndrome. *Rheumatol Int* 2001;21: 58–61.

205. Zubieta JK, Heitzeg MM, Smith YR, et al. COMT val158met genotype affects (micro)-opioid neurotransmitter responses to a pain stressor. *Science* 2003;299:1240–1243.

206. Gursoy S, Erdal E, Herken H, et al. Significance of catechol-O-methyltransferase gene polymorphism in fibromyalgia syndrome. *Rheumatol Int* 2003;23:104–107.

6

Neurotransmitters, Cytokines, Hormones, and the Immune System in Chronic Nonneuropathic Pain

I. Jon Russell

The purpose of this chapter is to present some of the evidence in support of a neurochemical, neuroendocrine, and immune cytokine-mediated pathogenesis for the fibromyalgia syndrome (FMS) as one of several clinically important, chronic, central soft tissue pain (STP) conditions. Before doing so, a background must be laid for the taxonomy of STP among other painful disorders, for the relationship of neuropathology to FMS, and for the criteria that any theory or model of FMS pathogenesis should satisfy before it can be considered acceptable.

CLASSIFICATION

For the practicing clinician and for the investigator working in the field, it is useful to have at ready disposal a working classification of the condition under study that helps to distinguish it from similar conditions and from other members of its own lineage. For that purpose a contemporary outline of the relevant disorders was developed more than 10 years ago (1) and was updated more recently (2). As shown in Table 6-1, FMS is one of several STP conditions, but it is not a form of arthritis, as is often misstated. The STP syndromes differ from arthritic disorders in that the synovial joints are not necessarily involved. On the other hand, an STP condition or syndrome can accompany an arthritic condition and can cause confusion about which condition is the cause of current symptoms. The anatomic structures that appear to be symptomatic in STP syndromes can include ligaments, tendons, fascia, bursae, muscles, and nerves. The anatomic structure can be directly affected by some active process or can be indirectly involved by virtue of referred pain. These soft tissue structures are known to

facilitate mechanical functions of the diarthrodial joints. Movements of the extremities that involve the joints can be painful even if the joints are functioning normally. This observation helps to explain the confusion about the nature of the two classifications relating to arthritic disorders and disorders of STP. Any of the typically involved STP structures can become painful and dysfunctional alone or in association with distinct inflammatory, autoimmune, arthritic, or endocrine disorders. The physical dysfunction and compromise in quality of life that results from STP syndromes can be as severe as arthritic diseases, so these STP syndromes are not benign.

The main subheadings shown in Table 6-1 divide the syndromes into localized, regionalized, and generalized categories.

Most of the "localized" conditions are believed to result from repetitive mechanical injury to inadequately conditioned tissues. They are often named anatomically and are disclosed by a typical history plus the exquisite tenderness elicited by digital palpation of the affected structures. Examples include biceps tendinitis, subacromial bursitis, and enthesopathies.

The "regionalized" syndromes can also result from "overuse" and may involve more than one type of body structure, but they are still limited in anatomic scope to a region or body quadrant. For example, the term myofascial pain syndrome (MPS) encompasses a family of conditions characterized by "trigger points" (TrPs, contrasted with the tender points, TePs, of FMS) in skeletal muscles and has traditionally been managed by physiatrists and neurologists. The masticatory myofascial pain dysfunction syndromes (MPDSs) comprise another family of conditions of the head and neck that can involve a dysfunctional temporomandibular joint and/or MPS TrPs in the muscles of mastication, so dental specialists typically treat these conditions. Several types of visceral pain can be referred to a single musculoskeletal

TABLE 6-1	A Contemporary Classification of Soft Tissue Pain Disorders

Localized
- Bursitis (subacromial, olecranon, trochanteric, prepatellar, anserine)
- Tenosynovitis (biceps, supraspinatus, infrapatellar, Achilles)
- Enthesopathies (39 total, lateral epicondylitis, medial epicondylitis)
- Entrapment syndrome (carpal tunnel, tarsal tunnel, cubital tunnel)

Regionalized
- Myofascial pain syndrome (MPS, e.g., piriformis, iliopsoas, trapezius)
- Masticatory myofascial pain syndrome (TMJ, MPS muscles of mastication)
- Referred pain (angina or subphrenic abscess to shoulder, hip to thigh)
- Complex regional pain syndrome
    Type 1—no objective neural injury (replaces reflex sympathetic dystropy)
    Type 2—objective neural injury (replaces causalgia)

Generalized
- Polymyalgia rheumatica
- Hypermobility syndrome
- Fibromyalgia syndrome
- Chronic fatigue syndrome (when widespread pain is present)

From Russell IJ. A new journal. *J Musculoskelet Pain* 1993;1(1):1–7; Russell IJ. Fibromyalgia. In: Loeser JD, ed. *Bonica's management of pain.* New York: Williams & Wilkins, 2000:543–559, with permissions.

structure or to a region of the body (e.g., angina felt in the shoulder or jaw). The recently renamed complex regional pain syndromes (CRPS Type 1 and Type 2, formerly reflex sympathetic dystrophy and causalgia, respectively) would be classified in this category as well.

The purpose of this discussion about classification in a chapter on neurochemicals is to state that the "generalized" category of STP implies a systemic process that affects the musculoskeletal system globally. That fact should say something about the pathogenesis of these disorders, which is different from what we would assume when considering localized or regionalized conditions.

People with FMS report chronic widespread pain. They are characterized by symmetrical pain and low pain thresholds to palpation pressure-induced tenderness at many of the same anatomic sites that can become symptomatic with some of the localized pain syndromes (3). The chronic fatigue syndrome (CFS) was originally characterized by persistent idiopathic fatigue and a number of other constitutional symptoms. It initially presented in epidemics, but more recently that diagnosis has been applied to sporadic cases as well. In a proportion of CFS patients, a widespread pain comorbidity resembles that of FMS. Adding to the confusion, the current criteria for CFS no longer exclude FMS as a concomitant diagnosis (4). The apparent overlap between FMS and CFS has led to speculation that they are identical, but there are important historical and clinical differences that support the hypothesis that they are really separate family members within the category of generalized STP syndromes. Full discussions of the criteria for the

classification and diagnosis of FMS and the clinical features of this disorder are the topics of other chapters in this book. The same applies to MPS, CRPS, and CFS.

SUBGROUPS OF FIBROMYALGIA SYNDROME

It has become increasingly relevant to discussions of FMS pathogenesis to consider the possibility that FMS is not homogeneous. Rather, FMS seems to be composed of a number of related conditions that are all identified clinically by the same research classification criteria (3). It is as if a few distinct initiating factors, working in fertile environments, have initiated processes that eventually follow the same (or a similar) final common pathway to produce the clinical features now recognized as FMS. Figure 6-1 shows a hypothetical model of a sequence of events that begins with one or more predisposing factors acted upon at some point by an event or agent to initiate a sequence of events that involve chemical changes in the central nervous system (CNS). The neurochemical abnormalities understandably lead to clinical manifestations that result in a very compromised individual with chronic clinical and emotional findings.

Differences in the initiating pathogenesis of FMS subgroups could be responsible for the observed heterogeneity

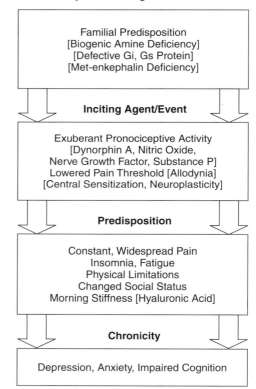

Figure 6-1. A hypothetical model showing a sequence of events leading to the fibromyalgia syndrome (FMS). The sequence begins with one or more predisposing factors acted upon at some point in time by an event or agent to initiate a sequence of events that involve neurochemical changes in the central nervous system (CNS). The neurochemical abnormalities understandably lead to clinical manifestations that cause collateral damage in many clinical systems. The result is a very compromised individual with chronic clinical and emotional findings.

with respect to clinical presentation, to neurochemical abnormalities, and to responsiveness to potent medications. For example, one research group (5,6) divides people meeting American College of Rheumatology (ACR) criteria for the research classification of FMS (3) into two clinical groups—those who have sought care for their pain are called "FMS patients" and those who have not are called "FMS nonpatients." The point is that they then find a number of clinical and biological differences between these subpopulations. Some would argue that those who meet the ACR criteria for FMS are really normal people who choose to be sick. The critics see the affected persons as having deluded themselves into a self-induced pain perception state, but in fact the people who meet those criteria are biochemically different from healthy normal controls (HNCs) in exactly the ways that would fit a chronic pain state.

The observer's viewpoint can have an important influence on how FMS patients are perceived. Clinicians would generally prefer to be "lumpers," hoping that the limited therapeutic resources available to them will work similarly in all of the apparently similar conditions. In contrast, students of pathogenesis would rather be "splitters," hoping to have the subgroup under study be as homogeneous as possible before seeking evidence for specific patterns of pathophysiology or pathochemistry, or both, that most of the affected individuals have in common.

NEUROPATHIC VERSUS NONNEUROPATHIC

One clinical approach to the classification of painful disorders is to view them as either neuropathic or nonneuropathic. Typical examples of well-known neuropathic conditions include diabetic peripheral neuropathy and postherpetic neuralgia. These conditions exhibit dramatic lesions of peripheral nerves. In fact, the term neuropathic has nearly become synonymous with peripheral neuropathic lesions. The reason that FMS might be defined as being nonneuropathic, then, is that it does not exhibit a pathogenesis involving the peripheral nervous system (PNS). It does not seem to have been initiated by or perpetuated by a pathologic lesion in the PNS.

So in common parlance many consider FMS to be nonneuropathic, but is that designation really correct? The *American Heritage Dictionary* defines neuropathy as "a disease or condition of the nervous system." The nervous system is properly viewed as being composed of two highly integrated parts, the CNS and the PNS. The apparently misleading title for this chapter is based on the contemporary rather than the classical dictionary application of neuropathic terminology. In contrast, if the neurochemical evidence in this chapter is found to be convincing, then FMS must be viewed as a painful condition involving pathologic function of the CNS. On that basis, FMS could be viewed as a central neuropathic condition.

To better understand this distinction, one must have some understanding of nociception and the concept of acute versus chronic pain.

The study of nociception is an attempt to understand the process of pain signal transmission from the source of a peripheral noxious stimulus (such as an injured toe) to the interpretative centers of the CNS. In that process, unique peripheral, and then central, neurons carry the painful signal electrically (see Figure 6-2). A critical site for the regulation of this process is in the region of the dorsal horn of the spinal cord. In that location afferent neurons relay the information from the periphery in the form of neurochemicals. At the same time regulatory neurons from the brain stem (caudally directed neuroinhibition) release other neurochemicals whose role is to control the magnitude of the signal sent on to the brain.

At the synaptic junctions between the participant neurons (e.g., an afferent axon of a dorsal root ganglion neuron interacting with an interneuron located in the dorsal horn of the spinal cord), the signal is relayed by neurotransmitters such

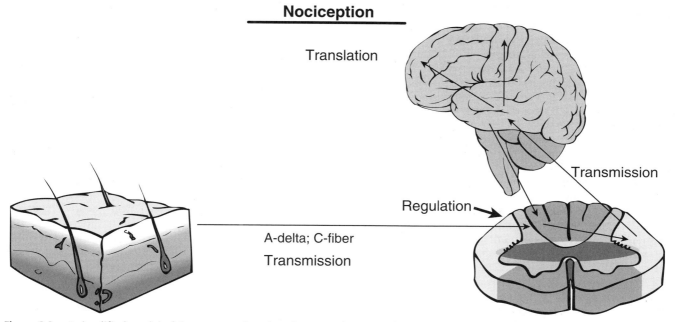

Nociception

Translation

Transmission

Regulation

A-delta; C-fiber

Transmission

Figure 6-2. A simplified model of the process of nociception. A noxious stimulus delivered to a peripheral tissue will send an electrical signal via A-δ and C-fiber to the dorsal horn of the spinal cord. There the message is transmitted by excitatory amino acids (EAA), but it is also regulated there by inhibitory neurochemicals relayed to the scene by neurons from the brain stem. The regulated signal crosses to the contralateral side and ascends to the thalamus, the sensory cortex, and the frontal mood cortex of the brain.

Balanced Nociception

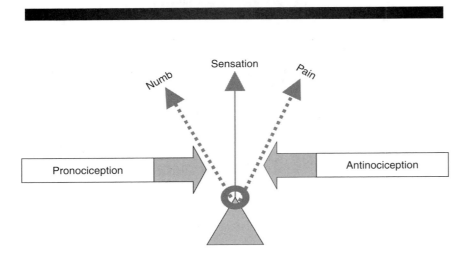

Figure 6-3. The proper balance between the forces regulating nociception. The normal process involves detecting pain when tissue injury is present and not feeling pain when no tissue injury exists. The distortion of this effect by too much pronociception can cause a nonnoxious signal to mimic the pain of true tissue injury. In contrast, too much antinociceptive activity could cause the affected individual to ignore a damaging noxious tissue injury that should be identified quickly and properly interpreted in time to prevent progressive damage.

as excitatory amino acids (EAAs) like glutamate and aspartate. These chemical carriers of the pain signal must be distinguished from other specialized neurochemicals that do not actually transmit the painful signal but, rather, modulate its magnitude. They either facilitate nociception (amplify the signal, i.e., pronociceptive) or inhibit nociception (suppress the signal, i.e., antinociceptive). The perception of a signal sent to the brain is a combination of these influences. As shown in Figure 6-3, the normal process involves detecting pain when tissue injury is present and not feeling pain when no tissue injury exists. The distortion of this effect by too much pronociception can cause a nonnoxious signal to mimic the pain of true tissue injury. In contrast, too much antinociceptive activity could cause a person to ignore a damaging noxious tissue injury that should be quickly perceived to prevent progressive damage.

Examples of pronociceptive neurochemicals include nerve growth factor (NGF), substance P (SP) the carboxy-terminal of SP, certain amino acids, and perhaps nitric oxide (NO). Antinociceptive neurochemicals include the amino terminal fragment of SP, serotonin, norepinephrine, endogenous opioids, certain amino acids, some minerals such as zinc, and perhaps NO. The antinociceptive neuroregulatory molecules accomplish their designated task by interacting with receptors on the afferent dorsal horn neurons to inhibit the release of the signal neurotransmitters (one mechanism of serotonin and norepinephrine) or by interfering with the process of pronociception (one mechanism attributed to the amino terminal fragment of SP).

The investigation of pain processing in FMS has benefited tremendously from decades of research on normally regulated nociception in animals and man. The pain component of FMS is now viewed as resulting from a pathologic amplification (pronociception) of normal incoming signals from the periphery. The result is an enhanced central (cognitive) interpretation of pain even when the signal from the periphery would have been perceived as nonnoxious (nonnociceptive, i.e., not painful) for a normal person without FMS. By definition, this means that people with FMS exhibit a lower than normal pain threshold. They meet the neurophysiologist's definition for allodynia (the experience of pain perceived from a nonnoxious stimulus) (7), so FMS could properly be renamed as "chronic widespread allodynia." This is different from the concept of hyperalgesia, which is defined as an abnormally aggressive response to a noxious (painful for a normal person) stimulus. Logically, the allodynia of FMS could result from too much pronociceptive neurochemical influence or from too little antinociceptive neurochemical influence or from a combination of both (the two-hit hypothesis). Fortunately, these hypotheses provide testable models and they identify specific neurochemical agents that can be assayed in patients with FMS.

It is also important to understand the difference between conditions characterized clinically as exhibiting acute pain and those with chronic pain. Acute pain usually results from a recent noxious stimulus, an injury that has a known cause, a clearly perceived severity, and a predictable prognosis. Acute pain would be understood as occurring by the process of nociception. In contrast, chronic pain usually has developed gradually over a period of many months (at least 3 months), often without an apparent direct cause; its severity is hard to objectively quantify and it has an uncertain prognosis. Chronic pain is usually viewed as nonnociceptive even though the pain that the affected person experiences may be more severe than many forms of acute pain. Acute pain can be characterized by the traumatic injury that causes a compound fracture. The dramatic lesion focuses the resources of orthopedic surgery and medicine to correct the problem, with a reasonable expectation that the effort will be rewarded by a decrease in the pain. In contrast, many chronic pain conditions lack a defined cause, are more difficult to diagnose, and are often associated with mood effects that stifle the interest of many clinicians. Also, the anticipated outcomes are less likely to be favorable.

The cause of FMS is still unknown. Theories regarding its etiology have undergone a gradual transition from a psychiatric process, as some still view it, to a muscle disorder, as it is currently classified in the Medline Index, to a genetically determined CNS disorder of nociception, neuroendocrine function, and cytokine participation, as it should now be considered. The evidence for neurochemical abnormalities, neuroendocrine abnormalities, and immune system abnormalities has been reviewed elsewhere (2,8,9) and will be summarized below. The interested reader is encouraged to read the original sources for more information.

NEUROCHEMICALS AND NEUROTRANSMITTERS

The roles of neurochemicals as neurotransmitters and modulators of the nociceptive process have been studied extensively in animals (10), and the findings are now at least theoretically relevant to human FMS with allodynia (11). This line of reasoning has led to the measurement of neurotransmitter levels in biological fluids obtained from FMS patients. Several major classes of biochemical participants in the nociceptive process are the biogenic amines (serotonin, norepinephrine, and dopamine), EAAs (glutamic acid, glutamine, aspartic acid, asparagine, glycine, arginine, etc.), neurokinins (substance P, calcitonin gene-related protein, arginine vasopressin, neuropeptide Y, etc.), NGF, and probably NO. The biogenic amines are generally considered to be antinociceptive while the EAAs, substance P, NGF, and perhaps even NO would more likely be pronociceptive. Both animal and human data are available. Some of the human data comes directly from studies of patients with FMS.

Serotonin (5HT)

Animal studies have provided some fascinating clues regarding the function of 5HT in the mammalian CNS. Dietary protein is digested in the gut, and the resulting amino acid, tryptophan (TRP), is absorbed through the intestinal mucosae. Albumin carries it to the blood brain barrier (BBB), where TRP is taken up by an energy-dependent process in competition with other aromatic amino acids. It is then delivered to the brain stem raphe nucleus where TRP is oxidatively decarboxylated to 5HT and packaged for axonal delivery at synapses in brain and spinal cord locations. For example, raphe axons release 5HT into the caudate nucleus and within the dorsal horn region at all levels of the spinal cord. In the spinal cord 5HT is known to inhibit the release of substance P by afferent neurons responding to peripheral stimuli. In this regard it is interesting to note that raphe neurons also contain substance P in concentrations inversely proportional to the 5HT concentration. The role of 5HT in the caudate nucleus is less clear, but it most likely is involved in regulating the magnitude of the signal relayed on the cerebral cortex.

A surprising observation from a murine model is that increased SP in the brain increases 5HT levels in the spinal cord, which in turn decreases release of SP into the spinal cord. There seems to be an inverse relationship between brain SP and spinal cord SP concentrations. If these observations are applicable to human FMS, one would expect low brain tissue levels of both 5HT and SP, while spinal cord 5HT concentrations would be low and spinal cord SP would be high.

Serotonin in Fibromyalgia Syndrome

Moldofsky et al. (12) were the first to suggest that 5HT might be involved in the pathogenesis of FMS, both in failing to attenuate persistent pain and to correct the chronic deficiency in slow wave sleep. They found a clinical correlate between FMS pain and the plasma concentration of TRP. More recently, the serum and cerebrospinal fluid (CSF) of FMS patients were found to exhibit low concentrations of TRP (13,14). Other investigators (15) supported early findings

of a low serum concentration of 5HT (16). It is now apparent that the low serum 5HT in FMS is due to low levels of 5HT in their peripheral platelets (17).

The levels of 5HT have not yet been reported in FMS CSF, but the levels of its immediate precursor 5-hydroxy-TRP (5HTP) and its metabolic product 5-hydroxyindole acetic acid (5HIAA) have been. Both were found to exhibit lower than normal concentrations in FMS CSF relative to the CSF of HNC (14,18). In addition, 5HIAA was measured in the 24-hour urine samples of patients with FMS and compared to the results from HNC (19). The rate of 5HIAA excretion was significantly lower in FMS than in the HNC, lower in female FMS than in male FMS, and lower in female FMS than in female HNC (19). Even the numbers of active FMS TePs correlated with the concentration of 5HT in FMS sera (20).

A Canadian positron-emission tomography (PET) study of HNCs indicated that normal women make substantially less 5HT in their brains than men do, but FMS was not considered in the study (21). A potentially important experiment would be to determine whether this gender difference in 5HT production, rather than the obvious differences in hormonal milieu, might predispose women to develop FMS. These findings are only indirect evidence to suggest that something is really amiss bodywide with the production or metabolism, or both, of 5HT in FMS. Perhaps the most critical location for such a deficiency would be in the CNS.

Norepinephrine in Fibromyalgia Syndrome

The role of α-adrenergic agonists like NE in the antinociception system of FMS patients may be similar to that of 5HT, but a number of unique features of this biogenic amine have attracted attention (22). The concentration of methoxy-hydroxy-phenylglycol (MHPG), the inactive metabolite of NE, is significantly lower than normal in FMS CSF (18). Considering the possibility that the elevated CSF substance P (SP) level might be lowered by an α-2-adrenergic agonist, tizanidine was given to people with FMS before drug and after 2 months of therapy while still taking the drug (23). The result was a significant lowering of the CSF SP (although not to normal levels) and simultaneous improvement in the clinical symptoms. Unfortunately, the two changes did not correlate significantly.

Dopamine in Fibromyalgia Syndrome

The concentration of homovanillic acid, the inactive metabolite of DA, was found to be significantly lower than normal in FMS CSF (18). This finding, which would imply low CNS levels of DA in FMS, was complemented by a study of the role of DA receptors in the function of the hypothalamus and pituitary in FMS (24). The investigators examined the physiologic response to buspirone (a DA antagonist and 5HT1A agonist). Buspirone is known to induce a unique hypothermic response through stimulation of a 5HT autoreceptor (5HT1A) and subsequent growth hormone (GH) release. The prolactin response to buspirone, however, appears to be mediated through a DA receptor (D2). On the basis of the assumption that FMS is more strongly related to stress and anxiety than to affective spectrum disorders, the authors predicted that FMS patients would exhibit an increased prolactin response (DA related) to a buspirone challenge test but would not produce hyperthermia or an increase in GH release (5HT1A related). They gave a 60-mg oral dose of buspirone to 22 premenopausal women with FMS and 14 age-matched and sex-matched healthy controls. The FMS patients showed an augmented prolactin response to buspirone compared to controls, but temperature and GH responses did not differ from controls. The authors hypothesized that these results favored a dysfunction of dopaminergic (D2) responsiveness resulting from increased numbers of or hypersensitivity of D2 receptors in FMS. Increased sensitivity or numbers of receptors might be the expected physiologic servomechanism consequence of low DA levels, as found earlier (18).

Excitatory Amino Acids

A number of amino acids are known to play a role in the nociceptive process (25–39). Since the first to be recognized (glutamic acid, glutamine, aspartic acid, asparagine) were found to be pronociceptive or excitatory, they were referred to as EAAs. To illustrate how this process involves these simple molecules, the following is a recognized sequence of events: A noxious stimulus in the periphery causes afferent nociceptive neurons to release glutamic acid into synapses within the dorsal horn of the spinal cord, where it activates *N*-methyl-*D*-aspartate (NMDA) receptors that then relay the message of peripheral pain to the brain. Several amino acids (such as glycine) are suspected of modulating (suppressing, antinociceptive) rather than facilitating the process of nociception. An important role of the amino acid arginine is to undergo cleavage by the enzyme NO synthase to produce citrulline and release the potent modulator NO.

The potential importance of these EAAs to the symptoms of FMS was highlighted by a sequence of several studies (40–42) in which patients with FMS were treated with drugs that inhibited the activation of the NMDA receptors by the EAAs. The evidence suggests that ketamine, an NMDA inhibitor, is able to substantially reduce the severity of FMS pain in about one-third to one-half of FMS patients.

A study of the concentrations of EAAs in the spinal fluid of primary fibromyalgia syndrome (PFMS) compared to HNC was conducted in order to explore their role in the processing of pain in FMS patients (29). Two disease controls also included in the study were FMS associated with other conditions [secondary fibromyalgia syndrome (SFMS)], or other painful conditions not exhibiting fibromyalgia (Other). It was hypothesized that CSF EAAs may be involved in pain processing in FMS in ways similar to their effects on nociception in experimental animals. It was found that the mean concentrations of most EAAs in the PFMS CSF did not differ from normal or from the disease controls. However, individual measures of pain intensity, determined using an examination-based measure of pain intensity, the tender point index (TPI), and CSF SP levels, covaried with their concentrations of glutamine and asparagine, metabolites of glutamate and aspartate, respectively. That suggested that reuptake and biotransformation may mask pain-related increases in EAAs. Individual concentrations of glycine and taurine also correlated with their respective TPI values in patients with PFMS.

Although a variety of excitatory manipulations affect taurine, glycine is an inhibitory transmitter as well as a positive modulator of the NMDA receptor. In both PFMS and SFMS patients, TPI covaried with arginine, the precursor to NO, whose concentrations, in turn, correlated with those of citrulline, a by-product of NO synthesis. These events predicted involvement of NO, a potent signaling molecule thought to be involved in pain processing (see below). Together these metabolic changes that covary with the intensity of pain and CSF SP in patients with FMS may reflect increased EAA release and a positive modulation of NMDA receptors by glycine, perhaps resulting in enhanced synthesis of NO. They also support patients' complaints that they perceive body pain.

Substance P

Substance P is an 11 amino acid neuropeptide that has several important roles in the process of nociception. Activated, small, thinly myelinated A-δ and C-fiber afferent neurons respond to noxious peripheral stimuli by releasing SP into laminae I and V (A-δ) and laminae II (C-fiber) of the spinal cord dorsal horn. With random interstitial diffusion, SP or its C-terminal peptide fragment makes contact with its neurokinin-1 (NK1) effector receptor. The mechanism of SP action in the dorsal horn of the spinal cord is not entirely clear, but it appears not to be a signal transporter like glutamic acid. Rather, SP apparently facilitates nociception by "arming" or "alerting" spinal cord neurons to incoming nociceptive signals from the periphery. Of course, SP released by the afferent nerve fibers into the dorsal horn of the spinal cord can also diffuse out into the extracellular space and from there to the CSF, where it can be measured as CSF SP.

Substance P in Animal Systems

Data from a murine system indicates that there is an inverse relationship between brain and spinal cord concentrations of SP. An increase of SP in the brain leads to an increase of 5HT in the spinal cord, which in turn inhibits the release of SP into the spinal cord. This inhibition of SP release in response to 5HT (or NE) in the area of the dorsal horn neurons is referred to as descending inhibition of nociception.

It is likely that potent biogenic amine agonists, like 5HT or NE, can lower SP in the spinal cord environment of FMS patients, but both may be necessary to completely normalize the levels of CSF SP before the desired clinical benefits will be achieved and will correlate with the biological change. Meanwhile, it may be useful to experimentally combine biogenic amine inhibitors with NK1 inhibitors for their predicted synergy.

It should be noted that 5HT, NE, and SP participate in the regulation of the hypothalamus and pituitary (43), which will be important to the concept of neuroendocrine abnormalities in FMS.

Substance P can be manipulated to induce allodynia in animal models. German investigators (44) examined the effects of administering SP intrathecally to rats. They observed a SP dose-dependent increase in the number of peripheral nerves and/or fiber types that were effective in driving the dorsal horn neuron to relay a nociceptive message to the brain. Substance P caused an increase in the size or number of mechanosensitive receptive fields involving nociceptive neurons, and it induced a lowering of the threshold for postsynaptic potentials. All these effects were consistent with the model that views SP as a facilitator of nociception.

Substance P in Fibromyalgia Syndrome

Vaeroy et al. (45), working in Norway, were the first to recognize that the concentration of SP was elevated (average = threefold) in the CSF of FMS patients compared to HNC subjects. Their findings have now been reproduced in three other clinical studies (46–48), as shown in Figure 6-4.

In the author's first study of CSF SP in FMS patients (46), age and gender had no influence on the measured CSF SP levels, but minor differences were related to ethnicity. In an attempt to further characterize the nature of the CSF SP abnormality, a number of lumbar-level CSF samples were collected in three sequential numbered fractions. The CSF SP concentrations in these samples failed to define a cranial to caudal gradient of CSF SP concentration. Another experiment involved inducing noxious pressure on the lower body TePs to see if it would have any effect on the lumbar-level CSF SP concentration. There was no significant increase in the levels of CSF SP, as might have been expected if the CSF SP were coming primarily from local afferent dorsal horn neurons. The elevation of CSF SP in FMS is not due to lowered activity of CSF SP esterase because the rate of cleavage of labeled SP by FMS CSF was normal (49).

The concentration of SP is normal in the serum of FM patients, and recent evidence suggests that SP levels in FMS serum correlate conversely with serum TRP and 5HIAA levels (50). Recent evidence (50) suggests, however, that SP levels in FMS serum correlate inversely with TRP levels and 5HIAA levels in FMS serum.

Relevance of Elevated Cerebrospinal Fluid Substance P in Fibromyalgia Syndrome

The biological relevance of substance P in CSF to the pain of PFMS is clearly supported by the fact that the EAA glutamic acid in PFMS correlates with the level of CSF SP in this patient group (29). This point is illustrated in Figure 6-5, where there is a linear relationship between CSF glutamine and SP levels in patients with PFMS. The same relationship was not exhibited by CSF samples from the HNC or subjects with inflammatory diseases without FMS or subjects with inflammatory diseases in addition to their FMS.

In each of the first four studies on the concentrations of SP in CSF, the conclusions were based on only a single sample of CSF from each subject. It was not possible to know from such data whether the abnormal CSF SP levels were stable or were fluctuating with variations in the patients' symptoms. To answer that question, 28 lumbar-level CSF samples were collected from the same medication-free patients an average of 12 months after the first medication-free sample had been obtained (51). "Medication-free" means that on both occasions the FMS patients discontinued for 2 weeks all medications believed to be helpful in the treatment of FMS symptoms. In many cases the CSF SP level did not change measurably over the span of 12 months; some exhibited a small increase, but none showed a decrease of CSF SP with time. On average, there was a slight increase in the concentration of CSF SP over time. In the subgroup that did exhibit an increase in CSF SP, that change correlated directly with a small clinical change in pain/tenderness that occurred over the same period. These findings imply that CSF SP may be integrally related to changes in the severity of the symptomatic pain of FMS.

An important question that must eventually be answered is whether elevated CSF SP is unique to FMS. An earlier report (52) indicated that CSF SP concentrations were lower than normal in a variety of chronic painful conditions. For example, CSF SP levels were found to be lower than normal in diabetic neuropathy (53) and chronic low back pain (54). In contrast, elevated levels of CSF SP have been found in patients with painful rheumatic diseases, whether or not they have concomitant FMS. In painful osteoarthritis of the hip, the elevated CSF SP prior to surgical treatment returned to normal after successful total hip arthroplasty (complete replacement of the hip joint with mechanical components), which left the patients nearly free from hip pain (55).

Experience with spinal fluid neuropeptides in San Antonio now includes analysis of SP in CSF collected from over 500 clinical subjects. Among them have been over 170 PFMS patients and over 75 HNC. Disease control groups have included more than 30 subjects with FMS associated with another painful condition (SFMS). A smaller group of 14 subjects had other painful conditions but lacked FMS. The group average CSF SP concentration for the PFMS was numerically higher than any other group; the next lower group mean was for the SFMS. Even lower was the group mean for painful rheumatic diseases without FMS. The

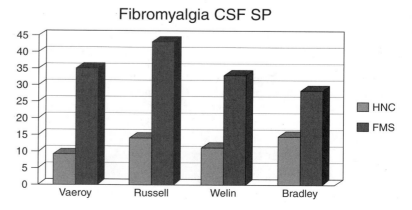

Figure 6-4. Cerebrospinal fluid substance P (CSF SP) levels in patients with fibromyalgia syndrome (FMS). The study by Vaeroy et al. in Norway (3) was the first to observe dramatically higher CSF SP levels in fibromyalgia syndrome (FMS) patients than in healthy normal controls (HNC). The studies by three other investigative groups (4–6) confirmed that finding with the involvement of subjects from a total of three ethnic groups.

Excitatory Amino Acids

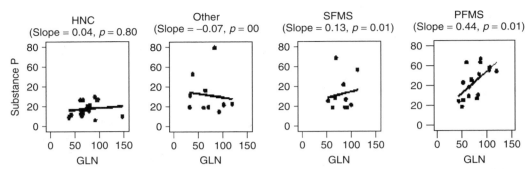

Figure 6-5. Relationship of spinal fluid glutamine levels to spinal fluid substance P (SP) levels in patients with primary fibromyalgia syndrome (PFMS). Cerebrospinal fluid (CSF) was obtained from three clinical groups that were designated as follows: Healthy Normal Controls (HNC); patients with inflammatory rheumatic diseases but not fibromyalgia syndrome (FMS) were designated Other; patients with inflammatory rheumatic diseases but also meeting criteria for FMS were designated Secondary FMS (SFMS); and patients with FMS who lacked any other painful condition were designated Primary FMS (PFMS). Each of the CSF samples was used to measure CSF glutamine (GLN) and cerebrospinal fluid substance P (CSF SP). The measures levels were graphed by subject group as shown above. The level of CSF GLN correlated with the level of CSF SP (the ordinate scale) only for the PFMS group.

lowest group mean values were with the HNC. Only the HNC CSF SP values were statistically significantly different from those found in the PFMS patients. In the SFMS group and in the Other Diseases Lacking FMS group, the CSF SP levels were not significantly different from either the HNC or the PFMS groups, perhaps, in part, because these SFMS and Other disease groups were composed of small numbers of subjects.

The FMS study group at the University of Alabama at Birmingham (48) has shown that the higher CSF SP levels in FMS correlated inversely with the regional cerebral blood flow (rCBF) within the caudate nucleus and thalamus of the same FMS patients. The reason for this relationship is not yet clear. It is not likely that the high levels of SP caused the apparent vasoconstriction because SP is known to be a potent dilator of cerebral vessels, provided that the vascular endothelium of those vessels is intact. It is possible that the decrease in blood flow could have been caused by neuropeptide Y (NPY) (56) or dynorphin A (57), since both are known to be potent vasoconstrictors and both are elevated [NPY in serum, DynA in CSF] in FMS. One could speculate, then, that the excess SP is produced in response to tissue hypoxia as an attempt by the CNS to restore more normal blood flow. That explanation seems unlikely, however, because major brain hypoxic injury in experimental animals (ligation of an internal carotid artery in rats) causes a substantial decrease in brain tissue levels of SP. Of course, not being able to immediately explain a biological finding does not negate it. As with many past observations, this finding may need to hibernate for awhile until further research discloses the key to understanding it.

Nerve Growth Factor

The elevated CSF SP in FMS prompted much speculation about what might be the cause. NGF was known to stimulate

the production of substance P in small, afferent, unmyelinated neurons. It was therefore an exciting development in the study of CSF SP in FMS to have found elevated levels of NGF in the CSF of PFMS patients, but not in FMS with an associated painful inflammatory condition (SFMS) (58). This finding, illustrated in Figure 6-6, provides clear neurochemical evidence for different etiologic subgroups of FMS patients in those two settings, even though the clinical presentations of the FMS symptoms and the examination signs may not be clinically distinguishable in the two groups (3). That observation would suggest that elevated CSF SP could be a common link between primary and SFMS but that the groups differ in the mechanism responsible for the elevated SP. In PFMS, NGF seems to induce the elevated CSF SP, while in SFMS the cause of the elevated CSF SP may be inflammation in the periphery.

Normally, NGF facilitates the production of SP primarily in nociceptive neurons. In PFMS and perhaps other situations involving central sensitization, it is believed that NGF may even induce the production of SP in large myelinated neurons that are not normally nociceptive. To complicate the model even further, evidence now suggests that CSF SP in FMS may be produced primarily by CNS interneurons rather than in neurons afferent to the dorsal horn of the spinal cord. In SFMS it is logical to believe that the peripheral inflammation so characteristic of the underlying rheumatic or infectious conditions may be responsible for the elevated CSF SP (59). For these reasons, NGF could be critical to the initiation or perpetuation of the painful symptoms of PFMS but not SFMS. In patients with PFMS, the focus of investigative study should perhaps be to learn why NGF would be pathologically elevated and how to reduce its effect on the pathologic production of CSF SP. In FMS associated with an inflammatory rheumatic disease, the substance P is most likely caused by the inflammation (60–63) and

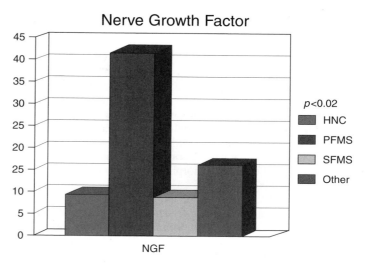

Figure 6-6. Cerebrospinal fluid nerve growth factor (NGF) levels in patients with primary fibromyalgia syndrome (FMS). Cerebrospinal fluid (CSF) was obtained from three clinical groups that were designated as follows: Healthy Normal Controls, HNC; patients with inflammatory rheumatic diseases but not fibromyalgia syndrome (FMS) were designated Other; patients with inflammatory rheumatic diseases but also meeting criteria for FMS were designated Secondary FMS (SFMS); and patients with FMS who lacked any other painful condition were designated Primary FMS (PFMS). Each CSF sample was used to measure nerve growth factor by radioimmunoassay (RAI). The measures levels were graphed by subject group as shown here. The level of CSF NGF was dramatically elevated only in the PFMS group.

does not require the mediation of NGF. In that situation the most critical task of therapy for both the rheumatic disease and the FMS would be to reduce or eliminate the inflammation. Again, this is an illustration of the importance of recognizing a subgroup and directing therapy accordingly.

Calcitonin Gene-Related Peptide

This neuropeptide is currently something of an enigma because it colocalizes with SP in afferent neural pathways, but the only function attributed to calcitonin gene-related peptide (CGRP) is competitive inhibition of the peptidase enzymes that degrade SP. In patients with diabetic neuropathy, CSF CGRP correlated highly with the concentration of CGRP in the peripheral nerves undergoing ischemic injury due to occlusion of the vasanervorum. In FMS CSF, CGRP was found to be numerically but not significantly higher than in HNC CSF. Considering that, it was surprising that CGRP in FMS CSF correlated inversely with the pain threshold, directly with the number of TePs by dolorimetry, directly with depression, and indirectly with the CSF 5HIAA concentration. The inverse correlation with 5HIAA ties the 5HT pathway to peptide mediators at the spinal cord level CSF. No such clinical correlations were found with CGRP in the HNC CSF samples.

Antinociceptive Activities

The data from one study suggested that there might be a weak negative correlation between CSF SP levels and pain in FMS (46). That is the opposite of the strong direct correlative relationship that was predicted, and it begs for explanation. The sample size was not large, so a weak correlation may not be very meaningful. On the other hand, an intriguing hypothetical explanation related to a proteolytic product of SP. SP endopeptidase can cleave intact SP to produce two main peptide fragments, the C-terminal (SP_{5-11}) and the N-terminal (SP_{1-7}) (64). Intact SP and its C-terminal peptide bind to the NK_1 receptor to facilitate nociception. The N-terminal fragment of enzymatically cleaved SP activates another receptor to effect potent antinociception that works by decreasing nerve cell surface NK1

receptors. As the measured concentration of SP increases, activation of the N-terminal receptor could progressively counteract the pronociceptive effect of the C-terminal portion of SP (65,66).

On the other hand, the concentration of met-enkephalin-arg-phe, which is supposed to exert an antinociceptive effect in the spinal cord, was found to be significantly decreased among a group of Swedish FMS patients when compared with HNC (47). This is the expected finding if one were to predict that an enkephalin deficiency would increase the magnitude of nociception.

Other antinociceptive mediators that have been studied include endogenous endorphins (57). Neither CSF-endorphin (μ-opioid receptor) nor dynorphin A (κ-opioid receptor) were low in FMS CSF. Actually, the surprise was that the concentration of dynorphin A in FMS CSF was actually elevated. That finding could indicate an attempt on the part of the endogenous opioid system to balance the increased nociception. Alternatively, it could have very different implications (see next paragraph) that could not have been predicted in 1991.

Dynorphin A and Fibromyalgia Syndrome Pathogenesis

Recent data from animal systems has led this author to hypothesize a very important role for CSF dynorphin A in FMS (67) that must be followed up with a prospective study. Dynorphin A is a κ-opioid receptor agonist, but it also can affect NMDA receptors. When high concentrations of dynorphin A were administered intrathecally to rats, the animals developed a flaccid paralysis. Intermediate concentrations of dynorphin A were less damaging but caused a persistent allodynia (68). The mechanism responsible for these effects appeared to involve NMDA receptors rather than the expected κ-opioid receptors. Increased production of dynorphin A has been known to occur in animal experiments in which the spinal cord was constricted or otherwise injured. Under those circumstances, administered antibodies to dynorphin A reduced the severity of the deficit resulting from such injury. On the other hand, when dynorphin A was allowed to induce spinal cord injury, the damage appeared to be irreversible.

A study conducted in Israel (69) showed that previously healthy people who suffered a whiplash injury in an automobile accident were much more likely (21% vs. 2%) to develop symptomatic FMS than were people who broke a lower extremity bone in an industrial accident. One could speculate that the reason for the differential effect on development of FMS was that the whiplash-induced cervical spine injury led to the production of neurotoxic dynorphin A levels. One could imagine a situation in which an emergency trauma physician examining a whiplash injury victim would be aware of FMS as a potential complication and would routinely inject antibodies to dynorphin A intrathecally as preventive prophylaxis.

Another puzzle that must be explained was that in one study (57) SP and dynorphin A were both elevated in the same FMS CSF samples. Dynorphin A can inhibit the release of SP after an acute noxious stimulus. More information is needed on this subject.

Nitric Oxide

Nitric oxide (NO) is a potent neuromodulator that is known to reduce the pain threshold in animals (70). NO is produced by the enzymatic action of nitric oxide synthase (NOS) on arginine. After a very brief half-life, the potent NO is inactivated by metabolism to stable nitrite (NO_2^-) or nitrate (NO_3^-). A study was conducted to quantify NO production in FMS by measuring NO_2^- and NO_3^- in CSF, plasma, and urine and to determine whether NO in FMS relates to the clinical and laboratory abnormalities that are typical for this condition. When averaged over all ages, the concentrations of CSF NO_2^- and of CSF, plasma, and 24-hour urine NO_3^- in FMS were not significantly different from HNC. It was discovered, however, that there were significant correlations between age and NO_3^- in plasma and urine of both groups but that their slopes were opposite (positive in HNC, negative in FMS). Stratification by age (above and below the mean of 42 years) revealed significantly elevated plasma and urinary NO_3^- levels in the younger FMS subjects. Correlations were found between CSF NO metabolites and the duration of FMS symptoms. Among the young FMS subjects, CSF NO_2^- and 24-hour urine NO_3^- correlated with body tenderness. The elevated production of NO in younger FMS patients represents an abnormal pattern of NOS activity early in the course of FMS that may cause the characteristically lowered pressure pain threshold. As the clinical symptoms persisted or gradually worsened with time, the abnormal NO levels fell to subnormal levels. If NO initiates the painful processes in FMS, the early changes may be more readily reversible than those exhibited with chronicity. Thus, it may be important to identify FMS early in its course so this sequence of events can be aborted.

Genetic Predisposition Model

Evidence for familial aggregation and a genetic basis for the disorder is also receiving more attention. About one-third of FMS patients report that another family member, usually a female, has a similar, chronic pain condition or has already been given the diagnosis of FMS. Several published studies have documented familial patterns and some have predicted an autosomal dominant mode of inheritance for FMS (71,72). There is growing evidence for an autosomal dominant mode of inheritance for FMS (73). A recent study by Yunus et al. (74) found probable linkage of FMS with the histocompatability locus examined by the sibship method.

A complete genome scan of family members with two or more FMS affected members is currently underway (Olson et al., 2004, unpublished), using samples of deoxyribonucleic acid (DNA) from a large number of FMS multicase families for comparison with clinical and laboratory genotypic features. Meanwhile, several candidate genes have been proposed to directly explain specific metabolic abnormalities that have been consistently observed in FMS.

A recent study of 80 multicase FMS families has already examined a total of eight markers spanning the genomic regions for the serotonin transporter (HTTLPR, three regional markers) on chromosome 17, the serotonin receptor 2A (HTR2A, three regional markers) on chromosome 13, and the histocompatability locus antigen (HLA, two regional markers) region of chromosome 6 (75). No evidence for linkage was found in the HTTLPR region. Families with an older age of onset were linked to the HLA region (lod = 3.02, $p = 0.00057$), suggesting an immune-mediated pathogenesis. In the HTR2A region the results indicated a moderately strong linkage to families with a younger age of onset, less severe pain, lower levels of depression, and absence of the irritable bowel syndrome (lod = 5.56, $p = 0.000057$). The HTR2A genome is polymorphically imprinted, so the issue of parent-of-origin will need to be considered in future studies. Bioinformatics mining and further sequencing of the genes in the HTR2A region will need to be utilized to identify specific polymorphisms for further clinical association testing.

Another appealing gene candidate for a role in causing FMS would be the catechol-O-methyltransferase (COMT) enzyme that physiologically inactivates catecholamines such as dopamine, norepinephrine, endorphins, and catecholamine-containing drugs. Polymorphism (really dimorphism) in the gene encodes for variations in the activity of the COMT enzyme. The COMT gene exists in two forms (low, L and high, H) that make copies differing by a single amino acid (either valine or methionine) at the variable site. This small variation has a big effect on the activity of COMT. Subjects with the LL (homozygous, one L gene from each parent) phenotype, who have two copies of the methionine version, make threefold to fourfold less COMT than the HH variants, which contain valine at the variable site.

The significance of COMT polymorphism (LL, LH, or HH) in FMS was assessed by Gursoy et al. (76). The analysis of COMT polymorphism was performed using polymerase chain reaction (PCR). Sixty-one patients with FMS and 61 HNC were included in the study. Although no significant difference was found between LL and LH separately, the LL and LH genotypes together were more highly represented in FMS patients than in the HNC ($p = 0.024$). In addition, HH genotypes in FMS were significantly lower than in the HNC groups ($p = 0.04$). There was no significant relationship between COMT polymorphism and the patients' psychiatric status, as assessed by several psychiatric tests ($p > 0.05$).

It has been hypothesized (77) that COMT functions by metabolizing dopamine and freeing receptors in the brain for the binding of endorphins to the μ-opioid receptors, which lead to pain relief. The more potent the COMT enzyme that is functioning in the body, the more dopamine that gets metabolized and the more endorphins that are allowed to bind. The LL genotype has been associated with an increased pain susceptibility.

The findings of these and other studies of genetic linkage to FMS clinical patterns have provided strong support for the concept that there are subgroups of FMS that present with unique but overlapping clinical manifestations. It is likely that genetic characterization of FMS subgroups will do more than any of the previous clinical and laboratory studies to move FMS from its current classification as a "syndrome" to that of a "disease." If that is true, it will likely come at the expense of subdividing the currently large clinical population of FMS into many subgroups. The advantage may be that the pathogenesis of those subgroups will be more apparent and the development of strategic chemical therapies will be substantially facilitated.

Gender Differences Model

The much higher prevalence of FMS among women than among men has led to speculation regarding a gender-specific cause. For example, in an epidemiologic study of a Midwestern community (78), the curves representing pain thresholds (sensitivity to a pressure stimulus) in men and women consistently showed lower values for women. Since the examination component of the ACR criteria for FMS involves the response to a fixed pressure stimulus of 4 kg, it is not surprising that the ACR criteria have identified more women than men with FMS.

Our understanding of the mechanisms responsible for this gender-related difference in pain thresholds is incomplete. Measurements of female hormones have not been very fruitful. A highly probable explanation for gender-related differences in pain perception has come from an unlikely source—PET of the brain. This concept was mentioned earlier in the serotonin subsection but bears brief repeating for its apparent influence on the gender-related differences to painful stimuli. A group of Canadian neuroradiologists (21) who were studying the CNS synthesis and metabolism of 5HT administered a radionucleotide-tagged analog of TRP (5-methyl TRP) to healthy adults of both sexes and measured the rate of its conversion to methyl-5HT. This reaction mimicked and paralleled the natural synthesis of serotonin in the brain. The ligand conversion rate was significantly lower (by about sevenfold) in women than in men, indicating a much lower rate of 5HT in women. Since 5HT is antinociceptive, this finding provides a logical nonendocrine basis for a gender-related differential in antinociceptive activity and could potentially explain why women might be at greater risk for developing chronic widespread allodynia (think FMS) in response to painful injury.

Neuroendocrine Models

Many symptoms of FMS resemble those observed in patients with hormone deficiencies. That observation has led to the study of neuroendocrine function in FMS (56). Subsets of people with FMS exhibit functional abnormalities in the hypothalamic-pituitary-adrenal (HPA) axis, in the sympathoadrenal (autonomic nervous) system, in the hypothalamic-pituitary-thyroid (HPT) axis, in the hypothalamic-pituary-gonadal (HPG) axis, or in the hypothalamic-pituitary-growth hormone (HGH) axis (79).

Hypothalamic-Pituitary-Adrenal Axis

The HPA axis is known to play an important role in coordinating the body's physiologic responses to physical and emotional stressors. Some have considered the FMS to be a stress-related syndrome because dysregulation of the normal stress response can produce symptoms mimicking those of FMS (79). The HPA axis exhibits a circadian rhythm related to the day and night or the sleep and awake 24-hour cycles. There is a low level of produced cortisol activity in the evening and a peak in the early morning hours. In addition, stress-induced secretion of cortisol can be superimposed on this basal circadian rhythm. Regulation of this HPA axis depends on the right balance of biochemicals in the hypothalamus, anterior pituitary, and the cortex of the adrenal gland. Key substances in this regulation are corticotropin-releasing hormone (CRH) and arginine vasopressin (VAP) from the hypothalamus. They induce the release of adrenocorticotropic hormone (ACTH) from the anterior pituitary, which facilitates glucocorticoid (cortisol) release from the adrenal cortex. The cortisol, then, feeds back on the hypothalamus to inhibit the cycle. Other mediators that regulate the HPA include serotonin, norepinephrine, substance P, and IL-6 (43,80).

In FMS patients the HPA axis exhibits an exaggerated ACTH response to insulin-induced hypoglycemia or to stressful exercise. Despite this dramatic rise in serum ACTH, the level of cortisol does not rise commensurately. It is possible that the stressors used to induce the rise in ACTH in these experiments also decreased the circulating levels of glucocorticoid binding protein (GBP), since GBP is a negative phase reactant (81–83) (meaning that its concentration goes down with physiologic stress such as inflammation), resulting in more of the available glucocorticoid being free (unbound to GBP in its active state) and therefore more potent in all its effects.

The picture reads quite differently with highly controlled hypoglycemic hyperinsulinemic clamp procedures, which show inadequate responsiveness (or excessive response to feedback inhibition) of the hypothalamic-pituitary portion of the axis (84). A loss of the circadian fluctuation of plasma cortisol has been reported in some FMS patients with elevated evening levels and with reduced cortisol excretion in 24-hour urine (56,85). Over one-third of FMS patients exhibit abnormal suppression of glucocorticoid production after dexamethasone administration (86,87).

The reader might logically interpret the preceding discussion to indicate adrenal insufficiency in FMS and wonder if FMS symptoms might be responsive to glucocorticoid therapy. That seems not to be the case, since administration of glucocorticosteroid medications to people with PFMS does not seem to improve their symptoms (88). Conversely, substantial improvement of FMS symptoms may result from otherwise indicated corticosteroid treatment of patients with rheumatoid arthritis (RA) or systemic lupus erythematosus (SLE) who also have FMS. Tapering the corticosteroid dosage too rapidly might exacerbate fibromyalgia-like symptoms in such inflammatory disorders. Whether that happens only in persons who carry an underlying predisposition to develop FMS is unknown.

In neurally mediated hypotension, which occurs in some FMS patients, the adrenergic (epinephrine, norepinephrine) response to physiologic stress, including postural changes, may be blunted. Some clinicians have found that administration of mineralocorticoids can reduce the severity of the neurally mediated hypotension and the attendant fatigue (89).

Hypothalamic-Pituitary-Human Growth Hormone Axis

HGH was studied in FMS because it was known to be produced during δ-wave sleep, which many FMS patients fail to achieve normally. HGH is difficult to measure because its release is pulsatile and its plasma half-life is very short. An alternative means of monitoring HGH production has been to measure the plasma levels of insulinlike growth factor-1 (IGF1, previously known as somatomedin C), which has a long half-life. An age-adjusted deficiency of IGF1 has been documented in a large number of FMS patients relative to normal controls (90).

In one well-designed study, parenteral therapy (daily injections) with HGH was effective in reducing the severity of FMS symptoms (91), but regular injection therapy with this hormone is not universally appealing to FMS patients. Also, IGF1 levels must be regularly monitored to adjust the HGH dosage, and the cost of such therapy is currently prohibitive.

Deficient function of the HGH axis could contribute to symptoms in FMS patients, particularly decreased psychological well-being and reduced exercise capacity. Another insight is that HGH is normally produced during exercise but FMS patients fail to produce HGH during aerobic exercise (92). It was proposed that the release of HGH during exercise might be suppressed in FMS by somatostatin and that administration of pyridostigmine before exercise can disinhibit HGH production. Indeed, 30 mg of pyridostigmine given before exercise resulted in increased release of HGH with exercise among FMS patients. It will be interesting to learn the results of the long-term studies of FMS exercise facilitated by preexercise dosing FMS patients with 30 mg of pyridostigmine or by daily therapy using 60 mg of sustained release pyridostigmine. Certainly, both of those approaches will be less expensive than parenteral replacement of HGH.

Hypothalamic-Pituitary-Gonadal Axis

The HPG axis was implicated in FMS primarily because women are about 3 to 5 times more commonly affected than men and because the onset of FMS often seems to be in the perimenopausal years. About 30% of female FMS patients are prematurely menopausal due to surgery (hysterectomy or oopherecomy) or insufficient estrogen therapy (93). A disproportionally large number of FMS patients (44%) suffer from premenstrual syndrome, and their pain relates to the phase of their menstrual cycle (94). Although estrogen deficiency might be a promoting or a permissive factor in female FMS patients, the hypothesis that there are gender-related differences in CNS 5HT production is frankly more appealing (21).

The reasons why these endocrinopathies would be associated with a chronic pain syndrome are not entirely clear. It

may be that CNS abnormalities in the availability of biogenic amines such as serotonin, norepinephrine, or dopamine are responsible for the abnormal regulation of the neuroendocrine system (18). Since these systems interact and are interdependent, in susceptible individuals a partial failure of one system may lead to subtle malfunctions of others.

IMMUNE ABNORMALITIES

A comprehensive review of this topic is available (95), but newer information is available to update it.

One of the earliest clinical findings to suggest an immune-mediated pathogenesis in FMS was livedo in some of the patient's extremities (96,97) and cutaneous hyperreactivity consistent with neurogenic inflammation (98). The finding of immunoglobulin deposits in the skin, particularly in the dermal epidermal junction, prompted speculation that immune mechanisms may be contributing to the pathogenesis of FMS (96,97,99,100). More recently, support for a role of immune mediators in the skin comes from a study of 53 female FMS patients and 10 HNC (101). Reverse transcription-polymerase chain reaction (RT-PCR) and immunohistochemistry were used to identify IL-1β in 38%, IL-6 in 27%, and tumor necrosis factor-α (TNF-α) in 32% of the skin tissues obtained from FMS patients respectively, compared to none of the HNC exhibiting these potent immune mediators.

An early epidemiologic search for serum antinuclear antibodies (ANA) disclosed that nearly one-third of FMS patients exhibit low titers of these autoantibodies (102), but more recent reports have reduced that value to 14% (103) or as low as 8.8% in FMS compared to 8.9% in patients with osteoarthritis (104).

During the era in which silicone breast implants (SBIs) were blamed for a variety of clinical disorders, a search for humoral immunity to polymeric antigens disclosed a family of antibodies (called antipolymer antibodies, or APA) to a high molecular weight, nonprotein, synthetic polymer (105). It is important to note that the relationship between the presumed inciting antigen and the detection antigen was unclear. The presence of these antibodies began to assume some importance when it was shown that their serum levels correlated with the severity of the symptoms in SBI recipients. When it was recognized that many clinical similarities existed between symptomatic SBI recipients and FMS patients without SBI, sera obtained from FMS patients were tested for APA (106). The assay for APA was positive in 47% of FMS patients, while the positivity in rheumatic disease patients ranged from 3% to 19%. In addition, APA correlated with the severity of symptoms in FMS patients.

A subsequent series of APA studies in FMS examined sera from PFMS and HNC by an enzyme-linked immunosorbant assay (ELISA). Using optical density (OD) units to represent APA levels, the assay was shown to be highly reproducible. Elevated levels of APA OD were found in PFMS relative to HNC ($p<0.001$). On the basis of an abnormal cut point of OD >0.03, 58.1% (79/136) of the PFMS patients were positive while only 25.8% (16/62) of the HNC were positive (sensitivity = 58.1%, specificity = 74.2%, $p<0.001$). Using APA OD as a continuous variable, significant correlations were found in PFMS patients between

APA OD and scores for stiffness, fatigue severity, limitation in physical activity, headache, anxiety, and depression. In HNC a significant correlation was found between APA OD and average pain threshold.

It is not yet clear how these findings should be interpreted relative to the pathogenesis of FMS. There are certainly environmental antigens that could induce an immune response in exposed individuals. One could postulate that APA-positive individuals were genetically poised to develop antibodies when exposed to such antigens and that the resultant immune process contributed in some way to the symptoms. Certainly, it would seem useful to identify the APA positive and negative subgroups to facilitate further study of the phenomenon and to suggest therapy focused on the underlying mechanism.

CYTOKINES IN FIBROMYALGIA SYNDROME

In the past there were intermittent reports of lymphocyte immune abnormalities in people with FMS, but the outcomes of the studies were quite variable and hard to interpret in light of the clinical picture (95). More recently, two studies have critically evaluated the possible role of cytokines in patients with FMS (107,108). Although most of the cytokines explored in these investigations did not differ between FMS and HNC, there were some dramatic, consistent, and relevant exceptions. The serum interleukin-8 (IL-8) and the interleukin-6 (IL-6) from in vitro stimulated peripheral blood mononuclear leukocytes (PBMC) cultures were significantly higher for the FMS subjects. There were also correlates with comorbidities. The serum IL-8 was most dramatically elevated in FMS patients who were also depressed, but it also correlated with pain intensity and the duration of FMS symptoms. Since IL-8 promotes sympathetic pain and IL-6 induces hyperalgesia, fatigue, and depression, it is hypothesized that they both may play a role in modulating the symptoms of FMS. Interleukin-8 is a monocyte-derived 8.0 kilodalton chemokine that promotes neutrophil chemotaxis and degranulation. Its signaling of other cells is mediated by high-affinity G protein-coupled receptors. Its production in vitro is stimulated by substance P, so that may help to explain the elevation of both of these cytokines even in different fluid compartments of FMS patients.

In this light, it is of interest that IL-6 has been successfully administered to people with FMS with the finding that it substantially modulated the severity of the FMS-related symptoms (80). That experiment was undertaken because IL-6 can serve as a direct or at least indirect stimulus of the HPA axis, but the effects on FMS patients were rather global. It is certainly possible that FMS is an IL-6 deficiency state and that the production of IL-6 by PBMC during in vitro culture bears no relationship to in vivo production of IL-6 where it is needed in the CNS.

G PROTEIN-COUPLED RECEPTORS

A family of cell surface receptors known as G protein-coupled receptors allows molecules on the outside of the cell membranes to signal their presence to the inside of the cell and to direct selected intracellular functions. When the effect is to be a *stimulation*, the receptor is designated a "Gs" protein-coupled receptor. When the designated function is *inhibition* of an intracellular process, the receptor is known as a "Gi" protein-coupled receptor. In both cases the intracellular target is control of the production of cyclic adenosine monophosphate (cAMP); Gs receptor activation increases intracellular cAMP, and Gi receptor activation prevents intracellular increases in cAMP. One of the characteristics of a specific Gi protein receptor on the surface membranes of human PBMC is its susceptibility to be blocked or inactivated by pertussis toxoid.

In a controlled experiment involving PBMC from HNC and from FMS patients, the FMS cells without pertussis exposure behaved like HNC cells poisoned by pertussis toxoid (109). Note that the FMS leukocytes were dysfunctional without exposure to the toxoid. The failure of the Gi protein-coupled receptor in FMS leukocytes to exert its normal inhibition of intracellular cAMP production by adenyl cyclase resulted in higher baseline and increased functional intracellular levels of cAMP. The investigators have proposed this defect as a sufficient cause for the allodynia that is so characteristic of FMS. It was also proposed as a diagnostic test for FMS. The natural ligand for this specific Gi protein-coupled receptor is still uncertain, but there is a 5HT receptor that is known to exhibit many of the phenotypical features attributed to this defective receptor in FMS.

Another group of investigators (110) examined the function of a Gs protein-coupled receptor in the PBMC of FMS patients and documented a defect in the response to β-adrenergic ligand. To investigate this receptor, the functions of PBMC from 18 female FMS patients were compared with that of nine demographically matched HNC. Aliquots of 10^6 (one million) cells were incubated with or without stimulation of β-agonist isoproterenol for 5 minutes. Basal and stimulated intracellular cAMP levels were determined by enzyme immunoassay. Two different concentrations of the isoproterenol (10^{-3} M and 10^{-5} M) were utilized. The basal levels of cAMP in FMS patients were numerically but not significantly elevated compared with the HNC ($p = 0.124$). In contrast, isoproterenol, at 10^{-5} M, significantly increased cAMP in the HNC cells ($p = 0.012$), but did not increase the mean intracellular cAMP levels in the FMS PBMC ($p = 0.74$). The authors concluded that these preliminary results imply diminished Gs protein-coupled β-adrenergic receptor function in FMS.

These two "first of their kind" experiments in FMS were performed to seek dysfunction in different G protein-coupled receptors that target cAMP production in FMS PBMC. The fact that both experiments were successful is of some concern because it becomes harder to explain with the involvement of two receptors from two or more different genetic locations. Both experiments need to be independently confirmed, but it is certainly possible that both receptors suffer from a common defect in FMS. The Gi or Gs designation is based on the α component of the G protein-coupled receptor, and perhaps there is a defect in the β component that is common to both. It is also possible that the α component of both the Gi and Gs suffers from a similar defect, which is being measured as two defects because of the experimental designs.

CONCLUSIONS REGARDING PATHOGENESIS

The FMS situation has changed dramatically in just a few years of concentrated research. In contrast to just two decades ago, when FMS patients were often viewed as healthy complainers without any real abnormalities, there are now criteria to aid in making the research classification diagnosis. Whereas the patients were once considered to be depressed somatizers, the psychiatric model is no longer adequate. Where the pathogenesis was once diligently sought in "painful muscles," the symptoms now appear to better fit a central neurosensitization model. Although it was said that there were no abnormal test findings in FMS, abnormalities in neurochemical mediators of CNS nociceptive function are clearly present in ways that are consistent with the patterns of symptoms.

The recognition of allodynia as a manifestation of abnormal central nociceptive processing has changed the collective view of FMS. It has led research in a new direction toward the study of nociceptive neurotransmission in FMS. Some of the abnormalities found in FMS, namely the low 5HT and the elevated SP, are logically consistent with a pain amplification syndrome. The extent to which these mechanisms are unique to FMS will be critical in determining the direction of future research. Certainly, a better understanding of the cause of FMS will represent an important step toward the development of more effective therapy.

REFERENCES

1. Russell IJ. A new journal. *J Musculoskelet Pain* 1993;1(1): 1–7.
2. Russell IJ. Fibromyalgia. In: Loeser JD, ed. *Bonica's management of pain*. New York: Williams & Wilkins, 2000: 543–559.
3. Wolfe F, Smythe HA, Yunus MB, et al. The American College of Rheumatology 1990 criteria for the classification of fibromyalgia. *Arthritis Rheum* 1990;33:160–172.
4. Fukuda K, Straus SE, Hickie I, et al. The chronic fatigue syndrome: a comprehensive approach to its definition and study. *Ann Intern Med* 1994;121:953–959.
5. Kersh BC, Bradley LA, Alarcon GS, et al. Psychosocial and health status variables independently predict health care seeking in fibromyalgia. *Arthritis Rheum* 2001;45:362–371.
6. Aaron LA, Bradley LA, Alarcon GS, et al. Psychiatric diagnoses in patients with fibromyalgia are related to health care-seeking behavior rather than to illness (see comment). *Arthritis Rheum* 1996;39:436–445.
7. Bonica JJ. Definitions and taxonomy of pain. In: Bonica JJ, Loeser JD Chapman CR et al., eds. *The management of pain*, Vol. I. Philadelphia, PA: Lea & Febiger, 1990:18–27.
8. Russell IJ. Fibromyalgia syndrome. In: Mense S, Simons DG, Russell IJ, eds. *Muscle pain: understanding its nature, diagnosis, and treatment*. Baltimore, MD: Lippincott Williams & Wilkins, 2001:289–337.
9. Bieber C, Russell IJ. Muscle and fibromyalgia. In: McMahon SB, Koltzenburg M, eds. *Wall and Melzack's textbook of pain*. London: Elsevier, 2004.
10. Malmberg AB, Yaksh TL. Hyperalgesia mediated by spinal glutamate or substance P receptor blocked by spinal cyclooxygenase inhibition. *Science* 1992;257:1276–1279.
11. Russell IJ. Neurochemical pathogenesis of fibromyalgia syndrome. *J Musculoskelet Pain* 1996;1(1-2):61–92.
12. Moldofsky H, Warsh JJ. Plasma tryptophan and musculoskeletal pain in nonarticular rheumatism ("fibrositis syndrome"). *Pain* 1978;5:65–71.
13. Russell IJ, Michalek JE, Vipraio GA, et al. Serum amino acids in fibrositis/fibromyalgia syndrome. *J Rheumatol Suppl* 1989;19:158–163.
14. Russell IJ, Vipraio GA, Acworth I. Abnormalities in the central nervous system (CNS) metabolism of tryptophan (TRY) to 3-hydroxy kynurenine (OHKY) in fibromyalgia syndrome (FS). *Arthritis Rheum* 1993;36(9):S222.
15. Hrycaj P, Stratz T, Muller W. Platelet 3H-imipramine uptake receptor density and serum serotonin in patients with fibromyalgia/fibrositis syndrome. *J Rheumatol* 1993;20: 1986–1987.
16. Russell IJ, Michalek JE, Vipraio GA, et al. Platelet 3H-imipramine uptake receptor density and serum serotonin levels in patients with fibromyalgia/fibrositis syndrome. *J Rheumatol* 1992;19:104–109.
17. Russell IJ, Vipraio GA. Serotonin (5HT) in serum and platelets (PLT) from fibromyalgia patients (FS) and normal controls (NC). *Arthritis Rheum* 1994;37(Suppl.):S214.
18. Russell IJ, Vaeroy H, Javors M, et al. Cerebrospinal fluid biogenic amine metabolites in fibromyalgia/fibrositis syndrome and rheumatoid arthritis. *Arthritis Rheum* 1992;35: 550–556.
19. Kang Y-K, Russell IJ, Vipraio GA, et al. Low urinary 5-hydroxyindole acetic acid in fibromyalgia syndrome: evidence in support of a serotonin-deficiency pathogenesis. *Myalgia* 1998;1:14–21.
20. Wolfe F, Russell IJ, Vipraio G, et al. Serotonin levels, pain threshold, and fibromyalgia symptoms in the general population. *J Rheumatol* 1997;24:555–559.
21. Nishizawa S, Benkelfat C, Young SN, et al. Differences between males and females in rates of serotonin synthesis in human brain. *Proc Natl Acad Sci USA* 1997;94:5308–5313.
22. Bennett RM, Clark SR, Campbell SM, et al. Symptoms of Raynaud's syndrome in patients with fibromyalgia. A study utilizing the Nielsen test, digital photoplethysmography, and measurements of platelet alpha 2-adrenergic receptors. *Arthritis Rheum* 1991;34:264–269.
23. Russell IJ, Michalek JE, Xiao Y, et al. Therapy with a central alpha-2-agonist (tizanidine) decreases cerebrospinal fluid substance P, and may reduce serum hyaluronic acid as it improves the clinical symptoms of the fibromyalgia syndrome. *Arthritis Rheum* 2002;46:S614.
24. Malt EA, Olafsson S, Aakvaag A, et al. Altered dopamine D2 receptor function in fibromyalgia patients: a neuroendocrine study with buspirone in women with fibromyalgia compared to female population based controls. *J Affect Disord* 2003;75(1):77–82.
25. Terman GW, Bonica JJ. Spinal mechanisms and their modulation. In: Loeser JD, Butler SH, Chapman CR et al., eds. *Bonica's management of pain*. Philadelphia, PA: Lippincott Williams & Wilkins, 2001:73–152.
26. Smullin DH, Skilling SR, Larson AA. Interactions between substance P, calcitonin gene-related peptide, taurine and excitatory amino acids in the spinal cord. *Pain* 1990;42: 93–101.
27. Okano K, Kuraishi Y, Satoh M. Pharmacological evidence for involvement of excitatory amino acids in aversive responses induced by intrathecal substance P in rats. *Biol Pharm Bull* 1993;16:861–865.
28. Okano K, Kuraishi Y, Satoh M. Involvement of substance P and excitatory amino acids in aversive behavior elicited by intrathecal capsaicin. *Neurosci Res* 1994;19:125–130.
29. Larson AA, Giovengo SL, Russell IJ, et al. Changes in the concentrations of amino acids in the cerebrospinal fluid that

correlate with pain in patients with fibromyalgia: implications for nitric oxide pathways. *Pain* 2000;87:201–211.

30. King AE, Lopez-Garcia JA. Excitatory amino acid receptor-mediated neurotransmission from cutaneous afferents in rat dorsal horn in vitro. *J Physiol* 1993;472:443–457.

31. Aanonsen LM, Lei S, Wilcox GL. Excitatory amino acid receptors and nociceptive neurotransmission in rat spinal cord. *Pain* 1990;41:309–321.

32. Cotman CW, Iversen LL. Excitatory amino acids in the brain—focus on NMDA receptors. *Trends Neurosci* 1987; 10:263–265.

33. Westlund KN, McNeill DL, Coggeshall RE. Glutamate immunoreactivity in rat dorsal root axons. *Neurosci Lett* 1988;96:13–17.

34. Aanonsen LM, Wilcox GL. Nociceptive action of excitatory amino acids in the mouse: Effects of spinally administered opioids, phencyclidine and sigma agonists. *J Pharmacol Exp Ther* 1987;243:9–19.

35. Sorkin LS, McAdoo DJ, Willis WD. Raphe magnus stimulation-induced antinociception in the cat is associated with release of amino acids as well as serotonin in the lumbar dorsal horn. *Brain Res* 1993;618:95–108.

36. Panter SS, Yum SW, Faden AI. Alteration in extracellular amino acids after traumatic spinal cord injury (see comments). *Ann Neurol* 1990;27:96–99.

37. Long JB, Rigamonti DD, Oleshansky MA, et al. Dynorphin A-induced rat spinal cord injury: evidence for excitatory amino acid involvement in a pharmacological model of ischemic spinal cord injury. *J Pharmacol Exp Ther* 1994;269: 358–366.

38. Mao J, Price DD, Hayes RL, et al. Differential roles of NMDA and non-NMDA receptor activation in induction and maintenance of thermal hyperalgesia in rats with painful peripheral mononeuropathy. *Brain Res* 1992;598:271–278.

39. Miller BA, Woolf CJ. Glutamate-mediated slow synaptic currents in neonatal rat deep dorsal horn neurons in vitro. *J Neurophysiol* 1996;76:1465–1476.

40. Graven-Nielsen T, Aspegren KS, Henriksson KG, et al. Ketamine reduces muscle pain, temporal summation, and referred pain in fibromyalgia patients. *Pain* 2000;85:483–491.

41. Oye I, Rabben T, Fagerlund TH. Analgesic effect of ketamine in a patient with neuropathic pain (Norwegian). *Tidsskrift for Den Norske Laegeforening* 1996;116:3130–3131.

42. Sorensen J, Bengtsson A, Backman E, et al. Pain analysis in patients with fibromyalgia. Effects of intravenous morphine, lidocaine, and ketamine. *Scand J Rheumatol* 1995;24:360–365.

43. Pillemer SR, Bradley LA, Crofford LJ, et al. The neuroscience and endocrinology of fibromyalgia. *Arthritis Rheum* 1997;40:1928–1939.

44. Hoheisel U, Mense S, Ratkai M. Effects of spinal cord superfusion with substance P on the excitability of rat dorsal horn neurons processing input from deep tissues. *J Musculoskeletal Pain* 1996;3(3):23–43.

45. Vaeroy H, Helle R, Forre O, et al. Elevated CSF levels of substance P and high incidence of Raynaud's phenomenon in patients with fibromyalgia: new features for diagnosis. *Pain* 1988;32:21–26.

46. Russell IJ, Orr MD, Littman B, et al. Elevated cerebrospinal levels of substance P in patients with fibromyalgia syndrome. *Arthritis Rheum* 1994;37:1593–1601.

47. Welin M, Bragee B, Nyberg F, et al. Elevated substance P levels are contrasted by a decrease in met-enkephalin-arg-phe levels in csf from fibromyalgia patients. *J Musculoskeletal Pain* 1995;3(Suppl. 1):4.

48. Bradley LA, Alberts KR, Alarcon GS, et al. Abnormal brain regional cerebral blood flow (rCBF) and cerebrospinal fluid (CSF) levels of substance P (SP) in patients and non-patients with fibromyalgia (FM). *Arthritis Rheum* 1996;39(Suppl.): S212.

49. Russell IJ, Orr MD, Michalek JE, et al. Substance P (SP), SP endopeptidase activity, and SP N-terminal peptide fragment (SP1-7) in fibromyalgia syndrome cerebrospinal fluid. *J Musculoskelet Pain* 1995;3(Suppl. 1):5.

50. Schwarz MJ, Spath M, Muller-Bardow H, et al. Substance P, 5-HIAA and tryptophan in serum of fibromyalgia patients. *Neurosci Lett* 1999;259:196–198.

51. Russell IJ, Fletcher EM, Vipraio GA, et al. Cerebrospinal fluid (CSF) substance P (SP) in fibromyalgia: changes in CSF SP over time parallel changes in clinical activity. *J Musculoskelet Pain* 1998;6(Suppl. 2):77.

52. Sjostrom S, Tamsen A, Hartvig P, et al. Cerebrospinal fluid concentrations of substance P and (met)enkephalin-Arg6-Phe7 during surgery and patient-controlled analgesia. *Anesth Analg* 1988;67:976–981.

53. Tsigos C, Diemel LT, Tomlinson DR, et al. Cerebrospinal fluid levels of substance P and calcitonin-gene-related peptide: correlation with sural nerve levels and neuropathic signs in sensory diabetic polyneuropathy. *Clin Sci* 1993;84:305–311.

54. Sjostrom S, Tamsen A, Hartvig P, et al. Cerebrospinal fluid concentrations of substance P and (met)enkephalin-Arg6-Phe7 during surgery and patient-controlled analgesia. *Anesth Analg* 1988;67:976–981.

55. Nyberg F, Liu Z, Lind C, et al. Enhanced CSF levels of substance P in patients with painful arthrosis but not in patients with pain from herniated lumbar discs. *J Musculoskelet Pain* 1995;3(Suppl. 1):2.

56. Crofford LJ, Pillemer SR, Kalogeras KT, et al. Hypothalamic-pituitary-adrenal axis perturbations in patients with fibromyalgia. *Arthritis Rheum* 1994;37:1583–1592.

57. Vaeroy H, Nyberg F, Terenius L. No evidence for endorphin deficiency in fibromyalgia following investigation of cerebrospinal fluid (CSF) dynorphin A and Met-enkephalin-Arg6-Phe7. *Pain* 1991;46:139–143.

58. Giovengo SL, Russell IJ, Larson AA. Increased concentrations of nerve growth factor in cerebrospinal fluid of patients with fibromyalgia. *J Rheumatol* 1999;26:1564–1569.

59. Matucci-Cerinic M, Partsch G, Marabini S, et al. High levels of substance P in rheumatoid arthritis synovial fluid. Lack of substance P production by synoviocytes in vitro [Letter]. *Clin Exp Rheumatol* 1991;9:440–441.

60. Hartung HP, Toyka KV, Substance P. the immune system and inflammation. *Int Rev Immunol* 1989;4:229–249.

61. Marabini S, Matucci-Cerinic M, Geppetti P, et al. Substance P and somatostatin levels in rheumatoid arthritis, osteoarthritis, and psoriatic arthritis synovial fluid. *Ann N Y Acad Sci* 1991; 632:435–436.

62. Menkes CJ, Renoux M, Laoussadi S, et al. Substance P levels in the synovium and synovial fluid from patients with rheumatoid arthritis and osteoarthritis. *J Rheumatol* 1993;20: 714–717.

63. Walsh DA, Mapp PI, Wharton J, et al. Localisation and characterisation of substance P binding to human synovial tissue in rheumatoid arthritis. *Ann Rheum Dis* 1992;51: 313–317.

64. Nyberg F, LeGreves P, Sundqvist C, et al. Characterization of substance P(1-7) and (1-8) generating enzyme in human cerebrospinal fluid. *Biochem Biophys Res Commun* 1984; 125:244–250.

65. Skilling SR, Smullin DH, Larson AA. Differential effects of C- and N-terminal substance P metabolites on the release of amino acid neurotransmitters from the spinal cord: potential role in nociception. *J Neurosci* 1990;10:1309–1318.

66. Yukhananov Ryu, Larson AA. An N-terminal fragment of substance P, Substance P(1-7), down-regulates neurokinin-1 binding in the mouse spinal cord. *Neuroscience* 1994;178: 163–166.

67. Russell IJ. Advances in fibromyalgia: possible role for central neurochemicals. *Am J Med Sci* 1998;315:377–384.

68. Vanderah TW, Laughlin T, Lashbrook JM, et al. Single intrathecal injections of dynorphin A or des-tyr-dynorphins produce long-lasting allodynia in rats: blockade by MK-801 but not naloxone. *Pain* 1996;68:275–281.

69. Buskila D, Neumann L, Vaisberg G, et al. Increased rates of fibromyalgia following cervical spine injury: a controlled study of 161 cases of traumatic injury. *Arthritis Rheum* 1997; 40:446–452.

70. Sarma J, Tandan SK, Hajare SW, et al. Effect of centrally administered nitric oxide modulators in Brewer's yeast-induced nociception in rats. *Indian J Exp Biol* 2000;38(11): 1123–1128.

71. Buskila D, Neumann L, Hazanov I, et al. Familial aggregation in the fibromyalgia syndrome. *Semin Arthritis Rheum* 1996;26:605–611.

72. Pellegrino MJ, Waylonis GW, Sommer A. Familial occurrence of primary fibromyalgia (see comments). *Arch Phys Med Rehabil* 1989;70:61–63.

73. Buskila D, Neumann L, Hazanov I, et al. Familial aggregation in the fibromyalgia syndrome. *Semin Arthritis Rheum* 1996;26:605–611.

74. Yunus MB, Rawlings KK, Khan MA, et al. Genetic studies of multicase families with fibromyalgia syndrome (FMS) with HLA typing. *Arthritis Rheum* 1995;38(Suppl.):S247.

75. Arnold LM, Iyengar S, Khan MA, et al. Genetic linkage of fibromyalgia to the serotonin receptor 2A region on chromosome 13 and the HLA region on chromosome 6: a report from the Fibromyalgia Family Study Group (FFSG). *Arthritis Rheum* 2003;48(9):S228.

76. Gursoy S, Erdal E, Herken H, et al. Significance of catechol-O-methyltransferase gene polymorphism in fibromyalgia syndrome. *Rheumatol Int* 2003;23(3):104–107.

77. Zubieta JK, Heitzeg MM, Smith YR, et al. COMT val158-met genotype affects mu-opioid neurotransmitter responses to a pain stressor. *Science* 2003;299(5610):1240–1243.

78. Wolfe F, Ross K, Anderson J, et al. The prevalence and characteristics of fibromyalgia in the general population. *Arthritis Rheum* 1995;38:19–28.

79. Crofford LJ. Neuroendocrine abnormalities in fibromyalgia and related disorders [Review] (45 refs). *Am J Med Sci* 1998; 315:359–366.

80. Torpy DJ, Papanicolaou DA, Lotsikas AJ, et al. Responses of the sympathetic nervous system and the hypothalamic-pituitary-adrenal axis to interleukin-6: a pilot study in fibromyalgia. *Arthritis Rheum* 2000;43:872–880.

81. Deak T, Meriwether JL, Fleshner M, et al. Evidence that brief stress may induce the acute phase response in rats. *Am J Physiol* 1997;273:R1998–R2004.

82. Fleshner M, Deak T, Spencer RL, et al. A long-term increase in basal levels of corticosterone and a decrease in corticosteroid-binding globulin after acute stressor exposure. *Endocrinology* 1995;136:5336–5342.

83. Fleshner M, Silbert L, Deak T, et al. TNF-alpha-induced corticosterone elevation but not serum protein or corticosteroid binding globulin reduction is vagally mediated. *Brain Res Bull* 1997;44:701–706.

84. Adler GK, Kinsley BT, Hurwitz S, et al. Reduced hypothalamic-pituitary and sympathoadrenal responses to hypoglycemia in women with fibromyalgia syndrome. *Am J Med* 1999;106: 534–543.

85. McCain GA. Nonmedicinal treatments in primary fibromyalgia [Review] (67 refs). *Rheum Dis Clin North Am* 1989;15:73–90.

86. Hudson JI, Pliner LF, Hudson MS, et al. The dexamethasone suppression test in fibrositis. *Biol Psychiatry* 1984;19: 1489–1493.

87. Ferraccioli G, Cavalieri F, Salaffi F, et al. Neuroendocrinologic findings in primary fibromyalgia and in other chronic rheumatic conditions. *J Rheumatol* 1990;17:869–873.

88. Clark S, Tindall E, Bennett RM. A double blind crossover trial of prednisone versus placebo in the treatment of fibrositis. *J Rheumatol* 1985;12:980–983.

89. Bou-Holaigah I, Calkins H, Flynn JA, et al. Provocation of hypotension and pain during upright tilt table testing in adults with fibromyalgia. *Clin Exp Rheumatol* 1997;15: 239–246.

90. Bennett RM, Clark SR, Campbell SM, et al. Low levels of somatomedin C in patients with the fibromyalgia syndrome. A possible link between sleep and muscle pain. *Arthritis Rheum* 1992;35:1113–1116.

91. Bennett RM, Clark SC, Walczyk J. A randomized, double-blind, placebo-controlled study of growth hormone in the treatment of fibromyalgia. *Am J Med* 1998;104: 227–231.

92. Paiva ES, Deodhar A, Jones KD, et al. Impaired growth hormone secretion in fibromyalgia patients: evidence for augmented hypothalamic somatostatin tone. *Arthritis Rheum* 2002;46(5):1344–1350.

93. Waxman J, Zatzkis SM. Fibromyalgia and menopause. Examination of the relationship. *Postgrad Med* 1986;80:165–167.

94. Anderberg UM, Marteinsdottir I, Hallman J, et al. Variability in cyclicity affects pain and other symptoms in female fibromyalgia syndrome patients. *J Musculoskelet Pain* 1998; 6(4):5–22.

95. Caro XJ. Is there an immunologic component to the fibrositis syndrome? *Rheum Dis Clin North Am* 1989;169–186.

96. Caro XJ. Immunofluorescent detection of IgG at the dermal-epidermal junction in patients with apparent primary fibrositis syndrome. *Arthritis Rheum* 1984;27:ll74–ll79.

97. Caro XJ, Wolfe F, Johnston WH, et al. A controlled and blinded study of immunoreactant deposition at the dermal-epidermal junction of patients with primary fibrositis syndrome. *J Rheumatol* 1986;13:1086–1092.

98. Littlejohn GO, Weinstein C. Helme Rd. Increased neurogenic inflammation in fibrositis syndrome. *J Rheumatol* 1987; 14: 1022–1029.

99. Enestrom S, Bengtsson A, Lindstrom F, et al. Attachment of IgG to dermal extracellular matrix in patients with fibromyalgia. *Clin Exp Rheumatol* 1990;8:127–135.

100. Enestrom S, Bengtsson A, Frodin T. Dermal IgG deposits and increase of mast cells in patients with fibromyalgia—relevant findings or epiphenomena? *Scand J Rheumatol* 1997;26(4):308–313.

101. Salemi S, Rethage J, Wollina U, et al. Detection of interleukin-1beta (IL-1beta), IL-6, and tumor necrosis factor-alpha in skin of patients with fibromyalgia. *J Rheumatol* 2003;30(1):146–150.

102. Yunus MB, Masi AT. Prevalence of antinuclear antibodies and connective tissue disease symptoms in primary fibromyalgia syndrome. *Clin Res* 1985;33:924A.

103. Dinerman H, Goldenberg DL, Felson DT. A prospective evaluation of 118 patients with the fibromyalgia syndrome: prevalence of Raynaud's phenomenon, sicca symptoms, ANA, low complement, and Ig deposition at the dermal-epidermal junction. *J Rheumatol* 1986;13:368–373.

104. Al Allaf AW, Ottenwell L, Puller T. The prevalence and significance of positive antinuclear antibodies in patients with fibromyalgia syndrome: 2–4 years' follow-up. *Clin Rheumatol* 2002;21(6):472–477.

105. Tenenbaum SA, Rice JC, Espinoza LR, et al. Use of antipolymer antibody assay in recipients of silicone breast implants (see comments). *Lancet* 1997; 349:449–454 [published erratum appears in *Lancet* 1997 May 24;349(9064): 1558].

106. Wilson RB, Gluck OS, Tesser JR, et al. Antipolymer antibody reactivity in a subset of patients with fibromyalgia correlates with severity. *J Rheumatol* 1999;26:402–407.

107. Gur A, Karakoc M, Nas K, et al. Cytokines and depression in cases with fibromyalgia. *J Rheumatol* 2002;29(2):358–361.

108. Wallace DJ, Linker-Israeli M, Hallegua D, et al. Cytokines play an aetiopathogenetic role in fibromyalgia: a hypothesis and pilot study. *Rheumatology* 2001;40:743–749.

109. Galeotti N, Ghelardini C, Zippi M, et al. A reduced functionality of Gi proteins as a possible cause of fibromyalgia. *J Rheumatol.* 2001;28(10):2298–2304.

110. Maekawa K, Twe C, Lotaif A, et al. Function of beta-adrenergic receptors on mononuclear cells in female patients with fibromyalgia. *J Rheumatol* 2003;30:364–368.

7

Dysfunction of the Autonomic Nervous System in Chronic Pain Syndromes

Manuel Martinez-Lavin

The autonomic nervous system (ANS) is the main regulatory system of the body in charge of maintaining essential involuntary functions, such as the so-called *vital signs* (blood pressure, pulse, respiration, and temperature), among many other variables (1). Dysfunction of the ANS has been associated with chronic pain syndromes. This chapter describes the basic concept of the ANS, discusses experimental models linking autonomic dysfunction to chronic pain, and presents emerging evidence suggesting that such dysfunction may play a key role in the pathogenesis of fibromyalgia (FM).

AUTONOMIC NERVOUS SYSTEM BASIC CONCEPTS

The ANS is the portion of the nervous system that controls the function of the different organs and systems of the body. It is "autonomic" because it works below the level of consciousness. One striking characteristic of this system is the rapidity and intensity of the onset and dissipation of its action. The ANS is activated by centers located in the spinal cord, brain stem, hypothalamus, and thalamus. These centers also receive input from the limbic system and other higher brain areas. These connections enable the ANS to serve as the principal part of the stress response system in charge of the fight-or-flight reactions.

The ANS works closely with the endocrine system, particularly with the hypothalamic-pituitary-adrenal axis. The adrenal glands are rich in autonomic neurotransmitters. Another endocrine axis closely related to the ANS involves growth hormone secretion.

The peripheral autonomic system is divided into two branches: sympathetic and parasympathetic. These two branches have antagonistic actions on most bodily functions, and thus their proper balance preserves homeostasis. The action of these two branches is mediated by neurotransmitters. Catecholamines are the sympathetic neurotransmitters, whereas acethylcoline acts in the parasympathetic periphery (1).

The naturally occurring sympathetic catecholamines are norepinephrine, epinephrine, and dopamine. The three substances act as neurotransmitters within the central nervous system. Norepinephrine acts also in peripheral postganglionic nerve endings and exerts its effects locally in the immediate vicinity of its release (2), whereas epinephrine is the circulating hormone of the adrenal medulla and influences processes throughout the body. The major metabolic transformation of catecholamines involves methylation and oxidative deamination. Methylation is catalyzed by the enzyme catechol-O-methyltransferase (COMT), whereas oxidative deamination is promoted by monoamine oxidase (MAO). There is an abundant functional polymorphism in the COMT gene with a guanine-to-adenosine transition at codon 158, resulting in a valine-to-methionine substitution (COMT, val-158-met). This polymorphism results in important functional alterations of the corresponding enzyme. Val/val genotype gives rise to an effective enzyme, whereas met/met genotype produces a "lazy" enzyme unable to effectively clear catecholamines from the system. The heterozygous val/met genotype results in an intermediate action enzyme. Met/met genotype is frequent, affecting 23% of the general population. This abundant polymorphism has a profound impact on autonomic regulation. Emerging evidence suggests that COMT polymorphism may also affect intensity of pain perception. Normal individuals with val/val genotype (thus having an effective catecholamine-clearing enzyme) are pain-resistant, whereas individuals with met/met genotype have a low pain threshold (3).

CLINICAL ASSESSMENT OF AUTONOMIC NERVOUS SYSTEM FUNCTION

The function of the ANS has been difficult to evaluate in clinical practice. Changes in breathing pattern, mental stress, or even posture immediately and completely alter the sympathetic/parasympathetic balance. Consequently, this dynamic system cannot be properly studied by "static" tests, such as levels of circulating neurotransmitters, and less so by their urinary catabolites. Useful bedside maneuvers to assess ANS function include measurements of supine and standing pulse and blood pressure. Sustained drops in systolic (>20 mm Hg) or diastolic (>10 mm Hg) blood pressure after standing for 3 minutes that are not associated with an increase in pulse rate of >30 beats per minute suggest autonomic deficit (4).

Fortunately, two clinical research instruments have been recently introduced to aid in the clinical research of cardiovascular autonomic function: heart rate variability analysis and the tilt table test.

HEART RATE VARIABILITY ANALYSIS

This method is based on the well-known fact that the heart rate is not fixed but varies constantly and at random from beat to beat. The antagonistic effects of the sympathetic and parasympathetic branches of the ANS on the sinus node dictate the periodic components of this constant variability. Heart rate variability can be studied in the time domain in which the basic units are milliseconds. Time domain mathematical calculations include, among others, the standard deviation of all R-R intervals duration as well as the percentage of adjacent pairs of R-R intervals that differ by more than 50 milliseconds from each other in a given time period. The higher time domain variability indexes signify the more parasympathetic influx on the sinus node.

Heart rate variability can also be studied in the frequency domain using spectral analysis where the basic units are Hertz (cycles per second). Pharmacologic and clinical studies have established that the high frequency band spectral power reflects parasympathetic activity on the heart, whereas low frequency band power is modulated mostly by sympathetic impulses. Since the two branches of the ANS have antagonistic effects on the sinus node, the ratio low frequency band/high frequency band is regarded as reflection of sympathetic activity (5).

This new method has several advantages. Because it is noninvasive, patients are subjected to no discomfort whatsoever. The equipment is portable, which means that recording can be done while subjects perform their routine activities. And lastly, the method is based on cybernetics—therefore it has boundless development potential.

TILT TABLE TEST

The tilt table test is another useful tool for studying orthostatic intolerance and syncope. It is based on the physiologic changes that occur after adopting upright posture with pooling of approximately 700 mL of blood in the lower parts of the body. In normal circumstances the ANS quickly compensates for this relative volume loss by increasing vascular tone and cardiac output. This mechanism avoids hypotension and inadequate cerebral perfusion. Tilt table testing examines this response in a controlled environment. With passive orthostasis, additional stress is exerted on the sympathetic nervous system by blocking the influence of muscle contraction that could increase venous return. In the first step subjects are supine for 30 minutes. Then the subject is tilted upright for 30 to 45 minutes at an angle of 60 to 80 degrees. Pharmacologic stimulation with isoproterenol is sometimes used as an additional step.

The normal response to tilting consists of an increase of heart rate of 10 to 15 beats per minute, an elevation of diastolic blood pressure of about 10 mm Hg, and little change in systolic pressure. There are two types of abnormal responses: orthostatic hypotension (defined as a reduction of systolic blood pressure of at least 20 mm Hg) or a reduction of diastolic blood pressure of at least 10 mm Hg. This hypotension may induce syncope. Another type of abnormal response is postural orthostatic tachycardia (POTS), which consists of a sustained increase of heart rate of at least 30 beats per minute or a sustained pulse rate of 120 beats per minute. Tilt table testing has been used mostly to study syncope in patients with no evidence of structural heart disease (6).

AUTONOMIC NERVOUS SYSTEM AND PAIN

For more than a century it has been assumed that abnormal activity of the sympathetic nervous system may be involved in the pathogenesis of protracted pain syndromes. This assumption was based mainly on the observations that the pain is spatially correlated with signs of autonomic dysfunction and that blocking the efferent sympathetic supply to the affected region relieves the pain. This latter premise led to the clinical concept of *sympathetically maintained pain*, which is applied to those neuropathic pain cases that respond to sympatholytic maneuvers (7). Sympathetically maintained pain has strong and ample foundations in the animal model; in contrast, the clinical information sustaining this pathogenesis is mostly anecdotal and usually does not fulfill the strict current evidence-based medicine criteria. The reason for this paradox is that most clinical evidence of sympathetically maintained pain comes from battlefield medicine, which in most instances does not fulfill the criteria for evidence-based medicine.

ANIMAL STUDIES OF SYMPATHETICALLY MAINTAINED PAIN

Under normal circumstances, primary afferent nociceptors do not have catecholamine sensitivity; however, under pathologic conditions, particularly after trauma, a sympathetic-afferent interaction can be established at both the peripheral and central levels.

In a rabbit model, after peripheral nerve injury, sympathetic stimulation and norepinephrine are excitatory for a subset of skin C-fibers nociceptors that express α-2 adrenergiclike receptors (8). Perhaps more germane to the pathogenesis of sympathetically maintained pain are the experimental models that have been extensively reproduced in which after nerve injury, sympathetic sprouting at the dorsal root ganglia becomes apparent and forms basketlike structures around large-diameter axotomized sensory neurons; sympathetic stimulation can activate such neurons repetitively (9).

Another site of abnormal posttraumatic connections occurs in the dorsal horn of the spinal cord, where there is an A-fibers sprouting into the superficial layers, thus causing tactile stimuli to be felt as painful. This mechanism may explain the allodynia.

HISTORY OF THE CONCEPT OF SYMPATHETICALLY MAINTAINED PAIN IN CLINICAL PRACTICE

For over a century military physicians have reported cases of persistent burning pain in soldiers who sustained traumatic partial peripheral nerve injury. Typically in such cases the pain is accompanied by hyperalgesia (currently defined as "an increased response to a stimulus which is normally painful"), allodynia (currently defined as "pain due to a stimulus which does not normally provoke pain"), and distal extremity swelling. In 1865, Mitchell coined the term *causalgia* (literally "burning pain") to describe such cases (10). Leriche reported in 1916 that sympathectomy dramatically relieves causalgia (11). This procedure was found to be effective in large series reports from military physicians in wars throughout the 20th century, including the Iran-Iraq war (12).

Later it became apparent that sympathetically maintained pain can also affect civilians and that it may develop after injuries not involving nerve trauma, such as bone fractures, and also after diverse illnesses, such as severe infection, stroke, and myocardial infarction. Those cases also found relief with sympathetic blockade. Evans in 1946 coined the term *reflex sympathetic dystrophy* to diagnose such cases (13).

The International Association for the Study of Pain introduced the term "complex regional pain syndrome" (CRPS) in 1994 to replace the terms causalgia and reflex sympathetic dystrophy. One of the arguments for the taxonomic change was the inconstant evidence of sympathetic hyperactivity in such instances. CRPS type 1 was introduced to substitute reflex sympathetic dystrophy, and CRPS type 2 was to be used instead of causalgia (14).

CONTROVERSY OVER THE SYMPATHETICALLY MAINTAINED PAIN CONCEPT

The clinical observations in favor of the sympathetically maintained pain concept can be summarized as follows: (a) Pain is spatially correlated with autonomic alterations, (b) sympatholytic maneuvers diminish the pain intensity, and (c) application of norepinephrine, the sympathetic neurotransmitter, rekindles the pain (7).

(a) *Pain is spatially correlated with autonomic alterations.* In CRPS type I temperature changes occur in the affected limb. In early stages, vasodilation induces increased local temperature. Later, the vasculature may develop sensitivity to catecholamines, possibly related to up-regulation of adrenoceptors, and decreased local temperature may supervene. Hyperhidrosis typically accompanies the temperature changes.

(b) *Sympatholytic maneuvers diminish pain intensity.* As described above, historically this has been the main

argument in favor of the sympathetically maintained pain concept. Different techniques are used to accomplish this task: surgical interruption of the sympathetic nerves proximal to the affected site, injection of local anesthetic around the sympathetic paravertebral ganglia that project to the affected body part, regional intravenous application of adrenergic blocking agents such as guanethidine or reserpine, or systemic intravenous infusion of phentolamine.

(c) *Local application of catecholamines rekindles the pain.* This phenomenon has been described in different types of neuropathic pain. After limb amputation, injection of epinephrine around the stump neuroma is intensely painful. Similar response has been observed in posttraumatic or postherpetic neuralgias (7).

A more physiologic adrenergic stimulus has been recently used. Baron et al. reported that whole body cooling induces endogenous catecholamines production and also worsens the pain and hyperalgesia in CRPS (15).

ARGUMENTS AGAINST THE SYMPATHETICALLY MAINTAINED PAIN CONCEPT

Several authorities in the field seriously doubt the sympathetically maintained pain concept, pointing to the scarcity of controlled clinical studies supporting this idea, the lack of specificity of sympathetic blockade procedures that involve not only sympathetic fibers but also somatic nerves, and the lack of correlation between pain and sympathetic dysfunction. Another argument used against this concept is the prominent psychiatric component that some patients with this diagnosis display (16).

AUTONOMIC NERVOUS SYSTEM DYSFUNCTION IN FIBROMYALGIA

Bengtssong and Bengtssong published in 1988 the first study of autonomic dysfunction in fibromyalgia (17). It was a controlled therapeutic trial of stellate ganglion blockade. They reported marked improvement of regional pain and tenderness in response to this maneuver, in contrast to the lack of effect to a sham injection in the neck area. Subsequently, Vaeroy et al., using Doppler probes to measure skin blood flow in the hands, found that FM patients have less vasoconstrictory response to acoustic stimulation and cooling. They concluded that the cutaneous manifestations of FM previously interpreted as Raynaud phenomenon should be reconsidered (18). These two seminal studies raised the possibility of sympathetic nervous system involvement in the pathogenesis of FM. Later, Elam et al. recorded muscle sympathetic activity with microelectrodes placed at the peroneal nerve level (19). They found no exaggerated sympathetic activity in FM subjects; nevertheless, these patients displayed less pronounced sympathetic activity in response to muscle contraction.

Since the publication of these seminal studies, little attention was paid to dysautonomia in FM until recently, with the introduction of heart rate variability and tilt table testing in the study of FM pathogenesis.

HEART RATE VARIABILITY ANALYSIS AND TILT TABLE TESTING IN FIBROMYALGIA

Our group has used heart rate variability analysis to assess ANS function in patients with FM. Our first study was short term and was intended primarily to define the response of the ANS to a simple active orthostatic stress (to stand up). Our main result showed that when compared to controls, patients with FM failed to increase low frequency ("sympathetic") band power as a response to the upright posture (20). This orthostatic sympathetic derangement has been confirmed by Kelemen et al. (21) and by Raj et al. (22), using the same method. Bou-Holaigah et al. used tilt table testing to assess the response of FM patients to passive orthostatic stress. They found that during upright tilt 12 of 20 FM patients (60%), but no controls, had abnormal drop in systolic blood pressure of at least 25 mm Hg and no associated increase in heart rate (23).

Therefore, this body of evidence strongly suggests that there is an orthostatic sympathetic derangement in patients with FM.

As technology and knowledge of heart rate variability evolved, we undertook a long-term study in patients with FM. This was intended to assess the circadian behavior of the ANS. Patients and controls wore a Holter monitor for 24 hours while performing their routine daily activities. Both time domain and frequency domain analyses demonstrated that patients with FM have changes consistent with relentless sympathetic hyperactivity during 24 hours. This alteration was particularly evident at night (24). This sympathetic hyperactivity in FM has been confirmed by Cohen et al. in both women and men using short-term (20 minutes) frequency domain analysis (25,26) and by Raj et al. using both time and frequency domain analyses during 24 hours (22).

Therefore, we can conclude that some patients with FM display prominent dysautonomia when studied by means of heart rate variability analysis or tilt table test, or both. This dysautonomia can be characterized as a sympathetic nervous system that is persistently *hyperactive* but *hyporeactive* to stress. This apparent paradox (sympathetic hyperactivity with hyporeactivity), nevertheless agrees with the basic physiologic principle demonstrating that chronic hyperstimulation of the beta-adrenergic receptors leads to receptor desensitization and down-regulation.

The hyporeactivity to stress concurs with the early reports of Vaeroy et al. (18) and Elam et al. (19), showing that FM patients have less peripheral sympathetic response to acoustic stimulation, cooling, or muscle contraction.

DYSAUTONOMIA MAY HELP EXPLAIN THE MULTISYSTEM FEATURES OF FIBROMYALGIA SYNDROME

FM is a multisystem illness. The multicenter study that led to the American College of Rheumatology (ACR) diagnostic criteria for FM stated that, besides its defining features (chronic widespread pain and tenderness at palpation in specific locations), patients with FM have significantly higher rates of diverse clinical manifestations when compared to patients with other rheumatic diseases. Such distinctive features are sleep disorders, fatigue, paresthesias, headache, anxiety, sicca symptoms, Raynaud phenomenon, morning stiffness, and irritable bowel (27). So any valid theory attempting to explain the pathogenesis of FM should first give a coherent explanation for the presence of these disparate features in the same patient.

ANS dysfunction may explain the diverse clinical manifestations of FM. It is suggested that due to a ceiling effect, the hyperactive sympathetic nervous system of such patients becomes unable to further respond to different stressors, thus explaining the constant fatigue and morning stiffness these patients have. Relentless sympathetic hyperactivity may explain sleep disorders, anxiety, pseudo-Raynaud phenomenon, sicca symptoms, and intestinal irritability (28). We recently performed concurrent analyses of heart rate variability and polysomnography in ten subjects with FM and compared them to an age/sex-matched control group. We confirmed our original electrocardiographic findings showing changes consistent with nocturnal sympathetic hyperactivity. Such changes coincided with increased nocturnal arousal-awakening episodes (29). Other investigators have shown that in normal sleeping persons, electrocardiographic signs of sympathetic surge precede arousal/awakening episodes. This body of evidence suggests that in FM, sympathetic hyperactivity causes the excessive arousal/awakening episodes (29).

FIBROMYALGIA AS A SYMPATHETICALLY MAINTAINED NEUROPATHIC PAIN SYNDROME

The defining FM features (widespread pain plus tenderness at palpation on specific anatomical points), as well as the paresthesias that these patients have, could theoretically be explained by the pathogenesis known as "sympathetically maintained pain" (30). The clinical manifestations of this type of neuropathic pain are characterized by its frequent posttraumatic onset and by the presence of stimuli-independent pain perception that is accompanied by paresthesias and allodynia. These are precisely FM pain features: Different controlled studies have determined that subjects with FM have higher rates of physical or emotional trauma prior to the onset of their symptoms. FM is clearly a stimulus-independent pain state since there is no underlying structural damage and inflammatory signs are conspicuously absent. Most patients with FM have paresthesias, as demonstrated in the original study that led to the ACR criteria. In this study over 80% of patients with FM had such sensory alteration. Simms and Goldenberg corroborated the extremely high prevalence of paresthesias (30). We used a questionnaire that is part of the Leeds Assessment of Neuropathic Symptoms and Signs Pain Scale. This instrument was developed to recognize neuropathic pain and set it apart from nociceptive pain. The questionnaire contains five items exploring five domains within the paresthesia syndrome. Our study showed that the overwhelming majority of patients with FM give assenting responses to questions pertaining to dysesthetic, evoked, paroxysmal, and thermal domains. This response rate was markedly different from that given by patients with active rheumatoid arthritis (31). Several groups of investigators have found that the typical FM tender points (TePs) reflect a state of generalized hyperalgesia (32). Hyperalgesia in the absence of underlying tissue damage strongly suggests a neuropathic etiology of the pain. It is interesting to note that most FM TePs are located in the neck area, a zone with a very rich sympathetic ganglia network. Nowhere else in the body are the sympathetic ganglia so near to the skin.

Experimental evidence now supports the clinical impression of FM as sympathetically maintained neuropathic pain syndrome. A prospective double-blind study demonstrated that 80% of subjects with FM have norepinephrine-evoked pain, compared to 30% of patients with rheumatoid arthritis or normal controls (33).

A prototype of sympathetically maintained pain syndrome is reflex sympathetic dystrophy (nowadays named CRPS type I). There are important points of coincidence between reflex sympathetic dystrophy and FM. We propose that FM is a generalized form of reflex sympathetic dystrophy (34).

MANAGEMENT OF DYSAUTONOMIA IN PATIENTS WITH FIBROMYALGIA

When discussing the management of dysautonomia in FM, it is important to first emphasize several points. The ANS is the main homeostatic system; therefore it regulates the function of most organs and systems of the body. As a consequence, a great variety of therapeutic modalities have secondary autonomic side effects. Several drugs already tested in FM, such as antidepressants and tranquilizing agents, have clear autonomic consequences. It is also important to note that the recognition of dysautonomia in FM is recent; therefore there are no controlled studies assessing the efficacy of drugs that directly affect autonomic neurotransmitters on the diverse manifestations of this painful syndrome. What will be discussed in this section deals with theoretically promising therapies focused on correcting autonomic abnormalities. Again, it is important to note that, unless otherwise stated, these are unproven remedies that should first be tested by appropriate clinical research before they are considered for clinical use (35).

NONPHARMACOLOGIC THERAPIES

Since sympathetic hyperactivity is prevalent in FM, it seems wise to ask patients to avoid the intake of sympathomimetic products such as nicotine, caffeine-containing soft drinks, and coffee. Graded aerobic exercise has a proven benefit for FM symptoms (36); this type of exercise also improves resting vagal tone (37). Biofeedback, a mind-body therapy technique that improves sympatho/vagal balance, when analyzed by heart rate variability studies (38) has been found to enrich

self-efficacy for function as well as to improve TeP score in patients with FM (36).

As discussed before, many patients with FM have orthostatic hypotension. Based on what is recommended for patients with idiopathic orthostatic hypotension (39), we suggest that patients with FM have a liberal intake of water with a high mineral content. It is my impression that this simple therapy may improve patients' well-being, particularly their chronic fatigue. The use of fitted stockings to the waist is another measure that may decrease blood pooling in the legs.

PHARMACOLOGIC THERAPIES

The use of medications should be reserved for those cases in which the intensity of the symptoms markedly constrains patients' quality of life. It is clear that in this chronic illness with dramatic manifestations in diverse organs and systems of the body, polypharmacy should be avoided.

Mounting evidence suggests that FM patients lose their autonomic circadian rhythmicity with nocturnal sympathetic hyperactivity; this alteration likely induces the sleep disorders. When insomnia is prominent, we recommend beginning with low dosages of sleep-inducing medications—that is, clonazepam 0.25 to 0.5 mg HS. When anxiety is also evident during the day, we add clonazepam 0.125 mg after breakfast and lunch.

We seldom use tricyclic antidepressants unless there is associated depression. Although this type of medication has proven its short-term efficacy in FM when assessed by double-blind studies, in our experience side effects such as anxiety, dizziness, and xerostomia limit its usefulness.

In view of the relentless sympathetic hyperactivity that these patients have, it seems logical to use adrenergic blocking agents. We have used, in selected cases (young patients with prominent autonomic manifestations such as palpitations, clammy hands, orthostatic tachycardia, and/or profound fatigue), low dosages of the β blocking agent propranolol (i.e., 10 mg t.i.d.). α-Adrenergic blocking agents would theoretically be useful in FM pain, since in sympathetically maintained pain syndromes primary nociceptors start to express α adrenoceptors. Nevertheless, current available α blocking agents have profound cardiovascular effects that will probably make them unfit for this type of clinical use.

Fludrocortisone with a starting dose of 1 mg per day may help to increase blood volume, thus avoiding orthostatic hypotension. It should be noted, however, that a double-blind study found that this medication given as monotherapy to patients with chronic fatigue syndrome failed to improve their symptoms (40).

Serotonin has a similar chemical structure and colocalizes with norepinephrine in different receptor sites. Low dosages (5 mg) of tropisetron, a highly selective and competitive 5-HT3-receptor antagonist, were found to be effective in FM in a double-blind short-term (10 days) study. Higher dosages lost their therapeutic benefit, suggesting a bell-shaped dose response curve (41). Interestingly, in a different study by the same research group, in which they measured circulating catecholamines, those patients with elevated basal dopamine tended to show a higher response rate to tropisetron (42).

Since FM pain has been proposed to have a neuropathic etiology (31), drugs used in diverse types of neuropathies could theoretically have a beneficial effect for FM subjects. Gabapentin is being used as an off-label indication. We prescribe this compound in escalating dosages in patients with marked paresthesias. We start with 300 mg at night and slowly increase it to no more than 1,500 mg in three divided doses. Xylocaine is a potent sodium channel blocker. Raphael et al. used lignocaine intravenously in an open study. They injected up to 550 mg $\times$ day per 6 days as an in-hospital treatment. Most of their patients reported pain relief that lasted a mean of 11 weeks (43). This provocative investigation should be further evaluated in controlled studies. It is worth noting that new types of antineuropathic medications are in development, such as sodium channel blockers with greater analgesic than anticonvulsant index, new GABA-enhancing drugs, and N-methyl-D-aspartate (NMDA) antagonists, among others (44). Therefore, it will be important to follow closely the developments in antineuropathic therapies, as this knowledge may be also useful for FM treatment.

Dysautonomia provides a different perspective on the mechanisms that lead to FM. This new approach offers a coherent explanation for FM's multisystem symptoms, including its psychological component. The proposal of FM as a sympathetically maintained neuropathic pain syndrome may serve two purposes; on the one hand it validates FM pain as real, and on the other it provides an opportunity to examine the unfolding neuropathic pain research knowledge and apply it to the understanding of FM.

Of course, more research is needed to consolidate this paradigm.

SUMMARY POINTS

- In animal models sympathetic nervous system dysfunction is involved in the pathogenesis of chronic pain syndromes.
- Considerable data suggest that some individuals with FM and other central pain syndromes may have dysfunction of the autonomic nervous system.
- Such dysautonomia is characterized by ongoing sympathetic overactivity (which may be especially prominent at night) and an inability to respond appropriately to stressors.
- It is proposed that autonomic dysfunction explains FM multisystem features, and that FM is a sympathetically maintained pain syndrome.

▪ IMPLICATIONS FOR PRACTICE

- Individuals with central pain syndromes with symptoms suggestive of dysautonomia may respond to specific therapies aimed at improving such autonomic dysfunction.

REFERENCES

1. Lefkowitz RJ, Hoffman BB, Taylor P. Neurotransmission. The autonomic and somatic nervous system. In: Hardman JG, Limbird LE, eds. *Goodman & Gilman's The pharmacological basis of therapeutics*, 9th ed. New York: McGraw-Hill, 1996: 105–140.
2. Landsberg L, Young JB. Physiology and pharmacology of the autonomic nervous system. In: Braunwald E, Fauci AS, Kasper DL et al., eds. *Harrison's Principles of Internal Medicine*, 15th ed. New York: McGraw-Hill, 2001:438–450.
3. Zubieta JK, Heitzeg MM, Smith YR, et al. COMT val158met genotype affects mu-opioid neurotransmitter responses to a pain stressor. *Science* 2003;299:1240–1243.
4. Hermosillo AG, Marquez MF, Jauregui-Renau K, et al. Orthostatic hypotension 2001. *Cardiol Rev* 2001;9:339–341.
5. Task force of the European Society of Cardiology and the North American Society of Pacing and Electrophysiology. Heart rate variability standards of measurement, physiological interpretation, and clinical use. *Circulation* 1996;93: 1043–1065.
6. Lamarre-Cliche M, Cusson J. The fainting patients: value of the head-upright tilt-table test in adult patients with orthostatic intolerance. *CMAJ* 2001;164:372–376.
7. Baron R, Levina JD, Fields HL. Causalgia and reflex sympathetic dystrophy: does the sympathetic nervous system contribute to the generation of pain? *Muscle Nerve* 1999;22: 678–695.
8. Sato J, Perl ER. Adrenergic excitation of cutaneous pain receptors induced by peripheral nerve injury. *Science* 1991; 251:1608–1610.
9. McLachlan EM, Jäning W, Devor M, et al. Peripheral nerve injury triggers noradrenergic sprouting within dorsal root ganglia. *Nature* 1993;363:543–546.
10. Mitchell SW. *Injuries of nerves and their consequence*. New York: Dover, 1865.
11. Leriche R. De la causalgia envisagee comme une nevrite du sympathique et de son traitement par la denudation et l'excision des plexus nerveus peri-arteriels. *Presse Med* 1916;24: 178–180.
12. Hassantash SA, Maier RV. Sympathectomy for causalgia: experience with military injuries. *J Trauma* 2000;49: 266–271.
13. Evans JA. Reflex sympathetic dystrophy. *Surg Clin North Am* 1946;26:435–448.
14. Merskey H, Boyduk N, eds. *Classification of chronic pain*. Seattle, WA: IASP Task Force on Taxonomy, IASP Press, 1994.
15. Baron R, Schattschneider J, Binder A, et al. Relationship between sympathetic vasoconstrictor activity and pain and hyperalgesia in complex regional pain syndrome: a case-control study. *Lancet* 2002;359:1655–1660.
16. Ochoa JL, Verdugo RJ. Reflex sympathetic dystrophy. A common clinical avenue for somatoform expression. *Neurol Clin* 1995;13:351–363.
17. Bengtsson A, Bengtsson M. Regional sympathetic blockade in primary fibromyalgia. *Pain* 1988;33:161–167.
18. Vaeroy H, Qiao Z, Morkrid L, et al. Altered sympathetic nervous system response in patients with fibromyalgia. *J Rheumatol* 1989;16:1460–1465.
19. Elam M, Johansson G, Wallin BG. Do patients with primary fibromyalgia have an altered muscle sympathetic nerve activity? *Pain* 1992;48:371–375.
20. Martinez-Lavin M, Hermosillo AG, Mendoza C, et al. Orthostatic sympathetic derangement in subject with fibromyalgia. *J Rheumatol* 1997;24:714–718.
21. Kelemen J, Lang E, Balint G, et al. Orthostatic sympathetic derangement of baroreflex in patients with fibromyalgia. *J Rheumatol* 1998;25:823–825.
22. Raj RR, Brouillard D, Simpsom CS, et al. Dysautonomia among patients with fibromyalgia: a noninvasive assessment. *J Rheumatol* 2000;27:2660–2665.

23. Bou-Holaigah I, Calkins H, Flynn JA, et al. Provocation of hypotension and pain during upright tilt table testing in adults with fibromyalgia. *Clin Exp Rheumatol* 1997;15: 239–246.

24. Martinez-Lavin M, Hermosillo AG, Rosas M, et al. Circadian studies of autonomic nervous balance in patients with fibromyalgia. A heart rate variability analysis. *Arthritis Rheum* 1998;42:1966–1971.

25. Cohen H, Neumann L, Shore M, et al. Autonomic dysfunction in patients with fibromyalgia: application of power spectral analysis of heart rate variability. *Semin Arthritis Rheum* 2000;29:217–227.

26. Cohen H, Neumann L, Alhosshle A, et al. Abnormal sympathovagal balance in men with fibromyalgia. *J Rheumatol* 2001;28:581–589.

27. Wolfe F, Smythe HA, Yunus MB, et al. The American College of Rheumatology 1990 criteria for the classification of fibromyalgia: report of the Multicenter Criteria Committee. *Arthritis Rheum* 1999;33:160–171.

28. Martinez-Lavin M, Hermosillo AG. Autonomic nervous system dysfunction may explain the multisystem features of fibromyalgia. *Semin Arthritis Rheum* 2000;29:197–199.

29. Kooh M, Martínez-Lavin M, Meza S, et al. Concurrent heart rate variability and polysomnography analyses in fibromyalgia patients. *Clin Exp Rheumatol* 2003;21:529–530.

30. Simms RW, Goldenberg DL. Symptoms mimicking neurologic disorders in fibromyalgia syndrome. *J Rheumatol* 1988;15:1271–1273.

31. Martinez-Lavin M, Lopez S, Medina M, et al. Use of the Leeds Assessment of Neuropathic Symptoms and Signs questionnaire in patients with fibromyalgia. *Semin Arthritis Rheum* 2003;32:407–411.

32. Russell J. Hyperalgesia. Advances in fibromyalgia: possible role for central neurochemicals. *Am J Med Sci* 1998;315: 377–384.

33. Martínez-Lavín M, Vidal M, Barbosa RE, et al. Norepinephrine-evoked pain in fibromyalgia. A randomized pilot study. ISCRTN 70707830. *BMC Musculoskelet Disord* 2002;3:2.

34. Martinez-Lavin M. Is fibromyalgia a generalized reflex sympathetic dystrophy? *Clin Exp Rheumatol* 2001;19:1–3.

35. Martínez-Lavín M. Management of dysautonomia in fibromyalgia. *Rheum Dis Clin North Am* 2002;28:379–387.

36. Hadhazy VA, Ezzo J, Creamer P, et al. Mind-body therapies for the treatment of fibromyalgia. A systematic review. *J Rheumatol* 2000;27:2911–2918.

37. O'Sullivan SE, Bell C. The effects of exercise and training on human cardiovascular reflex control. *J Auton Nerv Syst* 2000;81:16–24.

38. Cowan MJ, Kogan H, Burr R, et al. Power spectral analysis of heart rate variability after biofeedback training. *J Electrocardiol* 1990;23:85–94.

39. Jordan J. New trends in the treatment of orthostatic hypotension. *Curr Hypertens Rep* 2001;3:216–226.

40. Rowe PC, Calkins H, DeBusk K, et al. Fludrocortisone acetate to treat neurally mediated hypotension in chronic fatigue syndrome: a randomized controlled trial. *JAMA* 2001;285:52–59.

41. Farber L, Stratz T, Bruckle W et al., German Fibromyalgia Study Group. Efficacy and tolerability of tropisetron in primary fibromyalgia—a highly selective and competitive 5-HT3 receptor antagonist. *Scand J Rheumatol Suppl* 2000; 113:49–54.

42. Hochert K, Farber L, Landenburger S, et al. Effect of tropisetron on circulating catecholamines and other putative biochemical markers in serum of patients with fibromyalgia. *Scand J Rheumatol Suppl* 2000;113:46–48.

43. Raphael JH, Southall JL, Treherne GJ, et al. Efficacy and adverse effects of intravenous lignocaine therapy in fibromyalgia syndrome. *BMC Musculoskelet Disord* 2002;3: 21.

44. Woolf CJ, Mannion RJ. Neuropathic pain: etiology, symptoms, mechanisms, and management. *Lancet* 1999;353:1959–1964.

8

Functional Imaging of Pain

Richard H. Gracely and Laurence A. Bradley

Fibromyalgia (FM) is a significant medical problem characterized by chronic, widespread pain. Among rheumatology disorders, FM is second in prevalence only to rheumatoid arthritis, afflicting 2% to 4% of the U.S. population. In contrast to many other prevalent conditions, the mechanisms that initiate and maintain the symptoms of FM are largely unknown and treatment options are few and only modestly effective.

Recent advances in methods that assess the location and time course of neural activity in the brain have provided considerable evidence for supraspinal mechanisms that mediate a wide range of medical conditions. This chapter describes the recent use of functional brain imaging techniques in studies of FM. It begins with a brief description of the peripheral pain nervous system, describes the development and application of functional brain imaging methods, and reviews the application of these methods to patients with this prevalent, painful disorder.

THE AFFERENT PAIN SYSTEM: FROM RECEPTOR TO BRAIN

Sensory fibers (primary afferents) that innervate all body tissues respond to heat, cold, and mechanical pressure, as well as to chemical and metabolic (e.g., bradykinin, low pH) stimuli. These fibers include nociceptors that respond to noxious stimuli that are associated with potential or actual tissue damage. Signals from these nociceptors are transmitted to the spinal cord and brain. These primary afferents are composed of thinly myelinated Aδ and unmyelinated C fibers that differ in function. Some Aδ fiber nociceptors respond specifically to noxious mechanical stimuli, noxious thermal stimuli, or both. However, Aδ afferents are rapidly activated and transmit signals that tend to produce perceptions of relatively sharp pain that is referred to as "first pain." First pain serves as a warning to avoid tissue-damaging stimuli that may threaten the individual's integrity. In contrast, most C fiber nociceptors respond to a range of noxious mechanical, thermal, and chemical stimuli—in some cases not unless they are first sensitized by inflammatory agents. C fiber afferents conduct more slowly than the Aδ afferents and tend to produce perceptions of aching or burning pain that is referred to as "second pain." Second pain is diffuse, prolonged, and aversive and is the main component of pain associated with chronic medical conditions (1).

Nociceptor afferents enter the spinal cord (1) via the dorsal roots and terminate in lamina I, II, and V of the superficial dorsal horn. Activity in these nociceptors releases at their terminals excitatory neurotransmitters that activate secondary projection neurons. Excitatory transmitters include glutamate, which activates postsynaptic N-methyl-D-aspartate (NMDA) receptors, and Substance P and neurokinin A (NK), which activate postsynaptic NK receptors. NK receptors are also activated by calcitonin gene-related peptide (CGRP), nerve growth factor (NGF), and dynorphin A (2). Neurons in lamina I and II respond to specific noxious stimuli within small receptive fields (e.g., in muscle or joint). These second order neurons are termed "nociceptive specific" (NS) and are dominated by Aδ fiber input. Nociceptive neurons in lamina V respond to both noxious and nonnoxious mechanical stimuli and are termed "wide-dynamic range" (WDR) neurons.

The secondary neurons that originate within the dorsal horn ascend in three primary contralateral tracts that project to the thalamus and reticular formation. The largest input is from the spinothalamic tract, which provides a major nociceptive input to lateral, medial, and posterior thalamic nuclei (3). Direct spinothalamic tract projections to the ventroposterior lateral (VPL) and ventroposterior inferior (VPI) nucleus activate thalamic neurons that in turn project to the primary (S1) and secondary (S2) somatosensory cortices. These cortical regions are involved in sensory-discriminative aspects of pain as well as in the anticipation of painful stimuli (4). Spinothalamic tract projections to the posterior thalamic nuclei (i.e., pulvinar oralis, suprageniculate nucleus) activate neurons that project to the insular cortex, which has interconnections with the amygdala, prefrontal cortex, and cingulate cortex, forming a network involved in affective, cognitive, and autonomic responses to nociception. The insular and prefrontal cortices likely integrate nociceptive signals with memory of previous events, providing meaning and identifying potential threats associated with sources of painful stimuli (5).

89

A group of fibers in the anterior part of the anterolateral spinothalamic tract project to the gigantocellular part of the medulla and pons and to the lateral reticular nucleus, and third order neurons from these regions terminate in the medial geniculate body, the posterior group, and the intralaminar nuclei of the thalamus (3). The intralaminar nuclei are considered to be a cranial extension of the brain stem reticular formation and interconnect with both the prefrontal cortex and the cingulate cortex. The anterior cingulate cortex is a limbic region that is involved in the integration of cognition, affect, and response selection. A circuit from anterior cingulate cortex to the medial thalamic nuclei and to the periaqueductal gray (PAG) in the brainstem suggests that anterior cingulate cortex may also be involved in the modulation of reflex responses to noxious stimuli.

In addition to the major spinothalamocortical projection system, there are at least two other prominent pathways from the spinal cord to the brain (6). One pathway projects to the ventromedian nucleus of the thalamus and the dorsolateral frontal lobes via the dorsocaudal medulla (subnucleus reticularis dorsalis) (7). Another system projects to the parabrachial nucleus. The parabrachial nucleus, in turn, projects to the hypothalamus and amygdala (8), to the frontal cortices via intralaminar thalamus, and to the central nucleus of the amygdala and on to the basal forebrain (9,10). These pathways likely help mediate the interactions between pain and the cognitive and emotional responses observed in humans.

EVALUATION OF PAIN PROCESSING IN THE BRAIN

METHODOLOGY

A number of methods can be used to evaluate neural activity in the human brain. The simplest and oldest method is based on the use of scalp recording electrodes to assess a stimulus-evoked synchronized response in the electroencephalogram (EEG), which is almost always embedded in nonsynchronized EEG activity. Averaging the response to multiple stimuli reduces the random effects of nonsynchronized activity and results in a characteristic wave form of positive and negative peaks termed the cortical evoked potential (CEP). Analgesic agents often modify the magnitudes of specific components of the CEP, and this method has been proposed to be a nonverbal correlate of subjective pain (11). Although this association may be valid under specific circumstances, CEPs and verbal reports can be dissociated in a number of situations, including simple active or passive movement (12). CEPs recorded from the scalp by a single active electrode provide exceptional temporal resolution but no spatial information. Using this method, functional neuroimaging of the human brain can be accomplished to some degree by use of a large number of electrodes distributed over the scalp and by use of source analysis to locate the origins of the evoked activity (13). Alternatively, activity in cortical structures can be recorded directly by application of electrode arrays to brain tissue during neurosurgical procedures (14).

Electrical currents generate magnetic fields, and the minute magnetic fields generated by the neural activity associated with CEPs can be imaged by specialized devices that use supercooled detectors to measure these magnetic fields. The magnetoencephalograph (MEG) is measured using a Superconducting QUantum Interference Device, (SQUID). The SQUID neuromagnetometer is very sensitive to stray magnetic fields, so this elaborate piece of equipment must be housed in specially shielded rooms. Thus, in terms of expense and complexity, MEG is in the same class as other elaborate neuroimaging systems described below. Operationally, the use of MEG to image brain function is very similar to CEP methods. Evoked neural activity is measured with multiple sensors. Both methods provide the highest temporal resolutions of about 1 ms, but spatial localization requires software that solves the inverse problem of modeling the neural generators responsible for the pattern of evoked activity. MEG may provide better resolution than CEPs, in the range of a few millimeters.

Both CEP and MEG methods assess responses to brief stimuli with temporally precise onsets, such as provided by electrical, laser, and acoustic sources, or by well-controlled mechanical stimulation. These methods are not useful for stimuli that do not have such characteristics, such as blunt pressure used for assessment of tenderness in FM. In contrast, methods that analyze the spontaneous EEG can be used to assess the effects of all types of stimuli, including stimuli that are poorly controlled or stimuli without precise onsets. Thus the effects of blunt pressure, exercising an ischemic limb, or immersion of a limb in cold water, which cannot be assessed by the methods such as CEPs, can be assessed in terms of alterations in spontaneous EEG. These types of responses appear to be modulated by the presence of chronic pain syndromes (15), including FM (16).

The majority of recent interest has been in methods that do not measure neural activity directly but use specialized equipment to infer neural activity from highly localized increases in regional cerebral blood flow (rCBF) that occur in response to anticipated neural metabolic demand. The local increase in rCBF can be imaged by infusion of radioactive tracers with methods such as single-photon-emission computed tomography (SPECT) or positron-emission tomography (PET). In the case of functional magnetic resonance imaging (fMRI), the different magnetic properties of oxygenated and deoxygenated blood serve as an intrinsic tracer. Ferrous metal objects interfere with the MRI signal; a hairpin can cause a black region in a head MRI. Deoxygenated blood is paramagnetic and causes a similar, slight depression of fMRI signal from nearby tissue. Localized increases in rCBF in response to neural activity overcompensate for the amount of required oxygen. The result is a localized increase in the concentration of oxygenated blood and a decrease in the concentration of deoxygenated blood, which in turn results in decreased suppression (decreased hairpin effect) of the fMRI signal from nearby tissue. This effect produces the "blood oxygen level dependent" (BOLD) fMRI signal.

The various imaging methods differ in their ability to assess baseline rCBF and in temporal and spatial resolution. One advantage of the early methods of SPECT and PET is that they can assess static rCBF—for example, comparing the baseline neural activity among different patient populations. Relative disadvantages are the need to infuse radioactive tracers and modest temporal and spatial resolution. The time needed for a single image of the entire brain is approximately 30 minutes with SPECT, 1 minute with PET, and 2 seconds with fMRI. Localization improves accordingly; fMRI methods now allow visualization of activity in discrete regions such as thalamic nuclei. However, fMRI designs must repeatedly switch between conditions since the magnitude of the differential signal is relatively small and, in some cases, similar to the magnitude of longitudinal signal changes caused by drifts in scanner sensitivity. Thus AB designs, such as imaging before and after a long-lasting drug, are more appropriately performed with methods such as PET.

APPLICATION

The first demonstration of pain-induced changes in rCBF were made by Ingvar et al. (17), who demonstrated low-resolution increases in frontal cortex produced by painful electrical stimulation of the fingers of eight subjects. The modern era of pain functional neuroimaging began in the early 1990s with two studies using PET imaging to painful heat. Talbot et al. (18) demonstrated heat pain-related activity in primary (S1) and secondary (S2) somatosensory cortex and in the anterior cingulate cortex. Jones et al. (19) showed heat pain-related activity also in anterior cingulate cortex, and in the lateral thalamus and basal ganglion. In the following decade most of the neuroimaging studies of healthy individuals have replicated and elaborated on these patterns of pain-evoked activity. The accumulated evidence shows that phasic thermal nociceptive stimuli tend to increase activity in a network of structures in the contralateral hemisphere, including S1, S2, thalamus, and insular and anterior cingulate cortices.

On the basis of these first-generation studies, recent experiments have begun to examine issues such as the coding of changes in stimulus intensity, neural representations of individual differences in pain sensitivity, effects of experimental manipulations of pain-related affect, and brain activity associated with analgesic responses. For example, a recent PET study found that graded thermal stimuli (35°C to 50°C) resulted in associated increases in activity in contralateral S1, ipsilateral premotor area, and contralateral and ipsilateral cerebellum, putamen, thalamus, insular cortex, anterior cingulate cortex, and S2 (5). In a subsequent study these investigators also found a significant effect for perceived pain intensity across subjects. The pain rating to a constant 49°C painful heat stimulus was associated with activity in S1, prefrontal cortex, and in anterior cingulate cortex (20). These findings suggest specialization in processing the sensory and cognitive-affective dimensions of pain, with the processing of pain intensity distributed across multiple regions in both cerebral hemispheres.

A series of studies using hypnosis to selectively modify specific components of the pain experience supports the concept of separate processing systems for the sensory discriminative and affective dimensions of pain. Hypnotic suggestions to increase or decrease the perceived unpleasantness of noxious, tonic heat stimuli altered numerical ratings of unpleasantness without changing ratings of pain intensity (21). These suggestions also resulted in altered activity in the anterior cingulate cortex, rostral insular cortex, and S1. The changes in activity in the anterior cingulate cortex were correlated ($r = 0.42$) with

hypnosis-induced changes in pain unpleasantness ratings. Subsequent studies showed a complementary effect. Hypnotic suggestions of increased sensory intensity produced significant increases in ratings of both pain intensity and pain unpleasantness (22); altered pain intensity ratings were associated only with significant increases in activation in S1 (23).

EVALUATION OF PAIN PROCESSING IN FIBROMYALGIA

The pioneering application of brain functional imaging to patients with FM used SPECT; Mountz et al. (24) used SPECT to evaluate baseline levels of rCBF in ten patients with FM and in seven healthy control subjects. In this initial study, patients received infusions of approximately 25 m Ci of ^{99m}Tc-HMPAO, a radioactive tracer that permits imaging rCBF with this method. After the infusion the subjects underwent a 32-minute SPECT scan. This method resulted in a semiquantitative measure of rCBF with a resolution of about 8.5 mm. The analysis examined overall activity in larger areas of regions of interest (ROI) corresponding to the right and left thalamus and right and left head of the caudate nucleus. The results showed that patients, relative to controls, had lower rCBF, indicating lower neural activity during a quiescent resting state. Reduced neural activity was found both in the right and left thalamus and in the right and left caudate nucleus.

This initial investigation in ten patients was followed by a similar study by another group of investigators. Kwiatek et al. (25) used SPECT to assess resting rCBF in 17 patients with FM and in 22 healthy control subjects. These investigators observed decreased rCBF in the right thalamus but no decreases in either the left thalamus or in the caudate nuclei. These investigators also observed decreased rCBF in the inferior pontine tegmentum and near the right lentiform nucleus. In an example of correlational analyses over subjects described below for fMRI studies, these investigators also found no association between resting rCBF and a number of clinical variables, including psychometric measures of pain, depression, and anxiety; visual analog scale (VAS) measures of pain, sleep, stiffness, lethargy, and work difficulties; and experimental pressure pain sensitivity determined at ACR-defined tender points (TePs) and control points and the TeP count.

The consistent finding of reduced rCBF in the right thalamus was also observed in a second study by the Mountz group (26), who examined the influence of additional factors on the SPECT results. These authors divided the sample of patients with fibromyalgia into those with a traumatic etiology ($n = 11$) and those with a more gradual onset ($n = 21$). Both patient groups, compared to 29 healthy controls, showed significantly decreased rCBF in the left and right thalamus. However, only patients with a gradual, atraumatic etiology showed reduced rCBF in the left and right caudate.

The finding of decreased rCBF in the thalamus and in the caudate nucleus is not unique to FM. Low rCBF has been observed in patients with pain due to traumatic peripheral neuropathy (27) and to metastatic breast cancer (28). The thalamus plays an important role in early pain processing and has extensive interconnections with sensory, motor, and limbic systems. Studies of the human thalamus during neurosurgical procedures, in which discrete regions are activated by electrical stimulation, have evoked entire experiences of acute clinical pain, including emotional dimensions of fear and panic (29,30). These studies emphasize the role of the thalamus in pain perception and also indicate a role in memory processes. The thalamus is also the last synaptic relay between the spinal cord and higher brain structures, providing the final opportunity to modulate pain signals before they spread to multiple neuronal and humoral systems.

Abnormally low rCBF levels in the caudate nucleus have been documented in patients with pain related to spinal cord injury (31) and restless leg syndrome (32). The caudate nucleus receives a large input from spinal pain pathways, including both NS neurons that signal the presence of pain and WDR neurons that provide graded responses throughout the range of innocuous and painful stimulation (33–35). The caudate nucleus may also be involved in intrinsic analgesia systems; electrical stimulation of the caudate evokes analgesia in both primate and human studies (36,37).

Although the cause of thalamic and caudate abnormalities in rCBF is unknown, inhibition of activity in these regions is associated with, and may likely result from, prolonged excitatory nociceptive input (27). Demonstration of a prolonged state of excitatory input in FM would provide a critical link between the clinical findings and neural mechanisms such as central sensitization (38).

A series of recent studies have applied the high-resolution of fMRI to address these hypotheses and further specify brain regions involved in the pain abnormalities associated with FM. The first study by Gracely et al. (39) developed measures of pressure sensitivity that were relatively immune to the biases shown to affect traditional clinical measures of tenderness such as the TeP count or even dolorimeter measures of tenderness (40,41). These methods were used before the fMRI scans to fully characterize the pressure pain sensitivity in patients and control subjects and also during the fMRI experiments. For each of 16 FM patients, these investigators determined the amount of pressure required to evoke a pain sensation described as near "slightly intense" on a 0 to 20 combined numerical-verbal pain scale that has been shown to be very sensitive in this population (42). Two pressures were determined for a matched group of 16 healthy control subjects. In the *equal pressure condition*, these subjects received close to the same pressures delivered to the patients. However, since the patients are by definition sensitive to pressure, these stimulus pressures did not produce these same intense pain sensations in the controls and were rated as faintly painful or as nonpainful pressure sensations. In the *equal pain condition*, the pressures delivered to the healthy control subjects were increased to levels (4.2 kg) that evoked the same ratings of slightly intense pain that were produced by significantly less pressure (2.4 kg, $p<0.05$) in the patients.

Unlike other studies that apply pressure to specific FM TePs, these studies applied blunt pressure (1-cm diameter hard rubber probe) to the thumbnail. This site was chosen for the dense innervation of the thumb and the large representation of the thumb in primary somatosensory cortex. In addition, this site implicitly acknowledges that the tenderness observed in FM is not confined to classical TePs; these are simply regions in which everyone is more tender, and

thus they more convenient for manual testing. The use of the thumb also implicitly implies that the tenderness observed in FM is not due to muscle sensitivity or confined to muscles, but rather is a property of deep tissue. The use of the thumb also assumes that this sensitivity is not localized to specific regions but is generally expressed over the entire body.

All subjects in this study first received a conventional MRI of the head to assist in the anatomical localization of evoked changes in rCBF, followed by fMRI. Each fMRI scanning session lasted a little over 10 minutes. During the session complete functional images of the entire brain and cerebellum were obtained every 5 seconds, with a resolution of 3 mm in all three dimensions. The experiment began after three scans, which serve to bring the tissue response to equilibrium and are discarded. Subjects received ten 1-minute cycles of stimulation. Each cycle consisted of 30 seconds of nonpainful pressure stimulation (typically 0.5 kg) followed by 30 seconds of painful stimulation. Since the fMRI scans are delivered at 5-second intervals, six scans were obtained for both the innocuous and the painful stimulation in each cycle, for a total of 60 innocuous and 60 painful scans for the ten cycles. For each subject, these scans are subjected to a number of preprocessing steps (correction for head motion, intensity normalization, spatial smoothing, and high pass filtering, reslicing to 2 mm^3 voxels [voxel is a three-dimensional equivalent of a two-dimensional pixel]), and then for each voxel, the magnitudes of the signal generated during the 60 innocuous and 60 painful scans are compared by a standard statistical t-test and the results are expressed as a Z-statistic. The result is a statistical volume, or map, of each subject's brain that represents the statistical results of the difference in stimulus conditions. To perform group analyses, each of these volumes is converted to standard coordinate space (43).

The 16 FM patients participated in a single 10-minute fMRI scanning session, while the healthy controls participated in both an equal pressure and an equal pain scanning session. These conditions are shown in the upper-left panel of Figure 8-1, which shows the relationship of stimulus pressure and evoked pain during the fMRI scans. The mean data for the patients is shown at the upper left; a moderate amount of pressure produced a high level of pain. The results for the controls are shown by the remaining two points; pressures similar to those delivered to the patients evoked only faint pain in the controls, while nearly twice the pressure delivered to the patients produced the same level of pain in the controls that the patients experienced. The purpose of the study was to compare the effects in the patients to the two control conditions. A result in which the effects in patients were similar to those in controls receiving the same pressure would suggest that there is no physiologic augmentation and supports psychological mechanisms such as hypervigilence or a change in labeling behavior. The alternative result in which the effects in patients matched those in controls experiencing the same level of pain would be consistent with mechanisms involving physiologic augmentation of pain sensitivity. The results shown in Figure 8-1 clearly support the latter hypothesis. Equally painful stimulation, produced by significantly less pressure in the patients, produced similar increases in neural activity in a network of brain structures implicated in pain processing. These increases were observed in structures

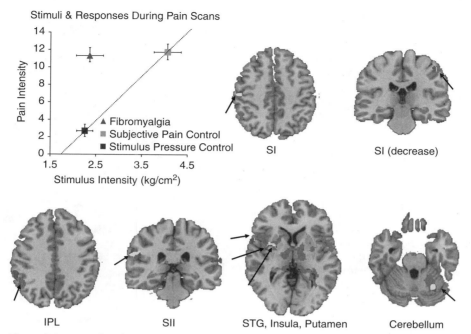

Figure 8-1. Functional magnetic resonance imaging (fMRI) responses to painful pressure applied to the left thumb in patients with fibromyalgia (FM) and healthy control subjects. The top left graph shows mean pain rating plotted against stimulus intensity for the experimental conditions. In the *Patient* condition, a relatively low stimulus pressure (2.4 kg/cm²) produced a high pain level (11.30 ± 0.90), shown by the triangle. In the *stimulus pressure control* condition, shown by the black square, administration of a similar stimulus pressure (2.33 kg/cm²) to control subjects produced a very low level of rated pain (3.05 ± 0.85). In the *subjective pain control* condition, shown by the gray square, administration of significantly greater stimulus pressures to the control subjects (4.16 kg/cm²) produced levels of pain (11.95 ± 0.94) similar to the levels produced in patients by lower stimulus pressures. The remainder of the figure shows common regions of activation in patients and in the *subjective pain control* condition, in which the effects of pressure applied to the left thumb sufficient to evoke a pain rating of 11 (moderate) is compared to the effects of innocuous pressure. Significant increases in the fMRI signal resulting from increases in regional cerebral blood flow (rCBF) are shown in standard space superimposed on an anatomical image of a standard brain (SPM96). Images are shown in radiologic view with the right brain shown on the left. Overlapping activations are shown by white shading. The similar pain intensities, produced by significantly less pressure in the patients, resulted in overlapping or adjacent activations in contralateral primary somatosensory cortex (SI), inferior parietal lobule (IPL), secondary somatosensory cortex (SII), superior temporal gyrus (STG), insula, putamen, and in ipsilateral cerebellum. The fMRI signal was significantly decreased in a common region in ipsilateral SI. (From Gracely RH, Petzke F, Wolf JM, et al. Functional MRI evidence of augmented pain processing in fibromyalgia. *Arthritis Rheum* 2002;46:1333–1343, with permission.)

involved in sensory discriminative processing (contralateral S1, S2), sensory association (contralateral superior temporal gyrus, inferior parietal lobule), motor response (contralateral putamen and ipsilateral cerebellum), and affective processing (contralateral insula). The two groups also shared a similar region of decreased signal in ipsilateral primary somatosensory cortex.

In contrast to the extensive common activations observed when comparing the equal pain conditions, there were no common activations when the equal pressure conditions were compared. Applying this low stimulus pressure to the healthy controls resulted in only two significant activations (in comparison to 12 in the patients), in the ipsilateral precentral gyrus and superior temporal gyrus. The effects of the low stimulus pressures in the patient and control groups

were also compared statistically by a t-test of the mean differences in signal between the two groups. The results further support an effect of pain augmentation in the FM patient group. The level of neural activity evoked by similar pain stimuli produced 13 regions of statistically greater activation in the patient group and only one region of greater activation in the control group (ipsilateral medial frontal gyrus). The regions of greater response in the patient group were in contralateral S1 cortex, inferior parietal lobule, insula, anterior and posterior cingulate cortex; ipsilateral S2 cortex; bilateral superior temporal gyrus; and cerebellum.

Neuroimaging of subjects' responses to stimulation revealed that, consistent with their verbal pain responses, both patients and controls exhibited significant increases in fMRI signal in the same brain regions (e.g., somatosensory cortices, insular cortex, putamen, cerebellum) in response to the stimulation. However, when the controls received pressure stimulation at the same low intensity levels delivered to patients, they showed significant signal increases in only two brain regions; neither of these regions overlapped with those activated within the patient group. These findings suggest that enhanced pain perception in persons with FM is associated with central augmentation of sensory input from the periphery.

This pivotal result indicates that the brain activations in patients and control subjects are consistent with verbal reports of pain magnitude. In each group of subjects reports of slightly intense pain are accompanied by activation in a network of brain structures implicated in pain processing. In addition, these results also show that in certain regions the response in FM patients was actually reduced in comparison to controls. The increased response in the caudate nucleus and in the thalamus observed in the control subjects was not found in FM. This lack of evoked responses is at first glance consistent with results observed in the resting state, in which FM showed reduced basal rCBF in caudate and thalamus (24). However, Gracely et al. (39) point out that this apparent consistency is not necessarily expected:

> Experimental determination of rCBF in the resting state should have little predictive value for evoked responses. Rather, comparison of both baseline flow and changes evoked by an intervention may provide more information about underlying mechanisms than can be provided by either result in isolation. For example, reduced baseline flow could permit a larger evoked response due to the classic physiological law of initial values, in which the reduced baseline permits a larger possible response up to a physiologic ceiling. Alternatively, reduced baseline flow might result from inhibitory processes that also attenuate evoked responses from the same region. The present findings of an attenuated increase of rCBF in contralateral (and possibly bilateral) caudate and in bilateral thalamus in patients with FM in this study along with previous findings of lowered resting rCBF in these structures in FM patients are consistent with a mechanism of tonic inhibition maintained by persistent excitatory input associated with ongoing and spontaneous pain.

The main result of augmented sensitivity to painful pressure in FM has been replicated recently by another laboratory using contact heat. Cook et al. (44) showed that similarly painful 10-second heat stimuli applied to the left hand—evoked by less heat in patients (mean 47.4°C) versus controls (48.3°C)—resulted in no significant differences in brain activation between a group of nine female FM patients and nine female healthy controls. In contrast, Figure 8-2 shows that similar painful stimulus temperatures resulted in significantly greater activations in the FM patients in contralateral insular cortex ($p < 0.01$). In addition, these authors compared responses to nonpainful heat stimuli and observed that random warm stimuli between 34°C and 42°C evoked significantly greater activity in patients in bilateral prefrontal cortex and in the supplemental motor area and in contralateral anterior cingulate cortex. These differences were found after statistical control for differences in depression and clinical pain; however, only the contralateral effects retained statistical significance.

These initial fMRI studies found evidence for increased pain sensitivity to either heat or pressure with designs that

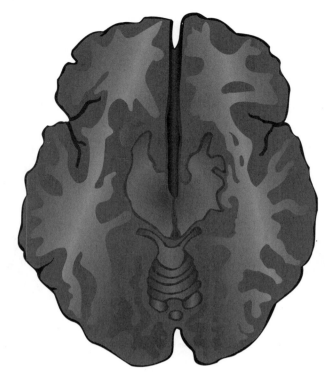

Heat-induced activity in contralateral insula is greater in patients with fibromyalgia

Figure 8-2. Functional magnetic resonance imaging (fMRI) analysis of painful heat applied to the left hand. This horizontal slice shows a region of significantly greater blood oxygen level dependent (BOLD) signal in the contralateral anterior insular cortex of patients with fibromyalgia (FM) compared to control participants. Significance ($p < 0.01$) is based on a region of interest (ROI) analysis of a specific region of the anterior insula. (From Cook DB, Lange G, Ciccone DS, et al. Functional imaging of pain in patients with primary fibromyalgia. *J Rheumatol* 2004;31:364–378, with permission.)

compared the effects of two different painful stimulus intensities delivered to each control subject to the effect of only one painful stimulus intensity delivered to patients with FM. To more fully explore the mechanisms of mechanical hyperalgesia, Grant et al. (45) used fMRI to compare the effects of multiple stimulus pressures delivered to the left thumb of 13 FM patients and 13 control subjects. Within each 10-minute scan, the subjects received 25 seconds of pressure alternating with 25 seconds of no pressure. The magnitude of the stimulus pressure was adjusted for each subject to produce a nonpainful touch sensation and painful pressure sensations rated as faint, very mild, and between moderate and slightly intense. In each scan the subjects received each of the four stimulus pressures three times in a random sequence. Similar to the study described above, the amount of stimulus pressure needed to evoke the various subjective levels of pain was significantly lower in the patients. The results showed that despite the differences in stimulus pressures, both patients and controls showed graded responses to stimulus pressure in regions involved in processing the sensory-discriminative dimension of pain sensation, including contralateral (right) thalamus, S1, and S2. Patients also showed activation of these regions in the side of the brain (left) ipsilateral to the side stimulated (left thumb), and control subjects showed graded responses in right insula and anterior cingulate that were not found in the patients. These results indicate common sensory-discriminative functions in both groups. If this system's dynamic range is limited, this result would be consistent with a central augmentation of the input into this system, an effect that must be substantiated by additional studies with an increased number of subjects. The small number of subjects also hinders interpretation of the differences between groups, but the results are consistent with a spatial, as well as intensive, augmentation of pain in the patient group and a reduced affective response in the patients, possibly due to adaptation to prolonged pain.

FM patients do not form a homogenous group but vary in terms of clinical pain, tenderness, and psychological variables such as anxiety, depression, and perceived control over pain. A recent study identified three distinct clusters of patients (46). In one of these groups the somatic symptoms appear to be related to psychological distress. Second-generation functional imaging studies can explore the possible role of such variables in the expression of experimental pain sensitivity. These experiments identify brain regions in which pain-evoked activity is modulated over a population of subjects by subject-specific variables. For example, Farrell et al. (47) investigated the role of pain locus of control on brain responses to painful pressure applied to the thumb. Pain locus of control is divided into several major scales: "internal locus of control" refers to perceived personal control over pain and "external, powerful doctors, locus of control" refers to the belief system that only trained healthcare professionals are capable of controlling a patient's pain. Another "external" scale described beliefs that such control is up to chance and not under the control of either the patient or healthcare professionals. In an analysis across subjects, Farrell et al. (47) found that internal locus of control was associated ($r = 0.84$) with the degree of pain-evoked activity in the contralateral secondary somatosensory cortex, while the external, powerful doctors locus of control was associated ($r = 0.82$, right; $r = 0.75$, left) with pain-related activity in posterior parietal cortex on both sides of the brain. Since the secondary somatosensory area may be related to stimulus labeling and the parietal cortex may be related to integration of sensations and higher cortical activity, these results suggest that cognitive factors such as attitudes about pain control may modulate perceived pain by engaging brain regions involved in interpretation and evaluation of sensory input.

Another common cognitive factor known to modulate pain reports is catastrophizing, a style in which pain is characterized as awful, horrible, and unbearable. Catastrophizing appears to play a substantial role in development of pain chronicity, Burton et al. (48) found that catastrophizing accounted for more than half (57%) of the variance in predicting the onset of a chronic pain condition from an acute pain event. Catastrophizing was once thought to be a symptom of depression, but it is now recognized as an independent factor that is, nevertheless, associated with depression. A recent fMRI study of the influence of catastrophizing on cerebral responses to blunt pressure pain in 29 FM patients statistically controlled for depression and suggested that this cognitive style modulated pain-evoked activity in a number of brain structures related to the anticipation of (contralateral medial frontal cortex, ipsilateral cerebellum) and attention to [contralateral anterior cingulate cortex (ACC), bilateral dorsolateral prefrontal cortex] pain, and to both emotional (ipsilateral claustrum, interconnected to the amygdala) and motor (contralateral lentiform nuclei) responses (49). Figure 8-3 shows the results for the contralateral anterior cingulate cortex, which were significant for both correlational and between-groups analyses. These results suggest that the deleterious effects of catastrophizing are mediated through a number of separate cognitive mechanisms. Modification of specific malleable mechanisms, such as interpretation of perceived threat or focused attention, might provide efficacious treatment for catastrophizing chronic pain patients and may prevent the transition from acute to chronic in susceptible individuals.

Although preliminary evidence suggests that the cognitive style of catastrophizing modulates pain reports independent of associated depression, depressed mood has been continually linked with chronic pain and may exert independent effects on pain processing. Giesecke et al. (50) recently examined the effects of depression in FM using an experimental design similar to the above investigations of locus of control and catastrophizing. Thirty patients with FM received fMRI scans during administration of painful blunt pressure to the left hand. Symptoms of depression, as measured by the Center for Epidemiological Studies Depression Scale (CES-D), were not associated with either pressure pain sensitivity or the level of pain-evoked activity in brain regions associated with processing the sensory-discriminative dimensions. CES-D scores, however, were

Activity Evoked by Painful Pressure

Figure 8-3. Influence of catastrophizing on functional magnetic resonance imaging (fMRI) activity evoked by painful pressure in patients with fibromyalgia (FM). Activity in anterior cingulate cortex (Brodman Area 32) evoked by painful pressure to the left thumb is significantly associated with catastrophizing in the entire sample of patients (left), and significantly more active in a high-catastrophizing group compared to a low-catastrophizing group (right, all p's <0.05, corrected for multiple comparisons). (From Gracely RH, Geisser ME, Giesecke T, et al. Pain catastrophizing and neural responses to pain among persons with fibromyalgia. *Brain* 2004; 127:835–843, with permission.)

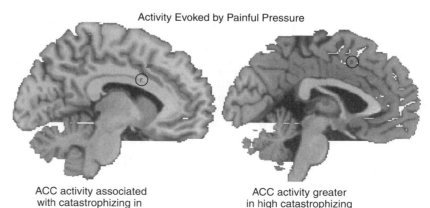

ACC activity associated with catastrophizing in correlational analysis

ACC activity greater in high catastrophizing group

significantly associated with pain-evoked activity in brain regions implicated in processing the motivational-affective dimensions of pain experience, specifically the contralateral anterior insula and bilateral amygdala. In a further analysis these authors identified seven FM patients who met diagnostic criteria for major depressive disorder (MDD) and compared the results of pressure pain testing in an age–gender match of seven FM patients without MDD and seven age and gender matched healthy control subjects. Equally painful stimuli, produced by significantly less stimulus pressures in the FM patients, resulted in similar activations in all three groups. These activations were in regions implicated in processing the sensory-discriminative dimension of pain, including contralateral S1 and S2. Only the patients with MDD showed additional activations in bilateral amygdala and in a specific region of the contralateral anterior insula. These results, which are consistent with the correlational analysis among a larger group of patients with FM, further support the concept that depression modulated pain-evoked activity in structures involved in processing affective characteristics of pain experience.

All the above neuroimaging studies of FM focus on the cerebral processing of acute pain evoked by brief blunt pressure or contact heat stimulation. The studies of the cognitive variables of pain locus of control (47) and catastrophizing (49) evaluated the interaction of these cognitions with evoked pain response—that is, they assessed the cognitive modulation of supraspinal pain processing. In addition to these known effects of cognition on pain, there is considerable evidence for the complementary effect of the chronic pain condition on cognition. The constellation of symptoms in FM also includes self-reports of cognitive difficulties. Patients report a number of problems, resulting in an overall impaired cognitive state that has been referred to as "fibro fog."

The cognitive deficits observed in FM resemble those found in aging—for example, the performance on measures of working memory tasks is similar to the performance from controls 20 years older (51,52). Neuroimaging studies of working memory in aged populations suggest that older subjects can show levels of performance that approach the levels of younger control subjects by utilizing relatively more cognitive resources. Bangert et al. (52) used fMRI to assess brain activity during a working memory task in 12 FM patients and nine age and education-matched control subjects. The specific task consisted of two conditions: a control condition in which subjects were presented four letters in alphabetical order and a manipulation condition in which the alphabetical order of the four letters was jumbled and the subject had to mentally alphabetize the letters. After a 3-second delay, the subjects were presented with a stimulus consisting of three blanks and a single letter of the four shown previously and they had to determine if the letter was in the correct alphabetized position. The results showed that both FM patients and healthy controls showed similar performance in both tasks. However, the imaging results suggest that, like the effects found with age, this similar performance was achieved by recruitment of greater brain resources. FMs showed more extensive neural activation in frontal and parietal regions, including bilateral activation in the middle frontal gyrus and right side activation in medial frontal

gyrus, superior parietal lobe, and precentral gyrus. These results support the hypothesis that FM patients show an age effect, using increasing cognitive resources to maintain levels of performance that require less resources in younger subjects. These initial results are provocative and naturally lead to further neuroimaging studies of cognitive deficits in FM and the means by which FM patients cope with such deficits.

SUMMARY AND FUTURE STUDIES

At present, functional brain imaging in FM has identified possible baseline changes in neural activity. Administration of a noxious pressure or heat stimulus results in changes in brain activity consistent with verbal reports of subjective pain magnitude; FM patients feel the same range of pain as do healthy controls, albeit at a significantly reduced level and range of stimulation. Variations of stimulus level within this reduced range results in similar encoding of stimulus intensity as observed with higher levels of stimuli in healthy controls. In individual patients the direction and magnitude of responses in specific structures are associated with at least two cognitive styles: pain locus of control and catastrophizing. This association suggests that these cognitive styles modulate the responses to painful stimulation, although the design of these studies cannot distinguish between this mechanism and other possibilities, such as a difference in pain processing that results in altered cognitive behaviors or a mechanism in which both the response to painful stimuli and cognitive behaviors represent parallel effects of a variable disease process. Of these possibilities, the cognitive modulation of pain processing is a likely hypothesis that future longitudinal experiments can verify. Since cognitive-behavioral therapeutic techniques can modify pain locus of control, a parallel appropriate change in brain processing in those with changed cognitive style would support a causal model in which pain locus of control modulates brain responses to painful stimulation.

This type of longitudinal, interventional study is one of many next-generation experiments using functional brain imaging of FM. The focus on individual differences is an important issue that will be examined in several types of new studies that range from subgrouping of similar patients to the use of techniques such as fMRI in the single individual for purposes such as diagnosis, monitoring of treatment efficacy, and medico-legal decision making. Studies of individuals promise to bridge the gap between the results of mechanistic studies in groups and individual clinical case management.

Future studies of FM will examine the response to pharmacologic and nonpharmacologic treatments and the individual differences in treatment response. Current studies using opiates have found increased activation in the basal ganglia and other regions (53) and have evaluated the reduction of pain-evoked activity in insula and other regions (54), including using the temporal resolution of fMRI to assess the time course of these effects (55). Studies of acupuncture have found reduced activity in a number of brain regions (including insula, putamen, superior temporal gyrus, and cingulate cortex) following manual manipulation of acupuncture needles (56,57) and an increase in activity in regions such as precentral and post central gyrus, inferior parietal lobule, and putamen/insula during electroacupuncture (57). In a PET study of opioid analgesia, Petrovic et al. (58) showed that administration of both a μ-opioid agonist (remifentanil) and placebo in healthy individuals evoked reduced reports of pain intensity and activation of the rostral anterior cingulate cortex, a region that is rich in opiate receptors and that receives input from cortical and limbic system regions. Placebo analgesia also evoked increased activation of the orbitofrontal cortex. More recently, an extensive fMRI study of placebo analgesia to both heat and electrical stimulation found both reductions in pain activity in regions associated with pain processing (thalamus, S2, anterior cingulate cortex, insula) and increased activity in orbitofrontal and dorsolateral prefrontal cortex, regions hypothesized to be involved in the anticipation of analgesia (59). The time course of these effects and the wide variety of regions activated suggest that placebo analgesia is more than just a simple verbal relabeling of unaltered experience. These results strongly suggest that administration of a placebo evokes a number of physiologic processes. These results also suggest that putative placebo mechanisms involving activation of intrinsic opioid analgesic systems may be involved in certain aspects of placebo analgesia but cannot account for the variety and extent of the observed effects.

All the functional brain imaging methods described above infer neural activity from changes in rCBF. In these types of studies the effects of opioids on neural activity are assessed by comparing rCBF before and after the administration of an opioid. Another type of brain imaging can infer opioid mechanisms at the receptor level. These receptor binding studies use PET to trace the effect of specific compounds that are labeled with a radioactive tag, and the binding of these tagged compounds can be imaged in the same manner that radioactive labeled blood is imaged in studies of rCBF. In an example of such a study, Zubieta et al. (60) showed that tonic pain produced by infusion of hypertonic saline into a facial (masseter) muscle induced regional release of endogenous opioids that bound to mu-type opioid receptors in several cortical and subcortical brain regions.

The opioid receptor binding methodology has been applied to the evaluation of genetic influences on pain responsivity. Zubieta et al. examined the relationship between μ-opioid receptor-mediated neurotransmission and a common functional polymorphism of the cathechol-O-methyltransferase (COMT) gene (61). This gene is involved in metabolizing catecholamines, which influences adrenergic/noradrenergic neurotransmission involved in pain modulation. In this procedure healthy subjects with one of three COMT genotypes underwent PET neuroimaging during infusion of hypertonic saline in the masseter and completed a standardized pain measure, the McGill Pain Questionnaire (62), which required them to choose quantified verbal descriptors (e.g., aching, miserable) to describe the sensory and affective dimensions of their subjective pain experience. Subjects with one extreme (met/met) genotype showed lower μ-opioid system activation in the striatopallidal regions (nucleus accumbens, ventral pallidum, and subthalamic nucleus) and in the amygdala in comparison to subjects with an intermediate (met/val) genotype. Subjects with the third (val/val) genotype displayed significantly higher μ-opioid system activation in the

dorsal anterior cingulate, anterior thalamus, and cerebellar vermis in comparison to subjects with the intermediate genotype. These findings were associated with subjective pain ratings; the met/met subjects reported the highest levels of pain, followed by the val/met and the val/val subjects, who reported the lowest levels of pain. Conversely, the volume of hypertonic saline required to produce pain was lowest in the met/met subjects, intermediate in the met/val subjects, and highest in the val/val subjects. These findings strongly suggest that the met/met genotype of COMT is associated with diminished μ-opioid system activation and enhanced pain responses in healthy persons. Additional studies are necessary to determine whether this genotype is also associated with disorders characterized by abnormalities in pain sensitivity or pain modulation.

PET, despite its relatively poor temporal and spatial resolution, has other advantages over conventional neural activation studies using fMRI. PET, and also SPECT, can provide a measure of baseline blood flow at rest and can be used to compare changes in inferred neural activity in specific regions between groups of subjects or within groups of subjects over time. PET can also be used to assess long-term processes such as an oral analgesic that, once activated, persists for an hour or more. In contrast, fMRI activation studies can assess only the effects of short interventions that can be turned on and off repeatedly within seconds to a minute. Conventional fMRI, for example, cannot directly assess the effect of an oral analgesic but can assess the interaction of the analgesic with a repeated brief stimulus, such as painful heat or pressure. However, new MRI methodologies are changing this limitation and expanding the types of physiologic variables that can be evaluated by functional brain imaging. Magnetic resonance perfusion (MR Perfusion) can assess cerebral blood flow and cerebral blood volume, providing measures of baseline differences similar to that currently provided by PET. Diffusion tensor imaging (DTI) provides a noninvasive, in vivo assessment of water molecular diffusion that reflects tissue configuration at a microscopic level in white matter regions. Quantification of water diffusion will improve the neuroradiologic assessment of a variety of gray and white matter disorders, including altered pain processing. Magnetic resonance spectroscopy (MRS) obtains spectra of multiple selected regions and determines the ratio of concentrations of metabolites such as N-acetyl-aspartate, creatine, choline, lactate, glucose, and glutamate. Usually a particular stable metabolite (creatine) is used as a standard and the concentration of the test metabolites are expressed as a ratio to this standard. Abnormalities in the levels of these metabolites are associated with a number of pathologic changes in brain tissue. This method has been applied to patients with chronic low back pain, showing reductions of N-acetyl-aspartate and glucose in dorsolateral prefrontal cortex (63) in this patient group compared to control subjects, and an association of levels of N-acetyl-aspartate in the orbitofrontal cortex with anxiety within the patient group (64).

SUMMARY POINTS

- A number of imaging modalities (SPECT, functional MRI, PET, spectroscopy) can be used to objectively image brain function.

- Many studies using a variety of these modalities have identified differences in functional imaging of the brain in FM and related conditions.
- The most recent of these studies have used functional MRI and have corroborated patients' self-report of increased pain sensitivity in FM by demonstrating activity in pain-related neural structures with normally nonpainful stimuli.
- The most recent of these imaging studies has also shown that how individuals perceive their pain (e.g., whether they feel that they can control their pain or whether they "catastrophize"—that is, have a pessimistic view of what their pain is doing to them) can markedly influence how pain is neurally processed in conditions such as FM.

■ IMPLICATIONS FOR PRACTICE

- Functional imaging studies leave little doubt that the pain experienced in conditions such as FM is "real."
- These studies also point out how important cognitions such as locus of control and catastrophizing are in chronic pain, in that these thoughts and attributions fundamentally alter pain processing. This may provide a basis for the efficacy of treatments such as cognitive-behavioral therapy.

REFERENCES

1. Price DD, Hu JW, Dubner R, et al. Peripheral suppression of first pain and central summation of second pain evoked by noxious heat pulses. *Pain* 1977;3:57–68.
2. Pillemer SR, Bradley LA, Crofford LJ, et al. The neuroscience and endocrinology of fibromyalgia. *Arthritis Rheum* 1997;40:1928–1937.
3. Jones AKP. The contribution of functional imaging techniques to our understanding of rheumatic pain. *Rheum Dis Clin North Am* 1999;25:123–152.
4. Sawamoto N, Honda M, Okada T, et al. Expectation of pain enhances responses to nonpainful somatosensory stimulation in the anterior cingulate cortex and parietal operculum/posterior insula: an event-related functional magnetic resonance imaging study. *J Neurosci* 2000;20:7438–7445.
5. Coghill RC, Sang CN, Maisog JM, et al. Pain intensity processing within the human brain: a bilateral distributed mechanism. *J Neurophysiol* 1999;82:1934–1943.
6. Rainville P. Brain mechanisms of pain affect and pain modulation. *Curr Opin Neurobiol* 2002;12:195–204.
7. Koyama T, Kato K, Mikami A. During pain-avoidance neurons activated in the macaque anterior cingulate and caudate. *Neurosci Lett* 2000;283:17–20.
8. Bester H, Chapman V, Beeson JM, et al. Physiological properties of the lamina I spinoparabrachial neurons in the rat. *J Neurophysiol* 2000;83:2239–2259.
9. Desbos C, Villanueva L. The organization of lateral ventromedial thalamic connections in the rat: a link for the distribution of nociceptive signals to widespread cortical regions. *Neuroscience* 2001;102:885–898.
10. Bourgeais L, Gauriau O, Bernard JF. Projections from the nociceptive area of the central nucleus of the amygdala to the forebrain: a PHA-L study in the rat. *Eur J Neurosci* 2001;14:229–255.
11. Gracely RH. Studies of pain in human subjects. In: Wall PD, Melzack R, eds. *Textbook of pain*, 4th ed. London: Churchill Livingstone, 1999:385–407.
12. Kakigi R, Matsuda Y, Kuroda Y. Effects of movement-related cortical activities on pain-related somatosensory evoked potentials following CO_2 laser stimulation in normal subjects. *Acta Neurol Scand* 1993;88:376–380.
13. Tarkka IM, Treede RD. Equivalent electrical source analysis of pain-related somatosensory evoked potentials elicited by a CO_2 laser. *J Clin Neurophysiol* 1993;10:513–519.
14. Lenz FA, Rios M, Chau D, et al. Painful stimuli evoke potentials recorded from the parasylvian cortex in humans. *J Neurophysiol* 1998;80:2077–2088.
15. Chen AC. New perspectives in EEG/MEG brain mapping and PET/fMRI neuroimaging of human pain. *Int J Psychophysiol* 2001;42:147–159.
16. Stevens A, Batra A, Kotter I, et al. Both pain and EEG response to cold pressor stimulation occurs faster in fibromyalgia patients than in control subjects. *Psychiatry Res* 2000;97:237–247.
17. Ingvar DH, Rosen I, Elmquist D. Activation patterns induced in the dominant hemisphere by skin stimulation. In: Zimmerman Y, ed. *Sensory functions of the skin*. Oxford: Pergamon Press, 1976:549–559.
18. Talbot JD, Marrett S, Evans AC, et al. Multiple representations of pain in the human cerebral cortex. *Science* 1991;251:1355–1358.
19. Jones AKP, Brown WD, Friston KJ, et al. Cortical and subcortical localization of response to pain in man using positron emission tomography. *Proc R Soc London B* 1991;244:39–44.
20. Coghill RC, McHaffie JG, Yen YF. Neural correlates of interindividual differences in the subjective experience of pain. *Proc Natl Acad Sci USA* 2003;100:8538–8542.
21. Rainville P, Duncan GH, Price DD, et al. Pain affect encoded in human anterior cingulate but not somatosensory cortex. *Science* 1997;277:968–971.
22. Rainville P, Carrier B, Hofbauer RK, et al. Dissociation of sensory and affective dimensions of pain using hypnotic modulation. *Pain* 1999;82:159–171.
23. Hofbauer RK, Rainville P, Duncan GH, et al. Cortical representation of the sensory dimension of pain. *J Neurophysiol* 2001;86:402–411.
24. Mountz JM, Bradley LA, Modell JG, et al. Fibromyalgia in women. Abnormalities of regional cerebral blood flow in the thalamus and the caudate nucleus are associated with low pain threshold levels. *Arthritis Rheum* 1995;38:926–938.
25. Kwiatek R, Barnden L, Rowe S. Pontine tegmental regional cerebral blood flow is reduced in fibromyalgia. *Arthritis Rheum* 1997;40:S43.
26. Bradley LA, Sotolongo A, Alberts KR, et al. Abnormal regional cerebral blood flow in the caudate nucleus among fibromyalgia patients and non-patients is associated with insidious symptom onset. *J Musculoskel Pain*, 1999;7:285–292.
27. Iadarola MJ, Max MB, Berman KF, et al. Unilateral decrease in thalamic activity observed with positron emission tomography in patients with chronic neuropathic pain. *Pain* 1995;63:55–64.
28. Di Piero V, Jones AKP, Iannotti F, et al. Chronic pain: a PET study of the central effects of percutaneous high cervical cordotomy. *Pain* 1991;46:9–12.
29. Lenz FA, Gracely RH, Hope EJ, et al. The sensation of angina pectoris can be evoked by stimulation of the human thalamus. *Pain* 1994;59:119–125.
30. Lenz FA, Gracely RH, Romanmoski AJ, et al. Stimulation in the human somatosensory thalamus can reproduce both the affective and sensory dimensions of previously experienced pain. *Nat Med* 1995;1:910–913.
31. Ness TJ, San Pedro EC, Richards JS, et al. A case of spinal cord injury-related pain with baseline rCBF brain SPECT imaging and beneficial response to gabapentin. *Pain* 1998;78:139–143.

32. San Pedro EC, Mountz JM, Liu HG, et al. Familial painful restless leg syndrome correlates with a pain-dependent variation of blood flow to the caudate nucleus, thalamus, and anterior cingulate gyrus. *J Rheumatol* 1998;25:2270–2275.

33. Sorkin LS, McAdoo DJ, Willis WD. Stimulation in the ventral posterior lateral nucleus of the primate thalamus leads to release of serotonin in the lumbar spinal cord. *Brain Res* 1992;581:307–310.

34. Chudler EH, Swigiyama K, Dong WK. Nociceptive responses in the neostriatum and globus pallidus of the anesthetized rat. *J Neurophysiol* 1993;69:1890–1903.

35. Diorio D, Viau V, Meaney MJ. The role of the medial prefrontal cortex (cingulate gyrus) in the regulation of hypothalamic-pituitary-adrenal response to stress. *J Neurosci* 1983;13:3839–3847.

36. Lineberry CG, Vierck CJ. Attenuation of pain reactivity by caudate nucleus stimulation in monkeys. *Brain Res* 1975;9:119–134.

37. Acupuncture Anesthesia Coordinating Group. Observations on electrical stimulation of the caudate nucleus of human brain and acupuncture in treatment of intractable pain. *Chin Med J* 1977;3:117–124.

38. Weigent DA, Bradley LA, Blalock JE, et al. Current concepts in the pathophysiology of abnormal pain perception in fibromyalgia. *Am J Med Sci* 1998;315:405–412.

39. Gracely RH, Petzke F, Wolf JM, et al. Functional MRI evidence of augmented pain processing in fibromyalgia. *Arthritis Rheum* 2002;46:1333–1343.

40. Petzke F, Gracely RH, Park KM, et al. What do tender points measure? Influence of distress on 4 measures of tenderness. *J Rheumatol* 2003;30:567–574.

41. Gracely RH, Grant MA, Giesecke T. Evoked pain measures in fibromyalgia. *Best Pract Res Clin Rheumatol* 2003;17:593–609.

42. Gendreau RM, Williams DA, Clauw DJ. Comparison of several pain measurement tools in fibromyalgia patients. *Arthritis Rheum* 2003;48:S616.

43. Talairach P, Tournoux J. *A stereotactive coplanar atlas of the human brain*. Stuttgart, Germany: Thieme Medical Publishers, 1988.

44. Cook DB, Lange G, Ciccone DS, et al. Functional imaging of pain in patients with primary fibromyalgia. *J Rheumatol* 2004;31:364–378.

45. Grant MAB, Farrell MJ, Kumar R, et al. FMRI evaluation of pain intensity coding in fibromyalgia patients and controls. *Arthritis Rheum* 2001;44:S394.

46. Giesecke T, Williams DA, Harris RE, et al. Subgroupings of fibromyalgia patients on the basis of pressure-pain thresholds and psychological factors. *Arthritis Rheum* 2003;48:2916–2922.

47. Farrell MJ, VanMeter JW, Petzke F, et al. Supraspinal activity associated with painful pressure in fibromyalgia is associated with beliefs about locus of pain control. *Arthritis Rheum* 2001;44:S394.

48. Burton AK, Tillotson MK, Main CJ, et al. Psychosocial predictors of outcome in acute and sub-chronic low back trouble. *Spine* 1995;20:722–728.

49. Gracely RH, Geisser ME, Giesecke T, et al. Pain catastrophizing and neural responses to pain among persons with fibromyalgia. *Brain* 2004;127:835–843.

50. Giesecke T, Clauw DJ, Ambrose KR, et al. Does depression influence mechanical hyperalgesia/allodynia in patients with fibromyalgia (FM)? *Arthritis Rheum* 2003;48:S86.

51. Park DC, Glass JM, Minear M, et al. Cognitive function in fibromyalgia patients. *Arthritis Rheum* 2001;44:2125–2133.

52. Bangert AS, Glass JM, Welsh RC, et al. Functional magnetic resonance imaging of working memory in fibromyalgia. *Arthritis Rheum* 2003;48:S90.

53. Lorenz IH, Kolbitsch C, Hormann C, et al. The influence of nitrous oxide and remifentanil on cerebral hemodynamics in conscious human volunteers. *Neuroimage* 2002;17:1056–1064.

54. Wise RG, Rogers R, Painter D, et al. Combining fMRI with a pharmacokinetic model to determine which brain areas activated by painful stimulation are specifically modulated by remifentanil. *Neuroimage* 2002;16:999–1014.

55. Wise RG, Williams P, Tracey I. Using fMRI to quantify the time dependence of remifentanil analgesia in the human brain. *Neuropsychopharmacology* 2004;29:626–635.

56. Hui KK, Liu J, Makris N, et al. Acupuncture modulates the limbic system and subcortical gray structures of the human brain: evidence from fMRI studies in normal subjects. *Hum Brain Mapp* 2000;9:13–25.

57. Kong J, Ma L, Gollub RL, et al. A pilot study of functional magnetic resonance imaging of the brain during manual and electroacupuncture stimulation of acupuncture point (LI-4 Hegu) in normal subjects reveals differential brain activation between methods. *J Altern Complement Med* 2002;8:411–419.

58. Petrovic P, Kalso E, Petersson KM, et al. Placebo and opioid analgesia—imaging a shared neuronal network. *Science* 2002;295(5560):1737–1740.

59. Wager TD, Rilling JK, Smith EE, et al. Placebo-induced changes in FMRI in the anticipation and experience of pain. *Science* 2004;303:1162–1167.

60. Zubieta JK, Smith YR, Bueller JA, et al. Regional mu opioid receptor regulation of sensory and affective dimensions of pain. *Science* 2001;293:311–315.

61. Zubieta JK, Heitzeg MM, Smith YR, et al. COMT val158met genotype affects mu-opioid neurotransmitter responses to a pain stressor. *Science* 2003;299:1240–1243.

62. Melzack R. The McGill pain questionnaire: major properties and scoring methods. *Pain* 1975;1:277–299.

63. Grachev ID, Fredrickson BE, Apkarian AV. Abnormal brain chemistry in chronic back pain: an in vivo proton magnetic resonance spectroscopy study. *Pain* 2000;89:7–18.

64. Grachev ID, Fredrickson BE, Apkarian AV. Brain chemistry reflects dual states of pain and anxiety in chronic low back pain. *J Neural Transm* 2002;109:1309–1334.

9

Muscles and Peripheral Abnormalities in Fibromyalgia

Haiko Sprott

Studies investigating the pathogenesis of fibromyalgia (FM) concentrate on different areas: muscular and microcirculatory changes (hypoxia), changes in pain modulating molecules, neuroendocrinological changes, changes in function of the autonomic nervous system, sleep disturbances, and psychological and psychiatric aberrations (1). Several clinical observations suggest that there is a focal muscle origin to the pain in FM (2). Most FM patients describe muscle as the possible source of their discomfort, and during repetitive muscular activity patients experience increasing pain (3). There is, for example, a reduction of the pain after these locations are injected with local anesthetic agents (4), though one must not exclude the fact that the input from the skin is also anesthetized. This gives some indication that nociceptive input exists or previously existed in FM patients. Nociceptors can also act as effectors—that is, they are able to secrete pain mediators such as cytokines (5,6), neuropeptides such as calcitonin gene-related peptide (CGRP) (7,8) and substance P (SP) (9,10), as well as other pain amplifying substances such as nitric oxide, serotonin, and nerve growth factor (11,12). Consideration of the phenomenon of "neurogenic inflammation" is necessary because of the potential role it may play in peripheral nociceptive mechanisms as well as in the initiation of peripheral sensitization in FM patients. Hypoxia is also involved in the onset of peripheral nociception. Hypoxia-induced adenosine release activates adenosine A_2 receptors and stimulates unmyelinated afferent fibers (13). Similar processes may also activate other peripheral afferent nociceptors (14). Endothelin is known to be an important vasoconstrictor and thus responsible for local hypoxic conditions (15). Furthermore, endothelin is fibrogenic (16). Interestingly, Pache et al. demonstrated increased concentrations of endothelin in the plasma of FM patients (17).

The hypothesis that a localized painful injury can result in the development of FM must be considered from a nociceptive starting point. Within the concept of a chronic pain disease, there is also the possibility that subsequent changes (neuronal plasticity) result in the self-perpetuation of pain in FM, even long after the initial nociceptive input has subsided.

We hypothesize that the origin of FM is based on peripheral nociceptive stimuli, which initiate the process of peripheral and central sensitization (see Figure 9-1). Insights into the development of this hypothesis are discussed in the following paragraphs; they focus primarily on the muscle but also give consideration to abnormalities of the skin and the blood.

THE ROLE OF MUSCLES IN PAIN DEVELOPMENT IN FIBROMYALGIA

Twenty years ago, Henriksson and his group described muscle abnormalities in biopsies from the trapezius muscle of FM patients: Degeneration or regeneration of fibers, perivascular collections of mononuclear inflammatory cells, moth-eaten fibers, and ragged red fibers were all observed (18,19). Although these light microscopic and ultrastructural findings are nonspecific, they nonetheless indicate that the muscle fibers are abnormal. Pathologic changes have also been described by Yunus et al. (20). These studies have shown that microcirculation is disturbed, mitochondria are damaged, and there is a reduced content of high-energy phosphates (see also ^{31}P magnetic resonance spectroscopy). Thus, in FM painful muscles may be in an energy-deficient state, even at rest. Pain analysis has supported the idea that there is a nociceptive origin to the pain. The biopsy findings described may be of diagnostic importance.

STRUCTURAL ABNORMALITIES

Structural abnormalities in the muscle tissue of patients with FM may be the effect of the production of several intracellular second messengers—that is, nitric oxide (NO) (21). Indeed, our laboratory and other investigators have provided evidence to show that, compared to controls, patients with FM characteristically have an increase in the synthesis of

> ## Primary fibromyalgia is a chronic painful disease caused by a strong or long-lasting nociceptive input activating a putative susceptibility resulting in and maintaining a central sensitization.

Figure 9-1. Hypothesis of the pathogenesis of fibromyalgia.

NO (22). Prolonged release of high levels of NO (23,24) may induce abnormal cell death in muscle tissue, which, in turn, might contribute to the structural and metabolic defects that have been identified in the muscle of FM patients [see also "DNA fragmentation" (25)].

In 1973, Fassbender et al. (26) published a morphologic study of the muscle of FM patients and hypothesized that local hypoxia caused degenerative changes. In 1986 the findings of Bengtsson et al. supported this hypothesis (27). Both reported decreased levels of adenosine diphosphate and phosphoryl creatine together with increased levels of adenosine monophosphate and creatine. Furthermore, they described discrete histopathologic and histochemical changes identified in muscle biopsies (28).

Electron microscopy analysis found that the muscle tissue of FM patients is characterized by high frequencies of "rubber band" morphology, mild myofibrillar separation, papillary projections, and subsarcolemmal accumulation of glycogen (29–31) (see Figure 9-2).

Muscle Fiber Typing

The fiber type and fiber size of muscles from FM patients are unremarkable compared to those of the healthy control population. The distribution of fibers showed about 2/3 type IA fibers; the majority of the remaining fibers were type IIA. Morphometry of the fibers using light microscopy has generally revealed no type II atrophy as described in the literature (25). We did not find any atrophic regions in our own biopsy samples from FM patients (32). Muscle fibers with cytopathologic findings such as core fibers, moth-eaten fibers, or target cells as examined with cytochrome *c* oxidase staining were rare: Moth-eaten fibers were found in approximately 25% of FM patients, which is of no relevance, as it is not specific for any disease. Fiber type grouping, an indication of reinnervation, was not found (32).

Deoxyribonucleic Acid Fragmentation

There is evidence of abnormal DNA fragmentation in the muscle tissue of individuals with FM (see Figure 9-3). Enzymatic DNA fragmentation assays revealed positive results, but in nuclei of FM muscle cells positive DNA fragmentation did not reflect apoptosis as identified by electron microscopy (33). Using electron microscopy several abnormalities were found in the muscle tissue of the subjects with FM. In all investigated FM samples, myofibers and actin filaments appeared disorganized; none of the tissue samples presented any features of apoptosis (34–38). Interfibrillar lipid and lipofuscin deposits have also been observed in these tissues. Interfibrillar glycogen was found in the tissue of at least 50% of the subjects with FM, and moth-eaten destruction of muscle fibers also appeared in several tissues of these subjects. In contrast, no myofiber or actin filament disorganization could be observed in the tissues of healthy controls (33). Electron microscopy revealed substantial differences between subjects with FM and healthy controls in both the number and shape of the mitochondria observed in the muscle tissue specimens. Specifically, the mean number of mitochondria found in the muscle tissue of the subjects with FM was significantly lower than that observed in the muscle tissue of healthy controls. Moreover, the mitochondria found in the tissue of the subjects with FM were substantially larger than those in the tissue of the controls (33).

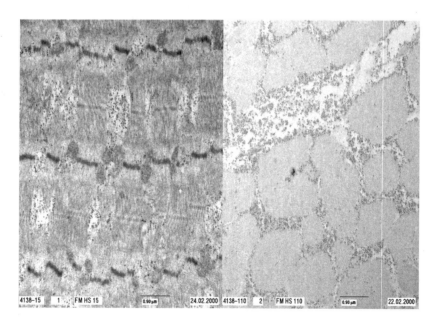

Figure 9-2. Ultrastructural abnormalities in muscle of fibromyalgia patients with disturbed microarchitecture and accumulation of glycogen.

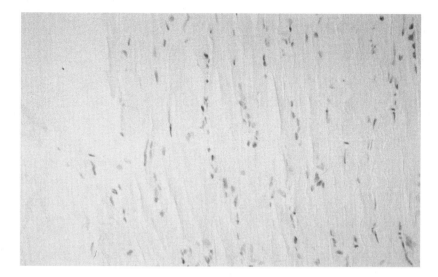

Figure 9-3. Deoxyribonucleic acid fragmentation (*dark dots*) in nuclei of fibromyalgic muscle fibers, stained with a DNA fragmentation detection kit (Klenow). Nuclei without DNA fragmentation appear brighter. Compared to healthy muscle tissue, there is an increased DNA fragmentation in fibromyalgic muscle. (From Sprott H, Salemi S, Gay RE, et al. Increased DNA fragmentation and ultrastructural changes in fibromyalgic muscle fibers. *Ann Rheum Dis* 2004;63:245–251, with permission.)

Neuropeptides and the Opioid System

Neuropeptides and the opioid system also appear to play an important role in the perception of pain (39). Neuropeptides, like SP, are released in neurogenic inflammation and influence the opioid system (40). The importance of these peripheral changes has become more relevant with regard to accessibility for analysis and targets for therapy (41).

Neuropeptides do not appear to play a prominent role in the nociception of FM muscle. We did not find any differences between the levels of serotonin, SP, galanin, pituitary adenylyl cyclase-activating polypeptide, and secretoneurin in the muscle tissue of FM patients and healthy controls (42). However, our findings are not consistent with the literature. For example, De Stefano et al. reported increased SP levels in the trapezius muscle of FM patients compared to healthy controls but also could show this elevation in patients with myofascial pain syndrome (43), leading them to conclude that the afferent nervous system might be involved in the development and perception of myofascial pain.

Three families of opioid peptides have been well characterized: the endorphins, enkephalins, and dynorphins. Immune cells are the most extensively examined source of opioids outside the central nervous system that interact with peripheral opioid receptors (44). In conditions of painful inflammation, met-enkephalin and dynorphin-A, among other pain modulating molecules, are found in circulating cells and in lymph nodes (45,46). In chronic inflammation local injections of μ-, δ- and κ-agonists produce a dose-dependent and stereospecific analgesia. This is reversible by selective antagonists, thus indicating the activation of peripheral μ-, δ- and κ-agonists receptors (47). κ-agonists receptor agonists produce both peripheral analgesic and anti-inflammatory effects (48–52). Possible underlying mechanisms of the latter include reduced release of proinflammatory neuropeptides (53–56) or cytokines (57), as well as the diminished expression of adhesion molecules (58,59).

Compared to healthy controls, opioid receptors in the muscle tissue of FM patients may be activated as a result of microtrauma to the muscle fibers and chronic pain (32). Tissue damage stimulates the expression of peripheral opioid receptors, which likely leads to a concomitant increase of

their function (41). In comparing the muscle tissues of FM patients to those of healthy subjects, no significant differences in the mRNA or protein expression of the δ- and κ-opioid receptors were detected (32). Interestingly, the μ-opioid receptor was not detectable in any of the muscle specimens. The enhancement of intracellular calcium may control δ- and κ-receptor-mediated antinociception (60,61), whereas the activation of ATP-gated potassium channels mediates the antinociception induced by μ-opioid receptor agonists (62,63).

In the muscle tissue of FM patients the expression of mRNA encoding for the δ-opioid receptors, as well as the specific opioid receptor protein, was found to be located around certain muscle fibers in muscle satellite cells (32). This was demonstrated using double staining with antibodies against human CD34, a marker staining for stem cells and also satellite cells (64,65) (see Figure 9-4). Muscle satellite cells are quiescent precursors interposed between myofibers and a sheath of external lamina. Thus far it is known that, following damage to skeletal muscle, satellite cells become activated, migrate toward the injured area, proliferate, and fuse with one another to form myotubes, which ultimately mature into myofibers (64,66). The results show that opioid receptors are present in muscle satellite cells (outside the central nervous system) on both the mRNA and protein level. The function of these receptors in satellite cells remains to be elucidated. The quantity of opioid receptor mRNA did not differ between healthy subjects and FM patients. Thus, the data do not necessarily support the concept that chronic pain in FM patients is related to an activation of the opioid receptor system in the muscles. These results might be of some therapeutic interest.

Age Dependency of Ultrastructural Changes

Age is an important demographic variable, given that it might be associated with changes in DNA fragmentation, muscle tissue structure, and mitochondrial oxidative metabolism (67). In our study the age range of our subjects was wide, and there was no significant difference in the mean age between the FM and healthy controls (33). Thus, it is

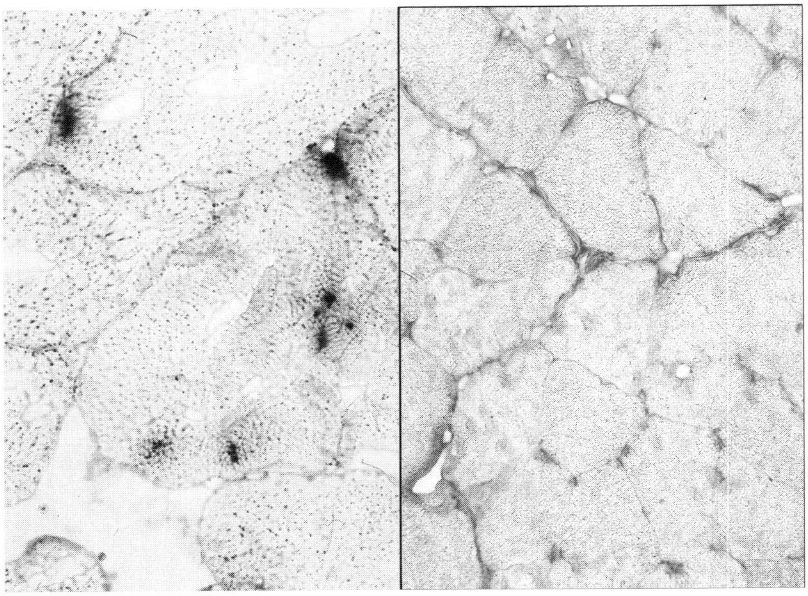

Figure 9-4. Example of opioid receptor mRNA (dark dots), Investigated by in-situ RT-PCR experiments in fibromyalgic muscle (left panel). Staining of muscle satellite cells with anti-CD34 (dark) and nuclei (bright) in fibromyalgic muscle (right panel).

unlikely that the abnormalities in DNA fragmentation and muscle ultrastructure of our subjects with FM were a result of age-related factors.

Physical Activity and Ultrastructural Changes

One cannot rule out the potential influence that physical inactivity may contribute to the ultrastructural changes in the muscle tissue of subjects with FM. It is unlikely, however, that low physical activity levels of FM patients alone can produce enhanced DNA fragmentation, particularly since this phenomenon tends to be associated with high levels of activity in healthy individuals (68,69). It appears that the enhanced DNA fragmentation and ultrastructural abnormalities seen in the muscle tissue of subjects with FM are not directly correlated to aging or low levels of physical activity (33).

The grounds for ultrastructural abnormalities in FM muscle are not clear. However, these abnormalities may be produced in part by the high levels of "muscle stress," for example, due to local hypoxic conditions. Furthermore, persistent focal contractions in muscle may contribute to ultrastructural tissue abnormalities as well as to the induction and/or chronicity of nociceptive transmission from muscle to the central nervous system (33). Increased electrical activity of the erector spinae muscle (see also ^{31}P Magnetic Resonance Spectroscopy below) in resting FM patients was measured by electromyogram (EMG) mapping (70) (see Figure 9-5).

FUNCTIONAL ABNORMALITIES

^{31}P Magnetic Resonance Spectroscopy

Studies using ^{31}P magnetic resonance imaging have reliably identified several abnormalities in the muscle tissue of FM patients. Park et al. found metabolic abnormalities in the quadriceps muscle tissue of patients with FM. Levels of phosphocreatine and ATP were relatively low at rest, and phosphorylation potential and total oxidative capacity were low during both rest and exercise (71). Our group found significantly higher levels of phosphodiesters and inorganic phosphate in the spectra of FM patients compared to controls (72), confirming the findings of Jubrias et al. (73).

Subjects were investigated only during the resting state. The comparison between FM and healthy subjects, independent of age, indicates significant increases of the relative signal intensity of inorganic phosphate and phosphodiesters and to a lesser extent an increase of phosphomonoesters. A significant decrease was found for the α-nucleoside triphosphate values in FM patients, whereas no significant differences were observed for phosphocreatin and in pH values. In a resting muscle, decreased concentrations of nucleoside triphosphate and increased values of inorganic phosphate are generally signs of a disturbance in energy metabolism. These changes are not specific enough to make a diagnosis and have been observed in several muscle diseases (inflammatory, mitochondrial, or metabolic myopathies) (74–76). These changes can also be caused by lowered perfusion (77). Increased phosphomonoester and phosphodiester values are often the result of higher membrane conversions, indicating disturbances in phospholipid metabolism.

The results of our laser fluxmetry studies of peripheral microcirculation in FM patients have revealed a higher concentration, a decreased speed, and a decreased flux of erythrocytes as well as a lower skin temperature at the examined tender points (TePs) (78,79). Lund et al. (80) reported abnormal oxygen pressure on the muscle surface above trigger points. Local hypoxia occurring with a decrease of high-energy phosphate levels results in morphologic changes. Fassbender et al. examined muscle biopsies from FM patients and reported a step-by-step destruction of myofilaments and swollen endothelial cells. These changes are probably associated with the relative hypoxia of the muscle cells in FM patients (26). It is not known whether the swollen endothelial cells are the cause or the result of hypoxia!

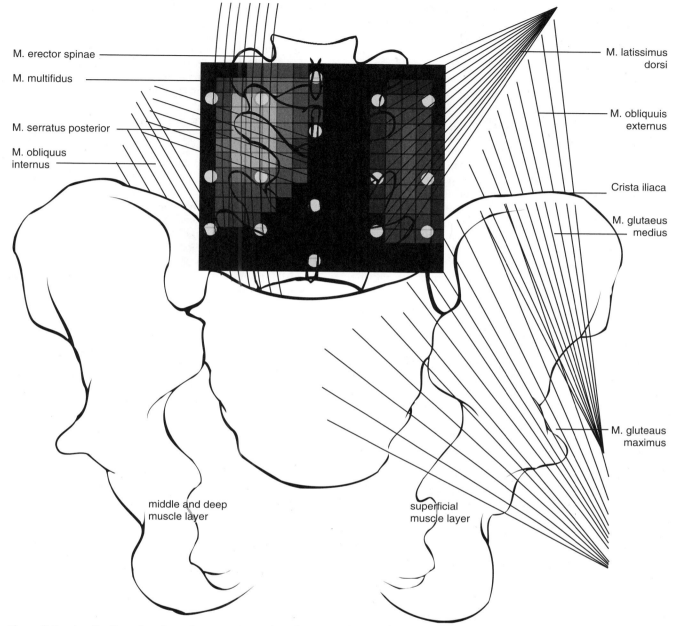

M. erector spinae

M. multifidus

M. serratus posterior

M. obliquus internus

M. latissimus dorsi

M. obliquuis externus

Crista iliaca

M. gluteaus medius

M. gluteaus maximus

middle and deep muscle layer

superficial muscle layer

Figure 9-5. Application of surface electromyogram (EMG)-mapping in the low back region. Schematic superposition of a calculated EMG map and muscles of investigated area. Dark stainings: low activity; bright stainings: high activity. The circles indicate the electrode positions. L2–L5 indicate the spinous processes. (From Anders C, Sprott H, Scholle HC, et al. Surface EMG of the lumbar part of the erector trunci muscle in patients with fibromyalgia. *Clin Exp Rheumatol* 2001;19:454, with permission.)

Bengtsson et al. found "moth-eaten" fibers in biopsies taken from trapezius muscle. Capillary density was ruled out as a potential cause, as it was the same in healthy controls and FM patients; therefore they also suggested that hypoxia may be the cause of altered morphologic findings (28). The same investigators found decreased levels of adenosine triphosphate, adenosine diphosphate, and phosphoryl creatine, together with increased levels of adenosine monophosphate and creatine. They described discrete changes in muscle morphology and concluded that there were two possible explanations for these findings. First, the chemical changes are secondary to hypoxia, and second, there might be a metabolic change that leads to either a defective synthesis

of energy-rich-phosphates or an increased degradation of these substances (27,81).

With regard to capillary density on the nailfolds, Morf et al. showed a lowered capillary density in FM than in healthy controls (79). Furthermore, in her study she describes morphologic abnormalities of nailfold capillaries (79). Frodin et al. examined nailfold capillary morphology and blood flow in FM patients and also found slight morphologic abnormalities (82).

Larsson et al. (83) found a correlation between pain and reduced blood flow supporting the hypothesis that localized muscle pain might be related to temporary hypoxia at the location of pain. Vaeroy et al. (84) recorded low levels of skin blood flow. A similarly reduced blood flow in FM was recorded by Bennett (85) and Backman (86). The question that arises from these findings is, what is the reason for the reduced blood flow? One reason could be that it results from vasoconstriction of unknown pathophysiology—for example, the local metabolic factors in the muscle, the sympathetic nerve activity, or hormonal factors control regulation of the microcirculation (87). The studies of Backman et al. illustrate the importance of the sympathetic nervous system activity in patients with FM. They found lower handgrip strength in FM patients compared to healthy controls before, as well as after, sympathetic blockade. A lower muscle relaxation rate was found in FM patients. The relaxation rate increased in FM patients during the sympathetic blockade (86). The efficiency of the stellate ganglion blockade was evaluated by measuring blood flow, temperature, and conductance responses of the skin. Bengtsson et al. concluded that the reduction of pain and TePs by a sympathetic blockade might be due to an improvement in microcirculation. Furthermore, they hypothesized that sympathetic activity contributes to the pathogenesis of FM (88). Bennett et al. found an increased density of α-2 receptors in FM patients, predisposing them to cold-induced and emotionally induced vasospasm. In the same study, they recorded a decreased blood flow before the start of the test (85). Coffman et al. showed that the α-2 receptors are predominant in controlling sympathetic vasoconstriction (89). Vaeroy et al. observed that the vasoconstrictory response to the cold pressure test was significantly lower in FM patients versus healthy controls. However, they were not able to rule out the possibility that the basal sympathetic tone was increased in the FM patients (84). If the stimulation for noradrenaline secretion is at the maximum, blood flow through the muscle can decrease to about 25% of normal flow volume (88). One explanation for this could be an increase in sympathetic nervous activity. It has been shown that sympathetic nervous activity is increased during static muscle contraction (90).

Based on these facts, it could be hypothesized that in FM patients afferent physical and psychological stimuli produce efferent motorial and sympathetic responses. The result of the efferent motorial response is an increase in muscle tension. The result of efferent sympathetic response is a sympathetic nervous overactivity. The increased sympathetic nervous activity also induces greater muscle tension and localized vasoconstriction in the arterioles and precapillary sphincters in FM muscle. Local vasoconstriction results in an increased concentration and speed of erythrocytes. The flux decreases (78). As a consequence, oxygen demand outweighs oxygen supply. Localized hypoxia, with a decrease of high-energy phosphate levels, occurs, resulting in morphologic changes, ischemia, and pain.

Several factors are thought to interact: muscle overload, bad posture of the spine (91), disturbed sleep (92), psychogenic factors (93), local hypoxia (26,80), or reduced high-energy phosphate levels (27). Thus, the results of these studies support the hypothesis that localized muscle pain in FM might be related to a localized transient hypoxic environment. Vasoconstriction occurs in the slightest amount at the TePs. The involvement of the sympathetic nervous system in the pathogenesis of pain in FM should be given extraordinary consideration.

ABNORMALITIES BESIDES THE MUSCLE

In addition, to the description of muscular changes, there is evidence for the involvement of the skin in the pathophysiology of FM (94). Skin tissue appears to be of particular importance in the development and perception of pain in FM patients. There is a diminished threshold for pain in patients with FM, especially at the anatomical region of TePs. The current opinion is that the TeP is the source of nociception, and several indications support this hypothesis. Nonetheless, from a clinical standpoint, there is no way of determining if the sensitivity of the structures above the TeP, under pressure, are indeed the source of nociception. One could also argue that the nociceptive input is localized in the skin and only becomes prominent above TePs because of the hard layer of the tendon-bone-junction. This hypothesis is unproven. However, some interesting abnormalities in the skin tissue of FM patients have been observed, as outlined below.

First of all, we could demonstrate highly ordered collagen cuffs around terminal nerve fibers in skin biopsies of FM patients (see Figure 9-6), whereas this was not found in any of the healthy controls (95). Moreover, both the urine excretion and serum levels of collagen crosslinks, a degradation product of collagen metabolism, were significantly lower than in healthy controls. One might speculate that these collagen crosslinks are needed to maintain the collagen cuffs around the nerves in the skin. This we termed as "micro scars" and compared them to macroscopic scars on the skin surface, which are in part characterized by lowered pain thresholds (and also sensitivity to changes in the weather). One of the reasons for collagen formation could be "neurogenic inflammation," which we also could demonstrate in the skin (96). To investigate whether proinflammatory cytokines are produced in FM patients, interleukin-1β, interleukin-6, and TNF-α were studied for their expression in the skin of FM patients. Positive signals for these cytokines on the mRNA level were detected in approximately one-third of the examined FM patients. None of the cytokines could be detected in the skin of healthy controls. Consistent with the mRNA data, immunoreactivity for the above mentioned cytokines could be detected on FM skin tissues in fibroblast-like cells. However, the number of positive cells and the intensity of staining were low.

Certain studies suggest that cytokines may play a role in FM, but their origin and localization has not yet been shown. Cytokines are able to activate fibroblasts and stimulate them to produce extracellular matrix (97). In order to detect neurogenic inflammation at sites of cytokine expression, slides were double labeled with a nerve marker, which shows the expression of cytokines at the site of nerves. In previous studies Wallace et al. reported significantly higher levels of interleukin-1 receptor antibodies (IL-1Ra) and interleukin-8 in sera (98). IL-1Ra and interleukin-6 were shown to be significantly higher in stimulated and unstimulated FM peripheral blood mononuclear cells (PBMC) compared to controls. Serum interleukin-6 levels were comparable to those in controls, but were elevated in supernatants of in vitro-activated PBMCs derived from patients with >2 years of symptoms. In the presence of phorbol myristate acetate, there were additional increases in IL-1Ra, interleukin-8, and interleukin-6 over control values.

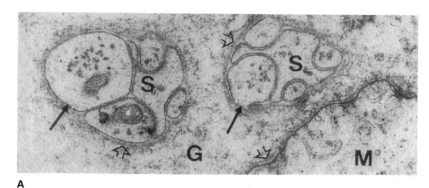

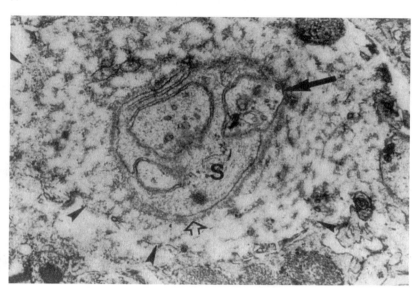

Figure 9-6. Subepidermal connective tissue in representative skin samples from a healthy control subject and a patient with fibromyalgia. **(A)** Uninvolved skin: cross section of 2 preterminal "naked" nerve fibers. Axons (*arrows*) are partly unfolded from Schwann's cell sheath (S). A basal lamina (*open arrow*) surrounds the nerve fibers. G, ground substance (extracellular matrix); M, myofibroblast. **B:** Subepidermal connective tissue of fibromyalgia skin from a trapezius TeP. Cross section of a nearly unmyelinated preterminal sensitive nerve with three axons. One of these is partly unfolded (*arrow*) from the Schwann's cell sheath. A clearly visible collagen cuff (*arrow heads*) sheaths the preterminal nerve fibers. (From Sprott H, Muller A, Heine H. Collagen crosslinks in fibromyalgia. *Arthritis Rheum* 1997;40:1452, with permission.)

Therefore, it was suggested that cytokines such as interleukin-8 act as a promotor of sympathetic pain and interleukin-6 as an inducer of hyperalgesia (98).

These results suggest an inflammatory component in some FM patients. Neurogenic inflammation may occur when SP and other neuropeptides released from sensory nerve fibers produce an inflammatory response (99). However, there is no proof as to whether these observations are either components of a given pathway or are unrelated epiphenomena.

Various investigators independent of one another have carried out extensive examinations of the neurotransmitter serotonin and the neuropeptide SP in FM (100–103). It is apparent that there are differences in concentration of serotonin and SP in the cerebrospinal fluid as well as in the serum of FM patients compared to the healthy control group.

An association exists between endogenous opioids and cytokines. Endorphins and enkephalins can increase the production of proinflammatory cytokines, including interleukin-1, interleukin-2, and interferon-gamma (104–107).

In preceding years, the opioid system distant from the nervous system has been the focus of our research. We know that endogenous opioids (endorphins, enkephalins, and dynorphins) and their receptors (μ-, δ-, and κ-opioid receptors) exist, but there is little compelling evidence of their consequences. From the scientific literature we do know the

following: Dynorphin-autoantibodies have been shown to be elevated in the serum of FM patients (108).

Endorphins seem to be decreased in the FM blood (109,110). The endogenous opioid peptides are not specific to one receptor (111). An interaction between endogenous opioids and their opioid receptor is essential for analgesia. They have been found in dorsal root ganglia on central and peripheral terminals of primary afferent neurons in animals as well as in humans (112,113). Our group has provided evidence that opioid receptors are present in skin tissue of FM patients (94). Skin tissues have detectable gene and protein expression levels of δ- and κ-opioid receptors (see Figure 9-7). The μ-opioid receptor was not detectable at either level. Other molecules and autoantibodies are currently under investigation (98,108,114–118).

The opioid system in combination with previously described mechanisms present in FM (e.g., elevated NO levels, peripheral opioid receptors, local hypoxic conditions, abnormalities of mitochondria, increased DNA fragmentation, increased endothelin levels, abnormal and spastic vessels, reduced microcirculation) provides a foundation for an explanatory model of the development of chronic pain in this disease. Chronic nociceptive stimuli result, as well as peripheral and central sensitization, chronic pain, and allodynia. Interestingly, it has always

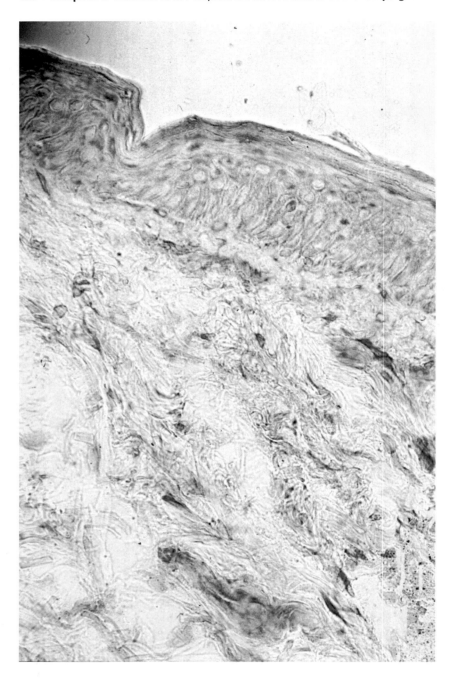

Figure 9-7. Example of opioid receptor protein (dark signals) in skin of fibromyalgia patients.

been possible to demonstrate all these abnormalities in a certain percentage of FM patients. This may be due to the heterogeneity of the FM population, may result from diagnostic errors (insufficient and subjective criteria to diagnose FM), and/or may be due to the existence of FM subgroups—for example, those demonstrated by the cytokine experiments (96,98).

In summary, there are some abnormalities in the peripheral system of FM patients—for example, in the muscle (see Table 9-1), in the blood (serotonin, cytokines), and in the skin (neurogenic inflammation, reduced microcirculation with changes of capillaries and collagen deposits around terminal nerves, resulting hypoxia). These abnormalities may not be specific to FM and thus do not justify an explanation of the origin of FM. However, they may explain sources of

nociception in FM patients which can initiate the cascade of neuroplastical changes in the central nervous system. Therefore, maintenance of sensitization, resulting in hypersensitivity and allodynia, appears to take place. Not every subject with a history of a strong or long-lasting stimulus will develop FM; thus there must also be some "susceptibility factors" (Figure 9-1).

Unambiguous diagnostic criteria to distinguish FM from other chronic widespread pain diseases have yet to be defined. Furthermore, there is a need to develop criteria to define and distinguish the various subsets of FM. This will enable clinicians to customize treatment to the individual's diagnosis (119). It should be added that in order for these advances to be made, it is critical that there is an integration of basic research and clinical investigation.

TABLE 9-1	Putative Muscle Abnormalities in Fibromyalgia	
OBSERVED MUSCLE ABNORMALITY	**LIKELIHOOD**	**REFERENCES**
Morphologic changes, such as		
• Degeneration or regeneration of muscle fibers	Confirmed	(18,19,28–31,34–38)
• Ragged red fibers	Confirmed	(18,19,28–31)
• Accumulation of glycogen, lipid	Confirmed	(29–31,33)
• Damaged mitochondria	Probable	(20,33)
• Increased DNA fragmentation	Probable	(25,33)
• Activation of opioid receptors	Speculative	(32,41)
• Moth-eaten fibers	Speculative	(18,19,28–32)
• Perivascular collections of inflammatory cells	Unlikely	(18,19)
• Type II fiber atrophy	Unlikely	(25,32)
Disturbed microcirculation	Confirmed	(20,77–80,82–86,88)
Local hypoxia	Confirmed	(26–28,80)
Increased NO levels and prolonged release	Confirmed	(21–24)
Reduced ATP levels	Confirmed	(20,26,27,71,73,81)
Increased electrical myographic activity	Probable	(70)
Increased levels of neuropeptides	Speculative	(32,41)

All the described muscle abnormalities are probably not specific for fibromyalgia (FM), as far as we know. DNA, deoxyribonucleic acid; NO, nitric oxide; ATP, adenosine triphosphate.

THERAPEUTIC APPROACHES

The aim for future therapeutic strategies should take into account some of these observations and target symptomatic relief in FM (120,121). There is evidence that targeting peripheral opioid receptors may be useful in the management of chronic pain diseases (122). Local pain therapy with selective opioids that interact with their specific opioid receptors in case of chronic painful syndromes appears to be an attractive alternative to the systemic application of opioids. Early local and sufficient analgesic interventions on the δ-opioid system in the skin of FM are an interesting therapeutic target to avoid neuroplastical changes in the region of the spinal cord (116,119).

Antagonistic interactions in both the induction of pain and inflammatory responses occur between pain modulating molecules and opioid peptides—for example, receptor-selective δ- or κ-opioid agonists attenuate the bradykinin effects, in contrast to selective μ-opioid agonists that do not (123). In order to reduce the risk of adverse effects that results from systemic treatment, new routes (e.g., local) of opioid administration have to be established. It has been suggested that the local application of opioids in the vicinity of peripheral nerve terminals prevents central side effects such as respiratory depression, addiction, nausea, and/or sedation (124). Recent data suggest that the activation of opioid receptors outside the central nervous system can initiate opioid antinociception. This indicates that targeting peripheral opioid receptors might be useful in the management of chronic pain diseases (122,125). These findings have expanded the field of knowledge in pain control and have led to suggestions for new approaches in the development of peripherally acting opioid analgesics with little to no central side effects.

Other physiologic systems, such as serotonin metabolism, may be further influenced, not only by the administration of tricyclics and/or selective serotonin reuptake inhibitors (SSRIs) but also by acupuncture (102,126,127). The serum serotonin level immediately increases after this intervention. In a clinical study of the effects of acupuncture treatment in FM patients, we observed a decrease in pain and number of TePs, normalization of the serum serotonin level, and an increase of serum SP (102). This suggests that acupuncture may also be a treatment option in pain therapy to reduce the symptoms in patients with FM (119).

The detection of cytokines in FM skin suggests the presence of inflammatory foci in the skin of certain FM patients (about 30%) and may explain the response to NSAID therapy in this particular subset of FM patients.

The endothelin-1 receptor antagonist bosentan is used for treating disturbed microcirculation in scleroderma patients with Raynaud phenomenon (128). This may be a potential treatment option for FM patients with disturbed microcirculation and elevated plasma endothelin-1 (17).

In conclusion, it is hypothesized that the peripheral abnormalities presented in FM come about in the following sequence. First there is a local injury that acts as a nociceptive input and results in acute pain. Under certain circumstances, neurogenic inflammation then maintains local permanent stimuli to the nervous system and leads to spreading of more nociceptive fields. Cytokines then activates skin fibroblasts that produce extracellular matrix. This mechanism ("micro scarification"), as well as the release of NO and endothelin, acts as chronic stimuli. Muscle tissue is now under hypoxic conditions and reacts with swelling of endothelial cells, muscular hypertension, mitochondrial changes, and satellite cell activation. This may be indicated by an increase in DNA fragmentation and elevated endothelin levels. Peripheral sensitization then leads to central sensitization. Neuroplastical changes in the nervous system can be observed. Receptive fields further increase. Efferent mechanisms and the involvement of the vegetative nervous system contribute to the amplification of the initial peripheral input signal. Microtrauma of muscle fibers can be objectified but may already be a secondary phenomenon. Nevertheless, they can react as nociceptive stimuli, which may amplify this vicious peripheral cycle. At a later stage of the disease the periphery becomes less important because central processes are then autonomous and can maintain a pathologic response to painless stimuli and also pain without stimuli (Figure 9-1). Central phenomena like depression, fatigue, and psychological disturbances are then inevitable in FM patients. Therapeutical intervention at this late stage of FM may be difficult or unsuccessful, or both.

There is still a need for improved understanding of the origin of FM, and effective treatment options must be developed to deal with each individual patient's symptoms (119,129,130). Research in this area is ongoing, but more comprehensive and progressive research is required to identify the factors that cause and perpetuate FM (131,132).

SUMMARY POINTS

- Although FM and related conditions have classically been considered to be "central" rather than "peripheral" processes, accumulating data now suggests that, at least in a subset of patients, peripheral factors may play a role.

■ IMPLICATIONS FOR PRACTICE

- If there is a subset of patients who have a peripheral rather than (or in addition to) a central cause for the pain or other symptoms of fibromyalgia, these individuals may respond to pharmacologic agents such as NSAIDs or selective opioids.

REFERENCES

1. Henriksson KG. Chronic muscular pain: aetiology and pathogenesis. *Baillieres Clin Rheumatol* 1994;8:703–719.
2. Bennett RM. Fibromyalgia and the disability dilemma. A new era in understanding a complex, multidimensional pain syndrome. *Arthritis Rheum* 1996;39:1627–1634.
3. Bennett RM. Fibromyalgia: the commonest cause of widespread pain. *Compr Ther* 1995;21:269–275.
4. Jaeger B, Skootsky SA. Double blind, controlled study of different myofascial trigger point injection technique. *Pain* 1987;31:S292.
5. Rajora N, Boccoli G, Burns D, et al. alpha-MSH modulates local and circulating tumor necrosis factor-alpha in experimental brain inflammation. *J Neurosci* 1997;17:2181–2186.
6. Leem JG, Bove GM. Mid-axonal tumor necrosis factor-alpha induces ectopic activity in a subset of slowly conducting cutaneous and deep afferent neurons. *J Pain* 2002;3:45–49.
7. Kilo S, Harding-Rose C, Hargreaves KM, et al. Peripheral CGRP release as a marker for neurogenic inflammation: a model system for the study of neuropeptide secretion in rat paw skin. *Pain* 1997;73:201–207.
8. Lawson SN, Crepps B, Perl ER. Calcitonin gene-related peptide immunoreactivity and afferent receptive properties of dorsal root ganglion neurones in guinea-pigs. *J Physiol* 2002;540:989–1002.
9. Harmar A, Keen P. Synthesis and central and peripheral axonal transport of substance P in a dorsal root ganglion-nerve preparation in vitro. *Brain Res* 1982;231:379–385.
10. Tegeder L, Zimmermann J, Meller ST, et al. Release of algesic substances in human experimental muscle pain. *Inflamm Res* 2002;51:393–402.
11. Woolf CJ. Phenotypic modification of primary sensory neurons: the role of nerve growth factor in the production of persistent pain. *Philos Trans R Soc London B Biol Sci* 1996;351:441–448.
12. Saade NE, Massaad CA, Ochoa-Chaar CI, et al. Upregulation of proinflammatory cytokines and nerve growth factor by intraplantar injection of capsaicin in rats. *J Physiol* 2002;545:241–253.
13. Taiwo YO, Levine JD. Direct cutaneous hyperalgesia induced by adenosine. *Neuroscience* 1990;38:757–762.
14. Konttinen YT, Kemppinen P, Sergerberg M, et al. Peripheral and spinal neural mechanisms in arthritis, with particular reference to treatment of inflammation and pain. *Arthritis Rheum* 1994;37:965–982.
15. Filippi S, Marini M, Vannelli GB, et al. Effects of hypoxia on endothelin-1 sensitivity in the corpus cavernosum. *Mol Hum Reprod* 2003;9:765–774.
16. Flamant M, Tharaux PL, Placier S, et al. Epidermal growth factor receptor trans-activation mediates the tonic and fibrogenic effects of endothelin in the aortic wall of transgenic mice. *FASEB J* 2003;17:327–329.
17. Pache M, Ochs J, Genth E, et al. Increased plasma endothelin-1 levels in fibromyalgia syndrome. *Rheumatology (Oxford)* 2003;42:493–494.
18. Henriksson KG, Bengtsson A, Larsson J, et al. Muscle biopsy findings of possible diagnostic importance in primary fibromyalgia (fibrositis, myofascial syndrome). *Lancet* 1982;2:1395.
19. Bengtsson A, Henriksson KG. The muscle in fibromyalgia—a review of Swedish studies. *J Rheumatol* 1989;19(Suppl.):144–149.
20. Yunus MB, Masi AT, Calabro JJ, et al. Primary fibromyalgia (fibrositis): clinical study of 50 patients with matched normal controls. *Semin Arthritis Rheum* 1981;11:151–171.
21. Choi YB, Lipton SA. Redox modulation of the NMDA receptor. *Cell Mol Life Sci* 2000;57:1535–1541.
22. Larson AA, Giovengo SL, Russell IJ, et al. Changes in the concentrations of amino acids in the cerebrospinal fluid that correlate with pain in patients with fibromyalgia: implications for nitric oxide pathways. *Pain* 2000;87:201–211.
23. Bradley LA, Weigent DA, Sotolongo A, et al. Blood serum levels of nitric oxide (NO) are elevated in women with fibromyalgia (FM): possible contributions to central and peripheral sensitization. *Arthritis Rheum* 2000;43:S173.
24. Graven-Nielsen T, Aspegren Kendall S, Henriksson KG, et al. Ketamine reduces muscle pain, temporal summation, and referred pain in fibromyalgia patients. *Pain* 2000;85:483–491.
25. Yunus MB, Kalyan-Raman UP, Kalyan-Raman K, et al. Pathologic changes in muscle in primary fibromyalgia syndrome. *Am J Med* 1986;81(Suppl. 3A):38–42.
26. Fassbender HG, Wegner K. Morphologie und Pathogenese des Weichteilrheumatismus [Morphology and pathogenesis of the soft-tissue rheumatism]. *Z Rheumaforsch* 1973;32:355–374.
27. Bengtsson A, Henriksson KG, Larsson J. Reduced high-energy phosphate levels in the painful muscles of patients with primary fibromyalgia. *Arthritis Rheum* 1986;29:817–821.

28. Bengtsson A, Henriksson KG, Larsson J. Muscle biopsy in primary fibromyalgia. Light-microscopical and histochemical findings. *Scand J Rheumatol* 1986;15:1–6.

29. Yunus MB, Kalyan-Raman UP, Masi AT, et al. Electron microscopic studies of muscle biopsy in primary fibromyalgia syndrome: a controlled and blinded study. *J Rheumatol* 1989;16:97–101.

30. Yunus MB, Kalyan-Raman UP. Muscle biopsy findings in primary fibromyalgia and other forms of nonarticular rheumatism. *Rheum Dis Clin North Am* 1989;15:115–134.

31. Jacobsen S, Bartels EM, Danneskiold-Samsoe B. Single cell morphology of muscle in patients with chronic muscle pain. *Scand J Rheumatol* 1991;20:336–343.

32. Salemi S, Aeschlimann A, Gay RE, et al. Expression and localization of opioid receptors in muscle satellite cells: no difference between fibromyalgia patients and healthy subjects. *Arthritis Rheum* 2003;48:3291–3293.

33. Sprott H, Salemi S, Gay RE, et al. Increased DNA fragmentation and ultrastructural changes in fibromyalgic muscle fibers. *Ann Rheum Dis* 2004;63:245–251.

34. Wyllie AH, Kerr JFR, Currie AR. Cell death. The significance of apoptosis. *Int Rev Cytol* 1980;68:251.

35. Wyllie AH. Glucocorticoid-induced thymocyte apoptosis is associated with endogenous endonuclease activation. *Nature* 1980;284:555–556.

36. Duke RC, Chervenak R, Cohen JJ. Endogenous endonuclease-induced DNA fragmentation: an early event in cell mediated cytolysis. *Proc Natl Acad Sci USA* 1983;80:6361.

37. Fawthrop DJ, Boobis AR, Davies DS. Mechanisms of cell death. *Arch Toxicol* 1991;65:437–444.

38. Gavrieli Y, Sherman Y, Ben-Sasson SA. Identification of programmed cell death in situ via specific labeling of nuclear DNA fragmentation. *J Cell Biol* 1992;119:493–501.

39. Kalso E, Smith L, McQuay HJ, et al. No pain, no gain: clinical excellence and scientific rigour—lessons learned from IA morphine. *Pain* 2002;98:269–275.

40. Stein C. Immune mechanisms in pain control. *J Neurochem* 2003;85(Suppl. 2):12.

41. Stein C, Schafer M, Machelska H. Attacking pain at its source: new perspectives on opioids. *Nat Med* 2003;9:1003–1008.

42. Sprott H, Bradley LA, Oh SJ, et al. Immunohistochemical and molecular studies of serotonin, substance P, galanin, pituitary adenylyl cyclase-activating polypeptide, and secretoneurin in fibromyalgic muscle tissue. *Arthritis Rheum* 1998;41:1689–1694.

43. De Stefano R, Selvi E, Villanova M, et al. Image analysis quantification of substance P immunoreactivity in the trapezius muscle of patients with fibromyalgia and myofascial pain syndrome. *J Rheumatol* 2000;27:2906–2910.

44. Machelska H, Stein C. Immune mechanisms in pain control. *Anesth Analg* 2002;95:1002–1008.

45. Cabot PJ, Carter L, Gaiddon C, et al. Immune cell-derived beta-endorphin. Production, release, and control of inflammatory pain in rats. *J Clin Invest* 1997;100:142–148.

46. Cabot PJ, Carter L, Schafer M, et al. Methionine-enkephalin- and dynorphin A-release from immune cells and control of inflammatory pain. *Pain* 2001;93:207–212.

47. Stein C, Millan MJ, Shippenberg TS, et al. Peripheral opioid receptors mediating antinociception in inflammation. Evidence for involvement of mu, delta and kappa receptors. *J Pharmacol Exp Ther* 1989;248:1269–1275.

48. Fields H. In: Borsook D, ed. *Molecular neurobiology of pain.* Seattle, WA: IASP, 1997:307–317.

49. Yaksh TL. Spinal systems and pain processing: development of novel analgesic drugs with mechanistically defined models. *Trends Pharmacol Sci* 1999;20:329–337.

50. Gunji N, Nagashima M, Asano G, et al. Expression of kappa-opioid receptor mRNA in human peripheral blood lymphocytes and the relationship between its expression and the inflammatory changes in rheumatoid arthritis. *Rheumatol Int* 2000;19:95–100.

51. Wetzel MA, Steele AD, Eisenstein TK, et al. μ-opioid induction of monocyte chemoattractant protein-1, RANTES, and IFN-γ-inducible protein-10 expression in human peripheral blood mononuclear cells. *J Immunol* 2000; 165:6519–6524.

52. Binder W, Machelska H, Mousa S, et al. Analgesic and anti-inflammatory effects of two novel kappa-opioid peptides. *Anesthesiology* 2001;94:1034–1044.

53. Yaksh TL. Substance P release from knee joint afferent terminals: modulation by opioids. *Brain Res* 1998;458:319–324.

54. Sprott H, Pap T, Rethage J, et al. Expression of the precursor of secretoneurin, secretogranin II, in the synovium of patients with rheumatoid arthritis and osteoarthritis. *J Rheumatol* 2000;27:2347–2350.

55. Averbeck B, Reeh PW, Michaelis M. Modulation of CGRP and PGE2 release from isolated rat skin by alpha-adrenoceptors and kappa-opioid-receptors. *NeuroReport* 2001;12: 2097–2100.

56. Delgado M, Leceta J, Ganea D. Vasoactive intestinal peptide and pituitary adenylate cyclase-activating polypeptide promote in vivo generation of memory Th2 cells. *FASEB J* 2002;16:1844–1846.

57. Chao CC, Molitor TW, Close K, et al. Morphine inhibits the release of tumor necrosis factor in human peripheral blood mononuclear cell cultures. *Int J Immunopharmacol* 1993;15: 447–453.

58. Wilson JL, Walker JS, Antoon JS, et al. Intercellular adhesion molecule-1 expression in adjuvant arthritis in rats: inhibition by kappa-opioid agonist but not by NSAID. *J Rheumatol* 1998;25:499–505.

59. Walker JS. Anti-inflammatory effects of opioids. *Adv Exp Med Biol* 2003;521:148–160.

60. Spampinato S, Speroni E, Govoni P, et al. Effect of omega-conotoxin and verapamil on antinociceptive, behavioural and thermoregulatory responses to opioids in the rat. *Eur J Pharmacol* 1994;254:229–238.

61. Ohsawa M, Nagase H, Kamei J. Role of intracellular calcium in modification of mu and delta opioid receptor-mediated antinociception by diabetes in mice. *J Pharmacol Exp Ther* 1998;286:780–787.

62. Carpenter E, Gent JP, Peears C. Opioid receptor independent inhibition of Ca^{2+} and K^+ currents in NG108-15 cells by kappa opioid receptor agonist U-50, 488H. *NeuroReport* 1996;7:1809–1812.

63. Ohsawa M, Nagase H, Kamei J. Role of intracellular calcium in modification of mu and delta opioid receptor-mediated antinociception by diabetes in mice. *J Pharmacol Exp Ther* 1998;286:780–787.

64. Beauchamp JR, Heslop L, Yu DS, et al. Expression of CD34 and Myf5 defines the majority of quiescent adult skeletal muscle satellite cells. *J Cell Biol* 2000;151:1221–1234.

65. Salemi S, Aeschlimann A, Gay RE, et al. Expression of opioid receptors in chronic pain patients with fibromyalgia, osteoarthritis, psychosis, rheumatoid arthritis and healthy controls. *Ann Rheum Dis* 2001;60(Suppl. 1):246.

66. Bischoff R. The satellite cell and muscle regeneration. In: Engel AG, Franzini-Armstrong C, eds. *Myology*, Vol. 1. New York: McGraw-Hill, 1994:97–118.

67. Wei YH, Kao SH, Lee HC. Simultaneous increase of mitochondrial DNA deletions and lipid peroxidation in human aging. *Ann NY Acad Sci* 1996;786:24–43.

68. Sandri M, Carraro U, Podhorska-Okolov M, et al. Apoptosis, DNA damage and ubiquitin expression in normal and mdx muscle fibers after exercise. *FEBS Lett* 1995;373: 291–295.

69. Kirtava Z, Mdinaradze-Kirtava DK, Jacobsson L, et al. Fibromyalgia and disability. *Scand J Rheumatol* 1995;24: 395–396.

70. Anders C, Sprott H, Scholle HC. Surface EMG of the lumbar part of the erector trunci muscle in patients with fibromyalgia. *Clin Exp Rheum* 2001;19:453–455.

71. Park JH, Phothimat P, Oates CT, et al. Use of P-31 magnetic resonance spectroscopy to detect metabolic abnormalities in muscles of patients with fibromyalgia. *Arthritis Rheum* 1998;41:406–413.

72. Sprott H, Rzanny R, Reichenbach JR, et al. 31P Magnetic resonance spectroscopy in fibromyalgic muscle. *Rheumatology* 2000;39:1121–1125.

73. Jubrias SA, Bennett RM, Klug GA. Increased incidence of a resonance in the phosphodiester region of 31P nuclear magnetic resonance spectra in the skeletal muscle of fibromyalgia patients. *Arthritis Rheum* 1994;37:801–807.

74. Matthews PM, Allaire C, Shoubridge EA, et al. In vivo muscle magnetic resonance spectroscopy in the clinical investigation of mitochondrial disease. *Neurology* 1991;41: 114–120.

75. Kemp GJ, Tayler DJ, Dunn JF, et al. Cellular energetics of dystrophic muscle. *J Neurol Sci* 1993;116:201–206.

76. Argov Z, Taivassalo T, De Stefano N, et al. Intracellular phosphates in inclusion body myositis—a 31P magnetic resonance spectroscopy study. *Muscle Nerve* 1998;21:1523–1525.

77. Toissaint JF, Kwong KK, M'Kparu F, et al. Interrelationship of oxidative metabolism and local perfusion demonstrated by NMR in human skeletal muscle. *J Appl Physiol* 1996;81: 2221–2228.

78. Jeschonneck M, Grohmann G, Hein G, et al. Abnormal microcirculation and temperature in tender points in patients with fibromyalgia (FM). *Rheumatology* 2000;39:917–921.

79. Morf S, Amann-Vesti B, Forster A, et al. Microcirculation abnormalities in patients with fibromyalgia measured by capillary microscopy and laser fluxmetry. *Arthritis Res Ther* 2005;7: R209–R216.

80. Lund N, Bengtsson A, Thorborg P. Muscle tissue oxygen pressure in primary fibromyalgia. *Scand J Rheumatol* 1986; 15:165–173.

81. Bengtsson A, Henriksson KG, Jorfeldt L, et al. Primary fibromyalgia. A clinical and laboratory study of 55 patients. *Scand J Rheumatol* 1986;15:340–347.

82. Frodin T, Bengtsson A, Skogh M. Nail fold capillaroscopy findings in patients with primary fibromyalgia. *Clin Rheumatol* 1988;7:384–388.

83. Larsson SE, Bodegard L, Henriksson KG, et al. Chronic trapezius myalgia. Morphology and blood flow studied in 17 patients. *Acta Orthop Scand* 1990;61:394–398.

84. Vaeroy H, Qiao ZG, Morkrid L, et al. Altered sympathetic nervous system response in patients with fibromyalgia (fibrositis syndrome). *J Rheumatol* 1989;16:1460–1465.

85. Bennett RM, Clark SR, Campbell SM, et al. Symptoms of Raynaud's syndrome in patients with fibromyalgia. A study utilizing the Nielsen test, digital photoplethysmography, and measurements of platelet alpha 2-adrenergic receptors. *Arthritis Rheum* 1991;34:264–269.

86. Backman E, Bengtsson A, Bengtsson M, et al. Skeletal muscle function in primary fibromyalgia. Effect of regional sympathetic blockade with guanethidine. *Acta Neurol Scand* 1988;77:187–191.

87. Schmidt RF, Thews G. [Local regulation of blood flow and microcirculation] Lokale Durchblutungsregulation und Mikrozirkulation. In: Schmidt RF, Thewes G, eds. *Physiologie des menschen*. Berlin, Heidelberg, New York: Springer, 1997;514–534.

88. Bengtsson A, Bengtsson M. Regional sympathetic blockade in primary fibromyalgia. *Pain* 1988;33:161–167.

89. Coffman JD, Cohen RA. Role of alpha-adrenoceptor subtypes mediating sympathetic vasoconstriction in human digits. *Eur J Clin Invest* 1988;18:309–313.

90. Mark AL, Victor RG, Nerhed C, et al. Microneurographic studies of the mechanisms of sympathetic nerve responses to static exercise in humans. *Circ Res* 1985;57:461–469.

91. Gallatie M, Bruckle W, Muller W. [X-ray changes of the lumbal spine in patients with fibromyalgia as compared with healthy controls] Radiologische LWS-Veränderungen bei Patienten mit generalisierter Tendomyopathie im Vergleich zu einer gesunden Kontrollgruppe. *Z Rheumatol* 1988;4(Suppl. P26): 280.

92. Moldofsky H. Sleep and fibrositis syndrome. *Rheum Dis Clin North Am* 1989;15:91–103.

93. Hell D, Balmer R, Battegay R, et al. [Generalized fibrositis syndrome and personality: a controlled study] Weichteilrheumatismus und Persönlichkeit: eine kontrollierte Studie. *Schweiz Rundsch Med Prax* 1982;71:1014–1021.

94. Sprott H, Salemi S, Gay RE, et al. Elevation of opioid receptor (OR) expression in skin tissues of fibromyalgia (FMS) patients. *J Musculoskelet Pain* 2001;9(Suppl. 5):77.

95. Sprott H, Muller A, Heine H. Collagen crosslinks in fibromyalgia. *Arthritis Rheum* 1997;40:1450–1454.

96. Salemi S, Rethage J, Wollina U, et al. Detection of interleukin 1beta (IL-1beta), IL-6, and tumor necrosis factor-alpha in skin of patients with fibromyalgia. *J Rheumatol* 2003;30:146–150.

97. Dasu MR, Barrow RE, Spies M, et al. Matrix metalloproteinase expression in cytokine stimulated human dermal fibroblasts. *Burns* 2003;29:527–531.

98. Wallace DJ, Linker-Israeli M, Hallegua D, et al. Cytokines play an aetiopathogenetic role in fibromyalgia: a hypothesis and pilot study. *Rheumatology (Oxford)* 2001;40:743–749.

99. Meggs WJ. Neurogenic switching: a hypothesis for a mechanism for shifting the site of inflammation in allergy and chemical sensitivity. *Environ Health Perspect* 1995;103:54–56.

100. Russell IJ, Michalek JE, Vipraio GA, et al. Platelet 3H-imipramine uptake receptor density and serum serotonin levels in patients with fibromyalgia/fibrositis syndrome. *J Rheumatol* 1992;19:104–109.

101. Wolfe F, Russell IJ, Vipraio G, et al. Serotonin levels, pain threshold, and fibromyalgia symptoms in the general population. *J Rheumatol* 1997;24:555–559.

102. Sprott H, Franke S, Kluge H, et al. Pain treatment of fibromyalgia by acupuncture. *Rheumatol Int* 1998;18:35–36.

103. Russell IJ, Orr MD, Littman B, et al. Elevated cerebrospinal fluid levels of substance P in patients with the fibromyalgia syndrome. *Arthritis Rheum* 1994;37:1593–1601.

104. Brown SL, van Epps DE. Opioid peptides modulate production of interferon-γ by human mononuclear cells. *Cell Immunol* 1986;103:19.

105. Mandler RN, Biddison WE, Mandler R, et al. β-Endorphin augments the cytolytic activity and interferon production of natural killer cells. *J Immunol* 1986;136:934.

106. Bessler H, Sztein MB, Serrate SA. β-Endorphin modulation of IL-1 induced IL-2 production. *Immunopharmacology* 1990; 19:5.

107. van den Bergh P, Rozing J, Nagelkeren L. Two opposing modes of action of β-endorphin on lymphocyte function. *Immunology* 1991;72:537.

108. Fasy TM, Russell IJ, McElroy KMT, et al. Autoantibodies binding enkephalin, historphin and other opioid peptides in a subset of fibromyalgia patients. *J Musculoskelet Pain* 2001; 5(Suppl.):24.

109. Tsigos C, Chrousos GP. Hypothalamic-pituitary-adrenal axis, neuroendocrine factors and stress. *J Psychosom Res* 2002;53: 865–871.

110. Panerai AE, Vecchiet J, Panzeri P, et al. Peripheral blood mononuclear cell beta-endorphin concentration is decreased in

chronic fatigue syndrome and fibromyalgia but not in depression: preliminary report. *Clin J Pain* 2002;18:270–273.

111. Kosterlitz HW. The Wellcome Foundation lecture, 1982. Opioid peptides and their receptors. *Proc R Soc London B Biol Sci* 1985;225:27–40.

112. Ji RR, Zhang Q, Law PY, et al. Expression of mu-, delta-, and kappa-opioid receptor-like immunoreactivities in rat dorsal root ganglia after carrageenan-induced inflammation. *J Neurosci* 1995;15:8156–8166.

113. Mansour A, Fox CA, Akil H, et al. Opioid-receptor mRNA expression in the rat CNS: anatomical and functional implications. *Trends Neurosci* 1995;18:22–29.

114. Russell IJ. Neurochemical pathogenesis of fibromyalgia syndrome. *J Musculoskelet Pain* 1999;7:183–191.

115. Fasy TM, Russell IJ, Lambert P. Nocistatin-binding autoantibodies are present in the sera of a subset of fibromyalgia patients. *J Musculoskelet Pain* 2001;5(Suppl.):25.

116. Fasy TM. The enkephalin-delta opioid receptor signalling pathway is a promising therapeutic target in the fibromyalgia syndrome. *J Musculoskelet Pain* 2001;5(Suppl.):26.

117. Kuan TS, Vukmirovic Z, Xiao YM, et al. Discrimination of fibromyalgia patients from normal controls using the levels of cerebrospinal chemicals. *J Musculoskelet Pain* 2001;5(Suppl.):39.

118. Kuan TS, Vukmirovic Z, Xiao YM, et al. Correlations of clinical variables with cerebrospinal chemical levels among fibromyalgia patients and healthy normal controls. *J Musculoskelet Pain* 2001;5(Suppl.):40.

119. Sprott H. What can rehabilitation interventions achieve in patients with primary fibromyalgia? *Curr Opin Rheumatol* 2003;15:145–150.

120. Sprott H, Muller W. Functional symptoms in fibromyalgia—monitored by an electronic diary. *Clin Bull Myofascial Ther* 1998;3:61–67.

121. Sprott H, Kopp G. Fibromyalgie-syndrom. In: Domschke W, Hohenberger W, Meinertz T et al., eds. *Therapie-handbuch.*

München, Wien, Baltimore,: Urban & Schwarzenberg, 2002: 9–12.

122. Stein C. Peripheral mechanisms of opioid analgesia. *Anesth Analg* 1993;76:182–191.

123. Lotz M. Neuropeptides, free radicals and nitric oxide. In: Hochberg MC, Silman AJ, Smolen JS et al., eds. *Rheumatology*. St. Louis: Mosby. An imprint of Elsevier Limited, 2003: 135–146.

124. Stein C. Peripheral analgesic actions of opioids. *J Pain Symptom Manage* 1991;6:119–124.

125. Salemi S, Bradley LA, Alarcón GS, et al. Expression of opioid receptors in human muscle and skin tissues detected by real time PCR. *Arthritis Rheum* 2000;43:S356.

126. Sprott H. Efficiency of acupuncture in patients with fibromyalgia. *Clin Bull Myofascial Ther* 1998;3:37–43.

127. Sprott H, Jeschonneck M, Grohmann G, et al. Microcirculatory changes over the tender points in fibromyalgia patients after acupuncture therapy (measured with laser-Doppler flowmetry). *Wien Klin Wochenschr* 2000;112:580–586.

128. Humbert M, Cabane J. Successful treatment of systemic sclerosis digital ulcers and pulmonary arterial hypertension with endothelin receptor antagonist bosentan. *Rheumatology (Oxford)* 2003;42:191–193.

129. Baumgartner E, Finckh A, Cedraschi C, et al. A six year prospective study of a cohort of patients with fibromyalgia. *Ann Rheum Dis* 2002;61:644–645.

130. Noller V, Sprott H. Prospective epidemiological observations on the course of the disease in fibromyalgia patients. *J Negat Results Biomed* 2003;2:4.

131. Wolfe F. The fibromyalgia problem. *J Rheumatol* 1997;24: 1247–1249.

132. Yunus MB. Primary fibromyalgia syndrome: a critical evaluation of recent criteria developments. *Z Rheumatol* 1989;48: 217–222.

10

Sleep and Its Potential Role in Chronic Pain and Fatigue

Harvey Moldofsky and James G. MacFarlane

Chronic fatigue syndrome (CFS) and fibromyalgia (FM) are chronic clinical conditions characterized by a variety of nonspecific somatic complaints. The two most prominent are intractable fatigue and unrefreshing sleep. In FM prominent diffuse musculoskeletal discomfort is the differentiating symptom. However, in terms of demographics and general clinical features, these two conditions cannot be clearly distinguished. That is, the prevalent symptoms of each disorder are present in the other (1).

The common complaint of sleep disturbances has kept these conditions within the purview of sleep disorders medicine. The combination of perceived sleep disturbance and chronic fatigue often prompts referrals to a sleep disorders clinic. It is then up to the sleep disorders specialist to sort out whether there is evidence for a primary sleep disorder that could explain the daytime impairment. The subjective experience of feeling "tired" is most often the focal point of the clinical evaluation.

What is tiredness? "Tired" is a troublesome complaint that is commonly used to describe an unpleasant ill-defined subjective experience that brings people to their physicians. Because the word has a variety of meanings, what the patient means by "tired" must be defined (2).

The description "tired" has several attributions. Fatigue may imply any of the following descriptive categories:

1. *Central fatigue.* The person may describe mental exhaustion with impairment in concentration or thinking that occurs as the result of intellectually demanding activities. The person may be unmotivated, bored, disinterested, or fed up with a particular task. If the lack of motivation is affecting all aspects of the personality, the complaint of tiredness may be a mask for abulia that characterizes a negative symptom of chronic schizophrenia or the presence of a degenerative brain disease—for example, Alzheimer, Huntington, or Parkinson disease. Tiredness is often used in the context of a mood disorder where the additional symptoms of sadness, irritability, guilt, and poor self-image may indicate a major depressive disorder. Other psychiatric disorders that have tiredness as a symptom may include general anxiety disorder, dysthymic disorder, and somatoform disorder, including neurasthenia.

2. *Physical fatigue.* A sense of overall physical exhaustion or depletion of energy as the result of physical effort can occur with or without any medical disease. Such chronic diseases as cancer; neuroendocrine, metabolic, infectious, rheumatic disease; and chronic painful diseases all have an adverse effect upon energy. Various drugs, radiation, and immune suppressants may induce profound physical exhaustion. On the other hand, where there is no evidence for a primary medical disease or psychiatric disorder and the fatigue is accompanied by unrefreshing sleep, such patients may be diagnosed with CFS or FM. Physical fatigue may be more specific, such as in conditions of muscular weakness, or progressive loss of strength may occur because of such neuromotor diseases as amyotrophic lateral sclerosis, postpolio syndrome, or myasthenia gravis.

3. *Sleepiness.* The implication is that the person feels an urge to return to sleep in the absence of central or physical fatigue. This person may actually avoid the sedentary situations preferred by those with FM and CFS, since to be inactive is to increase the propensity for falling asleep. Whereas rest or withdrawal from mental activities may relieve or reduce fatigue to some extent, only sleep relieves sleepiness.

The scientific literature provides further semiotic confusion where the word *fatigue* (i.e., driver fatigue) may be used to describe operational impairment in task performance or sleepiness. Given the confusion of language in the medical literature and various meanings and interpretations by patients, a careful clinical dissection of what the patient means by being tired is mandatory. The neglect of this clinical task may result in the physician prescribing unnecessary and expensive diagnostic procedures or inappropriate treatments.

Various chapters in this volume address the diagnostic features and management of those sleep disorders in which tiredness is a synonym for sleepiness. Moreover, the evaluations of the various medical and psychiatric conditions that result in tiredness are outside the scope of this chapter. Rather, this chapter will focus upon the assessment and management of those chronically tired patients who complain of unrefreshing sleep, chronic mental and physical fatigue in the absence of physical or laboratory evidence for a primary medical disease, or behavioral evidence for a primary psychiatric disorder. Often these people acquire such descriptive labels as "chronic fatigue syndrome" (3) or "fibromyalgia," where generalized ill-defined musculoskeletal pain and tenderness in specific anatomical regions accompany the fatigue (4).

EPIDEMIOLOGY

Epidemiologic studies reveal that 23% of the adult population in the United States report having experienced the symptom of persistent fatigue sometime during their lives (5). A cross-national epidemiologic study of primary care physicians shows that unexplained substantial fatigue occurring for more than 1 month affects approximately 8% of patients, with a range from 12% to 15% in Berlin, Santiago, and Manchester to a low prevalence between 2% and 4% in Ibadan, Verona, Shanghai, Seattle, and Bangalore (1). Within these variable prevalence clusters of patients with unexplained fatigue lay smaller groups of overlapping primary diagnoses, which include CFS and FM. In CFS, where patients complain of persistent fatigue for more than 6 months, between 0.4% and 1.5% of people are affected in the United States and Japan (6,7). In fibromyalgia syndrome (FMS), a disorder that affects approximately 2% of the population, more than 80% being women, debilitating fatigue affects between 76% and 81% of patients (4,8). Because of their symptom similarities, there is considerable overlap in diagnoses between CFS and FMS, which are also comorbid with such regional pain syndromes as temporomandibular joint disorder, irritable bowel syndrome, migraine, or tension headaches (9).

PATHOGENESIS

There are no known specific causes for CFS and FMS. Various hypotheses, including genetic factors, infectious agents, neurotransmitter, neuroendocrine, neuroimmune, and autonomic disturbances, and psychological stress factors, have been proposed for the etiology of these disorders. The fatigue and bodily hypersensitivity are thought to be the result of disturbances in central nervous system (CNS) functions (10). In particular, the myalgia and tender points (TePs) in specific anatomic regions and fatigue have been associated with unrefreshing sleep. The poor quality of sleep is related to the number of TePs in patients with FM, but not to psychological factors (11). The importance of disturbances in sleep physiology for the symptoms of these patients has been shown in four types of experiments:

1. Experimental disruption of slow wave sleep with noise in healthy subjects artificially induces both the musculoskeletal pain and fatigue symptoms (12–14). One of

these studies failed to show significant differences in TeP threshold after sleep disruption. Procedural differences, including the absence of an adaptation night, may have accounted for this discrepancy. The other study showed altered pain thresholds, but there was no associated increase in α-electroencephalogram (EEG) activity (14). However, α-EEG activity was quantified by computer generated frequency analysis rather than by visual scoring techniques previously described (12).

2. Experimental pain induction during sleep with infusion of 6% hypertonic saline resulted in increased sleep disturbance, with the appearance of increased α- and reduced δ-EEG sleep (15).

3. Experimental sleep deprivation of 40 hours duration was shown to reduce pain thresholds, which returned to baseline values specifically after slow wave sleep recovery (16).

4. Quantification of sleep disruption in patients with a clear diagnosis of FM.

Various studies have shown protracted sleep latencies (17,18), a reduced sleep efficiency index, a reduction of slow wave sleep and rapid eye movement (REM) sleep (17–20), increased motor activity during sleep and generalized restlessness (17–19,21–25), and an increase in α-EEG activity during non-REM sleep (12,18,20,26–29). The α-EEG non-REM sleep anomaly is the most extensively studied correlate of nonrestorative sleep, especially as it applies to CFS and FM. However, it is not specific to these conditions, and some studies have reported a low sensitivity (30).

Electrocardiographic analyses of FMS subjects show that sympathetic activity increases overnight when, normally, sympathetic activity declines during sleep (31). This finding is consistent with the autonomic disturbances with symptoms, including faintness, unsteadiness, palpitations, paresthesias, and blurring of vision that occur in some patients.

Some studies have shown changes in circadian sleep/wake-related autonomic, neuroendocrine, and immune functions of the body and alterations in neurotransmitter functions that affect substance P, catecholamine, serotonin, and neuroendocrine metabolism (10,32). However, disturbances in sleep physiology, pain, psychological distress, and physical deconditioning may confound many of these changes (33). Although no specific neuroendocrine, cytokine, or neuroimmune dysfunctions have been directly related to FMS, the abnormalities that have reported provide further evidence for the importance of disturbances in the sleeping/waking brain in the pathogenesis of the syndrome (10,32,34–40).

CLINICAL FEATURES

The clinical criteria for CFS are shown in Table 10-1; criteria for FMS are shown in Table 10-2. The emphasis placed upon pain and tenderness for the diagnosis of FMS by American College of Rheumatology (ACR) criteria may actually limit sensitivity and specificity (41). Other potential determinants for FM should include an evaluation of complaints of chronic fatigue, unrefreshing sleep, cognitive difficulties, and psychological distress, which are common.

TABLE 10-1	U.S. Centers for Disease Control (CDC) 1994 Criteria for Chronic Fatigue Syndrome (CFS)

A. Fatigue: severe, unexplained fatigue that is not relieved by rest, which can cause disability, and which has an identifiable onset (i.e., not lifelong fatigue). It must be persistent or relapsing fatigue that lasts for at least 6 or more consecutive months.

B. Four or more of the following symptoms:
- Impaired memory or concentration problems
- Tender cervical or axillary lymph nodes
- Sore throat
- Muscle pain
- Multijoint pain
- New onset headaches
- Unrefreshing sleep
- Postexertional malaise

From Fukuda K, Straus SE, Hickie I, et al. International Chronic Fatigue Syndrome Study Group. The chronic fatigue syndrome: a comprehensive approach to its definition and study. *Ann Intern Med* 1994;121:953–959, with permission.

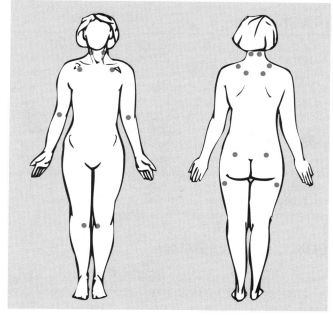

Figure 10-1. Anatomical distribution of 18 TePs in fibromyalgia syndrome (FMS).

Whereas fatigue and postexertional malaise along with impairment in cognitive functioning are the focus of attention in CFS, unrefreshing sleep, chronic muscular pain, and tenderness also prevail. These symptoms may follow a viral illness or a physical or psychological traumatic event—for example, an automobile whiplash injury or a work-related soft tissue injury—or they may appear for no apparent reason. FMS may occur in the context of potentially disabling arthritic disease (e.g., rheumatoid arthritis) or connective tissue disease (e.g., systemic lupus erythematosis), HIV, or Lyme disease.

In both CFS and FMS the quality of sleep is usually impaired. More than 80% of chronic fatigue patients describe significant impairment in their sleep quality (42). Patients commonly complain of light or superficial sleep in which they are sensitive to noise or are unable to turn off their thinking during their sleep, so that when they awaken they typically describe their sleep as unrefreshing. Their mental fatigue results in word lapses, word

TABLE 10-2	The American College of Rheumatology (ACR) 1990 Criteria for the Classification of Fibromyalgia Syndrome (FMS)

1. A history of widespread musculoskeletal pain for at least 3 months.
2. Tenderness is found in at least 11 of the 18 anatomical sites with the application of 4 kg pressure by palpation at the bilateral anatomical regions shown in Figure 10-1.

From Wolfe F, Smythe HA, Yunus MB, et al. The American College of Rheumatology 1990 criteria for the classification of fibromyalgia. Report of the Multicenter Criteria Committee. *Arthritis Rheum* 1990;33:160–172, with permission.

confusions, and problems in multitasking so that they are slower in performing such tasks but do not make more errors than normal (43). Their sensory sensitivities may extend to intolerance of noise, noxious smells, strong perfumes, and bright light. In addition to external sensory hypersensitivities they may describe internal sensitivities with intolerance to certain foods and symptoms of irritable bowel syndrome or irritable bladder.

The symptom of fatigue that characterizes FM and CFS shows a different diurnal variation compared to the symptoms of sleepiness that are featured in disorders of excessive daytime sleepiness. Upon morning awakening from light and unrefreshing sleep, patients with CFS and FMS rate their pain and fatigue as high. These symptoms may improve during the interval that varies between 10 AM and 3 PM, depending on the severity of the symptoms, followed by feeling exhausted and having more pain during the latter part of the afternoon and evening. Typically, the patients feel no better when they awaken or they have more aching, stiffness, and fatigue in the morning, which indicates that their sleep is nonrestorative (44).

By contrast, in those medical conditions characterized by muscular weakness, the motor tiredness increases coincident with physical activity over the course of the day and improves with rest. The tiredness associated with major depressive disorder is increased upon awakening, when the depression is more severe than in the evening, when both mood and tiredness improve. In dysthymic disorder the tiredness progressively increases over the course of the day (45). Sleepiness as the result of sleep restriction or disruption leaves the person feeling drowsy in the morning and again in mid-afternoon. However, there is reduced late afternoon and early evening sleepiness as a result of circadian variations in alertness. In narcolepsy the sleepiness is prevalent throughout the day.

DIAGNOSES

Although the diagnoses of CFS and FMS are based upon clinical criteria, sleep physiological analyses provide an added dimension of understanding and possibly a rationale for treatment. Neuropsychiatric assessment may be required to determine whether there is a brain or peripheral neuromotor disease that could explain the fatigue and weakness or whether there is a primary psychiatric disorder—for example, major depressive disorder, general anxiety disorder, dysthymia, or somatoform pain disorder. Such psychosocial concerns as current stressors and interpersonal, economic, insurance, or medicolegal problems need to be assessed as part of the overall management strategy.

CLINICAL ASSESSMENT

Specific enquiry about the quality of sleep is essential (i.e., the presence of light and unrefreshing sleep). The sleep–wake habits can be assessed with the aid of a sleep diary. Attention should be directed to potential agents that could interfere with sleep—for example, excessive use of caffeine, alcohol, nicotine, and certain classes of drugs. Some patients may have loud snoring and interruptions of breathing that may be indicative of sleep apnea (46–48). Others may describe dysesthesia and uncontrollable leg movements in the evening and restlessness or kicking during sleep that characterize restless legs syndrome and periodic involuntary limb movements disorder (49,50). Tiredness as the result of excessive daytime sleepiness should be differentiated from physical and central fatigue. Routine lab tests will help to exclude a primary medical disease. The routine use of expensive tests—imaging studies, for example—is not required. However, FM and CFS patients may be accompanied by concomitant rheumatic or connective tissue disease that requires careful medical diagnostic appraisal. Furthermore, because unrefreshing sleep, fatigue, and cognitive impairment are often accompanied by anxiety or depression, or both, an assessment of psychological disturbances is required as part of an overall plan of management.

SLEEP–WAKE DIARY

A self-monitored sleep/wake diary is a simple instrument that will reveal whether faulty habits result in insufficient or improper timing of sleep causing sleepiness from physical fatigue where there is no problem with scheduling or duration of sleep. The diary helps to clarify behaviors that may contribute to the tiredness—for example, excessive use of stimulants, alcohol, sedatives, hypnotics, or consumption of street drugs. This simple, inexpensive tool may save costly and unrewarding investigative procedures. Moreover, the diary can assist in reeducation to correct faulty habits and poor sleep hygiene that contribute to the complaint of tiredness.

CLINICAL RATING SCALES FOR VARIOUS ATTRIBUTES OF "TIREDNESS"

Self-rating Scales

"Tiredness" that is a symptom of depression is included in the Beck Depression Inventory (51). Fatigue scales that provide information about various aspects of fatigue include the following:

The Multidimensional Fatigue Inventory (MFI-20) (52) is a 20-item five-point Likert scale questionnaire that comprises five subscales, which include general fatigue, physical fatigue, reduced activity, reduced motivation, and mental fatigue.

The fatigue scale by Chalder et al. (53) has 11 items that measure fatigue intensity and separates mental and physical fatigue.

The Fatigue Severity Scale (54) includes nine items that provide a measure of fatigue severity. This simple scale was originally standardized on patients with fatigue related to multiple sclerosis and systemic lupus erythematosis.

These fatigue instruments, however, do not evaluate or exclude sleepiness. Sleepiness scales are commonly used in sleep research and clinical sleep laboratories. These include the Stanford Sleepiness Scale, which measures sleepiness at the time of the test. This instrument was originally developed for narcolepsy and comprises seven categories, ranging from "1," indicating alert—wide awake to "7," indicating almost asleep (55). The Epworth Sleepiness Scale, which measures an ongoing tendency for sleepiness, inquires about the chance of dozing in eight different situations (56). The chance of dozing is ranked from "0," meaning never, to "3," where there is a high chance of dozing. These passive situations include sitting and reading; watching TV; sitting inactive in a public place, such as a theater or meeting; sitting as a passenger in a car; lying down to rest in the afternoon; sitting or talking to someone; sitting quietly after a lunch without alcohol; and, finally, being in a car while stopped for a few minutes in traffic. The numbers of the eight situations are added together to give a global score from 0 to 24 with obviously higher ratings related to pathologic sleepiness. Interestingly, the Epworth does not include a question regarding irresistible daytime sleepiness.

Qualitative and Quantitative Self-rating Scales of Sleep

In addition to a subscale rating of subjective sleep quality, the Pittsburgh Sleep Quality Index (SQI) questionnaire provides subscale measures of sleep latency, sleep duration, and habitual sleep efficiency. There are also components that relate to sleep disturbances, use of sleeping medication, and daytime dysfunction. The sum of scores for these seven components yields one global score, which is a composite of sleep quality and quantity (57).

Nonrestorative sleep is a specific sleep factor within the 17-item, four-point Likert scale Sleep Assessment Questionnaire (SAQ), which includes five other factors: insomnia/hypersomnia, restless leg/motility, sleep schedules, excessive daytime sleeping, and sleep apnea. Importantly, this instrument has been validated against data obtained from polysomnography—for example, the α-EEG sleep disorder in patients with FM and CFS. The SAQ shows favorable sensitivity and specificity as a simple screening instrument for nonrestorative sleep disorders and other sleep pathologies. It has been found to be useful in screening for sleep pathologies in an epidemiologic study of a chronic fatigued population (58).

The Karolinska Sleep Diary (59) consists of seven self-rated items on a five-point Likert scale that yields two factors: (a) the SQI has items on sleep quality, ease of falling asleep, maintenance, and calmness of sleep; (b) a second factor comprises items on sufficiency of sleep, ease of awakening, and feeling refreshed. The amount of slow wave sleep and sleep efficiency were found to be predictors for the SQI.

Performance Tasks

The difficulty with self-rating estimates of fatigue is that they are not necessarily related to the observed behavior. Therefore, performance tasks consisting of behavioral assessments of vigilance are employed, especially if daytime sleepiness is being assessed, for example, as the result of sleep deprivation or a primary sleep disorder. This psychomotor vigilance task involves a 10-minute computerized assessment battery, which is sensitive to the effects of sleep loss and circadian rhythmicity and is devoid of practice effects (60,61). Efforts are underway to objectively measure performance in specific tasks—driving a car or truck, for example (62,63). Motor vehicle accidents are a common outcome of so-called "driver fatigue," where there are inattention or lapses in alertness as symptoms of sleepiness (64).

Many of these assessment tools are too cumbersome for routine use within the context of the sleep disorders clinic. At this time the most practical tools are: (a) the sleep–wake diary to assess scheduling and behavioral factors that may be compounding existing symptoms; (b) the Beck Depression Inventory to rule out comorbid depression; and (c) the SAQ, or other screening questionnaires, to rule out comorbid sleep disorders.

POLYSOMNOGRAPHY

When the diagnosis is uncertain or a primary sleep disorder is suspect, overnight polysomnography can provide objective evidence for the unrefreshing sleep and a rationale for treatment of the underlying sleep disorder.

These sleep disorders include the α-EEG sleep disorder, which is often associated with poor quality sleep or light and unrefreshing sleep (65). Initially, this sleep disorder, originally termed α-δ sleep, was described in a heterogeneous group of psychiatric patients with somatic malaise and fatigue (66). Subsequently α-EEG sleep was found in stages 2, 3, and 4 non-REM sleep in adults and children with FMS (12,67–71) and in some patients with CFS or unexplained chronic fatigue (72,73).

The α-EEG anomaly is not specific to CFS and FM. Other disorders in which α-EEG sleep, nonrestorative sleep, pain,

and fatigue symptoms may occur include rheumatoid arthritis (74–76) and systemic lupus erythematosis (77). Furthermore, it may be found in patients with psychophysiologic insomnia with unrefreshing sleep and fatigue (78) or in some patients with various primary sleep disorders—for example, periodic limb movement disorder, non 24-hour sleep–wake syndrome, sleep apnea, and narcolepsy—and occasionally in normal people (77–84). Studies examining the sensitivity of the α-EEG intrusion as a marker for FM and CFS have been equivocal. Also, the relative presence of the α-EEG anomaly is not always correlated with symptom severity (30). Unfortunately, variations in methodology, including frequency analysis techniques and inclusion and exclusion criteria, certainly hamper valid comparison between many studies. Still, this common but as yet unexplained EEG finding provides an opportunity for additional research into the mechanisms of disease. More recent studies have attempted to clarify the exact nature of the α-EEG anomaly and its permutations. Frequency analyses show that there is a progressive decline in the α EEG over the night. Detailed EEG frequency analyses differentiate three types of α-EEG sleep:

1. Tonic α-EEG sleep occurs throughout stages 2, 3, and 4 sleep where global ratings show 3 or more, that is, >40% prevalence of the α frequency (84).
2. Phasic α-EEG sleep, where the α frequency coincides with stage 3 and stage 4 sleep (α-δ sleep) and has maximal frontal α power localized symmetrically in the left and right anterior cingulum (67).
3. Periodic K-α and periodic polyphasic EEG burst activity (K-α/polyphasic burst variety of cyclical alternating pattern) is recorded when four or more consecutive K complexes, immediately followed by α-EEG activity of 0.5- to 5.0-second duration, or four or more polyphasic bursts occur in a sequence of approximately 20- to 40-second intervals. A rapid frequency, with an index of >15 per hour of sleep, is associated with unrefreshing sleep, fatigue, and muscular symptoms (85).

Other sleep disorders include restless legs and sleep-related periodic limb movement, which occurs in about 20% of FMS patients; 5% of FMS patients have significant obstructive sleep apnea (86).

The multiple sleep latency test aids in the differentiation of types of tiredness. Physical and mental fatigue may not be accompanied by rapid onset to sleep on the daytime naps, whereas those who have a problem remaining alert, which interferes with concentration, may show excessive daytime sleepiness. The test is especially important in some patients who, in addition to FMS or CFS, have hypersomnolence (87) or in some cases narcolepsy (88,89).

TREATMENT

Despite clinical criteria for recognizing these fatigue and pain syndromes, there is no satisfactory effective treatment for improving sleep quality, fatigue, and debilitating somatic symptoms. Treatment is either nonspecific—aiming to improve sleep habits—or employs medications that aim to relieve symptoms or aspects of sleep disorder.

NONSPECIFIC TREATMENT METHODS

Sleep Hygiene

Overall, sleep hygiene and nonspecific methods provide a suitable background regimen that is helpful for regularizing and facilitating sleep (90). On the basis of the principle that there is a dysregulation of the sleep and of the rhythms of the body, the fundamental principle of management involves regularizing both the patient's behavioral and physiologic functions. The psychological methods for improving circadian sleep–wake behavior are central to any cognitive behavioral approach in the management of FM. Sleep hygiene enables regulation of the circadian rhythm of sleep–wakefulness in which the pattern is disorganized because of faulty sleep habits. Two of the most common faulty habits are variable bedtimes and inadequate nocturnal sleep time, which result in disorganization of circadian rhythms and sleep deprivation with sleepiness and fatigue. Efforts should be directed to stabilizing the regulatory functions of sleep by going to bed and awakening at suitable specific times to assure adequate duration of sleep. The establishment of a regular daily routine not only includes meeting the body's sleep requirements but also requires a regular daily schedule of eating nutritious meals and engaging in a suitable exercise program. The exercise program involves following a gentle, graded aerobic fitness routine during that part of the day when there is least fatigue and pain—that is, commonly between 10 AM and 3 PM. Vigorous physical activities should be avoided before bedtime because their stimulating effect interferes with sleep. Frequently patients are sensitive to the effects of caffeine and alcohol so they often avoid their use because they interfere with sleep.

There is a need to attend to the sleep environment. That is, the aim is to reduce any psychological or environmental disturbances that are disruptive to sleep. Other behavioral methods that reduce psychological distress, such as hypnosis and biofeedback treatments, are helpful in modulating symptoms. Hypnotherapy results in improvement in muscle pain, fatigue, and sleep disturbance (91). Electromyographic biofeedback therapy helps to improve pain, TePs, and stiffness upon awakening in the morning (92).

Physical methods, which include massage and acupuncture, provide temporary improvement (93). Ultrasound and interferential current treatment decrease unrefreshing sleep, fatigue, pain, TePs, and tenderness, while increasing slow wave sleep and decreasing the percentage of stage 1 sleep (94). On the basis of the postulate that cardiovascular fitness training should improve sleep and symptoms of FM, a daily gentle graded aerobic fitness program that is tailored to individual needs reduces pain threshold measures and improves symptoms (95).

SPECIFIC TREATMENT METHODS

Sleep-promoting Agents

Medications that aim to improve sleep appear to help in some patients but have not been demonstrated to provide lasting benefit for pain. Tricyclic antidepressant agents, which facilitate CNS serotonin metabolism—cyclobenzaprine and amitriptyline, for example—may result in favorable effects on sleep up to 2 or 3 months and 5 months, respectively (96,97). However, sleep EEG studies show that neither amitriptyline nor cyclobenzaprine reduces the α-EEG sleep disorder (30,98). Selective serotonin reuptake inhibitors—fluoxetine, for example—provide no consistent benefits (99,100).

It would be expected that agents that increase slow wave sleep and reduce α-EEG sleep would benefit the quality of sleep, the pain, and the fatigue symptoms of FM.

Traditional sedatives/hypnotic benzodiazepines alone do not provide any specific benefit. Nonbenzodiazepine hypnotic drugs such as zopiclone (101) and zolpidem (102) improve subjective sleep and daytime tiredness but do not modify α-EEG sleep; nor do they benefit pain symptoms. Over-the-counter sedatives such as antihistamines and herbal agents—for example, valerian—have not been systematically assessed. L-tryptophan facilitates sleep, but there is no effect on α-EEG sleep, pain, and mood symptoms in patients with FM (103). However, 5-hydroxytryptophan, a direct precursor of brain serotonin, tends to improve pain and sleep quality (104), but its effect on the sleep physiology of FM patients is unknown. Although chlorpromazine has been shown to decrease pain and improve sleep physiology by reducing α-EEG sleep and by increasing slow wave sleep, the risk for long-term adverse effects does not make this a desirable drug (103). Agents that have been classified as anticonvulsants, such as gabapentin, pregabalin, and carbamazepine, have sedative properties and antinociceptive effects but have not been systematically assessed in terms of sleep physiology. Sodium oxybate improves sleep quality and symptoms of FMS while reducing α- and increasing δ-sleep (105). These findings require further large-scale confirmation. If confirmed, the research should help provide for a better understanding of CFS/FMS and pave the way for devising and testing specific molecules that would help to improve sleep quality and illnesses where fatigue problems prevail.

An important consideration when employing any medication for the management of symptoms related to FM or CFS is that these patients are most often exquisitely sensitive to any pharmacologic agent and are thus more likely to report troublesome side effects. It is not uncommon for these patients to derive a therapeutic benefit from a fraction of the recommended adult starting dose. Such a minimal dose will, in turn, minimize side effects.

Sleep-related Neuroendocrine Substances

No consistent abnormalities have been reported in the secretion of melatonin in either FMS or CFS, nor has its administration been found to be useful in controlled studies (33). Furthermore, the use of morning bright light treatment, which tends to modify the timing of the nocturnal secretion of melatonin and is helpful in seasonal affective disorder, does not benefit sleep, pain, or mood symptoms in patients with FM (106). On the other hand, growth hormone, which is found to be reduced in FMS, improves the symptoms of FM (36), but the high costs and daily injections of this hormone make its use impractical for the treatment of the disorder.

Management of Primary Sleep Disorders

For those patients who are found to have specific primary sleep disorders—for example, restless legs and periodic limb movement during sleep (PLMS) or sleep apnea—specific remedial measures that have been demonstrated to provide relief for these conditions should be considered. Unfortunately, there are no systematic studies of their benefits on sleep pathologies for the pain and fatigue symptoms in patients with FM (90).

CLINICAL COURSE AND PREVENTION

Long-term outcome studies indicate that CFS patients rarely return to their premorbid levels of energy prior to the acute onset of their fatigue. Similarly, the prognosis for CFS with current limitations of treatment remains poor, and symptoms may persist for an extended time. Current treatments are equivocal in efficacy. There are no known remedial measures to prevent these illnesses.

KEY CLINICAL POINTS

Whereas clinical criteria exist for CFS and FMS, the subjective nature of these nonspecific pain and fatigue disorders may become confounded by psychological distress experienced by patients involved with insurance and medicolegal matters related to disability claims. Their need to provide proof of disability and the symptoms of distress may serve to magnify the sleep, fatigue, and pain symptoms, resulting in controversy about whether the symptoms are indications of medical illnesses or illness behavior.

Also, symptoms are not specific. Similar fatigue, pain, and unrefreshing sleep symptoms appear with other diagnostic labels that have emerged in various medical specialties in order to address these unexplained symptoms in patients that populate their specialties—for example, Gulf War syndrome, multiple chemical sensitivity syndrome or sick building syndrome (allergy, clinical immunology), and chronic pain in somatoform disorder (psychiatry). These fatigue, pain, and sleep symptoms also occur with other unexplained illnesses, such as irritable bowel syndrome, temporomandibular pain syndrome, interstitial cystitis, migraine, chronic headache, and atypical chest pain (107). Furthermore, FMS is not distinctive because the symptoms may accompany rheumatic or connective tissue disease (osteoarthritis, for example) and rheumatoid arthritis, and they occur commonly in patients with systemic lupus erythematosis, Lyme disease, endocrine disorder [for example, myxedema (108,109)], and such psychiatric illnesses as major depression, general anxiety disorder, and posttraumatic stress disorder (110).

The accurate diagnosis of FM and CFS must begin with a clear definition of the most common symptomatic descriptor: "feeling tired." This must be differentiated from excessive daytime sleepiness. Comorbid sleep disorders must be ruled out. Given the multidisciplinary nature of sleep disorders medicine, this differentiation is aided with the assistance of a *comprehensive* sleep disorders clinic. Even though treatment for these syndromes is limited, diagnosis remains essential, as validation for the patient is often the critical first step toward self-management or rehabilitation, or both.

SUMMARY POINTS

- Although insomnia and other sleep complaints are very common in FM and related conditions, no sleep abnormalities are specific for FM.

■ IMPLICATIONS FOR PRACTICE

- Polysomnography is indicated in the patient with chronic pain or fatigue, or both, when there are symptoms suggesting a primary sleep disorder (e.g., sleep apnea, restless legs syndrome, etc.).
- Both pharmacologic and nonpharmacologic therapies can be useful in treating the sleep disturbances seen in FM and related conditions.
- Many of these therapies may improve sleep, but not pain or the other cardinal symptoms of FM.

REFERENCES

1. Skapinakis P, Lewis G, Mavreas V. Cross-cultural differences in the epidemiology of unexplained fatigue syndromes in primary care. *Br J Psychiatry* 2003;182:205–209.
2. Lindberg CA, ed. Tired, adjective. *The Oxford American thesaurus of current English.* Oxford University Press, 1999.
3. Fukuda K, Straus SE, Hickie I et al., International Chronic Fatigue Syndrome Study Group. The chronic fatigue syndrome: a comprehensive approach to its definition and study. *Ann Intern Med* 1994;121:953–959.
4. Wolfe F, Smythe HA, Yunus MB, et al. The American College of Rheumatology 1990 criteria for the classification of fibromyalgia. Report of the Multicenter Criteria Committee. *Arthritis Rheum* 1990;33:160–172.
5. Price RK, North CS, Wessely S, et al. Estimating the prevalence of chronic fatigue syndrome and associated symptoms in the community. *Public Health Rep* 1992;107:514–522.
6. Jason LA, Richman JA, Rademaker AW, et al. A community-based study of chronic fatigue syndrome. *Arch Intern Med* 1999;159(18):2129–2137.
7. Kawakami N, Iwata N, Fujihara S, et al. Prevalence of chronic fatigue syndrome in a community population in Japan. *Tohoku J Exp Med* 1998;186(1):33–41.
8. Wolfe F, Hawley DJ, Wilson K. The prevalence and meaning of fatigue in rheumatic disease. *J Rheumatol* 1996;23:1407–1417.
9. Aaron LA, Burke MM, Buchwald D. Overlapping conditions among patients with chronic fatigue syndrome, fibromyalgia, and temporomandibular disorder. *Arch Intern Med* 2000; 24(160):221–227.
10. Pillemer SR, Bradley LA, Crofford LJ, et al. The neuroscience and endocrinology of fibromyalgia. Conference summary. *Arthritis Rheum* 1991;34:15–21.
11. Yunus MB, Ahles TA, Aldag JC, et al. The relationship of the clinical features with psychological status in primary fibromyalgia. *Arthritis Rheum* 1991;34:15–21.
12. Moldofsky H, Scarisbrick P, England R, et al. Musculoskeletal symptoms and non-REM sleep disturbance in patients

with "fibrositis syndrome" and healthy subjects. *Psychosom Med* 1975;37:341–351.

13. Older SA, Battafarano DF, Danning CL, et al. The effects of delta wave sleep interruption on pain thresholds and fibromyalgia-like symptoms in healthy subjects; correlations with insulin-like growth factor I. *J Rheumatol* 1998;25:1180–1186.

14. Lentz MJ, Landis CA, Rothermel J, et al. Effects of selective slow wave sleep disruption on musculoskeletal pain and fatigue in middle aged women. *J Rheumatol* 1999;26:1586–1592.

15. Drewes AM, Nielson KD, Arendt-Nielson L, et al. The effect of cutaneous and deep pain on the electroencephalogram during sleep: an experimental study. *Sleep* 1997;20:632–640.

16. Onen SH, Alloui A, Gross A, et al. The effects of total sleep deprivation, selective sleep interruption and sleep recovery on pain tolerance thresholds in healthy subjects. *J Sleep Res* 2001;10:35–42.

17. Horne JA, Shackell BS. Alpha-like EEG activity in non-REM sleep and the fibromyalgia (fibrositis) syndrome. *Electroencephalogr Clin Neurophysiol* 1991;79:271–276.

18. Branco J, Atalaia A, Paiva T. Sleep cycles and alpha-delta sleep in fibromyalgia syndrome. *J Rheumatol* 1994;21:1113–1117.

19. Touchon J, Besset A, Billiard M, et al. Fibrositis syndrome: polysomnographic and psychological aspects. In: Koella WP, Obál F, Schulz H et al., eds. *Sleep '86.* New York: Gustav Fischer Verlag, 1988:445–447.

20. Drewes AM, Nielsen KD, Taagholt SJ, et al. Sleep intensity in fibromyalgia: focus on the microstructure of the sleep process. *Br J Rheumatol* 1995;34:629–635.

21. Shaver JLF, Lentz M, Landis CA, et al. Sleep, psychological distress, and stress arousal in women with fibromyalgia. *Res Nurs Health* 1997;20:247–257.

22. Wittig RM, Zorick FJ, Blumer D, et al. Disturbed sleep in patients complaining of chronic pain. *J Nerv Ment Dis* 1982;70:429–431.

23. Molony RR, MacPeek DM, Schiffman PL, et al. Sleep, sleep apnea, and fibromyalgia syndrome. *J Rheumatol* 1986;13:797–800.

24. Clauw D, Blank C, Hiltz R, et al. Polysomnography in fibromyalgia patients [Abstract]. *Arthritis Rheum* 1994;37 (Suppl. 9):S348.

25. Staedt J, Windt H, Hajaki G, et al. Cluster arousal analysis in chronic pain-disturbed sleep. *J Sleep Res* 1993;2:134–137.

26. Roizenblatt S, Tufik S, Goldenberg J, et al. Juvenile fibromyalgia: clinical and polysomnographic aspects. *J Rheumatol* 1977;24:579–585.

27. Drewes AM, Gade J, Nielsen KD, et al. Clustering of sleep electroencephalographic patterns in patients with the fibromyalgia syndrome. *Br J Rheumatol* 1995;34:1151–1156.

28. Perlis ML, Giles DE, Bootzin RR, et al. Alpha sleep and information processing, perception of sleep, pain and arousability in fibromyalgia. *Int J Neurosci* 1997;89:265–280.

29. Ware JC, Russell IJ, Campos E. Alpha intrusions into the sleep of depression and fibromyalgia syndrome (fibrositis) patients [Abstract]. *Sleep Res* 1986;15:210.

30. Carette S, Oakson G, Guimont C, et al. Sleep electroencephalography and the clinical response to amitriptyline in patients with fibromyalgia. *Arthritis Rheum* 1995;38(9):1211–1217.

31. Martinez-Lavin M, Hermosillo AG, Rosas M, et al. Circadian studies of autonomic nervous balance in patients with fibromyalgia: a heart rate variability analysis. *Arthritis Rheum* 1998;41:1966–1971.

32. Landis CA, Lentz MJ, Rothermel J, et al. Decreased nocturnal levels of prolactin and growth hormone in women with fibromyalgia. *J Clin Endocrinol Metab* 2001;86(4):1672–1678.

33. Geenen R, Jacobs JWG, Bijlsma JWJ. Evaluation and management of endocrine dysfunction in fibromyalgia. *Rheum Dis Clin North Am* 2002;28:389–404.

34. Bennett RM, Clark SC, Campbell SM, et al. Low levels of somatomedin C in patients with the fibromyalgia syndrome. A possible link between sleep and muscle pain. *Arthritis Rheum* 1992;35:1113–1116.

35. Paiva ES, Deodhar A, Jones KD, et al. Impaired growth hormone secretion in fibromyalgia patients: evidence for augmented hypothalamic somastatin. *Arthritis Rheum* 2002;46:440–450.

36. Bennett RM, Clark SC, Walczyk J. A randomized, double-blind, placebo-controlled study of growth hormone in the treatment of fibromyalgia. *Am J Med* 1998;104:227–231.

37. Demitrack MA, Crofford LJ. Evidence for and pathophysiologic implications of the hypothalamic-pituitary-adrenal axis dysregulation in fibromyalgia and chronic fatigue syndrome. *Ann N Y Acad Sci* 1998;840:684–697.

38. Adler GK, Kinsley BT, Hurwitz S, et al. Reduced hypothalamic-pituitary-adrenal and sympathoadrenal responses to hypoglycaemia in women with fibromyalgia syndrome. *Am J Med* 1999;106:534–543.

39. Klerman EB, Goldenberg DL, Brown EN, et al. Circadian rhythms of women with fibromyalgia. *J Clin Endocrinol Metab* 2001;86:1034–1039.

40. Moldofsky H, Lue FA, Dickstein J, et al. Disordered circadian sleep-wake neuroendocrine and immune functions in chronic fatigue/fibromyalgia syndrome. *Arthritis Rheum* 1998;41(Sept Suppl):S255.

41. Schochat T, Raspe H. Elements of fibromyalgia in an open population. *Rheumatology* 2003;42:829–835.

42. Unger ER, Nisenbaum R, Moldofsky H, et al. Sleep assessment in a population-based study of chronic fatigue syndrome. *BMC Neurol* 2004 (Apr 19);4(1):6.

43. Coté KA, Moldofsky H. Sleep, daytime symptoms, and cognitive performance in patients with fibromyalgia. *J Rheumatol* 1997;24:2014–2023.

44. Moldofsky H. Sleep and pain. *Sleep Med Rev* 2001;5:387–398.

45. Moldofsky H. The contribution of sleep medicine to the assessment of the tired patient. *Can J Psychiatry* 2000;45:51–55.

46. Carette S, Oakson G, Guimont C, et al. Sleep EEG and clinical response to amitriptyline in patients with fibromyalgia. *Arthritis Rheum* 1995;38(9):1211–1217.

47. May KP, West SG, Baker MR, et al. Sleep apnea in male patients with fibromyalgia syndrome. *Am J Med* 1993;94:505–508.

48. Alvarez LB, Alonso Valdivielso JL, Alegre Lopez J, et al. Fibromyalgia syndrome: overnight falls in arterial oxygen saturation. *Am J Med* 1997;101:54–60.

49. Yunus MB, Aldag JC. Restless legs syndrome and leg cramps in fibromyalgia: controlled study. *Br Med J* 1996;312:1339.

50. Tayag-Kier CE, Keenan GF, Scalzi LV, et al. Sleep and periodic limb movements in sleep in juvenile fibromyalgia. *Pediatrics* 2000;106:E70.

51. Beck AT, Ward CH, Mendelson M, et al. An inventory for measuring depression. *Arch Gen Psychiatry* 1961;4:561–567.

52. Smets EMA, Garssen B, Bonke B, et al. The multidimensional fatigue inventory (MFI): psychometric qualities of an instrument to assess fatigue. *J Psychosom Res* 1995;39:315–325.

53. Chalder T, Berelowitz G, Pawlikowska T, et al. Development of a fatigue scale. *J Psychosom Med* 1993;37:147–153.

54. Krupp LB, La Rocca NG, Muir-Nash J, et al. The fatigue severity scale: application to patients with multiple sclerosis and systemic lupus erythematosis. *Arch Neurol* 1989;46:1121–1123.

55. Hoddes E, Zarcone V, Smythe H, et al. Quantification of sleepiness: a new approach. *Psychophysiology* 1973;10:431–436.

56. John MW. A new method for measuring daytime sleepiness: the Epworth sleepiness scale. *Sleep* 1991;14:540–545.

57. Buysse DJ, Reynolds CF III, Monk TH, et al. The Pittsburgh sleep quality index: a new instrument for psychiatric practice and research. *Psychiatr Res* 1989;28:193–213.

58. Unger ER, Nisenbaum R, Moldofsky H, et al. Sleep assessment in a population-based study of chronic fatigue syndrome. *BMC Neurol* 2004;4:6.

59. Keklund G, Akerstedt T. Objective components of individual differences in subjective sleep quality. *J Sleep Res* 1997;6: 217–220.

60. Dinges DF, Powell JW. Microcomputer analyses of performance on a portable simple visual RT task during sustained operations. *Behav Res Methods Instrum Comput* 1985;17: 652–655.

61. Van Dongen HP, Dinges DF. Investigating the interaction between the homeostatic and circadian processes of sleep-wake regulation for the prediction of waking neurobehavioural performance. *J Sleep Res* 2003;12:181–187.

62. Horne JA, Reyner LA. Sleep related vehicle accidents. *Br Med J* 1995;310:565–567.

63. Mitler MM, Miller JC, Lipsitz JJ, et al. The sleep of long-haul drivers. *N Engl J Med* 1997;337:755–761.

64. Aldrich MS. Automobile accidents in patients with sleep disorders. *Sleep* 1989;12:487–494.

65. Benca R, Moldofsky H, Ancoli Israel S. Special considerations in insomnia diagnosis and management: depressed, elderly, and chronic pain populations. *J Clin Psychiatry* 2004;65(Suppl. 8):26–35.

66. Hauri P, Hawkins D. Alpha delta sleep. *Electroencephalogr Clin Neurophysiol* 1973;34:233–237.

67. Anch AM, Lue FA, MacLean AW, et al. Sleep physiology and psychological aspects of the fibrositis (fibromyalgia) syndrome. *Can J Psychol* 1991;45:178–184.

68. Branco J, Atalaia A, Paiva T. Sleep cycles and alpha-delta sleep in fibromyalgia syndrome. *J Rheumatol* 1994;21:1113–1117.

69. Drewes AM, Nielsen KD, Taagholt SJ, et al. Sleep intensity in fibromyalgia: focus on the microstructure of the sleep process. *Br J Rheumatol* 1995;34:629–635.

70. Roizenblatt S, Tufik S, Goldenberg J, et al. Juvenile fibromyalgia. Clinical and polysomnographic aspects. *J Rheumatol* 1997;24:579–585.

71. Roizenblatt S, Moldofsky H, Benedito-Silva AA, et al. Alpha sleep characteristics in fibromyalgia. *Arthritis Rheum* 2001;44:222–230.

72. Whelton CL, Salit I, Moldofsky H. Sleep, Epstein-Barr virus infection, musculoskeletal pain, and depressive symptoms in chronic fatigue syndrome. *J Rheumatol* 1992;19: 939–943.

73. Manu P, Lane TJ, Matthews Castriotta RJ, et al. Alpha-delta sleep in patients with a chief complaint of chronic fatigue. *South Med J* 1994;87:465–470.

74. Moldofsky H, Lue FA, Smythe HA. Alpha EEG and morning symptoms in rheumatoid arthritis. *J Rheumatol* 1983;10: 373–379.

75. Drewes AM, Svendsen L, Taagholt SJ, et al. Sleep in rheumatoid arthritis: a comparison with healthy subjects and studies of sleep/wake interactions. *Br J Rheumatol* 1998;37:71–81.

76. Mahowald MW, Mahowald ML, Bundlie SR, et al. Sleep fragmentation in rheumatoid arthritis. *Arthritis Rheum* 1989;32:974–978.

77. Bruce IN, Fraser K, Gladman DD, et al.: Sleep abnormalities in patients with SLE and fatigue. *Arthritis Rheum.* 1998; 41(Sept Suppl):1802.

78. Schneider-Helmert D, Kumar A. Sleep, its subjective perception and daytime performance in insomniacs with a pattern of alpha sleep. *Biol Psychiatry* 1995;37:99–105.

79. Saskin P, Moldofsky H, Lue FA. Periodic movements in sleep and sleep-wake complaint. *Sleep* 1985;8:318–324.

80. Honda M, Koga E, Ishikawa T, et al. Alpha-delta sleep in a case of non 24h sleep-wake syndrome: quantitative electroencephalogram analysis of alpha and delta band waves. *Psychiatry Clin Neurosci* 1997;51:387–392.

81. Pivik RT, Harman KA. Reconceptualization of EEG alpha activity during sleep: all alpha activity is not equal. *J Sleep Res* 1995;4:131–137.

82. Scheuler W, Kubicki S, Marquardt J, et al. The sleep pattern—quantitative analysis and functional aspects. In: Koella WP, Obál F, Schulz H et al., eds. *Sleep'86.* New York: Gustav Fischer Verlag, 1988:284–286.

83. Connemann BJ, Mann K, Pacual-Marki RD, et al. Limbic activity in slow wave sleep in a healthy subject with alpha-delta sleep. *Psychiatry Res Neuroimaging* 2001;107:165–171.

84. MacLean AW, Lue FA, Moldofsky H. The reliability of visual scoring of alpha EEG sleep. *Sleep* 1995;18:565–569.

85. MacFarlane JG, Shahal B, Moldofsky H. Periodic K-alpha sleep EEG activity and periodic leg movements during sleep: comparisons of clinical features and sleep parameters. *Sleep* 1996;19:200–204.

86. Moldofsky H, Cesta A, Mously C, et al. Prevalence of sleep disorders in fibromyalgia. *Sleep* 2002;25(Suppl):A501.

87. Sarzi-Puttini P, Rizzi M, Andreoli A, et al. Hypersomnolence in fibromyalgia syndrome. *Clin Exp Rheumatol* 2002;20:69–72.

88. Disdier P, Genton P, Harle JR, et al. Fibromyalgia and narcolepsy. *J Rheumatol* 1993;20:888–889.

89. Disdier P, Genton P, Bolla G, et al. Clinical screening for narcolepsy/cataplexy in patients with fibromyalgia. *Clin Rheumatol* 1994;13(1):132–134.

90. Moldofsky H. Management of sleep disorders in fibromyalgia. *Rheum Dis Clin North Am* 2002;28:353–365.

91. Haanen HCM, Hoenderdos HTW, Van Romunde LKJ, et al. Controlled trial of hypnotherapy in the treatment of refractory fibromyalgia. *J Rheumatol* 1991;18:72–75.

92. Ferraccioli G, Ghirelli L, Scita F, et al. EMG biofeedback training in fibromyalgia syndrome. *J Rheumatol* 1987;14(4): 820–825.

93. Deluze C, Bosia L, Zirbs A, et al. Electroacupuncture in fibromyalgia: results of a controlled trial. *Br Med J* 1992; 305(6864):1249–1252.

94. Almeida TF, Roizenblatt S, Benedito-Silva AA, et al. The effect of combined therapy (ultrasound and interferential current) on pain and sleep in fibromyalgia. *Pain* 2003;104: 665–672.

95. Burckhardt CS, Mannerkorpi K, Hedenberg L, et al. A randomized, controlled clinical trial of education and physical training for women with fibromyalgia. *J Rheumatol* 1994; 21(4):714–720.

96. Bennett RM, Gatter RA, Campbell SM, et al. A comparison of cyclobenzaprine and placebo in the management of fibrositis: a double blind controlled study. *Arthritis Rheum* 1988;3:1535–1542.

97. Carette S, Bell MV, Reynolds WJ, et al. Comparison of amitriptyline, cyclobenzaprine and placebo in the treatment of fibromyalgia: a randomized double blind clinical trial. *Arthritis Rheum* 1994;37:32–40.

98. Reynolds WJ, Moldofsky H, Saskin P, et al. The effects of cyclobenzaprine on sleep physiology and symptoms in patients with fibromyalgia. *J Rheumatol* 1991;18:452–454.

99. Goldenberg D, Mayskiy M, Mossey C, et al. A randomized, double-blind crossover trial of fluoxetine and amitriptyline in the treatment of fibromyalgia. *Arthritis Rheum* 1996;39: 1852–1859.

100. Wolfe F, Cathey MA, Hawley DJ. A double blind placebo controlled trial of fluoxetine in fibromyalgia. *Scand J Rheumatol* 1994;23(5):255–259.

101. Drewes AM, Andreasen A, Jennum P, et al. Zopiclone in the treatment of sleep abnormalities in fibromyalgia. *Scand J Rheumatol* 1991;20:288–293.

102. Moldofsky H, Lue FA, Mously C, et al. The effect of zolpidem in patients with fibromyalgia: a dose ranging, double blind, placebo controlled, modified crossover study. *J Rheumatol* 1966;23:529–533.

103. Moldofsky H, Lue FA. The relationship of alpha and delta EEG frequencies to pain and mood in 'fibrositis' patients treated with chlorpromazine and L-tryptophan. *Electroencephalogr Clin Neurophysiol* 1980;50:71–80.

104. Caruso I, Sarzi Puttini P, Cazzola M, et al. Double-blind study of 5-hydroxytryptophan versus placebo in the treatment of primary fibromyalgia syndrome. *J Int Med Res* 1990;18: 201–209.

105. Scharf MB, Baumann M, Berkowitz DV. The effects of sodium oxybate on clinical symptoms and sleep patterns in patients with fibromyalgia. *J Rheumatol* 2003;30:1070–1074.

106. Pearl SJ, Lue F, MacLean AW, et al. The effects of bright light treatment on the symptoms of fibromyalgia. *J Rheumatol* 1996;23:896–902.

107. Silver DS, Wallace DJ. The management of fibromyalgia-associated syndromes. *Rheum Dis Clin North Am* 2002;28: 405–417.

108. Golding DN. Hypothyroidism presenting with musculoskeletal symptoms. *Ann Rheum Dis* 1970;29:10–14.

109. Bland JH, Frymoyer JW. Rheumatic syndromes of myxedema. *N Engl J Med* 1970;282:1171–1174.

110. Yunus M. A comprehensive medical evaluation of patients with fibromyalgia. *Rheum Dis Clin NA* 2003;28:201–217.

11

Symptoms and Signs of Fibromyalgia Syndrome: An Overview

Muhammad B. Yunus

DEFINITION AND CLASSIFICATION OF FIBROMYALGIA SYNDROME

Fibromyalgia syndrome (FMS), also called fibromyalgia, is a common condition that is characterized by widespread musculoskeletal aches and pain as well as exaggerated pain on pressure, called tender points (TePs) (1–7). Fibromyalgia may be called primary if there are no associated or concurrent pathologic conditions that may partly explain the symptoms—for example, arthritis, a connective tissue disease, a neurologic disease, or hypothyroidism. A patient with FMS who has these conditions may be said to have concomitant fibromyalgia. In the Multicenter Criteria study for classification of fibromyalgia, the term "concomitant or secondary" fibromyalgia has been used (6), but use of the term "secondary" in this context is confusing. For example, fibromyalgia may coexist with hypothyroidism or rheumatoid arthritis (RA), but it is not secondary to these diseases. Symptoms or TePs of FMS do not go away when hypothyroidism or coexisting RA is adequately treated. The features of primary FMS and concomitant FMS are similar (2). Thus, both concomitant and primary FMS may simply be called fibromyalgia or FMS.

Myofascial pain syndrome (MPS) is a regional soft tissue pain (RSTP) syndrome (in contrast to widespread pain in FMS) that is characterized by local or regional muscle pain and palpated tenderness. Other features of MPS have been suggested—for example, referred pain on palpation, palpable band, and twitch response of the affected muscle (8). However, the validity and significance of any other feature besides regional pain and tenderness have not been established (9). No convincing data exist that MPS is uniquely different from RSTP that requires only regional pain and TeP(s) for its diagnosis (10). We believe that MPS is a forme fruste FMS. We had found that a substantial proportion of our RSTP patients had a significantly higher frequency of systemic symptoms as compared to normal controls—for example, fatigue (44%), poor sleep (57%), paresthesia (30%), and tension-

type headache (26%)—although these features were significantly less frequent than in FMS (10). In our preliminary study we found that 40% of patients with RSTP developed widespread musculoskeletal pain after a mean period of 6 years (11), and, conversely, most patients with FMS started with localized or regional pain. Lapossy et al. also reported that 25% of their 53 patients who had initially presented with low back pain later developed fibromyalgia (12). MPS (RSTP) and FMS are overlapping syndromes clinically (10), psychologically (10), and biophysiologically (13,14).

CLINICAL FEATURES OF FIBROMYALGIA SYNDROME

SYMPTOMS

FMS, more common among females in the 40–60 age group, is an illness or disease of protean manifestations (see Table 11-1). Besides widespread pain and stiffness, the systemic nature of FMS with fatigue, poor sleep, headaches, and anxiety was first described, although anecdotally, by Traut in 1968 (15). Yunus et al. later confirmed all these symptoms in the first controlled clinical study of FMS using normal controls (2). A few additional symptoms were also found to be more common in FMS than controls—for example, swollen feeling in soft tissues, paresthesia, tension-type headaches, migraine, and irritable bowel syndrome (2). TePs were also showing for the first time to be significantly more common than in the normal controls, and this study provided the first data-based criteria for fibromyalgia (2). Other studies that included chronic pain controls subsequently confirmed these FMS features (3–7,10,16,17). The onset of fibromyalgia symptoms often follows infection (particularly viral infection), trauma, and mental stress (18–21).

Pain in many locations is the integral symptom of fibromyalgia. It is usually present in all four limbs, as well as the upper or lower back. About two-thirds of the patients

TABLE 11-1	Symptoms in Fibromyalgia Syndrome Based on Four Large Series with N of More than 100[a]

SYMPTOMS	MEAN (%)
Musculoskeletal	
Pain at multiple sites	100
Stiffness	76
"Hurt all over"	62
Swollen feeling in tissues	52
Nonmusculoskeletal	
General fatigue	87
Morning fatigue	75
Sleep difficulties	72
Paresthesia	54
Dizziness/vertigo (23,24)	59
Tinnitus (24)	17
Sicca symptoms[b] (25,26)	15
Raynaud phenomenon[c] (6,25)	14
Anxiety[d]	60
Mental stress	61
Depression	37
Cognitive dysfunction[e] (27)	61
Selected Associated Syndromes	
Headaches	54
Dysmenorrhea	43
Irritable bowel syndrome	38
Restless legs syndrome (28)	31
Female urethral syndrome (29,30)	15

[a] N = 118 (4); N = 113 (5); N = 293 (6); N = 536 (22) (combined male and female patients). The figures are the average of % symptoms in a particular series of four when reported (not all the studies reported all symptoms). For some symptoms, other references were used as shown and average calculated if applicable.

[b] Includes patients who were not on an antidepressant drug.

[c] Definition specified as "dead white pallor on exposure to cold."

[d] Anxiety, mental stress, and depression were evaluated by a single item question.

[e] Note that cognitive dysfunctions in FMS may be present irrespective of medications or psychiatric disorders (31).

From Goldenberg DL. Fibromyalgia syndrome. An emerging but controversial condition. *JAMA* 1987;257:2782–2787; Yunus MB, Masi AT, Aldag JC. A controlled study of primary fibromyalgia syndrome: clinical features and association with other functional syndromes. *J Rheumatol* 1989;19(Suppl.):62–71; Wolfe F, Smythe HA, Yunus MB, et al. The American College of Rheumatology 1990 criteria for the classification of fibromyalgia. Report of the Multicenter Criteria Committee. *Arthritis Rheum* 1990;33:160–172; Yunus MB, Inanici F, Aldag JC, et al. Fibromyalgia in men: comparison of clinical features with women. *J Rheumatol* 2000;27:485–490, with permissions.

state that they "hurt all over," and this symptom has been found to be useful in differentiating fibromyalgia from other conditions, such as RA (5,6,32). FMS patients use multiple words in describing their pain. Leavitt et al. used an adapted McGill Pain Questionnaire to compare the pain characteristics in 50 patients with FMS and 50 patients with RA and found that pain in fibromyalgia had a wider spatial distribution and involved a greater number of pain descriptors—for example, aching, hurting, sore, exhausting, nagging, annoying, shooting, radiating, miserable, unbearable, and throbbing (33). Several words—radiating, steady, spasm, spreading, and gnawing, for example—were employed more frequently by patients with FMS than by those with RA.

Common sites of pain or stiffness are low back, neck, shoulder region, arms, hands, hips, thighs, knees, legs, and feet (5,6). However, many other areas, including the anterior chest (2,34), may be affected. Chest pain in fibromyalgia may be a presenting symptom and mimic cardiopulmonary disease (34). The presence of local tenderness (TePs) in the chest wall as well as other parts of the body (see the section entitled "Physical Examination" below) suggests FMS, but concomitant cardiopulmonary diseases cannot be ruled out. Some patients complain mostly of joint, rather than muscle, pain (35). Pain in metacarpophalangeal and proximal interphalangeal joints may raise the question of arthritis, for example, RA, particularly when accompanied by a complaint of swelling in these joints (2,5,35). On rare occasions some patients complain of pain predominantly or exclusively in one side of the body (2). The reason for such unilateral pain is not clear, but we have noted that the involved side is often predominantly used in performing mechanical tasks.

Stiffness is a common accompaniment of pain and reported by about 85% of patients (2). It is usually worse in the morning but may be experienced at other times—for example, in the evening and particularly after a period of physical inactivity. Unlike RA, morning stiffness does not correlate with disease severity in FMS—for example, pain, fatigue, and TePs (5). Pain and stiffness sites strongly correlate with each other (our unpublished data).

Pain and stiffness are often aggravated by cold or humid weather, anxiety, stress, overuse (including occupational use), inactivity, poor sleep (2–6,16,17,36), and noise (6) (see Table 11-2). Many patients are also sensitive to smell and noise (21). Psychological distress is associated with severity of pain and other symptoms (37–39). Many patients report moderate physical activity, local heat, massage, rest and relaxation, and stretching exercises to be beneficial (2,5,17) (Table 11-2). We had observed a correlation between smoking and pain, global severity, functional disability, and numbness in FMS (40). Body mass index was correlated with functional disability with a weaker association with fatigue and number of TePs (41). These studies make another

TABLE 11-2	Modulating Factors of Fibromyalgia Syndrome Pain (Mean %) Based on Four Series as in Table 11-1[a]

Aggravating Factors	
Weather (cold/humid)	65
Poor sleep	70
Anxiety/stress	61
Physical inactivity	49
Noise (6,44)	22
Relieving Factors	
Local heat	58
Rest	54
Moderate activities	46
Massage	40
Stretching exercise	43

[a] The figures are the average of % factors in a particular series of four studies when reported (not all the studies reported all the modulating factors).

case for the patients to stop smoking and lose weight to help their pain and functions. Most patients state that their pain and stiffness are worse in the morning and the evening (2,42). In studies of chronobiological influences on FMS, Moldofsky reported that the worst times for a fibromyalgia patient are in the morning, the later half of the afternoon, and the evening (42). During these periods patients feel more achy, stiff, and lethargic, experience more emotional distress, and show decreased cognitive performance. Unlike normal controls, the FMS patients feel their best between 10 AM and 2 PM, the peak time being around noon (42). A physician should inquire about such diurnal variation of symptoms in a patient and, if such variation is present, advise that patient to use this window of feeling relatively well to accomplish important daily activities. In the same paper, Moldofsky also described seasonal effect in FMS. By self-report, patients experience worse mood, pain, and energy level during November and March. This is consistent with our earlier report that 44% of our patients felt better during summer and spring; only one of our 50 patients had preferred the winter (2). Similar findings have also been reported among the patients with low pain threshold (43).

Fatigue is quite common in fibromyalgia; moderate or severe fatigue occurs in about 75% to 90% of patients (1–7,19). A typical patient describes it by saying, "I am always tired." It is variously described as exhaustion, tiredness, lack of energy, fatigue, being "drained out," and sometimes as a global feeling of general weakness. It is aggravated by physical activities, psychological distress, poor sleep, infections, and medication side effects, and it may cause significant dysfunctions in daily living (2,5). Fatigue, rather than pain or stiffness, may be the presenting feature in some patients. In some, fatigue is the major symptom during a flare-up. As is the case with pain, fatigue in FMS is likely of central origin, similar to chronic fatigue syndrome (45). Fatigue is associated with pain, global severity, and functional disability (22), as well as poor sleep (46).

Swollen feeling and paresthesia are common symptoms, being reported by about half the patients (2–6). In some patients these are significantly troubling complaints. Although these symptoms may involve any site, they are predominantly present in the extremities. Objective joint swelling or sensory deficits are, however, absent on physical examination (see below). Paresthesia is described as pins and needles, tingling, or numbness. Patients may complain of these symptoms at numerous sites, but they are reported most frequently in the extremities. Similar to pain, paresthesia may have a radiating quality that may be confused with radiculopathy due to an anatomic pathology.

A careful neurologic examination is therefore important (47). Such an examination is mandatory if the intensity or the quality of paresthesia changes. The frequency of this symptom is around 40% to 60% but has been reported to be as high as 84% (48). Paresthesia, with or without radiating distribution, along with other neurologic symptoms, such as weakness, vertigo, headaches, and fatigue, may mimic a neurologic disorder, and some patients may consult a neurologist before a diagnosis of FMS is made. It is important to take a good history and do a proper neurologic examination so that concomitant neurologic diseases are not missed. To evaluate a patient fully, one may have to request laboratory tests and X-rays if indicated by clinical findings (47). We have seen

several patients who had numbness on presentation with normal neurologic findings who later developed spinal stenosis and peripheral neuropathies. The quality of paresthesia became different (more unpleasant and constant) and the severity was worse with abnormal neurologic findings.

The mechanisms of paresthesia and subjective swelling are not clearly understood. We had reported a significant intercorrelation between these two symptoms, as well as correlation between both of them and total pain sites (5). It seems quite likely that these phenomena of subjective swelling and paresthesia result from abnormal sensory perception due to central sensitization. These symptoms did not correlate with psychological factors (5,38). Electromyograph and nerve conduction velocity studies in primary fibromyalgia are normal (48,49).

Neurootologic symptoms are common in fibromyalgia. Taking an average figure from two uncontrolled studies (23,50), dizziness/vertigo was reported in about 60%, and hearing loss (mostly asymptomatic) was present in 18% (23,24,50). Additionally, 17% complained of tinnitus (24) and 20% of discomfort and hypersensitivity to loudness, as well as aggravation of their pain by noise (50). I agree with the authors' opinion in these papers that the cause of such neurootologic abnormalities in FMS is most likely a dysfunction of the central nervous system, including the brain stem.

Nonrestorative sleep is common in fibromyalgia (1–7, 10,22). A review of the literature suggests that about 70% of the FMS patients describe sleep problems and 75% to 80% have morning fatigue. They complain of difficulty falling asleep with tossing and turning, of difficulty obtaining deep sleep during the night, and of waking up tired. They wake up frequently during sleep, sometimes with pain. FMS patients complain of light sleep, and it has been said that they are even aware of a cat's movements in the room. Morning fatigue is likely an indicator of nonrestorative sleep. Sleep quality and increased morning pain were associated with phasic α-sleep activity by sleep electroencephalogram in one study (51). A number of factors may contribute to poor sleep in FMS: restless legs syndrome, periodic limb movement disorder, other conditions causing night pain, pulmonary or cardiac diseases with cough and shortness of breath, gastroesophageal reflux disease, psychological distress (anxiety, depression, and mental stress), coffee and alcohol intake or smoking prior to several hours of bedtime, medications, light, noise, a lack of exercise, and irregular sleep habits. Poor sleep is correlated with fatigue and psychological distress (2,5,22), as well as pain (52). Poor sleep may aggravate pain and fatigue (2,5,6,22). There is a relationship between poor sleep and pain as well as attention to pain, and poor sleep the previous night predicts pain the next day, which is then followed by a poor night's sleep (52).

Psychological symptoms—anxiety, stress, and depression evaluated by a single item question were present in about 60% (5,6), and depression evaluated in a similar manner was present in 37% (5).

Several *associated symptoms and conditions* have been described in fibromyalgia (Table 11-1). They include irritable bowel syndrome, headaches, chronic fatigue syndrome, restless legs syndrome, periodic limb movement disorder, temporomandibular dysfunction, primary dysmenorrhea, depression, female urethral syndrome, and multiple chemical sensitivity (5,14,28–30,53,54). More than one study has shown that these associated conditions, as well as other chronic pain conditions such as RA, are more common in FMS than in healthy controls (3,5,6,14,28–30,54). The recognition of the associated conditions is important for comprehensive diagnosis, avoidance of unnecessary investigations, and management of FMS. Collectively, these conditions have been called central sensitivity syndromes (CSS) (14,53), and they will be further discussed in another chapter.

Sicca symptoms are reported by many patients and have been found to be significantly more common in fibromyalgia than in normal and other disease controls (6,25,55–57). A subgroup of FMS patients has also been reported to have primary Sjögren syndrome in one study (57) but not in others. What causes these symptoms is not well understood. This symptom was not related to drugs (such as an antidepressant medication) or to psychological symptoms of anxiety, stress, or depression among our patients (25). None of our patients with dry mouth had evidence of Sjögren syndrome or other connective tissue diseases—systemic lupus erythematosus (SLE) or RA, for example—on their first visit or during subsequent follow-up in our study (25). Sicca symptoms may be due to an autonomic dysfunction or an abnormal sensory perception, or both. However, one should be aware that several connective tissue diseases—for example, RA (44,58,59), SLE (60–64), and Sjögren syndrome (65,66)—have been reported to be associated with fibromyalgia.

Raynaud (or Raynaud-like) phenomenon (RP) has been reported by several investigators (3,25,26,67,68). The prevalence has varied from 3% (67) to 53% (68); the varying occurrence is likely explained by different definitions of RP, age, and number of patients studied. Only three studies have appropriately used normal controls (6,25,67). Yunus et al. defined RP as "clear description of reversible dead white pallor of an acral structure, precipitated by cold exposure or emotion" (25). Wolfe et al. (6) used a similar definition. RP was present in 8.8% of 160 female patients versus 2.3% of 80 female controls ($p<0.07$) (25) and in 16.7% of 293 patients versus 9.6% of 265 controls ($p<0.01$) (6). The occurrence of physician-diagnosed RP was low at 3% (however, digital color change in cold was reported by 13% of patients) in the study of Bennett et al. (67). This study showed a significant cold-induced vasospasm and elevated α-2 adrenergic receptors in platelets as compared to normal controls. There was no correlation between RP symptoms and cold-induced vasospasm. The mechanism of vasospasm in FMS may be due to increased vasoconstrictor response to catecholamines, resulting from elevated α-2 receptor density or sensitivity (67). It has been suggested that the vasodilatory phase of RP may be related to increased local substance P (68).

Cognitive dysfunctions in FMS have been reported by many investigators using control groups and a validated battery of neuropsychological testing (27,31,69–72). The findings included poor memory, difficulty in information processing, attention deficit, and decreased verbal fluency. Memory may be affected by age, pain, stress, depression, poor sleep, education level, and medications. However, a well-designed study controlled for age, education, and depression showed that FMS patients (not taking psychoactive medications) had significant cognitive problems, mostly in working memory, free recall, and verbal fluency, compared to normal controls (31).

PHYSICAL EXAMINATION

Physical examination is vital in full evaluation of FMS. In primary fibromyalgia without concomitant disease, patients look healthy, although sometimes anxious or depressed. Physical examination is unremarkable, except for the findings in the soft tissues and the skin. Examination of the joints shows no objective swelling, but in a subgroup of patients there is articular tenderness, most likely a part of generalized tenderness due to central sensitization. The most important examination in FMS is the assessment of TePs in soft tissues. Like many other physical signs—enlarged liver or a heart murmur, for example—eliciting TePs requires skill and needs to be learned. TePs are best palpated by the pulp of one of the first three fingers, depending on the comfort and preference of the examiner, using approximately 4 kg of pressure. A distinct perception of pain as compared to mere pressure qualifies for a TeP. I start with gentle pressure on a TeP site and gradually increase it until the patient perceives the pressure to be painful. This degree of pressure is best learned by using a dolorimeter (algometer). The capped part of the instrument is pushed at a rate of 1 kg per second on a TeP location. The examiner asks the patient to remember the amount of pressure the patient had felt by the dolorimeter and then the examiner manually palpates the other side, again asking the patient if this manual pressure is equivalent to the degree of pressure that was perceived by the dolorimeter on the other side. A few varieties of algometers are commercially available, but the one used by the FMS Criteria Committee was a Chattilon dolorimeter (Chattilon Instruments, Kew Gardens, NY) having a 1.54 cm^2 area on the stopper (6). Another way is to put pressure on a fairly firm surface—for example, the upper border of the trapezius or the suboccipital region—and then to observe how much pressure is needed to blanch the nailbed of the palpating finger. One must realize that this is only approximate, but with practice one gets a good idea of 4 kg pressure. Another useful way to learn proper TeP examination is to approach under the supervision or with the help of a mentor who is experienced in FMS evaluation. For teaching purposes, I ask my patient to "remember" the amount of pressure I put on one side of a TeP—for example, midtrapezius—and have the student or the resident (or another physician) apply manual force on the other side. I am always impressed by the fact that patients always know if the learner has applied the mentor's correct degree of pressure. Since an important parameter of TeP examination is to have the patient differentiate between pain and pressure, I often start with gentle pressure on a TeP site and gradually increase it until the patient can perceive the pressure to be painful (mild or greater pain will count as a TeP) (6).

For research purposes, tenderness may be graded as mild, moderate, or severe, as was done in the Multicenter FMS Criteria study (6). A sensation of pain without any observed pain behavior is graded mild. A visible sign of involuntary grimacing, flinching, and a sudden withdrawal of a body part would qualify for moderate or severe pain, depending on the severity of response. The "jump sign" is characterized by an unexpected brisk and accentuated jerky movement with an upward motion simulating a jump. TeP may also be quantitated using a 0 to 10 scale that may provide greater sensitivity of change in a drug study (73).

It is important to remember that 18 sites of TeP in the American College of Rheumatology (ACR) criteria were derived statistically in order to obtain a manageable number of TePs that would give optimal sensitivity and specificity. Fibromyalgia patients may have tenderness on pressure in a large number of sites, including various muscles, tendons, ligaments, chest wall, shin, and other bones. TePs in 75 sites have been reported (74). An aphorism to remember is that a FMS patient may be tender on palpation virtually everywhere. One of my patients had tenderness on the eyelids! Her eye examination by an ophthalmologist within the next few days was completely normal. Many patients are tender in the so-called control points. Control points are useless in the diagnosis or treatment of FMS (75). A subgroup of patients is, in fact, diffusely tender all over on palpation.

The number of TePs was found to correlate with psychological distress in community studies (76), where all TePs were counted showing a larger dispersal of data (unlike studies that used ACR criteria for inclusion). However, studies employing FMS patients in the clinic and using ACR classification criteria failed to show such correlation (16,38). This may be due to a difference in subjects studied [clinic patients are different from nonpatients in the population (77) and a limited range of TePs (11–18) analyzed in clinic patients (16,22)].

TePs have been found to be significantly consistent in the same patient over a period of time when examined by the same examiner (78), and there is significant intraobserver and interobserver reliability (79,80).

Allodynia is defined as pain on a normally innocuous stimulus—touch, massage, or normally innocuous heat, for example—and has been well demonstrated in FMS compared to normal controls (81). Many woman patients complain that they cannot hug their spouses because of pain caused by gentle pressure, and a subset of patients is sensitive to massage in addition to touch. The underlying mechanism is most likely marked central sensitization with aberrant neurochemicals that may be modulated by multiple factors, including genetics, previous sensitization by a stimulus (e.g., mental or physical trauma), and psychological distress.

Other physical signs in fibromyalgia are cutaneous hyperemia and skin fold tenderness (6,32). *Cutaneous hyperemia* is seen at the sites of TePs within seconds to 2 to 3 minutes of mechanically palpating these sites. Although uncommon, some patients display spontaneous hyperemia without palpation. The mechanism for such phenomenon is unknown. *Skin fold tenderness* is elicited by pinching a fold of skin and subcutaneous tissues by moderate pressure. It is more likely to be elicited at the TeP sites, although such tenderness may be diffusely present in many patients. TePs and skin fold tenderness most likely share the same pathophysiological mechanism, that is, central sensitization. Cutaneous hyperemia may be explicable on the basis of "neurogenic inflammation" (82). Skin fold tenderness correlates with TePs (32) and has been shown to have a sensitivity of 60% and a specificity of 83% in the Multicenter ACR Criteria study (6). Hyperemia had limited sensitivity (50%) and specificity (31%) in this study.

Reticular discoloration of skin is a net-like bluish or pinkish mottled discoloration of skin that is usually seen in the legs or thighs. It was first described by Caro (83), and we have observed the same finding in some of our patients. Reticular discoloration may resemble livedo retucularis found in vasculitis. In the Multicenter study (6) only 15% of patients were observed to have this finding but had a high specificity (95%).

For practical purposes, the only finding that is useful in diagnosis of FMS is multiple TePs.

The so-called *fibrositic nodules* were described in earlier literature as firm, mobile, globular, or spindle-shaped tender structures consisting of fatty tissue, fibrous cords, and muscles (with globular density in certain areas), generally of 3 to 6 mm in diameter (15,65,84,85). None of these observations had a control group. Some of the nodules have the consistency of being ropey. They are sore to the touch and more often than not, patients draw attention to these "nodules." We had also observed these tender "nodules," mostly in the lumbo-sacral region (2). One such nodule was biopsied and showed fibrofatty tissue without any inflammatory cells. Subsequently we had recorded them by protocol in FMS and normal healthy controls and found no significant difference between the patients and the controls in number of nodules; nodules in FMS were distinctly tender as compared to those among the normal controls (our unpublished data). It is the tenderness, we believe, that draws the attention of the patients who then report them to their physicians.

Finally, it is important that a physician diagnoses concomitant diseases by careful history and physical examination. A comprehensive evaluation of an FMS patient, including physical examination, has been described elsewhere (47). Physical findings in FMS are shown in Table 11-3.

FIBROMYALGIA SYNDROME AMONG MEN

Clinical features of fibromyalgia among men seen in a rheumatology clinic in the United States were compared to those in women (22). A number of features were significantly less common or fewer in the male patients, for example, fatigue, morning fatigue, "hurt all over," irritable bowel syndrome, and the number of total symptoms as well as number of TePs. Stepwise logistical regression showed significant differences in the number of TePs between men and women. However, global severity, pain severity, and functional disabilities were similar in the two groups. These findings among men are quite similar to those found in a population study (86). Another study of gender differences

TABLE 11-3 Physical Signs (%) in Fibromyalgia Syndrome[a]

Tender points (11+ among ACR 18 sites)	100
Skin fold tenderness	60
Cutaneous hyperemia	50
Reticular skin discoloration	15

ACR, American College of Rheumatology.
[a]It is important to look for signs of concomitant diseases.
From Wolfe F, Smythe HA, Yunus MB, et al. The American College of Rheumatology 1990 criteria for the classification of fibromyalgia. Report of the Multicenter Criteria Committee. *Arthritis Rheum* 1990;33:160–172, with permission.

in fibromyalgia from Israel showed unexpected results. Men had significantly greater or more frequent fatigue, pain, morning stiffness, depression, and irritable bowel syndrome; there was no difference in TePs (87). The different findings among Israeli men may, at least, be due to possible cultural differences. Assessment of the psychological distress by validated questionnaires showed similar results between men and women (86–88), as was the case in headaches, an FMS-related syndrome (89).

DIAGNOSIS OF FIBROMYALGIA SYNDROME

Diagnosis and differential diagnosis of FMS have been covered in detail elsewhere in this text. Since diagnosis of FMS is a clinical one based on history and TeP examination, this section provides an overview of FMS diagnosis. For classification of FMS by ACR criteria, a patient must have widespread pain and 11+ TePs in 18 specified sites (see Chapter 23). To qualify for widespread pain, a patient must have pain in all these areas: above the waist, below the waist, right side, left side, and the lower side of the body. Again, proper assessment of TePs is important. A substantial number of clinically diagnosed FMS do not fulfill the classification criteria of ACR. These patients have incomplete FMS, defined by either having 11+ TePs and no widespread pain or having widespread pain with 5 to 10 TePs, in association with typical FMS symptoms (90). Those without widespread pain had pain in at least three noncontiguous areas. FMS is purely a clinical diagnosis and does not need any laboratory or X-ray investigation, unless a concomitant disease requires such investigations. It is also important to know that the presence of another disease does not exclude the diagnosis of FMS (6). It is clear that the examiner should be adroit in TeP examination, knowing exactly where to palpate and how much pressure to apply in order to make a diagnosis of FMS.

SUMMARY POINTS

- Although fibromyalgia is defined on the basis of pain and tenderness, studies among various ethnic groups have shown a consistent pattern of multiple symptoms that include widespread pain and stiffness, fatigue, poor sleep, morning fatigue, paresthesia, dizziness, a subjective swollen feeling, cognitive difficulties, psychological distress, and sensitivity to environmental factors, such as weather and noise, as well as many associated conditions, for example, headaches, irritable bowel syndrome, and restless legs syndrome.

■ IMPLICATIONS FOR PRACTICE

- Core symptoms of FMS are widespread pain (often "hurt all over"), fatigue, and poor sleep.
- Other common symptoms are swollen feeling, paresthesia, dizziness, cognitive difficulties, and mental distress (anxiety, stress, depression).

- Associated conditions include headaches, irritable bowel syndrome, chronic fatigue syndrome, pelvic pain, chronic fatigue syndrome, restless legs syndrome, and female urethral syndrome.
- The most important physical sign is the presence of multiple TePs.
- Many patients have clinical FMS without fulfilling ACR criteria.

REFERENCES

1. Smythe HA. Non-articular rheumatism and psychogenic musculoskeletal syndromes. In: McCarty DJ, ed. *Arthritis and allied conditions*. Philadelphia: Iea & Febiger, 1979; 881–891.
2. Yunus M, Masi AT, Calabro JJ, et al. Primary fibromyalgia (fibrositis): clinical study of 50 patients with matched normal controls. *Semin Arthritis Rheum* 1981;11:151–171.
3. Bengtsson A, Henriksson KG, Jorfeldt L, et al. Primary fibromyalgia. A clinical and laboratory study of 55 patients. *Scand J Rheumatol* 1986;15:340–347.
4. Goldenberg DL. Fibromyalgia syndrome. An emerging but controversial condition. *JAMA* 1987;257:2782–2787.
5. Yunus MB, Masi AT, Aldag JC. A controlled study of primary fibromyalgia syndrome: clinical features and association with other functional syndromes. *J Rheumatol* 1989; 19(Suppl):62–71.
6. Wolfe F, Smythe HA, Yunus MB, et al. The American College of Rheumatology 1990 criteria for the classification of fibromyalgia. Report of the Multicenter Criteria Committee. *Arthritis Rheum* 1990;33:160–172.
7. White KP, Speechley M, Harth M, et al. The London fibromyalgia epidemiology study: the prevalence of fibromyalgia syndrome in London, Ontario. *J Rheumatol* 1999;26:1570–1576.
8. Travell J, Simons DG. *Myofascial pain and dysfunction: the trigger point manual*. Baltimore, MD: Williams & Wilkins, 1983.
9. Wolfe F, Simons DG, Fricton J, et al. The fibromyalgia and myofascial pain syndromes: a preliminary study of tender points and trigger points in persons with fibromyalgia, myofascial pain syndrome and no disease. *J Rheumatol* 1992; 19:944–951.
10. Inanici F, Yunus MB, Aldag JC. Clinical features and psychologic factors in regional soft tissue pain: comparison with fibromyalgia syndrome. *J Musculoskelet Pain* 1999;7: 293–301.
11. Inanici F, Yunus MB, Castillo LD, et al. Prognosis of regional fibromyalgia: comparison with fibromyalgia syndrome. *J Musculoskelet Pain* 1998;6:97.
12. Lapossy E, Maleitzke R, Hrycaj P, et al. The frequency of transition of chronic low back pain to fibromyalgia. *Scand J Rheumatol* 1995;24:29–33.
13. Bendtsen L, Jensen R, Olesen J. Qualitatively altered nociception in chronic myofascial pain. *Pain* 1996;65:259–264.
14. Yunus MB. Central sensitivity syndromes: a unified concept for fibromyalgia and other similar maladies. *J Indian Rheumatol Assoc* 2000;8:27–33.
15. Traut EF. Fibrositis. *J Am Geriatr Soc* 1968;16:531–538.
16. Choudhury AK, Yunus MB, Haq SA, et al. Clinical features of fibromyalgia in a Bangladeshi population. *J Musculoskelet Pain* 2001;9(2):25–33.
17. Campbell SM, Clark S, Tindall EA, et al. Clinical characteristics of fibrositis. I. A "blinded," controlled study of symptoms and tender points. *Arthritis Rheum* 1983;26:817–824.

18. Buskila D, Neumann L, Vaisberg G, et al. Increased rates of fibromyalgia following cervical spine injury. A controlled study of 161 cases of traumatic injury. *Arthritis Rheum* 1997; 40:446–452.
19. Wolfe F. Fibromyalgia. *Rheum Dis Clin North Am* 1990;16: 681–698.
20. Greenfield S, Fitzcharles MA, Esdaile JM. Reactive fibromyalgia syndrome. *Arthritis Rheum* 1992;35:678–681.
21. Prince A, Bernard AL, Edsal PA. A descriptive analysis of fibromyalgia from the patients' perspective. *J Musculoskelet Pain* 2000;8:35–47.
22. Yunus MB, Inanici F, Aldag JC, et al. Fibromyalgia in men: comparison of clinical features with women. *J Rheumatol* 2000;27:485–490.
23. Rosenhall U, Johansson G, Orndahl G. Otoneurologic and audiologic findings in fibromyalgia. *Scand J Rehabil Med* 1996;28:225–232.
24. Bayazit YA, Gursoy S, Ozer E, et al. Neurotologic manifestations of the fibromyalgia syndrome. *J Neurol Sci* 2002;196: 77–80.
25. Yunus MB, Hussey FX, Aldag JC. Antinuclear antibodies and "connective tissue disease features" in fibromyalgia syndrome: a controlled study. *J Rheumatol* 1993;20: 1557–1560.
26. Dinerman H, Goldenberg DL, Felson DT. A prospective evaluation of 118 patients with the fibromyalgia syndrome: prevalence of Raynaud's phenomenon, sicca symptoms, ANA, low complement, and Ig deposition at the dermal-epidermal junction. *J Rheumatol* 1986;13:368–373.
27. Dick B, Eccleston C, Crombez G. Attentional functioning in fibromyalgia, rheumatoid arthritis, and musculoskeletal pain patients. *Arthritis Rheum* 2002;47:639–644.
28. Yunus MB, Aldag JC. Restless legs syndrome and leg cramps in fibromyalgia syndrome: a controlled study. *Br Med J* 1996;312:1339.
29. Wallace DJ. Genitourinary manifestations of fibrositis: an increased association with the female urethral syndrome. *J Rheumatol* 1990;17:238–239.
30. Paira SO. Fibromyalgia associated with female urethral syndrome. *Clin Rheumatol* 1994;13:88–89.
31. Park DC, Glass JM, Minear M, et al. Cognitive function in fibromyalgia patients. *Arthritis Rheum* 2001;44:2125–2133.
32. Yunus MB, Masi AT, Aldag JC. Preliminary criteria for primary fibromyalgia syndrome (PFS): multivariate analysis of a consecutive series of PFS, other pain patients, and normal subjects. *Clin Exp Rheumatol* 1989;7:63–69.
33. Leavitt F, Katz RS, Golden HE, et al. Comparison of pain properties in fibromyalgia patients and rheumatoid arthritis patients. *Arthritis Rheum* 1986;29:775–781.
34. Pellegrino MJ. Atypical chest pain as an initial presentation of primary fibromyalgia. *Arch Phys Med Rehabil* 1990;71: 526–528.
35. Reilly PA, Littlejohn GO. Peripheral arthralgic presentation of fibrositis/fibromyalgia syndrome. *J Rheumatol* 1992;19: 281–283.
36. Wolfe F, Ross K, Anderson J, et al. The prevalence and characteristics of fibromyalgia in the general population. *Arthritis Rheum* 1995;38:19–28.
37. Benjamin S, Morris S, McBeth J, et al. The association between chronic widespread pain and mental disorder: a population-based study. *Arthritis Rheum* 2000;43:561–567.
38. Yunus MB, Ahles TA, Aldag JC, et al. Relationship of clinical features with psychological status in primary fibromyalgia. *Arthritis Rheum* 1991;34:15–21.
39. White KP, Nielson WR, Harth M, et al. Chronic widespread musculoskeletal pain with or without fibromyalgia: psychological distress in a representative community adult sample. *J Rheumatol* 2002;29:588–594.
40. Yunus MB, Arslan S, Aldag JC. Relationship between fibromyalgia features and smoking. *Scand J Rheumatol* 2002; 31:301–305.
41. Yunus MB, Arslan S, Aldag JC. Relationship between body mass index and fibromyalgia features. *Scand J Rheumatol* 2002;31:27–31.
42. Moldofsky H. Chronobiological influences on fibromyalgia syndrome: theoretical and therapeutic implications. *Baillieres Clin Rheumatol* 1994;8:801–810.
43. Bellamy N, Sothern RB, Campbell J. Aspects of diurnal rhythmicity in pain, stiffness and fatigue with fibromyalgia. *J Rheumatol* 2004;31:379–389.
44. Wolfe F, Cathey MA, Kleinheksel SM. Fibrositis (Fibromyalgia) in rheumatoid arthritis. *J Rheumatol* 1984;11:814–818.
45. Kent-Braun JA, Sharma KR, Weiner MW, et al. Central basis of muscle fatigue in chronic fatigue syndrome. *Neurology* 1993;43:125–131.
46. Nicassio PM, Moxham EG, Schuman CE, et al. The contribution of pain, reported sleep quality, and depressive symptoms to fatigue in fibromyalgia. *Pain* 2002;100:271–279.
47. Yunus MB. A comprehensive medical evaluation of patients with fibromyalgia syndrome. *Rheum Dis Clin North Am* 2002;28:201–217.
48. Simms RW, Goldenberg DL. Symptoms mimicking neurologic disorders in fibromyalgia syndrome. *J Rheumatol* 1988; 15:1271–1273.
49. Ersoz M. Nerve conduction tests in patients with fibromyalgia: a comparison with normal controls. *Rheumatol Int* 2003; 23:166–170.
50. Gerster JC, Hadj-Djilani A. Hearing and vestibular abnormalities in primary fibrositis syndrome. *J Rheumatol* 1984; 11:678–680.
51. Roizenblatt S, Moldofsky H, Benedito-Silva AA, et al. Alpha sleep characteristics in fibromyalgia. *Arthritis Rheum* 2001;44:222–230.
52. Affleck G, Urrows S, Tennen H, et al. Sequential daily relations of sleep, pain intensity and attention to pain among women with fibromyalgia. *Pain* 1996;68:363–368.
53. Arslan S, Yunus MB. Fibromyalgia: making a diagnosis, understanding its pathophysiology. *Consultant* 2003;43:1233–1244.
54. Slotkoff AT, Radulovic DA, Clauw DJ. The relationship between fibromyalgia and multiple chemical sensitivity syndrome. *Scand J Rheumatol* 1997;26:364–367.
55. Gunaydin I, Terhorst T, Eckstein A, et al. Assessment of keratoconjunctivitis sicca in patients with fibromyalgia: results of a prospective study. *Rheumatol Int* 1999;19:7–9.
56. Rhodus NJ, Frikcton J, Carlson P, et al. Oral symptoms associated with fibromyalgia syndrome. *J Rheumatol* 2003;30: 1841–1845.
57. Bonafede RP, Downey DC, Bennett RM. An association of fibromyalgia with primary Sjogren's syndrome: a prospective study of 72 patients. *J Rheumatol* 1995;22:133–136.
58. Arslan S, Yunus MB, Aldag JC. Fibromyalgia syndrome in rheumatoid arthritis [Abstract]. *Arthritis Rheum* 2001; 44(Suppl):S71.
59. Wolfe F, Michaud K. Severe rheumatoid arthritis (RA), worse outcomes, comorbid illness, and sociodemographic disadvantage characterize RA patients with fibromyalgia. *J Rheumatol* 2004;31:695–700.
60. Middleton GD, McFarlin JE, Lipsky PE. The prevalence and clinical impact of fibromyalgia in systemic lupus erythematosus. *Arthritis Rheum* 1994;37:1181–1188.
61. Friedman AW, Tewi MB, Ahn C, et al., LUMINA Study Group. Systemic lupus erythematosus in three ethnic groups: XV. Prevalence and correlates of fibromyalgia. *Lupus* 2003; 12(4):274–279.
62. Handa R, Aggarwal p, Wali JP, et al. Fibromyalgia in Indian patients with SLE. *Lupus* 1998;7:475–478.

63. Valencia-Flores M, Cardiel MH, Santiago V, et al. Prevalence and factors associated with fibromyalgia in Mexican patients with systemic lupus erythematosus. *Lupus* 2004;13:4–10.

64. Buskila D, Press J, Abu-Shakra M. Fibromyalgia in systemic lupus erythematosus: prevalence and clinical implications. *Clin Rev Allergy Immunol* 2003;25:25–28.

65. Vitali C, Tavoni A, Neri R, et al. Fibromyalgia features in patients with primary Sjogren's syndrome. Evidence of a relationship with psychological depression. *Scand J Rheumatol* 1989;18:21–27.

66. Ostuni P, Botsios C, Sfriso P, et al. Fibromyalgia in Italian patients with primary Sjogren's syndrome. *Joint Bone Spine* 2002;69:51–57.

67. Bennett RM, Clark SR, Campbell SM, et al. Symptoms of Raynaud's syndrome in patients with fibromyalgia. A study utilizing the Nielsen test, digital photoplethysmography, and measurements of platelet alpha 2-adrenergic receptors. *Arthritis Rheum* 1991;34:264–269.

68. Vaeroy H, Helle R, Forre O, et al. Elevated CSF levels of substance P and high incidence of Raynaud phenomenon in patients with fibromyalgia: new features for diagnosis. *Pain* 1988;32:21–26.

69. Grisart J, Van der Linden M, Masquelier E. Controlled processes and automaticity in memory functioning in fibromyalgia patients: relation with emotional distress and hypervigilance. *Clin Exp Neuropsychol* 2002;24:994–1009.

70. Sephton SE, Studts JL, Hoover K, et al. Biological and psychological factors associated with memory function in fibromyalgia syndrome. *Health Psychol* 2003;22:592–597.

71. Sletvold H, Stiles TC, Landro NI. Information processing in primary fibromyalgia, major depression and healthy controls. *J Rheumatol* 1995;22(1):137–142.

72. Grace GM, Nielson WR, Hopkins M, et al. Concentration and memory deficits in patients with fibromyalgia syndrome. *J Clin Exp Neuropsychol* 1999;21:477–487.

73. Okifuji A, Turk DC, Sinclair JD, et al. Development and determination of a threshold point for the identification of positive tender points in fibromyalgia syndrome. *J Rheumatol* 1997;24:377–383.

74. Simms RW, Goldenberg DL, Felson DT, et al. Tenderness in 75 anatomic sites. Distinguishing fibromyalgia patients from controls. *Arthritis Rheum* 1988;31:182–187.

75. Wolfe F. What use are fibromyalgia control points? *J Rheumatol* 1998;25:546–550.

76. McBeth J, Macfarlane GJ, Benjamin S, et al. The association between tender points, psychological distress, and adverse childhood experiences: a community-based study. *Arthritis Rheum* 1999;42:1397–1404.

77. Aaron LA, Bradley LA, Alarcon GS, et al. Psychiatric diagnoses in patients with fibromyalgia are related to health care-seeking behavior rather than to illness. *Arthritis Rheum* 1996;39:436–445.

78. Yunus MB, Masi AT, Aldag JC. Short-term effects of ibuprofen in primary fibromyalgia syndrome: a double blind, placebo controlled trial. *J Rheumatol* 1989;16:527–532.

79. Cott A, Parkinson W, Bell MJ, et al. Interrater reliability of the tender point criterion for fibromyalgia. *J Rheumatol* 1992;19:1955–1959.

80. Turk DC, Okifuji A, Sinclair JD, et al. Pain, disability, and physical functioning in subgroups of patients with fibromyalgia. *J Rheumatol* 1996;23:1255–1262.

81. Kosek E, Ekholm J, Hansson P. Sensory dysfunction in fibromyalgia patients with implications for pathogenic mechanisms. *Pain* 1996;68:375–383.

82. Littlejohn GO, Weinstein C, Helme RD. Increased neurogenic inflammation in fibrositis syndrome. *J Rheumatol* 1987;14:1022–1025.

83. Caro XJ. Immunofluorescent detection of IgG at the dermal-epidermal junction in patients with apparent primary fibrositis syndrome. *Arthritis Rheum* 1984;27:1174–1179.

84. Llewellyn LJ, Jones AB. *Fibrositis*. London: Heinemann, 1915.

85. Valentine V. Aetiology of fibrositis. A review. *Ann Rheum Dis* 1947;6:241–249.

86. Wolfe F, Ross K, Anderson J, et al. Aspects of fibromyalgia in the general population: sex, pain threshold, and fibromyalgia symptoms. *J Rheumatol* 1995;22:151–156.

87. Buskila D, Neumann L, Alhoashle A, et al. Fibromyalgia syndrome in men. *Semin Arthritis Rheum* 2000;30:47–51.

88. Inanici F, Yunus MB, Aldag JC. Psychological features in men with fibromyalgia syndrome: comparison with women. *Ann Rheum Dis* 2000;59(Suppl. 1):62.

89. Marcus DA. Gender differences in treatment-seeking chronic headache sufferers. *Headache* 2001;41:698–703.

90. Yunus MB, Inanici F, Aldag JC. Incomplete fibromyalgia syndrome: clinical and psychological comparison with fibromyalgia syndrome. *Arthritis Rheum* 1998;41(Suppl. 9): S258.

12

Neurologic Features of Fibromyalgia

Robert Bennett

Patients with fibromyalgia (FM) have a multiplicity of symptoms that also occur in many other disorders. The contemporary concept of symptom generation, now supported by many carefully conceived studies, embraces the concept of central sensitization (1,2). The term *central sensitization* refers to an abnormality in sensory processing in which impulses from the periphery are amplified at the level of the spinal cord and above. In this way sensations arising in peripheral tissues, which would be of no concern to a healthy individual, may become symptoms that need medical evaluation. Because of this multiplicity of symptoms, FM patients are often mislabeled as having a somatizing disorder or being hypochondriacs. As most symptoms that FM patients experience can be traced directly to having FM, they are at a significant risk of having potentially serious nonfibromyalgia-related problems overlooked or misdiagnosed. This is particularly true of FM patients presenting with symptoms of apparent neurologic origin.

RESTLESS LEGS

Restless legs syndrome (RLS) was first described by Willis in 1672 and given its name in 1945 by Ekbom (it is sometimes still referred to as Ekbom syndrome). It is the most common sleep-related movement disorder and has a prevalence of 5% to 15% in the adult white population. It is commonly associated with periodic limb movements during sleep, which leads to nonrestorative sleep and daytime sleepiness. However, a discordance of restless legs symptomatology and periodic limb movement disorder is reported in about 20% of subjects.

ASSOCIATION WITH FIBROMYALGIA

The association of FM with RLS was first described over 20 years ago in the seminal paper by Yunus et al. that described many of the clinical features of fibrositis (3). The syndrome is by far the most common cause of neurologic symptoms in FM patients. In the author's academic rheumatology clinic, RLS is seen in about 60% of FM patients using a standardized questionnaire. In a 1996 study, 135 female patients with FM, 54 with rheumatoid arthritis, and 87 healthy controls reported symptoms of RLS in 31%, 8%, and 2% respectively (4). A diagnosis of RLS should be considered in any FM patient with symptoms suggesting a peripheral neuropathy or radiculopathy.

The critical differences between a peripheral neuropathy and RLS are that neuropathies are not associated with either restlessness, nocturnal worsening, or relief by movement. Indeed, RLS is one of the few sensorimotor disorders that is provoked by rest and that also follows a nocturnal pattern.

DIAGNOSIS OF RESTLESS LEGS SYNDROME

The diagnosis of RLS is based on the patient history and is supported by a normal neurologic examination and a clinical response to levodopa (L-dopa) (see Table 12-1). It is important to note that the term *restless legs syndrome* is somewhat misleading as the same symptoms can occur less commonly in the upper limbs, trunk, and skull. The finding of a periodic limb movement disorder on polysomnography is strongly supportive of this diagnosis, but about 20% of patients with RLS do not have periodic limb movement disorder. Another useful clue in diagnosing RLS is reduction of symptoms by physical and emotional stimulation and their aggravation by conditions of reduced arousal. For instance, exacerbation of symptoms may occur in relation to use of sedating substances, attempting to sit still at a performance, and postprandial drowsiness. The differential diagnosis of RLS includes leg cramps (5,6), drug-induced akathisia (7), and the painful legs and moving toes syndrome (8,9).

PATHOPHYSIOLOGY

The strong association of RLS with FM begs the question as to whether they have a common neurophysiologic basis. One common finding on electrophysiologic testing is an increased excitability of the spinal flexion reflex (10). Interestingly, in unmedicated RLS patients, this increased excitability only

TABLE 12-1	Restless Legs Syndrome

Diagnostic Features of Restless Legs Syndrome

A distressing need or urge to move the legs (akathisia), usually accompanied by an uncomfortable, deep-seated sensation in the legs that is:

1. Brought on by rest (sitting or lying down)
2. Relieved with moving or walking
3. Worse at night or in the evening
4. Improved by the use of L-dopa

Features Frequently Associated with the Syndrome

1. Involuntary limb movements while patient is awake
2. Periodic limb movements while patient is asleep

occurs during sleep, whereas in healthy controls the spinal flexion reflex is decreased during sleep (11). This suggests that RLS involves a reversal of the normal circadian inhibition of this reflex. Contemporary studies using functional magnetic resonance imaging (fMRI) and single-photon-emission computed tomography (SPECT) scanning have shown small but consistent decreases in dopaminergic function in the striatum for RLS patients compared to controls (12,13).

There is a long list of literature linking iron deficiency with RLS, although most patients do not show the typical clinical features of a deficiency. However, low levels of iron have been reported in the cerebrospinal fluid (CSF) (14). Brain iron content can now be accurately measured using magnetic resonance imaging (MRI) techniques. Interestingly, the iron content varies considerably from area to area and is found in greatest amounts in the dopaminergic brain areas such as the substantia nigra and striatum (15). RLS symptoms have shown strong inverse correlations with the MRI-assessed iron content in these areas (16). Furthermore, treatment with intravenous iron (200 mg iron every few days for five treatments) was reported to effect a complete remission of symptoms in 82% of patients (most of whom did not have anemia). In a study using oral iron supplements, there was an improvement in RLS symptoms in those patients who had serum ferritin levels <45 mg per L, but not for those with higher levels (17). The reasons why a reduced iron content in dopaminergic brain areas might be related to the symptomatology of RLS is the observation that tyrosine hydroxylase, a molecule involved in the rate-limiting step for the synthesis of dopamine, requires iron as a cofactor. Clinically it is important to note that the relationship between RLS symptomatology and iron deficiency is much stronger for brain iron stores than peripheral body stores.

TREATMENT

There is a great variability in the symptoms of RLS (18). In many patients the symptoms are relatively mild and often intermittent; such patients may never require medications. The first-line treatment for RLS is the prescription of L-dopa or levodopa/carbidopa in the early evening. A beneficial response basically confirms the diagnosis of RLS without resort to polysomnography. However, long-term treatment with levodopa/carbidopa at more than 2 tablets of 25 mg/100 mg/d fails in about 80% of patients due to rebound (recurrence of symptoms during the latter part of the night and during the day) or augmentation (occurrence of symptoms before the usual time for the evening dose). In such cases, use of the direct dopamine receptor agonists (which have a long half-life) provides effective long-lasting relief for the majority of patients.

Pergolide, pramipexole, ropinirole, and cabergoline have all been shown to alleviate RLS symptoms in 70% to 100% of patients (19). The most common side effect of dopamine agonists is a dose-related nausea; some patients develop increased somnolence, dizziness, constipation, and dyskinesias. As already noted, there is persuasive evidence that reduced brain levels of iron are relevant to the generation of RLS symptomatology. Thus, the prescription of an oral iron supplement is recommended in patients with a ferritin level of <45 mg per L and continued until the level is >50 mg per L (17). Clonazepam is still frequently prescribed for the treatment of RLS. However, polysomnographic studies have failed to show a therapeutic efficacy in reducing periodic limb movements. It would appear that the apparent benefit from clonazepam and other sedatives is a continuation of sleep despite any disturbance from periodic limb movements.

PARESTHESIAE

Sensations of numbness and tingling are common complaints in FM patients. In the majority of such patients, these symptoms turn out to be due to RLS. However, the possibility of a peripheral neuropathy or less commonly a central lesion, such as a herniated disc, spinal stenosis, multiple sclerosis, Chiari malformation, or a brain tumor, needs to be considered.

A diagnosis of a peripheral neuropathy should be considered in those patients who have a slowly progressive sensory loss in the lower limbs with dysthetic symptoms such as numbness, burning, or pain. These symptoms are typically symmetric and spread proximally in a typical stocking distribution. They do not usually compromise motor strength. With progression of the neuropathy, mild gait disturbances may occur. Examination of the deep tendon reflexes is the most important test to distinguish between peripheral and central lesions. An absent or reduced tendon reflex suggests a peripheral neuropathy, whereas a brisk reflex, especially when associated with a positive Hoffman or Babinski sign, suggests a central pathology. However, it should be noted that many FM patients have brisk reflexes without ancillary evidence of upper motor neuron lesions. The reason for this is not entirely clear but may relate to enhanced spinal reflexes as result of central sensitization or anxiety.

Compression mononeuropathies are common findings in FM patients and must be distinguished from polyneuropathies. There have been no studies exploring the cause of compression neuropathies in FM patients. However, it seems likely that their increased prevalence may be related to weight gain, biomechanical factors secondary to musculoskeletal pain, hypermobility (20), and heightened sensitivity as a consequence of central sensitization. The major clinical features of the compression enteropathy are pain (usually distal to the entrapment side but may also be retrograde), paresthesiae, and weakness distal to the entrapment site.

By far the most common entrapment neuropathy in FM patients is a carpal tunnel syndrome (21–23). In one report, some 30% of FM patients had symptoms compatible with carpal tunnel syndrome, and 55% of these had abnormal nerve conduction tests. In some patients there is a marked diurnal variation in median nerve compression symptomatology that may be related to the tendency for FM subjects to develop a cyclical fluid retention (24); this may be helped by reduction of carbohydrate intake. Having FM has been associated with a poor response to carpal tunnel release surgery (25). In the author's experience, other entrapment neuropathies, especially tarsal tunnel syndrome, ulna neuropathy, meralgia paresthetica, and Morton neuroma (interdigital neuroma), are important considerations during the neurologic evaluation of FM patients.

Is not uncommon for FM patients to be given a diagnosis of thoracic outlet syndrome. There have been no published studies of this association. However, this diagnosis should be considered in those FM patients who have prominent symptoms when using the arms above the head. The symptoms of thoracic outlet syndrome are caused by compression of the neurovascular bundle as it passes from the thorax to the axilla. The potential sites for obstruction are compression by the scalene muscles in the first rib, the costoclavicular space, and the pectoralis minor coracoid process. The most common cause of thoracic outlet syndrome is shoulder muscle weakness related to the effects of pain, obesity, poor posture, and heavy breasts. This diagnosis should be considered in patients who have numbness in an ulnar distribution, arm weakness, and the sensation of upper limb swelling. When vascular obstruction is prominent, patients may note mottling discoloration of the skin, dilated veins, and diffuse pain in the forearm and hand. On examination provocative testing such as Adson maneuver, shoulder hyperabduction, and an exaggerated military position will strengthen the clinical impression but should not be a basis for diagnosis. Currently, the most useful noninvasive test is Doppler ultrasound with the patient's arm in both a neutral and abducted position (26,27). Carpal tunnel syndrome often coexists with thoracic outlet syndrome and may cause diagnostic confusion due to retrograde (i.e., symptoms proximal to the side of entrapment) pain and paresthesiae. Other conditions causing similar symptoms that need to be considered are Pancoast syndrome, syringomyelia, cervical radiculopathy, spinal tumors, and adhesive capsulitis.

Myofascial trigger points in the muscles of the shoulder girdle often give rise to pain when the arms are used above the head and thus need to be considered in the differential diagnosis of thoracic outlet symptoms. Commonly involved muscles are the latissimus dorsi, teres major, deltoid, and pectoralis minor (28). It should be noted that myofascial trigger points can be the sole cause of symptoms or an associated finding.

hypersensitivity (i.e., central sensitization). Problems with hearing loss are an infrequent complaint in FM patients. By far, the most common symptom that may be related to otoneurologic problems is the complaint of dizziness. In one study, 72% of female FM patients complained of vertigo/dizziness. A sensorineural hearing loss was found in 15% of subjects, and abnormal auditory brainstem responses (ABR) were found in 30% of subjects (29).

In another study of FM subjects, dizziness was the most common complaint, followed by tinnitus, hearing loss, and vertigo. All but one patient had normal audiometry testing. The Dix–Hallpike maneuver was positive for rotary vertigo in 20.8% of subjects. None of the patients had abnormal bithermal caloric testing. The ABR results of the patients with and without cochleovestibular symptoms were not significantly different. It was concluded that FM patients can complain of otologic symptoms even though they do not have any clinically or audiologically detectable ear disease. The authors hypothesized that a neural disintegration, or some other event-related disordered neurophysiology, could be the mechanism involved in the pathogenesis of otoneurologic and other symptoms of the disease that leads to abnormal perception of stimuli coming from the patient's internal or external environment (30).

Event-related potentials (ERPs) are a powerful tool to investigate the real-time course of brain electrical mass activation during cognitive processing. During the waking state, a late component of the auditory event-related potential, the P300, is elicited when subjects detect a rare "target" stimulus. It is usually not elicited when subjects either ignore or fail to detect the stimulus. The presence of P300 is therefore thought to reflect conscious processing of the stimulus. The P300 auditory ERPs were evaluated in 13 untreated female FM patients and 10 healthy controls. The FM group was further evaluated before and after treatment with sertraline. FM subjects had significantly lower P300 amplitudes, but not significantly different P300 latencies, than controls. Anxiety and depression scores did not correlate significantly with P300 latencies or amplitudes at the study entry. After treatment with sertraline, the P300 auditory ERP amplitudes of the FM group were almost the same as the control group. It was hypothesized that the lower amplitude ERPs in FM patients was result of a dysfunction in higher order cognitive processing and that this could be reversed by treatment with sertraline.

Another ERP study evaluated the auditory brainstem response and found it to be abnormal in 31% of FM subjects (31). Unlike the P300 event-related potentials, which measure conscious awareness of sound, an abnormal brainstem response is more suggestive of an anatomic neurophysiologic deficit. Disordered brainstem function in FM was also supported by an investigation using oculomotor testing in 36 FM patients compared to 71 healthy controls. Saccadic movements were found to be abnormal in 42%, and the smooth pursuit eye movements were abnormal in 18.9%, of FM subjects (32).

AUDITORY SYMPTOMS

Increased sensitivity to loud noise is a common complaint of FM patients and is assumed to be a feature of generalized

VISUAL SYMPTOMS

FM patients frequently complain of blurred vision without any significant findings on ophthalmologic testing. There have been no formal studies of this symptom, but in the author's experience the first consideration should be a medication-related side effect. The most likely culprit is an antidepressant with a powerful antagonism of muscarinic receptors (e.g., amitriptyline).

As in the case of all new symptoms in FM patients, it is critical to consider the broad differential diagnosis (33). This includes errors of refraction, migraine headaches, glaucoma, macular degeneration, giant cell arteritis, cerebral tumors and infections, diabetes, retinal detachment, corneal ulcers, uveitis, vitreal hemorrhage, the toxic effects of drugs on the retina, and medications that affect the accommodation reflex.

AUTONOMIC DYSFUNCTION

There is now persuasive evidence that many FM patients have autonomic dysfunction. Findings consistent with this dysfunction include dry eyes and dry mouth, increased cold sensitivity, neurally mediated hypotension, and impaired variation of the R–R interval on electrocardiography (34–40). Some physicians hypothesize that autonomic dysfunction is the prime cause of FM symptomatology (41).

A particular manifestation of autonomic dysfunction called "neurally mediated hypotension" occurs in about 30% of FM patients (38). The classic symptoms of neurally mediated hypotension are lightheadedness and feelings of faintness. This problem should be considered in any patient who complains of severe fatigue lasting 20 to 72 hours after a minor physical activity or fatigue that is precipitated by standing upright for more than about 15 minutes. Feelings of faintness may be minimal or absent in some patients with this problem. Other symptoms ascribed to neurally mediated hypotension are headaches, mental confusion, cognitive dysfunction, panic attacks, visual blurring, nausea, and increased muscle aching. Symptoms of dysautonomia are often aggravated by hot weather, unaccustomed exertion, the beginning of menses, large meals, inadequate fluid intake, and stressful situations. Some medications, particularly α-1-adrenoceptor blockers and dopamine agonists, exacerbate symptoms.

A diagnosis of neurally mediated hypotension cannot be ruled out just because the patient has a normal blood pressure or even an absence of orthostatic changes. Thus, a high index of suspicion needs to be entertained for this diagnosis in all FM patients. Confirmation is usually made with a three-stage upright tilt table test. This involves tilting the patient to 70 degrees for 45 minutes (stage 1), followed by 70 degrees of tilt with an infusion of isoproterenol at a rate of 1 to 2 µg per minute (stage 2), and, lastly, 10 minutes at 70 degrees of tilt with isoproterenol at a rate of 3 to 4 µg per minute. An abnormal response to upright tilt is defined by syncope or presyncope in association with a drop in systolic blood pressure of at least 25 mm Hg and no associated increase in heart rate (42).

In adolescents with FM, consideration should be given to variation of orthostatic intolerance that has been called the "postural orthostatic tachycardia syndrome" (POTS) (43).

These patients typically have symptoms of lightheadedness, disabling fatigue, exercise intolerance, dizziness, and near syncope. During tilt table testing they have a heart rate increase of >30 beats per minute (or a maximum heart rate of 120 beats per minute) without any significant change in blood pressure. This usually occurs within the first 10 minutes of testing and is accompanied by a triggering of the patient symptoms. These patients also exhibit an exaggerated response to isoproterenol infusions (44,45).

The successful management of autonomic dysfunction is dependent on the patient being educated regarding the basics of its underlying physiology. In the first instance, it is necessary to stress the importance of increased sodium and fluid intake. There is a general perception that "salt is bad for you." This has led to general dietary recommendations to reduce salt intake as it may contribute to high blood pressure and associated cerebral and cardiac disease. This general dictum is bad advice for individuals with neurally mediated hypotension. Thus the first tier of treatment is to ensure adequate intake of salt and fluid (46).

The next tier of treatment is to reduce situations likely to cause orthostatic changes. These include hot baths, hot tubs, saunas, standing for long periods, rush-hour shopping, sunbathing, and unnecessary psychological stressors. Many patients are intolerant of alcohol and some find that caffeinated drinks aggravate the symptoms (46).

Furthermore, there are certain actions that the patient can employ to reduce symptoms. One simple adaptation, which helps to minimize fluid loss during the night, is to raise the head of the bed 6 to 9 inches. Other maneuvers include sitting in a cross-legged position, sitting in a knee chest position, and, if one has to stand for a prolonged period, resting one leg on a stool or chair. A general increase in physical fitness is also considered to be beneficial as a long-term benefit. However, as symptoms of neurally mediated hypotension are usually aggravated by unaccustomed exertion, the increments in exercise need to be very gradual.

The third tier of treatment is the judicious use of medications. The first medication that is usually employed is fludrocortisone (Florinef) to enhance sodium retention. Over-the-counter pseudoephedrine preparations (e.g., nonsedating Sudafed) taken before situations that might be expected to result in symptoms is often a simple and effective strategy. In more recalcitrant cases, the use of midodrine (ProAmatine) needs to be considered (47), but concerns regarding an elevation of supine blood pressure also need to be considered. Beta blockers (e.g., metoprolol, pinadol) supposedly reduce the reflex from the left ventricles to the carotid baroreceptors that mediates the fall in blood pressure; the evidence for their efficacy is variable (48,49). The author uses them as a last resort as they often cause more fatigue and impair exercise tolerance.

DIZZINESS

Dizziness is another common complaint of FM patients that has a potential neurologic basis. Dizziness is a patient descriptive term that encompasses numerous disorders including vertigo, orthostatic hypotension, psychiatric disorders, hyperventilation, muscle imbalance, and medication side effects. In most cases a carefully taken history will distinguish between these various possibilities.

Vertigo arises from an asymmetry of information arising in the vestibular system. It is usually described in terms of motion of the environment or self. Patients often describe themselves spinning, tilting, or moving. Making a distinction between peripheral causes (e.g., benign positional vertigo, labyrinthitis, Ménière disease, otitis media) and central lesions (brainstem strokes, cerebellopontine tumors) is usually dependent on the physical examination, audiometry, and imaging studies. The physical examination should concentrate on positional changes in symptoms (benign positional vertigo), asymmetric hearing loss, orthostatic blood pressure and pulse changes, the observation of nystagmus, and gait disturbance.

If the patient complains of impaired hearing in one ear, a Weber test should be performed. When a tuning fork is placed in the midline of the forehead, a sensorineural hearing loss is suggested by a louder sound on the "good" side; if a conductive hearing loss is present, the sound is louder on the "bad" side. This can be confirmed with the Rinne test, which involves placing the tuning fork on the mastoid bone behind the ear of the affected side. In conduction deafness the sound should be at least as loud, or louder, when the fork is placed on the mastoid as compared to holding the fork just adjacent to the auditory meatus. A sensorineural hearing loss on one side suggests Ménière disease or an acoustic neuroma, whereas a conduction deafness suggests middle ear disease.

The finding of nystagmus always suggests vestibular disorder. Peripheral vestibular lesions tend to produce a horizontal nystagmus whereas central lesions usually produce a nystagmus that is vertical and oblique in addition to being horizontal. Benign positional vertigo is demonstrated by the Dix–Hallpike maneuver. This involves moving the patient rapidly from the sitting to the lying position with the head tilted downward off the table at 45 degrees and rotated 45 degrees to one side. Reproduction of the patient's vertiginous symptoms and the development of nystagmus after a latency of 5 to 15 seconds are diagnostic of positional vertigo.

Many FM patients end up being given a diagnosis of "nonspecific dizziness." This should be considered in patients who have difficulty in describing their symptoms and simply insist that "I am dizzy or lightheaded." There have been no studies looking at causes for dizziness in FM patients. If the patient has poorly defined symptoms suggestive of nonspecific dizziness, studies done and other populations would suggest a high likelihood of a psychiatric disorder, especially depression and anxiety/panic disorder.

Presyncope is the prodromal symptom of fainting. It is a near faint that typically lasts for seconds to minutes and is recognized by the patient as "nearly blacking out" or "nearly fainting." The evaluation of presyncope is the same as for syncope. Neurally mediated hypotension, cardiac arrhythmias, and vasovagal attacks are some of the more common causes. Neurally mediated hypotension has been described in up to 30% of FM patients and is always a major consideration when an FM patient complains of dizziness. This subject is covered in the section on "autonomic dysfunction."

Symptoms of vertigo/dizziness have been ascribed to myofascial trigger points in the sternocleidomastoid and upper trapezius muscles by Travell and Simons (50). This presumably should be a common cause of these symptoms in FM patients, but there have been no definitive studies concerning this association. However, temporomandibular pain disorder is a common association with FM and there are several studies indicating that 30% to 70% of these patients have complaints of vertigo/dizziness (51–53).

Many medications can cause or enhance the sensation of dizziness (54). These include antianxiety drugs, tricyclic antidepressants, antihypertensive drugs, antituberculous drugs, polypeptide antibiotics, local anesthetics, and nonsteroidal anti-inflammatory drugs.

RADICULOPATHY

It is not uncommon for FM patients to report radiating pain down an arm or leg, suggestive of a radiculopathy. In most cases, a careful and expert examination will reveal myofascial trigger points to be the most likely cause. For instance, myofascial trigger points in the supraspinatus and teres major muscles often have a pain referral distribution along the ulnar side of the arm, sometimes as far as the little finger (28). Myofascial pain syndromes of the upper limb are often misdiagnosed as frozen shoulder, cervical radiculopathy, or thoracic outlet syndrome (55). Myofascial trigger points in the gluteus medius/minimus and the piriformis muscles often refer pain in a sciatic distribution (56). The recognition and effective treatment of myofascial pain generators is an important skill in the comprehensive management of FM patients (57).

The defining clinical characteristic of myofascial pain is the finding of a trigger point. This is a well-defined point of focal tenderness within a muscle. Palpation of this focus usually elicits pain in a referred distribution that reproduces the patient's symptoms. Importantly, referred pain from a trigger point does not follow a nerve root distribution (i.e., it is not dermatomal). Palpation usually reveals a ropelike induration of the associated muscle fibers, often referred to as the "taut band." Sometimes, snapping this band or needling the trigger point produces a localized twitch response of the involved muscle. This twitch response can only be reproducibly elicited in fairly superficial muscles. Importantly, trigger points produce functional consequences in terms of a restriction of range of movement and weakness (probably a reflex inhibition secondary to pain), which is usually associated with easy fatigability of the involved muscle.

A critical element in the effective management of myofascial pain syndromes is the correction of predisposing factors such as deconditioning, poor posture, repetitive mechanical stress, mechanical imbalance (e.g., leg-length inequality), joint disorders, and nonrestorative sleep. These interfere with the ability of the muscle to fully recover and are the most common reason for treatment failures.

Stretching the involved muscles needs to be done daily as the basis of a myofascial trigger point is a focal contraction of sarcomeric units (55). This results in a prolonged adenosine triphosphate (ATP) consumption, and the restoration of a muscle to its full stretch length breaks the link between the energy crisis and contraction of sarcomeric units (55). Effective stretching is most commonly achieved through the technique of spray and stretch (58). This involves the cutaneous application, along the axis of the muscle, of ethyl chloride spray while at the same time passively stretching the involved muscle. Other techniques to enhance effective stretching include trigger point to pressure release, postisometric relaxation, reciprocal inhibition, and deep stroking massage (55). Furthermore, muscles harboring trigger points usually become weak due to the inhibitory effects of pain. A program of slowly progressive strengthening is essential to restore full function and minimize the risk of recurrence and the perpetuation of satellite trigger points.

Injection of trigger points is generally considered to be the most effective means of direct inactivation. A peppering technique using a fine needle to inactivate all the foci within a trigger point locus is the critical element of successful trigger point therapy (59). Accurate localization of the trigger point is confirmed if a local twitch response is obtained; however, this may not be obvious when needling deeply lying muscles. Successful elimination of the trigger point usually results in a relaxation of the taut band. Although dry needling is effective, the use of a local anesthetic (1% lidocaine or 1% procaine) helps confirm the accuracy of the injection and provides instant gratification for patients (60). There is no evidence that the injection of corticosteroids provides any enhanced effect.

MOTOR WEAKNESS

FM patients commonly complain of muscle weakness and increased muscle fatigability. However, electromyographic studies that have used the technique of twitch interpolation have reported different results. In one twitch interpolation electromyographic study, a reduction of "true" quadriceps muscle strength per unit area of about 35% was found (61), and in another study no changes were noted (62).

In an attempt to assess both peripheral and central components of muscle fatigue of the elbow flexor muscles, maximal voluntary activation and strength of elbow flexors were quantified using twitch interpolation during attempted maximal isometric contractions both in unfatigued muscles and during fatigue (produced by 45 minutes of submaximal exercise) in FM patients compared to healthy controls. Maximal voluntary strength before and during exercise was within the normal range. Central fatigue did not develop to a greater extent in the patient group. No patient had a decline in twitch amplitude during exercise below the 95% confidence limit for the decline in control subjects. However, the increment in perceived effort (Borg Scale) was abnormally large in five FM patients during the fatiguing exercise. It was concluded that neither poor motivation, reflex pain inhibition, nor muscle contractile failure are important in the pathogenesis of fatigue in patients with FM. However, the subjective response to exercise is commonly excessive (63). Many FM patients become deconditioned with resulting loss of strength due to declining muscle mass (64), and several recent studies have reported benefits from gently progressive strength training (65–67). Focal muscle weakness can often be traced to a particularly painful myofascial trigger point. Another consideration for reduced muscle mass in some FM patients is an associated growth hormone deficiency (68); this is best screened for by a plasma IGF-1 level (69). In one study, supplemental growth hormone therapy was of general benefit (70).

HEADACHES

Headache is one of the most common symptoms associated with FM (3,71,72). In some cases there is an increased prevalence of some types of headache in FM, but the possibility of unrelated problems needs to be constantly monitored (see Table 12-2). Tension-type headaches seemed to be the most common presentation, but there is also a well-documented association with vascular headaches (3,73–75). In the 1990 American College of Rheumatology Classification study, headaches were reported in just over 50% of FM subjects (76). This figure needs to be considered in the context of headache as one of the most common medical symptoms affecting about 15% of the population at any one time. Both migraine and tension-type headaches affect women predominantly, while cluster headache is much more common in men. When a careful chronological history is taken from FM patients with migraine headaches, it is often apparent that the vascular headaches started in their teenage years. Conversely, FM has been reported in 36% of subjects with transformed migraine (77).

Many tension-type headaches in FM patients can be traced to myofascial trigger points in the head and neck (78). In this respect, patients with an associated temporomandibular pain disorder invariably complain of prominent headache symptoms (79). Temporomandibular pain disorder has been described in 75% to 90% of FM patients (80).

The common association of FM and headaches can easily lead to the assumption that all headaches in FM patients are related to having this disorder. Of course, about 90% of the time this assumption will be correct, but in the other 10% it can lead to serious misdiagnosis.

Over the last two years, the author has encountered headaches in FM patients related to cerebral aneurysms, tumors, and Chiari I malformation. Carefully listening to the patient's description of the headache and paying attention to "danger signs" indicative of infection, a vascular lesion, metabolic disturbance, or a space-occupying lesion will provide the initial clues as to a possibly serious underlying problem. For instance, a headache with an acute onset that reaches its maximum intensity within a few minutes could be due to a subarachnoid hemorrhage or a rapidly expanding berry aneurysm. In contrast, the typical migraine headache may start acutely but does not reach maximum intensity for several hours. On the other hand, cluster headaches may

TABLE 12-2	Causes of Headache in Fibromyalgia Patients

MORE COMMON IN FIBROMYALGIA	UNRELATED TO FIBROMYALGIA
Tension headaches	Chiari I malformation
Vascular headaches	Sinus headache
Chronic daily headache	Intracerebral tumors
Referred myofascial pain	Posttraumatic
Dysautonomia	Cervical spine disease
Medication-induced headache	Glaucoma

reach full intensity within a few minutes but may be distinguished from more serious causes by the autonomic features of rhinorrhea and tearing, as well as their relatively short duration of <2 hours. A brain tumor should be suspected in patients with a headache that is worsened by changing posture or maneuvers that raise intrathoracic pressure such as coughing or straining, especially if there is associated nausea or vomiting. Other alerting features to a brain tumor are new onset seizures or a change in personality, mental status, or level of consciousness.

The treatment of migraine headaches in FM patients follows the same general principles as in non-FM patients (81). Patients should be warned about avoiding precipitating circumstances and foods, the use of ergotamine preparations, and 5-HT(1B/1D) receptor agonists. There is increasing evidence for the use of antiepileptic agents in migraine prophylaxis, and, in this respect, topiramate is proving to be particularly efficacious (82–84).

Many FM patients are found to have mixed tension/vascular headaches. In these patients, trigger point therapy with local anesthetic injections may reduce the frequency of migraine headaches.

Another problem that needs to be considered in FM patients is a diagnosis of "chronic daily headache" (77). Chronic daily headache and chronic (transformed) migraine (TM) patients represent more than one third of the subjects seen in specialized headache centers.

"Transformed migraine" is the name given to a group of patients who start out with typical migraine headaches and develop chronic daily headaches (85). The typical clinical presentation is that of a daily noncontinuous bilateral pressure or tightening involving the frontotemporal areas. Other common symptoms are photophobia, phonophobia, nausea, insomnia, and emotional disturbances (85). Most of these patients continue to develop typical full-blown migraine attacks. There is good evidence that many of these patients overuse symptomatic headache remedies on a daily basis and that this medication misuse is a factor in the etiology of their headaches. In a recent study of the patients with chronic daily headaches, the average intake of symptomatic medications was three to four tablets per patient per day. Most of the patients overused simple analgesics (isolated or in combination with other substances) (75.2%), caffeine-containing drugs (71.4%), drugs containing ergotamine derivatives (26.1%), triptans (alone or combined) (15.5%), drugs with narcotics (13%), and anti-inflammatory drugs (3.7%) (86).

The effective management of patients with chronic deadly headaches involves education regarding the causative role of the overuse of symptomatic remedies and their discontinuation while starting on an increasing dose regimen of prophylactic medications. In this respect, tizanidine, an antispasmodic, is proving particularly useful (87). In very recalcitrant cases, a combination of medications and behavioral therapy may be required (88).

CHIARI

Many of the symptoms of the Chiari I malformation are similar to those experienced by FM patients and thus this disorder needs to be considered in comprehensive evaluation of FM. The Chiari I malformation is defined in part as tonsillar herniation of at least 3 mm below the foramen magnum; it may or may not be associated with a syringomyelia. This causes an overcrowding of the cranio-cervical junction with obstruction of the normal flow of CSF. The clinical manifestations, including an associated syringomyelia, are related to compression of neural tissues resulting from the abnormal CSF dynamics.

CLINICAL FEATURES

In a study of 364 patients with symptoms related to Chiari I malformation (238 had an associated syringomyelia), Milhorat et al. described the symptoms and physical findings (89). The most common problem (81% of subjects) was suboccipital headache. This was described as a heavy, crushing, or pressurelike sensation at the back of the head that radiated to the vertex and behind the eyes and below to the neck and shoulders. A distinctive feature of the headaches was their tendency to be accentuated by physical exertion, Valsalva maneuvers, head dependency, and sudden changes in posture. Female patients of menstrual age tended to experience an accentuation of symptoms during the week preceding menses. Visual disturbances were reported by 78% of subjects. In most cases the symptoms were intermittent and consisted of retro-orbital pressure or pain, visual phenomena such as floaters or flashing lights, blurred vision, photophobia, diplopia, and visual field cuts. Most of these symptoms were accentuated by the same factors that affected suboccipital headaches. Neuro-ophthalmologic examinations were usually normal. It was noted that an erroneous diagnosis of multiple sclerosis was common in young women with the symptoms. Oto-neurologic symptoms were reported by 74% of subjects. These comprised symptoms of dizziness, disequilibrium, pressure in the ears, tinnitus, decreased hearing or hyperacusis, vertigo, and oscillopsia. Like ocular disturbances, most of these symptoms were accentuated by the same factors that affected suboccipital headaches. There were very few objective findings except for nystagmus. In 16 patients, audiometric testing revealed low-frequency sensorineural hearing loss in association with two types of vestibulopathy: a peripheral type characterized by impaired caloric responses and the absence of central abnormalities and a central type characterized by normal caloric responses and distinct neural abnormalities, such as impaired opticokinetic nystagmus; impaired smooth pursuit; saccadic dysmetria; and downbeat, positional, or periodic alternating nystagmus. Symptoms indicative of spinal cord involvement were present in 223 of 238 subjects who had an associated syringomyelia. The most common symptoms in the subgroup were weakness, paresthesia or hyperesthesia, nonradicular segmental pain, analgesia or anesthesia, spasticity, trophic phenomena, burning dysesthesia, and poor position sense. Objective findings included impaired fine-motor function of the hands (48 patients), muscular weakness (25 patients), analgesia or anesthesia (18 patients), and hyperreflexia (18 patients). Nonspecific disturbances in the study population included chronic fatigue (210 patients), impaired recent memory (142 patients), cervicogenic pain (125 patients), low back pain (87 patients), and episodic nausea or vomiting (65 patients). Skeletal anomalies, especially at the skull base, were a frequent finding. These included scoliosis in 40% to 60% of patients, basilar invagination in 25% to 50% of patients, and Klippel-Feil syndrome in 5% to 10% of patients. It is evident from this wide array of presentations that the diagnosis of Chiari I malformation should be considered in the differential diagnosis of many neurologic disorders as well as poly-symptomatic disorders such as FM. Indeed, Milhorat commented that common misdiagnoses in this series of 364 Chiari I patients included migraine, FM, and multiple sclerosis, and that by the time of definitive diagnosis, 59% had been told by at least one physician that they suffered from a psychogenic disorder. It is important to understand that the MRI finding of a Chiari malformation may be entirely without symptoms (90,91).

THE ASSOCIATION OF CHIARI I MALFORMATION FIBROMYALGIA

Alarcón et al. published an abstract of the preliminary findings of an investigation that evaluated the presence of Chiari I malformation in 30 rheumatology patients with FM, 12 nonpatients with FM, and 16 healthy controls. Blinded MRI readings revealed that the Chiari malformation tended to be identified most frequently (20%) in the patients with FM ($p = 0.07$) (92). Thimineur also reported an increased prevalence of FM and temporomandibular pain in subjects with Chiari malformations (93). On the other hand, another MRI study described a prospective comparison of 39 consecutive FM patients seen in two tertiary care centers with 23 gender-matched asymptomatic controls (18). All patients underwent extensive neurologic examination and underwent an MRI of the posterior fossa and cervical spine. The MRIs were assessed by two blinded radiologists who evaluated the diameter of the cervical canal from C1 to C7 and the level of the cerebellar tonsils relative to the foramen magnum. Significant tonsillar herniation was found in 31% of the FM patients and 73% of controls! Significant cervical spinal stenosis was not found in either group. A neurosurgeon who reviewed the MRIs in a blinded fashion considered that 47% of the FM and 50% of the controls were possible surgical candidates. As the overall prevalence of Chiari I malformation is about 0.5%, most rheumatologists can be expected to see a few cases each year. However, it should be noted that about 30% of patients with MRI findings of Chiari I malformation are completely asymptomatic (90,91).

DIAGNOSIS

The limits of the foramen magnum are defined as a line drawn from the basion to the opisthion. In healthy individuals, the tip of the cerebellar tonsils are about 3 mm above this line. The Chiari I malformation is usually defined radiologically as ≥3 mm caudal descent of the cerebellar tonsils below this line. More complex guidelines have also been developed that provide an index of hindbrain overcrowding in the posterior fossa. As about one third of patients with MRI evidence of Chiari I are completely asymptomatic, clinical features must also be reviewed, taking into

consideration the possible relationship of a patient's symptoms to the presence of Chiari malformation. In the case of FM patients, this is especially important, as there is a considerable overlap of symptoms between the two disorders.

TREATMENT

Surgical intervention to correct the defect of Chiari I malformation involves the decompression of the tonsillar compression at the cervico-medullary junction with or without cervical laminectomy (94,95). This is not a minor surgical procedure, especially in FM patients who often experience a flare after any operation. If an FM patient is found to have a symptomatic Chiari malformation with appropriate physical and radiologic findings, the author recommends a consultation with a neurologist and two independent neurosurgeons. Having FM considerably complicates the decision as to whether an operation for a Chiari I malformation will be beneficial as there is no evidence that it helps the basic problem of central sensitization, and, hence, most symptoms can be expected to be unchanged. However, I have personally seen several FM patients who have benefited from this surgery in terms of headaches and cognitive function.

■ IMPLICATIONS FOR PRACTICE

- Think of the diagnosis of RLS in all FM patients who are complaining of paresthesiae. If in doubt, give a 5 day trial of levodopa/carbidopa.
- Reduced hearing is not a feature of FM and always requires a careful workup. Dizziness in FM is seldom due to inner ear disease. Phonophobia is probably a manifestation of the central sensitization.
- Neurally mediated hypotension occurs in about one third of FM patients. Think of this diagnosis in patients with prominent postexertional fatigue, unexplained dizziness, fluctuating cognitive dysfunction, and descriptions of light-headedness and faintness.
- Dizziness is a common nonspecific symptom. Apart from the usual differential diagnosis, major considerations in FM are dysautonomia, hyperventilation, the heightened awareness of central sensitization, medications, orthostasis, and trigger points in the sternocleidomastoid muscles.
- Always consider the possibility that radicular symptoms, in the absence of hard neurologic signs, are due to referred pain/dysthesia from a myofascial trigger point in the shoulder or pelvic girdle musculature.
- Muscle weakness is a common complaint in FM patients. In many cases it is a result of reflex inhibition of maximal muscle contraction due to pain emanating from a myofascial trigger point.
- Vascular and tension headaches are the "norm" in FM. They often antedate the onset of generalized pain. Always consider the possibility that migraine has been "transformed" to the entity of chronic daily headaches. Do not assume that all headaches are secondary to having FM.
- Chiari I malformation occurs in about 1 in every 200 people, and, thus, several of these patients will be seen by rheumatologists each year. Many of the symptoms of Chiari are similar to FM. It is not uncommon for

Chiari I to be asymptomatic and thus a very careful cross specialty evaluation is necessary before advising surgery.

REFERENCES

1. Staud R. Evidence of involvement of central neural mechanisms in generating fibromyalgia pain. *Curr Rheumatol Rep* 2002;4(4):299–305.
2. Bennett RM. Emerging concepts in the neurobiology of chronic pain: evidence of abnormal sensory processing in fibromyalgia. *Mayo Clin Proc* 1999;74(4):385–398.
3. Yunus M, Masi AT, Calabro JJ, et al. Primary fibromyalgia (fibrositis): clinical study of 50 patients with matched normal controls. *Semin Arthritis Rheum* 1981;11:151–171.
4. Yunus MB, Aldag JC. Restless legs syndrome and leg cramps in fibromyalgia syndrome: a controlled study. *Br Med J* 1996;312:1339.
5. Butler JV, Mulkerrin EC, O'Keeffe ST. Nocturnal leg cramps in older people. *Postgrad Med J* 2002;78(924):596–598.
6. Kanaan N, Sawaya R. Nocturnal leg cramps. Clinically mysterious and painful—but manageable. *Geriatrics* 2001;56(6): 34, 39–42.
7. Young WB, Piovesan EJ, Biglan KM. Restless legs syndrome and drug-induced akathisia in headache patients. *CNS Spectr* 2003;8(6):450–456.
8. Dressler D, Thompson PD, Gledhill RF, et al. The syndrome of painful legs and moving toes. *Mov Disord* 1994;9(1):13–21.
9. Walters AS, Hening WA, Shah SK, et al. Painless legs and moving toes: a syndrome related to painful legs and moving toes? *Mov Disord* 1993;8(3):377–379.
10. Bara-Jimenez W, Aksu M, Graham B, et al. Periodic limb movements in sleep: state-dependent excitability of the spinal flexor reflex. *Neurology* 2000;54(8):1609–1616.
11. Aksu M, Bara-Jimenez W. State dependent excitability changes of spinal flexor reflex in patients with restless legs syndrome secondary to chronic renal failure. *Sleep Med* 2002;3(5):427–430.
12. Turjanski N, Lees AJ, Brooks DJ. Striatal dopaminergic function in restless legs syndrome: 18F-dopa and 11C-raclopride PET studies. *Neurology* 1999;52(5):932–937.
13. Ruottinen HM, Partinen M, Hublin C, et al. An FDOPA PET study in patients with periodic limb movement disorder and restless legs syndrome. *Neurology* 2000;54(2):502–504.
14. Earley CJ, Connor JR, Beard JL, et al. Abnormalities in CSF concentrations of ferritin and transferrin in restless legs syndrome. *Neurology* 2000;54(8):1698–1700.
15. Connor JR, Boyer PJ, Menzies SL, et al. Neuropathological examination suggests impaired brain iron acquisition in restless legs syndrome. *Neurology* 2003;61(3):304–309.
16. Allen RP, Barker PB, Wehrl F, et al. MRI measurement of brain iron in patients with restless legs syndrome. *Neurology* 2001;56(2):263–265.
17. O'Keeffe ST, Gavin K, Lavan JN. Iron status and restless legs syndrome in the elderly. *Age Ageing* 1994;23(3): 200–203.
18. Clauw DJ, Petzke F, Rosner MJ, et al. Prevalence of Chiari malformation and cervical spine stenosis in fibromyalgia. *Arth Rheum* 2000;43(9 Suppl):S173.
19. Happe S, Trenkwalder C. Role of dopamine receptor agonists in the treatment of restless legs syndrome. *CNS Drugs* 2004;18(1):27–36.
20. Grahame R. Pain, distress and joint hyperlaxity. *Joint Bone Spine* 2000;67(3):157–163.
21. Perez-Ruiz F, Calabozo M, Alonso-Ruiz A, et al. High prevalence of undetected carpal tunnel syndrome in patients with fibromyalgia syndrome. *J Rheumatol* 1995;22: 501–504.
22. Sarmer S, Yavuzer G, Kucukdeveci A, et al. Prevalence of carpal tunnel syndrome in patients with fibromyalgia. *Rheumatol Int* 2002;22(2):68–70.
23. Perez-Ruiz F, Calabozo M, Alonso-Ruiz A, et al. Fibromyalgia and carpal tunnel syndrome. *Ann Rheum Dis* 1997;56(7): 438–439.
24. Deodhar AA, Fisher RA, Blacker CV, et al. Fluid retention syndrome and fibromyalgia. *Br J Rheumatol* 1994;33(6): 576–582.
25. Akkus S, Kutluhan S, Akhan G, et al. Does fibromyalgia affect the outcomes of local steroid treatment in patients with carpal tunnel syndrome? *Rheumatol Int* 2002;22(3): 112–115.
26. Gillard J, Perez-Cousin M, Hachulla E, et al. Diagnosing thoracic outlet syndrome: contribution of provocative tests, ultrasonography, electrophysiology, and helical computed tomography in 48 patients. *Joint Bone Spine* 2001;68(5): 416–424.
27. Ouriel K. Noninvasive diagnosis of upper extremity vascular disease. *Semin Vasc Surg* 1998;11(2):54–59.
28. Gerwin RD. Myofascial pain syndromes in the upper extremity. *J Hand Ther* 1997;10(2):130–136.
29. Rosenhall U, Johansson G, Orndahl G. Otoneurologic and audiologic findings in fibromyalgia. *Scand J Rehabil Med* 1996;28(4):225–232.
30. Bayazit YA, Gursoy S, Ozer E, et al. Neurotologic manifestations of the fibromyalgia syndrome. *J Neurol Sci* 2002; 196(1-2):77–80.
31. Rosenhall U, Johansson G, Orndahl G. Neuroaudiological findings in chronic primary fibromyalgia with dysesthesia. *Scand J Rehabil Med* 1987;19:147–152.
32. Rosenhall U, Johansson G, Orndahl G. Eye motility dysfunction in chronic primary fibromyalgia with dysesthesia. *Scand J Rehabil Med* 1987;19:139–145.
33. Shingleton BJ, O'Donoghue MW. Blurred vision. *N Engl J Med* 2000;343(8):556–562.
34. Martinez-Lavin M, Hermosillo AG, Rosas M, et al. Circadian studies of autonomic nervous balance in patients with fibromyalgia: a heart rate variability analysis [In Process Citation]. *Arthritis Rheum* 1998;41(11):1966–1971.
35. Martinez-Lavin M, Hermosillo AG, Mendoza C, et al. Orthostatic sympathetic derangement in subjects with fibromyalgia. *J Rheumatol* 1997;24(4):714–718.
36. Martinez-Lavin M, Vidal M, Barbosa RE, et al. Norepinephrine-evoked pain in fibromyalgia. A randomized pilot study [ISRCTN70707830]. *BMC Musculoskelet Disord* 2002;3(1):2.
37. Martinez-Lavin M, Lopez S, Medina M, et al. Use of the Leeds Assessment of Neuropathic Symptoms and Signs questionnaire in patients with fibromyalgia. *Semin Arthritis Rheum* 2003;32(6):407–411.
38. Bou-Holaigah I, Calkins H, Flynn JA, et al. Provocation of hypotension and pain during upright tilt table testing in adults with fibromyalgia. *Clin Exp Rheumatol* 1997;15(3): 239–246.
39. Schondorf R, Benoit J, Wein T, et al. Orthostatic intolerance in the chronic fatigue syndrome. *J Auton Nerv Syst* 1999; 75(2-3):192–201.
40. Andersson M, Bagby JR, Dyrehag L, et al. Effects of staphylococcus toxoid vaccine on pain and fatigue in patients with fibromyalgia/chronic fatigue syndrome. *Eur J Pain* 1998; 2(2):133–142.
41. Martinez-Lavin M, Hermosillo AG. Autonomic nervous system dysfunction may explain the multisystem features of fibromyalgia [Editorial; Comment]. *Semin Arthritis Rheum* 2000;29(4):197–199.
42. Perez-Paredes M, Pico-Aracil F, Florenciano R, et al. Head-up tilt test in patients with high pretest likelihood of neurally

mediated syncope: an approximation to the "real sensitivity" of this testing. *Pacing Clin Electrophysiol* 1999;22(8): 1173–1178.

43. Grubb BP, Kosinski DJ, Boehm K, et al. The postural orthostatic tachycardia syndrome: a neurocardiogenic variant identified during head-up tilt table testing. *Pacing Clin Electrophysiol* 1997;20(9 Pt 1):2205–2212.

44. Stewart JM, Gewitz MH, Weldon A, et al. Patterns of orthostatic intolerance: the orthostatic tachycardia syndrome and adolescent chronic fatigue. *J Pediatr* 1999;135(2 Pt 1): 218–225.

45. Tanaka H, Yamaguchi H, Matushima R, et al. Instantaneous orthostatic hypotension in children and adolescents: a new entity of orthostatic intolerance. *Pediatr Res* 1999;46(6): 691–696.

46. Nair N, Padder FA, Kantharia BK. Pathophysiology and management of neurocardiogenic syncope. *Am J Manag Care* 2003;9(4):327–334.

47. Kaufmann H, Saadia D, Voustianiouk A. Midodrine in neurally mediated syncope: a double-blind, randomized, crossover study. *Ann Neurol* 2002;52(3):342–345.

48. Mahanonda N, Bhuripanyo K, Kangkagate C, et al. Randomized double-blind, placebo-controlled trial of oral atenolol in patients with unexplained syncope and positive upright tilt table test results. *Am Heart J* 1995;130(6):1250–1253.

49. Madrid AH, Ortega J, Rebollo JG, et al. Lack of efficacy of atenolol for the prevention of neurally mediated syncope in a highly symptomatic population: a prospective, double-blind, randomized and placebo-controlled study. *J Am Coll Cardiol* 2001;37(2):554–559.

50. Travell JG, Simons DG. *Myofascial pain and dysfunction: the trigger point manual.* Baltimore, MD: Williams & Wilkins, 1983.

51. Parker WS, Chole RA. Tinnitus, vertigo, and temporomandibular disorders. *Am J Orthod Dentofacial Orthop* 1995; 107(2):153–158.

52. Lam DK, Lawrence HP, Tenenbaum HC. Aural symptoms in temporomandibular disorder patients attending a craniofacial pain unit. *J Orofac Pain* 2001;15(2):146–157.

53. Tuz HH, Onder EM, Kisnisci RS. Prevalence of otologic complaints in patients with temporomandibular disorder. *Am J Orthod Dentofacial Orthop* 2003;123(6):620–623.

54. Wennmo K, Wennmo C. Drug-related dizziness. *Acta Otolaryngol Suppl* 1988;455:11–13.

55. Simons DG. Myofascial pain caused by trigger points. In: Mense S, Simons DG, Russel IJ, eds. *Muscle pain: understanding its nature, diagnosis, and treatment.* Philadelphia, PA: Lippincott Williams & Wilkins, 2001:205–288.

56. Simons DG, Travell JG. Myofascial origins of low back pain. 3. Pelvic and lower extremity muscles. *Postgrad Med* 1983; 73:99.

57. Borg-Stein J. Management of peripheral pain generators in fibromyalgia. *Rheum Dis Clin North Am* 2002;28(2):305–317.

58. Rudin NJ. Evaluation of treatments for myofascial pain syndrome and fibromyalgia. *Curr Pain Headache Rep* 2003; 7(6):433–442.

59. Hong C-Z. Considerations and recommendations regarding myofascial trigger point injection. *J Musculoskelet Pain* 1994;2(1):29–59.

60. Hong CZ. Lidocaine injection versus dry needling to myofascial trigger point. The importance of the local twitch response. *Am J Phys Med Rehabil* 1994;73(4):256–263.

61. Norregaard J, Bulow PM, Vestergaard-Poulsen P, et al. Muscle strength, voluntary activation and cross-sectional muscle area in patients with fibromyalgia. *Br J Rheumatol* 1995;34: 925–931.

62. Jacobsen S, Wildschiodtz G, Danneskiold-Samsoe B. Isokinetic and isometric muscle strength combined with transcutaneous electrical muscle stimulation in primary fibromyalgia syndrome. *J Rheumatol* 1991;18:1390–1393.

63. Miller TA, Allen GM, Gandevia SC. Muscle force, perceived effort, and voluntary activation of the elbow flexors assessed with sensitive twitch interpolation in fibromyalgia. *J Rheumatol* 1996;23:1621–1627.

64. Bennett RM, Clark SR, Goldberg L, et al. Aerobic fitness in patients with fibrositis. A controlled study of respiratory gas exchange and 133-xenon clearance from exercising muscle. *Arthritis Rheum* 1989;32:454–460.

65. Rooks DS, Silverman CB, Kantrowitz FG. The effects of progressive strength training and aerobic exercise on muscle strength and cardiovascular fitness in women with fibromyalgia: a pilot study. *Arthritis Rheum* 2002;47(1):22–28.

66. Hakkinen A, Hakkinen K, Hannonen P, et al. Strength training induced adaptations in neuromuscular function of premenopausal women with fibromyalgia: comparison with healthy women. *Ann Rheum Dis* 2001;60(1):21–26.

67. Jones KD, Burckhardt CS, Clark SR, et al. A randomized controlled trial of muscle strengthening versus flexibility training in fibromyalgia. *J Rheumatol* 2002;29(5):1041–1048.

68. Bennett RM. Adult growth hormone deficiency in patients with fibromyalgia. *Curr Rheumatol Rep* 2002;4(4):306–312.

69. Bennett RM, Cook DM, Clark SR, et al. Hypothalamic-pituitary-insulin-like growth factor-I axis dysfunction in patients with fibromyalgia. *J Rheumatol* 1997;24(7):1384–1389.

70. Bennett RM, Clark SR, Walczyk J. A randomized, double-blind, placebo-controlled study of growth hormone in the treatment of fibromyalgia. *Am J Med* 1998;104(3):227–231.

71. Arnold LM, Keck PE Jr, Welge JA. Antidepressant treatment of fibromyalgia. A meta-analysis and review. *Psychosomatics* 2000;41(2):104–113.

72. Okifuji A, Turk DC, Marcus DA. Comparison of generalized and localized hyperalgesia in patients with recurrent headache and fibromyalgia. *Psychosom Med* 1999;61(6):771–780.

73. Peres MF, Young WB, Kaup AO, et al. Fibromyalgia is common in patients with transformed migraine. *Neurology* 2001; 57(7):1326–1328.

74. Nicolodi M, Volpe AR, Sicuteri F. Fibromyalgia and headache. Failure of serotonergic analgesia and N-methyl-D-aspartate-mediated neuronal plasticity: their common clues [In Process Citation]. *Cephalalgia* 1998;18(Suppl. 21): 41–44.

75. Peres MF. Fibromyalgia, fatigue, and headache disorders. *Curr Neurol Neurosci Rep* 2003;3(2):97–103.

76. Wolfe F, Smythe HA, Yunus MB, et al. The American College of Rheumatology 1990 criteria for the classification of fibromyalgia: Report of the Multicenter Criteria Committee. *Arthritis Rheum* 1990;33:160–172.

77. Peres MF, Young WB, Kaup AO, et al. Fibromyalgia is common in patients with transformed migraine. *Neurology* 2001; 57(7):1326–1328.

78. Davidoff RA. Trigger points and myofascial pain: toward understanding how they affect headaches. *Cephalalgia* 1998; 18(7):436–448.

79. Hallberg LR, Carlsson SG. Psychosocial vulnerability and maintaining forces related to fibromyalgia. In-depth interviews with twenty-two female patients. *Scand J Caring Sci* 1998;12(2):95–103.

80. Hedenberg-Magnusson B, Ernberg M, Kopp S. Presence of orofacial pain and temporomandibular disorder in fibromyalgia. A study by questionnaire [In Process Citation]. *Swed Dent J* 1999;23(5-6):185–192.

81. Brandes JL. Treatment approaches to maximizing therapeutic response in migraine. *Neurology* 2003;61(8 Suppl. 4):S21–S26.

82. Pappagallo M. Newer antiepileptic drugs: possible uses in the treatment of neuropathic pain and migraine. *Clin Ther* 2003;25(10):2506–2538.

83. Edwards KR, Potter DL, Wu SC, et al. Topiramate in the preventive treatment of episodic migraine: a combined analysis from pilot, double-blind, placebo-controlled trials. *CNS Spectr* 2003;8(6):428–432.

84. Mathew NT, Kailasam J, Meadors L. Prophylaxis of migraine, transformed migraine, and cluster headache with topiramate. *Headache* 2002;42(8):796–803.

85. Krymchantowski AV, Moreira PF. Clinical presentation of transformed migraine: possible differences among male and female patients. *Cephalalgia* 2001;21(5):558–566.

86. Krymchantowski AV. Overuse of symptomatic medications among chronic (transformed) migraine patients: profile of drug consumption. *Arq Neuropsiquiatr* 2003;61(1):43–47.

87. Freitag FG. Preventative treatment for migraine and tension-type headaches: do drugs having effects on muscle spasm and tone have a role? *CNS Drugs* 2003;17(6):373–381.

88. Grazzi L, Andrasik F, D'Amico D, et al. Behavioral and pharmacologic treatment of transformed migraine with analgesic overuse: outcome at 3 years. *Headache* 2002;42(6): 483–490.

89. Milhorat TH, Chou MW, Trinidad EM, et al. Chiari I malformation redefined: clinical and radiographic findings for 364 symptomatic patients. *Neurosurgery* 1999;44(5): 1005–1017.

90. Elster AD, Chen MY. Chiari I malformations: clinical and radiologic reappraisal. *Radiology* 1992;183(2):347–353.

91. Meadows J, Kraut M, Guarnieri M, et al. Asymptomatic Chiari type I malformations identified on magnetic resonance imaging. *J Neurosurg* 2000;92(6):920–926.

92. Alarcón GS, Bradley LA, Hadley MN, et al. Does Chiari malformation contribute to fibromyalgia symptoms? *Arthritis Rheum* 1997;40:S190.

93. Thimineur M, Kitaj M, Kravitz E, et al. Functional abnormalities of the cervical cord and lower medulla and their effect on pain: observations in chronic pain patients with incidental mild Chiari I malformation and moderate to severe cervical cord compression. *Clin J Pain* 2002;18(3): 171–179.

94. Taylor FR, Larkins MV. Headache and Chiari I malformation: clinical presentation, diagnosis, and controversies in management. *Curr Pain Headache Rep* 2002;6(4):331–337.

95. Chang CZ, Howng SL. Surgical outcome of Chiari I malformations—an experience sharing and literature review. *Kaohsiung J Med Sci* 1999;15(11):659–664.

13

Myofascial Pain Syndromes of the Head and Face

Eli Eliav and Rafael Benoliel

Pain syndromes of the head and face comprise a wide range of diagnostic entities including primary and secondary headaches (HA) (1) (see Table 13-1), with a number of syndromes particular to the orofacial complex (2–4). One of the most common orofacial pain syndromes is a group termed *temporomandibular disorders* (TMDs). TMD is essentially an all-encompassing term that includes disorders of the temporomandibular joint (TMJ) and the masticatory muscles. The International Headache Society (IHS), in its most recent classification (1), clearly classifies TMJ related pain and describes to masticatory muscle myofascial pain (MMP) as a possible initiating factor in tension-type headache (TTH). For orofacial pain and particularly TMDs the IHS classification is limiting, and orofacial pain specialists have tended to use alternative widely accepted systems (5,6). The American Academy of Orofacial Pain (AAOP) classification (6) is based on the IHS system and logically expands it. In this classification, TMDs are subclassified into TMJ articular disorders and masticatory-muscle disorders (see Table 13-2).

This chapter will focus on craniofacial myofascial pain, particularly masticatory MMP, but will cover basic features of TTH. Additionally, we will examine their relationships to other headache entities and to widespread pain syndromes such as fibromyalgia (FM).

hypotheses. The continued lack of evidence base for these unicausal theories led to the proposition of new theories combining stress and occlusal disharmonies (10,11) and later multifactorial (6) and biopsychosocial (12) theories.

Unfortunately, from the first description of this entity (13) and the emphasis on tooth-loss as a major etiological factor in TMDs, two problems were created. First was the concept that regional musculoskeletal pain was invariably associated with anatomic factors such as the dental occlusion or the TMJ itself—a misconception that proved difficult to change. Secondly, there has been a separation of masticatory MMP from other chronic regional pain syndromes such as TTH. Perhaps in view of early etiologic theories it seemed natural that dentists treat TMDs while the other medical specialties cared for additional chronic craniofacial pains. However, data expressing common ground between TTH and MMP is available suggesting that we need to reexamine the justification for the present nosological separation. Encouraging such change, the 1994 International Association for the Study of Pain (IASP) classification (14) combines temporomandibular pain and dysfunction with tension headache under the same category of "craniofacial pain of musculoskeletal origin."

The definition of internal derangements (ID) of the TMJ (15–17) conceptually separated the joint from MMP and led to modern classifications of joint and muscle-related disorders (5,6).

BACKGROUND ON TEMPOROMANDIBULAR DISORDERS

Pain in the temporomandibular region appears to be relatively common, occurring in approximately 10% of the population over age 18 (7). Diagnosis of pain associated with TMDs has been approached under more than a dozen names reflecting the confusion surrounding its etiology and often its therapy. The historical development of etiologic theories has been reviewed elsewhere (8,9), but in general early theories were similar in that they offered "one cause—one disease"

DIAGNOSIS OF MASTICATORY MYOFASCIAL PAIN

At present, diagnosis of masticatory myofascial pain is based largely on the history and clinical examination of the patient. However, clinical signs are difficult to measure with consistency (18,19), and interrater reliability for some signs of MMP is not good (20). In spite of these limitations, the AAOP (6) lists practical clinical criteria for diagnosis (see Table 13-3).

TABLE 13-1	Headache Classification

Primary Headaches
- Migraine
- Tension-type
- Cluster and other trigeminal autonomic cephalalgias (TACs)
- Other primary
  - Primary stabbing
  - Primary cough
  - Primary exertional
  - Primary associated with sexual activity
    - Preorgasmic
    - Orgasmic
  - Hypnic
  - Primary thunderclap
  - Hemicrania continua
  - New daily persistent

Secondary Headaches
- Head and/or neck trauma
- Cranial or cervical vascular disorder
- Nonvascular intracranial disorder
- Substance or its withdrawal
- Infection
- Disorders of homeostasis
- Disorders of cranium, neck, eyes, ears, nose, sinuses, teeth, mouth, or other facial or cranial structure
- Psychiatric disorder

From Goadsby PJ, Headache Classification Subcommittee of the International Headache Society. The international classification of headache disorders. *Cephalalgia* 2004;24(Suppl. 1):24–136, with permission.

MMP is characterized by a regional, dull, aching muscle pain and the presence of localized tender sites and trigger points in muscle, tendon, or fascia. When palpated, these trigger points (21,22) may produce a characteristic pattern of regional referred pain and/or autonomic symptoms on

TABLE 13-2	Classification of Temporomandibular Disorders

TMJ Articular Disorders
- Congenital
- Disc derangements
- Dislocation
- Inflammatory
- Osteoarthritis
- Ankylosis
- Fracture

Masticatory-Muscle Disorders
- Myofascial pain
- Myositis
- Myospasm
- Local myalgia—unclassified
- Myofibrotic contracture
- Neoplasia

TMJ, temporomandibular joint.
From Okeson, JP, The American Academy of Orofacial Pain. *Orofacial pain: guidelines for assessment, classification, and management.* Chicago: Quintessence Publishing Co., Inc, 1996, with permission.

TABLE 13-3	Masticatory Muscle Myofascial Pain

Diagnostic Criteria
- Regional dull, aching pain
  - Aggravated by mandibular movement involving the muscles of mastication
- Hyperirritable sites or trigger points
  - Frequently found within a taut band of muscle or tissue
  - Provocation of these trigger points alters the pain complaint and reveals a pattern of referral
- >50% reduction of pain with vapocoolant spray or local anesthetic injection to the trigger point followed by muscle stretch

From Okeson, JP, The American Academy of Orofacial Pain, *Orofacial pain: guidelines for assessment, classification, and management.* Chicago: Quintessence Publishing Co., Inc, 1996, with permission.

provocation (6). Indeed, MMP often refers to intraoral, auriculotemporal, supraorbital, and maxillary areas depending on the muscles involved and the intensity of the pain (22–24). At times the pain refers diffusely throughout one side of the face (25), compounding diagnosis. Usually, however, patients localize the pain to areas around the ear, the angle of the mandible, and the temporal region. Although MMP is typically a unilateral pain syndrome it may also occur bilaterally, with some evidence that bilateral pain is more commonly associated with underlying psychogenic factors (26). The temporal pain pattern varies considerably, with some patients experiencing the most intense pain in the morning or late afternoon and others having no fixed pattern (27,28), but fortunately the pain rarely wakes the patient from sleep. Typically, MMP is characterized by chronicity with reported onset weeks to several years previously. Pain may be aggravated during function, with transient spikes of pain occurring spontaneously or induced by jaw movements (6); indeed, pain on function may be the patient's primary complaint.

In addition to pain there may be deviation of the mandible on opening, fullness of the ear, dizziness, and soreness of the neck (29–33). Dizziness has been associated with pain in the sternocleidomastoid muscle (29,32) and ear stuffiness with spasm of the medial pterygoid (34).

Examination usually reveals limited mouth opening (<40 mm, interincisal). The masticatory and neck muscles may be tender to palpation (31,32,35), leading to referred areas of pain (23,24,29).

NEUROPHYSIOLOGIC STUDIES AND DIAGNOSTIC TOOLS

Neurophysiologic methods and quantitative sensory testing (QST) offer excellent tools in assessing trigeminal somatosensory function. Combining various techniques (e.g., electrical, mechanical, and thermal) allows accurate diagnosis of nerve function and of the contribution of the central nervous system (CNS) in orofacial pain conditions. Excellent reviews are available on the applicability of these methods in chronic orofacial pain (36) and in TMDs in particular (37).

There have been numerous studies documenting neurophysiologic characteristics of TMD patients (38–40), and some relevant examples are described below. Downward tapping on the chin may induce a myotatic reflex (the "jaw jerk") in the jaw-closing muscles (41). TMD patients have significant differences in reflex amplitude and latency between painful and nonpainful sides (42). During active clenching, the interruption of sustained electromyography (EMG) activity of the masseter by a tap to the chin (the so called "silent period") is longer in patients than in controls (43–45). This has been an inconsistent finding (46) and has been attributed to experimental methodological variations. Shorter masseteric inhibitory periods were found in patients than in controls when evoked by tooth-pulp stimulation (47) and in response to tooth tapping (46), suggesting increased excitability of the central motor neuron pool in these patients (47). No difference was found, however, in the duration of the masseteric inhibitory period between the painful and the nonpainful sides (47). A further demonstration of an association between hyperactivity of masticatory muscles and TMDs is that EMG inhibitory responses following initial tooth contact are either absent or reduced, and that EMG activity, not normally detected when the mouth is open, is found in 50% of TMD patients (48). Several other studies report that patients with MMP have higher resting masseter and temporalis EMG activity than nonpatients (49), and their significance is discussed under the section on etiology. Comparison of the bilateral activity in the anterior temporalis and the masseter muscles during clenching shows that subjects with muscle pain demonstrate asymmetric recruitment of these muscles in contrast to the more symmetric recruitment seen in normal subjects (50). In summary, neurophysiologic tests, although offering insight into TMD-related CNS changes and possible pathophysiology, are at present not an applicable diagnostic tool for TMDs.

Recently, we described patients with TMD that were characterized by QST of the trigeminal nerve (51). Our data clearly demonstrated large myelinated fiber hypersensitivity in the skin overlying TMJs with clinical pain and pathology, but patients with MMP demonstrated large myelinated nerve fiber hyposensitivity. Hagberg et al. (52) used electrical stimuli to evaluate patients with orofacial joint and muscle pain. In comparison to control subjects, patients showed higher detection, discomfort, and pain thresholds (decreased sensitivity) to stimuli applied to the skin over the masseter muscle. Within the patient group, those with the greatest spontaneous pain had the lowest threshold values. Lowered electrical pain thresholds (increased sensitivity) have also been observed in similar patients at both trigger points and areas of referred pain (53) and in patients with chronic tension-type headache (CTTH) (54). Tonic muscular pain has been shown to induce an elevation of detection threshold to graded monofilaments both in the affected and in the contralateral side, suggesting involvement of central mechanisms (55).

Although the QST methodology described is in its early stages, it is clear that this methodology may be a useful addition to the clinician's diagnostic armamentarium.

Thermography has been widely employed as a noninvasive diagnostic test for various conditions. Its applicability in craniomandibular disorders has been assessed with relatively nonspecific findings (56).

EPIDEMIOLOGY

TMD is recognized as the most common chronic orofacial pain condition (57). However, many studies on the prevalence of TMD signs and symptoms focus on samples of patients seeking treatment, on convenience samples, or other nonrepresentative portions of the population (9). Standardization of methods and reliability data are rarely provided and are prerequisites in dental epidemiologic studies; indeed, poor interrater reliability challenges the validity of comparing data across studies (20). A further major problem is the definition of criteria: diverse inclusion and exclusion criteria have been used by different groups (58). As previously defined, TMD refers to a group of pain conditions and dysfunctions, and not all epidemiologic studies have used the same classification or inclusion and exclusion criteria. LeResche et al. (59) demonstrate the problems of assessing the prevalence of TMJ disorders using two different classification schemes on the same population sample. Indeed, the criteria employed to include patients in studies prior to modern classifications were such that they encompassed a number of disorders into one entity, and under today's concepts (5,6) these patients would be diagnosed differently. This questions the current validity of much of the epidemiologic research performed before criteria and diagnoses were standardized.

Because epidemiologic studies of TMD address a number of symptoms, conclusions as to the behavior of any one sign or symptom should be arrived at with due consideration. In Agerberg and Carlsson's (60) classic cross-sectional study, about half of the 15- to 44-year-old population had at least one symptom of dysfunction and one third had two or more symptoms. Many studies have shown a large percentage of subjects reporting signs and symptoms of mandibular dysfunction in the general population, ranging from 28% to 86% (61).

In a population of patients over 18 years old a prevalence of 48.8% was observed with need for treatment estimated at 3.5% to 9.7% (62). In a subgroup that was examined clinically, the prevalence of clinical signs was 81.8% with a calculated estimate that the overall sample would have a sign prevalence of 78.7% (62), extremely high figures. In a critical review Greene and Marbach (9) state: "epidemiological studies suggest that as many as three fourths of the population may, to some degree, be affected by this disorder"; a prevalence suggestive of an epidemic. They continue: "there are serious doubts, however, about whether the findings of these studies should be accepted without first raising critical questions regarding their validity." Therefore, the data available must be carefully analyzed and applied while appreciating the inherent limitations of these studies.

Wanman and Agerberg (63,64) reported a symptom and sign prevalence of 20% in a 17-year-old study group. They followed up this group for 2 years and found that although the incidence was 8% there was no general increase in the severity or number of symptoms in this study period. The conclusion is that there is extreme symptom fluctuation: new symptoms appear as often as old ones disappear. Studying the onset and progression of TMDs over a 20-year period, it was concluded that in addition to fluctuation of symptoms, progression to severe pain and dysfunction was extremely rare (65). Solberg et al. (66) examined 739 university students and found that 76% had signs or symptoms of dysfunction; they only rated 5% as needing treatment. There is also good compatibility between the figure of Solberg et al. (66) and the data on the percentage of individuals who seek treatment (3% to 7%) (61). Unfortunately, data is lacking on the significance of signs and symptoms. We cannot reliably predict which signs and symptoms will deteriorate and therefore justify early treatment. Clinical judgment alone is relied upon to decide which signs and symptoms will be treated, but clinical judgment varies and in the absence of clear criteria this alone cannot be relied upon. Clear indications for early treatment would therefore seem to be limited to pain and serious dysfunction.

Signs and symptoms of mandibular dysfunction have been found in all age groups (67,68), with a tendency to increase with age (61,69). Dworkin et al. (57) report that TMJ pain, however, is less common among elderly patients, and Rugh and Solberg (61) review accumulated evidence suggesting that in the elderly symptoms may be lower or the same than in the general population, with some studies showing only a slight elevation in the prevalence of some signs in this age group. Signs of mandibular dysfunction have been described in children and adolescents with a higher prevalence than was previously suspected (27,68). The syndrome occurs also in edentulous patients (70,71).

In the available epidemiologic studies of the general population, TMD signs and symptoms appear to be equally distributed between the sexes (67,72) or with a female preponderance (7,62), especially for TMD of muscular origin (i.e., MMP) (73). The majority (up to 80%) of patients who seek treatment, however, are females (7,27,32,35,61,67).

The association between certain skeletal morphological features and the prevalence of TMD has been the focus of much controversy. Data presented in Greene and Marbach's review (9) indicate that the distribution of major occlusal categories in a patient group does not differ significantly from the normal population.

CHRONIC MASTICATORY MUSCLE MYOFASCIAL PAIN

The interplay between a peripheral nociceptive source in muscle and a faulty CNS component (sensitization) probably underlies most myofascial disorders, including masticatory myofascial pain, TTH, and FM (74,75). Lowered pressure-pain thresholds have been consistently reported in TMD patients (76,77), suggesting peripheral sensitization of muscle nociceptors. What exactly activates the peripheral muscle nociceptor and induces muscle hyperalgesia is unclear. Stimuli may include peripheral chemical and mechanical agents in addition to reactive or even primary central mechanisms (78,79), which may lead, for example, to neurogenic inflammation. Experimental inflammatory conditions of the TMJ and pericranial muscles lead to changes classically associated with central sensitization (80), which can be reversed with central delivery of N-methyl-D-aspartate (NMDA) antagonists. This finding implicates central neuroplasticity in initiating and maintaining chronic muscle pain

and may lead to novel treatment approaches. What affects the transition from acute to chronic MMP? It has been suggested that this process involves neuroplastic changes in medullary dorsal horn, including functional and morphologic changes, while endogenous factors working to attenuate these changes (e.g., descending inhibition) vary in effect between patients (75). Attempts at designing models for predicting chronicity in TMD patients have revealed that high characteristic pain intensity and the presence of myofascial pain were the most significant predictors of chronicity (81). Patients developing chronicity differed significantly in numerous biopsychosocial variables (e.g., they suffered from more current anxiety disorders, mood disorders, and somatization disorders). Similar findings were reported by Garofalo et al. (82) who found that high pain intensity, high disability score, higher depression and somatization scores, and being female with myofascial pain were predictors of chronicity. These findings are consistent with the theory that prolonged and intense nociceptive input is one of the initiating factors for chronicity with biopsychosocial variables possibly acting as perpetuating factors.

Altered pain regulation is suggested by findings of significantly more prevalent generalized body pain (e.g., FM and back pain) and headache in TMD patients (83). In support of this theory, TMD patients exhibit lower pain thresholds, greater temporal summation of mechanically evoked pain, stronger after-sensations, and multisite hyperalgesia (84,85). These indicate generalized hyperexcitability of the CNS and generalized upregulation of nociceptive processing (decreased inhibition or increased facilitation) and have been suggested as important pathophysiologic mechanisms (85). In support of this hypothesis, pain from TMDs was not attenuated after peripheral noxious stimuli (ischemic tourniquet test), which would normally activate noxious inhibitory modulation (86), suggesting differential or faulty recruitment of inhibitory controls.

We will briefly review etiologic factors in the induction of MMP that may be involved in the induction of a persistent peripheral muscular lesion, altered pain modulation, or decreased coping abilities. Etiologic theory of TMDs is probably the area where most controversy exists. Much has been written on the etiology of MMP, only attesting to how little we still know. We are aware that a very complex assortment of intrinsic and extrinsic factors act together to induce MMP in patients (87). Some may be statistically significant at the group level, but the exact contribution of individual parameters in each clinical case is still difficult to assess (87). An interesting approach is to identify individual factors in patients and attempt to recognize their roles as possible predisposing factors, initiating factors, and perpetuating factors (6). Individual factors may serve any or all of these roles in different patients.

PERSISTENT PERIPHERAL MUSCULAR LESION

Trauma

It has been increasingly recognized that traumatic events in the craniofacial region lead to cases of chronic TMD pain, as is seen in chronic posttraumatic headache (1). In considering the etiology of TMDs, trauma can be classified as macrotrauma (e.g., head injury) or microtrauma (e.g., para-functional jaw habits and overloading of muscles). Trauma history is present in significant numbers of patients with TMD (88) and has been documented to cause regional myofascial pain (89). Indirect trauma, as in hyperextension-flexion injury to the cervical complex (whiplash), has not enough substantial clinical data to support a causative role.

Muscle Hyperactivity and Microtrauma

Sustained or repeated abnormal loading of the masticatory apparatus has been postulated as a source of microtrauma that may lead to chronic TMDs. In this context, the most widespread belief is that MMP is induced by repetitive teeth clenching, grinding, or abnormal posturing of the jaw. These habits are, however, extremely common and statistically have not been proven to induce MMP (90). The theory that muscle hyperactivity can cause pain is based on accumulated data that prolonged and unaccustomed exercise in the hand, leg, and back is followed by transient local muscle soreness (91–95). Exercise-induced muscle soreness appears on the following day and, in the absence of repeated vigorous exercise, gradually disappears in 1 week (22,94). These exercises usually involve eccentric lengthening (isotonic) contractions of the involved muscle with subsequent injury suggested as the mechanism. Damage was found, however, to be less likely following isometric and shortening exercises, a situation most likely to occur in tooth clenching and tooth grinding. Histochemical and histologic research on rodents has also supported the hypothesis that lengthening contractions produce more damage than shortening contractions (96–98). Initially, muscle spasticity was thought to be the underlying cause of masticatory muscle pain, but no evidence has been found to reveal maintained muscular activity (99), and EMG studies have shown that muscle activity in the jaw-closing muscles occurs when the patient attempts to open the mouth (38). Indeed, activity in muscle nociceptors tends to induce inhibition of the α motorneuron pool of the muscle during contraction (100). During painful mastication, EMG activity of jaw-closing muscles is decreased in the agonist phase and slightly increased in the antagonist phase (101,102). Moreover, TMD patients have a substantially reduced biting force compared to controls, which has been attributed to muscle pain and tenderness (103,104). These findings are likely to reflect a protective mechanism that avoids further tissue damage.

However, evidence of a damage process in the human masticatory muscles is largely indirect and based mostly on experimental tooth clenching. Christensen (105) measured a prolonged increase in tissue fluid pressure following experimental tooth clenching in humans, suggesting an inflammatory response. Based on intramuscular blood flow studies (106) and on thermography studies (56) that show an immediate postcontraction hyperemia, the transient pain has been postulated to be due to a contraction-induced ischemia (107).

Masticatory-muscle pain can be induced in normal volunteers by sustained high force jaw contractions, by tooth grinding as an isotonic exercise (105,108), and by tooth clenching as an isometric exercise (109–113). These models of experimental pain have been termed *endogenous* (79). Protrusive exercises (114) induced soreness that occurred on the same day and lasted till evening; however, no documentation was

provided on delayed muscle soreness or jaw movement restriction. Indeed much of the work on clenching-induced experimental jaw pain has not reported on the presence of delayed muscle pain or soreness. Pain is, however, difficult to induce following sustained isometric protrusive contractions (115), and no significant postexperimental changes were found in maximum active pain-free opening, lateral excursion, and jaw pain for up to 7 days following the experiment (107, 115), contradicting previous findings. Replication of some of these studies (116) revealed that the five methods used did not consistently produce pain, and no significant site specificity was found—even when the exercise was intended to cause such specificity. Some subjects appeared to be very susceptible to developing a bilateral muscle pain during or after most of these unilateral stressful exercises, while other subjects did not. The authors suggest that this may be due to the extensive "coactivation" of many muscles (117–119). Patients with a diagnosis of MMP are, however, characterized by unilateral muscle pain that has only been reproduced following unilateral stressful exercise (120), with the contralateral side involved significantly more often than the ipsilateral side.

Obviously, these experimental exercises, which are not identical to the parafunctional activities that occur in patients, produce complex masticatory-muscle responses that are not yet well understood. The conflicting evidence available may indicate that susceptibility or other cofactors [e.g., relative hypoperfusion; see (107)] may play a role. There is further support for this susceptibility theory in experiments on muscle-pain patients versus healthy controls. Jaw muscle-pain patients are able to do only a fraction of the work performed by healthy subjects (115), and a reduced endurance capacity was found in those with either active or past jaw muscle pain when compared to controls (121). While the models described have not totally elucidated the mechanisms underlying MMP, they have consistently shown that pain following muscle contraction is of short duration and self-limiting. Thus, sustained or repeated abnormal loading of the masticatory apparatus as in these experiments is of a doubtful primary role in chronic MMP. The role of overloading in TMJ disorders is not within the scope of this chapter.

Experimental muscle-pain models induced by external stimuli are referred to as exogenous. These external stimuli include the injection of algesic substances such as hypertonic saline (122–125), neuropeptides (e.g., serotonin, bradykinin) (126–129), and capsaicin (130) and induce reliable models of muscle pain. The potential contribution of these models is great and will no doubt shed light on the neuropharmacology and sensorimotor mechanisms underlying MMP. Relevant examples of such experiments are specifically discussed below in the section on gender.

In summary, available data do not support the traditional concept of myofascial pain induced or maintained by muscle hyperactivity (40). The pain-adaptation model (40) based on data from chronic musculoskeletal pain conditions (including that of temporomandibular myofascial pain) suggests that the observed changes in motor function are secondary to chronic pain and mediated at the spinal level. Changes in masticatory-muscle function—secondary to experimental muscle pain—support this model and confirm clinical complaints of dysfunction in muscular TMD patients (78,79).

BRUXISM AND OCCLUSAL DERANGEMENT

Bruxism may be defined as the subconscious, nonfunctional grinding of teeth and may occur during the day or at night. The association between bruxism and MMP, however, is not entirely clear. A specific relationship between bruxism and MMP is based on the vicious cycle theory where an occlusal interference or a painful lesion of a muscle is supposed to induce a spasm in the affected muscle, which in turn leads to ischemia because of the compression of blood vessels. Ischemic contractions are painful and activate muscle nociceptors; by this mechanism, the vicious cycle is closed. While the extent of the occlusal "interference" may be minute, the important fact is that such interference can upset proprioceptive feedback and thus cause bruxism and spasm of masticatory muscles (131). These assumptions have been refuted by experiments demonstrating that artificial occlusal discrepancies tend to reduce bruxism rather than enhance it (132). Moreover, γ-motorneuron activity of an experimentally inflamed muscle was lower than in animals with an intact muscle (133) not supporting injury-induced muscle hyperactivity.

In recent meta-analyses (134,135), no evidence base was found to justify occlusal adjustment as a treatment for TMD. Furthermore, a prerequisite for such an etiology would be persistently elevated activity of masticatory muscles at rest in MMP patients. Although EMG activity recorded from masticatory muscles in patients is higher (49), later studies have shown that this activity fails to accurately define patients versus controls (136).

Thus, bruxism is not any more perceived as related to occlusal "disharmonies" but rather as a physiologic behavior that may sometimes be associated with MMP (137). Indeed, some view bruxism as an arousal phenomenon (138) or a sleep parasomnia (139). Bruxism occurs most often when the sleep stage is suddenly shifted to a lighter one: mostly during stage 1 or 2 of sleep, and rarely at the deep stages (3 and 4) of sleep. Bruxism is never initiated during the rapid eye movement (REM) bursts of REM sleep, when the arousal threshold is quite high (138). It appears that light sleep or lightening of sleep, either externally applied or internally originated, is important for the occurrence of bruxism (138). The majority of masseteric EMG "disturbances" (defined as activity >4 times the general background voltage) are found in stage 2, but additionally also in the REM sleep stage (140). When "bruxers" were compared to controls, it was found that bruxers had significantly higher masseter muscle activity when bruxism lasted longer than a 5-second duration (141). No significant difference was found, however, in activities of 3 to 5-second durations. Furthermore, the recorded differences between bruxers and controls were detected only in stage 2 of sleep but not in stages 3 or 4. Some preliminary results suggest that a majority of patients with bruxism have pain levels and sleep quality comparable with MMP patients (142). On the other hand, patients having bruxism without muscle pain do not show differences in any of the sleep variables compared to matched controls (142). So far there seem to be no studies examining whether bruxism meets the criteria for sleep disorders associated with FM, such as α-wave intrusions in non-rapid eye movement (N-REM) and particularly stage 4 sleep (143).

In summary, the etiology of nocturnal bruxism is currently thought to be related to changes in the central/autonomic nervous system, and the role of peripheral inputs (e.g., occlusal prematurities and the periodontium) is considered secondary (144). The precise association between bruxism and MMP is unclear at this stage (142,145). However, if muscle hyperactivity secondary to bruxism or some other parafunction is not the cause of pain but rather a "pain-adaptation" response (40), then essentially bruxism can no longer be considered as a primary etiologic mechanism of pain in MMP.

THE TEMPOROMANDIBULAR JOINT AND MASTICATORY MYOFASCIAL PAIN

Theoretically, trauma or noxious stimulation of TMJ tissues can produce a sustained excitation of masticatory muscles that may serve to protect the masticatory system from potentially damaging movements and stimuli (146). Clinically, the comorbidity of arthralgia and myalgia has led to such hypotheses linking their etiologies, but these have not been proven (147). Such comorbidity may reflect sensitization mediated by primary afferents in the TMJ and muscles of mastication cosynapsing on a dorsal horn neuron (convergence). Moreover, experimental injection into the TMJ of algesic chemicals resulted in sustained reflex increase in EMG activity of jaw-opening muscles; excitatory effects were also seen in jaw-closing muscles but were generally weaker (148). While such effects may be related to clinically based concepts of myofascial dysfunction (e.g., splinting, myospastic activity, and trigger points), the weak effects in muscles that are invoked clinically to show such dysfunction (jaw-closing) and the stronger effects in antagonist muscles (jaw-closing) suggest associations more in keeping with protective, withdrawal-type reflexes (146). Based upon the present available data, it seems that pain originating in the TMJ contributes minimally to the development of MMP.

DECREASED COPING ABILITY AND ALTERED PAIN MODULATION

Stress

Stress is difficult to accurately describe and define and therefore to measure. Several methods have been designed to attempt to measure the emotional results of stress or the intensity of environmental stress. The three major theories of stress each have methods for their measurement. Patient selection is important to consider in all studies and a factor decisively influential to the results obtained (149). Furthermore, chronic pain is a common problem in the community and those that finally do seek treatment usually have more severe pain and a poorer prognosis.

Stimulus-orientated theories emphasize the demanding or disorganizing influences of the environment. In such theories, when a threshold level is reached, the individual's ability to withstand stress is overcome and symptoms develop. Whether employing the Social Readjustment Rating Scale of Holmes and Rahe (150,151), a semistructured psychiatric interview (152), or a life events questionnaire (153), craniomandibular disorder patients were consistently shown to suffer from significantly more stress. These studies did not, however, differentiate between TMJ disorders and MMP.

The emotional reaction of the individual to stress is emphasized in response-oriented theories. These responses are thought to be mediated by the neuroendocrine system. The Subjective Stress Scale, a response-oriented test, demonstrated significantly higher scores in craniomandibular disorder patients (154). Using the Minnesota Multiphasic Personality Inventory (MMPI), various authors (10) have shown a mild degree of emotional disturbance in craniomandibular disorder patients. However, the MMPI has been widely criticized because it confuses physical symptoms (which may be organic) with the assessment of hypochondriasis, hysteria, and depression. Almost all populations with chronic pain show mild changes in the MMPI, but it does not mean that the findings indicate emotional change. The inadequacy of the MMPI in studies is stressed by Smythe (155), who considers the MMPI "an especially poor scale to use if there is interest in the presence and nature of a psychological component in a condition with somatic symptoms."

The third theory, termed *interactive*, proposes that the impact of stressors is tempered by the interaction between the environment and the individual's perceptual and cognitive processes. None of the tests available in this area seem very useful in assessing craniomandibular patients. The Derogatis Stress Profile has been applied to characterize a population of craniomandibular patients (156). Comparing muscle-pain patients to joint- pain patients, it was found that the muscle-pain group had higher stress ratings with more pain and impaired activity and a nonsignificant trend of an inability to cope with stress (156).

Patients with muscle pain are frequently found to suffer from other stress-related disorders such as migraine and backache, nervous stomach, and ulcers (157–160). Elevated urinary concentrations of catecholamines and 17-hydroxy steroids in these patients suggest higher stress levels (161,162). A positive relationship was also found between increased urinary epinephrine and high levels of nocturnal masseter muscle activity, implying that nocturnal bruxism is stress related (163). However, the relationship between bruxism and MMP is unclear and, therefore, one cannot deduce from this that MMP patients suffer from stress.

Marbach et al. (164) attempted to identify potential risk factors for the temporomandibular pain and dysfunction syndrome (TMPDS). They investigated the relationship of personal social and recent experiential factors, especially health behaviors and physical illnesses and injuries that contribute to life stress and TMPDS. Their key finding was that cases have strikingly higher rates of recent serious illness and injury events, even after adjustment for levels of illness attitudes that may have affected reporting (164). However, when they compared childhood onset (before age 13) of the three most common physical problems, they found no case-control difference.

Experimental stress in normal individuals increases masticatory muscle EMG activity (38,165,166), supporting the theory that stress induces muscular hyperactivity and leads to MMP (167). However, more recent studies (81,82) suggest that stress-related disorders may be more related to the development of TMD chronicity and may therefore be viewed more as perpetuating rather than initiating factors.

Psychosocial Correlates

Early studies emphasize the contribution of psychological factors to MMP (30,168). A background of depressive illness has been described in facial-pain patients (169), and a significantly large number of MMP patients are depressed compared to controls (170). However, on the basis of an extensive literature review, Rugh and Solberg (58) concluded that there was little evidence suggesting that MMP is related to any specific personality trait. Thus, Marbach et al. (171) found no significant difference in either state-anxiety or trait-anxiety between patients with intractable facial pain and groups of general dental and general medical patients. No difference in depression and anhedonia has been noted between MMP patients and controls (172), and only a minority of chronic facial-pain patients are cortisol nonsuppressors on the Dexamethasone Suppression Test (173). The hypothesis that MMP patients represent a population whose pain results from their emotional state has been challenged (174). Comparing MMP patients to patients with facial pain and lesions or pathophysiologic disorders showed little evidence of neuroticism in either group (174). Furthermore, examining the premorbid characteristics of MMP patients did not reveal abnormal parental bonding attitudes in this group (174), nor did they show any other measures of previous premorbid personality traits (175). Schnurr et al. (176) subclassified their TMD patients as myogenic (i.e., MMP) and TMJ facial pain and compared these to nonfacial injury "pain controls" and healthy controls. The results suggest that MMP and TMJ pain patients do not appear to be significantly different from other pain patients or healthy controls in personality type, response to illness, attitudes toward health care, or ways of coping with stress.

These results indicate that not all MMP patients suffer from psychosocial disorders, and the role of such influences as initiating or perpetuating factors is unclear.

Genes, Gender, and Susceptibility

The sequencing of the human genome has elucidated the presence of 30,000 to 40,000 human genes. Some of these genes and protein end products will emerge as new therapeutic targets for chronic pain. Information concerning genetically controlled drug toxicity and common adverse drug reactions will be available on an individual basis. Genetically governed interindividual differences are also found in the drug-transport proteins and drug targets (receptors), altering the pharmacokinetics and pharmacodynamics of a variety of drugs. For example, the analgesic potency of morphine will be dictated partly by any variation in the expression of μ-opioid receptors. Polymorphisms in this receptor lead to interindividual differences in responses to pain and its relief by opioid drugs (177). Thus, although no genetic influence has been proven in TMDs, host susceptibility probably plays a role in MMP at a number of levels. Susceptibility is governed at any given time by such "permanent" factors as genetics of injury response and pain modulation, pharmacogenomics and gender, and such "temporary" factors as concomitant illness or serious life events. Thus, any of the etiologic agents discussed may contribute to MMP in one patient but not in another, who may require a single or a combination of etiologic factors to develop MMP.

GENDER AND TEMPOROMANDIBULAR DISORDERS

The effects of gender on the epidemiology of pain syndromes and on pain thresholds have been extensively reported. Women suffer significantly more from migraines (178), TTHs (179), facial pains (180), FM (181), and TMDs (182,183). Under experimental conditions, women consistently demonstrate a lowered pain threshold (184), often affected by the stage of the menstrual cycle and by exogenous hormones such as oral contraceptives (185). Both hormone replacement therapy and use of oral contraceptives have been associated with increased risk of TMD (186,187), although a recent report failed to confirm this association (188). In a study examining progression to chronicity in acute TMD patients, significant differences between men and women were observed (189). Overall, more psychosocial stress was present in all patients progressing to chronicity, but specifically women with a muscle disorder were extremely likely to become chronic pain sufferers. There is evidence that estrogen and nerve growth factor (NGF) may interact in the regulation of nociceptive processes. When NGF was systemically administered to healthy human subjects, muscle pain, particularly in the craniofacial region, was observed but was more pronounced in women than in men (190). Interactions between NGF and estrogen have been shown (191), but the mechanisms involved in TMDs are unclear.

The injection of glutamate into the masseter muscle or the TMJ of the rat induced significantly greater muscle activity in female rats (192,193). Gonadectomy significantly reduced the magnitude of muscle activity in female rats following glutamate injection into the TMJ, a phenomenon partially reversible by the delivery of estrogen (192). These studies clearly demonstrate that there are sex-related differences in glutamate-evoked jaw muscle activity that are female sex hormone dependent.

The practical applications of gender differences in TMDs are still unclear. However, in addition to gender specific interactions between neuropeptides and hormones, the continued accumulation of knowledge pertaining to menstrually related changes in pain sensitivity and increased analgesic use, epidemiologic data concerning pain syndromes in women, and pharmacologic traits particular to each gender may elucidate pathophysiologic mechanisms.

TREATMENT OF MMP

The management of TMDs falls into four categories: physical, pharmacologic, psychological, and surgical (194). Most pain physicians with experience in the field of TMD will attest to the success of conservative physical therapy, including muscle exercise, thermal packs, and oral splints. However, few, if any, of these therapies have been unequivocally proven in controlled trials (195). Often, reassurance and education of the patient, combined with simple muscle exercises for masticatory and neck muscles, will result in pain alleviation and restored mandibular function (196–199), although the evidence base for prolonged relief is lacking (195). Muscle tenderness may be treated with vapocoolant sprays and injections of local anesthetics into identified "trigger points" (22,200).

The historic importance of occlusion in the etiology of TMDs, although largely unproven, led to the extensive use of occlusal adjustment and oral splints. Although occlusal adjustment does not have enough of an evidence base, oral splints seem to be beneficial in TMJ arthralgia (201), and recent meta-analyses demonstrated marginal benefit for TMDs in general (134,135). Forssell (135) calculated the number needed to treat (NNT) for occlusal appliances in the treatment of TMDs based on two high quality studies (202,203). NNT calculates the number of patients that need to be treated to obtain one patient ≥50% reduction of worst pain. For oral splints, an NNT of 6 was obtained for TMJ pain and of 4.3 for MMP. The exact mode of action of splints is unproven so that, to date, splints are regarded as adjunct therapy.

Nonsteroidal anti-inflammatory drugs (NSAIDs) are used extensively in the management of pain and disability associated with joint disease. The discovery of the subtypes of the cyclo-oxygenase enzyme (COX) led to the release of drugs specifically targeting the inflammation-induced form of COX (COX-2). Although the antiplatelet and gastrointestinal safety profile of selective COX-2 inhibitors is superior, they still have potentially serious side effects on the renal and cardiovascular systems. Desirable effects of NSAIDs are attained by the inhibition of inflammatory cytokines and prostaglandins. This has peripheral and central effects, including the reduction in peripheral sensitization and plasma extravasation, as well as reduction in central production of prostaglandins. For the treatment of TMDs, calculations of NNTs for drugs versus placebo reveal the encouraging figures of 2.7 and 3.5 (135).

In myofascial-pain patients, NSAIDs (ibuprofen) combined with diazepam are superior to an NSAID alone (204). Amitriptyline at low doses (10 mg per day to 30 mg per day) is superior to placebo (173) and has been consistently reported as beneficial for patients with craniofacial myofascial pain, including predominantly muscular TMDs (205), posttraumatic myofascial pain (89), and CTTHs (206). The use of clonazepam, a long-acting benzodiazepine with anticonvulsant properties, has been beneficial (207), but cyclobenzaprine has proven superior to clonazepam in a recent study (208). Still, quality drug trials in myofascial-pain and arthralgic-pain patients are lacking, and treatment remains somewhat empiric [for review see (209)].

Like other chronic-pain syndromes, MMP is a complex entity associated with behavioral changes, secondary psychological gains, changes in mood and attitudes to life, and drug abuse. The measured endpoints of treatment outcomes largely concentrate on changes in pain intensity and frequency. However, other outcomes need to be assessed—including restoration of functional activity, eradication of drug abuse and dependency, and rehabilitation of residual emotional distress. These parameters are greatly influenced by the psychosocial makeup of each patient and, therefore, need to be addressed. Cognitive-behavioral treatment is an option in addressing such problems and aims at altering negative overt behavior, thoughts, or feelings in chronic-pain patients and to diminish distress and suffering. These aims are achieved with a program that teaches personal skills such as relaxation, goal-setting, problem-solving, communication, and the ability to alter emotional responses to pain. Whether separately or combined with other pain treatments, cognitive-behavioral therapy produced significantly decreased pain, emotional distress, and disability (210). These findings stress the need for an evaluation and treatment plan that accounts for both the physical and emotional dimensions of chronic pain.

Present day pain therapies remain problematic and have limited success. Under these circumstances, patient interest and demand for complementary or alternative medicine (CAM) is increasing. Chronic-pain patients are, in general, more likely to seek CAM treatments (211). Approximately 20% of facial-pain patients in a referral center had attended a CAM specialist previously (212), and up to 36% of TMD patients reported treating their symptoms with CAM techniques (213). The existing evidence supports the value of acupuncture for the management of idiopathic HA (214) and has shown promise in the management of TMDs (213). However, well-planned studies need to assess the clinical effectiveness and cost-effectiveness of acupuncture and other CAM therapies for facial pain.

Fortunately, although our knowledge of etiology is limited, prognosis in the majority of MMP patients is good, and remission of pain and dysfunction is readily achieved for long periods (215–219).

TENSION-TYPE HEADACHE

TTH is extremely common with a lifetime prevalence of approximately 80% (179). Based on clinical and temporal characteristics, the IHS subclassifies TTH into episodic (infrequent and frequent), chronic, and probable TTH (see Table 13-4) (1).

EPISODIC TENSION-TYPE HEADACHE

Pain is usually mild to moderate in intensity (220), but increases with an increase in headache frequency (221). Episodic tension-type headache (ETTH) is almost exclusively bilateral (>90%) (222) and is usually described as "bandlike" and affects, in order of frequency, the occipital, parietal, temporal, or frontal areas (223,224). Quality of

TABLE 13-4	Tension-Type Headache

- Infrequent episodic TTH
  - With pericranial tenderness
  - Without pericranial tenderness
- Frequent episodic TTH
  - With pericranial tenderness
  - Without pericranial tenderness
- Chronic TTH
  - With pericranial tenderness
  - Without pericranial tenderness
- Probable TTH

TTH, tension-type headache.
From Goadsby PJ, Headache Classification Subcommittee of the International Headache Society. The international classification of headache disorders. *Cephalalgia* 2004; 24(Suppl. 1):24–136, with permission.

TABLE 13-5	Diagnostic Criteria: Episodic Tension-Type Headache[a]

Infrequent ETTH
A. At least 10 episodes occurring <1 d/mo on average (<12 d/yr) and fulfilling criteria B—D
Frequent ETTH
A. At least 10 episodes occurring ≥1 but <15 d/mo for at least 3 mo (≥12 and <180 d/yr) and fulfilling criteria B—D

B. Headache lasting from 30 min to 7 d
C. Headache has at least two of the following characteristics:
   a. Bilateral location
   b. Pressing/tightening (nonpulsating) quality
   c. Mild or moderate intensity
   d. Not aggravated by routine physical activity such as walking or climbing stairs
D. Both of the following:
   a. No nausea or vomiting (anorexia may occur)
   b. No more than one of photophobia or phonophobia
E. Not attributed to another disorder

ETTH, episodic tension-type headache.
[a]With or without pericranial tenderness.
From Goadsby PJ, Headache Classification Subcommittee of the International Headache Society. The international classification of headache disorders. *Cephalalgia* 2004; 24(Suppl. 1):24–136, with permission.

pain is usually described as pressurelike, dull, or as a sensation of tightness and is rarely aggravated by physical activity (224). Accompanying symptoms are rare in the less frequent forms of TTH, but mild to moderate anorexia is reported by 18% of cases (222), and mild photophobia (10%) or phonophobia (7%) has been observed (222,224). Sleep disturbances are reported frequently by TTH sufferers in general, and fatigue is reported in up to 80% of cases.

Based on temporal features the IHS (1) subclassifies ETTH into infrequent or frequent, both with or without pericranial muscle tenderness. The IHS classification lists five diagnostic criteria for ETTH (listed A–E) with the first criterion (A) distinguishing, by temporal features, between infrequent and frequent ETTH (see Table 13-5).

CHRONIC TENSION-TYPE HEADACHE

Classically, the patient with CTTH (see Table 13-6) is middle-aged with a more or less continuous daily headache beginning years previously. Pain quality is similar to that reported in ETTH and is mostly pressurelike and bilateral (222). The location of CTTH is usually frontal, temporal, or frontotemporal (223,225), and HA are often accompanied (32% of cases) by photo- or phonophobia (225). TTH sufferers report a lack of sufficient and restorative sleep.

ETIOLOGY

The etiology of TTH is uncertain and it is unclear whether the presence of pericranial muscle tenderness is the cause or the result of the headache. TTH induced by prolonged tooth

TABLE 13-6	Diagnostic Criteria: Chronic Tension-Type Headache[a]

A. Headache occurring on ≥15 d/mo on average for >3 mo (≥180 d/yr) and fulfilling criteria B—D
B. Headache lasts hours or may be continuous.
C. Headache has at least 2 of the following:
   a. Bilateral location
   b. Pressing/tightening (nonpulsating) quality
   c. Mild or moderate intensity
   d. Not aggravated by routine physical activity such as walking or climbing stairs
D. Both of the following:
   a. No more than one of photophobia or phonophobia or mild nausea
   b. Neither moderate or severe nausea nor vomiting
E. Not attributed to another disorder

---

[a]With or without pericranial tenderness.
From Goadsby PJ, Headache Classification Subcommittee of the International Headache Society. The international classification of headache disorders. *Cephalalgia* 2004;24(Suppl. 1):24–136, with permission.

clenching produced muscle tenderness that preceded onset of headache by several hours (226), while many patients with TTH present without pericranial myofascial tenderness. In TTH patients with muscle tenderness, it has been suggested that the mechanisms involve persistent nociceptive input leading to central sensitization that is negatively affected by faulty central modulation (227). This hypothesis is very similar to that proposed for MMP.

TREATMENT OF TENSION-TYPE HEADACHE

The management of TTH may be subdivided into abortive (individually treat the acute attack) or prophylactic approaches depending on headache frequency. Abortive approaches are largely pharmacologic while psychologic (228), physiotherapeutic (229), and TMD-aimed (230) treatments have all been employed in the prophylactic treatment of TTH with varying degrees of success.

As abortive therapy, NSAIDs have been consistently proven efficacious and are considered the first choice (231). Mild HA may respond favorably to 1 g of paracetamol or aspirin, but in general the NSAIDs of choice are high dose ibuprofen (800 mg) or naproxen sodium (825 mg) (231,232). Caffeine at doses from 130 to 200 mg has been proven to increase the efficacy of ibuprofen and other mild analgesics in the treatment of TTH (233).

Tricyclic antidepressants have been extensively studied and have been consistently the most efficacious drugs in prophylactically reducing both frequency and severity of CTTH (206,234). Amitriptyline was shown to be effective in CTTH but not in ETTH, suggesting different pathophysiologic mechanisms (235). Based on the high frequency at which pericranial muscle tenderness is observed in TTH, investigators have attempted treatment employing muscle

relaxants, including the use of botulinum toxin [see (236)]. Large trials are needed to confirm early reports of success.

HEADACHE, MYOFASCIAL PAINS, AND FIBROMYALGIA

INTRODUCTION

Many investigators (237–240) believe primary headache syndromes represent a continuum of clinical severity presentations with a common pathophysiologic mechanism (241). Similarly, masticatory muscle pain has been suggested to be a localized expression of a spectrum of myofascial disorders with many similarities between TMD, TTH, and FM (242,243). Indeed, the segregation of MMP from other myofascial pain disorders of a more generalized type such as FM has been questioned by others (244).

There are great similarities, and possible overlap, between patients suffering from headache and MMP (245). The sex ratio is similar—about 75% females in both groups; age distribution and contributing psychophysiologic mechanisms are shared (58,246). Muscle tenderness is a frequent finding in headache patients (246), the distribution of which may be distinctly similar to that in MMP patients (247). Thus, two of the fundamental symptoms of MMP, pain of daily occurrence and tenderness of muscles to palpation, fail to properly differentiate between headache and MMP patients. Presently, we will examine the possibility that a continuum exists between TTH, MMP, and generalized myofascial disorders such as FM.

MIGRAINE AND MASTICATORY MYOFASCIAL PAIN

The association between migraine and temporomandibular dysfunction was studied by Watts et al. (248). Fifty patients with mixed headache syndromes were compared to 50 MMP patients. The authors stated that the rate of migraine in the MMP group did not differ from that in the general population and concluded that MMP and migraine patients are two segregated groups. The role that vascular mechanisms, related to other craniofacial pains (e.g., migraine, cluster headache, paroxysmal hemicrania), play in MMP is not entirely clear. While the importance of vascular mechanisms may not yet be fully appreciated, one should not dismiss its contribution to MMP. Vascular headache is REM-locked (249), and some data (250) point to a REM-locked destructive form of bruxism that may link certain forms of MMP with vascular mechanisms.

TENSION-TYPE HEADACHE AND MASTICATORY MYOFASCIAL PAIN

In spite of stated similarities, most MMP patients have pain and muscle tenderness on palpation unilaterally (32,35), while TTH causes pain bilaterally. Comparison of EMG activity in the anterior temporalis and the masseter muscles during clenching demonstrates that MMP subjects with unilateral muscle pain asymmetrically recruit these muscles, while a more symmetric recruitment was seen in normal subjects (50). TTH and FM are therefore more similar, both being predominantly syndromes of a bilateral nature (251).

MMP is thought of as an initiating or perpetuating factor in TTH (1,226,252). TMD patients report HA significantly more frequently and of higher severity (253,254), and, specifically, MMP patients report a significantly higher incidence of tension headache than controls (245,248). In spite of these findings, the exact connection between MMP and TTH remains unclear.

Recently, HAs occurring on a daily basis have been classified together as chronic daily headache (CDH) (1). Primary CDH is a frequent entity that probably affects 4% to 5% of the population and can be subdivided into transformed migraine, CTTH, new daily persistent headache, and hemicrania continua. Comparison of MMP patients to CDH patients revealed high levels of similarity in psychological distress parameters (255), but these may be secondary to pain duration and severity, which were similar between groups.

HEADACHE AND FIBROMYALGIA

Similarities have been observed in the distribution of muscle tender points (TePs) between recurrent headache patients and FM patients (256). In patients with concomitant CDH and FM, there was significantly more insomnia and more incapacitating HA than in HA patients without FM (257). Within CDH, both migrainous and nonmigrainous HA have been similarly associated with generalized muscle pains (258). The most significant headache parameter associated with muscle pain was headache frequency and not HA diagnosis. The authors suggest that their findings may indicate that musculoskeletal pains and chronic HA (irrespective of diagnosis) may share central sensitization as a common etiologic factor (258). In this and further studies (259,260), a highly significant correlation was found between HA and muscle pain in the upper body area, which may suggest segmental effects.

TEMPOROMANDIBULAR DISORDERS AND FIBROMYALGIA

Similarly, pain outside the craniofacial region is common amongst TMD patients (261). Female patients with widespread pain are at significantly increased risk of developing TMDs (83), suggesting that TMDs may be related, and in continuum, to generalized muscle disorders. Indeed, patients with FM, regional myofascial pain such as MMP, and chronic fatigue syndrome (CFS) share many clinical features including myalgia, fatigue, and disturbed sleep, suggesting a common etiology. Between 20% and 70% of patients with FM meet criteria for CFS, and, conversely, 35% to 70% of CFS patients seem to have comorbid FM (262–265). Moreover, 18% of patients with TMD have signs suggestive of FM, and up to 75% of FM patients demonstrate comorbid MMP (266–268). In a recent study (158), patients with FM, TMD, and CFS demonstrated significantly elevated prevalence rates of irritable bowel syndrome, sleep disturbances, and concentration difficulties. However, TMD patients were distinguishable in that they suffered from a much higher rate of masticatory muscle tenderness (expected) and a reduced

prevalence of fatigue, muscle weakness, migratory arthralgias, and burning or shooting muscle pains.

Much controversy still surrounds FM as a disease entity and how it should be classified (269,270). Moreover, the boundaries between FM and regional myofascial pain (MP) are at times poorly demarcated in spite of established criteria (271,272). A major differentiating feature between FM and MP is the presence of trigger points and a palpable band of tight muscle in MP as opposed to multiple TePs in FM (273,274). By definition, trigger points, on palpation, refer pain to a distant site, but this condition for trigger points has been suggested as unnecessary (275); trigger points may be considered active or latent (25), further fogging the boundaries between MP and FM. The other basic difference is the proposed chronic, widespread, systemic character of FM (271) as opposed to the acute, localized nature of MP. However, this distinction has been termed *artificial* (276) in the light of the possibility that, on the one hand, FM may begin as a localized pain disorder and later become widespread and, on the other hand, that persistent MP may involve multiple sites and cause systemic symptoms (273,277). Many of the "perpetuating factors" in MP are termed *modulating factors* of FM: physical activity, cold, stress, and weather changes (273,275). Indeed, it has been suggested that FM and regional MP represent an overlapping spectrum (243).

Considering the diagnosis of MMP, there are many cases where muscle tenderness affects many sites in the head and neck, and trigger points are hard to find. These patients have TePs and characteristics associating them with FM, for example, disturbed sleep, anxiety, and general fatigue. When the symptoms of FM patients are compared with those of patients with MMP, no symptoms are specific to MMP (244), suggesting that such local "syndromes" of myofascial pain should be compiled to form one entity. Should these patients be diagnosed separately or compiled? Focusing on the one region in which pain is greatest may account for a restricted diagnosis such as MMP, when in effect this disorder can be a local symptom of a more generalized condition (244). Findings of faulty pain processing in MMP patients would seem to support this contention (278,279). Others believe that generalized syndromes should be separately classified (280).

Blasberg and Chalmers (33) retrospectively reviewed a series of MMP patients for evidence of generalized musculoskeletal pain. Their controls were a group of patients seen over the same time period but with other orofacial pains. A greater proportion of patients with MMP had complaints outside the jaw. These findings were statistically significant for neck muscles and for back muscles but not so for headache or pain in the extremities. The patient group also reported significantly more bilateral pain than controls. They conclude that there are great similarities between these FM patients. In eight patients with FM, six had severe signs of mandibular dysfunction using the Helkimo Anamnestic Dysfunction Index (281), thus promoting the hypothesis that a connection may exist between these entities. FM, by definition, is characterized by a widespread pain in 97.6% of patients throughout both sides and in both the upper and the lower parts of the body (251). It is therefore not surprising that many have signs of MMP. More recently (282), 162 female patients with a previous diagnosis of MMP were reexamined 7 years later to elicit a history of comorbid FM.

Thirty-eight patients (23.5%) had a positive history of FM but showed no difference in presenting signs and symptoms relating to the MMP. However, patients with a positive history of FM reported more MMP symptoms accompanied by more severe pain, increased depression, and somatization symptoms. In conclusion, increased chronicity was observed for MMP patients with comorbid FM that also seem to be more resistant to treatment (283).

The data suggests both similarities and salient differences between TMD and generalized muscle disorders. Although it is clear that in many cases MMP is a local pain syndrome with minimal complaints in other areas of the body, many cases present with complaints suggestive of a generalized widespread disorder. However, there could be other characteristics of MMP beyond its "locality" that make MMP into a discrete entity from FM.

THE TRIGEMINOVASCULAR SYSTEM

Some of the thinking on vascular craniofacial pain could be quite useful when applied to the study of chronic facial pain and, in particular, MMP. While the cascade of vascular changes and muscle contraction and spasm may contribute to craniofacial pain, findings strongly propose that neurogenic inflammation may play the major role in vascular headache (284). In view of the cardinal role of the trigeminal system in conveying vascular headache (285), the possibility of interrelated central mechanisms of headache and facial pain cannot be discounted. A continuum, as suggested for headache, may exist for facial pain, spanning from clearly vascular facial pains such as cluster headache to some "combination" and "muscle contraction" (i.e., MMP) facial pains. Research in the area of MMP should concentrate more on central generators and modulators of pain mechanisms rather than peripheral inputs such as occlusal interferences and "muscle hyperactivity." One attractive way to better understand MMP is to study the role of trigeminal neurogenic inflammation (286) and the contribution of the sympathetic nervous system (287) to orofacial pain mechanisms.

SUMMARY POINTS

- Pain in the temporomandibular region appears to be relatively common, occurring in approximately 10% of the population.
- Individuals with these conditions are more likely to be female and to have other regional and widespread pain conditions.
- Cohorts with both temporomandibular disorder and TTH have been shown to have lowered pain thresholds, not only in the region of pain but in areas of referred pain and distant regions.
- The muscle hyperactivity seen in these conditions (e.g., bruxism) is currently thought to be related to changes in the central/autonomic nervous system and/or a result of pain, and mediated at the spinal level, rather than this being the primary cause of the pain.

■ IMPLICATIONS FOR PRACTICE

- Most physicians with experience in the field of TMD will attest to the success of conservative physical therapy, including muscle exercise, thermal packs, and oral splints. However, few, if any, of these therapies have been unequivocally proven in controlled trials.
- Studies comparing the efficacy of different therapies for both TMD and prophylaxis against TMD suggest that tricylic compounds (e.g., amitriptyline, cyclobenzaprine) may be slightly more effective than NSAIDs, which are somewhat more effective than local therapies (e.g., occlusal splints).
- Psychological factors play a role in symptom expression in these conditions, and therapies such as cognitive-behavioral therapy could be helpful as a primary or adjunct management strategy.

REFERENCES

1. Goadsby PJ, Headache Classification Subcommittee of the International Headache Society. The international classification of headache disorders. *Cephalalgia* 2004;24(Suppl. 1): 24–136.
2. Sharav Y, Benoliel R. Primary vascular-type craniofacial pain. *Compend Contin Educ Dent* 2001;22(2):119–122,124–126, 128.
3. Benoliel R, Sharav Y. Craniofacial pain of myofascial origin: temporomandibular pain & tension-type headache. *Compend Contin Educ Dent* 1998;19(7):701–704,706,708–710.
4. Benoliel R, Sharav Y. Neuropathic orofacial pain. *Compend Contin Educ Dent* 1998;19(11):1099–1102,1104.
5. Dworkin SF, LeResche L. Research diagnostic criteria for temporomandibular disorders: review, criteria, examinations and specifications [Critique]. *J Craniomandib Disord* 1992; 6(4):301–355.
6. Okeson JP, The American Academy of Orofacial Pain. *Orofacial pain: guidelines for assessment, classification, and management.* Chicago, IL: Quintessence Publishing, 1996.
7. LeResche L. Epidemiology of temporomandibular disorders: implications for the investigation of etiologic factors. *Crit Rev Oral Biol Med* 1997;8(3):291–305.
8. McNeill C. History and evolution of TMD concepts. *Oral Surg Oral Med Oral Pathol Oral Radiol Endod* 1997;83(1):51–60.
9. Greene CS, Marbach JJ. Epidemiologic studies of mandibular dysfunction: a critical review. *J Prosthet Dent* 1982; 48(2):184–190.
10. Solberg WK, Flint RT, Brantner JP. Temporomandibular joint pain and dysfunction: a clinical study of emotional and occlusal components. *J Prosthet Dent* 1972;28(4):412–422.
11. Ramfjord SP, Ash MM. *Occlusion*, 3rd ed. Philadelphia, PA: WB Saunders, 1983.
12. Dworkin SF, Burgess JA. Orofacial pain of psychogenic origin: current concepts and classification. *J Am Dent Assoc* 1987;115(4):565–571.
13. Costen JB. A syndrome of ear and sinus symptoms dependent upon disturbed function of the temporomandibular joint. *Ann Otol Rhinol Laryngol* 1934;43(1):1–15.
14. Merskey H, Bogduk N, International Association for the Study of Pain. *Classification of chronic pain: descriptions of chronic pain syndromes and definition of pain terms*, 2nd ed. Seattle, WA: IASP Press, 1994:68–71.
15. Eversole LR, Machado L. Temporomandibular joint internal derangements and associated neuromuscular disorders. *J Am Dent Assoc* 1985;110(1):69–79.

16. Westesson PL. Double-contrast arthrography and internal derangement of the temporomandibular joint. *Swed Dent J Suppl* 1982;13(Suppl):1–57.

17. Dolwick MF, Riggs RR. Diagnosis and treatment of internal derangements of the temporomandibular joint. *Dent Clin North Am* 1983;27(3):561–572.

18. Kopp S, Wenneberg B. Intra- and interobserver variability in the assessment of signs of disorder in the stomatognathic system. *Swed Dent J* 1983;7(6):239–246.

19. Carlsson GE, Egermark-Eriksson I, Magnusson T. Intra- and inter-observer variation in functional examination of the masticatory system. *Swed Dent J* 1980;4(5):187–194.

20. Dworkin SF, LeResche L, DeRouen T, et al. Assessing clinical signs of temporomandibular disorders: reliability of clinical examiners. *J Prosthet Dent* 1990;63(5):574–579.

21. Krauss H. *Clinical treatment of back and neck pain.* New York: McGraw-Hill, 1970:57–59.

22. Travell J, Simons D. *Myofascial pain and dysfunction: the trigger point manual.* Baltimore, MD: Williams & Wilkins, 1983:165–182.

23. Wright EF. Referred craniofacial pain patterns in patients with temporomandibular disorder. *J Am Dent Assoc* 2000;131(9):1307–1315.

24. Fricton JR, Kroening R, Haley D, et al. Myofascial pain syndrome of the head and neck: a review of clinical characteristics of 164 patients. *Oral Surg Oral Med Oral Pathol* 1985;60(6):615–623.

25. Campbell SM. Regional myofascial pain syndromes. *Rheum Dis Clin North Am* 1989;15(1):31–44.

26. Gerschman JA, Reade PC, Hall W, et al. Lateralization of facial pain, emotionality and affective disturbance. *Pain* 1990;41(Suppl. 1):S19.

27. Perry HT Jr. The symptomology of temporomandibular joint disturbance. *J Prosthet Dent* 1968;19(3):288–298.

28. Laskin DM. Etiology of the pain-dysfunction syndrome. *J Am Dent Assoc* 1969;79(1):147–153.

29. Travell J. Referred pain from skeletal muscle; the pectoralis major syndrome of breast pain and soreness and the sternomastoid syndrome of headache and dizziness. *N Y State J Med* 1955;55(3):331–340.

30. Schwartz L. *Disorders of the temporomandibular joint.* Philadelphia, PA: WB Saunders, 1959:223–231.

31. Gelb H, Tarte J. A two-year clinical dental evaluation of 200 cases of chronic headache: the craniocervical-mandibular syndrome. *J Am Dent Assoc* 1975;91(6):1230–1236.

32. Sharav Y, Tzukert A, Refaeli B. Muscle pain index in relation to pain, dysfunction, and dizziness associated with the myofascial pain-dysfunction syndrome. *Oral Surg Oral Med Oral Pathol* 1978;46(6):742–747.

33. Blasberg B, Chalmers A. Temporomandibular pain and dysfunction syndrome associated with generalized musculoskeletal pain: a retrospective study. *J Rheumatol Suppl* 1989;19:87–90.

34. Block SL. Possible etiology of ear stuffiness (barohypoacusis) in MPD syndrome. *J Dent Res* 1976;55(752):B250.

35. Butler JH, Folke LE, Bandt CL. A descriptive survey of signs and symptoms associated with the myofascial pain-dysfunction syndrome. *J Am Dent Assoc* 1975;90(3):635–639.

36. Jaaskelainen SK. Clinical neurophysiology and quantitative sensory testing in the investigation of orofacial pain and sensory function. *J Orofac Pain* 2004;18(2):85–107.

37. De Laat A, Svensson P, Macaluso GM. Are jaw and facial reflexes modulated during clinical or experimental orofacial pain? *J Orofac Pain* 1998;12(4):260–271.

38. Yemm R. Neurophysiological studies of temporomandibular joint dysfunction. In: Zarb GA, Carlsson GE, eds. *The temporomandibular joint.* Copenhagen: Munksgaard, 1979:215–237.

39. Dubner R, Sessle BJ, Storey AT. *The neural basis of oral facial function.* New York: Plenum, 1978:160–171.

40. Lund JP, Donga R, Widmer CG, et al. The pain-adaptation model: a discussion of the relationship between chronic musculoskeletal pain and motor activity. *Can J Physiol Pharmacol* 1991;69(5):683–694.

41. Lund JP, Lamarre Y, Lavigne G, et al. Human jaw reflexes. *Adv Neurol* 1983;39:739–755.

42. Cruccu G, Frisardi G, van Steenberghe D. Side asymmetry of the jaw jerk in human craniomandibular dysfunction. *Arch Oral Biol* 1992;37(4):257–262.

43. Bessette R, Bishop B, Mohl N. Duration of masseteric silent period in patients with TMJ syndrome. *J Appl Physiol* 1971;30(6):864–869.

44. Bailey JO Jr, McCall WD Jr, Ash MM Jr. Electromyographic silent periods and jaw motion parameters: quantitative measures of temporomandibular joint dysfunction. *J Dent Res* 1977;56(3):249–253.

45. Widmalm SE. The silent period in the masseter muscle of patients with TMJ dysfunction. *Acta Odontol Scand* 1976;34(1):43–52.

46. Zulqarnain BJ, Furuya R, Hedegard B, et al. The silent period in the masseter and the anterior temporalis muscles in adult patients with mild or moderate mandibular dysfunction symptoms. *J Oral Rehabil* 1989;16(2):127–137.

47. Sharav Y, McGrath PA, Dubner R. Masseter inhibitory periods and sensations evoked by electrical tooth pulp stimulation in patients with oral-facial pain and mandibular dysfunction. *Arch Oral Biol* 1982;27(4):305–310.

48. Munro RR. Electromyography of the masseter and anterior temporalis muscles in the open-close-clench cycle in temporomandibular joint dysfunction. *Monogr Oral Sci* 1975;4:117–125.

49. Glaros AG, McGlynn FD, Kapel L. Sensitivity, specificity, and the predictive value of facial electromyographic data in diagnosing myofascial pain-dysfunction. *Cranio* 1989;7(3):189–193.

50. Nielsen IL, McNeill C, Danzig W, et al. Adaptation of craniofacial muscles in subjects with craniomandibular disorders. *Am J Orthod Dentofacial Orthop* 1990;97(1):20–34.

51. Eliav E, Teich S, Nitzan D, et al. Facial arthralgia and myalgia: can they be differentiated by trigeminal sensory assessment? *Pain* 2003;104(3):481–490.

52. Hagberg C, Hellsing G, Hagberg M. Perception of cutaneous electrical stimulation in patients with craniomandibular disorders. *J Craniomandib Disord* 1990;4(2):120–125.

53. Vecchiet L, Giamberardino MA, Saggini R. Myofascial pain syndromes: clinical and pathophysiological aspects. *Clin J Pain* 1991;7(Suppl. 1):S16–S22.

54. Bendtsen L, Jensen R, Olesen J. Decreased pain detection and tolerance thresholds in chronic tension-type headache. *Arch Neurol* 1996;53(4):373–376.

55. Stohler CS, Kowalski CJ, Lund JP. Muscle pain inhibits cutaneous touch perception. *Pain* 2001;92(3):327–333.

56. Mongini F, Caselli C, Macri V, et al. Thermographic findings in cranio-facial pain. *Headache* 1990;30(8):497–504.

57. Dworkin SF, Huggins KH, LeResche L, et al. Epidemiology of signs and symptoms in temporomandibular disorders: clinical signs in cases and controls. *J Am Dent Assoc* 1990;120(3):273–281.

58. Rugh JD, Solberg WK. Psychological implications in temporomandibular pain and dysfunction. In: Zarb GA, Carlsson GE, eds. *The temporomandibular joint.* Copenhagen: Munksgaard, 1979:239–268.

59. LeResche L, Dworkin SF, Sommers EE, et al. An epidemiologic evaluation of two diagnostic classification schemes for temporomandibular disorders. *J Prosthet Dent* 1991;65(1):131–137.

60. Agerberg G, Carlsson GE. Functional disorders of the masticatory system. I. Distribution of symptoms according to age

and sex as judged from investigation by questionnaire. *Acta Odontol Scand* 1972;30:597–613.

61. Rugh JD, Solberg WK. Oral health status in the United States: temporomandibular disorders. *J Dent Educ* 1985; 49(6):398–406.

62. Locker D, Slade G. Prevalence of symptoms associated with temporomandibular disorders in a Canadian population. *Commun Dent Oral Epidemiol* 1988;16(5):310–313.

63. Wanman A, Agerberg G. Two-year longitudinal study of symptoms of mandibular dysfunction in adolescents. *Acta Odontol Scand* 1986;44(6):321–331.

64. Wanman A, Agerberg G. Two-year longitudinal study of signs of mandibular dysfunction in adolescents. *Acta Odontol Scand* 1986;44(6):333–342.

65. Magnusson T, Egermark I, Carlsson GE. A longitudinal epidemiologic study of signs and symptoms of temporomandibular disorders from 15 to 35 years of age. *J Orofac Pain* 2000; 14(4):310–319.

66. Solberg WK, Woo MW, Houston JB. Prevalence of mandibular dysfunction in young adults. *J Am Dent Assoc* 1979;98(1): 25–34.

67. Helkimo M. Epidemiologic surveys of dysfunction of the masticatory system. In: Zarb GA, Carlsson GE, eds. *The temporomandibular joint*. Copenhagen: Munksgaard, 1979:175–192.

68. Nielsen L, Melsen B, Terp S. Prevalence, interrelation, and severity of signs of dysfunction from masticatory system in 14-16-year-old Danish children. *Commun Dent Oral Epidemiol* 1989;17(2):91–96.

69. Tervonen T, Knuuttila M. Prevalence of signs and symptoms of mandibular dysfunction among adults aged 25, 35, 50 and 65 years in Ostrobothnia, Finland. *J Oral Rehabil* 1988; 15(5):455–463.

70. Carlsson GE. Symptoms of mandibular dysfunction in complete denture wearers. *J Dent* 1976;4(6):265–270.

71. Agerberg G. Mandibular function and dysfunction in complete denture wearers—a literature review. *J Oral Rehabil* 1988;15(3):237–249.

72. Christensen LV. Facial pains and the jaw muscles: a review. *J Oral Rehabil* 1981;8(3):193–201.

73. List T, Wahlund K, Wenneberg B, et al. TMD in children and adolescents: prevalence of pain, gender differences, and perceived treatment need. *J Orofac Pain* 1999;13(1):9–20.

74. Bendtsen L. Sensitization: its role in primary headache. *Curr Opin Investig Drugs* 2002;3(3):449–453.

75. Mense S. The pathogenesis of muscle pain. *Curr Pain Headache Rep* 2003;7(6):419–425.

76. Svensson P, Arendt-Nielsen L, Nielsen H, et al. Effect of chronic and experimental jaw muscle pain on pain-pressure thresholds and stimulus-response curves. *J Orofac Pain* 1995;9(4):347–356.

77. Svensson P, List T, Hector G. Analysis of stimulus-evoked pain in patients with myofascial temporomandibular pain disorders. *Pain* 2001;92(3):399–409.

78. Graven-Nielsen T, Mense S. The peripheral apparatus of muscle pain: evidence from animal and human studies. *Clin J Pain* 2001;17(1):2–10.

79. Svensson P, Graven-Nielsen T. Craniofacial muscle pain: review of mechanisms and clinical manifestations. *J Orofac Pain* 2001;15(2):117–145.

80. Sessle BJ. The neural basis of temporomandibular joint and masticatory muscle pain. *J Orofac Pain* 1999;13(4): 238–245.

81. Epker J, Gatchel RJ, Ellis E III. A model for predicting chronic TMD: practical application in clinical settings. *J Am Dent Assoc* 1999;130(10):1470–1475.

82. Garofalo JP, Gatchel RJ, Wesley AL, et al. Predicting chronicity in acute temporomandibular joint disorders using the research diagnostic criteria. *J Am Dent Assoc* 1998; 129(4):438–447.

83. John MT, Miglioretti DL, LeResche L, et al. Widespread pain as a risk factor for dysfunctional temporomandibular disorder pain. *Pain* 2003;102(3):257–263.

84. Sarlani E, Grace EG, Reynolds MA, et al. Evidence for up-regulated central nociceptive processing in patients with masticatory myofascial pain. *J Orofac Pain* 2004;18(1): 41–55.

85. Sarlani E, Greenspan JD. Evidence for generalized hyperalgesia in temporomandibular disorders patients. *Pain* 2003; 102(3):221–226.

86. Maixner W, Sigurdsson A, Fillingham RB, et al. Regulation of acute and chronic orofacial pain. In: Fricton JR, Dubner R eds. *Orofacial pain and temporomandibular disorders*. Seattle, WA: IASP press, 1995:85–102.

87. Greene, CS. The etiology of temporomandibular disorders: implications for treatment. *J Orofac Pain* 2001;15(2):93–105; discussion 106–116.

88. Pullinger AG, Seligman DA. Trauma history in diagnostic groups of temporomandibular disorders. *Oral Surg Oral Med Oral Pathol* 1991;71(5):529–534.

89. Benoliel R, Eliav E, Elishoov H, et al. Diagnosis and treatment of persistent pain after trauma to the head and neck. *J Oral Maxillofac Surg* 1994;52(11):1138–1147; discussion 1147–1148.

90. Scholte AM, Steenks MH, Bosman F. Characteristics and treatment outcome of diagnostic subgroups of CMD patients: retrospective study. *Commun Dent Oral Epidemiol* 1993;21(4):215–220.

91. Friden J, Sjostrom M, Ekblom B. A morphological study of delayed muscle soreness. *Experientia* 1981;37(5): 506–507.

92. Friden J, Sjostrom M, Ekblom B. Myofibrillar damage following intense eccentric exercise in man. *Int J Sports Med* 1983;4(3):170–176.

93. Brendstrup P. Late edema after muscular exercise. *Arch Phys Med Rehabil* 1962;43:401–405.

94. Jones DA, Newham DJ, Clarkson PM. Skeletal muscle stiffness and pain following eccentric exercise of the elbow flexors. *Pain* 1987;30(2):233–242.

95. Friden J. Muscle soreness after exercise: implications of morphological changes. *Int J Sports Med* 1984;5(2):57–66.

96. Stauber WT, Fritz VK, Vogelbach DW, et al. Characterization of muscles injured by forced lengthening. I. Cellular infiltrates. *Med Sci Sports Exerc* 1988;20(4):345–353.

97. Fritz VK, Stauber WT. Characterization of muscles injured by forced lengthening. II. Proteoglycans. *Med Sci Sports Exerc* 1988;20(4):354–361.

98. Armstrong RB, Ogilvie RW, Schwane JA. Eccentric exercise-induced injury to rat skeletal muscle. *J Appl Physiol* 1983;54(1):80–93.

99. Moller E, Sheik-Ol-Eslam A, Lous I. Deliberate relaxation of the temporal and masseter muscles in subjects with functional disorders of the chewing apparatus. *Scand J Dent Res* 1971;79(7):478–482.

100. Lund JP, Stohler CS. Effects of pain on muscular activity in temporomandibular disorders and related conditions. In: Stohler CS, Carlson DS, eds. *Biological and psychological aspects of orofacial pain*. Ann Arbor, MI: University of Michigan, 1994:74–91.

101. Svensson P, Arendt-Nielsen L, Houe L. Sensory-motor interactions of human experimental unilateral jaw muscle pain: a quantitative analysis. *Pain* 1996;64(2):241–249.

102. Turp JC, Schindler HJ, Pritsch M, et al. Antero-posterior activity changes in the superficial masseter muscle after exposure to experimental pain. *Eur J Oral Sci* 2002;110(2): 83–91.

103. Shiau YY, Peng CC, Wen SC, et al. The effects of masseter muscle pain on biting performance. *J Oral Rehabil* 2003; 30(10):978–984.

104. Molin C. Vertical isometric muscle forces of the mandible. A comparative study of subjects with and without manifest mandibular pain dysfunction syndrome. *Acta Odontol Scand* 1972;30(4):485–499.

105. Christensen LV. Facial pain and internal pressure of masseter muscle in experimental bruxism in man. *Arch Oral Biol* 1971;16(9):1021–1031.

106. Moller E, Rasmussen BK, Bonde-Peterson F. Mechanism of ischemic pain in human muscles of mastication: pressure, EMG, force and blood flow of the temporal and masseter muscles during biting. In: Bonica JJ, ed. *Advances in pain research and therapy*. New York: Raven Press, 1979.

107. Clark GT, Adler RC, Lee JJ. Jaw pain and tenderness levels during and after repeated sustained maximum voluntary protrusion. *Pain* 1991;45(1):17–22.

108. Christensen LV. Facial pain from the masticatory system induced by experimental bruxism: a preliminary report. *Tandlaegebladet* 1967;71(12):1171–1181.

109. Christensen LV. Facial pain from experimental tooth clenching. *Tandlaegebladet* 1970;74(2):175–182.

110. Christensen LV. Some subjective-experiential parameters in experimental tooth clenching in man. *J Oral Rehabil* 1979; 6(2):119–136.

111. Christensen LV. Some electromyographic parameters of experimental tooth clenching in adult human subjects. *J Oral Rehabil* 1980;7(2):139–146.

112. Christensen LV. Effects of an occlusal splint on integrated electromyography of masseter muscle in experimental tooth clenching in man. *J Oral Rehabil* 1980;7(4):281–288.

113. Christensen LV. Progressive jaw muscle fatigue of experimental tooth clenching in man. *J Oral Rehabil* 1981;8(5): 413–420.

114. Scott DS, Lundeen TF. Myofascial pain involving the masticatory muscles: an experimental model. *Pain* 1980;8(2): 207–215.

115. Clark GT, Beemsterboer PL, Jacobson R. The effect of sustained submaximal clenching on maximum bite force in myofascial pain dysfunction patients. *J Oral Rehabil* 1984; 11(4):387–391.

116. Bowley JF, Gale EN. Experimental masticatory muscle pain. *J Dent Res* 1987;66(12):1765–1769.

117. Gibbs CH, Mahan PE, Wilkinson TM, et al. EMG activity of the superior belly of the lateral pterygoid muscle in relation to other jaw muscles. *J Prosthet Dent* 1984;51(5):691–702.

118. Wood WW. Medial pterygoid muscle activity during chewing and clenching. *J Prosthet Dent* 1986;55(5):615–621.

119. Wood WW, Takada K, Hannam AG. The electromyographic activity of the inferior part of the human lateral pterygoid muscle during clenching and chewing. *Arch Oral Biol* 1986; 31(4):245–253.

120. Kydd WL, Choy E, Daly C. Progressive jaw muscle fatigue and electromyogram activity produced by isometric unilateral biting. *Cranio* 1986;4(1):17–21.

121. Choy E, Kydd WL. Bite force duration: a diagnostic procedure for mandibular dysfunction. *J Prosthet Dent* 1988; 60(3):365–368.

122. Graven-Nielsen T, Arendt-Nielsen L, Svensson P, et al. Quantification of local and referred muscle pain in humans after sequential i.m. injections of hypertonic saline. *Pain* 1997;69(1-2):111–117.

123. Graven-Nielsen T, Fenger-Gron LS, Svensson P, et al. Quantification of deep and superficial sensibility in saline-induced muscle pain—a psychophysical study. *Somatosens Mot Res* 1998;15(1):46–53.

124. Graven-Nielsen T, McArdle A, Phoenix J, et al. In vivo model of muscle pain: quantification of intramuscular chemical, electrical, and pressure changes associated with saline-induced muscle pain in humans. *Pain* 1997;69(1-2): 137–143.

125. Graven-Nielsen T, Arendt-Nielsen L, Svensson P, et al. Stimulus-response functions in areas with experimentally induced referred muscle pain—a psychophysical study. *Brain Res* 1997;744(1):121–128.

126. Babenko V, Graven-Nielsen T, Svensson P, et al. Experimental human muscle pain and muscular hyperalgesia induced by combinations of serotonin and bradykinin. *Pain* 1999; 82(1):1–8.

127. Babenko VV, Graven-Nielsen T, Svensson P, et al. Experimental human muscle pain induced by intramuscular injections of bradykinin, serotonin, and substance P. *Eur J Pain* 1999;3(2):93–102.

128. Ernberg M, Lundeberg T, Kopp S. Pain and allodynia/hyperalgesia induced by intramuscular injection of serotonin in patients with fibromyalgia and healthy individuals. *Pain* 2000; 85(1-2):31–39.

129. Jensen K, Tuxen C, Pedersen-Bjergaard U, et al. Pain and tenderness in human temporal muscle induced by bradykinin and 5-hydroxytryptamine. *Peptides* 1990;11(6): 1127–1132.

130. Marchettini P, Simone DA, Caputi G, et al. Pain from excitation of identified muscle nociceptors in humans. *Brain Res* 1996;740(1-2):109–116.

131. Krogh-Poulsen WG, Olsson A. Occlusal disharmonies and dysfunction of the stomatognathic system. *Dent Clin North Am* 1966;11:627–635.

132. Rugh JD, Barghi N, Drago CJ. Experimental occlusal discrepancies and nocturnal bruxism. *J Prosthet Dent* 1984; 51(4):548–553.

133. Mense S. Considerations concerning the neurobiological basis of muscle pain. *Can J Physiol Pharmacol* 1991;69(5): 610–616.

134. Forssell H, Kalso E, Koskela P, et al. Occlusal treatments in temporomandibular disorders: a qualitative systematic review of randomized controlled trials. *Pain* 1999;83(3): 549–560.

135. Forssell H and Kalso E. Application of principles of evidence-based medicine to occlusal treatment for temporomandibular disorders: are there lessons to be learned? *J Orofac Pain* 2004;18(1):9–22; discussion 23–32.

136. Glaros AG, Glass EG, Brockman D. Electromyographic data from TMD patients with myofascial pain and from matched control subjects: evidence for statistical, not clinical, significance. *J Orofac Pain* 1997;11(2):125–129.

137. Rugh JD, Harlan J. Nocturnal bruxism and temporomandibular disorders. *Adv Neurol* 1988;49:329–341.

138. Satoh T, Harada Y. Electrophysiological study on tooth-grinding during sleep. *Electroencephalogr Clin Neurophysiol* 1973;35(3):267–275.

139. Association ASD. *International classification of sleep disorders: diagnosis and coding manual*. Rochester MN: American Sleep Disorder Association, 1990:181–185.

140. Dettmar DM, Shaw RM, Tilley AJ. Tooth wear and bruxism: a sleep laboratory investigation. *Aust Dent J* 1987;32(6): 421–426.

141. Wieselmann G, Permann R, Korner E, et al. Distribution of muscle activity during sleep in bruxism. *Eur Neurol* 1986; 25(Suppl. 2):111–116.

142. Lavigne GJ, Velly-Miguel AM, Montplaisir J. Muscle pain, dyskinesia, and sleep. *Can J Physiol Pharmacol* 1991;69(5): 678–682.

143. Moldofsky H. Sleep and fibrositis syndrome. *Rheum Dis Clin North Am* 1989;15(1):91–103.

144. Kato T, Thie NM, Huynh N, et al. Topical review: sleep bruxism and the role of peripheral sensory influences. *J Orofac Pain* 2003;17(3):191–213.

145. Lavigne GJ, Kato T, Kolta A, et al. Neurobiological mechanisms involved in sleep bruxism. *Crit Rev Oral Biol Med* 2003;14(1):30–46.

146. Sessle BJ, Hu JW. Mechanisms of pain arising from articular tissues. *Can J Physiol Pharmacol* 1991;69(5):617–626.

147. Schiffman EL, Anderson GC, Fricton JR, et al. The relationship between level of mandibular pain and dysfunction and stage of temporomandibular joint internal derangement. *J Dent Res* 1992;71(11):1812–1815.

148. Broton JG, Sessle BJ. Reflex excitation of masticatory muscles induced by algesic chemicals applied to the temporomandibular joint of the cat. *Arch Oral Biol* 1988;33(10):741–747.

149. Merskey H. Chronic pain syndromes and their treatment. In: Kennard C, ed. *Recent advances in clinical neurology*. Edinburgh: Churchill Livingstone, 1988:87–107.

150. Stein S, Hart DL, Loft G, et al. Symptoms of TMJ dysfunction as related to stress measured by the social readjustment rating scale. *J Prosthet Dent* 1982;47(5):545–548.

151. Fearon CG, Serwatka WJ. Stress: a common denominator for nonorganic TMJ pain-dysfunction. *J Prosthet Dent* 1983; 49(6):805–808.

152. Feinmann C, Harris M. Psychogenic facial pain. Part 1: The clinical presentation. *Br Dent J* 1984;156(5):165–168.

153. Speculand B, Hughes AO, Goss AN. Role of recent stressful life events experience in the onset of TMJ dysfunction pain. *Commun Dent Oral Epidemiol* 1984;12(3):197–202.

154. Moody PM, Calhoun TC, Okeson JP, et al. Stress-pain relationship in MPD syndrome patients and non-MPD syndrome patients. *J Prosthet Dent* 1981;45(1):84–88.

155. Smythe HA. Problems with the MMPI. *J Rheumatol* 1984; 11(4):417–418.

156. Lundeen TF, Sturdevant JR, George JM. Stress as a factor in muscle and temporomandibular joint pain. *J Oral Rehabil* 1987;14(5):447–456.

157. Aaron LA, Buchwald D. Chronic diffuse musculoskeletal pain, fibromyalgia and co-morbid unexplained clinical conditions. *Best Pract Res Clin Rheumatol* 2003;17(4):563–574.

158. Aaron LA, Burke MM, Buchwald D. Overlapping conditions among patients with chronic fatigue syndrome, fibromyalgia, and temporomandibular disorder. *Arch Intern Med* 2000; 160(2):221–227.

159. Krogstad BS, Dahl BL, Eckersberg T, et al. Sex differences in signs and symptoms from masticatory and other muscles in 19-year-old individuals. *J Oral Rehabil* 1992; 19(5): 435–440.

160. Turp JC, Kowalski CJ, Stohler CS. Temporomandibular disorders—pain outside the head and face is rarely acknowledged in the chief complaint. *J Prosthet Dent* 1997;78(6): 592–595.

161. Vanderas AP, Menenakou M, Papagiannoulis L. Emotional stress and craniomandibular dysfunction in children. *Cranio* 2001;19(2):123–129.

162. Evaskus DS, Laskin DM. A biochemical measure of stress in patients with myofascial pain-dysfunction syndrome. *J Dent Res* 1972;51(5):1464–1466.

163. Clark GT, Rugh JD, Handelman SL. Nocturnal masseter muscle activity and urinary catecholamine levels in bruxers. *J Dent Res* 1980;59(10):1571–1576.

164. Marbach JJ, Lennon MC, Dohrenwend BP. Candidate risk factors for temporomandibular pain and dysfunction syndrome: psychosocial, health behavior, physical illness and injury. *Pain* 1988;34(2):139–151.

165. Perry HT, Lammie GA, Main J, et al. Occlusion in a stress situation. *J Am Dent Assoc* 1960;60:626–633.

166. Yemm R. Temporomandibular dysfunction and masseter muscle response to experimental stress. *Br Dent J* 1969; 127(11):508–510.

167. Haber JD, Moss RA, Kuczmierczyk AR, et al. Assessment and treatment of stress in myofascial pain-dysfunction syndrome: a model for analysis. *J Oral Rehabil* 1983;10(2): 187–196.

168. Moulton RE. Psychiatric considerations in maxillofacial pain. *J Am Dent Assoc* 1955;51(4):408–414.

169. Lascelles RG. Atypical facial pain and depression. *Br J Psychiatry* 1966;112(488):651–659.

170. Fine EW. Psychological factors associated with non-organic temporomandibular joint pain dysfunction syndrome. *Br Dent J* 1971;131(9):402–404.

171. Marbach JJ, Lipton JA, Lund PB, et al. Facial pains and anxiety levels: considerations for treatment. *J Prosthet Dent* 1978;40(4):434–437.

172. Marbach JJ, Lund P. Depression, anhedonia and anxiety in temporomandibular joint and other facial pain syndromes. *Pain* 1981;11(1):73–84.

173. Sharav Y, Singer E, Schmidt E, et al. The analgesic effect of amitriptyline on chronic facial pain. *Pain* 1987;31(2):199–209.

174. Salter M, Brooke RI, Merskey H, et al. Is the temporomandibular pain and dysfunction syndrome a disorder of the mind? *Pain* 1983;17(2):151–166.

175. Merskey H, Lau CL, Russell ES, et al. Screening for psychiatric morbidity. The pattern of psychological illness and premorbid characteristics in four chronic pain populations. *Pain* 1987;30(2):141–157.

176. Schnurr RF, Brooke RI, Rollman GB. Psychosocial correlates of temporomandibular joint pain and dysfunction. *Pain* 1990;42(2):153–165.

177. Uhl GR, Sora I, Wang Z. The mu opiate receptor as a candidate gene for pain: polymorphisms, variations in expression, nociception, and opiate responses. *Proc Natl Acad Sci USA* 1999;96(14):7752–7755.

178. Breslau N, Rasmussen BK. The impact of migraine: epidemiology, risk factors, and co-morbidities. *Neurology* 2001; 56(6 Suppl 1):S4–S12.

179. Rasmussen BK. Epidemiology of headache. *Cephalalgia* 1995;15(1):45–68.

180. Rauhala K, Oikarinen KS, Jarvelin MR, et al. Facial pain and temporomandibular disorders: an epidemiological study of the Northern Finland 1966 Birth Cohort. *Cranio* 2000;18(1): 40–46.

181. Yunus MB. Gender differences in fibromyalgia and other related syndromes. *J Gend Specif Med* 2002;5(2):42–47.

182. Jensen R, Rasmussen BK, Pedersen B, et al. Prevalence of oromandibular dysfunction in a general population. *J Orofac Pain* 1993;7(2):175–182.

183. Huang GJ, LeResche L, Critchlow CW, et al. Risk factors for diagnostic subgroups of painful temporomandibular disorders (TMD). *J Dent Res* 2002;81(4):284–288.

184. Fillingim RB, Maixner W, Kincaid S, et al. Sex differences in temporal summation but not sensory-discriminative processing of thermal pain. *Pain* 1998;75(1):121–127.

185. Fillingim RB, Ness TJ. Sex-related hormonal influences on pain and analgesic responses. *Neurosci Biobehav Rev* 2000; 24(4):485–501.

186. Dao TT, Knight K, Ton-That V. Modulation of myofascial pain by the reproductive hormones: a preliminary report. *J Prosthet Dent* 1998;79(6):663–670.

187. LeResche L, Saunders K, Von Korff MR, et al. Use of exogenous hormones and risk of temporomandibular disorder pain. *Pain* 1997;69(1-2):153–160.

188. Hatch JP, Rugh JD, Sakai S, et al. Is use of exogenous estrogen associated with temporomandibular signs and symptoms? *J Am Dent Assoc* 2001;132(3):319–326.

189. Phillips JM, Gatchel RJ, Wesley AL, et al. Clinical implications of sex in acute temporomandibular disorders. *J Am Dent Assoc* 2001;132(1):49–57.

190. Petty BG, Cornblath DR, Adornato BT, et al. The effect of systemically administered recombinant human nerve growth factor in healthy human subjects. *Ann Neurol* 1994;36(2): 244–246.

191. Gollapudi L, Oblinger MM. Estrogen and NGF synergistically protect terminally differentiated, ER alpha-transfected PC12 cells from apoptosis. *J Neurosci Res* 1999;56(5): 471–481.

192. Cairns BE, Sim Y, Bereiter DA, et al. Influence of sex on reflex jaw muscle activity evoked from the rat temporomandibular joint. *Brain Res* 2002;957(2):338–344.

193. Cairns BE, Gambarota G, Svensson P, et al. Glutamate-induced sensitization of rat masseter muscle fibers. *Neuroscience* 2002;109(2):389–399.

194. Benoliel R, Sharav Y, Tal M, et al. Management of chronic orofacial pain: today and tomorrow. *Compend Contin Educ Dent* 2003;24(12):909–920, 922–924, 926–928.

195. Feine JS, Widmer CG, Lund JP. Physical therapy: a critique. *Oral Surg Oral Med Oral Pathol Oral Radiol Endod* 1997; 83(1):123–127.

196. Michelotti A, Steenks MH, Farella M, et al. The additional value of a home physical therapy regimen versus patient education only for the treatment of myofascial pain of the jaw muscles: short term results of a randomized clinical trial. *J Orofac Pain* 2004;18(2):114–125.

197. De Laat A, Stappaerts K, Papy S. Counseling and physical therapy as treatment for myofascial pain of the masticatory system. *J Orofac Pain* 2003;17(1):42–49.

198. Di Fabio RP. Physical therapy for patients with TMD: a descriptive study of treatment, disability, and health status. *J Orofac Pain* 1998;12(2):124–135.

199. Selby A. Physiotherapy in the management of temporomandibular disorders. *Aust Dent J* 1985;30(4):273–280.

200. Murphy GJ. Physical medicine modalities and trigger point injections in the management of temporomandibular disorders and assessing treatment outcome. *Oral Surg Oral Med Oral Pathol Oral Radiol Endod* 1997;83(1): 118–122.

201. Ekberg EC, Vallon D, Nilner M. Occlusal appliance therapy in patients with temporomandibular disorders. A double-blind controlled study in a short-term perspective. *Acta Odontol Scand* 1998;56(2):122–128.

202. Ekberg E, Vallon D, Nilner M. The efficacy of appliance therapy in patients with temporomandibular disorders of mainly myogenous origin. A randomized, controlled, short-term trial. *J Orofac Pain* 2003;17(2):133–139.

203. Ekberg EC, Vallon D, Nilner M. Occlusal appliance therapy in patients with temporomandibular disorders. A double-blind controlled study in a short-term perspective. *Acta Odontol Scand* 1998;56(2):122–128.

204. Singer E, Sharav Y, Dubner R, et al. The efficacy of diazepam and ibuprofen in the treatment of chronic myofascial orofacial pain. *Pain* 1987;21(Suppl. 4):583.

205. Plesh O, Curtis D, Levine J, et al. Amitriptyline treatment of chronic pain in patients with temporomandibular disorders. *J Oral Rehabil* 2000;27(10):834–841.

206. Bendtsen L, Jensen R. Amitriptyline reduces myofascial tenderness in patients with chronic tension-type headache. *Cephalalgia* 2000;20(6):603–610.

207. Harkins S, Linford J, Cohen J, et al. Administration of clonazepam in the treatment of TMD and associated myofascial pain: a double-blind pilot study. *J Craniomandib Disord* 1991;5(3):179–186.

208. Herman CR, Schiffman EL, Look JO, et al. The effectiveness of adding pharmacologic treatment with clonazepam or cyclobenzaprine to patient education and self-care for the treatment of jaw pain upon awakening: a randomized clinical trial. *J Orofac Pain* 2002;16(1):64–70.

209. Moulin DE. Systemic drug treatment for chronic musculoskeletal pain. *Clin J Pain* 2001;17(Suppl. 4):S86–S93.

210. McCracken LM, Turk DC. Behavioral and cognitive-behavioral treatment for chronic pain: outcome, predictors of outcome, and treatment process. *Spine* 2002;27(22): 2564–2573.

211. Eisenberg DM, Kessler RC, Foster C, et al. Unconventional medicine in the United States. Prevalence, costs, and patterns of use. *N Engl J Med* 1993;328(4):246–252.

212. Turp JC, Kowalski CJ, Stohler CS. Treatment-seeking patterns of facial pain patients: many possibilities, limited satisfaction. *J Orofac Pain* 1998;12(1):61–66.

213. Myers CD, White BA, Heft MW. A review of complementary and alternative medicine use for treating chronic facial pain. *J Am Dent Assoc* 2002;133(9):1189–1196.

214. Melchart, D, Linde K, Fischer P, et al. *Acupuncture for idiopathic headache (Cochrane Review).* Oxford: The Cochrane Library, 2003, Update Software.

215. Magnusson T, Carlsson GE, Egermark I. Changes in subjective symptoms of craniomandibular disorders in children and adolescents during a 10-year period. *J Orofac Pain* 1993; 7(1):76–82.

216. Skeppar J, Nilner M. Treatment of craniomandibular disorders in children and young adults. *J Orofac Pain* 1993;7(4): 362–369.

217. Brown DT, Gaudet EL Jr. Outcome measurement for treated and untreated TMD patients using the TMJ scale. *Cranio* 1994;12(4):216–222.

218. Mejersjo C, Carlsson GE. Long-term results of treatment for temporomandibular joint pain-dysfunction. *J Prosthet Dent* 1983;49(6):809–815.

219. Okeson JP, Hayes DK. Long-term results of treatment for temporomandibular disorders: an evaluation by patients. *J Am Dent Assoc* 1986;112(4):473–478.

220. Gobel H, Petersen-Braun M, Soyka D. The epidemiology of headache in Germany: a nationwide survey of a representative sample on the basis of the headache classification of the International Headache Society. *Cephalalgia* 1994;14(2): 97–106.

221. Rasmussen BK, Jensen R, Schroll M, et al. Interrelations between migraine and tension-type headache in the general population. *Arch Neurol* 1992;49(9):914–918.

222. Rasmussen BK, Jensen R, Olesen J. A population-based analysis of the diagnostic criteria of the International Headache Society. *Cephalalgia* 1991;11(3):129–134.

223. Friedman AP. Characteristics of tension headache: a profile of 1,420 cases. *Psychosomatics* 1979;20(7):451–7–461.

224. Iversen HK, Langemark M, Andersson PG, et al. Clinical characteristics of migraine and episodic tension-type headache in relation to old and new diagnostic criteria. *Headache* 1990;30(8):514–519.

225. Langemark M, Olesen J, Poulsen DL, et al. Clinical characterization of patients with chronic tension headache. *Headache* 1988;28(9):590–596.

226. Jensen R and Olesen J. Initiating mechanisms of experimentally induced tension-type headache. *Cephalalgia* 1996; 16(3):175–182; discussion 138–139.

227. Jensen R, Bendtsen L, Olesen J. Muscular factors are of importance in tension-type headache. *Headache* 1998;38(1): 10–17.

228. Holroyd KA, Martin PR. Psychological treatments of tension-type headache. In: Olesen J, Tfelt-Hansen P, Welch KWA, eds. *The headaches.* Philadelphia, PA: Lippincott Williams & Wilkins, 2000.

229. Carlsson JY, Jensen R. Physiotherapy of tension-type headache. In: Olesen J, Tfelt-Hansen P, Welch KWA, eds. *The headaches.* Philadelphia, PA: Lippincott Williams & Wilkins, 2000.

230. Graff-Radford SB, Forssell H. Oromandibular treatment of tension-type headache. In: Olesen J, Tfelt-Hansen P, Welch KWA, eds. *The headaches.* Philadelphia, PA: Lippincott Williams & Wilkins, 2000.

231. Mathew NT, Scoenen J. Acute pharmacotherapy of tension-type headache. In Olesen J, Tfelt-Hansen P, Welch KWA, eds. *The headaches.* Philadelphia, PA: Lippincott Williams & Wilkins, 2000.

232. Schoenen J. Tension-type headache. In: Diener HC, ed. *Drug treatment of migraine and other headaches.* Basel: Karger, 2000:314–321.

233. Diamond S, Freitag FG. The use of ibuprofen plus caffeine to treat tension-type headache. *Curr Pain Headache Rep* 2001;5(5):472–478.

234. Tomkins GE, Jackson JL, O'Malley PG, et al. Treatment of chronic headache with antidepressants: a meta-analysis. *Am J Med* 2001;111(1):54–63.

235. Cerbo R, Barbanti P, Fabbrini G, et al. Amitriptyline is effective in chronic but not in episodic tension-type headache: pathogenetic implications. *Headache* 1998;38(6):453–457.

236. Stillman MJ. Pharmacotherapy of tension-type headaches. *Curr Pain Headache Rep* 2002;6(5):408–413.

237. Viswanathan V, Bridges SJ, Whitehouse W, et al. Childhood headaches: discrete entities or continuum? *Dev Med Child Neurol* 1998;40(8):544–550.

238. Schulman EA. Overview of tension-type headache. *Curr Pain Headache Rep* 2001;5(5):454–462.

239. Spierings EL. Headache continuum: concept and supporting evidence from recent study of chronic daily headache. *Clin J Pain* 2001;17(4):337–340.

240. Schade AJ. Quantitative assessment of the tension-type headache and migraine severity continuum. *Headache* 1997;37(10):646–653.

241. Nelson CF. The tension headache, migraine headache continuum: a hypothesis. *J Manipulative Physiol Ther* 1994;17(3):156–167.

242. Sharav Y, Benoliel R. Temporomandibular pain. In: Vaeroy H, Merskey H, eds. *Progress in fibromyalgia and myofascial pain.* Amsterdam: Elsevier Science, 1993:237–252.

243. Meyer HP. Myofascial pain syndrome and its suggested role in the pathogenesis and treatment of fibromyalgia syndrome. *Curr Pain Headache Rep* 2002;6(4):274–283.

244. Widmer CG. Chronic muscle pain syndromes: an overview. *Can J Physiol Pharmacol* 1991;69(5):659–661.

245. Magnusson T, Carlsson GE. Comparison between two groups of patients in respect of headache and mandibular dysfunction. *Swed Dent J* 1978;2(3):85–92.

246. Raskin NH, Appenzeller O. Headache. *Major Probl Intern Med* 1980;19:1–244.

247. Tfelt-Hansen P, Lous I, Olesen J. Prevalence and significance of muscle tenderness during common migraine attacks. *Headache* 1981;21(2):49–54.

248. Watts PG, Peet KM, Juniper RP. Migraine and the temporomandibular joint: the final answer? *Br Dent J* 1986;161(5):170–173.

249. Dexter JD, Weitzman ED. The relationship of nocturnal headaches to sleep stage patterns. *Neurology* 1970;20(5):513–518.

250. Ware JC, Rugh JD. Destructive bruxism: sleep stage relationship. *Sleep* 1988;11(2):172–181.

251. Henriksson KG, Bengtsson A. Fibromyalgia—a clinical entity? *Can J Physiol Pharmacol* 1991;69(5):672–677.

252. Graff-Radford SB, Newman AC. The role of temporomandibular disorders and cervical dysfunction in tension-type headache. *Curr Pain Headache Rep* 2002;6(5):387–391.

253. Ciancaglini R, Radaelli G. The relationship between headache and symptoms of temporomandibular disorder in the general population. *J Dent* 2001;29(2):93–98.

254. Pettengill C. A comparison of headache symptoms between two groups: a TMD group and a general dental practice group. *Cranio* 1999;17(1):64–69.

255. Vazquez-Delgado E, Schmidt J, Carlson C, et al. Psychological and sleep quality differences between chronic daily headache and temporomandibular disorders patients. *Cephalalgia* 2004;24(6):446–454.

256. Okifuji A, Turk DC, Marcus DA. Comparison of generalized and localized hyperalgesia in patients with recurrent headache and fibromyalgia. *Psychosom Med* 1999;61(6):771–780.

257. Peres MFP, Kaup A, Zukerman OE, et al. Fibromyalgia and chronic daily headache. *Cephalalgia* 2000;20(4):302–303.

258. Hagen K, Einarsen C, Zwart JA, et al. The co-occurrence of headache and musculoskeletal symptoms amongst 51,050 adults in Norway. *Eur J Neurol* 2002;9(5):527–533.

259. Blau JN, MacGregor EA. Migraine and the neck. *Headache* 1994;34(2):88–90.

260. Lipchik GL, Holroyd KA, Talbot F, et al. Pericranial muscle tenderness and exteroceptive suppression of temporalis muscle activity: a blind study of chronic tension-type headache. *Headache* 1997;37(6):368–376.

261. Hagberg C. General musculoskeletal complaints in a group of patients with craniomandibular disorders (CMD). A case control study. *Swed Dent J* 1991;15(4):179–185.

262. Goldenberg DL, Simms RW, Geiger A, et al. High frequency of fibromyalgia in patients with chronic fatigue seen in a primary care practice. *Arthritis Rheum* 1990;33(3):381–387.

263. Buchwald D, Garrity D. Comparison of patients with chronic fatigue syndrome, fibromyalgia, and multiple chemical sensitivities. *Arch Intern Med* 1994;154(18):2049–2053.

264. Hudson JI, Goldenberg DL, Pope HG Jr, et al. Comorbidity of fibromyalgia with medical and psychiatric disorders. *Am J Med* 1992;92(4):363–367.

265. Wysenbeek AJ, Shapira Y, Leibovici L. Primary fibromyalgia and the chronic fatigue syndrome. *Rheumatol Int* 1991;10(6):227–229.

266. Hedenberg-Magnusson B, Ernberg M, Kopp S. Symptoms and signs of temporomandibular disorders in patients with fibromyalgia and local myalgia of the temporomandibular system. A comparative study. *Acta Odontol Scand* 1997;55(6):344–349.

267. Plesh O, Wolfe F, Lane N. The relationship between fibromyalgia and temporomandibular disorders: prevalence and symptom severity. *J Rheumatol* 1996;23(11):1948–1952.

268. Rhodus NL, Fricton J, Carlson P, et al. Oral symptoms associated with fibromyalgia syndrome. *J Rheumatol* 2003;30(8):1841–1845.

269. Crofford LJ, Clauw DJ. Fibromyalgia: where are we a decade after the American College of Rheumatology classification criteria were developed? *Arthritis Rheum* 2002;46(5):1136–1138.

270. Wolfe F. Stop using the American College of Rheumatology criteria in the clinic. *J Rheumatol* 2003;30(8):1671–1672.

271. Wolfe F, Smythe HA, Yunus MB, et al. The American College of Rheumatology 1990 criteria for the classification of fibromyalgia. Report of the Multicenter Criteria Committee. *Arthritis Rheum* 1990;33(2):160–172.

272. Scudds RA, Trachsel LC, Luckhurst BJ, et al. A comparative study of pain, sleep quality and pain responsiveness in fibrositis and myofascial pain syndrome. *J Rheumatol Suppl* 1989;19:120–126.

273. Wolfe F. Fibrositis, fibromyalgia, and musculoskeletal disease: the current status of the fibrositis syndrome. *Arch Phys Med Rehabil* 1988;69(7):527–531.

274. Sheon RP. Regional myofascial pain and the fibrositis syndrome (fibromyalgia). *Compr Ther* 1986;12(9):42–52.

275. Simons DG. Myofascial pain syndrome due to trigger points. In: Goodgold J, ed. *Rehabilitation medicine.* St Louis, MO: Mosby, 1988:686–723.

276. Thompson JM. Tension myalgia as a diagnosis at the Mayo Clinic and its relationship to fibrositis, fibromyalgia, and myofascial pain syndrome. *Mayo Clin Proc* 1990;65(9): 1237–1248.

277. Bennett RM. Current issues concerning management of the fibrositis/fibromyalgia syndrome. *Am J Med* 1986;81(3A): 15–18.

278. Maixner W, Fillingim R, Sigurdsson A, et al. Sensitivity of patients with painful temporomandibular disorders to experimentally evoked pain: evidence for altered temporal summation of pain. *Pain* 1998;76(1-2):71–81.

279. Fillingim RB, Fillingim LA, Hollins M, et al. Generalized vibrotactile allodynia in a patient with temporomandibular disorder. *Pain* 1998;78(1):75–78.

280. McCain GA, Scudds RA. The concept of primary fibromyalgia (fibrositis): clinical value, relation and significance to other chronic musculoskeletal pain syndromes. *Pain* 1988; 33(3):273–287.

281. Eriksson PO, Lindman R, Stal P, et al. Symptoms and signs of mandibular dysfunction in primary fibromyalgia syndrome (PSF) patients. *Swed Dent J* 1988;12(4): 141–149.

282. Raphael KG, Marbach JJ, Klausner J. Myofascial face pain. Clinical characteristics of those with regional vs. widespread pain. *J Am Dent Assoc* 2000;131(2):161–171.

283. Raphael KG, Marbach JJ. Widespread pain and the effectiveness of oral splints in myofascial face pain. *J Am Dent Assoc* 2001;132(3):305–316.

284. Moskowitz MA, Buzzi MG, Sakas DE, et al. Pain mechanisms underlying vascular headaches. Progress Report 1989. *Rev Neurol (Paris)* 1989;145(3):181–193.

285. Dostrovsky JO, Davis KD, Kawakita K. Central mechanisms of vascular headaches. *Can J Physiol Pharmacol* 1991; 69(5):652–658.

286. Basbaum AI, Levine JD. The contribution of the nervous system to inflammation and inflammatory disease. *Can J Physiol Pharmacol* 1991;69(5):647–651.

287. Benoliel R, Eliav E, Tal M. No sympathetic nerve sprouting in rat trigeminal ganglion following painful and non-painful infraorbital nerve neuropathy. *Neurosci Lett* 2001;297(3): 151–154.

14

Psychosocial Factors in Fibromyalgia

Laurence A. Bradley and Graciela S. Alarcón

Fibromyalgia (FM) is a chronic disorder characterized by persistent, widespread pain and abnormal pain sensitivity in response to a wide array of stimuli such as mechanical pressure, cold, heat, and ischemia (1,2). Individuals with FM also show a substantial number of other "medically unexplained" symptoms, including fatigue, sleep disturbance, impairments in attention and other cognitive functions, stiffness of muscles and joints, and subjective joint swelling. A large number of studies of patients recruited from tertiary care settings have shown that these individuals are characterized by relatively high levels of anxiety, depression, or other forms of emotional distress, as well as a large number of lifetime psychiatric diagnoses (3–5). In addition, patients with FM seen at tertiary care centers are characterized by high levels of health service utilization and medication usage. For example, patients undergo an average of nearly one radiographic examination and 2.5 laboratory evaluations per year, and they tend to undergo more surgical procedures than rheumatology patients with inflammatory disease and other "nonfibromyalgia" illnesses [e.g., back and neck surgery, abdominal surgery, gynecologic surgery (6,7)].

It has been shown that patients with FM are characterized by high levels of psychological distress and that additional psychosocial factors, such as stressful life events, as well as clinical pain intensity, are associated with seeking health care from physicians and complementary or alternative medicine practitioners (8,9). As a consequence, some health care providers and investigators view patients with FM as (a) hypervigilant about common, unpleasant sensory experiences or (b) somatizers who seek to "medicalize" their symptoms (10). In other words, they consider FM to be a functional somatic syndrome in which pain and other symptoms are magnified and perpetuated by patients' beliefs that they are due to a serious disease or condition that may eventually have a catastrophic outcome (10).

This book provides substantial and replicable evidence that FM is associated with abnormalities in several physiologic systems (e.g., neuroendocrine axes) that may contribute to abnormal pain perception as well as fatigue, sleep disturbance, cognitive dysfunction, and functional disability. Nevertheless, in order to best understand patients with FM and develop optimal treatments for them, it is critical to understand the psychosocial factors that interact with physiologic abnormalities and thus produce the symptoms and behavior of individuals with FM. This chapter will first present a model of abnormal pain sensitivity and behavior that acknowledges that a wide array of biologic and psychosocial variables influence pain perception and pain-related behavior. The key construct in this model, termed the body-self neuromatrix, provides a theoretical context for evaluating empirical evidence concerning the role of psychosocial variables in FM. The chapter will then review our present understanding of three important areas concerning the influence of psychosocial factors on the behavior and health status of patients with FM. First, it will examine the evidence concerning the extent to which psychosocial factors influence pain responses or other behaviors of persons with FM in controlled laboratory conditions. It then will evaluate the extent to which psychosocial factors, such as major stressful life events, may contribute to the development of FM. Finally, the chapter will examine the current literature concerning the extent to which psychosocial variables may contribute to treatment-related outcomes in pain and other dimensions of health status among patients with FM. This portion of the chapter will devote specific attention to relatively new psychosocial constructs in this area that are relevant to outcomes such as fear of pain and readiness to change.

THE BODY-SELF NEUROMATRIX

All current models of the etiopathogenesis of FM posit that a complex interaction between central and peripheral factors is responsible for producing the high levels of pain and abnormal pain sensitivity that characterize FM (11–13). Although a thorough discussion of these models is beyond the scope of this chapter, it is important to note that all the models are consistent with Melzack's recent revision of the gate control theory of pain transmission and modulation (14).

The revised theory is consistent with our current conceptualization of pain as a multidimensional, unpleasant experience that is associated with tissue damage or is described in terms of such damage. It suggests that multiple endogenous and exogenous influences may alter pain perception. The theory posits that the activity of a network of brain pathways linking the thalamus, cortex, and limbic system forms a neuromatrix that generates patterns of neural activity. The synaptic links within this network initially are genetically determined, but over time they are shaped by sensory input. This pattern-generating mechanism underlies the awareness that one's body is distinct from the environment (i.e., "self") as well as perceptions of pain and pain behavior. In addition, the mechanism underlies stress-regulation functions of the central nervous system (CNS), including hypothalamic-pituitary-adrenal (HPA) axis activity, immune function, and the release of endorphins as well as proinflammatory and anti-inflammatory cytokines in peripheral soft tissues and the CNS.

Figure 14-1 shows that the function of the neuromatrix is influenced by multiple inputs, including (a) endocrine, immune, and autonomic system activity; (b) sources of afferent input (somatosensory, viscerosensory); (c) medullary descending inhibition; (d) pathologic input (e.g., from damaged afferents or musculoskeletal defects); (e) CNS plasticity (e.g., central sensitization); (f) attention; and (g) psychosocial and health status factors (e.g., environmental stressors, depression, anxiety, coping strategies). In addition, pain perception, pain behavior, and stress-regulation functions may influence one another as well as the inputs noted above. For example, coping strategies may influence attention and thus alter pain perception through effects on limbic system activity. Moreover, any factor (e.g., change in sex-related hormones, treatment interventions) that changes the function of pain transmission or pain modulation pathways within the neuromatrix may influence pain sensitivity. Therefore, it is possible for psychosocial variables to contribute to variations in pain sensitivity, overt behavior, or stress regulation over brief time periods, such as a laboratory experiment in which an investigator assesses participants' ratings of the intensity and unpleasantness of thermal heat under different experimental conditions. We will examine the results of this type of experiment in the next section of this chapter. Moreover, the model also suggests that psychosocial variables, such as repeated or prolonged exposure to stressors, may produce profound changes in one or more of the inputs that influence the function of the neuromatrix. These changes may evoke relatively stable changes in pain perception and behavior as well as in stress-regulation function. We will examine the evidence concerning the influence of psychosocial variables on the development of the widespread pain and abnormal pain sensitivity associated with FM and alterations in health status later in this chapter.

INFLUENCE OF ALTERATIONS IN COGNITION AND AFFECT ON LABORATORY-BASED MEASURES OF PAIN SENSITIVITY

Numerous studies have shown that persons with FM display generalized tenderness in response to pressure stimulation of both tender points (TePs) in muscle tissue and a wide array of "control" points such as the midulna, midtibia, and the thumbnail (15–19). Persons with FM exhibit the same levels of tenderness whether they have sought medical treatment for their symptoms or not (16,17). These individuals also show relatively low pain thresholds and tolerance levels in response to thermal heat and cold as well as electrocutaneous stimulation (20–22). Staud et al. have produced an elegant series of studies that have shown that persons with FM, compared to controls, report higher levels of "second pain" in response to phasic thermal and mechanical stimulation (23–25). In addition, the perceptions of second pain, or "windup," decay much more slowly among the patients with FM after the stimulation is terminated. These studies suggest that the mechanism underlying abnormal windup responses involves CNS hyperexcitability of spinal dorsal horn neurons produced by central sensitization. Moreover, these alterations in pain responses are observed independently of confounding

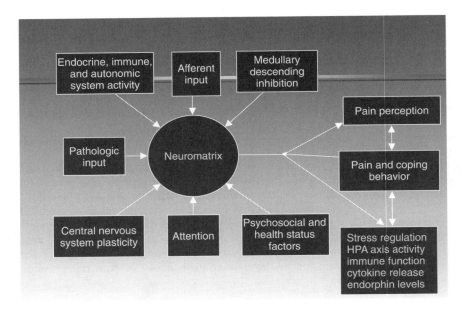

Figure 14-1. Model of the body-self neuromatrix. The neuromatrix is a construct that represents a widespread network of brain pathways linking the thalamus, cortex, and limbic system that generates patterns of neural activity responsible for perceptions of pain and reflexive and complex pain behaviors, as well as stress-regulation functions of the central nervous system (CNS). The function of the neuromatrix is initially influenced by genetic factors and subsequently is also influenced by multiple endogenous and exogenous factors. In addition, pain perception, pain behavior, and stress regulation may influence one another by altering the inputs to the neuromatrix.

psychological factors, such as expectancy effects or response biases for reporting pain even at low stimulus intensity levels (25,26).

Nevertheless, individual variations in cognitive or affective factors are associated with differences among individuals in pain sensitivity. Among healthy individuals, for example, hypnotic suggestions designed to either increase or decrease perceptions of pain unpleasantness alter healthy persons' ratings of tonic heat stimuli in the expected directions without changing ratings of pain intensity (27). Both types of hypnotic suggestion produce significant changes in the activity of the anterior cingulate cortex, rostral insular cortex, and primary somatosensory cortex (S1). Moreover, the hypnosis-induced changes in pain unpleasantness and increases in functional activity of the anterior cingulate cortex are strongly correlated with one another ($r = 0.42$). Similarly, hypnotic suggestions of increased stimulus intensity produce significant increases in ratings of both pain intensity and pain unpleasantness; however, altered pain intensity ratings are associated only with significant changes in activation of the S1 (28).

CATASTROPHIZING

This construct, which includes both cognitive and affective dimensions, is highly associated with the behavior of patients with chronic-pain conditions. Catastrophizing includes at least three components. These are: (a) helplessness—that is, perceived difficulty in coping effectively with pain; (b) magnification—that is, a tendency to consistently anticipate that pain will produce highly negative consequences; and (c) rumination—that is, perceived difficulty in distracting oneself from pain. Among patients with FM, high scores on a self-report measure of catastrophizing are strongly correlated with ratings of functional disability even after controlling for demographic and clinical variables as well as neuroticism (29). In addition, high levels of catastrophizing are associated with low pain threshold and tolerance responses and with high scores on the pain affect (i.e., unpleasantness) scale of the McGill Pain Questionnaire (MPQ) (30,31). The influence of catastrophizing on these measures of pain is independent of depression. Consistent with studies from other laboratories (32,33), depression is associated with lower levels of pain sensitivity among the patients with FM (30). Moreover, neuroimaging of brain responses to noxious stimulation in FM reveals that, after controlling for the influence of depression, high levels of catastrophizing are associated with increased activation in several brain regions involved in cognitive or emotional modulation of pain such as the anterior cingulate cortex and the prefrontal cortex (31).

NEGATIVE AFFECT

Staud et al. recently assessed the extent to which laboratory measures of pain sensitivity and pain-related negative affect (PRNA) predict patients' reports of the intensity of their FM pain (34). PRNA is a construct that, similar to catastrophizing, is associated with self-reports of anxiety, depression, frustration, and fear associated with persistent pain. It was found that windup responses and their decay, TeP count, and PRNA account for 49.7% of the variance in

patients' clinical pain intensity ratings. The two windup variables accounted for 28% of the variance in clinical pain scores whereas PRNA and the TeP count, both of which are associated with psychological distress, accounted for nearly 22% of the variance in the pain scores. These findings are consistent with those of independent investigations that have shown that self-reports of depressive symptoms are associated with patients' ratings of the intensity of mechanical pressure stimulation applied to the TePs included in standard TeP exams (17). A subsequent investigation performed by Staud et al. revealed that a measure of body pain area, derived from patients' responses to a body pain map, in combination with PRNA and TeP count, accounted for 45% of the variance in the clinical pain intensity ratings of patients with FM (35). The TeP count, however, accounted for only 4% of the variance in clinical pain ratings.

Three issues regarding the research described above are important to note. First, high levels of catastrophizing alone do not completely account for abnormal pain sensitivity in persons with FM. Indeed, some patients with FM display high levels of pain sensitivity despite reporting relatively low levels of catastrophizing (36).

Second, the relationship between catastrophizing and pain sensitivity is not unique to FM. For example, we have reported similar associations among patients with osteoarthritis (OA) of the knee (37). We compared patients with knee OA and age-matched healthy controls on their responses to the Pain Catastrophizing Scale (PCS) and the pain affect (unpleasantness) scale of the MPQ. The latter ratings were made in response to pressure stimulation of the knee that was tailored for each participant so that both patients and controls reported that the intensity of stimulation was approximately 50 on a 100 point scale. We found that the patients, compared to controls, produced significantly higher scores on the PCS and on the pain affect scale of the MPQ even though their pain intensity ratings did not differ from those of the controls. Moreover, catastrophizing mediated the association between status as a patient with knee OA and high pain affect ratings. In addition, compared to white patients, African-American patients tended to report higher levels of both catastrophizing and pain affect.

Finally, although the literature described above suggests that depression is highly associated with patients' reports of clinical pain intensity, it tends to be correlated with relatively low levels of pain sensitivity. However, recent studies of patients with temporomandibular joint disorder (TMD) suggest that it may be premature to conclude that depression does not influence experimental pain responses. TMD is a disorder that frequently overlaps with FM and is also associated with enhanced windup responses (38). It has been found that among patients with TMD, depression accounts for a modest, albeit statistically significant, proportion of the variance in patients' displays of ischemic pain threshold (11%) and tolerance (5%) (39). Depression also is associated with increased perception of postischemic parasthesias (40). The variation across studies in the association between depression and pain sensitivity may be due to several factors. These factors may include differences in the specific attributes of FM versus TMD as well as differences in type of experimental stimulation (i.e., ischemic vs. thermal or pressure) or in the measures used to assess depression. Thus, additional research is necessary to fully understand the relationship between depression and experimental pain responses in persons with FM.

ENVIRONMENTAL STRESSORS AND PAIN-RELATED AFFECT

The relationship between exposure to environmental stressors and the pain responses of patients with FM is an important issue that has not been extensively studied. There is some evidence that frequent exposure to daily stressors mediates the high levels of psychological distress reported by patients with FM (41). In addition, stressful life experiences, in combination with factors such as high levels of negative affect and pain, are highly related to seeking medical care for FM symptoms (8,42).

Until recently, however, there have been few attempts to document the effects of exposure to environmental stressors and changes in pain reports among patients with FM. Davis et al. exposed patients with FM and those with OA to either a negative mood induction or a neutral mood (control) condition prior to discussing a stressful interpersonal event from their own lives for 30 minutes (43). Stress-related increases in pain were exacerbated by negative mood induction among women with FM but not among women with OA. These findings suggest that among patients with persistent musculoskeletal pain, those with FM may be particularly vulnerable to the negative effects of social stressors.

Studies of healthy individuals suggest that exposure to stressors tends to produce higher levels of negative affect such as anger (44) as well as enhanced pain ratings in response to noxious stimuli such as capsaicin (45). Exposure to stressors also tends to enhance memory of the pain evoked by noxious stimulation (46). However, these studies generally have not distinguished between individuals' perceptions of pain intensity and pain unpleasantness. Thus, we do not fully understand the extent to which patients' reports of stress-related increases in their clinical pain may reflect increased perception of the affective dimension of pain.

We recently reported the preliminary findings of a study in which we asked patients with FM and healthy controls to vividly imagine for 4 minutes either highly stressful experiences or relatively neutral experiences from their lives prior to administration of a thermal heat stimulation procedure similar to that used by Staud et al. (24). Contrary to our expectations, we found that patients and controls did not differ in their cardiovascular responses (i.e., blood pressure, heart rate) to the stressful or control imagery conditions. Nevertheless, FM patients, compared to the healthy controls, produced significantly higher pain unpleasantness ratings when stressful imagery preceded the thermal stimulation [see Figure 14-2 (47)]. There was no difference between patients and controls in stress-evoked changes in their pain intensity ratings. In addition, the patients showed greater activation in brain regions involved in anticipation of and cognitive regulation of pain such as the cerebellum as well as the posterior temporal and premotor cortices. These findings are similar to those regarding neural activation associated with catastrophizing (31).

In summary, the findings reviewed above strongly suggest that negative cognitions and affect greatly influence patients'

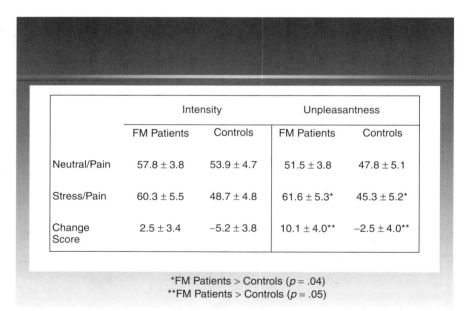

	Intensity		Unpleasantness	
	FM Patients	Controls	FM Patients	Controls
Neutral/Pain	57.8 ± 3.8	53.9 ± 4.7	51.5 ± 3.8	47.8 ± 5.1
Stress/Pain	60.3 ± 5.5	48.7 ± 4.8	61.6 ± 5.3*	45.3 ± 5.2*
Change Score	2.5 ± 3.4	−5.2 ± 3.8	10.1 ± 4.0**	−2.5 ± 4.0**

*FM Patients > Controls (*p* = .04)
**FM Patients > Controls (*p* = .05)

Figure 14-2. Mean (±SEM) pain intensity and unpleasantness ratings produced by patients with fibromyalgia (FM) and healthy control persons. We administered thermal heat stimulation that was tailored to individual participants in order to produce pain intensity ratings of approximately 50 on 100 cm visual analog scales during baseline conditions. We then assessed participants' pain intensity and unpleasantness ratings of thermal heat stimulation under two counterbalanced conditions. Under one condition participants vividly imagined a highly stressful event from their own lives prior to stimulation. Under the other condition participants vividly imagined a relatively neutral event from their own lives prior to stimulation. We then analyzed change in participants' ratings evoked by stressful versus neutral imagery. Patients with fibromyalgia (FM), compared to controls, showed significantly greater increases in thermal pain unpleasantness ratings as a function of stressful imagery. Patients and controls did not differ on change in pain intensity ratings.

affective responses to noxious stimulation in the laboratory as well as their ratings of pain affect or unpleasantness. Laboratory manipulations such as negative mood induction and exposure to personally relevant stressors also evoke increased ratings of clinical pain and pain unpleasantness, respectively. Two neuroimaging investigations suggest that the neural mechanisms underlying the influence of catastrophizing and exposure to laboratory stressors on pain affect are similar to one another. Depression also is associated with enhanced ratings of clinical pain among patients with FM. Current evidence suggests that depression is associated with diminished pain sensitivity among patients with FM. However, additional research is necessary to better understand the relationship between depression and pain sensitivity in these persons.

Finally, recent studies have examined the role that exposure to stressful events might play in the onset of FM. This issue will be examined below.

PSYCHOSOCIAL FACTORS AND THE ETIOPATHOGENESIS OF FIBROMYALGIA

FAMILIAL AND GENETIC FACTORS ASSOCIATED WITH PAIN SENSITIVITY AND AFFECTIVE/ANXIETY DISORDERS

The revised gate control theory suggests that genetic factors initially determine the pattern-generating mechanism of the neuromatrix. Indeed, recent animal and human research suggests that there are important genetic influences on pain transmission and modulation that may be relevant to the abnormal pain sensitivity among women with FM. For example, Mogil et al. demonstrated that the melanocortin-1 receptor (Mc1r) gene mediates kappa-opioid analgesia in female mice only (48). This finding suggested that individuals with variants of the human MC1R gene, associated in humans with red hair and fair skin, might also display altered κ-opioid analgesia. Indeed, it was found that women with two variant MC1R alleles displayed significantly greater analgesia from the κ-opioid pentazocine than their male counterparts as well as men and women without these variant alleles (48).

There also are human studies regarding genetic influences on μ-opioid analgesia. For example, Zubieta et al. found that healthy men and women who were homozygous for the met^{158} allele of the catechol-O-methyltransferase (COMT) polymorphism ($val^{158}met$) showed diminished regional μ-opioid system responses to a tonic pain challenge compared to heterozygotes (49). The diminished μ-opioid system responses were associated with higher sensory and affective ratings of pain and self-reports of a more negative internal affective state.

Diatchenko et al. recently examined the relationship between several haplotypes of the $val^{158}met$ polymorphism associated with enhanced pain sensitivity and the onset of TMD in healthy young women (50). It was found that the presence of these haplotypes was significantly associated with the onset of TMD over a 3-year period. In addition, the predictive power of these haplotypes was significantly enhanced when combined with baseline levels of somatization.

The relationship between COMT and FM has not yet been studied. However, two independent laboratories have reported that female patients with FM are significantly more likely than controls to show a functional polymorphism in the promoter region of the serotonin transporter gene that is also associated with affective disorders, anxiety-related traits, and migraine headaches (51,52). It is not yet known, however, whether this functional polymorphism is associated with enhanced pain sensitivity in FM patients or their female, first-degree relatives.

Finally, two recent studies have provided evidence of aggregation of depressive disorders among family members of women with FM (53,54). These relationships were especially pronounced among the female family members. In addition, similar to the results of an earlier study performed by Buskila and Neumann (55), the female relatives of the women with FM showed significantly greater pain sensitivity in response to mechanical pressure stimulation at the FM TePs than the male and female relatives of patients with rheumatoid arthritis (RA) (53). These investigations suggest that genetic and/or psychosocial influences within the family (i.e., social learning) related to affective or anxiety disorders may contribute to the etiopathogenesis of FM.

EXPOSURE TO ENVIRONMENTAL STRESSORS AND THE ONSET OF FIBROMYALGIA

Fourteen percent of patients who attend specialized rheumatology practices report that they began to experience FM symptoms after highly stressful, emotionally traumatic events (56). One type of stressful event that has received a great deal of attention from investigators is sexual or physical abuse and other forms of victimization, such as parental neglect. Several studies of patients with FM or persistent, widespread pain indicate that those who recall histories of sexual or physical abuse, compared to patients who do not recall abuse, report significantly higher levels of environmental stress, pain, fatigue, and functional disability (57–59). In addition, these abused patients with FM display a response bias toward perceiving a wide range of mechanical pressure stimuli as painful, regardless of their actual intensities (57). Studies of women with chronic pelvic pain suggest that abnormalities in the function of the HPA axis may in part mediate the effects of abuse on pain and other physical symptoms (60). The possible associations among abuse, HPA axis function, and pain responses have not yet been examined among women with FM.

Prospective studies have shown that the strong relationships between patients' self-reports of childhood abuse or victimization and their current levels of persistent pain generally are not supported when documented records of abuse among the patients are correlated with their current pain reports (61,62). Raphael's prospective study is especially noteworthy (62). She identified 676 children with documented histories of neglect or abuse and 520 control children with comparable demographic backgrounds and found no relationship between neglect or abuse and the number of medically explained or unexplained painful symptoms nearly 30 years later. However, when the participants were asked as adults to report memories of abuse or neglect, there was a significant association between these negative events and the presence of one or more medically unexplained pain symptoms.

Raphael also performed a prospective study of a community-based sample of residents in the New York City metropolitan area that produced similar findings concerning the effects of another major, stressful life event—the World Trade Center attacks in 2001 (63,64). She found that the likelihood of meeting criteria for probable posttraumatic stress disorder approximately 6 months after the attacks was 3 times greater in women who reported FM-like symptoms during this period than in those who did not report these symptoms (63). Nevertheless, the World Trade Center attacks were not associated with a significant increase in the number of women who reported FM-like symptoms during the 6-month, postattack period. It should be noted, however, that the presence of a major depression-like syndrome prior to the attacks was positively associated with the development of FM-like symptoms following the attacks (64).

Raphael has suggested that the negative findings of the prospective studies described above may be limited because these studies used individuals' self-reports of pain or other physical symptoms as criterion measures instead of performing physical examinations on the participants or directly evaluating their pain sensitivity responses (62,64). We agree that the use of these examinations or quantitative sensory testing procedures would be very useful. For example, the literature on abuse among women with irritable bowel syndrome (IBS), which frequently overlaps with FM, has established relationships between memories of abuse history and symptom intensity (65). However, recent studies in this area have shown consistently that retrospective reports of abuse history among women with IBS are not associated with enhanced pain sensitivity in response to rectal balloon distention (66). We conclude, then, that it is essential to use reliable records of abuse, victimization, or other major, stressful life events among patients with FM as well as direct examination of their health status and pain sensitivity in order to determine the extent to which these events may contribute to the development of the cardinal features of FM—that is, widespread pain and pain sensitivity.

PHYSICAL TRAUMA AND THE ONSET OF FIBROMYALGIA

Physical injuries represent another potential source of stressors that might influence the development of FM in some individuals. Indeed, between 14% and 23% of patients with FM report that their symptoms began following a physical injury or trauma, such as surgery (67–69). It is critically important to develop a better understanding of the physiologic mediators that may contribute to the development of FM after physical injury. One potential mediator is a set of events referred to as central sensitization. It has been established in animal models that prolonged nociceptive input from A-δ and C afferents evoked by tissue damage may depolarize the spinal dorsal horn neurons enough so that there is an exaggerated release of excitatory amino acids and substance P (SP) from presynaptic afferent terminals that causes the dorsal horn neurons to become hyperexcitable. As a consequence, low intensity stimulation of the skin or deep muscle tissue generates high levels of nociceptive input to the brain that, in turn, can produce perceptions of widespread pain or abnormal pain sensitivity, or both (70,71).

There also is evidence that following the initiation of central sensitization, spinal glia cells are activated by a wide array of factors that contribute to hyperalgesia, such as excitatory amino acids, SP, nitric oxide, and prostaglandins. Once activated, glia cells release several proinflammatory cytokines, SP, nitric oxide, and prostaglandins that further enhance the hyperexcitability of the dorsal horn neurons (72) and may produce abnormal pain sensitivity at sites distal to the original tissue injury (73).

Most investigators acknowledge that central sensitization, or a similar, centrally mediated process, contributes to the widespread pain and abnormal pain sensitivity associated with FM (74,75). There also is evidence that some physical trauma, such as whiplash injuries, are associated with diminished spinal reflex thresholds or other responses consistent with hyperexcitability of spinal cord neurons (76). However, not enough controlled prospective studies with positive findings exist to conclude that physical injuries may trigger the development of FM (77). Moreover, no investigation has identified a structural abnormality in the muscle or skin tissue of patients with FM that is reliably associated with FM (78). Nevertheless, one longitudinal study suggests that any causal association between injury and the development of FM is most likely to be found among women. Neumann et al. (79) examined 102 patients with acute cervical spine injuries and reported that 22 met criteria for FM. The investigators subsequently performed a 3-year follow-up evaluation of 20 of the patients with FM. They found that all the 11 women with FM still met criteria for the disorder at follow-up whereas only 1 of the 9 men remained positive for FM. It is possible, then, that there may be one or more sex-related variables that increase the likelihood that women will manifest the cardinal symptoms of FM for extended periods of time following cervical spine injury.

Goldenberg (56) has suggested that physical trauma among highly anxious persons may lead to development of FM symptoms as a consequence of maladaptive behavior patterns. For example, highly anxious individuals who experience a physical injury may display increased muscle tension levels over prolonged periods and avoid physical activity. The internal stressors associated with the chronically high levels of anxiety (e.g., negative cognition and affect), in combination with physical deconditioning, may lead to the neuroendocrine and other physiologic abnormalities associated with FM and thus contribute to its development.

Indeed, it generally has been shown that persons who develop FM following physical injury are characterized by significantly higher levels of disability, inactivity, or financial compensation than patients who do not identify injury-related triggers for the onset of their symptoms (80,81). These data also show that patients who report physical injury prior to the onset of FM are more likely to receive financial compensation than those who do not report injury prior to symptom onset even when the both groups of patients report the same levels of function on standardized assessment instruments (81). In addition, one meta-analytic study has shown that patients with chronic pain who receive financial compensation exhibit significantly poorer functional outcomes after treatment than patients without compensation (82). One might conclude, then, that psychological distress, as well as financial compensation or other possible social reinforcements for maladaptive illness behavior (e.g., inactivity), may play a larger role in the development or maintenance of FM symptoms than any pain-related, physiologic consequences of the injury.

However, the results of several prospective studies suggest that both the potential physiologic effects of injury and psychosocial factors contribute to the development of persistent widespread pain. For example, Harkness et al. studied nearly 900 newly employed workers over a 2-year period and found that several physical maneuvers that might cause tissue damage, as well as psychosocial factors, were associated with the onset of widespread body pain (83). The physical maneuvers included lifting more than 24 pounds with both hands, pulling more than 56 pounds, and prolonged working with hands at or above shoulder level. The psychosocial factors included low job satisfaction, low social support, and monotonous work. However, monotonous work and low social support were the two best independent predictors of symptom onset. In a similar study involving a population-based sample, McBeth et al. showed that even though low-level mechanical trauma, such as those experienced at work, may contribute to the onset of chronic widespread pain, the most consistent factor associated with the pain was a high score on a measure of abnormal illness behavior (84).

SOMATIZATION AND THE ONSET OF WIDESPREAD BODY PAIN

In addition to performing prospective studies of factors related to the onset of widespread pain in the workplace, McBeth et al. have also examined factors that may contribute to widespread pain in community-based samples. These investigators performed a prospective study of 1,658 adults and found that, after adjusting for age and sex, high scores on measures of somatization and maladaptive coping mechanisms were the strongest predictors of the development of chronic widespread pain (85). This is an especially interesting finding given the recent prospective study of the development of TMD in young adult women (50). As noted earlier, several haplotypes of the $val^{158}met$ polymorphism of the COMT gene that are associated with enhanced pain sensitivity, in addition to high levels of somatization, were significant predictors of the development of TMD over a 3-year period. These findings suggest that, as we learn more about genetic factors associated with pain sensitivity or with the development of disorders with medically unexplained symptoms (e.g., TMD), it will be especially useful to perform population-based studies of the onset of FM or persistent widespread pain in which (a) individual genotypes, (b) baseline measures of pain sensitivity, and (c) psychosocial factors (e.g., somatization, coping strategy usage) will be included in the multivariate prediction models.

In summary, several psychosocial factors appear to be associated with the etiopathogenesis of FM. First, family aggregation studies suggest that psychosocial influences within the family environment, perhaps in combination with specific genotypes associated with enhanced pain sensitivity and affective or anxiety disorders, are correlated with FM, primarily among women. Prospective studies of large samples of individuals in the community or workplace indicate that psychosocial variables, such as depression, somatization, or low job satisfaction, are associated with the onset of widespread body pain or other FM-like symptoms.

The investigations reviewed above also suggest that physical stressors, such as job-related physical trauma, may contribute to the onset of widespread body pain. Two important issues regarding these findings should be noted. First, the power of physical trauma to predict the onset of FM-like symptoms in the workplace tends to be weaker than that of somatization or the other affective and cognitive variables noted above. In addition, some physical trauma, such as cervical spine injury, may influence the onset or maintenance of FM, primarily in women. The second issue is that investigators and clinicians frequently assume that physical trauma may directly contribute to the development of FM by altering the firing thresholds of spinal dorsal horn neurons. However, clinical studies have not yet provided direct evidence of the structural abnormalities in muscle or other soft tissues that may generate the prolonged nociceptive transmission that contributes to centrally maintained abnormalities in pain perception (i.e., central sensitization).

Finally, sophisticated prospective studies of major life stressors, such as sexual abuse or exposure to terrorist attack, indicate that these events are not reliably associated with increases in pain levels or new cases of FM. These negative findings may be due in part to the methodologic limitations of (a) identifying persons with FM-like symptoms solely through questionnaire administration or interview and (b) relying upon retrospective memories of abuse or victimization that may not be entirely accurate. However, even if persons' memories of abuse are not accurate, the distress associated with these memories may enhance patients' perceptions of pain or illness behaviors (43,47).

PSYCHOSOCIAL VARIABLES AND TREATMENT OUTCOMES

Clinicians and investigators are keenly aware that current pharmacologic interventions for FM produce modest outcomes in health status. For example, Williams recently noted that pharmacologic interventions reduce the intensity of pain and other symptoms in <50% of patients and produce lasting improvement in functional status in only 12% of these persons (86). Although several new pharmacologic compounds for treatment of FM will soon be available (87), it is widely acknowledged that optimal treatment plans for most patients with FM should include interventions such as exercise and coping skills training, in addition to pharmacologic agents (86). This multidimensional approach to treating persons with FM is consistent with Melzack's revised gate control theory described earlier in this chapter (14). That is, multidimensional treatment programs may alter several physiologic and psychosocial factors that influence pain perception and behavior and therefore may be more likely than pharmacologic agents alone to produce meaningful improvements in symptoms and quality of life.

During the late 1980s investigators and clinicians began to include cognitive-behavioral therapy (CBT) interventions in their treatment plans for patients with FM (88). A variety of CBT interventions have been used successfully to help improve the quality of life among patients with behavioral or medical disorders, including those with RA (89) and knee OA (90). All these interventions are based on the premise that behaviors are influenced by social reinforcement from the environment as well as internal cognitive and emotional factors, such as beliefs about one's ability to control symptoms and affective states. In addition, they all include four essential components: (a) education, (b) acquisition of cognitive and behavioral coping skills, (c) rehearsal of coping skills in the clinic and in patients' home or work environments, and (d) prevention of relapse.

Since 1990 a large number of studies of the efficacy of CBT interventions for FM have shown that these interventions produce significant reductions in patients' ratings of pain, other clinical symptoms, functional disability, and in pain threshold measures or TeP counts (91–94). None of these studies, however, used attention-placebo comparison groups to control for the nonspecific effects of prolonged or frequent contact with concerned health professionals. Thus it is not possible to attribute the treatment gains documented in these studies to the specific components of CBT interventions. Moreover, three studies of the efficacy of CBT interventions that have included credible attention-placebo control conditions have produced negative findings (95–97). This suggests that the positive patient outcomes documented in the trials without attention-placebo controls may be due largely to the nonspecific components of CBT interventions, such as positive shifts in mood attributable to increased attention from health professionals or anticipation of improvement.

These negative findings have prompted investigators to begin to attempt to identify patient cognitions regarding pain that may either impede or enhance the efficacy of CBT interventions. One set of maladaptive cognitions involves maladaptive expectations that increased activity or similar behaviors will produce large increases in pain. The second set of cognitions includes potentially adaptive beliefs, such as readiness to adopt new health behaviors or to accept that medical treatment might not completely relieve pain.

MALADAPTIVE COGNITIONS

Melzack's revised gate control theory posits that preoccupation with pain or exaggerated expectations of activity-induced increases in pain are associated with enhanced pain experiences (14). Thus, several standardized instruments have been developed to measure these maladaptive cognitions, including (a) the Pain Anxiety Symptoms Scale (98), (b) the Tampa Scale for Kinesiophobia (99), (c) the Fear-Avoidance Beliefs Questionnaire (100), and (d) the Fear of Pain Scale-III (101). Using these scales, it has been shown that these maladaptive cognitions are associated with behaviors such as low lifting and carrying capacity during functional assessments (102), as well as self-reports of disability (103), depressed mood, and pain severity (104).

We recently suggested that CBT investigators should begin to examine the extent to which negative expectations regarding pain among patients with FM may influence their responses to treatment (105). If maladaptive expectations concerning pain do help mediate treatment outcomes, it will be necessary to include coping skills training components designed to modify these cognitions in CBT protocols. Maladaptive cognitions also are likely to influence the outcomes

of patients involved in exercise interventions for FM. Investigators in this area, then, should also begin to assess the influence of negative patient cognitions on treatment outcomes and develop effective methods for altering these cognitions.

A small number of studies, done primarily in Europe, have begun to examine methods for modifying maladaptive cognitions by demonstrating to patients that their expectations about pain are not valid. These investigations have shown that *in vivo* exposure of patients with persistent back pain to a series of physical movements that typically evoke expectations of enhanced pain produces stable (up to 1 year) improvements in self-reports of pain-related fear and disability as well as in physical activity level assessed by ambulatory monitors (106). The key factors in this intervention are that the movements are (a) highly relevant for each individual and (b) presented in a hierarchy beginning with movements that evoke expectations of relatively small increases in pain and ending with those associated with large increases in pain.

The effects of *in vivo* exposure for reducing negative expectations concerning pain have not yet been studied in CBT or exercise therapy interventions for persons with FM. However, Rooks et al. recently adopted a similar strategy in their evaluation of progressive strength training and aerobic exercise program for patients with FM (107). This program required all patients to begin with a low volume of water-based exercise performed at low intensity for 4 weeks. Next, patients began progressive, land-based training to improve cardiovascular endurance, strength, and flexibility over 16 weeks. It was anticipated that this program would minimize poor tolerance of, and noncompliance with, the exercise protocol. Indeed, the investigators reported the compliance rate was 81% with no reports of exercise-induced injuries. Moreover, the program produced significant improvements in upper and lower body muscle strength, 6-minute walk distance, and self-reports of functional ability.

READINESS TO CHANGE

This construct is the central component of the Transtheoretical Model of Behavior Change (108). The transtheoretical model has been used successfully to explain differences among individuals in success in altering behaviors associated with psychological and physical health, such as smoking, alcohol consumption, diabetes self-management, weight management, and contraception usage (109). The model posits that when people attempt to alter their health-related behavior they go through specific "stages of change" that represent variations in "readiness"—that is, how prepared they are to make behavioral changes. The stages usually are labeled (a) precontemplation (no intention to change in the near future), (b) contemplation (thinking about the possibility of change in the future without commitment to act), (c) preparation (actively considering making changes in behavior within the next month), (d) action (active work toward making desired behavioral change), and (e) maintenance (ongoing active work to maintain behavioral changes and avoid relapse) (110). A large body of research performed since the early 1980s suggests that persons who do make sustained changes in their health behavior use different behavior change strategies as they progress through the model's five stages (109). As a consequence, it has been suggested that attempts to tailor interventions for patients involved in treatment protocols, such as exercise or CBT interventions for pain management, might benefit from assessment of their readiness for change (110).

Kerns et al. developed the Pain Stages of Change Questionnaire in 1997 in order to produce reliable and valid measurements of readiness to change that could be used in treatment planning for patients with persistent pain (111). Most studies of this measure have been performed with heterogeneous samples of patients with persistent pain, including subgroups of patients with FM. Initial investigations revealed that patients' responses to the Pain Stages of Change Questionnaire are reliably associated with variations in their use of coping strategies (112,113). However, it was difficult to reliably classify patients in one of five specific stages of change using the questionnaire. In addition, examination of the responses of the patients with FM revealed that their responses were significantly associated with self-reports of depression but not with disability (113). Nevertheless, the most recent study in this area showed that among patients with FM (a) a multidisciplinary pain treatment program produced reliable changes in readiness to self-manage pain, (b) changes in readiness were associated with changes in the use of pain coping strategies, and (c) treatment-evoked increases in readiness to self-manage pain were positively associated with positive outcomes (114). Specifically, decreases in precontemplation and increases in maintenance were associated with improvements from baseline to 6-month follow-up in self-reports of depression, pain severity, and disability.

ACCEPTANCE OF PAIN

This relatively new construct represents a complex set of cognitions involving (a) acceptance that it is unlikely that medical or behavioral treatments will completely eliminate one's pain, (b) acceptance of the need to shift one's attention from pain to nonpain aspects of life, and (c) the realization that such acceptance does not signify personal failure. Indeed, it may be that acceptance of persistent pain is necessary for individuals to stop searching for treatments that provide complete relief of pain and to begin making changes in their behavior that may help them to better manage persistent pain and improve their quality of life. A study of a small group of patients with FM revealed that scores on a measure of acceptance, a subscale on the Illness Cognition Questionnaire (115), were negatively associated with ratings of pain severity and catastrophizing and were positively associated with mental health scores on the MOS 36-item Short Form Health Survey (SF-36) (116). A subsequent study of patients with chronic pain revealed that higher levels of acceptance were associated with less attention to pain, greater engagement with daily activities, higher motivation to complete activities, and higher self-efficacy regarding performance of daily activities (117).

In summary, much of the current research on psychosocial variables associated with treatment outcomes stems from the negative findings documented in studies of CBT interventions with credible attention-placebo control conditions. Although early studies of psychosocial variables tended to focus on maladaptive variables, such as expectations that movement will evoke higher levels of pain, greater emphasis is now being devoted to relatively positive variables such as readiness to change and acceptance of pain. In addition, the

focus of research in this area has begun to shift from exclusively measuring associations between psychosocial variables and health status (e.g., pain severity, mood, function) to evaluating change on these psychosocial and health status variables produced by CBT or other behavioral treatment interventions. The readiness to change construct may prove to be a key variable in producing positive treatment outcomes. However, it still is necessary to determine whether it is beneficial to tailor CBT or exercise programs in accord with individual patient responses to the Pain Stages of Change Questionnaire. In addition, we have previously suggested that the development of more effective pharmacologic interventions for pain associated with FM may indirectly enhance the outcomes produced by CBT or exercise interventions (105). The development of new measures of psychosocial variables, such as the Pain Stages of Change Questionnaire, may allow investigators to determine if (a) reductions in pain produced by pharmacotherapy evoke changes in pain-related cognitions and (b) these changes in cognition contribute to outcomes produced by CBT and exercise interventions.

■ IMPLICATIONS FOR PRACTICE

- Establishing a patient's psychological state is extremely important in the evaluation of FM, since treatment approaches are diverse and success often depends on an accurate emotional evaluation of the patient.
- In tertiary centers a sizable percentage of FM patients have comorbid psychiatric disorders, but this percentage is smaller in primary care practices.
- The most common psychological pathology patterns include depression, somatization, anxiety states, and mood disorders.
- Posttraumatic stress disturbance is reported in 20% to 50% of patients with FM, and its prevalence varies with practice settings. Physical, substance, alcohol, and sexual abuse are especially prevalent in this group.
- Even though comorbid psychiatric conditions are important to identify and treat, cognitions (ways that people view their pain and what they do about it—for example, catastrophizing—and external locus of control) and maladaptive illness behaviors (bad habits that patients develop that worsen or perpetuate their condition) might be even more important.
- Individuals who have these features might be those that benefit most from cognitive-behavior therapy programs.

ACKNOWLEDGMENT

This work is supported by the National Institute of Arthritis, Musculoskeletal, and Skin Diseases (1 RO1 AR43136; P60 P60 AR48095) and the American Fibromyalgia Syndrome Association.

REFERENCES

1. Wolfe F, Smythe HA, Yunus MB, et al. The American College of Rheumatology 1990 criteria for the classification of fibromyalgia. Report of the Multicenter Criteria Committee. *Arthritis Rheum* 1990;33:160–172.

2. Gibson JJ, Littlejohn GO, et al. Altered heat pain thresholds and cerebral event-related potentials following painful CO_2 laser stimulation in subjects with fibromyalgia syndrome. *Pain* 1994;58:185–193.

3. Wolfe F, Cathey MA, Kleinheksel SM, et al. Psychological status in primary fibrositis and fibrositis associated with rheumatoid arthritis. *J Rheumatol* 1984;11:500–506.

4. Ahles TA, Yunus MB, Riley SD, et al. Psychological factors associated with primary fibromyalgia syndrome. *Arthritis Rheum* 1984;27:1101–1106.

5. Payne TC, Leavitt F, Garron DC, et al. Fibrositis and psychological disturbance. *Arthritis Rheum* 1982;25:213–217.

6. Wolfe F, Anderson J, Harkness P, et al. A prospective, longitudinal, multicenter study of service utilization and costs in fibromyalgia. *Arthritis Rheum* 1997;40:1560–1570.

7. Ter Borg EJ, Gerards-Rociu E, Hannen HC, et al. High frequency of hysterectomies and appendectomies in fibromyalgia compared with rheumatoid arthritis: a pilot study. *Clin Rheumatol* 1999;18:1–3.

8. Kersh BC, Bradley LA, Alarcón GS, et al. Psychosocial and health status variables independently predict health care seeking in fibromyalgia. *Arthritis Rheum* 2001;45:362–371.

9. Dobkin PL, De Civita M, Bernatsky S, et al. Does psychological vulnerability determine health-care utilization in fibromyalgia? *Rheumatology* 2003;42:1324–1331.

10. Barsky AJ, Borus JF. Functional somatic syndromes. *Ann Intern Med* 1999;130:910–921.

11. Bennett RM. Emerging concepts in the neurobiology of chronic pain: evidence of abnormal sensory processing in fibromyalgia. *Mayo Clin Proc* 1999;74:385–398.

12. Yunus MB. Towards a model of pathophysiology of fibromyalgia: aberrant central pain mechanisms with peripheral modulation. *J Rheumatol* 1992;19:846–850.

13. Staud R. Evidence of involvement of central neural mechanisms in generating fibromyalgia pain. *Curr Rheumatol Rep* 2002;4:299–305.

14. Melzack R. Gate control theory: on the evolution of pain concepts. *Pain Forum* 1996;5:125–128.

15. Granges G, Littlejohn GO. A comparative study of clinical signs in fibromyalgia/fibrositis syndrome, healthy and exercising subjects. *J Rheumatol* 1993;20:344–351.

16. Bradley LA, Alarcón GS, Triana M, et al. Health care seeking behavior in fibromyalgia: associations with pain thresholds, symptom severity, and psychiatric morbidity. *J Musculoskelet Pain* 1994;2:79–87.

17. Aaron LA, Bradley LA, Alarcón GS, et al. Psychiatric diagnoses are related to health care seeking behavior rather than illness in fibromyalgia. *Arthritis Rheum* 1996;39:436–445.

18. Mountz JM, Bradley LA, Modell JG, et al. Fibromyalgia in women. Abnormalities of regional cerebral blood flow in the thalamus and the caudate nucleus are associated with low pain threshold levels. *Arthritis Rheum* 1995;38:926–938.

19. Granges G, Littlejohn G. Pressure pain threshold in pain-free subjects, in patients with chronic regional pain syndromes, and in patients with fibromyalgia syndrome. *Arthritis Rheum* 1993;36:642–646.

20. Gibson JJ, Littlejohn GO, Gorman MM, et al. Altered heat pain thresholds and cerebral event-related potentials following painful CO_2 laser stimulation in subjects with fibromyalgia syndrome. *Pain* 1994;58:185–193.

21. Arroyo JF, Cohen ML. Abnormal responses to electrocutaneous stimulation in fibromyalgia. *J Rheumatol* 1993;20:1925–1931.

22. Carli G, Suman AL, Biasi G, et al. Reactivity to superficial and deep stimuli in patients with chronic musculoskeletal pain. *Pain* 2002;100:259–269.

23. Staud R, Cannon RC, Mauderli AP, et al. Temporal summation of pain from mechanical stimulation of muscle tissue in normal controls and subjects with fibromyalgia syndrome. *Pain* 2003;102:87–95.

24. Staud R, Vierck CJ, Cannon RL, et al. Abnormal sensitization and temporal summation of second pain (wind-up) in patients with fibromyalgia syndrome. *Pain* 2001;91:165–175.

25. Staud R, Price DD, Robinson ME, et al. Maintenance of windup of second pain requires less frequent stimulation in fibromyalgia patients compared to normal controls. *Pain* 2004;110:689–696.

26. Petzke F, Clauw DJ, Ambrose K, et al. Increased pain sensitivity in fibromyalgia: effects of stimulus type and mode of presentation. *Pain* 2003;105:403–413.

27. Rainville P, Duncan GH, Price DD, et al. Pain affect encoded in human anterior cingulate but not somatosensory cortex. *Science* 1997;27:968–971.

28. Hofbauer RK, Rainville P, Duncan GH, et al. Cortical representation of the sensory dimension of pain. *J Neurophysiol* 2001;86:402–411.

29. Martin MY, Bradley LA, Alexander RW, et al. Coping strategies predict disability in patients with primary fibromyalgia. *Pain* 1996;68:45–53.

30. Geisser ME, Casey KL, Brucksch CB, et al. Perception of noxious and innocuous heat stimulation among healthy women and women with fibromyalgia: association with mood, somatic focus, and catastrophizing. *Pain* 2003;102:243–250.

31. Gracely RH, Geisser ME, Giesecke T, et al. Pain catastrophizing and neural responses to pain among persons with fibromyalgia. *Brain* 2004;127(Pt 4):835–843.

32. Dworkin RH, Clark WC, Lipsitz JD. Pain responsivity in major depression and bipolar disorder. *Psychiatry Res* 1995;56:173–181.

33. Cianfrini LR, McKendree-Smith NL, Bradley LA. Pain sensitivity and bilateral activation of brain structures during pressure stimulation of patients with fibromyalgia is not mediated by major depression (DEP). *Arthritis Rheum* 2001;44(Suppl. 9):S395.

34. Staud R, Robinson ME, Vierck CJ Jr, et al. Ratings of experimental pain and pain-related negative affect predict clinical pain in patients with fibromyalgia syndrome. *Pain* 2003;105:215–222.

35. Staud R, Price DD, Robinson ME, et al. Body pain area and pain-related negative affect predict clinical pain intensity in patients with fibromyalgia. *J Pain* 2004;5:338–343.

36. Giesecke T, Williams DA, Harris RE, et al. Subgrouping of fibromyalgia patients on the basis of pressure-pain thresholds and psychological factors. *Arthritis Rheum* 2003;48:2916–2922.

37. Bradley LA, Kersh BC, DeBerry JJ, et al. Lessons from fibromyalgia: abnormal pain sensitivity in knee osteoarthritis. *Novartis Found Symp* 2004;260:258–270.

38. Maixner W, Fillingim R, Sigurdsson A, et al. Sensitivity of patients with painful temporomandibular disorders to experimentally evoked pain: evidence for altered temporal summation of pain. *Pain* 1998;76:71–81.

39. Sherman JJ, Leresche L, Huggins KH, et al. The relationship of somatization and depression to experimental pain response in women with temporomandibular disorders. *Psychosom Med* 2004;66:852–860.

40. Suarez-Roca H, Pinerua-Shuhaibar L, Morales ME, et al. Increased perception of post-ischemic paresthesias in depressed subjects. *J Psychosom Res* 2003;55:253–257.

41. Uveges JM, Parker JC, Smarr KL, et al. Psychological symptoms in primary fibromyalgia syndrome: relationship to pain, life stress, and sleep disturbance. *Arthritis Rheum* 1990;33:1279–1283.

42. Aaron LA, Bradley LA, Alexander MT. Work stress, psychiatric history, and medication usage predict initial use of medical treatment for fibromyalgia symptoms: a prospective analysis. In: Jensen TS, Turner JA, Wiesenfeld-Hallin Z et al., eds. Proceedings of the 7th World Congress on Pain.

Progress in Pain Research and Management, Vol 8. Seattle, WA: IASP Press, 1997:683–691. The location of the Congress was Vancouver, Canada.

43. Davis MC, Zautra AJ, Reich JW. Vulnerability to stress among women in chronic pain from fibromyalgia and osteoarthritis. *Ann Behav Med* 2001;23:215–226.

44. Logan HL, Gedney JJ, Sheffield D, et al. Stress influences the level of negative affectivity after forehead cold pressor pain. *J Pain* 2003;4:520–529.

45. Logan H, Lutgendorf S, Rainville P, et al. Effects of stress and relaxation on capsaicin-induced pain. *J Pain* 2001;2:160–170.

46. Gedney JJ, Logan H. Memory for stress-associated acute pain. *J Pain* 2004;5:83–91.

47. Bradley LA, McKendree-Smith NL, Deutsch G, et al. Stressful imagery evokes enhanced thermal pain unpleasantness ratings and activation of cerebellum and motor, prefrontal, and posterior/temporal cortex in patients with fibromyalgia (FM). *Arthritis Rheum* 2004;50(Suppl):S493–S494.

48. Mogil JS, Wilson SG, Chesler EJ, et al. The melanocortin-1 receptor gene mediates female-specific mechanisms of analgesia in mice and humans. *Proc Natl Acad Sci USA* 2003;100:4867–4872.

49. Zubieta J-K, Heitzig MM, Smith YR, et al. COMT $val^{158}met$ genotype affects μ-opioid neurotransmitter responses to a pain stressor. *Science* 2003;299:1240–1243.

50. Diatchenko L, Slade GD, Nackley AG, et al. Genetic basis for individual variations in pain perception and the development of a chronic pain condition. *Hum Mol Genet* 2005;14:135–143.

51. Offenbaecher M, Bondy B, de Jonge S, et al. Possible association of fibromyalgia with a polymorphism in the serotonin transporter gene regulatory region. *Arthritis Rheum* 1999;42:2482–2488.

52. Cohen H, Buskila D, Neumann L, et al. Confirmation of an association between fibromyalgia and serotonin transporter promoter region (5-HTTLPR) polymorphism, and relationship to anxiety-related personality traits. *Arthritis Rheum* 2002;46:845–847.

53. Arnold LM, Hudson JI, Hess EV, et al. Family study of fibromyalgia. *Arthritis Rheum* 2004;50:944–952.

54. Raphael KG, Janal MN, Nayak S, et al. Familial aggregation of depression in fibromyalgia: a community-based test of alternate hypotheses. *Pain* 2004;110:449–460.

55. Buskila D, Neumann L. Fibromyalgia syndrome (FM) and nonaraticular tenderness in relatives of patients with FM. *J Rheumatol* 1997;24:941–944.

56. Goldenberg DL. Do infections trigger fibromyalgia [Editorial]? *Arthritis Rheum* 1993;36:1489–1492.

57. Alexander RW, Bradley LA, Alarcón GS, et al. Sexual and physical abuse in women with fibromyalgia: association with outpatient health care utilization and pain medication usage. *Arthritis Care Res* 1998;11:102–115.

58. Imbierowicz K, Egle UT. Childhood adversities in patients with fibromyalgia and somatoform pain disorder. *Eur J Pain* 2002;7:113–119.

59. Van Houdenhove B, Neerinckx E, Lysens R, et al. Victimization in chronic fatigue syndrome and fibromyalgia in tertiary care: a controlled study on prevalence and characteristics. *Psychosomatics* 2001;42:21–28.

60. Heiss C, Ehlert V, Hander JP, et al. Abuse-related posttraumatic stress disorder and alterations of the hypothalamic-pituitary-adrenal axis in women with chronic pelvic pains. *Psychsom Med* 1998;60:309–318.

61. McBeth J, Morris S, Benjamin S, et al. Associations between adverse events in childhood and chronic widespread pain in adulthood: are they explained by differential recall? *J Rheumatol* 2001;28:2305–2309.

62. Raphael KG, Widom CS, Lange G. Childhood victimization and pain in adulthood: a prospective investigation. *Pain* 2001;92:283–293.

63. Raphael KG, Janal MN, Nayak S. Comorbidity of fibromyalgia and posttraumatic stress disorder symptoms in a community sample of women. *Pain Med* 2004;5:33–41.

64. Raphael KG, Natelson BH, Janal MN, et al. A community-based survey of fibromyalgia-like pain complaints following the World Trade Center terrorist attacks. *Pain* 2002;100:131–139.

65. Scarinci IC, McDonald-Haile J, Bradley LA, et al. Altered pain perception and psychosocial features among women with gastrointestinal disorders and history of abuse: a preliminary model. *Am J Med* 1994;97:108–118.

66. Ringel Y, Whitehead WE, Toner BB, et al. Sexual and physical abuse are not associated with rectal hypersensitivity in patients with irritable bowel syndrome. *Gut* 2004;53:838–842.

67. Waylonis GW, Perkins RH. Post-traumatic fibromyalgia. A long-term follow-up. *Am J Phys Med Rehabil* 1994;73:403–412.

68. Greenfield S, Fitzcharles MA, Esdaile JM. Reactive fibromyalgia syndrome. *Arthritis Rheum* 1992;35:678–681.

69. Neumann L, Zeldets V, Bolotin A, et al. Outcome of posttraumatic fibromyalgia: a 3-year follow-up of 78 cases of cervical spine injuries. *Semin Arthritis Rheum* 2003;32:320–325.

70. Coderre TJ, Katz J, Vaccarino AL, et al. Contribution of central neuroplasticity to pathological pain: review of clinical experimental evidence. *Pain* 1993;52:259–285.

71. Schaible H-G, Ebersberger A, von Banchet GS. Mechanisms of pain in arthritis. *Ann N Y Acad Sci* 2001;966:343–354.

72. Watkins LR, Milligan ED, Maier SF. Glial activation: a driving force for pathological pain. *Trends Neurosci* 2001;24:450–455.

73. Milligan ED, Twining C, Chacur M, et al. Spinal glia and proinflammatory cytokines mediate mirror-image neuropathic pain in rats. *J Neurosci* 2003;23:1026–1040.

74. Bennett RM. Emerging concepts in the neurobiology of chronic pain: evidence of abnormal sensory processing in fibromyalgia. *Mayo Clin Proc* 1999;74:385–398.

75. Weigent DA, Bradley LA, Blalock JE, et al. Current concepts in the pathophysiology of abnormal pain perception in fibromyalgia. *Am J Med Sci* 1998;315:405–412.

76. Banic B, Petersen-Felix S, Andersen OK, et al. Evidence for spinal cord hypersensitivity in chronic pain after whiplash injury and in fibromyalgia. *Pain* 2004;107:7–15.

77. Buskila D, Neumann L. Musculoskeletal injury as a trigger for fibromyalgia/posttraumatic fibromyalgia. *Curr Rheumatol Rep* 2000;2:104–108.

78. Sprott H, Salemi S, Gay RE, et al. Increased DNA fragmentation and ultrastructural changes in fibromyalgic muscle fibres. *Ann Rheum Dis* 2004;63:245–251.

79. Neumann L, Zeldets V, Bolotin A, et al. Outcome of posttraumatic fibromyalgia: a 3-year follow-up of 78 cases of cervical spine injuries. *Semin Arthritis Rheum* 2003;32:320–325.

80. Turk DC, Okifuji A, Starz TW, et al. Effects of type of symptom onset on psychological distress and disability on fibromyalgia syndrome patients. *Pain* 1996;68:423–430.

81. Aaron LA, Bradley LA, Alarcón GS, et al. Perceived physical and emotional trauma as precipitating events in fibromyalgia: association with health care seeking and disability status but not pain severity. *Arthritis Rheum* 1997;40:453–460.

82. Rohling ML, Binder LM, Langhinrichsen-Rohling J. Money matters: a meta-analytic review of the association between financial compensation and the experience and treatment of chronic pain. *Health Psychol* 1995;14:537–547.

83. Harkness EF, Macfarlane GJ, Nahit E, et al. Mechanical injury and psychosocial factors in the work place predict the onset of widespread body pain: a two-year prospective study among cohorts of newly employed workers. *Arthritis Rheum* 2004;50:1655–1664.

84. McBeth J, Harkness EF, Silman AJ, et al. The role of workplace low-level mechanical trauma, posture and environment in the onset of chronic widespread pain. *Rheumatology* 2003;42:1–9.

85. McBeth J, Macfarlane GJ, Benjamin S, et al. Features of somatization predict the onset of chronic widespread pain: results of a large population-based study. *Arthritis Rheum* 2001;44:940–946.

86. Williams DA. Psychological and behavioural therapies in fibromyalgia and related syndromes. *Best Pract Res Clin Rheumatol* 2003;17:649–665.

87. Arnold LM, Lu Y, Crofford LJ, et al. A double-blind, multicenter trial comparing duloxetine with placebo in the treatment of fibromyalgia patients with or without major depressive disorder. *Arthritis Rheum* 2004;50:2974–2984.

88. Bradley LA. Cognitive-behavioral therapy for primary fibromyalgia. *J Rheumatol* 1989;19(Suppl):131–136.

89. Bradley LA, Young LD, Anderson KO, et al. Effects of psychological therapy on pain behavior of rheumatoid arthritis patients. Treatment outcome and six-month followup. *Arthritis Rheum* 1987;30:1105–1114.

90. Keefe FJ, Caldwell DS, Baucom D, et al. Spouse-assisted coping skills training in the management of knee pain in osteoarthritis: long-term followup results. *Arthritis Care Res* 1999;12:101–111.

91. White KP, Nielson WR. Cognitive-behavioral treatment of fibromyalgia syndrome: a follow-up assessment. *J Rheumatol* 1995;22:717–721.

92. Turk DC, Okifuji A, Sinclair JD, et al. Interdisciplinary treatment for fibromyalgia syndrome: clinical and statistical significance. *Arthritis Care Res* 1998;11:186–195.

93. Williams DA, Cary MA, Groner KH, et al. Improving physical functional status in patients with fibromyalgia: a brief cognitive behavioral intervention. *J Rheumatol* 2002;29:1280–1286.

94. Cedraschi C, Desmeules J, Rapiti E, et al. Fibromyalgia: a randomised, controlled trial of a treatment programme based on self management. *Ann Rheum Dis* 2004;63:290–296.

95. Buckelew SP, Conway R, Parker J, et al. Biofeedback/relaxation training and exercise interventions for fibromyalgia: a prospective trial. *Arthritis Care Res* 1998;11:196–209.

96. Nicassio PM, Radojevic V, Weisman MH, et al. A comparison of behavioral and educational interventions with fibromyalgia. *J Rheumatol* 1997;24:2000–2007.

97. Vlaeyen JWS, Teeken-Gruben NJG, Boosens MEJB, et al. Cognitive-educational treatment of fibromyalgia: a randomized clinical trial. I Clinical affects. *J Rheumatol* 1996;23:1237–1245.

98. McCracken LM, Zayfert C, Gross RT. The Pain Anxiety Symptoms Scale: development and validation of a scale to measure fear of pain. *Pain* 1992;50:67–73.

99. Roelofs J, Goubert L, Peters ML, et al. The Tampa Scale for Kinesiophobia: further examination of psychometric properties in patients with chronic low back pain and fibromyalgia. *Eur J Pain* 2004;8:495–502.

100. Waddell G, Newton M, Henderson I, et al. A Fear-Avoidance Beliefs Questionnaire (FABQ) and the role of fear-avoidance beliefs in chronic low back pain and disability. *Pain* 1993;52:157–168.

101. Kerns RD, Rosenberg R, Jamison RN, et al. Readiness to adopt a self-management approach to chronic pain: the Pain Stages of Change Questionnaire (PSOCQ). *Pain* 1997;72:227–234.

102. Burns JW, Mullen JT, Higdon LJ, et al. Validity of the Pain Anxiety Symptoms Scale (PASS): prediction of physical capacity variables. *Pain* 2000;84:247–252.

103. Ciccone DS, Just N. Pain expectancy and work disability in patients with acute and chronic pain: a test of the fear avoidance hypothesis. *J Pain* 2001;2:181–194.

104. Turk DC, Robinson JP, Burwinkle T. Prevalence of fear of pain and activity in patients with fibromyalgia syndrome. *J Pain* 2004;5:483–490.

105. Bradley LA, Alarcón GS. Fibromyalgia. In: Koopman WK, Moreland LW, eds. *Arthritis and allied conditions: a textbook of rheumatology*, 15th ed. Philadelphia, PA: Lippincott Williams & Wilkins, 2004:1869–1910.

106. Vlaeyen JW, de Jong J, Geilen M, et al. The treatment of fear of movement/(re)injury in chronic low back pain: further evidence on the effectiveness of exposure in vivo. *Clin J Pain* 2002;18:251–261.

107. Rooks DS, Silverman CB, Kantrowitz FG. The effects of progressive strength training and aerobic exercise on muscle strength and cardiovascular fitness in women with fibromyalgia: a pilot study. *Arthritis Rheum (Arthritis Care Res)* 2002;47:22–28.

108. Prochaska JO, DiClemente CC. Stages and processes of self-change of smoking: toward an integrative model of change. *J Consult Clin Psychol* 1983;51:390–395.

109. Prochaska JO, Velicer WF. The transtheoretical model of health behavior change. *Am J Health Promot* 1997;12:38–48.

110. Kerns RD, Habib S. A critical review of the pain readiness to change model. *J Pain* 2004;5:357–367.

111. Kerns RD, Rosenberg R, Jamison RN, et al. Readiness to adopt a self-management approach to chronic pain: the Pain Stages of Change Questionnaire (PSOCQ). *Pain* 1997;72:227–234.

112. Jensen MP, Nielson WR, Romano JM, et al. Further evaluation of the Pain Stages of Change Questionnaire: is the transtheoretical model of change useful for patients with chronic pain? *Pain* 2000;86:255–264.

113. Jensen MP, Nielson WR, Turner JA, et al. Readiness to self-manage pain is associated with coping and with psychological and physical functioning among patients with chronic pain. *Pain* 2003;104:529–537.

114. Jensen MP, Nielson WR, Turner JA, et al. Changes in readiness to self-manage pain are associated with improvement in multidisciplinary pain treatment and pain coping. *Pain* 2004;111:84–95.

115. Evers AW, Kraaimaat FW, van Lankveld W, et al. Beyond unfavorable thinking: the Illness Cognition Questionnaire for chronic diseases. *J Consult Clin Psychol* 2001;69:1026–1036.

116. Viane I, Crombez G, Eccleston C, et al. Acceptance of pain is an independent predictor of mental well-being in patients with chronic pain: empirical evidence and reappraisal. *Pain* 2003;106:65–72.

117. Viane I, Crombez G, Eccleston C, et al. Acceptance of the unpleasant reality of chronic pain: effects upon attention to pain and engagement with daily activities. *Pain* 2004;112:282–288.

15

Fibromyalgia in Children

David D. Sherry

A host of conditions exist in adults that are not generally thought of as typical childhood illnesses or conditions. Arthritis is a prime example, but pediatric rheumatology clinics all over the world are teeming with children with various forms of arthritis. Pain syndromes are no exception. Although children should not be burdened with chronic pain, there seems to be an explosion of children with a variety of chronic musculoskeletal pain syndromes, including fibromyalgia. These children suffer enormously, and the pain impairs their ability to develop and mature in order to reach their full potential. Family members also suffer due to the degree of dysfunction and disruption of normal family life.

Not only do these children suffer from pain but they frequently suffer from social isolation, sometimes to the point of being ostracized, even by the medical community. Physicians may tell them that they are faking or that it is all in their heads, or will, in frustration, tell family that they cannot help the child. However, the pain is real—as is the suffering. These children are not volunteers; they and their families are perhaps the most desperate patients we care for. Living with the unknown and the incurable is hardly bearable.

I hope in this chapter to explain some of what we know about these conditions in children, to show how to recognize them, and to offer a therapeutic approach.

THE NAME

The term fibromyalgia, when applied to children, presents problems since it is essentially a diagnosis of adults (1). Although there are similarities between adults and children who have widespread pain, the definition of fibromyalgia is different for children as is, perhaps, the treatment and outcome. There are few studies of children with fibromyalgia; what we know about fibromyalgia comes mostly from studies of adults, including the American College of Rheumatology (ACR) criteria of 1990 (2). Children have a variety of presentations that have been called fibromyalgia, including complex regional pain syndrome type 1 that spreads to include most of the body; chronic pain and 11 or 5 (or fewer),

depending on the criteria used, of 18 possible painful points; or severe pain to light touch over the entire body. The impact of merely labeling a child as having fibromyalgia is not known and may have long-lasting consequences, especially regarding health and disability insurance. When defining childhood fibromyalgia, authors typically use the criteria set forth by Yunus and Masi in 1985, which require only 5 painful trigger points and multiple related symptoms (see Table 15-1) (3) or the ACR criteria of 1990, which require 11 of the 18 possible painful trigger points. Both require chronic widespread pain, albeit somewhat differently defined. These criteria are not interchangeable as Reid et al. found that, of the children identified by the Yunus and Masi criteria as having fibromyalgia, only 78% were likewise identified by the ACR criteria (4). Most authors distinguish between children with regional pain syndromes, such as complex regional pain syndrome type 1, and children with diffuse pain, such as fibromyalgia. However, it has been my observation that many physicians will diagnose a child with prolonged widespread pain as having fibromyalgia without regard to either set of criteria. Malleson et al. make this point in their attempt to reclassify these pain syndromes as either localized idiopathic pain or diffuse idiopathic pain (5). Nevertheless, the term fibromyalgia will be used here to identify the subset of children with chronic amplified musculoskeletal pain, without clear autonomic dysfunction, and with widespread constant pain with painful tender or trigger points (6). The term widespread musculoskeletal pain will be used when discussing references that use this term since these children may or may not have fibromyalgia as defined above. We will not discuss children with localized pain syndromes or those with intermittent severe localized or diffuse musculoskeletal pain.

EPIDEMIOLOGY

There has been little research on the prevalence of fibromyalgia in children. Buskila, using the ACR criteria, found that 21 (6%) of a sample of 338 school children, aged 9 to 15, fulfilled criteria for fibromyalgia (7). An additional seven subjects (2%) had 11 or more tender points (TePs)

TABLE 15-1 The Yunus and Masi Criteria for Fibromyalgia in Children

MAJOR

1. Generalized musculoskeletal aching at three or more sites for 3 or more months
2. Absence of underlying condition or cause
3. Normal laboratory tests
4. Five or more typical tender points

MINOR

1. Poor sleep
2. Fatigue
3. Chronic anxiety or tension
4. Chronic headaches
5. Irritable bowel syndrome
6. Subjective soft tissue swelling
7. Numbness
8. Pain modulation by physical activities
9. Pain modulation by weather factors
10. Pain modulation by anxiety/stress

Fibromyalgia defined as present if the subject has:
all four major criteria and three minor criteria;
or first three major criteria, four tender points, and five minor criteria.
From Yunus MB, Masi AT. Juvenile primary fibromyalgia syndrome. A clinical study of thirty-three patients and matched normal controls. *Arthritis Rheum* 1985;28(2):138–145, with permission.

without widespread pain and so were not included in the fibromyalgia group. Fifteen children who had been classified as having fibromyalgia from this unique group were reevaluated 30 months later and 11 (78%) resolved their painful trigger points and pain (8). Since these children were not seeking medical care for musculoskeletal pain, it is unknown if this is indicative of the incidence of what we recognize as fibromyalgia in the clinic.

Compared to the 6% found in Israeli children above, Clark et al. reported a much lower prevalence of fibromyalgia in Mexican children (9). They examined 548 children between the ages of 9 and 15 and found that only 1.2% fulfilled the criteria for fibromyalgia. They speculated that this was due to cultural differences. It has been shown that there is more low back pain in developed nations than in developing nations (10).

In Finland, Mikkelsson et al. studied 1,756 children with a structured pain questionnaire and identified 7.5% reporting widespread pain (11). Physical examinations were not done.

Another way of approaching this question is to look at the percentage of children presenting to pediatric rheumatology clinics who are diagnosed with fibromyalgia. There are several reports of what diagnoses are made in pediatric rheumatology clinics, and fibromyalgia is diagnosed in approximately 3% of children; however, between two and five times as many children are given nebulous diagnoses such as limb pain, back pain, psychogenic pain, or idiopathic pain syndrome, and they probably include some children who have fibromyalgia (12–16).

It is the general consensus that the number of children with fibromyalgia and widespread musculoskeletal pain is increasing, but there are no epidemiologic data upon which to base this view. However, if one considers the pages dedicated to chronic pain syndromes in various editions of the *Textbook of Pediatric Rheumatology*, they have increased steadily from 2 pages in 1982, 3 pages in 1990, and 4 pages in 1995, to a chapter of 13 pages in 2000 (17–20).

SEX

Girls are overrepresented in all series of childhood fibromyalgia; a combination of reports from clinics suggests a girl-to-boy ratio of 5:1 (3–5,21–26). However, in studies not based in the clinic, a school survey revealed a girl-to-boy ratio of 2:1, and in children of women with fibromyalgia the female-to-male ratio was approximately 1.5:1 (7,27,28). This may be explained to a degree by the fact that girls more frequently report pain and have lower pain thresholds (7,29). However, concerning clinic patients, there is no difference in physician utilization between Dutch boys and girls reporting chronic pain (30).

RACE

Although no formal epidemiologic studies have been reported, a majority of children with fibromyalgia have been white (22,31). There is a suspicion that the majority of patients are from the upper socioeconomic level, but data is lacking and this could certainly represent access to healthcare rather than true differences in incidence. However, it is my impression that over the years this is changing and fibromyalgia is increasingly recognized in children of all races and socioeconomic levels.

AGE

Since fibromyalgia is frequently seen in adults, the mean age of childhood onset fibromyalgia is influenced by the maximum age that is seen in the pediatric clinics. Nevertheless, most report a mean age around 12 to 14. More important are the very young children, since below age 7 or 8 this is a rare condition. It is only with trepidation that one should make this diagnosis in the very young. However, it is not uncommon for parents to report that their adolescent has hurt ever since he or she could remember or talk. It is extremely unusual, even in these children, for medical help to have been sought below the age of 7. One exception is children who have had prior hypermobility pains, which are common in young children, before the onset of their fibromyalgia [and hypermobility has been associated with an increased incidence of fibromyalgia (32)].

ETIOLOGY

There is no known etiology. A host of possible factors may contribute to the development of fibromyalgia in children. In some children one factor may predominate, whereas in others it plays no role at all. Because the cause is unknown, there have been multiple associations made to a variety of disparate factors ranging from genetic to purely psychological. No one factor is uniformly present in children with fibromyalgia.

Several studies have pointed to genetic factors. Buskila et al., in studying 58 offspring from 20 mothers with fibromyalgia, found that 28% had fibromyalgia (27). Additionally, the authors noted a male-to-female ratio of 0.8 in the offspring and no difference in psychological variables studied, implying a genetic rather than a psychological cause. There are other reports that not only fibromyalgia, but also chronic pain, is more common in family members of children with fibromyalgia (26). However, the genetic influences are not overwhelmingly strong, and the vast majority of children with fibromyalgia are from families that do not have other members with it.

Hypermobility has been proposed as a cause of fibromyalgia. Gedalia et al. screened 338 schoolchildren for both hypermobility and fibromyalgia and found that 81% of those with fibromyalgia were also hypermobile (32). However, only a small percentage of children with hypermobility get fibromyalgia. Reid et al. found that none of 15 children with fibromyalgia were hypermobile, and Gedalia, later in a rheumatology clinic setting, found that only 14% were hypermobile (4,25). In adults there is a greater frequency of hypermobility among those with fibromyalgia; however, only 27% were hypermobile (33).

Very few studies have looked at hormonal causes in children with fibromyalgia—even though it is predominantly found in girls and its onset, in many, coincides with the onset of puberty. Prolactin levels were normal in 11 children with fibromyalgia (25).

Psychological causes of childhood fibromyalgia loom large in the experience of many, but good controlled studies are lacking. However, in a study of over 1,000 children who were pain free initially, girls with more psychosocial difficulties, who had headaches and who were more active in sports, were more likely to develop, over the next year, widespread musculoskeletal pain (34). Looking the other way round, Egger et al. found "girls with musculoskeletal pains, headaches, and abdominal pains were associated with anxiety disorders, and musculoskeletal pain, in both boys and girls, was associated with depression" (35). These two studies were population studies; no physical examinations were performed, so no subject was given a formal diagnosis.

In studies of children with idiopathic musculoskeletal pain, Aasland et al. found that children with chronic pain had more pain role models, more school stress, and more often lived with just one biological parent as compared to children with arthritis (36). Mikkelsson, also from Finland, found children with fibromyalgia had a higher depression score than did children with widespread musculoskeletal pain (37). Six of ten children with fibromyalgia evaluated by Vandvik and Forseth had psychiatric diagnoses, mostly depression and anxiety (24). In these children they found a very high rate of chronic pain in the family (seven mothers and three fathers). Although family clustering may reflect genetic cause or propensity, this is balanced by the theory that role models within the family and the family's psychological environment may predispose to fibromyalgia—that is, nurture versus nature. There is one report of both parents and four children who developed almost identical chronic pain after a motor vehicle crash and during prolonged litigation (38).

It is likely that there is a combination of both intrinsic factors, such as individual pain threshold, female sex, and intrinsic coping strategies, and extrinsic factors, such as previous pain experiences, social stresses, parental modeling of chronic-pain behaviors, poor sleep, and central and peripheral pain mechanisms, that work in concert to give rise to the constellation of signs and symptoms we call fibromyalgia. Regardless of the etiology, the tenacious feeling about the etiology frequently leads to a marked level of frustration in these children and their families. Clinically, this can be manifested by the host of reasons the family will put forward as causes of their child's fibromyalgia. These include "Lyme test negative Lyme disease," mononucleosis, connective tissue disease, muscle disease, lupus [in children with a benignly positive antinuclear antibodies (ANA) test], or injury (39). Many families will hear of a case of fibromyalgia that is cured with the treatment du jour, which will motivate them to try numerous allopathic and complementary treatments. Whatever the cause, these children's lives (and their families') are significantly disrupted and they are desperate for help.

CLINICAL MANIFESTATIONS

The presentation of children with fibromyalgia varies with each child, but unifying threads weave a pattern recognizable from child to child. Since this is a clinical diagnosis, careful attention needs to be heeded regarding these clinical clues. Having said this, there are some notable exceptions that will be discussed later.

Most children with fibromyalgia are preadolescent to adolescent girls with a chief complaint of body pain and fatigue. Some will limit their complaint to back pain. The pain starts insidiously but increases to the point of severe pain and marked disability. Uniformly, children who miss significant amounts of school due to musculoskeletal pain have fibromyalgia or another amplified musculoskeletal pain syndrome rather than an inflammatory or rheumatic illness. Not only have they missed school, but also they are usually engaged in multiple social activities that they are unable to do no matter how enjoyable.

It is rare to be the second doctor they have seen. Most have had multiple consultations with many physicians addressing every complaint. The neurologist evaluates the headache, the gastroenterologist the abdominal pain, the endocrinologist the fatigue, and finally, the rheumatologist, usually after the orthopedist, the musculoskeletal pain. Unlike most children who have rheumatic diseases, children with fibromyalgia frequently have a generally positive review of systems; they feel their bodies more than most. Additionally, the past history can reveal either episodes of prior prolonged pain or that the child heals very slowly after routine injuries and illnesses.

The social history is fairly typical. These are good children, high achieving, and very involved in sports and social activities, and they are generally viewed as helpers—mature children who like to please others. Not uncommonly there has been a series of major life events, but whether these occur more often than in controls is unknown. Although the pain and disability place increased stress upon them, they are thought to be handling it quite well.

Each of the criteria (Table 15-1) needs to be explored. The major criteria are uniformly present; however, the frequency of the minor criteria varies depending upon the study population (3,4,21). The 1990 ACR criteria are reviewed elsewhere (Chapter 10).

MAJOR CRITERIA

Generalized Musculoskeletal Aching at Three or More Sites for 3 or More Months

This usually will involve half of the body (in accordance with the adult criteria), but it can be more confined. Most often the pain is symmetric and, although constant, can include morning stiffness and evening pain.

Absence of Underlying Condition or Cause

Most serious conditions leading to the degree of pain and dysfunction present in these children will manifest themselves before the 3-month time period. Occasionally, a child with unrecognized musculoskeletal disease will be misdiagnosed with fibromyalgia. The most common condition, in my experience, is enthesitis. However, children with fibromyalgia can have enthesalgia, so a therapeutic trial of anti-inflammatory agents may be required before establishing the diagnosis.

Normal Laboratory Tests

Most children will have a screening of complete blood count, measurement of acute phase reactants, chemistry panels, and thyroid function tests. Imaging may be indicated, but it usually is not unless only one body region is affected (back). Significantly abnormal laboratory tests should put the diagnosis on hold until further investigations or therapeutic trials can be done or, if needed, enough time is allowed for the underlying illness to fully manifest itself. This is not to say that secondary fibromyalgia may not exist, but it precludes a diagnosis of primary fibromyalgia.

Five or More Typical Tender Points

This is a bit of a misnomer since the classic 18 points should be painful by report, not just tender or sore (3). Pain at these sites is usually elicited by applying approximately 4 kg of pressure with the thumb. In children, Buskila has argued that 3 kg may be a better discriminator between normal and abnormal sensitivity to pressure (40). Control points should not be painful to palpation; however, many authors either do not use control points to differentiate between fibromyalgia and widespread pain or fail to mention whether control points were tested.

MINOR CRITERIA

Poor Sleep

The most frequent complaint associated with childhood fibromyalgia is poor sleep. These children wake up tired and frequently remain tired all day. In the evenings they have a bit more energy—to the point that they find it hard to go to sleep. The one study of sleep in children with fibromyalgia studied 34 children with fibromyalgia, 10 children with diffuse pain, and 17 asymptomatic control children (23). In this report the mothers were also studied, and 71% of the mothers of the children with fibromyalgia also had fibromyalgia, whereas only 30% of the mothers of children with widespread pain did and none of the control mothers did. The mothers with fibromyalgia had the most abnormal sleep with decreased sleep efficiency, increase in arousal during sleep, and α-intrusion in slow wave sleep. Even though the children with fibromyalgia had less abnormal sleep, this did not lessen their sleep complaints. Most children with fibromyalgia who report very poor sleep—for example, "I only sleep 1 hour a night"—do not fall asleep during the day or have hypersomnolence. When observed, these children sleep much longer than they report.

Fatigue

Almost all these children will report fatigue. The fatigue can, at times, be more limiting than the pain, and if they go to school at all they may go late because of the morning fatigue. This can be very frustrating because they sometimes may be able to work through the pain but not the fatigue. There is an overlap between children who satisfy the criteria for juvenile chronic fatigue syndrome and fibromyalgia (41).

Chronic Anxiety or Tension

Most of these children do not feel particularly tense or anxious except as it relates to their illness. A few children will have overt free-floating anxiety prior to the onset of their fibromyalgia. This can be manifested by undue worry that the diagnosis is not correct and more studies need to be done.

Chronic Headaches

These are generally muscle contraction tension headaches. However, they can be described in hyperbolic terms. Occasionally the headache is the primary complaint and the fatigue and body pains are much less of a concern. Rarely are there migraine-associated symptoms. The headache does not respond well to standard migraine therapies. Headache, more than musculoskeletal pain, leads to the complaint of decreased ability to concentrate (42).

Irritable Bowel Syndrome

This is the least frequent minor criterion manifested by children with fibromyalgia. They may have abdominal pain but rarely the diarrhea or constipation associated with irritable bowel.

Subjective Soft Tissue Swelling

Swelling is also one of the less often reported minor criteria, but the number of children who report swelling of the lower back, the hip, or other deep structure is still surprising. Sometimes the child will point out swelling during the examination; however, the examiner is unable to appreciate any edema or soft tissue enlargement.

Numbness

This usually involves large parts of the body not along either dermatomal or peripheral nerve distributions. Hands and feet can become numb if the child is hyperventilating, which is not uncommon. This will be considered further below in the discussion of conversion reactions.

Pain Modulation by Physical Activities

This is a very common minor criterion. Most children will report that even if they force themselves to be active, they suffer for it the next day with extreme musculoskeletal pain and fatigue.

Pain Modulation by Weather Factors

Another common criterion is one usually manifested as feeling more pain during inclement weather and feeling better on hot, dry days. However, if the weather stays constant, the pain continues to get worse over time.

Pain Modulation by Anxiety/Stress

This is slightly less frequent than the modulation criteria of weather and activity. Some children will definitely identify stressors that will cause an increase in their symptoms. However, some are very defensive about any psychological factor playing any role at all and will not be able to identify any stressors in their life—much less an untoward effect of stress or anxiety.

OTHER FEATURES

Many noncriteria findings are common to many patients and are features of their fibromyalgia.

Allodynia

Allodynia is pain felt in response to normally nonpainful stimuli and is common. This is elicited by either light touch or by gently pinching a fold of skin. The area of allodynia is not dermatomal or innervated by a single peripheral nerve, and the border can, during repeated examinations, vary widely, come and go, or be quite vague. The allodynia frequently will cause the child not to wear tight clothes or any clothes at all when at home. Some girls will wear only a light nightgown because the weight of regular fabric causes pain.

Incongruent Affect and La Belle Indifference

The quality of pain and pain behavior is noteworthy. Most patients will have a cheerful affect while complaining of severe pain and an indifference to the pain and disability (43). This can lead to the feeling that the child is not experiencing much pain or is exaggerating, and the child is accused of faking or just seeking attention. However, one must take at face value the fact that the pain is real and severe since all pain is subjective and is known only to the sufferer (44).

Conversion Symptoms

It is not unusual for children with fibromyalgia to have overt conversion symptoms. Conversion symptoms do not hurt, but they involve motor and sensory nerve dysfunction. The numbness discussed above as a minor criterion may be a conversion symptom. Conversion symptoms may include paralysis, blindness, abnormal shaking, and pseudoseizures. Many children complain of dizziness. In one study of 12 children with fibromyalgia and dizziness, no abnormalities were found in vestibular function, rotary chair testing, and electronystagmography (45).

Waddell's Nonorganic Back Pain Signs

Waddell et al. described a set of signs that helps distinguish organic back pain from nonorganic (46). These include allodynia, passive rotation, axial loading, distracted straight leg raising, and overreaction. I have found the first three the most useful. Allodynia is described above. Passive rotation is the process of passively rotating the patient at the ankles and knees while keeping the pelvis, back, and shoulder in the same plane. This should not hurt the back since the back is not moving. The axial loading test is done by exerting downward pressure on the top of a standing patient's head. Neck pain may be reported, but it should not hurt the lower back. The distracted straight leg raising test is positive when flexion of the hip causes back pain when the subject is supine but not when sitting and attention is drawn away from the back. Overreaction is defined at excessive wincing, screaming, or collapsing with pain. This is very subjective but is overtly obvious to the experienced examiner. Song et al. have a somewhat modified Waddell checklist in which 77% of children with organic back pain had no inappropriate symptoms while 79% of children with nonorganic back pain had two or more inappropriate symptoms (47).

Children do not like to follow rules and so will present with overlapping amplified musculoskeletal pain syndromes. Therefore, a child may have complex regional pain syndrome type 1 of the foot and then the pain will spread to include most of the body. The child will have widespread allodynia so all 18 TePs are painful. This child could fit the definition of fibromyalgia. It is impossible to tell from the literature how often there are overlapping amplified pain syndromes, but in my experience this is not rare.

DIFFERENTIAL DIAGNOSIS

SPONDYLOARTHROPATHY

Spondyloarthropathy and enthesitis are the most frequent diagnoses I make in children referred for fibromyalgia. Referring physicians infrequently recognize enthesitis, and it is not often helped with the standard over-the-counter pain and anti-inflammatory medications (48). The salient features include a family history of low back pain (even if there is an alleged cause), morning pain and stiffness, tenderness at multiple entheses (especially the plantar fascial insertion on the calcaneous, the Achilles tendon insertion, the inferior pole of the patella, and over the sacroiliac joints), and, perhaps, a limited modified Schober's measurement (49).

THYROID DISEASE

Both hypothyroidism and hyperthyroidism can be associated with widespread body pain in children (50,51). Usually other features of thyroid disease are present. Most children, especially if fatigue is a major complaint, will have thyroid function tests done early in the course of their illness.

TUMOR

Most malignant diseases will cause more systemic illness and declare themselves relatively rapidly. However, the one exception is a spinal cord tumor, which can be associated with long-standing back pain and disability (52). Careful attention to the neurologic examination and spine mobility can usually identify these children.

OTHER

One mother who was diagnosed with fibromyalgia and her 10-year-old son with similar symptoms were found to have hyperkalemic periodic paralysis (53). The first patient referred to my chronic musculoskeletal pain clinic for fibromyalgia had widespread arthritis. It should give one pause before making a diagnosis of fibromyalgia since it is more than just a process of tallying up painful points.

ASSESSMENT OF DISEASE ACTIVITY

Both initially and during follow-up, some sort of ongoing assessment of disease activity should be made. Two major arenas need to be measured: pain and dysfunction. Since pain is subjective it is best measured by self-report. This is possible even in younger children using various scales that have been validated for younger children, which usually involve faces depicting different levels of pain (54). Functional measures can take a variety of forms, from direct measurement of standard activities to questionnaires. There are no fibromyalgia-specific measures for children, but general scales measuring activities of daily living, such as the Childhood Health Assessment Questionnaire, can be helpful (55).

In addition to pain and function, some assessment of the psychodynamics involved in the life of the child and family is warranted (26,43). Regardless of the premorbid psychological condition, the pain and dysfunction can have widespread psychological ramifications on the family members.

TREATMENT

Before discussing the variety of treatments per se, it is first paramount to establish a trusting and sincere rapport with the child and family. It is only upon this trust that any recommendations you may give will be taken seriously. Foremost is to believe that the child is in pain. Frequently children are given both verbal and nonverbal messages that the pain is all in their heads or that they are malingering. This accomplishes nothing but alienation. I have found it useful to explain the pain in terms of sympathetically mediated pain amplification; this makes the pain very real and can introduce the treatment strategies (6).

It is important to remember that the primary goal of therapy is to restore function, which we can do, and the secondary goal is to reduce pain, which we cannot directly treat. A corollary to the above is that the peripheral symptoms—sleep, fatigue, abdominal pains, numbness, headache, and such—are also not directly treated but most get better as function improves.

There have been no controlled studies of various therapies in children with fibromyalgia, a fact made evident by the plethora of disparate therapies that have been advanced. Therefore, most authors will recommend treating children with fibromyalgia in much the same manner as adults (3,21,22,25,56). Most of this treatment has centered on sleep (low-dose tricyclic antidepressants), pain control (nonsteroidal anti-inflammatory agents), education, and mild aerobic exercise (57). One report on the use of cyclobenzaprine in 15 children said that it helped 11, but the degree and durability of improvement was not reported (22). In another study, only 3 of 33 children treated with cyclobenzaprine would recommend it to other children with fibromyalgia (21).

Although sleep is a frequent theme in the descriptions of childhood fibromyalgia, no data address the benefit of treating sleep per se. Good sleep hygiene is advocated, but the degree to which it will be helpful is unknown. As with adults, it has been recommended to try a low-dose tricyclic antidepressant medication to facilitate sleep initiation (21,56).

Analgesics have not been studied in children with fibromyalgia but in my experience they do not work. Children may be on multiple agents because each helps "just a little," but the pain is still ranked as severe. It seems to me that these children suffer more untoward effects of medication than do children with inflammatory rheumatic diseases. Therefore, my approach is to discontinue as quickly as possible nonsteroidal anti-inflammatory agents, muscle relaxants, anticonvulsants, antidepressants (if used for pain rather than depression or anxiety), pain medications, including opioids, and nonallopathic remedies and treatments. Children with clinical depression or pervasive anxiety may benefit from an antidepressant such as a serotonin reuptake inhibitor.

Exercise therapy has not been formally studied in children but in our hands an intense aerobic exercise program—that is, 5 to 6 hours of physical and occupational daily for an average or 2 to 3 weeks—is associated with most children resolving their pain and almost all regaining full function (58). Using this intense exercise treatment program, 13 of 14 children with fibromyalgia resolved all back pain and trigger points, 10 of 12 resolved their initial sleep disturbance, and 6 of 7 resolved their depressive symptoms (59). This is the same program used very successfully in children with complex regional pain syndrome type 1 (60). In our program all medications and treatments are discontinued unless there is another indication for them, since the burden is on the children to fix themselves with exercise rather than to have us fix them with medication.

Many authors advocate mild aerobic training; however, it is imperative that minimal function be restored, such as attending school and engaging in normal social activities (21,56).

Psychological therapy for children with fibromyalgia has mostly taken the form of cognitive behavior therapy (61,62). Walco and Ilowite treated five girls with fibromyalgia with four to nine sessions of instruction in self-regulation of musculoskeletal pain (progressive relaxation and guided imagery); four reported no pain an average of 10 months later (63). Gedalia et al. reported that only two of five found cognitive-behavioral therapy to be of help (25). Others have recommended more formal psychotherapy based on the results of an initial psychological evaluation (24,26,58). It is my experience that children do benefit to a degree from cognitive behavior therapy but it does not lead to complete relief and they do not practice it often, even when the pain flares up; most children and families benefit more from more traditional psychotherapy.

Other nonallopathic treatments are frequently sought, but there is no data on their benefit. In addition to herbal therapy, massage, magnet therapy, homeopathy, reflexology, and aromatherapy, to name a few, have been tried, and, in the children I see, to no avail. None can be recommended.

OUTCOME

The long-term prognosis of children with fibromyalgia is not known. The outcome study of Buskila et al. reports that 11 of 15 schoolchildren previously found on screening to have fibromyalgia resolved their fibromyalgia after 30 months (8). These children, it can be argued, were very dissimilar to clinic patients since none had sufficient symptoms and dysfunction to be referred to specialty care. In a study of 12 children diagnosed with fibromyalgia and instructed to get counseling, biofeedback, and aerobic conditioning, after 15 to 60 months 11 still had significant pain (64). Siegel et al. treated 45 children with low-dose tricyclic antidepressant medication, mild exercise, and nonsteroidal mediation, and 94% of 33 subjects called 1 year later still had diffuse pain and poor sleep, although their overall well-being improved 1.8 points on a 1 to 10 point scale (21). As above, those treated by Walco and Ilowite with a cognitive behavior program fared better, but the sample size was extremely small, as was the sample treated with intense exercise therapy (59,63).

Nonpainful long-term outcomes have not been reported, although I have had patients who have had a variety of seemly related conditions develop, including pure conversion reactions, eating disorders, school avoidance, suicide attempts, and acting out behaviors. Others have developed nonfibromyalgia painful conditions, including incapacitating headache or abdominal pain, and amplified musculoskeletal pain such as complex regional pain syndrome type 1.

Substantial long-term outcome data should be evaluated based on the degree of involvement (pain and disability), psychological factors, and treatment used and should include fibromyalgia, other amplified musculoskeletal pains, and the nonpainful long-term outcome variables listed above.

SUMMARY POINTS

- Although good epidemiologic studies are lacking, chronic widespread pain and fibromyalgia are common in children and may be increasing in frequency.

■ IMPLICATIONS FOR PRACTICE

- Children with fibromyalgia suffer significant pain and disability and need compassionate care that should include accurate diagnosis as well as a consistent evaluative and therapeutic approach.
- At a minimum, normal function should be restored; school attendance should be mandatory and social and sports activities encouraged.
- If pain continues, either pain-coping skills via cognitive-behavioral therapy or more formal psychotherapy should be pursued.
- The use of pharmacologic agents should be limited to specific indications and not used just for pain control or just because the diagnosis is fibromyalgia.

REFERENCES

1. Schanberg LE. Widespread pain in children: when is it pathologic? *Arthritis Rheum* 2003;48(9):2402–2405.
2. Wolfe F, Smythe HA, Yunus MB, et al. The American College of Rheumatology 1990 criteria for the classification of fibromyalgia. Report of the Multicenter Criteria Committee. *Arthritis Rheum* 1990;33(2):160–172.
3. Yunus MB, Masi AT. Juvenile primary fibromyalgia syndrome. A clinical study of thirty-three patients and matched normal controls. *Arthritis Rheum* 1985;28(2):138–145.
4. Reid GJ, Lang BA, McGrath PJ. Primary juvenile fibromyalgia: psychological adjustment, family functioning, coping, and functional disability. *Arthritis Rheum* 1997;40(4):752–760.
5. Malleson PN, al-Matar M, Petty RE. Idiopathic musculoskeletal pain syndromes in children. *J Rheumatol* 1992;19(11):1786–1789.
6. Sherry DD. An overview of amplified musculoskeletal pain syndromes. *J Rheumatol* 2000;27(Suppl. 58):44–48.
7. Buskila D, Press J, Gedalia A, et al. Assessment of nonarticular tenderness and prevalence of fibromyalgia in children. *J Rheumatol* 1993;20(2):368–370.
8. Buskila D, Neumann L, Hershman E, et al. Fibromyalgia syndrome in children—an outcome study. *J Rheumatol* 1995;22(3):525–528.
9. Clark P, Burgos-Vargas R, Medina-Palma C, et al. Prevalence of fibromyalgia in children: a clinical study of Mexican children. *J Rheumatol* 1998;25(10):2009–2014.
10. Volinn E. The epidemiology of low back pain in the rest of the world. A review of surveys in low- and middle-income countries. *Spine* 1997;22(15):1747–1754.
11. Mikkelsson M, Salminen JJ, Kautiainen H. Non-specific musculoskeletal pain in preadolescents. Prevalence and 1-year persistence. *Pain* 1997;73(1):29–35.
12. Bowyer S, Roettcher P, Pediatric Rheumatology Database Research Group. Pediatric rheumatology clinic populations in the United States: results of a 3 year survey. *J Rheumatol* 1996;23(11):1968–1974.
13. Denardo BA, Tucker LB, Miller LC, et al. Demography of a regional pediatric rheumatology patient population. Affiliated

Children's Arthritis Centers of New England [Comment]. *J Rheumatol* 1994;21(8):1553–1561.

14. Malleson PN, Fung MY, Rosenberg AM. The incidence of pediatric rheumatic diseases: results from the Canadian Pediatric Rheumatology Association Disease Registry [Comment]. *J Rheumatol* 1996;23(11):1981–1987.

15. Rosenberg AM. Analysis of a pediatric rheumatology clinic population. *J Rheumatol* 1990;17(6):827–830.

16. Symmons DP, Jones M, Osborne J, et al. Pediatric rheumatology in the United Kingdom: data from the British Pediatric Rheumatology Group National Diagnostic Register. *J Rheumatol* 1996;23(11):1975–1980.

17. Ragsdale CG. Differential diagnosis: nonrheumatic conditions that present with rheumatic symptoms. In: Cassidy JT, ed. *Textbook of pediatric rheumatology*. New York: John Wiley and Sons, 1982:568–570.

18. Cassidy JT, Petty RE. *Textbook of pediatric rheumatology*, 2nd ed. New York: Churchill Livingstone, 1990:104–107.

19. Cassidy JT, Petty RE. *Textbook of pediatric rheumatology*, 3rd ed. Philadelphia, PA: WB Saunders, 1995:125–129.

20. Sherry DD, Malleson PN. Idiopathic musculoskeletal pain syndromes. In: Cassidy JT, Petty RE, eds. *Textbook of pediatric rheumatology*, 4th ed. Philadelphia, PA: WB Saunders, 2000:381–394.

21. Siegel DM, Janeway D, Baum J. Fibromyalgia syndrome in children and adolescents: clinical features at presentation and status at follow-up. *Pediatrics* 1998;101(3 Pt 1): 377–382.

22. Romano TJ. Fibromyalgia in children; diagnosis and treatment. *W V Med J* 1991;87(3):112–114.

23. Roizenblatt S, Tufik S, Goldenberg J, et al. Juvenile fibromyalgia: clinical and polysomnographic aspects. *J Rheumatol* 1997; 24(3):579–585.

24. Vandvik IH, Forseth KO. A bio-psychosocial evaluation of ten adolescents with fibromyalgia. *Acta Paediatr* 1994; 83(7):766–771.

25. Gedalia A, Garcia CO, Molina JF, et al. Fibromyalgia syndrome: experience in a pediatric rheumatology clinic. *Clin Exp Rheumatol* 2000;18(3):415–419.

26. Schanberg LE, Keefe FJ, Lefebvre JC, et al. Social context of pain in children with juvenile primary fibromyalgia syndrome: parental pain history and family environment. *Clin J Pain* 1998;14(2):107–115.

27. Buskila D, Neumann L, Hazanov I, et al. Familial aggregation in the fibromyalgia syndrome. *Semin Arthritis Rheum* 1996;26(3):605–611.

28. Buskila D, Neumann L. Fibromyalgia syndrome (FM) and nonarticular tenderness in relatives of patients with FM. *J Rheumatol* 1997;24(5):941–944.

29. Perquin CW, Hazebroek-Kampschreur AA, Hunfeld JA, et al. Pain in children and adolescents: a common experience. *Pain* 2000;87(1):51–58.

30. van Eekelen FC, Perquin CW, Hunfeld JA, et al. Comparison between children and adolescents with and without chronic benign pain: consultation rate and pain characteristics. *Br J Gen Pract* 2002;52(476):211–213.

31. Yunus MB, Berg BC, Masi AT. Multiphase skeletal scintigraphy in primary fibromyalgia syndrome: a blinded study. *J Rheumatol* 1989;16(11):1466–1468.

32. Gedalia A, Press J, Klein M, et al. Joint hypermobility and fibromyalgia in schoolchildren. *Ann Rheum Dis* 1993; 52(7):494–496.

33. Acasuso-Diaz M, Collantes-Estevez E. Joint hypermobility in patients with fibromyalgia syndrome. *Arthritis Care Res* 1998;11(1):39–42.

34. Jones GT, Silman AJ, Macfarlane GJ. Predicting the onset of widespread body pain among children. *Arthritis Rheum* 2003;48:2615–2621.

35. Egger HL, Costello EJ, Erkanli A, et al. Somatic complaints and psychopathology in children and adolescents: stomach aches, musculoskeletal pains, and headaches. *J Am Acad Child Adolesc Psychiatry* 1999;38(7):852–860.

36. Aasland A, Flato B, Vandvik IH. Psychosocial factors in children with idiopathic musculoskeletal pain: a prospective, longitudinal study. *Acta Paediatr* 1997;86(7):740–746.

37. Mikkelsson M, Sourander A, Piha J, et al. Psychiatric symptoms in preadolescents with musculoskeletal pain and fibromyalgia. *Pediatrics* 1997;100(2 Pt 1):220–227.

38. Mailis A, Furlong W, Taylor A. Chronic pain in a family of 6 in the context of litigation [Comment]. *J Rheumatol* 2000;27(5):1315–1317.

39. Sigal LH, Patella SJ. Lyme arthritis as the incorrect diagnosis in pediatric and adolescent fibromyalgia. *Pediatrics* 1992;90(4):523–528.

40. Buskila D. Fibromyalgia in children—lessons from assessing nonarticular tenderness. *J Rheumatol* 1996;23(12): 2017–2019.

41. Breau LM, McGrath PJ, Ju LH. Review of juvenile primary fibromyalgia and chronic fatigue syndrome. *J Dev Behav Pediatr* 1999;20(4):278–288.

42. Hunfeld JA, Perquin CW, Bertina W, et al. Stability of pain parameters and pain-related quality of life in adolescents with persistent pain: a three-year follow-up. *Clin J Pain* 2002;18(2):99–106.

43. Sherry DD, McGuire T, Mellins E, et al. Psychosomatic musculoskeletal pain in childhood: clinical and psychological analyses of 100 children. *Pediatrics* 1991;88(6):1093–1099.

44. Merskey DM, Bogduk N. *Classification of chronic pain. Descriptions of chronic pain syndromes and definitions of pain terms.* Seattle, WA: IASP Press, 1994.

45. Rusy LM, Harvey SA, Beste DJ. Pediatric fibromyalgia and dizziness: evaluation of vestibular function. *J Dev Behav Pediatr* 1999;20(4):211–215.

46. Waddell G, McCulloch JA, Kummel E, et al. Nonorganic physical signs in low-back pain. *Spine* 1980;5(2):117–125.

47. Song KM, Morton AA, Koch KD, et al. Chronic musculoskeletal pain in childhood. *J Pediatr Orthop* 1998;18(5): 576–581.

48. Sherry DD, Malleson PN. The idiopathic musculoskeletal pain syndromes in childhood. *Rheum Dis Clin North Am* 2002;28(3):669–685.

49. Sherry DD, Sapp LR. Enthesalgia in childhood: site-specific tenderness in healthy subjects and in patients with seronegative enthesopathic arthropathy. *J Rheumatol* 2003;30(6): 1335–1340.

50. Carette S, Lefrancois L. Fibrositis and primary hypothyroidism. *J Rheumatol* 1988;15(9):1418–1421.

51. Wilke WS, Sheeler LR, Makarowski WS. Hypothyroidism with presenting symptoms of fibrositis. *J Rheumatol* 1981; 8(4):626–631.

52. Parker AP, Robinson RO, Bullock P. Difficulties in diagnosing intrinsic spinal cord tumours. *Arch Dis Child* 1996;75(3): 204–207.

53. Gotze FR, Thid S, Kyllerman M. Fibromyalgia in hyperkalemic periodic paralysis. *Scand J Rheumatol* 1998;27(5): 383–384.

54. Hain RD. Pain scales in children: a review. *Palliat Med* 1997;11(5):341–350.

55. Singh G, Athreya BH, Fries JF, et al. Measurement of health status in children with juvenile rheumatoid arthritis. *Arthritis Rheum* 1994;37(12):1761–1769.

56. Anthony KK, Schanberg LE. Juvenile primary fibromyalgia syndrome. *Curr Rheumatol Rep* 2001;3(2):165–171.

57. Russell IJ. Fibromyalgia syndrome: approaches to management. *Bull Rheum Dis* 1996;45(3):1–4 [erratum appears in *Bull Rheum Dis* 1996;45(5):5].

58. Sherry DD. Pain syndromes. In: Isenberg DA, Miller JJI, eds. *Adolescent rheumatology*. London: Martin Duntz, Ltd, 1998:197–227.

59. Sherry DD, Wallace CA. Resolution of fibromyalgia with an intensive exercise program [Abstract]. *Clin Exp Rheumatol* 1992;10:196.

60. Sherry DD, Wallace CA, Kelley C, et al. Short- and long-term outcomes of children with complex regional pain syndrome type I treated with exercise therapy. *Clin J Pain* 1999; 15(3):218–223.

61. Eccleston C, Malleson PN, Clinch J, et al. Chronic pain in adolescents: evaluation of a programme of interdisciplinary cognitive behaviour therapy. *Arch Dis Child* 2003;88(10): 881–885.

62. Eccleston C, Yorke L, Morley S, et al. Psychological therapies for the management of chronic and recurrent pain in children and adolescents. *Cochrane Database Syst Rev* 2003(1):CD003968.

63. Walco GA, Ilowite NT. Cognitive-behavioral intervention for juvenile primary fibromyalgia syndrome. *J Rheumatol* 1992;19(10):1617–1619.

64. Rabinovich CE, Schanberg LE, Stein LD, et al. A follow up study of pediatric fibromyalgia patients [Abstract]. *Arthritis Rheum* 1990;33(Suppl. 9):S146.

16

Fibromyalgia in Inflammatory and Endocrine Disorders

David S. Hallegua

Fibromyalgia (FM) is a common painful musculoskeletal condition in which numerous neurotransmitter, hormonal, cytokine, and circulatory disturbances have been described. A large proportion of patients with various hormonal, neuropsychiatric, and autoimmune illnesses have been diagnosed with secondary FM. This may be due to the fact that the criteria used to diagnose FM are overly simplistic, which leads to overdiagnosis in these illnesses. Alternatively, this could represent pathophysiologic mechanisms of the evolution of FM and warrants closer scrutiny.

Chronic widespread pain (CWP) is estimated to occur in about 10% of the general population in epidemiologic studies (1). FM is a common painful musculoskeletal condition that is estimated to be present in 2% of the population (1). Patients fulfill criteria for FM based on the presence of pain for at least 3 months and at least 11 out of 18 designated tender points (TePs) being tender at a specified amount of pressure (2). The criteria do not take into account the presence of other well-defined syndromes such as irritable bowel syndrome (IBS) or temporomandibular joint dysfunction in a significant proportion of patients, giving a syndrome that is much more complex than just pain alone. Extensive investigation over the past decade has uncovered many cytokine, neurotransmitter, hormonal, and circulatory disturbances in FM. Conversely, a variable proportion of patients with various inflammatory conditions such as lupus, hormonal deficits such as growth hormone (GH) deficiency, neurotransmitter alterations such as chronic stress, and circulatory disturbances such as Raynaud syndrome are associated with the presence of FM (see Table 16-1). Whether this represents the overlap of a common illness with a widely prevalent condition such as CWP or FM is a subject of debate and active investigation.

AUTOIMMUNE DISORDERS AND FIBROMYALGIA SYNDROME

SYSTEMIC LUPUS

Different studies have found a 22% to 61% prevalence of FM in systemic lupus erythematosus (SLE). Pistiner et al. initially reported on 570 lupus patients in the 1980s and found the prevalence of fibrositis to be 22% (3). Most investigators, such as Middleton et al. and Morand et al. have found 22% to 35% of their lupus patients to have FM (4,5). A study by Romano found a FM prevalence of 61% in their lupus subset (6). They hypothesized that pain medications and anti-inflammatory medications may have raised the pain threshold and lowered the number of TePs detected in the other studies, thereby decreasing the percentage of patients with FM.

Another possible reason for a high prevalence of FM in lupus is that the musculoskeletal symptoms of FM overlap with those of lupus. Low titer false-positive antinuclear antibodies (ANA) are common in the general population and may be seen in primary FM, leading to an erroneous diagnosis of lupus in FMS. Wallace et al. reported on 44 consecutive patients seen to rule out an autoimmune illness in office consultation (7). Although an ANA was seen in all the patients at some point, 20% of patients tested negative for ANA using different methods of testing. After several confirmatory tests and follow up, the diagnosis was lupus in 43%, FM in 32%, RA in 9%, myasthenia gravis in 2%, and undiagnosed in 15%. Two hundred and sixty-six SLE patients with disease duration ≤5 years at study entry were evaluated longitudinally for the presence of FM (per ACR criteria) (8). Demographic and psychological variables, clinical features, autoantibodies, and level of functioning were assessed for association with the presence of FM. The prevalence of FM was 14 patients [5%; 9/92

TABLE 16-1	Conditions Associated with an Increased Prevalence of Fibromyalgia Syndrome	
NAME OF CONDITION	**PREVALENCE OF FIBROMYALGIA (%)**	**REFERENCES**
Definite Association		
Systemic lupus	1–61	(3–9)
Sjögren's syndrome	5–47	(9–12)
Hepatitis C	5–18.9	(13–16)
Lyme disease	8–25	(17–19)
Irritable bowel syndrome	20–65	(20–23)
Probable Association		
Growth hormone deficiency	40	(24)
Hyperprolactinemia	71	(25)
Possible Association		
Endometriosis	5.9	(26)
Hypothyroidism	5	(27)

Caucasians (C), 4/109 African Americans (AA), 1/65 Hispanics (H)]. No difference was seen between those with and without FM with respect to gender, education level, and income below poverty level, disease activity, or damage. The strongest association with FM was a self-reported history of anxiety or affective disorder ($p = 0.0237$, OR = 4.6 and $p = 0.0068$, OR = 3.4, respectively). Caucasian ethnicity was strongly associated with FM ($p = 0.0066$, OR = 7.5), and African American ethnicity was negatively associated with FM ($p = 0.0204$, OR = 0.3). Poorer self-reported physical functioning was associated with FM ($p = 0.0443$, OR = 0.96).

In summary, there is a high prevalence of FM in SLE patients. This is partly due to the overdiagnosis of SLE in patients with FM symptoms and a positive ANA. An increase in vigilance for this association should be maintained, since this could lead to the inappropriate use of corticosteroids and immunosuppressive drugs to treat the "lupus" symptoms. Corticosteroid use and withdrawal could also be a cause of the high prevalence of FM in SLE patients.

SJÖGREN'S SYNDROME

Studies have also demonstrated a high prevalence of secondary FMS in primary Sjögren's syndrome (PSS) (9–11,28). Ostoni found a prevalence of 22% in 100 patients with PSS, which was similar to the high prevalence (42%) reported by Dohrenbusch in ten patients with PSS. The prevalence of FM in secondary Sjögren's syndrome was lower in the Dohrenbusch article (5% of 20 patients). Vitali et al. found a prevalence of 47% of FM in 30 PSS syndrome patients. They found a prevalence of depression (47%) using a Hamilton Depression Rating Scale in FM compared to the controls with osteoarthritis (20%) and diabetes mellitus (7%) ($p<0.01$). FM symptoms correlated with the presence of depression in the PSS subset ($p<0.001$).

Bonafede et al. screened 72 patients with FM with a Schirmer test and biopsied a minor salivary gland in all the patients with abnormal Schirmer tests. Twenty-eight FM patients (38%) had a Schirmer test <15 mm wetting at 5 minutes; sicca symptoms were noted in only 19% of patients. Salivary gland biopsy in these 28 patients showed a focus score of ≥1 in 5, an ANA was found in 4, rheumatoid factor in 3, and anti-SSA/SSB antibodies in 2. Another eight patients had abnormal salivary gland lymphocytic foci with fewer than 50 cells or the density was <1 focus/4 mm^2, although all eight patients had a positive ANA. None of the eight patients developed systemic features of SS over a 6-year period. The prevalence of PSS on stringent testing is 6.9%, with a 11% prevalence for possible Sjögren's syndrome.

A tertiary center referral bias probably overestimates the true prevalence in FM. Tishler et al. studied the association and prevalence of sleep disturbances and FM in 65 patients with PSS syndrome using a ten-point Mini Sleep Questionnaire (MSQ) focusing on sleep complaints and compared the response to 67 patients with rheumatoid arthritis (RA), 53 patients with RA and sicca symptoms, and 31 patients with osteoarthritis (12). All patients with PSS were evaluated for the presence of FM. Sleep disturbances of a moderate to severe degree was reported by 49 out of 65 PSS patients (75%), which was significantly higher than the controls ($p<0.001$). FM was present in 36 out of 65 PSS patients (55%) and was associated with sleep disturbances. This suggests that an etiology other than joint pain or sicca symptoms may account for the increased incidence of FM in PSS syndrome.

Dry eye and dry mouth symptoms are seen in up to 18% of FM patients (29). These sicca symptoms may be due to sympathetic overactivity or to the anticholinergic side effects of medications used to treat FMS. They can also be due to the early PSS masquerading as FMS.

Other autoimmune diseases in which the prevalence of FM and CWP has been studied include inflammatory bowel disease (IBD) and endometriosis (26,30). Five hundred and twenty-one patients with IBD came in to be examined from a 5-year prospective survey on IBD. On exam, 18 patients were found to have FM (3.5%) and 38 (7.3%) were found to have CWP. These numbers reflect similar percentages to those found in the general and rheumatologic clinic populations. A cross-sectional survey in 3,680 patients with surgically diagnosed endometriosis revealed a slightly higher rate of coexisting FM than the rate commonly used for women in the general population (5.9 vs. 3.4%; $p<0.0001$).

The higher prevalence of FM in patients with SLE and Sjögren's suggests the potential importance of cytokine abnormalities that could lead to the pathogenesis of this illness. Cytokine levels have been investigated in FM and will be mentioned in the section on infections and FM.

HORMONAL DISTURBANCES AND FIBROMYALGIA

PROLACTIN

Buskila et al. assessed the prevalence of FM in hyperprolactinemia in 21 women seen in an infertility clinic over a period of 2 years (25). Forty-four women from the same clinic without hyperprolactinemia recruited in a consecutive manner served as controls. The prevalence of FM in the patients with high prolactin levels was 71%, versus 4.5% in the controls ($p<0.0001$). Thresholds for tenderness in FM patients in nine designated TePs using a dolorimeter was 5.0 SD 1.5, while it was 5.0 SD 1.4 in control patients ($p<0.0001$).

Prolactin levels have been studied in small groups of FM patients (31,32). Griep et al. investigated the release of prolactin and GH in response to insulin-induced hypoglycemia in ten female FM patients and compared them to matched controls. The basal levels of morning prolactin were significantly higher in FM patients when compared to the controls. The levels of prolactin after induction of hypoglycemia varied widely in patients and controls, and no conclusion could be drawn from the results.

Landis et al. studied the nocturnal secretion of GH and prolactin during the early sleep and sleep onset period in 25 female FM patients and 21 female controls. The mean serum concentration of prolactin in control patients was significantly higher than in FM patients during the early sleep period (controls—23.2 $+/-2.2$ µg/L vs. FM—16.9 $+/-2.0$ µg/L; $p<0.025$). The prolactin levels increased more in control patients than in FM patients at the onset of sleep (16.2 $+/-2.4$ vs. 9.4 $+/-1.5$; $p<0.025$). There was a direct relationship between prolactin levels and sleep efficiency ($r = 0.42$; $p<0.05$) and a modest inverse relationship between sleep latency and prolactin levels ($r = 0.48$; $p<0.05$).

The findings of disturbed prolactin levels may have pathophysiologic significance or may be a sign of stress or disturbances in dopamine secretion in the central nervous system (CNS).

GROWTH HORMONE

Hallegua et al. assessed the prevalence of FM in GH-deficient patients (24). Of the 19 patients who were examined, nine were on GH injections in a trial to assess the effects of GH on cardiac function and the remaining ten were on placebo injections. Of the ten patients on placebo, four fulfilled the ACR criteria for FM. One patient of the nine patients on active therapy fulfilled criteria for FM. Paresthesiae suggestive of restless legs syndrome appeared to predict which patients with GH deficiency would develop FM (60% in FM vs. 0% in non-FM; $p<0.05$).

Bennett et al. studied insulinlike growth factor (IGF-1) levels in 500 patients with FM and compared them to 152 control patients, of whom 74 were healthy blood donors and 26 had localized myofascial pain syndrome (33). The mean levels of IGF-1 were 138 $+/-56$ ng per mL compared to 215 $+/-86$ ng per mL in controls ($p = 0.00000000001$). The low levels of IGF-1 were not related to clinical variables such as obesity, deconditioning, pain, or depression. Patients with FM had a rapid decline of IGF-1 over 1 to 2 years if their levels were normal during initial testing.

Buchwald et al. performed a similar study in smaller numbers of FM patients and compared them with patients with chronic fatigue syndrome and healthy controls (34). The 27 FM patients had similar IGF-1 and IGF binding protein levels when compared to the 15 chronic fatigue patients, 15 patients with chronic fatigue and FM, and the normal controls. The disparate results could represent a referral bias to a tertiary care center or could be due to the smaller number of patients.

Leal-Cerro et al. studied the hypothalamic-pituitary-IGF-1 axis in a small number of FM patients (35). Spontaneous GH secretion was reduced in FM compared to healthy controls with respect to basal levels, pulse height, and pulse area (basal levels—controls: 2.5 $+/- 0.5$ µgm per L vs. 1.2 $+/- 0.1$ µgm per L; $p<0.05$). Upon stimulation with GH releasing hormone, the mean levels of growth hormone were very similar. Treatment with GH injections resulted in increase in the levels of IGF-1. In Sweden, Bagge et al. found similar results in a pilot study of ten patients with FM and ten controls (36). Landis et al. studied GH levels along with prolactin and found them lower in FM patients than in controls in the early sleep period (GH 1.6 $+/-0.4$ in controls vs. 0.6 $+/-0.4$ in FM) (32). The GH levels failed to rise during sleep in FM and an inverse relationship existed between age and GH levels. The IGF-1 levels were not different in the two groups. Similarly Griep et al. found lower levels of GH in FM and an exaggerated response to stimulation testing with insulin-induced hypoglycemia (31).

McCall-Hosenfeld et al. employed a similar procedure using a stepped hyperinsulinemic clamp to study change in GH levels due to hypoglycemia (37). IGF-1 levels were studied in 23 premenopausal FM patients and in 25 controls and were found to be very similar. IGF-1 was negatively associated with age ($p<0.0006$), body mass index (BMI) ($p <0.006$), and 24-hour urinary free cortisol ($p<0.007$) in healthy controls. The median peak level of GH was lower in FM (range 5 to 58 ng per mL, median 13) when compared to the controls (range 6 to 68, median 21; $p = 0.04$). BMI was a significant predictor for average GH levels in FM ($r = -0.62$; $p = 0.01$) and also in controls. When the effects of obesity were removed, there was no association between FM and the average peak of GH.

Paiva et al. investigated the reason for decreased GH secretion in FM patients (38). Twenty FM patients and ten healthy controls were exercised to voluntary exhaustion on a treadmill. The experiment was done once a month for two months with the addition of one dose of pyridostigmine 30 mg 1 hour prior to exercise during the second exercise protocol. Blood was drawn for GH and cortisol levels 1 hour before, just before and after the exercise, and 1 hour after exercise. Compared to the controls, FM patients did not increase their cortisol or GH levels after exercise ($p<0.003$). After pyridostigmine, the GH levels increased eightfold and approached the levels of that of the control patients ($p<0.001$). The cortisol levels did not vary with the pyridostigmine, which induces GH secretion by reducing the somatostatin tone in the CNS.

Bennett et al. performed a double-blind placebo controlled trial of GH replacement therapy in female patients with FM (39). Of the 50 women with FM and low IGF-1 levels, 22 patients on GH and 23 patients on placebo completed the 9-month trial. The FM patients in GH had a statistically significant improvement in their TeP score ($p<0.03$) and their FM Impact Questionnaire score ($p<0.04$). Carpal tunnel syndrome symptoms occurred in seven patients with

FM compared to one patient on placebo. The benefits were seen after 6 months of therapy with GH injections and appeared to wear off after stopping the injections.

In summary, the aggregate data suggest decreased secretion of GH in about 30% of patients with FM syndrome. A single double-blind trial showed modest efficacy in reducing pain and some other symptoms in FM. However, FM is an overlap of multiple functional disturbances with increasing support for central nervous sensitization for external stimuli.

THYROID HORMONE AND FIBROMYALGIA

Lack of thyroid hormone causes diffuse myalgia, arthralgia, and fatigue and mimics the symptoms of FM. Good clinical practice dictates checking for thyroid dysfunction in patients suspected to have primary or secondary FM. Carette et al. examined 100 patients with subclinical hypothyroidism for the presence of FM (27). Nineteen of the patients reported widespread body pain. Five patients had seven or more TePs on examination. The prevalence of fibrositis by criteria existing prior to the ACR criteria was 5%, indicating that FM was uncommon in primary subclinical or biochemical hypothyroidism. After treatment with thyroid hormone replacement, symptoms improved in 15 out of 19 patients with diffuse pain, although the TeP exam did not change. Wilke et al. treated eight FM patients with biochemical hypothyroidism with thyroid hormone replacement, and resolution of myalgic symptoms occurred in six of them (40).

Riedel et al. studied the effect of injecting a number of hypothalamic releasing hormones in 16 FM patients and 17 control patients (41). Although thyrotropin releasing hormone (TRH) showed no differences between the two groups, basal tri-iodothyronine levels was lower in FM patients than in controls. Neeck et al. stimulated 13 FM patients and 10 controls with 400 μgm of TRH and found that levels of thyroid stimulating hormone and thyroid hormones on stimulation were lower in FM when compared to controls (42). Basal levels were similar in both groups.

Thus there is no conclusive evidence of specific thyroid dysfunction in FMS syndrome, although it remains an important diagnosis to exclude when making the primary diagnosis.

CORTICOSTEROIDS AND FIBROMYALGIA

Disturbances in hormones associated with the stress response have been postulated to be important in the genesis of FM symptoms. Although there is no data on the prevalence of FM in clinical models of cortisol excess or deficiency, FM symptoms are commonly seen when corticosteroid therapy is rapidly tapered in some patients (43). There are isolated case reports of FM presenting itself after pituitary resection for Cushing disease (44).

McCain et al. studied the diurnal variation of cortisol secretion in FM and RA patients (45). Trough levels of cortisol were higher in FM than in RA patients (trough levels 347.3 +/−254.7 vs. 232.8 +/−70.0 nmol/L, $p < 0.001$). Seven out of 20 FM patients showed failure of suppression of cortisol on a dexamethasone suppression test (DST) compared to 1 out of 20 with RA ($p < 0.001$). An abnormal DST did not correlate with the presence of depression in FM or RA. Conversely, Ataoglu et al. found that the DST was abnormal only in FM patients with depression when compared to FM patients without depression and normal controls (46). Seven out of 20 FM patients with depression and 1 out of 26 FM patients without depression had an abnormal DST ($p < 0.014$). The difference in suppressed levels of cortisol in the depressed FM was significantly higher when compared to the levels in the normal controls ($p < 0.03$).

Several investigators have studied the effect on adenocorticotrophic hormone (ACTH) and cortisol levels by stimulating the pituitary-adrenal axis using either insulin-induced hypoglycemia or using corticotrophin releasing hormone (CRH). Adler et al. measured baseline 24-hour urinary cortisol and morning and evening ACTH and cortisol in 13 premenopausal FM patients (47). The patients had hormonal measurements done after the induction of graded insulin-induced hypoglycemia and in response to ACTH stimulation and saline control infusion. There was a 30% decrease in the response to hypoglycemia with respect to levels of ACTH and epinephrine, which was statistically significant. The epinephrine response correlated inversely with health status as measured by the FM Impact Questionnaire ($p = 0.01$). Patients with FM therefore have an impairment in activating the hypothalamic-pituitary axis and sympathetic-adrenal axis in response to hypoglycemia.

Riedel et al. injected 13 female FM patients and 13 control patients with 100 μgm of CRH (48). Basal and stimulated levels of ACTH, cortisol, somatostatin, and GH were assessed. CRH levels were also followed for 2 hours. The increase in CRH after injection was significantly higher at baseline in FM than in normal controls, suggesting a higher basal secretion of CRH in FM due to pain or stress. Somatostatin levels also increased after injection and lasted for about 45 minutes. GH levels, which were low at baseline, increased after 45 minutes, coincident with decreasing levels of somatostatin and CRH. There was no difference in the stimulated levels of ACTH and cortisol between the two groups. Griep et al. studied the hypothalamic-pituitary-adrenal (HPA) axis in 40 FM patients (F:M; 36:4) and compared it to 28 chronic low back pain patients (F:M; 12:2) and 14 healthy sedentary controls (F:M; 12:2) (49). Basal 24-hour urinary cortisol levels were lower in FM than in the controls ($p < 0.03$). A standard CRH challenge test showed an exaggerated ACTH response in both FM patients ($p < 0.001$) and low back pain patients ($p < 0.02$). An overnight DST revealed two and four nonsuppressors in the FM and low back pain, respectively. A low-dose and high-dose ACTH stimulation test revealed a normal cortisol response in both groups. This confirms the presence of mild hypocortisolemia, exaggerated ACTH response, and a cortisol feedback resistance in FM.

Clark et al. ascertained the response of 20 patients with FM to prednisone 15 mg versus placebo everyday in a double-blind crossover design (50). No benefit was seen with visual analogue scales or with dolorimeter measurements with this therapy.

Thus the studies indicate evidence of increased activity of CRH in FM, although the adrenal response to it is blunted and the feedback of cortisol on the brain is defective. This indicates that newer agents that block CRH activity and others that modulate glucocorticoid receptor activity are needed to treat the CRH-ACTH-cortisol axis in FM.

SEX HORMONES AND FIBROMYALGIA

The prevalence of FM increases with age and affects more women than men. Hence studies have attempted to look at the role, if any, that reproductive hormones play in the pathogenesis of this illness. Mcfarlane et al. performed a population postal survey on 1,178 female participants in northwest England (51). Although examinations were not conducted on any of the participants, the risk of CWP was unrelated to the length of the menstrual cycle, the length of the period, or contraceptive pill use. A relationship was found between the total score on a premenstrual symptom questionnaire and CWP. The age at menopause or the duration of menopause did not show any relationship with the risk for CWP. Current estrogen replacement use was associated with CWP, but this was most likely due to the use of this therapy more often in patients with CWP. Ostonsen et al. studied 40 pregnant FM patients with interviews in a retrospective manner (52). All but one patient reported worsening of symptoms of FM, particularly in the third trimester. Using oral contraceptives did not ameliorate symptoms. Premenstrual worsening of symptoms was reported in up to 72% of the patients interviewed.

Korszun et al. studied follicle stimulating hormone (FSH), lactate dehydrogenase (LDH), progesterone, and estradiol levels in nine premenopausal FM patients during a 12-hour period in the follicular phase (53). Pooled samples were used to assess hormonal levels, and a LDH pulse detection method was used to detect LDH pulses. No differences were seen between total hormone levels or LDH pulsatile function when these patients were compared to normal controls. Riedel et al. studied the effect of luteinizing hormone-releasing hormone (LH-RH) on the ovary in six patients and compared them to normal controls (41). The response to LH-RH was blunted in the FM patients, and the authors concluded that this was the effect of chronic stress on the ovary due to CRH. Dessien et al. studied the levels of adrenal androgens in 57 female FM patients and correlated the levels with impairment as assessed by the FM Impact Questionnaire (54). Levels of dihydroepiandrostenedione sulfate (DHEAS) and testosterone were significantly lower in premenopausal women with FM when compared to normal controls ($p<0.0001$ and $p<0.0001$, respectively). DHEAS levels, but not testosterone levels, were significantly lower in postmenopausal FM patients when compared to appropriate controls ($p<0.0005$ and $p<0.06$, respectively). DHEAS levels correlated inversely with pain score after being adjusted for age ($p<0.001$) but the correlation was not significant when adjusted for BMI. Testosterone levels correlated with physical functioning ($p<0.002$). Thus, low androgen levels can be found in FM patients—particularly if they are obese.

Hormonal abnormalities—especially low androgen levels—are present in female FM patients. It is unclear whether the levels are a primary abnormality in FM or secondary to other phenomena.

INFECTIONS AND FIBROMYALGIA

FM is reported to have a flulike illness at the onset in up to 50% of patients (55). Hence it is not much of a surprise that chronic viral illnesses such as hepatitis C and human immunodeficiency virus (HIV) infections have a higher prevalence of FM than that seen in the general population.

Using criteria in existence prior to ACR criteria, 15 out of 51 HIV patients tested positive for FM by examination of 14 TePs, compared to 34% with psoriatic arthritis and 57% of patients with RA (56). Buskila et al. investigated the prevalence of FM in 130 HIV-positive patients in a Boston acquired immune deficiency syndrome (AIDS) clinic (57). About 11% of the HIV positive patients met the ACR criteria for FM. Forty-seven percent of HIV patients with musculoskeletal symptoms had FM as a cause for their symptoms. When the HIV patients with FM were compared to the HIV patients without FM, a higher prevalence of depressed mood ($p = 0.01$) and a longer duration of HIV ($p = 0.01$) were noted. When the HIV patients with FM were compared to FM patients with no risk for factors for HIV, the HIV patients with FM were found to have a greater percentage of male patients ($p = 0.01$) and also reported depressed mood more often ($p = 0.0001$). It is possible that FM in HIV patients is related to the stress of being diagnosed with a potentially fatal and incurable illness.

Musculoskeletal symptoms are common in hepatitis C virus (HCV) infection and have been reported in up to 81% of patients with HCV infection (58,59). Of 58 patients with confirmed HCV infection, the prevalence of FM on examination was 10%. The presence of FM was related to the presence of musculoskeletal pain (50% of patients) but not to the degree of damage to the liver, liver function test elevation, or autoimmune markers. Buskila et al. found that 14 out of 90 patients infected by HCV ($p<0.001$) and one patient out of 32 patients with cirrhosis not related to alcoholic liver disease had the 1990 ACR examination criteria for FM (13). None of the 128 healthy controls had FM. Kozanaglu et al. examined 95 patients with chronic hepatitis C infection for the prevalence of FM and compared this to the prevalence in 95 healthy controls (14). FM was found in 18.9% of HCV infected patients and in 5.3% of controls.

Although chronic anxiety and stress could explain the increased prevalence of FM in HCV infection, the patients were not aware of being infected by hepatitis C in some of the prevalence studies when the diagnosis of FM was made. Another study looked at the mode of acquisition of HCV and its relationship to FM (15). Of 77 patients with hepatitis C in a Finnish clinic, 4 (5%) fulfilled criteria for FM. All were infected through contaminated anti-D immunoglobulin infection, as opposed to intravenous drug use (IVDU). Anxiety and depression symptoms were higher in both the anti-D HCV group ($p = 0.0001$) and the IVDU HCV group ($p = 0.005$).

One hundred and twelve FM patients were studied using an ELISA test and confirmed with a RIBA test for the prevalence of hepatitis C infection (16). When compared to RA, about 15.2 % of patients were positive by ELISA and 16 out of 17 had positive RIBA tests. About 47% of these FM patients never had a high ALT level to suggest the presence of HCV infection.

Thus about 10% to 20% of HCV infected patients have FM as an explanation of their musculoskeletal symptoms. Since up to 50% of HCV patients have positive autoimmune serologies that are nonspecific, the accurate diagnosis of FM is important in order to direct appropriate therapy. Alternatively, about 15% of FM may have underlying HCV infection, which may not cause any elevation of liver function tests to arouse clinical suspicion for testing for the virus.

Leventhal et al. reported that three patients with FM were found to have serological evidence of acute parvoviral infection 1 month after the onset of their symptoms (60). Berg et al. selected 15 female FM patients who recalled a viral prodrome preceding the onset of their FM and compared them to 11 patients who did not recall such symptoms, while excluding FM patients who reported trauma as a trigger for their FM (61). Twenty-six female medical workers served as controls. Serum IgG and IgM antibodies and polymerase chain reaction (PCR) for B19 deoxyribonucleic acid (DNA) were not different among the FM patients and the controls. Prior parvoviral infection was seen in 11 of 26 FM patients and 12 of 26 control patients. Eight out of fifteen patients with FM that had a viral prodrome at its onset had positive parvoviral IgG antibodies as opposed to

TABLE 16-2 Relationship of Abnormal Hormonal, Cytokine, Neurotransmitter, and Autonomic Disturbances Found in Fibromyalgia and the Prevalence of Fibromyalgia in Other Conditions with Similar Abnormalities

ABNORMALITY	ASSOCIATION WITH FIBROMYALGIA	PREVALENCE IN DISEASE HAVING THE SAME ANOMALY
Hormonal Growth hormone (GH), an anabolic hormone, is secreted mainly during deep sleep. Hypothalamic-pituitary-adrenal axis (HPA) mediates the stress response.	Strong association in FM with decreased GH levels. Positive results with replacement. Mild hypocortisolemia and increased CRH production and relative insensitivity of the pituitary to CRH and to cortisol feedback inhibition.	Small study showing an increased prevalence but having insufficient power to show a significant difference. Evidence for secondary FM in patients who have their corticosteroids rapidly tapered.
Cytokine IL-2, a T cell proliferation and differentiation cytokine.	IL-2 and IL-2 receptor increased at basal levels and upon stimulation.	Increased IL-2 may increase prevalence of FM in autoimmune diseases and infections.
IL-6 stimulates B-cells to produce antibodies, stimulates the HPA axis, and produces acute phase reactants.	IL-6 is elevated in primary and secondary FM patients at baseline or with stimulation.	IL-6 is important in Th2 mediated illnesses such as lupus and Sjögren's where the prevalence of FM is increased.
IL-8 influences chemotaxis of neutrophils and mediates sympathetic nerve pain.	IL-8 is increased in the serum of patients with primary and secondary FM of >2 yr duration.	IL-8 is important for attracting neutrophils in infectious and autoimmune diseases.
Neurotransmitter Serotonin levels important in maintaining pain threshold and normal mood.	Serotonin levels are low in the serum and in blood platelets and in the CSF of FM patients.	Depression, which is also associated with low serotonin levels, does not appear to have an increased prevalence of FM.
Norepinephrine is essential for normal alertness and in maintaining normal vasomotor function.	Norepinephrine levels are low in the CSF of FM patients. However there is evidence of sympathetic nervous system overactivity.	PTSD that is associated with high norepinephrine levels in the CSF has an increase in FM prevalence.
Substance P is an important mediator of sympathetic pain.	Increased levels of substance P levels found consistently in FM.	Chronic pain models such as low back pain have not been found to have elevated levels of substance P.
Autonomic Nervous System Irritable bowel syndrome may be caused partly due to disturbed motility.	An increase in the prevalence of IBS is seen in FM in multiple studies.	Conversely, studies on the prevalence of FM in IBS have shown an increase in prevalence.
Migraine headache may be partly explained by autonomic nerve disturbances.	Up to 50% of FM patients have headache—with the majority having migraine type headaches.	The prevalence of FM in transformed migraine is very high, suggesting a common etiology.

GH, growth hormone; HPA, hypothalamic-pituitary-adrenal axis; FM, fibromyalgia; CRH, corticotrophin releasing hormone; PTSD, posttraumatic stress disorder; CSF, cerebrospinal fluid; IBS, irritable bowel syndrome.

3 of 11 without such a prodrome. Although this was not statistically significant, a better study would look at the presence of parvovirus IgM antibody levels within 3 months of the onset of FM that has viral prodrome at its commencement.

A retrospective chart review of 800 patients referred for nonspecific musculoskeletal and neurologic symptoms in possible chronic Lyme disease patients suggested that 77 patients had FM as the cause of their symptoms (17). Many had received multiple courses of antibiotic therapy. When treatment for FM was instituted, most, if not all, symptoms responded. In a university hospital, 22 of 287 patients (8%) with Lyme disease seen over a 3.5-year period had FM on examination (18). Of these, 15 out of 22 FM formed an observational cohort and were followed for a mean of 2.5 years (range 1 to 4 years). Most of the FM patients (9 out of 15) developed their symptoms within a mean of 1.7 months after their Lyme diagnosis. Of the 15 patients with chronic Lyme disease and FM, 11 had a positive ELISA test for Lyme disease. The remaining four patients had either a positive Western blot (1) or cellular immune responses to Borrelia antigens (3). All CNS abnormalities and physical signs of chronic Lyme (except for a swollen knee in one patient) resolved with treatment with antibiotics. Symptoms and signs fulfilling criteria for FM persisted in 14 out of 15 patients in spite of successful treatment with antibiotics for Lyme disease. Sigal reported on the first 100 patients referred to the Lyme Disease Center at the Robert Wood Johnson Medical School (19). Of these, only 37 had previous or current Lyme disease as the cause of their symptoms. Twenty-five of the 100 patients had FM on evaluation. Of the 25, 3 had concurrent Lyme and 17 had a history suggesting Lyme infection that had been treated. Five FM patients were misdiagnosed as having Lyme infection.

In areas endemic for Lyme disease, it is important to entertain FM as a possible differential diagnosis in the absence of a response to antibiotics when chronic symptoms are present.

The increase in prevalence of FM in infections and autoimmune illnesses can be attributed to induction of abnormalities in cytokine levels and function. Investigations of cytokine levels and function in FM has been hampered by the lack of homogeneity of subjects studied and the uncertainty of how to study cytokines best—through serum levels, tissue staining, or stimulating immune cells. FM patients were reported to have elevated levels of IL-1ra, IL-2, IL-2r, IL-6, and IL-8 and increased secretion of IL-2 by stimulated T-lymphocytes when compared to controls (62–65). Skin biopsies of FM patients had positive immunostaining for cytokines significantly more often than in control patients (66). These important observations suggest mechanisms by which FM may evolve in autoimmune illnesses and infections. Further study of cytokines in various subsets of patients with primary and secondary FM may help to further elucidate the pathogenic significance of these cytokines in FM. Further detail on cytokine abnormalities are discussed in the basic science section of the text.

CONCLUSION

A plethora of conditions are associated with an increased prevalence of FM. Of interest, some of the presumed pathogenetic mechanisms in these conditions are found in primary FM as well (see Table 16-2). It is very likely that each

of these underlying mechanisms for disease form a separate subset of patients with FM. Sophisticated testing, as well as separating FM patients into different subsets based on symptoms and test results, will enhance our understanding of the syndrome and lead to directed therapies.

SUMMARY POINTS

- FM is seen more commonly in individuals with a variety of inflammatory and neuroendocrine disorders.

▪ IMPLICATIONS FOR PRACTICE

- Even though an individual may have an inflammatory or neuroendocrine disorder, that person may also have FM.
- In individuals with comorbid FM it is sometimes difficult to determine if current symptoms are due to the FM or to the concurrent disorder. A therapeutic trial of treatment(s) known to work in FM is imperative in this setting because the morbidity associated with therapy for FM is significantly less than for inflammatory or neuroendocrine disorders.

REFERENCES

1. Wolfe F, Ross K, Anderson J, et al. The prevalence and characteristics of fibromyalgia in the general population. *Arthritis Rheum* 1995;38:19–28.
2. Wolfe F, Smythe HA, Yunus MB, et al. The American College of rheumatology criteria for the classification of fibromyalgia. Report of the Multicenter Criteria Committee. *Arthritis Rheum* 1990;33:160–172.
3. Pistiner M, Wallace DJ, Nessim S, et al. Lupus erythematosus in the 1980s: a survey of 570 patients. *Semin Arthritis Rheum* 1991;37:1181–1188.
4. Middleton GD, MacFarlane JE, Lipsky PE. The prevalence and clinical impact of fibromyalgia in systemic lupus erythematosus. *Arthritis Rheum* 1994;37:1181–1188.
5. Morand EF, Miller MH, Whittingham S, et al. Fibromyalgia syndrome and disease activity in systemic lupus erythematosus. *Lupus* 1994;3:187–191.
6. Romano TJ. Coexistence of fibromyalgia with systemic lupus erythematosus. *Am J Pain Manage* 1992;2:211–214.
7. Wallace DJ, Schwartz E, Chi-Lin H, et al. The "rule out lupus" consultation: clinical outcomes and perspectives. *J Clin Rheumatol* 1995;1:158–164.
8. Friedman AW, Tewi MB, Ahn C et al., LUMINA Study Group. Systemic lupus erythematosus in three ethnic groups: XV. Prevalence and correlates of fibromyalgia. *Lupus* 2003;12(4):274–279.
9. Ostuni P, Botsios C, Sfriso P, et al. Prevalence and clinical features of fibromyalgia in systemic lupus erythematosus, systemic sclerosis and Sjögren's syndrome. *Minerva Med* 2002;93(3):203–209.
10. Bonafede RP, Downey DC, Bennett RM. An association of fibromyalgia with primary Sjögren's syndrome: a prospective study of 72 patients. *J Rheumatol* 1995;22:133–136.
11. Vitali C, Tavoni A, Neri R, et al. Fibromyalgia features in patients with primary Sjögren's syndrome. Evidence of a relationship with psychological depression. *Scand J Rheuamtol* 1989;18:21–27.

12. Tishler M, Barak Y, Paran D, et al. Sleep disturbances, fibromyalgia and primary Sjögren's syndrome. *Clin Exp Rheumatol* 1997;15(1):71–74.
13. Buskila D, Shnaider A, Neumann L, et al. Fibromyalgia in hepatitis C virus infection. Another infectious disease relationship. *Arch Intern Med* 1997;157(21):2497–2500.
14. Kozanoglu E, Canataroglu A, Abayli B, et al. Fibromyalgia syndrome in patients with hepatitis C infection. *Rheumatol Int* 2003;23(5):248–251.
15. Goulding C, O'Connell P, Murray FE. Prevalence of fibromyalgia, anxiety and depression in chronic hepatitis C virus infection: relationship to RT-PCR status and mode of acquisition. *Eur J Gastroenterol Hepatol* 2001;13(5):507–511.
16. Rivera J, de Diego A, Trinchet M, et al. Fibromyalgia-associated hepatitis C virus infection. 1. *Br J Rheumatol* 1997; 36(9):981–985.
17. Hsu VM, Patella SJ, Sigal LH. "Chronic Lyme disease" as the incorrect diagnosis in patients with fibromyalgia. *Arthritis Rheum* 1993;36(11):1493–1500.
18. Dinerman H, Steere AC. Lyme disease associated with fibromyalgia. *Ann Intern Med* 1992;117(4):281–285.
19. Sigal LH. Summary of the first 100 patients seen at a Lyme disease referral center. *Am J Med* 1990;88(6):577–581.
20. Lubrano E, Iovino P, Tremolaterra F, et al. Fibromyalgia in patients with irritable bowel syndrome. An association with the severity of the intestinal disorder. *Int J Colorectal Dis* 2001 Aug;16(4):211–215.
21. Veale D, Kavanagh G, Fielding JF, et al. Primary fibromyalgia and the irritable bowel syndrome: different expressions of a common pathogenetic process. *Br J Rheumatol* 1991 Jun;30(3):200–202.
22. Sperber AD, Atzmon Y, Neumann L, et al. Fibromyalgia in the irritable bowel syndrome: studies of prevalence and clinical implications. *Am J Gastroenterol* 1999 Dec;94(12):3541–3546.
23. Sivri A, Cindas A, Dincer F, et al. Bowel dysfunction and irritable bowel syndrome in fibromyalgia patients. *Clin Rheumatol* 1996 May;15(3):283–286.
24. Hallegua DJ, Wallace DJ, Silverman S, et al. Prevalence of fibromyalgia in growth hormone deficient adults. *J Musculoskelet Pain* 2001;9(3):35–42.
25. Buskila D, Fefer P, Harman-Boehm I, et al. Assessment of nonarticular tenderness and prevalence of fibromyalgia in hyperprolactinemic women. *J Rheumatol* 1993;20(12):2112–2115.
26. Sinaii N, Cleary SD, Ballweg ML, et al. High rates of autoimmune and endocrine disorders, fibromyalgia, chronic fatigue syndrome and atopic diseases among women with endometriosis: a survey analysis. *Hum Reprod* 2002;17(10):2715–2724.
27. Carette S, Lefrancois L. Fibrositis and primary hypothyroidism. *J Rheumatol* 1988;15(9):1418–1421.
28. Dohrenbusch R, Gruterich M, Genth E. Fibromyalgia and Sjögren syndrome—clinical and methodological aspects. *Z Rheumatol* 1996;55(1):19–27.
29. Dinerman H, Goldenberg DL, Felson DT. A prospective evaluation of 118 patients with the fibromyalgia syndrome: prevalence of Raynaud's phenomenon, sicca symptoms, ANA, low complement, and Ig deposition at the dermal-epidermal junction. *J Rheumatol* 1986;13(2):368–373.
30. Palm O, Moum B, Jahnsen J, et al. Fibromyalgia and chronic widespread pain in patients with inflammatory bowel disease: a cross sectional population survey. *J Rheumatol* 2001; 28(3):590–594.
31. Griep EN, Boersma JW, de Kloet ER. Pituitary release of growth hormone and prolactin in the primary fibromyalgia syndrome. *J Rheumatol* 1994;21(11):2125–2130.
32. Landis CA, Lentz MJ, Rothermel J, et al. Decreased nocturnal levels of prolactin and growth hormone in women with fibromyalgia. *J Clin Endocrinol Metab* 2001;86(4):1672–1678.
33. Bennett RM, Cook DM, Clark SR, et al. Hypothalamic-pituitary-insulin-like growth factor-I axis dysfunction in patients with fibromyalgia. *J Rheumatol* 1997;24(7):1384–1389.
34. Buchwald D, Umali J, Stene M. Insulin-like growth factor-I (somatomedin C) levels in chronic fatigue syndrome and fibromyalgia. *J Rheumatol* 1996;23(4):739–742.
35. Leal-Cerro A, Povedano J, Astorga R, et al. The growth hormone (GH)-releasing hormone-GH-insulin-like growth factor-1 axis in patients with fibromyalgia syndrome. *J Clin Endocrinol Metab* 1999;84(9):3378–3381.
36. Bagge E, Bengtsson BA, Carlsson L, et al. Low growth hormone secretion in patients with fibromyalgia—a preliminary report on 10 patients and 10 controls. *J Rheumatol* 1998; 25(1):145–148.
37. McCall-Hosenfeld JS, Goldenberg DL, Hurwitz S, et al. Growth hormone and insulin-like growth factor-1 concentrations in women with fibromyalgia. *J Rheumatol* 2003;30(4):809–814.
38. Paiva ES, Deodhar A, Jones KD, et al. Impaired growth hormone secretion in fibromyalgia patients: evidence for augmented hypothalamic somatostatin tone. *Arthritis Rheum* 2002;46(5):1344–1350.
39. Bennett RM, Clark SC, Walczyk J. A randomized, double-blind, placebo-controlled study of growth hormone in the treatment of fibromyalgia. *Am J Med* 1998;104(3):227–231.
40. Wilke WS, Sheeler LR, Makarowski WS. Hypothyroidism with presenting symptoms of fibrositis. *J Rheumatol* 1981; 8(4):626–631.
41. Riedel W, Layka H, Neeck G. Secretory pattern of GH, TSH, thyroid hormones, ACTH, cortisol, FSH, and LH in patients with fibromyalgia syndrome following systemic injection of the relevant hypothalamic-releasing hormones. *Z Rheumatol* 1998;57(Suppl. 2):81–87.
42. Neeck G, Riedel W. Thyroid function in patients with fibromyalgia syndrome. *J Rheumatol* 1992;19(7):1120–1122.
43. Magiakou MA, Chrousos GP. Corticosteroid therapy, non-endocrine disease, and corticosteroid withdrawal. *Curr Ther Endocrinol Metab* 1994;5:120–124.
44. Disdier P, Harle JR, Brue T, et al. Severe fibromyalgia after hypophysectomy for Cushing's disease. *Arthritis Rheum* 1991;34(4):493–495.
45. McCain GA, Tilbe KS. Diurnal hormone variation in fibromyalgia syndrome: a comparison with rheumatoid arthritis. *J Rheumatol Suppl* 1989;19:154–157.
46. Ataoglu S, Ozcetin A, Yildiz O, et al. Evaluation of dexamethasone suppression test in fibromyalgia patients with or without depression. *Swiss Med Wkly* 2003;133(15-16):241–244.
47. Adler GK, Kinsley BT, Hurwitz S, et al. Reduced hypothalamic-pituitary and sympathoadrenal responses to hypoglycemia in women with fibromyalgia syndrome. *Am J Med* 1999;106(5):534–543.
48. Riedel W, Schlapp U, Leck S, et al. Blunted ACTH and cortisol responses to systemic injection of corticotrophin-releasing hormone (CRH) in fibromyalgia: role of somatostatin and CRH-binding protein. *Ann NY Acad Sci* 2002;966: 483–490.
49. Griep EN, Boersma JW, Lentjes EG, et al. Function of the hypothalamic-pituitary-adrenal axis in patients with fibromyalgia and low back pain. *J Rheumatol* 1998;25(7):1374–1381.
50. Clark S, Tindall E, Bennett RM. Double blind crossover trial of prednisone versus placebo in the treatment of fibrositis. *J Rheumatol* 1985;12(5):980–983.

51. Macfarlane TV, Blinkhorn A, Worthington HV, et al. Sex hormonal factors and chronic widespread pain: a population study among women. *Rheumatology (Oxford)* 2002;41(4): 454–457.

52. Ostensen M, Rugelsjoen A, Wigers SH. The effect of reproductive events and alterations of sex hormone levels on the symptoms of fibromyalgia. *Scand J Rheumatol* 1997;26(5): 355–360.

53. Korszun A, Young EA, Engleberg NC, et al. Follicular phase hypothalamic-pituitary-gonadal axis function in women with fibromyalgia and chronic fatigue syndrome. *J Rheumatol* 2000;27(6):1526–1530.

54. Dessein PH, Shipton EA, Joffe BI, et al. Hypo secretion of adrenal androgens and the relation of serum adrenal steroids, serotonin and insulin-like growth factor-1 to clinical features in women with fibromyalgia. *Pain* 1999;83(2):313–319.

55. Buchwald D, Goldenberg DL, Sullivan JL, et al. The "chronic, active Epstein-Barr virus infection" syndrome and primary fibromyalgia. *Arthritis Rheum* 1987;30:1132–1136.

56. Simms RW, Zerbini CA, Ferrante N, et al. Fibromyalgia syndrome in patients infected with human immunodeficiency virus. *Am J Med* 1992;92(4):368–374.

57. Buskila D, Gladman DD, Langevitz P, et al. Fibromyalgia in human immunodeficiency virus infection. *J Rheumatol* 1990;17(9):1202–1206.

58. Barkhuizen A, Bennett RM. Hepatitis C infection presenting with rheumatic manifestations. *J Rheumatol* 1997;24: 1238–1239.

59. Barkhuizen A, Rosen HR, Wolf S, et al. Musculoskeletal pain and fatigue are associated with chronic hepatitis C: a report of 239 hepatology clinic patients. *Am J Gastroenterol* 1999;94:1355–1360.

60. Leventhal LJ, Naides SJ, Freundlich B. Fibromyalgia and parvovirus infection. *Arthritis Rheum* 1991;34(10):1319–1324.

61. Berg AM, Naides SJ, Simms RW. Established fibromyalgia syndrome and parvovirus B19 infection. *J Rheumatol* 1993; 20(11):1941–1943.

62. Wallace DJ, Bowman RL, Wormsley SB, et al. Cytokines and immune regulation in patients with fibrositis. *Arthritis Rheum* 1989;32:1334–1335.

63. Gur A, Karakoc M, Nas K, et al. Cytokines and depression in cases with fibromyalgia. *J Rheumatol* 2002;29: 358–361.

64. Wallace DJ, Linker-Israeli M, Hallegua D, et al. Cytokines play an aetiopathogenetic role in fibromyalgia: a hypothesis and pilot study. *Rheumatology (Oxford)* 2001;40: 743–749.

65. Maes M, Libbrecht I, Van Hunsel F, et al. The immune-inflammatory pathophysiology of fibromyalgia: increased serum soluble gp130, the common signal transducer protein of various neurotrophilic cytokines. *Psychoneuroendocrinology* 1999;24:371–383.

66. Salemi S, Rethage J, Wollina U, et al. Detection of interleukin 1beta (IL-1beta), IL-6, and tumor necrosis factor-alpha in skin of patients with fibromyalgia. *J Rheumatol* 2003;30:146–150.

17

Chronic Fatigue Syndrome

Atul Deodhar

"Chronic fatigue syndrome" (CFS) is a relatively new term, first used in English-language scientific literature in 1987 (1). Some of the previous terms used to describe people with extreme, debilitating fatigue were "neurasthenia," "epidemic neuromyesthenia," "psychiasthenia," "general paresis," "anancastic condition," "Icelandic disease," "Royal Free disease," "postviral fatigue syndrome," and "myalgic encephalitis" (2–5).

"Neurasthenia" was a common diagnosis in the 19th century and in the 20th century before the First World War. It described an illness that for decades was thought to be nonpsychiatric and neurologic, predominantly affecting "successful people" and caused by environmental factors (6). It is argued that the popularity of "neurasthenia" declined with changes in contemporary explanations and attitudes involving mental illness, as it became clear that neurasthenia was in fact a "culturally sanctioned form of illness behavior" (7). Although one can only speculate whether patients with these various diagnoses indeed had CFS, it is safe to say that CFS was most probably a subset of these conditions.

In the mid-1980s the diagnostic label of "chronic EBV infection" or "postviral fatigue syndrome" became popular after Jones reported presence of high titers of Epstein-Barr virus (EBV) antibodies compatible with active infection lasting for at least 1 year in 39 out of 44 patients complaining of chronic fatigue (8). In a 1987 article, Buchwald et al. used the term "chronic fatigue syndrome" for the first time to describe one-fifth of all patients seeking primary care for any reason who were found to be suffering from a condition "consistent with" what the authors called "chronic active EBV infection" (1). The term "chronic fatigue syndrome" became globally accepted after the Centers for Disease Control and Prevention (CDC) in 1988 defined the original diagnostic criteria for this condition—criteria that an international working group modified in 1994 (9,10). In the mid-1990s researchers coined another new term, "chronic fatigue and immune dysfunction syndrome" (CFIDS), to stress the immunologic derangements seen in some patients with CFS, and the patient lobbies in the United States picked it up. Since the immune system perturbations seen in some patients with CFS are neither sensitive nor specific for this disorder (described later), "CFS" remains the most widely used nomenclature in the United States. The same disorder is termed "myalgic encephalitis" (ME) in the United Kingdom.

DEFINITION

For patients to be diagnosed with CFS, their fatigue needs to be of new onset, profound, disabling, and lasting up to 6 months, along with self-reported impairments in concentration, short-term memory, sleep disturbances, and musculoskeletal pain. To formally define the diagnostic criteria, researchers from the CDC proposed a "working case definition" for CFS in 1988 (9). An international CFS study group subsequently revised this original definition by adding features of cognitive dysfunction and postexercise fatigue to make it more inclusive (10). The 1994 revision of the original CDC definition—now accepted worldwide—still requires a new onset (or definite origin, as opposed to "lifelong") of disabling fatigue that lasts for more than 6 months and reduces the patient's functional capacity. No obvious medical cause for the fatigue should be apparent on thorough history, physical examination, and the routine blood tests, such as complete blood count, chemistry panel, sedimentation rate, and thyroid function tests. In addition, the patient needs to fulfill four out of the following eight symptoms: (a) self-reported impairment in short-term memory, (b) sore throat, (c) tender cervical or axillary nodes, (d) myalgias, (e) arthralgias, (f) new onset headache, (g) nonrefreshing sleep, and (h) postexertional malaise (see Table 17-1).

The 1994 International CFS Study Group definition of CFS, now the most widely used definition, has three important aspects worth noting. Firstly, the definition of CFS is based purely on expert consensus and symptoms described by the patient. No objective signs on examination or specific laboratory tests could diagnose CFS, although either could rule out CFS by finding a probable cause for long term fatigue secondary to a medical condition (e.g., hypothyroidism) or a psychiatric condition (psychosis). Secondly, it does not exclude patients with minor, "nonpsychotic" psychiatric disorders

TABLE 17-1	The International Chronic Fatigue Syndrome Study Group Definition

Main Criteria

1. Severe persistent or relapsing fatigue
   A. Lasting >6 consecutive mo
   B. New or definitive onset (not lifelong)
   C. Not the result of ongoing exertion
   D. Not alleviated by rest
   E. Results in a substantial reduction in previous levels of occupational, educational, social, and personal activities
2. Presence of at least four out of the following eight symptoms:
   A. Impairment in short-term memory or concentration
   B. Recurrent sore throat
   C. Tender cervical or axillary lymph nodes
   D. Myalgia
   E. Arthralgia (without joint swelling or redness)
   F. Headache of new type, pattern, or severity
   G. Unrefreshing sleep
   H. Postexertional malaise

Exclusionary Criteria

1. Active medical condition that could explain the chronic fatigue
2. Past or current diagnosis of major depressive disorder
3. Alcohol or substance abuse within 2 yr before the onset of CFS
4. Severe obesity (body mass index ≥45)

CFS, chronic fatigue syndrome.

such as anxiety and "nonmelancholic depression." The third important feature of this definition is that it also characterizes a separate group of patients—the "idiopathic chronic fatigue." These are the patients who do not fulfill all the criteria of CFS because of either lack of severity or because they do not have four out of eight of the symptoms described above (10).

EPIDEMIOLOGY

Even though fatigue is a common symptom among the general population, with up to 18% of the polled respondents to large surveys complaining of fatigue of 6 months duration or more, only 1.4% of them attributed their excessive tiredness to CFS (11). The prevalence of CFS diagnosed on the basis of the 1994 revised criteria varies in different studies depending upon the population studied. A community-based epidemiologic study from Chicago indicated that CFS occurred in 0.42% of general population, with the highest levels of CFS found among women, minority groups, and persons with lower levels of education and occupational status (12). This was in contrast to the original observation that CFS is predominantly a disease of young, white, successful women, somewhat similar to descriptions of 19th-century neurasthenia. However, this "white predominant" observation comes from a study done in New South Wales, Australia, with a bias relating to the population studied (13). Most epidemiologic studies would, however, indicate that

CFS indeed appears to be more common in women than in men (13,14).

Other studies from different parts of the United States, such as the Pacific Northwest and San Francisco, have shown a similar prevalence of 0.1% to 0.7% in the general population (14,15) but a much higher (up to 2.6%) prevalence in patients attending a primary care clinic for any cause (16). A recent study from Wichita, KS, using a random dialing technique estimated the prevalence of CFS to be 0.37% in women, 0.08% in men, and 0.23% in the general population.

CLINICAL FEATURES

As explained above, since the diagnosis of CFS is based purely on "patient described symptoms," history taking is the most important diagnostic tool available to clinicians to reach the correct diagnosis. Patients with CFS typically present with a wide spectrum of frustrating symptoms for which they have not received satisfactory explanations despite consulting a large number of health care providers. Their chief presenting complaint is extreme debilitating fatigue that interferes with normal day-to-day activities. Usually a host of other symptoms suggestive of possible infectious etiology are present, such as chronic pain and congestion in the ear, nose, and throat area; mild grade fever; cervical lymphadenopathy; and night sweats. Anorexia, nausea, sleep disturbances, heat, and/or cold intolerance are some of the other symptoms of CFS patients. Since CFS and fibromyalgia (FM) coexist in anywhere between 21% and 80% of such patients (17), generalized musculoskeletal pain for which no cause is found is also a common complaint. Symptoms suggestive of irritable bowel syndrome, temporomandibular disorders, and multiple chemical sensitivities—common overlapping conditions with FM—are also reported (18). Significant weight loss is not a common complaint in patients with CFS, and its presence should raise the possibility of another diagnosis.

There are no diagnostic signs on physical examination and no laboratory tests that can confirm the diagnosis of CFS. However, a detailed and thorough history, physical examination, and a set of common laboratory tests are indicated in a patient with CFS to evaluate for the presence of any significant medical or psychiatric causes that could explain the chronic fatigue. Viral antibody tests and exhaustive immunologic tests are not indicated for the diagnosis of CFS.

PATHOPHYSIOLOGY

THE "INFECTIOUS AGENT" ETIOLOGY

Since fatigue is a common occurrence during and after common viral infections such as flu or infectious mononucleosis, various researchers have proposed a chronic viral infection as the etiology for CFS. Earlier studies investigated chronic active infection with EBV as a possible cause of CFS (8,19). This was based on the finding that the mean titers of antibodies to viral capsid antigen and to early antigen were greater in the sera of patients with CFS than for healthy individuals. Subsequently, various other viral agents such as human herpesvirus 6 and 7, cytomegalovirus (CMV), group B coxsackie virus, enteroviruses, human T-cell lymphotrophic virus II, hepatitis C, retroviruses, and *Varicella zoster* virus were implicated in the pathogenesis of CFS (20,8,21). However, raised antibody titers alone could not prove the viral etiology since not all patients with raised antibody titers had chronic fatigue and not all patients with CFS had high antiviral antibody titers (22). Also, some patients with CFS have no clinical or laboratory evidence of any viral infection (23,24).

One large study of more than 500 chronically fatigued patients compared the seroprevalence and the antibody titers of 13 common viruses and found no differences in those with chronic fatigue compared to control subjects (25). When patients with chronic fatigue were divided into subsets that included CFS, the results were not different. Another study comparing CFS patients with and without serologic evidence of EBV infection found no difference in the physical findings, psychiatric assessment, or laboratory tests within the groups (26). The authors concluded that EBV serologic patterns had little clinical usefulness in evaluating patients with chronic fatigue. More recently, Koelle et al. conducted a co-twin control study of 22 monozygotic twin pairs, of which one twin met criteria for CFS and the other twin was healthy. Levels of antibodies to five common viruses implicated in the etiology of CFS were measured and polymerase chain reaction (PCR) assays for ten different viral deoxyribonucleic acids (DNA) were performed. For all assays the results did not differ between the group of twins with CFS and the healthy twins (27).

Patients treated with full antibiotic treatment for *Borrelia burgdorferi*, the spirochete that causes Lyme disease, frequently experience chronic fatigue and malaise that can persist for months after the treatment is over. One study of patients with chronic fatigue who were from a region endemic for Lyme disease, examined serologic reactivity to *B. burgdorferi* but failed to show positive serologies at a higher than expected rate for patients with chronic fatigue (28).

Mycoplasma and *Chlamydia* have also been implicated as causative pathogens for CFS (29–32). A PCR-based assay detected the presence of the *Mycoplasma* genus in 52% of CFS patients, as opposed to 14% of controls (29), and a recent study of a larger European patient population found that 69% of patients with CFS had evidence of infection by at least one *Mycoplasma* species compared to only 5% of controls (33). In the same study 17% of patients had evidence of infection by multiple *Mycoplasma* species. Compared to *Mycoplasma*, *Chlamydia* infection was seen in a smaller percentage (7.5%) of patients with CFS (32). These results indicate that at least a subset of CFS patients shows evidence of bacterial infections, but they do not prove a "cause and effect" relationship.

There is no evidence for the role of chronic yeast (candidiasis) infection in CFS, although the lay press and some "self-help" books promote the use of yeast-avoidance and sugar-free diets to combat *Candida albicans* overgrowth (34). A study of 100 consecutive patients with chronic fatigue failed to show any historical, physical, or laboratory evidence of candidiasis in patients with CFS (35).

THE "IMMUNE DYSFUNCTION" THEORY

CFIDS is a popular term among some researchers and patient support groups; however, the immune abnormalities found in patients with CFS are inconsistent and nonspecific. One confounding factor in the studies of immune derangement in CFS is the case definition. Several studies investigating the immunologic differences between patients with CFS and normal controls were done on patients fulfilling the original 1988 CDC criteria but prior to the development of the 1994 International Working Group's diagnostic criteria. The changes in the diagnostic criteria for CFS from 1988 to 1994 make the comparison of results across the studies difficult.

The data on CD4+ and CD8+ T lymphocytes number and function in patients with CFS are contradictory. Two earlier studies showed an increase in the percentage of suppressor-cytotoxic CD8+ T lymphocytes expressing the class II activation markers in patients fulfilling the 1988 CDC criteria of CFS. They also showed a reduction in the percentage of CD4+ T cells as well as the CD4,CD45RA, or naive T cells, and a reduced CD4+/CD8+ ratio (36,37). However, another study by Landay et al. contradicted these findings and showed that compared to healthy controls, patients with CFS had a reduced CD8+ suppressor cell population, although it confirmed that these cells did express increased class II activation markers (22). Another subset of T lymphocytes—the CD4,CD45RO, or the memory T cells—showed increased levels of adhesion markers (CD29, CD54, and CD58), indicating activation in a sample of CFS patients compared to controls (37). CFS patient lymphocytes showed reduced proliferative responses to various mitogens, but this finding was not specific for this syndrome since lymphocytes from fatigue patients not meeting the CDC definition also showed similar abnormalities (37).

Reports on the number of circulating natural killer (NK) cells in the peripheral blood of patients with CFS are also contradictory, with some investigators reporting increased (38,39), some reporting decreased (40,41), and some finding no differences when compared to healthy controls (22,37). These variations in the results may be related to the differences in the definition of NK cells (CD56+ cells vs. CD3-CD8-CD56+ cells) among different studies (42). Two studies also reported that the function of NK cells was suppressed in CFS (41,39).

At best, studies on immunologic derangement in patients with CFS show nonspecific chronic, low-level immune system activation, though their significance in the pathogenesis, and their relationship to the symptoms of fatigue, remains unresolved (43).

ROLE OF CYTOKINES

There has been a lot of interest in measuring circulating cytokines in patients with CFS since it is known that infusion of proinflammatory cytokines such as IL-1 can induce sickness behavior in rodents and flulike symptoms of fatigue and malaise (similar to those seen in patients with CFS) in humans (44). Also, many original studies on cytokines in CFS patients were done in the early 1990s, when chronic viral infections (e.g., EBV) were thought to be an etiologic factor in the pathogenesis of CFS and it was thought that the cytokine profiles in patients with CFS could give a clue to the viral etiology of this syndrome. Several studies have tried to compare and contrast the cytokine profile in patients with acute viral infections to that in patients with CFS (45–47).

Serum levels of transforming growth factor β (TGF-β) were found to be higher in patients with CFS than in control subjects, but when the peripheral blood mononuclear cells (PBMCs) from CFS patients were cultured the TGF-β release in response to lipopolysaccharide was depressed (38). Bennett et al. subsequently confirmed this finding (48). In contrast, levels of proinflammatory cytokines such as IL-1β, IL-6, and TNF-α tested in the peripheral blood from patients with CFS were not different compared to controls (45,38), but when the cultured PBMCs from patients with CFS were stimulated with lipopolysaccharide, IL-1β, IL-6, and TNF-α release were increased compared to control subjects (38). A significant increase in both spontaneous and mitogen-induced IL-6 secretion by PBMC was observed in CFS patients during a "natural" state of fatigue but not during an "experimental fatigue" induced by exercise (49).

When CFS patients with evidence of reactivation of EB virus infection were compared to those with acute infectious mononucleosis, the levels of interferon-γ were significantly increased during the acute infectious mononucleosis but not in patients with CFS (45). Neopterin, a marker of macrophage-monocyte activation, was found to be high in patients with CFS in two studies by Chao et al. (38,50) but not by Linde et al. (45).

More recently, with the similarities between CFS and myasthenia gravis, researchers have sought to investigate presence of immunologic abnormalities against neurotransmitter receptors in CFS. Using a sensitive radioligand assay, Tanaka et al. examined serum autoantibodies to recombinant human muscarinic cholinergic receptor 1 (CHRM1) in patients with CFS, in patients with various autoimmune diseases, and in healthy controls. The anti-CHRM1 antibody levels were higher in patients with CFS and autoimmune diseases than in healthy controls (51).

Elevated levels of 2 to 5A synthetase activity and RNaseL activity indicate a nonspecific stimulation of the immune system and have been shown to be present in several studies of CFS patients (52–54). Based on these observations, a 37 k Dalton 2 to 5A binding protein in extracts of PBMCs has been proposed as a marker of CFS, as it was not found in control FM or depression patients (55–57). Additional large follow-up studies on the sensitivity and specificity of this observation are required to confirm this test's stability before it could be recommended either to diagnose or to rule out CFS.

SLEEP DISTURBANCES IN CHRONIC FATIGUE SYNDROME

Sleep disturbances are common in CFS, and "nonrefreshing sleep" is part of the international diagnostic criteria (Table 17-1). However, a severe but treatable sleep disturbance such as the sleep apnea syndrome or narcolepsy can explain the etiology of chronic fatigue and hence rules out CFS as the diagnosis. Patients with CFS complain of difficulty in falling asleep, maintaining sleep, poor overall sleep quality, and daytime drowsiness (58–60). Earlier studies have shown disordered sleep physiology in CFS similar to FM, characterized by an α intrusion within non–rapid eye movement (non–REM) sleep on the electroencephalogram (EEG) (61). CFS patients also have decreased stage IV non–REM sleep, which is the deep and restorative sleep (62). This accompanies increased nocturnal vigilance and light, unrefreshing sleep.

Some authors question the significance and specificity of these sleep disturbances in the pathophysiology of CFS. In a study of 30 patients referred to a university hospital for assessment of their chronic fatigue, Manu et al. found that primary sleep disorders were relatively common but that α-δ sleep was not a specific marker of either FM or CFS (63). In a monozygotic co-twin control study, the CFS twins had worse subjective sleep than their healthy co-twins despite little objective data on the polysomnogram supporting this discrepancy (64). This suggests that the CFS patients suffer from an element of sleep-state misperception. In a study of 1,000 consecutive sleep disorder patients referred for polysomnogram, 5% were found to have the α-EEG sleep anomaly and less than half of those complained of chronic pain (65). Also, no correlation was found between this sleep disturbance and their psychological characteristics.

In an unselected population of CFS patients, polysomnogram and multiple sleep latency tests showed that 54% had no primary sleep disorder and nearly 70% had no sleepiness either (66). A comparison between CFS patient groups with and without primary sleep disorder showed no clinical differences in symptoms and severity of CFS (66). It is therefore unlikely that CFS is simply a somatic expression of any primary sleep disorder.

THE NEUROENDOCRINOLOGY OF CHRONIC FATIGUE SYNDROME

There has been a lot of interest in the neuroendocrinology of CFS. Studies showing abnormalities in the hypothalamic-pituitary-adrenal (HPA) axis as well as central nervous system (CNS) serotonin physiology have produced some of the strongest evidence by far to support a "biologic basis" for this condition. There appears to be no evidence for a specific or uniform dysfunction of the HPA axis in CFS; however, a recent comprehensive review concluded that multiple factors such as physical inactivity, sleep disturbances, psychiatric problems, medication, and ongoing stress can affect the HPA axis (67).

The commonest reported endocrine abnormality in up to one-third of all CFS patients appears to be hypocortisolism of CNS origin (rather than adrenal gland origin) (68). These patients have low circulating cortisol and disturbance of the relationship between cortisol and central neurotransmitter function (68). This HPA dysregulation differs from that seen in melancholic depression but shares some features with FM (69). Since physical and emotional stressors exacerbate the onset and course of CFS, the impaired activation of the HPA axis by stress seems to play a role in the pathophysiology of CFS (70). Apart from stress, serotonergic and noradrenergic input from hypothalamus stimulates HPA axis activity. Some authors have suggested deficient serotonergic activity in CFS (71). Administration of serotonergic drugs such as buspirone has been shown to increase serum prolactin levels in CFS patients in contrast to suppressed levels of prolactin in controls and also in patients with depression (72,68).

Decreased serum levels of insulinlike growth factor 1 (IGF-1) have been reported in patients with FM, a condition frequently associated with CFS (73). One small study of 20 patients reported that the serum IGF-1 levels and nocturnal secretion of growth hormone (GH) was significantly lower in patients with CFS than in controls, but peak GH responses to insulin-induced hypoglycemia and arginine administration did not differ significantly between the two groups (74). However, another study comparing four groups of patients with CFS, CFS with FM, FM alone, and controls found no difference in IGF-1 or in IGF binding protein 3 in the groups (75). Dehydroepiandrostenedione and its sulfate form (DHEA and DHEA-S)—hormones that are thought to play a role in mood and energy—have also been investigated in CFS patients. Despite inconsistency in the results, the majority of the studies found the levels of DHEA and DHEA-S to be low in CFS (67).

IS CHRONIC FATIGUE SYNDROME A PSYCHIATRIC DISORDER?

The medical profession commonly labels a disorder as "psychiatric" if no consistent physical finding or laboratory test is found to "prove" its physical existence. CFS is no exception (76). There may be an unfortunate tendency to trivialize such a disorder, and some researchers even predicted that CFS would meet the same fate as neurasthenia—"a decline in social value as majority of its sufferers have primary psychiatric disorders" (7). Others, however, have challenged the notion of dividing medical disorders into two distinct "physical" and "psychiatric" categories and have argued that every diagnosis should take into account the psychosocial factors along with the biological abnormalities (77,78).

One of the confounding factors in determining the prevalence of psychiatric disorders in CFS may be the type of instruments used in a study to ascertain the presence or absence of psychopathology (43). If unexplained symptoms in CFS patients are attributed to psychiatric cause, the prevalence of psychiatric disorders may be overestimated. It is argued that the Diagnostic Interview Schedule, a highly structured interview administered by lay personnel, may overestimate the prevalence of psychiatric disorders (79–81) whereas the Structured Clinical Interview for DSM-III-R, an instrument used by trained clinicians, may show lower rates (82). Also, the examiner's own attitude toward classifying the unexplained symptoms "psychiatric" versus "physical" plays an important role in labeling a patient with "somatization disorder" and affects the stated prevalence of that particular psychiatric diagnosis (83).

There is no denying that psychiatric disorders are common and can be found in up to two-thirds of CFS patients (79), although which comes first, the chronic fatigue or the psychiatric condition, is debated. For example, depression is common in CFS patients, and in one study the onset of the first depressive episode was found to precede the onset of chronic fatigue (84). However, another study found that the psychological disturbance is likely to be a consequence of, rather than an antecedent risk factor to, CFS (82). A recent study has shown that concurrent psychiatric illness reduces quality of life and emotional well being in CFS patients, and individuals with a psychiatric illness that predated the onset of CFS suffered the greatest emotional distress (85). Despite their coexistence, major depression and CFS have several differences, as summarized in Table 17-2 (43).

In a study of 200 patients with CFS, panic disorder was present in 13% of patients, a frequency 10-fold greater than that in the general population (86). Other studies showed that mood disorders were found in 47%, somatization disorders in 13%, and anxiety disorders in 9% of CFS patients (87,79). Hypochondriacal symptoms, diagnosed by self-reported questionnaires and interviews of CFS patients, were found to reduce the quality of life (88). A subgroup of patients with CFS may show winter exacerbation in their symptoms resembling seasonally affective disorder (89). However, not all psychiatric diagnoses are more common in

TABLE 17-2	Differences in Chronic Fatigue Syndrome and Major Depression	
	CHRONIC FATIGUE SYNDROME	**MAJOR DEPRESSION**
Sore throat, lymphadenopathy, arthralgias, postexertional fatigue	Common	Not common
Anhedonia, guilt, lack of motivation	Uncommon	Common
Hypothalamic-pituitary-adrenal axis perturbations	Central down-regulation	Central up-regulation with mild hypercortisolism
Sleep disturbances	Sleep-state misperception, alpha intrusion of non–REM sleep	Reduced REM latency, increased REM density
Coexistence	Many patients may not have major depression	Most do not have CFS
Treatment	Therapeutic doses of antidepressants do not work	Drugs of choice: antidepressants

REM, rapid eye movement; CFS, chronic fatigue syndrome.

CFS patients compared to controls. When patients with CFS were compared to fatigued controls not fulfilling the CFS criteria, patients with CFS were more likely to have somatization disorder and to attribute their illness to a physical cause, but their likelihoods of current psychiatric disorders, the active mood disorders, and the prevalence of pre-existing psychiatric disorders were comparable to fatigued controls (90). Another study from Australia found that the prevalence of major depression (12.5%) and of total psychiatric disorder (24.5%) was similar to the general community estimates (82).

COGNITIVE FUNCTION IN CHRONIC FATIGUE SYNDROME

CFS patients commonly complain of cognitive functional impairments in day-to-day activities that require concentration and memory, and these could be some of the most disabling symptoms for these patients. Because of the frequency of these symptoms, "self-reported impairment of short-term memory" is a part of the definition of CFS. However, studies suggest that on objective testing patients with CFS do not suffer gross deficits in cognitive functioning (91). General intellectual abilities and higher-order cognitive skills are intact in patients with CFS, and the measured impairments are relatively subtle and are related to speed and efficiency of complex information processing (92). Evidence also suggests that CFS patients have poor learning of information (93).

Even though CFS patients believe that their fatigue leads to the cognitive dysfunction, a review of neurocognitive studies in CFS patients found no evidence that fatigue is related to their performance on neuropsychological testing (93). It is known that emotional factors influence subjective report of cognitive difficulty as depressed patients make similar complaints with cognition. The effect of emotional distress on performance on objective testing remains uncertain, and the impairments are unlikely to be explained solely by the severity of the depression and anxiety (94). Contrary to the earlier studies showing a white matter involvement, no specific pattern of cerebral abnormalities has been found that uniquely characterizes CFS patients (92).

A longitudinal study of neurocognitive testing in patients with CFS indicated that after a mean of 42 months the objective and subjective attention abilities, mood, level of fatigue, and disability improved. Moreover, the baseline psychiatric status and age were significant predictors of outcome (95).

DYSAUTONOMIA IN CHRONIC FATIGUE SYNDROME

Patients with neurally mediated hypotension (NMH) often complain of fatigue, dizziness, diminished concentration, tremulousness, and nausea—symptoms common to CFS patients. Dysautonomia and NMH are also found in some patients with FM, Gulf War syndrome, and those who are generally physically deconditioned. Earlier studies from one group found evidence of significant hypotension on tilt-table testing in almost all patients with CFS (96,97), an observation not confirmed by others (98). Also, autonomic function,

as assessed by an analysis of heart rate variability on tilt-table test, was not different in patients with CFS and in healthy controls (99).

In small, uncontrolled studies patients with CFS showed rapid improvement in their fatigue with atenolol or disopyramide, agents used in the treatment of NMH, although a larger placebo-controlled trial using fludrocortisone, another agent used in the treatment of NMH, failed to show any improvement in symptoms of CFS patients (100).

It is now generally believed that a subset of CFS patients has features of dysautonomia, and their symptoms may improve with measures to increase the intravascular volume with fluid, salt, fludrocortisone, or compression stockings (101).

MANAGEMENT OF CHRONIC FATIGUE SYNDROME

A number of "pathogenesis-driven" therapies have been tried based on what many have thought to be important aspects of CFS etiology. These include acyclovir for presumed chronic EB viral infection, fludrocortisone for NMH, intravenous immunoglobulin (IVIG) for suspected immune dysfunction, and so on (102–104). Some of the initial small and uncontrolled trials showed promising results but larger, placebo-controlled trials failed to demonstrate improvement on a reproducible basis (see Table 17-3).

Two trials on antiviral medication (acyclovir and valacyclovir) in patients with CFS who also had persistent antibodies to EB virus not only failed to improve either symptoms or function (105,102) but in one trial patients withdrew because of acyclovir-induced nephrotoxicity (102). Therapy with transfer factor active against herpesviruses was unsuccessful in a small pilot study of CFS patients (106). High-dose monthly IVIG treatment has been tried in CFS with varying success (107,104,108). A double-blind placebo-controlled trial showed statistically significant improvement in symptoms and function but no change in quality of life and depression scores in patients treated with IVIG compared to patients on placebo infusions (107). Two other trials failed to reproduce these results and showed no benefit in using IVIG (104,108).

A small nonblinded trial of Interferon-α 2b in patients with CFS showed early promise with improvement in fatigue in 25% and complete remission in 15% of patients (109). However, a later, bigger, placebo-controlled double-blind trial of Interferon-α 2a in patients with CFS showed significant improvement in quality of life scores only in a small subset of patients but not in the whole group (110).

Fludrocortisone monotherapy was tried in a double-blind placebo-controlled trial in patients with CFS based on the hypothesis that NMH could be contributing to the major symptom of fatigue (103). It failed to produce any improvement in fatigue, and the tilt-table test results did not change either. Another randomized controlled trial of low-dose hydrocortisone treatment not only failed to improve symptoms but also caused significant adrenal suppression (111). A recent trial using a combination therapy with hydrocortisone and fludrocortisone also failed to produce any improvement (112).

TABLE 17-3 Controlled Clinical Trials in the Treatment of Chronic Fatigue Syndrome

AUTHOR (YEAR)	REFERENCE NO.	STUDY	RESULTS
Antiviral Studies			
Straus (1988)	(102)	Acyclovir vs. placebo	No difference
Lerner (2002)	(105)	Valacyclovir vs. placebo	No difference
De Vinci (1996)	(106)	Transfer factor vs. placebo	No difference
Immunologic			
Lloyd (1990)	(107)	IVIG vs. placebo	IVIG better
Peterson (1990)	(104)	IVIG vs. placebo	No difference
Vollmer-Conna (1997)	(108)	IVIG vs. placebo	No difference
Brook (1993)	(109)	Interferon-α 2b vs. placebo	Interferon-α 2b better
See (1996)	(110)	Interferon-α 2a vs. placebo	Interferon-α 2a better only in a subgroup with decreased NK cell function
Lloyd (1993)	(126)	Dialyzable leukocyte extract vs. placebo	No difference
Zachrisson (2002)	(127)	Staphylococcus toxoid vs. placebo	Staphylococcus toxoid injections better
Hormonal			
Peterson (1998)	(100)	Fludrocortisone vs. placebo	No difference
McKenzie (1998)	(111)	Hydrocortisone vs. placebo	No difference
Rowe (2001)	(103)	Fludrocortisone vs. placebo	No difference
Blockmans (2003)	(112)	Hydrocortisone plus fludrocortisone vs. placebo	No difference
Moorkens (1998)	(128)	Growth hormone vs. placebo	No difference
Sleep Related			
Williams (2002)	(129)	Melatonin plus phototherapy vs. placebo	No difference
Olson (2003)	(130)	Dexamphetamine vs. placebo	Dexamphetamine better
Dietary			
Brouwers (2002)	(131)	Polynutrient supplements vs. placebo	No difference
Exercise			
Powell (2001)	(115)	Patient education and exercise vs. standard medical care	Exercise group did better
Fulcher (1997)	(114)	Graded aerobic exercise vs. flexibility + relaxation therapy	Graded aerobic exercise better
Antidepressants			
Hartz (2003)	(132)	Citalopram vs. placebo	Citalopram better
Hickie (2000)	(133)	Moclobemide vs. placebo	No difference
Vercoulen (1996)	(134)	Fluoxetine vs. placebo	No difference
Psychological			
Lloyd (1993)	(126)	Cognitive behavioral therapy (CBT) vs. placebo	No difference
Sharpe (1996)	(117)	CBT vs. medical care	CBT better
Prins (2001)	(119)	CBT vs. support group vs. control	CBT better
Ridsdale (2001)	(120)	CBT vs. counseling	No difference

IVIG, intravenous immunoglobulin; NK, natural killer; CBT, cognitive behavioral therapy.

Because of the lack of a clear etiology and uncertainty on pathogenesis, pharmacologic treatments of CFS have been inadequate and unsatisfactory, as reported above. Since the conventional medicines fail to significantly improve symptoms, desperate patients often resort to complementary and alternative medicine (CAM) in search of relief. With the advent of the Internet, these unproven, uninvestigated, and unscientific therapies based on dubious claims have found a large audience. CAM includes vitamin and mineral supple-

mentations in supraphysiologic doses, herbal therapy, avoidance diets, energy healing, and "faith-based" therapies. Very little data are available in scientific literature on the efficacy or the toxicity, or both, with these agents, and hence their use is not recommended.

Patients with CFS complain of exercise intolerance, and "postexertional malaise" is part of the definition of CFS. One of the major causes of this symptom is physical deconditioning (113). Fulcher et al. compared graded aerobic exercises in CFS patients without psychiatric or sleep disorder to flexibility exercises combined with relaxation therapy in a randomized crossover trial (114). Graded exercise treatment was found to be more effective than the flexibility routine in improving the fatigue and physical function, although it was independent of the improvement in strength and peak aerobic capacity produced by the exercise. Another randomized controlled trial of an educational intervention encouraging patients to exercise showed that graded aerobic exercise was effective in reducing symptoms of fatigue, improved sleep and mood and also improved physical functioning (115).

Various psychological interventions, such as cognitive behavioral therapy (CBT), counseling, and antidepressant medication have been tried in the management of CFS. Gruber et al. reviewed studies of antidepressant medications in what they called "disorders on the interface of psychiatry and medicine" such as FM, CFS, irritable bowel syndrome, and so on (116). Their review concluded that these disorders benefit to varying degrees from antidepressant medications, although there was little correlation between improvement in psychological symptoms and physical symptoms of a given disorder. CBT, a nonpharmacologic treatment, is based on a hypothesis that certain cognitions and behavior could perpetuate symptoms and disability, as they may act as obstacles to recovery. CBT emphasizes self-help and aims to help by changing these unhelpful cognitions and behavior. In a randomized controlled trial, CBT improved physical functioning in 73% of patients with CFS when compared to 27% of patients who received only the routine medical care (117). CBT can also encourage graded exercise, which can facilitate recovery from CFS. However, resistance to accepting this therapeutic rationale or poor motivation to treatment adherence, as well as secondary gains, such as receiving monetary benefit from illness, predict poor outcome in CFS patients (118). In the same study, membership in a self-help group also predicted poor outcome, raising concerns that such groups may be reinforcing a sickness behavior. Another multicenter, randomized controlled study of CBT, support-group therapy, and the natural course of the disease confirmed the benefit of CBT in reducing fatigue severity and improving functional outcome compared to the other two groups (119). Membership in "support groups" had no benefit. Counseling was found to be as effective as CBT in a randomized trial based on general practices in England (120).

In conclusion, both graded exercise programs and CBT have been shown to be effective and should be offered to all patients with CFS. Treatment of accompanying ailments such as sleep disorders and NMH and psychiatric disorders such as depression would also help in improving the fatigue and functional capacity and hence should be individualized.

PROGNOSIS OF CHRONIC FATIGUE SYNDROME

The prognosis of CFS seems to vary with age (children vs. adults) and also with the stringency of the definition (121). A 13-year follow-up of children and adolescents with CFS found that nearly 80% had experienced improvement in their symptoms, with 37% experiencing complete resolution and another 42% experiencing partial resolution (122). Another study in the setting of a university pediatric clinic followed children with idiopathic chronic fatigue (3 months duration) for 4 years. At follow-up, 65% reported resolution of symptoms, 29% reported improvement, and 6% were unchanged (123). Compared to children, the prognosis in adults with CFS is not that good. An 18-month follow-up study of adult patients with CFS found only 3% reporting complete recovery and 17% reporting partial improvement. At follow-up, the patients were having considerable problems at work because of functional incapacity (124).

Joyce et al. carried out a systematic review of the prognosis of CFS from 26 published studies (125). They found that 54% to 94% of children recovered from CFS in follow-up studies compared to <10% of adults reporting return to premorbid level of functioning. The reported risk factors for poor prognosis were older age, more chronic illness, having a psychiatric disorder, and the belief that their CFS was secondary to physical causes (125).

SUMMARY POINTS

- Like FM, the symptom complex now known as CFS has clearly been described for centuries in the medical literature under a variety of terms.
- Like other conditions in this spectrum, CFS had been suspected to be due to a chronic infection. Unlike other conditions in this spectrum, both patients and credible investigators still maintain this hypothesis, although no consistent immunologic findings have been described and no pathogen has been identified.
- The evidence suggests that perhaps a subset of those with CFS might have an as-yet unidentified primary infection or immune disturbance, whereas the remainder has a condition very similar in pathogenesis to FM.

■ IMPLICATIONS FOR PRACTICE

- Because of the lack of a clear etiology and uncertainty on pathogenesis, randomized controlled trials of pharmacologic treatments of CFS have generally been inadequate and unsatisfactory.
- In contrast, both CBT and graded aerobic exercise have generally been efficacious in CFS, although the beneficial effects of these therapies are limited by adherence and compliance to treatments.

REFERENCES

1. Buchwald D, Sullivan JL, Komaroff AL. Frequency of 'chronic active Epstein-Barr virus infection' in a general medical practice. *JAMA* 1987;257(17):2303–2307.
2. Carlson ET. The nerve weakness of the 19th century. *Int J Psychiatry* 1970;9:50–54.
3. Steele J. The hysteria and psychiasthenia constructs as an alternative to manifest anxiety and conflict-free ego functions. *J Abnorm Psychol* 1969;74(1):79–85.

4. Storm-Mathisen A. General paresis; a follow-up study of 203 patients. *Acta Psychiatr Scand* 1969;45(2):118–132.

5. Skoog G. Onset of anancastic conditions. A clinical study. *Acta Psychiatr Scand Suppl* 1965;184:1–82.

6. Wessely S. Old wine in new bottles: neurasthenia and 'ME'. *Psychol Med* 1990;20(1):35–53.

7. Abbey SE, Garfinkel PE. Neurasthenia and chronic fatigue syndrome: the role of culture in the making of a diagnosis. *Am J Psychiatry* 1991;148(12):1638–1646.

8. Jones JF, Ray CG, Minnich LL, et al. Evidence for active Epstein-Barr virus infection in patients with persistent, unexplained illnesses: elevated anti-early antigen antibodies. *Ann Intern Med* 1985;102(1):1–7.

9. Holmes GP, Kaplan JE, Gantz NM, et al. Chronic fatigue syndrome: a working case definition. *Ann Intern Med* 1988; 108(3):387–389.

10. Fukuda K, Straus SE, Hickie I et al., International Chronic Fatigue Syndrome Study Group. The chronic fatigue syndrome: a comprehensive approach to its definition and study. *Ann Intern Med* 1994;121(12):953–959.

11. Pawlikowska T, Chalder T, Hirsch SR, et al. Population based study of fatigue and psychological distress. *Br Med J* 1994; 308(6931):763–766.

12. Jason LA, Richman JA, Rademaker AW, et al. A community-based study of chronic fatigue syndrome. *Arch Intern Med* 1999;159(18):2129–2137.

13. Lloyd AR, Hickie I, Boughton CR, et al. Prevalence of chronic fatigue syndrome in an Australian population. *Med J Aust* 1990;153(9):522–528.

14. Steele L, Dobbins JG, Fukuda K, et al. The epidemiology of chronic fatigue in San Francisco. *Am J Med* 1998;105(3A): 83S–90S.

15. Buchwald D, Umali P, Umali J, et al. Chronic fatigue and the chronic fatigue syndrome: prevalence in a Pacific Northwest health care system. *Ann Intern Med* 1995;123(2):81–88.

16. Wessely S, Chalder T, Hirsch S, et al. The prevalence and morbidity of chronic fatigue and chronic fatigue syndrome: a prospective primary care study. *Am J Public Health* 1997; 87(9):1449–1455.

17. Aaron LA, Buchwald D. Chronic diffuse musculoskeletal pain, fibromyalgia and co-morbid unexplained clinical conditions. *Best Pract Res Clin Rheumatol* 2003;17(4): 563–574.

18. Bennett R. Fibromyalgia, chronic fatigue syndrome, and myofascial pain. *Curr Opin Rheumatol* 1998;10(2):95–103.

19. Jones JF. Epstein-Barr virus and the chronic fatigue syndrome: a short review. *Microbiol Sci* 1988;5(12):366–369.

20. Ablashi DV, Eastman HB, Owen CB, et al. Frequent HHV-6 reactivation in multiple sclerosis (MS) and chronic fatigue syndrome (CFS) patients. *J Clin Virol* 2000;16(3): 179–191.

21. Komaroff AL. Chronic fatigue syndromes: relationship to chronic viral infections. *J Virol Methods* 1988;21(1-4):3–10.

22. Landay AL, Jessop C, Lennette ET, et al. Chronic fatigue syndrome: clinical condition associated with immune activation. *Lancet* 1991;338(8769):707–712.

23. Farrar DJ, Locke SE, Kantrowitz FG. Chronic fatigue syndrome. 1: Etiology and pathogenesis. *Behav Med* 1995; 21(1):5–16.

24. Greenberg DB. Neurasthenia in the 1980s: chronic mononucleosis, chronic fatigue syndrome, and anxiety and depressive disorders. *Psychosomatics* 1990;31(2):129–137.

25. Buchwald D, Ashley RL, Pearlman T, et al. Viral serologies in patients with chronic fatigue and chronic fatigue syndrome. *J Med Virol* 1996;50(1):25–30.

26. Matthews DA, Lane TJ, Manu P. Antibodies to Epstein-Barr virus in patients with chronic fatigue. *South Med J* 1991; 84(7):832–840.

27. Koelle DM, Barcy S, Huang ML, et al. Markers of viral infection in monozygotic twins discordant for chronic fatigue syndrome. *Clin Infect Dis* 2002;35(5):518–525.

28. Coyle PK, Krupp LB, Doscher C, et al. *Borrelia burgdorferi* reactivity in patients with severe persistent fatigue who are from a region in which Lyme disease is endemic. *Clin Infect Dis* 1994;18(Suppl. 1):S24–S27.

29. Vojdani A, Choppa PC, Tagle C, et al. Detection of mycoplasma genus and *Mycoplasma fermentans* by PCR in patients with chronic fatigue syndrome. *FEMS Immunol Med Microbiol* 1998;22(4):355–365.

30. Choppa PC, Vojdani A, Tagle C, et al. Multiplex PCR for the detection of Mycoplasma fermentans, M. hominis and M. penetrans in cell cultures and blood samples of patients with chronic fatigue syndrome. *Mol Cell Probes* 1998;12(5): 301–308.

31. Chia JK, Chia LY. Chronic *Chlamydia pneumoniae* infection: a treatable cause of chronic fatigue syndrome. *Clin Infect Dis* 1999;29(2):452–453.

32. Nicolson GL, Gan R, Haier J. Multiple co-infections (mycoplasma, chlamydia, human herpes virus-6) in blood of chronic fatigue syndrome patients: association with signs and symptoms. *APMIS* 2003;111(5):557–566.

33. Nijs J, Nicolson GL, De Becker P, et al. High prevalence of mycoplasma infections among European chronic fatigue syndrome patients. Examination of four mycoplasma species in blood of chronic fatigue syndrome patients. *FEMS Immunol Med Microbiol* 2002;34(3):209–214.

34. Morris DH, Stare FJ. Unproven diet therapies in the treatment of the chronic fatigue syndrome. *Arch Fam Med* 1993; 2(2):181–186.

35. Renfro L, Feder HM Jr, Lane TJ, et al. Yeast connection among 100 patients with chronic fatigue. *Am J Med* 1989; 86(2):165–168.

36. Klimas NG, Salvato FR, Morgan R, et al. Immunologic abnormalities in chronic fatigue syndrome. *J Clin Microbiol* 1990;28(6):1403–1410.

37. Straus SE, Fritz S, Dale JK, et al. Lymphocyte phenotype and function in the chronic fatigue syndrome. *J Clin Immunol* 1993;13(1):30–40.

38. Chao CC, Janoff EN, Hu SX, et al. Altered cytokine release in peripheral blood mononuclear cell cultures from patients with the chronic fatigue syndrome. *Cytokine* 1991;3(4): 292–298.

39. Morrison LJ, Behan WH, Behan PO. Changes in natural killer cell phenotype in patients with post-viral fatigue syndrome. *Clin Exp Immunol* 1991;83(3):441–446.

40. Gupta S, Vayuvegula B. A comprehensive immunological analysis in chronic fatigue syndrome. *Scand J Immunol* 1991;33(3):319–327.

41. Caligiuri M, Murray C, Buchwald D, et al. Phenotypic and functional deficiency of natural killer cells in patients with chronic fatigue syndrome. *J Immunol* 1987;139(10): 3306–3313.

42. Evengard B, Klimas N. Chronic fatigue syndrome: probable pathogenesis and possible treatments. *Drugs* 2002;62(17): 2433–2446.

43. Afari N, Buchwald D. Chronic fatigue syndrome: a review. *Am J Psychiatry* 2003;160(2):221–236.

44. Dantzer R. Current studies on the neurobiology of chronic fatigue syndrome. *Encephale* 1994;20 Spec No 3:597–602.

45. Linde A, Andersson B, Svenson SB, et al. Serum levels of lymphokines and soluble cellular receptors in primary Epstein-Barr virus infection and in patients with chronic fatigue syndrome. *J Infect Dis* 1992;165(6):994–1000.

46. Kerr JR, Tyrrell DA. Cytokines in parvovirus B19 infection as an aid to understanding chronic fatigue syndrome. *Curr Pain Headache Rep* 2003;7(5):333–341.

47. Levy JA. Viral studies of chronic fatigue syndrome. *Clin Infect Dis* 1994;18(Suppl. 1):S117–S120.

48. Bennett AL, Chao CC, Hu S, et al. Elevation of bioactive transforming growth factor-beta in serum from patients with chronic fatigue syndrome. *J Clin Immunol* 1997;17(2):160–166.

49. Gupta S, Aggarwal S, Starr A. Increased production of interleukin-6 by adherent and non-adherent mononuclear cells during 'natural fatigue' but not following 'experimental fatigue' in patients with chronic fatigue syndrome. *Int J Mol Med* 1999;3(2):209–213.

50. Chao CC, Gallagher M, Phair J, et al. Serum neopterin and interleukin-6 levels in chronic fatigue syndrome. *J Infect Dis* 1990;162(6):1412–1413.

51. Tanaka S, Kuratsune H, Hidaka Y, et al. Autoantibodies against muscarinic cholinergic receptor in chronic fatigue syndrome. *Int J Mol Med* 2003;12(2):225–230.

52. Suhadolnik RJ, Peterson DL, O'Brien K, et al. Biochemical evidence for a novel low molecular weight 2-5A-dependent RNase L in chronic fatigue syndrome. *J Interferon Cytokine Res* 1997;17(7):377–385.

53. Suhadolnik RJ, Reichenbach NL, Hitzges P, et al. Changes in the 2-5A synthetase/RNase L antiviral pathway in a controlled clinical trial with poly(I)-poly(C12U) in chronic fatigue syndrome. *In Vivo* 1994;8(4):599–604.

54. Snell CR, Vanness JM, Strayer DR, et al. Physical performance and prediction of 2-5A synthetase/RNase L antiviral pathway activity in patients with chronic fatigue syndrome. *In Vivo* 2002;16(2):107–109.

55. De Meirleir K, Bisbal C, Campine I, et al. A 37 kDa 2-5A binding protein as a potential biochemical marker for chronic fatigue syndrome. *Am J Med* 2000;108(2):99–105.

56. Demettre E, Bastide L, D'Haese A, et al. Ribonuclease L proteolysis in peripheral blood mononuclear cells of chronic fatigue syndrome patients. *J Biol Chem* 2002;277(38):35746–35751.

57. Tiev KP, Demettre E, Ercolano P, et al. RNase L levels in peripheral blood mononuclear cells: 37-kilodalton/83-kilodalton isoform ratio is a potential test for chronic fatigue syndrome. *Clin Diagn Lab Immunol* 2003;10(2):315–316.

58. Morriss R, Sharpe M, Sharpley AL, et al. Abnormalities of sleep in patients with the chronic fatigue syndrome. *Br Med J* 1993;306(6886):1161–1164.

59. Sharpley A, Clements A, Hawton K, et al. Do patients with "pure" chronic fatigue syndrome (neurasthenia) have abnormal sleep? *Psychosom Med* 1997;59(6):592–596.

60. Krupp LB, Jandorf L, Coyle PK, et al. Sleep disturbance in chronic fatigue syndrome. *J Psychosom Res* 1993;37(4):325–331.

61. Moldofsky H. Fibromyalgia, sleep disorder and chronic fatigue syndrome. *Ciba Found Symp* 1993;173:262–271.

62. Fischler B, Le Bon O, Hoffmann G, et al. Sleep anomalies in the chronic fatigue syndrome. A comorbidity study. *Neuropsychobiology* 1997;35(3):115–122.

63. Manu P, Lane TJ, Matthews DA, et al. Alpha-delta sleep in patients with a chief complaint of chronic fatigue. *South Med J* 1994;87(4):465–470.

64. Watson NF, Kapur V, Arguelles LM, et al. Comparison of subjective and objective measures of insomnia in monozygotic twins discordant for chronic fatigue syndrome. *Sleep* 2003;26(3):324–328.

65. Rains JC, Penzien DB. Sleep and chronic pain: challenges to the alpha-EEG sleep pattern as a pain specific sleep anomaly. *J Psychosom Res* 2003;54(1):77–83.

66. Le Bon O, Hoffmann G, Murphy J, et al. How significant are primary sleep disorders and sleepiness in the chronic fatigue syndrome? *Sleep Res Online* 2000;3(2):43–48.

67. Cleare AJ. The neuroendocrinology of chronic fatigue syndrome. *Endocr Rev* 2003;24(2):236–252.

68. Parker AJ, Wessely S, Cleare AJ. The neuroendocrinology of chronic fatigue syndrome and fibromyalgia. *Psychol Med* 2001;31(8):1331–1345.

69. Demitrack MA, Crofford LJ. Evidence for and pathophysiologic implications of hypothalamic-pituitary-adrenal axis dysregulation in fibromyalgia and chronic fatigue syndrome. *Ann NY Acad Sci* 1998;840:684–697.

70. Crofford LJ. The hypothalamic-pituitary-adrenal stress axis in fibromyalgia and chronic fatigue syndrome. *Z Rheumatol* 1998;57(Suppl. 2):67–71.

71. Neeck G, Crofford LJ. Neuroendocrine perturbations in fibromyalgia and chronic fatigue syndrome. *Rheum Dis Clin North Am* 2000;26(4):989–1002.

72. Bakheit AM, Behan PO, Dinan TG, et al. Possible upregulation of hypothalamic 5-hydroxytryptamine receptors in patients with postviral fatigue syndrome. *Br Med J* 1992;304(6833):1010–1012.

73. Bennett RM, Cook DM, Clark SR, et al. Hypothalamic-pituitary-insulin-like growth factor-I axis dysfunction in patients with fibromyalgia. *J Rheumatol* 1997;24(7):1384–1389.

74. Berwaerts J, Moorkens G, Abs R. Secretion of growth hormone in patients with chronic fatigue syndrome. *Growth Horm IGF Res* 1998;8(Suppl. B):127–129.

75. Buchwald D, Umali J, Stene M. Insulin-like growth factor-I (somatomedin C) levels in chronic fatigue syndrome and fibromyalgia. *J Rheumatol* 1996;23(4):739–742.

76. Matthews DA, Manu P, Lane TJ. Evaluation and management of patients with chronic fatigue. *Am J Med Sci* 1991;302(5):269–277.

77. Kendler KS. A psychiatric dialogue on the mind-body problem. *Am J Psychiatry* 2001;158(7):989–1000.

78. Oken D. Multiaxial diagnosis and the psychosomatic model of disease. *Psychosom Med* 2000;62(2):171–175.

79. Manu P, Matthews DA, Lane TJ. The mental health of patients with a chief complaint of chronic fatigue. A prospective evaluation and follow-up. *Arch Intern Med* 1988;148(10):2213–2217.

80. Manu P, Lane TJ, Matthews DA, et al. Screening for somatization disorder in patients with chronic fatigue. *Gen Hosp Psychiatry* 1989;11(4):294–297.

81. Escobar JI, Manu P, Matthews D, et al. Medically unexplained physical symptoms, somatization disorder and abridged somatization: studies with the diagnostic interview schedule. *Psychiatr Dev* 1989;7(3):235–245.

82. Hickie I, Lloyd A, Wakefield D, et al. The psychiatric status of patients with the chronic fatigue syndrome. *Br J Psychiatry* 1990;156:534–540.

83. Johnson SK, DeLuca J, Natelson BH. Assessing somatization disorder in the chronic fatigue syndrome. *Psychosom Med* 1996;58(1):50–57.

84. Manu P, Matthews DA, Lane TJ, et al. Depression among patients with a chief complaint of chronic fatigue. *J Affect Disord* 1989;17(2):165–172.

85. Tiersky LA, Matheis RJ, DeLuca J, et al. Functional status, neuropsychological functioning, and mood in chronic fatigue syndrome (CFS): relationship to psychiatric disorder. *J Nerv Ment Dis* 2003;191(5):324–331.

86. Manu P, Matthews DA, Lane TJ. Panic disorder among patients with chronic fatigue. *South Med J* 1991;84(4):451–456.

87. Manu P, Lane TJ, Matthews DA. Somatization disorder in patients with chronic fatigue. *Psychosomatics* 1989;30(4):388–395.

88. Manu P, Affleck G, Tennen H, et al. Hypochondriasis influences quality-of-life outcomes in patients with chronic fatigue. *Psychother Psychosom* 1996;65(2):76–81.

89. Terman M, Levine SM, Terman JS, et al. Chronic fatigue syndrome and seasonal affective disorder: comorbidity, diagnostic

overlap, and implications for treatment. *Am J Med* 1998; 105(3A):115S–124S.

90. Lane TJ, Manu P, Matthews DA. Depression and somatization in the chronic fatigue syndrome. *Am J Med* 1991;91(4): 335–344.

91. Wearden AJ, Appleby L. Research on cognitive complaints and cognitive functioning in patients with chronic fatigue syndrome (CFS): What conclusions can we draw? *J Psychosom Res* 1996;41(3):197–211.

92. Tiersky LA, Johnson SK, Lange G, et al. Neuropsychology of chronic fatigue syndrome: a critical review. *J Clin Exp Neuropsychol* 1997;19(4):560–586.

93. Michiels V, Cluydts R. Neuropsychological functioning in chronic fatigue syndrome: a review. *Acta Psychiatr Scand* 2001;103(2):84–93.

94. DeLuca J, Johnson SK, Natelson BH. Neuropsychiatric status of patients with chronic fatigue syndrome: an overview. *Toxicol Ind Health* 1994;10(4-5):513–522.

95. Tiersky LA, DeLuca J, Hill N, et al. Longitudinal assessment of neuropsychological functioning, psychiatric status, functional disability and employment status in chronic fatigue syndrome. *Appl Neuropsychol* 2001;8(1):41–50.

96. Rowe PC, Bou-Holaigah I, Kan JS, et al. Is neurally mediated hypotension an unrecognised cause of chronic fatigue? *Lancet* 1995;345(8950):623–624.

97. Bou-Holaigah I, Rowe PC, Kan J, et al. The relationship between neurally mediated hypotension and the chronic fatigue syndrome. *JAMA* 1995;274(12):961–967.

98. Poole J, Herrell R, Ashton S, et al. Results of isoproterenol tilt table testing in monozygotic twins discordant for chronic fatigue syndrome. *Arch Intern Med* 2000;160(22): 3461–3468.

99. Yataco A, Talo H, Rowe P, et al. Comparison of heart rate variability in patients with chronic fatigue syndrome and controls. *Clin Auton Res* 1997;7(6):293–297.

100. Peterson PK, Pheley A, Schroeppel J, et al. A preliminary placebo-controlled crossover trial of fludrocortisone for chronic fatigue syndrome. *Arch Intern Med* 1998;158(8): 908–914.

101. Gerrity TR, Bates J, Bell DS, et al. Chronic fatigue syndrome: what role does the autonomic nervous system play in the pathophysiology of this complex illness? *Neuroimmunomodulation* 2002;10(3):134–141.

102. Straus SE, Dale JK, Tobi M, et al. Acyclovir treatment of the chronic fatigue syndrome. Lack of efficacy in a placebo-controlled trial. *N Engl J Med* 1988;319(26):1692–1698.

103. Rowe PC, Calkins H, DeBusk K, et al. Fludrocortisone acetate to treat neurally mediated hypotension in chronic fatigue syndrome: a randomized controlled trial. *JAMA* 2001;285(1):52–59.

104. Peterson PK, Shepard J, Macres M, et al. A controlled trial of intravenous immunoglobulin G in chronic fatigue syndrome. *Am J Med* 1990;89(5):554–560.

105. Lerner AM, Beqaj SH, Deeter RG, et al. A six-month trial of valacyclovir in the Epstein-Barr virus subset of chronic fatigue syndrome: improvement in left ventricular function. *Drugs Today (Barc)* 2002;38(8):549–561.

106. De Vinci C, Levine PH, Pizza G, et al. Lessons from a pilot study of transfer factor in chronic fatigue syndrome. *Biotherapy* 1996;9(1-3):87–90.

107. Lloyd A, Hickie I, Wakefield D, et al. A double-blind, placebo-controlled trial of intravenous immunoglobulin therapy in patients with chronic fatigue syndrome. *Am J Med* 1990;89(5): 561–568.

108. Vollmer-Conna U, Hickie I, Hadzi-Pavlovic D, et al. Intravenous immunoglobulin is ineffective in the treatment of patients with chronic fatigue syndrome. *Am J Med* 1997; 103(1):38–43.

109. Brook MG, Bannister BA, Weir WR. Interferon-alpha therapy for patients with chronic fatigue syndrome. *J Infect Dis* 1993;168(3):791–792.

110. See DM, Tilles JG. Alpha-interferon treatment of patients with chronic fatigue syndrome. *Immunol Invest* 1996;25 (1-2):153–164.

111. McKenzie R, O'Fallon A, Dale J, et al. Low-dose hydrocortisone for treatment of chronic fatigue syndrome: a randomized controlled trial. *JAMA* 1998;280(12):1061–1066.

112. Blockmans D, Persoons P, Van Houdenhove B, et al. Combination therapy with hydrocortisone and fludrocortisone does not improve symptoms in chronic fatigue syndrome: a randomized, placebo-controlled, double-blind, crossover study. *Am J Med* 2003;114(9):736–741.

113. Riley MS, O'Brien CJ, McCluskey DR, et al. Aerobic work capacity in patients with chronic fatigue syndrome. *Br Med J* 1990;301(6758):953–956.

114. Fulcher KY, White PD. Randomised controlled trial of graded exercise in patients with the chronic fatigue syndrome. *Br Med J* 1997;314(7095):1647–1652.

115. Powell P, Bentall RP, Nye FJ, et al. Randomised controlled trial of patient education to encourage graded exercise in chronic fatigue syndrome. *Br Med J* 2001;322(7283): 387–390.

116. Gruber AJ, Hudson JI, Pope HG Jr. The management of treatment-resistant depression in disorders on the interface of psychiatry and medicine. Fibromyalgia, chronic fatigue syndrome, migraine, irritable bowel syndrome, atypical facial pain, and premenstrual dysphoric disorder. *Psychiatr Clin North Am* 1996;19(2):351–369.

117. Sharpe M, Hawton K, Simkin S, et al. Cognitive behaviour therapy for the chronic fatigue syndrome: a randomized controlled trial. *Br Med J* 1996;312(7022):22–26.

118. Bentall RP, Powell P, Nye FJ, et al. Predictors of response to treatment for chronic fatigue syndrome. *Br J Psychiatry* 2002;181:248–252.

119. Prins JB, Bleijenberg G, Bazelmans E, et al. Cognitive behaviour therapy for chronic fatigue syndrome: a multicentre randomised controlled trial. *Lancet* 2001;357(9259): 841–847.

120. Ridsdale L, Godfrey E, Chalder T, et al. Chronic fatigue in general practice: is counselling as good as cognitive behaviour therapy? A UK randomised trial. *Br J Gen Pract* 2001; 51(462):19–24.

121. Bombardier CH, Buchwald D. Outcome and prognosis of patients with chronic fatigue vs chronic fatigue syndrome. *Arch Intern Med* 1995;155(19):2105–2110.

122. Bell DS, Jordan K, Robinson M. Thirteen-year follow-up of children and adolescents with chronic fatigue syndrome. *Pediatrics* 2001;107(5):994–998.

123. Feder HM, Dworkin PH, Orkin C Jr. Outcome of 48 pediatric patients with chronic fatigue. A clinical experience. *Arch Fam Med* 1994;3(12):1049–1055.

124. Vercoulen JH, Swanink CM, Fennis JF, et al. Prognosis in chronic fatigue syndrome: a prospective study on the natural course. *J Neurol Neurosurg Psychiatry* 1996;60(5):489–494.

125. Joyce J, Hotopf M, Wessely S. The prognosis of chronic fatigue and chronic fatigue syndrome: a systematic review. *Q J Med* 1997;90(3):223–233.

126. Lloyd AR, Hickie I, Brockman A, et al. Immunologic and psychologic therapy for patients with chronic fatigue syndrome: a double-blind, placebo-controlled trial. *Am J Med* 1993;94(2):197–203.

127. Zachrisson O, Regland B, Jahreskog M, et al. Treatment with staphylococcus toxoid in fibromyalgia/chronic fatigue syndrome—a randomised controlled trial. *Eur J Pain* 2002; 6(6): 455–466.

128. Moorkens G, Wynants H, Abs R. Effect of growth hormone treatment in patients with chronic fatigue syndrome:

a preliminary study. *Growth Horm IGF Res* 1998;8(Suppl. B): 131–133.

129. Williams G, Waterhouse J, Mugarza J, et al. Therapy of circadian rhythm disorders in chronic fatigue syndrome: no symptomatic improvement with melatonin or phototherapy. *Eur J Clin Invest* 2002;32(11):831–837.

130. Olson LG, Ambrogetti A, Sutherland DC. A pilot randomized controlled trial of dexamphetamine in patients with chronic fatigue syndrome. *Psychosomatics* 2003;44(1): 38–43.

131. Brouwers FM, Van Der WS, Bleijenberg G, et al. The effect of a polynutrient supplement on fatigue and physical activity of patients with chronic fatigue syndrome: a double-blind randomized controlled trial. *Q J Med* 2002;95(10):677–683.

132. Hartz AJ, Bentler SE, Brake KA, et al. The effectiveness of citalopram for idiopathic chronic fatigue. *J Clin Psychiatry* 2003;64(8):927–935.

133. Hickie IB, Wilson AJ, Wright JM, et al. A randomized, double-blind placebo-controlled trial of moclobemide in patients with chronic fatigue syndrome. *J Clin Psychiatry* 2000;61(9): 643–648.

134. Vercoulen JH, Swanink CM, Zitman FG, et al. Randomised, double-blind, placebo-controlled study of fluoxetine in chronic fatigue syndrome. *Lancet* 1996;347(9005):858–861.

18

The Functional Bowel Disorder Spectrum

Lucinda A. Harris and Lin Chang

Functional gastrointestinal disorders (FGIDs) are quite common and are estimated to account for up to 40% of diagnoses made by gastroenterologists (1). There are over 20 functional bowel syndromes with different clinical features that are generally characterized by chronic or recurrent symptoms that are attributable to the gastrointestinal (GI) tract and not explained by any biochemical or structural abnormalities (2). The most common FGID is irritable bowel syndrome (IBS), which is found in 10% to 20% of the population (3). Other common FGIDs include globus, noncardiac chest pain, dyspepsia, functional constipation and diarrhea, gall bladder dysfunction, sphincter of Oddi dysfunction, functional abdominal pain, and functional anorectal disorders (4). It is beyond the scope of this chapter to discuss all FGIDs, therefore, the most commonly seen disorders—atypical chest pain, functional dyspepsia (FD), IBS, and chronic constipation—will be discussed in terms of their epidemiology, diagnosis, pathophysiology, and treatment.

There are a number of studies which have demonstrated elevated health care costs of IBS patients compared to non-IBS patients with indirect and direct annual costs estimated to be a total of up to 30 billion dollars (5,6). These studies similarly found that health care costs were increased particularly with regard to outpatient rather than inpatient services (7–9). Interestingly, one study found that the majority of excess total health care costs were due to non-lower GI-related services (10). This finding is supported by the increased physician visits by IBS patients not only for GI symptoms, but also for non-IBS related reasons (11). The increased health care costs and physician visits for non-GI complaints are due in large part to the fact that many patients with FGID, particularly IBS, also report extraintestinal symptoms such as fatigue (12,13), muscle pain (12,13), sleep disturbances (14), and sexual dysfunction (15). IBS patients are twice as likely as comparison groups to be diagnosed with a non-GI chronic-pain disorder (16). These non-GI chronic disorders include fibromyalgia (FM), chronic fatigue syndrome, chronic pelvic pain, and interstitial cystitis (17,18). These two syndromes share many similar clinical and physiologic features suggesting that there may be shared pathophysiologic mechanisms (16,19,20). Although the pathophysiology of IBS and FM are incompletely understood, several observations suggest that a similar pathophysiologic model integrating neurobiologic, behavioral, and psychological factors is operative in both. These observations will be discussed in more detail below.

FUNCTIONAL GASTROINTESTINAL DISORDERS

Although the pathophysiologic mechanisms underlying FGID are not well understood, the predominant mechanism is thought to be an altered brain-gut axis resulting in alterations of gut mechanoelastic properties, motility, secretion, and visceral hypersensitivity (21). These physiologic abnormalities are seen only in a subset of patients, and, therefore, there is no diagnostic biologic marker to diagnose these disorders. As a result, the diagnoses are made based on symptom criteria, which have in part been evidence based and also are agreed upon by expert opinion. Most recently, the Rome Committee, which is comprised of a group of experts specializing in FGID, have developed symptom-based diagnostic criteria to identify each of the FGIDs (22). There have been various versions over the years. The most recent definitions are known as the Rome II criteria and are included in the following diagnostic sections of each FGID (see Table 18-1).

ATYPICAL CHEST PAIN

Definition

Atypical chest pain is defined as midline pain or discomfort that is *not* burning in quality and is assumed to be of esophageal origin. It is also imperative that gastroesophageal reflux disease (GERD), achalasia, and all other motility disorders with a recognized pathologic basis must be absent. Structural or metabolic conditions, which may explain the chest pain (e.g., cardiac disease), must be excluded.

TABLE 18-1	The Spectrum of Functional Gastrointestinal Disorders[a]

Esophageal Disorders

Globus

Rumination syndrome

Functional chest pain of presumed esophageal origin

Functional heartburn

Functional dysphagia

Unspecified functional esophageal disorder

Gastroduodenal Disorders

Functional dyspepsia

Ulcer-like dyspepsia

Dysmotility-like dyspepsia

Unspecified (nonspecific) dyspepsia

Aerophagia

Functional vomiting

Bowel Disorders

Irritable bowel syndrome

Functional abdominal bloating

Functional constipation

Functional diarrhea

Unspecified functional bowel disorder

Functional Abdominal Pain

Functional abdominal pain syndrome

Unspecified functional abdominal pain

Functional Disorders of the Biliary Tract and Pancreas

Gallbladder dysfunction

Sphincter of Oddi dysfunction

Anorectal Disorders

Functional fecal incontinence

Functional anorectal pain

Levator ani syndrome

Proctalgia fugax

Pelvic floor dyssynergia

Functional Pediatric Disorders[b]

[a]As defined by the Rome II committee.
[b]Not outlined in detail.

Epidemiology

The exact prevalence of this disorder is difficult to assess but the literature suggests that one half to one third of patients with chest pain severe enough to undergo invasive workup have no evidence of coronary artery disease (23,24). Approximately 15% to 30% of patients undergoing cardiac catheterization have normal coronary angiograms, that is, there are about 100,000 new cases of noncardiac chest pain per year (25). This number may actually underestimate the actual number of cases of atypical chest pain because not all individuals with this condition undergo cardiac catheterization. Prior to the Rome II definition of functional chest pain of presumed esophageal origin, Locke et al. (26) compared the prevalence of noncardiac chest pain in male and female community residents using mailed questionnaires. Noncardiac chest pain was defined as "chest pain, any pain, or discomfort felt inside the chest but not including heartburn or any pain that is primarily in the abdomen." The overall prevalence of noncardiac chest pain was 23.1 per 100 (3.9 per 100 for frequent symptoms). No significant gender differences in the prevalence of "noncardiac chest pain" were found. However, there appears to be a female predominance in tertiary care referral populations with functional chest pain of esophageal origin. This condition is a subgroup of those with noncardiac chest pain, which has equal gender prevalence in the general population but a higher female-to-male ratio in tertiary care referral centers (27).

Pathophysiology

At least three mechanisms have been implicated in the etiology of this disorder: (a) stimulation of esophageal mechanoreceptors, (b) stimulation of acid-sensitive receptors, and (c) visceral hypersensitivity (28). Many patients with atypical chest pain seem to experience high-amplitude esophageal contractions with poor peristaltic progression and prolonged duration. These contractions have been observed during esophageal manometry, but the correlation of these high-amplitude contractions to episodes of pain has not been clearly demonstrated (29). Often, patients who have these contractions are asymptomatic at the time they are identified, and pharmacologic intervention during manometry does not correlate with symptom improvement (30). However, psychological stress has been demonstrated to increase the amplitude of esophageal contractions in patients with nutcracker esophagus, a condition where there are multiple high-amplitude contractions, particularly of the distal esophagus (31).

Esophageal exposure to acid also seems to play a role in atypical chest pain. Acid perfusion tests, ambulatory pH, and motility studies have confirmed that acid exposure can induce pain in patients with noncardiac chest pain (32). The mechanism by which acid induces atypical chest pain has not been clearly elucidated. No clear chemoreceptors have been identified for the detection of acid, but it is postulated that intraepithelial free nerve endings may act in this capacity (33).

Visceral hypersensitivity is the concept that seems to play a key role in most FGIDs. When abnormal motility failed to be the primary mechanism to explain the etiology of FGID, research in patients with IBS revealed that they perceived noxious and nonnoxious sensations in response to balloon distention in the rectosigmoid colon at pressures and volumes that were significantly lower than control subjects (34,35). Applying this same concept to patients with atypical chest pain, balloon distention in the esophagus was associated with significantly greater sensitivity to pain compared to healthy controls (36). The mechanisms of visceral hypersensitivity are not completely understood, and many factors (i.e., genetic, motility, inflammatory, psychosocial, and stress) have been proposed to contribute to alterations in enteric and afferent spinal neural function that results in central nervous system (CNS) modulation of this information, which in turn produces long-term sensitization of pathways involved in the transmission of visceral sensation. Evidence for this can be found in a study that shows that repeated esophageal balloon distentions in patients with noncardiac chest pain causes increasing pain perception compared to healthy controls and patients with nonstructural dysphagia (37).

Diagnostic Approach

According to the Rome II diagnostic criteria for functional chest pain of esophageal origin, the pain must be present for at least 12 weeks (need not be consecutive) during the past 12 months (38). The algorithm in Figure 18-1 outlines an approach to the diagnostic workup of atypical chest pain that is comprehensive in evaluating the possible etiologies of this disorder. It is clear that in the evaluation of atypical chest pain, coronary artery disease should be ruled out due to its life-threatening potential. An electrocardiogram and stress test are reasonable screening tools. However, a low threshold for performing cardiac catheterization is indicated, particularly in the case of an equivocal stress test or in an individual with family history of coronary artery disease. If biliary or pancreatic pathology is suspected due to timing of the pain (i.e., several hours postprandially/early morning) or radiation to the right upper quadrant of the abdomen, then proper laboratory evaluation of the blood for liver function tests (LFTs) and for amylase and/or lipase should be performed. Since the overall sensitivity of abdominal sonogram for detecting stone disease is very high, this too may prove useful. From a GI perspective, screening with upper endoscopy or barium swallow should be initiated.

Treatment

It is reasonable to begin empiric treatment with an 8-week course of proton pump inhibitor (PPI) therapy for the possibility of an underlying acid-sensitive disorder, for example,

GERD. More than 75% of patients with noncardiac chest pain, unselected for the presence or absence of ulcer disease, have responded to high dose acid suppression (39). The relief of noncardiac chest pain by PPIs is nearly equal to that of typical reflux symptoms and is not influenced by the presence of nonspecific motility disorders (40).

In patients believed to have an esophageal motility disorder underlying their atypical chest pain, a variety of medications aimed at relieving esophageal spasm have been tested with variable results. These include anticholinergic agents (41,42), nitrates (43,44), hydralazine (45), and calcium channel blockers (46,47). Calcium channel blockers have been the most well studied of these medications, but the results are inconclusive at best. The rationale behind their use was the fact that in normal individuals they are known to decrease esophageal pressures (48). The limitations of these studies include small number of study subjects, the fact that some patients were on smooth muscle relaxants, and that standard manometry was used to evaluate patients. Results may have been different had ambulatory manometry been used to select patients whose chest pain episodes correlated with abnormal motility. More recently, botulinum toxin injection has anecdotally been shown to help patients with esophageal motility disorders with symptoms of chest pain and dysphagia. However, the results are not long lasting (49).

Antidepressant drugs and behavioral therapies have demonstrated the most beneficial effect in patients with noncardiac chest pain. Tricyclic antidepressants (TCAs) have been shown to exert their beneficial effects independent of modifying depression or anxiety. In fact, the doses used to treat noncardiac chest pain are far lower than those used to treat psychiatric symptoms. However, trazadone, in doses of 100 to 150 mg daily, has been shown to improve global symptoms as well as distress ratings (50). The improvement was not correlated to changes in manometric parameters. TCAs appear to modulate visceral pain perception and affect GI motility, as well as help with sleep (51). Proposed mechanisms of action for the TCA in chronic-pain disorders include both central and peripheral actions. Central actions include suppression of the reuptake of amine neurotransmitters affecting ascending CNS arousal systems and central analgesic and mood effects. TCAs have a peripheral inhibitory effect on primary sensory afferent nerves, and, therefore, these medications would relieve GI symptoms in part by reducing visceral sensorimotor afferent information reaching higher centers of the CNS. They also exert a peripheral effect because of their noradrenergic action that increases GI transit time.

Studies evaluating the efficacy of behavioral therapy have usually employed combined relaxation techniques with breathing exercises and education. It has not only been shown to diminish chest pain but also anxiety and depression. In addition, several studies have also shown a sustained benefit (52,53).

FUNCTIONAL DYSPEPSIA

Definition

FD, also referred to as nonulcer dyspepsia (NUD), is a functional bowel disorder characterized by persistent epigastric

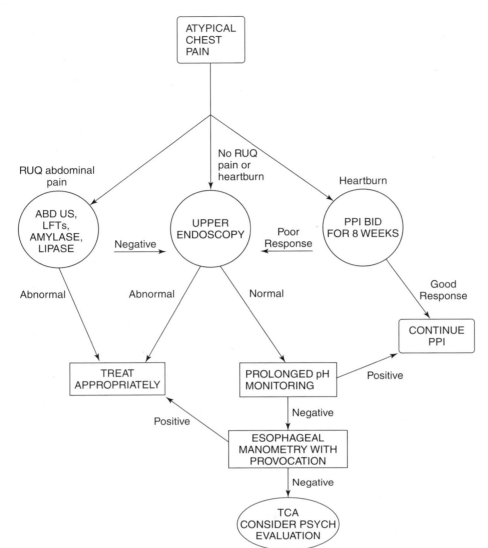

Figure 18-1. Algorithm for diagnosis of atypical chest pain. This algorithm provides a comprehensive approach to the diagnostic workup of atypical chest pain.

ABD US, abdominal ulterasound; LFTs, liver function; PPI, proton pump inhibitor; RUQ, right upper quadrant; TCA, tricyclic antidepressant.

discomfort or pain. FD is often classified into four clinical subgroups: (a) reflux-like with symptoms of heartburn and acid regurgitation; (b) ulcer-like with symptoms of epigastric pain; (c) dysmotility-like with symptoms of nausea, bloating, fullness, and early satiety; and (d) nonspecific—symptoms do not fit either ulcerlike or dysmotilitylike profile. The refluxlike dyspepsia is particularly controversial because it often overlaps with patients who have endoscopy negative esophageal reflux disease (NERD) (54).

Data on the prevalence of this disorder is fairly well established. Several studies have established that if the reflux-like group is eliminated, approximately 25% of the community population annually report epigastric or upper abdominal pain or discomfort (11,26,55,56). There is no clear gender prevalence in FD; however, prevalence may be slightly higher in men than in women overall and lower in the elderly.

Diagnosis

The Rome II diagnostic criteria for FD defines it as a condition with at least 12 weeks of persistent abdominal pain or discomfort, which need not be consecutive, over at least a 1-year period (22). Other features that need to be present are (a) no evidence of organic disease, particularly at upper endoscopy, that explains the symptoms; (b) no evidence that the dyspepsia is relieved by defecation or associated with the onset of change in stool form or frequency to suggest IBS; and (c) absence of predominant heartburn. In addition to abdominal pain, other symptoms, such as bloating, early satiety, belching, and nausea, are often present. To make a definitive diagnosis of FD, it is important to exclude structural causes which may explain GI symptoms, particularly if patients have alarm symptoms suggestive of organic and not functional GI disease, such as onset of symptoms at an age >45 years old, GI bleeding, dysphagia, weight loss, persistent vomiting, and prior or family history of an upper GI malignancy. Although it can be argued to start empiric treatment for dyspepsia prior to embarking on a diagnostic evaluation (see treatment section below), the best initial diagnostic test to perform is an upper endoscopy. Endoscopy should be considered particularly in patients with alarm symptoms. Evidence also exists that patients who undergo an upper endoscopy, particularly those with moderate or high anxiety, have greater satisfaction knowing they have a negative endoscopy, which results in a decreased preoccupation with health and fear of illness and death (57). An upper GI barium study is less sensitive and specific than an upper endoscopy and hence is not generally recommended. Testing for *Helicobacter pylori* is generally recommended because of its association with peptic ulcer disease and GI malignancy (58). Ultrasound of the abdomen, gastric emptying study, electrogastrogram (EGG, which can record electrical activity, that is, gastric rhythm in the stomach), gastroduodenal manometry or sensory testing, 24-hour esophageal pH testing, GI hormone assays, and gastric acid secretion studies are not routinely recommended unless the clinical situation warrants further testing (22). The significance of tests like gastroduodenal manometry and EGG may give objective evidence of neuromuscular dysfunction, but the role of these tests in the evaluation and management of FD requires further study (22).

Higher degrees of neuroticism, hypochondriasis, and conversion hysteria have all been reported in FD patients (59,60). In addition, depression, anxiety, and hypochondriasis have been found more often in patients with FD compared to healthy individuals (61,62). Patients with chronic or severe symptoms may benefit from a psychiatric history and appropriate psychometric testing to rule out depression, anxiety, or other psychological disorders.

Pathophysiology

The designations of the various subgroups of FD do not indicate the underlying pathophysiologic mechanisms. The basis for the current understanding of the pathophysiology of FD lies in understanding the two principal abnormalities that have been described and studied, namely, upper gut dysmotility and visceral sensory dysfunction. To understand these concepts, an understanding of the normal gut physiology is necessary. Primarily, the stomach serves as a reservoir for food as it enters the GI tract. Food entering the proximal stomach causes receptive relaxation and gastric accommodation. This process of relaxation is known to be mediated by the vagus nerve because it disappears in patients who have undergone a vagotomy. The stomach is equipped with a gastric pacemaker system that depolarizes at a rate of 3 cycles per minute. When the waves of depolarization spread out from the pacemaker, they create a circumferential electrical wave that migrates toward the pylorus and is associated with a tonic contraction (63). As measured by volume changes within an intragastric flaccid bag using a computerized distention device called a barostat, tonic contraction occurs at a nearly constant luminal pressure (64). Gastric emptying of solids seems to occur in two phases: (a) an initial lag phase—where food is redistributed from the proximal to the distal stomach, and (b) a nearly linear emptying phase—where food goes from the antrum to the small intestine.

The evidence for motor dysfunction in FD is supported by the following findings: (a) delayed gastric emptying with antral hypomotility, (b) gastric arrythmias, and (c) maldistribution of food within the stomach due to abnormal accommodation. However, these findings are seen in only a subgroup of patients with FD. Delayed gastric emptying can be found in 24% to 78% of patients with FD (65). The presence of gastric arrhythmias in FD has been measured using

an EGG. Electrodes are either placed cutaneously over the upper abdomen or attached directly to the mucosa lining the gastric cavity. Up to two thirds of patients with FD demonstrate gastric dysrhythmias (66,67). Tachygastria (>10 cycles per min) is the most frequent abnormality found. However, it is not a universal finding, and though it may be linked to delayed gastric emptying, it cannot account for symptoms in the majority of individuals with FD. A challenging aspect of FD is the lack of a correlation between antral hypomotility or delayed gastric emptying and symptoms of dyspepsia, which raises the question of the importance of these abnormal motility findings in the pathophysiology of FD symptoms. Lastly, in a subgroup of patients with dysmotilitylike FD, but without delayed gastric emptying, abnormal distribution of food to the distal stomach was found (68). This was thought to represent either a defect in proximal accommodation or increased distal gastric accommodation. Although defective meal-induced reduction in gastric tone has been shown in FD patients, this does not seem to correlate with dyspeptic symptoms in unselected patients (69). In a subgroup of patients with meal-related epigastric symptoms, 40% had impaired gastric accommodation associated with early satiety and a history of weight loss (70). These findings suggest that gastric relaxation is impaired in FD, particularly in patients with meal-related symptoms. Studies have shown that reflex relaxation of the stomach was reduced in response to food in the stomach and duodenal distention, but gastric and duodenal sensitivity was normal (71).

A subgroup of patients with FD has visceral hypersensitivity. A variety of studies have utilized balloon distention in the proximal stomach to assess visceral hypersensitivity as a marker for FD. They have shown heightened sensitivity to graded inflation of an intragastric balloon as a factor in pathogenesis (72,73). Approximately 34% to 65% of FD patients demonstrate gastric hypersensitivity to balloon distention (73–75). Furthermore, gastric hypersensitivity has also been demonstrated in individuals with FD who have not sought health care (76). Gastric hypersensitivity has correlated with specific symptoms of weight loss, belching, and pain. However, it does not appear to correlate with delayed gastric emptying or abnormal gastric tone or compliance. The fact that a significant proportion of patients have no sensitivity to distention indicates that other factors may be active in symptom production.

It is likely that visceral hypersensitivity in FD is due to improper processing of nociceptive information (74). Spinal afferent neurons transmit visceral afferent noxious information (77) that is relayed to brain regions including the anterior cingulate cortex (ACC) (limbic area) and the secondary somatosensory cortex (78,79). Descending pathways from the cortical and brainstem nuclei project to the level of the dorsal horn neurons within the spinal cord to modulate afferent sensory input. While peripheral mechanisms contribute to visceral hypersensitivity, alterations in central pain processing mechanisms play an important role in modulating incoming visceral sensory information. Functional neuroimaging studies using positron emission tomography (PET) in healthy individuals demonstrated that increases in gastric distention and symptoms were associated with progressive increases in activation of the thalamic nuclei, insula, ACC, caudate nuclei, periaqueductal gray in the brainstem, cerebellum, and occipital cortex (80). There are no published studies assessing alterations in cerebral blood flow in patients with FD to evaluate potential supraspinal processes, which may play a role in FD. While FD patients have visceral hypersensitivity, they have normal somatic perception in most studies (71,81,82), suggesting that altered pain processing in FD is mainly related to visceral events.

The role of *H. pylori*, the bacteria implicated in causing peptic ulcer disease and chronic gastritis, in dyspepsia not related to mucosal lesions has been much debated (83,84). Studies also dispute the symptomatic benefit of treating this organism in FD (85–87).

Treatment

The treatment of FD can be challenging as there is limited effective therapy. As in any FGID, reassurance and an education is the first line of therapy. In addition, lifestyle modifications, such as smoking cessation, decreasing alcohol, caffeine, and aspirin, or nonsteroidal anti-inflammatory drug use may be helpful. Patients should be urged to try five to six low-fat meals per day, especially if early satiety or postprandial fullness is a bothersome symptom.

Pharmacotherapy has been utilized and found to be efficacious in certain patients. These medications include prokinetics, serotonergic agents, acid suppression medication, pain modulating agents, and antiemetics. In addition, nonpharmacologic therapies such as behavioral treatments can be considered.

Prokinetic agents that have been used in the treatment of FD include cisapride (no longer available in the United States because of safety concerns), domperidone [not Food and Drug Administration (FDA) approved in the United States], and metoclopromide. For some, there is symptomatic benefit in taking these agents. It does not always correlate with delayed gastric emptying. The side effects of metoclopromide, such as sedation, irritability, and extrapyramidal effects, have limited its therapeutic use.

Serotonergic agents like $5HT_1$ receptor agonists (e.g., sumatriptan) and $5HT_3$ receptor antagonists (e.g., alosetron and ondanestron) have been tried with mixed results. Given subcutaneously, sumatriptan increased gastric accommodation and decreased sensitivity to mechanical distention (88). Alosetron had some beneficial effects in FD patients but did not effect gastric compliance or perception in healthy control subjects (89,90). Lastly, the $5HT_4$ agonist, tegaserod, which acts also as a prokinetic agent, was tested in healthy volunteers because of its ability to enhance gastric emptying of solids in humans. Gastric barostat studies in healthy controls demonstrated that the drug did not alter sensitivity to gastric perceptual thresholds, but it did increase gastric compliance. In addition, pre- and postprandial intraballoon volumes were significantly higher after a 6-mg twice daily dose of tegaserod compared to placebo (91). There is a preliminary study that has shown the efficacy of tegaserod in the treatment of FD patients (92). Tegaserod has also been shown to improve gastric emptying in the subgroup of patients with FD and delayed gastric emptying (93).

Acid suppressant therapies have been tried with mixed results in FD. Studies evaluating antacids and H_2 antagonists (e.g., ranitidine, famotidine, cimetitine, and nizatidine) have usually found that these agents are only slightly more effective than placebo (94). A meta-analysis of 22 randomized, placebo-controlled clinical trials evaluating the efficacy of H_2 antagonists in NUD was performed (95). Fourteen of these trials had a parallel design, three were crossover design, and six had multi-crossover design. Fifteen studies found that H_2 antagonists were superior to placebo although the quality of these studies was often suboptimal. Epigastric pain, but not global assessment of symptoms, was significantly relieved by H_2 antagonists. However, many of these studies included GERD patients, which may explain any potential benefit these agents may have had.

Two large trials compared the efficacy of omeprazole and placebo in patients with NUD (96,97). Patients with epigastric pain (ulcerlike) had 40% relief, but those with dysmotilitylike dyspepsia did not respond differently compared to placebo. Two other studies assessed the efficacy of lansoprazole compared to placebo in patients with FD. The first study was conducted in the United States and showed a positive effect with 15 or 30 mg of lansoprazole (98). However, a second study in China showed no difference with 15 and 30 mg doses of lansoprazole compared to placebo (99). Nonetheless, PPIs are often recommended as a first line of therapy in FD.

Patients with FD who are found to have *H. pylori* infection are often treated with a combined antibiotic and acid suppression regimen. Two meta-analyses evaluating the efficacy of *H. pylori* treatment in FD reported conflicting results, but they included different numbers of studies (100,101). The therapeutic gain of *H. pylori* treatment is only 5% to 10% over placebo, but benefit is sustained for at least 12 months (102). The benefits of this treatment may outweigh the risks (103). Currently, it is reasonable to check for *H. pylori* in patients with FD and treat if present. Patients need to be informed that the majority of patients will not have symptom relief, and other treatments may need to be considered (102).

Other agents have been tried in a relatively small number of FD patients. There is limited data with antidepressants, but low-dose TCA may be beneficial (104). Other medications that relax the gastric fundus may be of some benefit, but more studies are needed to determine their value in treating FD. These medications include buspirone ($5HT_{1A}$ agonist), sumatriptan ($5HT_1$ agonist), tegaserod ($5HT_4$ agonist), citalopram (selective serotonin reuptake inhibitor, SSRI), fluoxetine (SSRI), and clonidine ($\alpha 2$ adrenergic agonist) (105,106).

Nonpharmacologic treatments such as psychological treatments (e.g., hypnosis) and cognitive-behavioral therapy (CBT) have been evaluated in FD. A recent published review attempted to determine the effectiveness of psychological interventions including psychotherapy, psychodrama, CBT, relaxation therapy, and hypnosis in the improvement of either individual or global dyspepsia symptom scores and quality of life scores of patients with NUD (107). The investigators concluded that there was currently insufficient evidence to confirm the efficacy of psychological intervention in NUD. There was also no evidence on the combined effects of pharmacologic and psychological therapy. Nevertheless, if there were any benefits of psychological therapies, they were likely to persist long term. Psychological therapies may therefore be offered to patients with severe symptoms, particularly those who have not responded to pharmacologic therapies.

Other alternative treatment options, which have not been well studied in FD, are worth mentioning. Red chili pepper may be effective in the treatment of FD (108), and the effect of peppermint oil in FD is similar to that of the prokinetic agent cisapride (109). A multicenter, randomized trial assessed the efficacy and safety of an herbal preparation, STW 5-II, containing extracts from bitter candy tuft, matricaria flower, peppermint leaves, caraway, licorice root, and lemon balm for the treatment of patients with FD. GI symptom scores significantly decreased in subjects on active treatment compared to the placebo. After 8 weeks, 43.3% on active treatment and 3.3% on placebo reported complete relief of symptoms. Agents used in the treatment of nausea, such as ondansetron, perchlorperazine, and promethazine, and antihistamines used in the treatment of motion sickness, such as dimenhydrinate and cyclizine, may be helpful when nausea is a dominant symptom. Complementary alternative treatments such as acupuncture and acupressure had been shown to decrease nausea and vomiting in chemotherapy patients but have not been studied in patients with FD. However, the positive effects of this treatment may generalize to the treatment of FD (110) and could be considered in interested patients, but well-designed trials are needed.

IRRITABLE BOWEL SYNDROME

Definition

IBS is one of the most common FGIDs characterized by chronic or recurrent abdominal pain and/or discomfort associated with altered bowel habits not explained by biochemical or structural abnormalities. IBS has worldwide prevalence rates of 9% to 23% in the general population (21) and accounts for 12% of diagnoses made by primary care physicians and 36% of diagnoses made by gastroenterologists (111).

This condition appears to have a female predominance of 2 to 4:1 depending on whether studies were conducted in a community or tertiary setting (112). It is well established that a greater number of women seek health care services for symptoms of IBS than men. Reports of nausea, bloating, constipation, and extraintestinal symptoms seem more prevalent in women with IBS than in men. Furthermore, recent clinical trials suggest that gender differences in response to pharmacologic treatments also occur (113–116). Numerous factors need to be considered in the exploration of these differences. These factors include biologic, hormonal, behavioral, psychological, and sociocultural differences between men and women (112). Several studies indicate that the menstrual cycle influences GI symptoms, which are reportedly increased immediately before and during menses. In addition, brain-imaging studies have reported gender differences in the central processing of aversive information originating from pelvic viscera in IBS (117). Further studies are needed to provide additional insight into gender differences in the epidemiology, pathophysiology, symptom expression, and response to treatment in IBS.

IBS patients may present with diarrhea and/or constipation and therefore are often subgrouped by predominant bowel habit. These subgroups are referred to as diarrhea-predominant IBS (IBS-D: IBS associated with abdominal pain, fecal urgency, and diarrhea), constipation-predominant IBS (IBS-C: IBS associated with abdominal discomfort, bloating, and constipation), and IBS associated with alternating diarrhea and constipation (IBS-A).

Diagnosis

A thorough medical history and physical examination are essential to make a proper diagnosis of IBS. The differential diagnoses of IBS are shown in Table 18-2. These other conditions, which should be considered in patients who present with IBS symptoms, may be based on the predominant bowel habit (e.g., diarrhea and/or constipation). The diagnosis of IBS is based on the Rome II symptom criteria for IBS (see Table 18-3) (22). These criteria require that the abdominal pain or discomfort should be present for at least 12 weeks (not necessarily consecutive) over a 12-month period and be associated with at least two of the following features: (a) relief with defecation, (b) a change in stool consistency (e.g., watery/loose or lumpy/hard), and/or (c) a change in stool frequency (i.e., <3 stools per week or >3 stools per day). Supportive symptoms for the diagnosis of IBS include the following features at least 25% of the time: (a) abnormal stool form, (b) passage of mucus, (c) bloating or distention, (d) abnormal stool passage (feeling of strain, urgency, or feeling of incomplete evacuation), and/or (e) altered stool frequency [>3 bowel movements (BMs) or <3 BMs per day]. The approach to diagnosing IBS is to identify the dominant symptom complex and then eliminate "red flag" signs and symptoms that may indicate an organic disorder and not IBS. Table 18-4 outlines these "alarm signs," which need to be assessed in the evaluation of a patient with symptoms suggestive of IBS. When "alarm signs" such as weight loss, fever, anemia, GI bleeding, family history of colon cancer or onset of disease late in life are excluded, the Rome criteria reach a sensitivity of 65%, specificity of 100%, and a positive predictive value of 100%. In a recent study, 93% of patients diagnosed, based on Rome II criteria and the absence of red flags, were found to be true positive cases after 2 years (118). Hence, if the diagnosis of IBS is made properly, the risk of missing organic disease is low, and most patients have no change in diagnosis after initial evaluation (119–121). Recent guidelines by the American Gastroenterological Association (AGA) have advocated the following diagnostic tests be considered: (a) complete blood count (CBC), (b) thyroid stimulating hormone (TSH), (c) complete metabolic profile, (d) erythrocyte sedimentation rate (ESR) or C-reactive protein, (e) stool for ova and parasites (O and P), (f) fecal occult blood testing, (g) stool culture examination, and (h) celiac sprue panel (21). Other diagnostic tests including barium enema, flexible sigmoidoscopy, or colonoscopy, as well as hydrogen breath tests for bacterial overgrowth, can be considered on an individualized basis. However, it is important that in the medical evaluation of patients with IBS symptoms practitioners take an evidence-based medicine approach. The decision to perform many of the tests mentioned above must be made with a certain amount of discrimination. Evidence from studies of reasonably good quality has suggested that the diagnostic yield is not very high, particularly in the absence of alarm signs. In fact, for many, the yield of the tests is <2% (122). The presence of "red flag" symptoms would suggest a

TABLE 18-2	Differential Diagnosis of Irritable Bowel Syndrome Based on Predominant Symptom[a]

SYMPTOM	DIFFERENTIAL DIAGNOSES
Diarrhea	
Malabsorption	• Intestinal disorders
	• Pancreatic insufficiency
	• Postgastrectomy
Infection	• Bacteria
	• Parasites (e.g., *Giardia*)[b]
	• HIV-associated infections
Inflammatory bowel conditions	• Ulcerative colitis
	• Crohn disease[c]
	• Microscopic or collagenous colitis
Endocrinologic disorders	• Diabetes mellitus
	• Hyperthyroidism
Diet	• Lactose or fructose intolerance
	• Alcohol
	• Caffeine
	• Sorbitol
	• Wheat (in patients with celiac disease)
Malignancy	• Colon cancer
	• Endocrine neoplasm
Medications	• SSRIs
	• NSAIDs
	• Antibiotics
	• Chemotherapy
Constipation	
Neurologic	• Multiple sclerosis
	• Parkinson disease
	• Spinal cord lesion
Endocrinologic disorders	• Hypothyroidism
	• Hypercalcemia
Malignancy	• Colon cancer
Medications	• Calcium channel blockers
	• Opiates or other analgesics
	• Chemotherapy
	• TCAs
Abdominal Pain	
Gynecologic	• Endometriosis
	• Ovarian cancer
	• Dysmenorrhea
Psychiatric	• Somatization
	• Depression
	• Anxiety

[a]Not an all inclusive list.
[b]*Giardia* may cause symptoms of alternating constipation and diarrhea.
[c]Crohn disease can sometime cause obstructive symptoms of constipation, pain, and bloating.

SSRIs, Serotonin substance reuptake inhibitors; NSAIDs, Nonsteroidal anti-inflammatory drugs; TCAs, tricyclic antidepressants.

TABLE 18-3	Rome II Criteria for Irritable Bowel Syndrome

At least 12 weeks or more, which need not be consecutive, in the preceding 12 months of abdominal discomfort or pain that has two out of three features:

1. Relieved with defecation; *and/or*
2. Onset associated with a change in frequency of stool; *and/or*
3. Onset associated with a change in form (appearance) of stool.

From Drossman DA, Corazziari E, Talley NJ, et al. *ROME II. The functional gastrointestinal disorders. Diagnosis, pathophysiology and treatment: a multinational consensus*, 2nd ed. McLean, VA: Degnon Associates, 2000, with permission.

TABLE 18-4	Alarm Symptoms and Signs in Irritable Bowel Syndrome Patients Requiring Further Investigation

Medical History
Age of onset ≥50 y/o
Weight loss of ≥10 lb
Nocturnal or refractory diarrhea
Significant travel history suggestive of GI infection
Severe constipation or diarrhea
Rectal bleeding
Rashes/arthritis

Family History
Celiac disease
Colon cancer/polyps
Inflammatory bowel disease

Physical Examination
Oral ulcers
Fever
Guaiac positive stool
Abdominal or rectal mass
Rectal bleeding
Rash

Laboratory Data
Increased white blood cell count
Anemia
Elevated ESR or C-reactive protein
Abnormal blood chemistries

GI, gastrointestinal; ESR, erythrocyte sedimentation rate.

higher pretest probability of the presence of an organic disorder. Performing colonoscopy has resulted in identifying organic disease in only 1% to 2% of cases in patients with IBS-like symptoms (122). However, it has been recommended by the American College of Gastroenterology (ACG) that patients ≥50 years of age should undergo a routine colon examination (e.g., colonoscopy or barium enema with a flexible sigmoidoscopy) for screening purposes similar to the general healthy population (123). The threshold is lowered to 40 years of age if there is a significant family history of colon cancer.

Two medical conditions that have a relatively high pretest probability in IBS patients are lactose intolerance and celiac sprue. In the case of lactose intolerance, the prevalence is approximately 22% to 26% and is similar to that of the general population, which is 25% (122). In fact, documentation of lactase deficiency seldom leads to improvement in IBS symptoms (124). Furthermore, up to one third of patients with reported lactose intolerance actually absorb lactose normally (125), and some people with lactose malabsorption may consume moderate quantities of lactose without symptoms (e.g., 12.5 g per day) (126).

The prevalence of celiac sprue in patients with IBS-like symptoms ranges from 0% to 11.4% (127–131). A study done in the United Kingdom demonstrated a sevenfold increase in occurrence of celiac disease in patients suspected of having IBS seen in a gastroenterology practice (127). In general, the studies reporting a relatively higher prevalence of celiac sprue were performed in a GI specialty setting (127,131), while the other studies with the lower prevalence rates evaluated primary care patients (128–130) who probably had less severe GI symptoms. Cash et al. (122) found that the pretest probability for the presence of celiac disease in patients with IBS symptoms was significantly higher than that found in the general population (4.67% vs. 0.25% to 0.5%). Therefore, screening with celiac sprue-associated antibodies (e.g., antiendomysial antibody and anti-tissue transglutaminase) may be indicated. Additionally, 5% to 7% of patients with celiac disease are IgA deficient and, therefore, the clinician may want to also measure IgA levels. A recent study by Speigel et al. used decision analysis to determine if initial testing for celiac sprue might be a cost-effective diagnostic strategy in IBS compared to empiric IBS treatment (132). Under base-case conditions, testing for celiac sprue instead of starting empiric IBS therapy cost an incremental $11,000 to achieve one additional symptomatic improvement. Testing for celiac sprue in patients with IBS has an acceptable cost when the prevalence of celiac sprue is above 1% and was the dominant strategy when the prevalence exceeded 8%. The decision to test should be based upon a consideration of the population prevalence of underlying celiac sprue, the operating characteristics of the screening test employed, and the cost of proposed therapy for IBS (132).

Another condition to consider excluding in a patient with IBS symptoms is bacterial overgrowth. Two studies from the same research group found that 78% to 84% of patients with IBS had bacterial overgrowth (133,134). Those patients with bacterial overgrowth that were treated with neomycin had a ≥35% reduction (i.e., improvement in symptoms) compared with an 11% reduction in patients on placebo (134). However, these studies had methodologic limitations that prohibit routine hydrogen breath testing for bacterial overgrowth from being generally advocated. These investigators also recently found abnormal lactulose breath tests for bacterial overgrowth in all 42 patients with FM, suggesting similar underlying mechanisms in IBS and FM. However, the effect on GI symptoms was not evaluated and the significance of this finding is not clear (135).

Pathophysiology

Similar to the other FGIDs, the pathophysiology of IBS is not completely understood but is considered to be a biopsychosocial disorder. The key pathophysiologic mechanism underlying IBS is currently believed to be an altered brain-gut axis (21,136). Altered brain-gut interactions are associated with abnormal gut motility, visceral hypersensitivity, and altered neuroimmune responses. Stress is widely believed to play a major role in the pathophysiology and clinical presentation of IBS and may induce these altered physiologic responses via its effects on brain-gut interactions. In predisposed individuals, which may be due to genetic factors (137–139), they may experience permanent enhanced stress responsiveness of the central stress circuits under sustained stress and thereby increase their vulnerability to developing functional and affective disorders (140). Stress may be central (e.g., psychological distress) or peripheral (e.g., infection, surgery) in origin. Studies have indicated that patients with IBS report more lifetime and daily stressful events, including IBS, compared with patients with organic GI conditions or healthy individuals (21). Stress in IBS patients is also strongly associated with symptom onset, exacerbation, and severity. Despite the fact that the effects of stress on gut function are universal, patients with IBS appear to have a greater reactivity to stress compared with healthy individuals (141).

Gastrointestinal Motility

The concept of stress-induced alterations in GI motility dates back to the work of Thomas Almy (142), who demonstrated that gut motility was increased in both normal individuals and patients with IBS who were presented with a psychologically stressful situation. Subsequent research demonstrated that patients with IBS had increased motility related to meals, particularly after meals, compared with control subjects (143,144). Studies have also demonstrated that a variety of GI motility abnormalities, such as prolonged propagating contractions and high-amplitude propagating contractions, are more commonly seen in patients with IBS compared with healthy individuals (145–148). However, there does not seem to be a consistent motility abnormality to explain symptoms in all IBS patients, and, therefore, it cannot currently be used as a diagnostic marker for IBS. Nonetheless, in general, patients with IBS-D have more rapid GI transit times while patients with IBS-C have normal to slower GI transit. GI transit or motility has not been well studied in IBS patients with alternating bowel habits.

Visceral Hypersensitivity

The concept of visceral hypersensitivity evolved from the clinical findings of recurring abdominal pain, tenderness during palpation of the sigmoid colon on physical examination, and excessive pain during endoscopic evaluation of the sigmoid colon. Experimental evidence confirmed that a variety of perceptual alterations exist in patients with IBS. Patients with IBS have increased sensitivity to balloon distention in both the upper and lower GI tract as well as heightened perception of physiologic intestinal contractions compared to normal individuals (35,149–152). In contrast, most studies have demonstrated that IBS patients do not exhibit generalized hypersensitivity to noxious somatic stimulation (35,153,154). However, there was a recent study that found that patients with IBS had rectal hypersensitivity as well as somatic hypersensitivity to thermal stimuli applied to the foot and to a lesser extent to the hand (155). At least two mechanisms are thought to contribute to visceral hypersensitivity in IBS: a hypervigilance towards expected aversive events arising from the viscera and a hyperalgesia that is inducible by sustained noxious visceral stimulation (151,156).

Modulation of Central Nervous System Networks

In recent years, an appreciation for CNS modulation of the brain-gut axis has occurred, particularly with the growing number of functional neuroimaging studies. It is known that signals from the brain to the gut are important in ensuring optimal digestive function, reflex regulation of the GI tract, and modulation of mood states. Recent applications of functional brain-imaging techniques of Position Emission Tomography and functional magnetic resonance imaging (fMRI) have begun to more directly address the role of specific central networks in normal and altered processing of visceral-related input (79,157,158). In healthy subjects, the brain regions most consistently activated are the mid/anterior insula, subregions of the ACC, prefrontal cortex (PFC), thalamus, and, in some cases, pontine regions such as the dorsal pons and periaqueductal gray. These brain areas are consistently activated in response to visceral as well as somatic nociceptive stimuli (159).

There is growing evidence for altered visceral sensory, affective, and motor responses found in IBS to be associated with detectable differences in regional cerebral blood flow using functional brain imaging. Using distal colonic balloon distention, several studies have demonstrated alterations in regional brain activation in patients with IBS compared with healthy control subjects (157,158). The dorsal subregion of the ACC is an area that is consistently activated to a greater degree in patients with IBS compared to controls (157–159). This region is concerned with cognitive processing of sensory input, including attentional processes and response selection. Furthermore, dorsal ACC activation correlates with the subjective unpleasantness of visceral (160) as well as somatic pain (161). There is evolving evidence to suggest that IBS patients have altered activation of brain regions concerned with attentional processes and response selection (ACC and anterior midcingulate cortex) of cortical regions concerned with emotional and autonomic responses to stimuli (ventromedial PFC, perigenual ACC, and infragenual cingulate cortex), and of subcortical regions receiving cortical projections from the latter as well as afferent input from the viscera (hypothalamus, amygdala, dorsal pons) in response to *actual* or *anticipated but undelivered* colorectal distention. Some of these findings are consistent with exaggerated threat appraisal, enhanced anxiety responses, and hypervigilance toward GI sensations in IBS patients (158,159). These observations suggest that patients with IBS may fail to use CNS downregulating mechanisms in response to incoming or anticipated visceral pain. Furthermore, they show altered activation or deactivation of brain areas involved in the emotional or cognitive processing of visceral stimuli, ultimately resulting in the amplification of pain perception.

Supporting the significant influence of central factors on IBS symptomatology, it has been recently demonstrated that alterations in brain activation patterns are affected by treatment. It has recently been shown that in IBS patients who are treated with the 5HT$_3$ antagonist alosetron, which is an FDA-approved medication for women with IBS-D (162), there are decreases in regional cerebral blood flow in brain regions (including the ventromedial PFC, infragenual cingulate cortex, and amygdala) that are associated with improvement in IBS symptoms and emotional ratings (163,164). There is also a case report of a woman with severe IBS with psychological distress who had resolution of activations in the region of the anterior midcingulate cortex/dorsal ACC and primary somatosensory cortex measured by fMRI following termination of an abusive relationship, resolution of IBS symptoms, and normalization of psychological symptom scores (165). These findings support the clinically significant contribution of centrally mediated modulation of visceral pain in IBS.

Psychosocial Factors

As illustrated in the previous case study, many patients with IBS or other FGID may have concurrent psychological disturbances, particularly those with severe symptoms or those seen in tertiary care referral centers. A number of psychosocial factors have been recognized to modify the illness experience and influence health care utilization and treatment outcomes. These factors include a history of emotional, sexual, or physical abuse; stressful life events; chronic social stress; anxiety disorders; or maladaptive coping styles (21). A current conceptual model regarding the role of psychosocial factors and stress in IBS suggests that adverse life experiences (past and present) influence stress responsiveness, physiologic responses, and susceptibility to developing and exacerbating symptoms via amplification of brain-gut interactions. Given the importance of characterizing psychosocial factors in IBS, since they have the potential to modify the illness experience and influence patterns of pain reporting and health care utilization, a psychosocial interview may unveil associated symptoms and concerns that the patient may not have expressed previously and which may be contributing to the severity of the illness and its outcome (166).

Immune and Inflammatory Mediators

The strong influence of psychological distress on GI function is further illustrated by a more recent development in the understanding of the pathophysiology of IBS, which is the role of mucosal immune or inflammatory mediators. The impetus of this has been the observation that 7% to 30% of patients with recent history of proven bacterial gastroenteritis go on to develop IBS-like symptoms, that is, "postinfectious IBS" (PI-IBS) (167). It has been noted that a subset of patients with IBS can trace the development of their symptoms to an episode of infectious diarrhea, primarily bacterial or amebic, and possibly even viral (168–170). Risk factors for PI-IBS include duration of acute diarrheal illness, female sex, and the presence of significant life stressors occurring around the time of the infection (167). An additional observation has been that there are mucosal abnormalities in the colon of patients with PI-IBS. Rectal mucosal cellularity and intestinal permeability were compared in patients at 2, 6, and 12 weeks and 1 year after an acute infection with *Campylobacter* enteritis and a history of PI-IBS and normal controls (171). Patients with previous *Campylobacter* infection and PI-IBS were found to have an increased number of intraepithelial lymphocytes and enterochromaffin (EC) cells and increased intestinal permeability, even after 1 year compared to control. Further studies evaluated the secretory granules of the EC cells and found that patients with PI-IBS had granules containing mainly serotonin. EC cells in healthy control subjects had granules containing primarily PYY, a peptide associated with antisecretory effects. It is conceivable that these findings play a role in the GI symptoms that are seen in a subset of patients with IBS. A subsequent study by these investigators was performed to prospectively determine the relative importance of both psychological and histologic factors in the development of PI-IBS after *Campylobacter* infection (172). PI-IBS, predominantly of the diarrhea-predominant subtype, occurred in 103 of 747 (13.8%) of those infected. EC cell counts were higher in patients with PI-IBS compared with patient controls and healthy volunteers. Lamina propria T lymphocytes were significantly higher in patients with PI-IBS and patient controls in contrast to healthy volunteers. Anxiety, depression, and fatigue were significantly increased in patients with PI-IBS compared with patient controls. Increased EC cell counts and depression were equally important independent predictors of developing PI-IBS. There is another study which found that patients with PI-IBS have greater mRNA expression of the inflammatory mediator, interleukin-1β (IL-1β), both during and after the infection, compared with individuals who do not develop PI-IBS (173). There is also increasing evidence of increased mucosal immune markers in unselected IBS patients. Increased intraepithelial lymphocytes, T cells (174), and mast cells (175) have been noted. Approximately 40% of patients with IBS diagnosed by Rome criteria were found to have evidence of nonspecific microscopic colitis on colonic tissue biopsies (174).

Role of Serotonin in Gastrointestinal Function and Irritable Bowel Syndrome

The regulation of peristalsis and secretion within the gut is primarily under the control of the enteric nervous system (ENS), although gut function is also significantly influenced by extrinsic neural input from the parasympathetic and sympathetic nervous systems. Many neuropeptides are involved in the regulation of motility, sensation, and secretion. A key mediator of both of these functions is serotonin (176,177), 95% of which is in the gut. Ninety percent of serotonin in the gut is localized within the EC cells and 10% in the enteric neurons. The excitatory receptors 5HT$_{1P}$, 5HT$_3$, and 5HT$_4$ have been found to be particularly important in modulating gut activity (178). When the gut mucosa is stimulated, either mechanically or by chemical stimulation, serotonin is released from the EC cells (see Figure 18-2). Serotonin then acts on the 5HT$_{1P}$ receptor located on the terminals of the intrinsic primary afferent neurons (IPANs) within the submucosal plexus. 5HT$_4$ receptors are located on the presynaptic terminals of these afferent nerves and, when activated, facilitate the release of calcitonin gene-related peptide (CGRP)

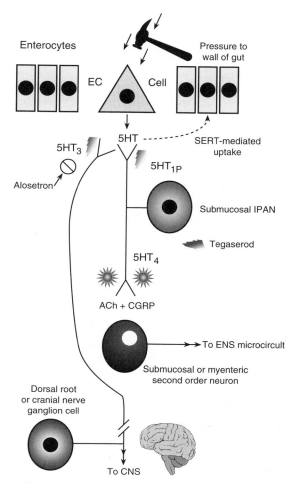

Figure 18-2. Peristaltic reflex and site of drug action. When the gut is stimulated, either mechanically or by chemical stimulation, serotonin (5HT) is released from the enterochromaffin (EC) cells. Serotonin then acts on the 5HT$_{1P}$ receptor located on the terminals of the intrinsic primary afferent neurons (IPANs) within the submucosal plexus. 5HT$_4$ receptors are located on the presynaptic terminals of theses afferent nerves and, when activated, facilitate the release of calcitonin-gene-related-peptide (CGRP) and acetylcholine (ACh). Activation of these interneurons within the enteric nervous system (ENS) results in the release of other neuropeptides that lead to the contractual response of the mucosa, that is, the peristaltic reflex. A 5HT$_4$ *receptor agonist*, such as tegaserod, thus promotes peristaltic activity by enhancing the release of transmitters in the reflex pathway and is thus used for constipation-type IBS. 5HT$_3$ *receptor antagonists*, such as alosetron and cilansetron, act on 5HT$_3$ receptors, located on enteric neurons within the myenteric plexus as well as on vagal and spinal afferents, to modulate painful stimuli and slow intestinal reflexes and are used to treat severe IBS-D. Serotonin reuptake transporter (SERT) is one of the primary mechanisms for determining availability of serotonin in the extracellular space. CNS, central nervous system. (From Gershon MD. Serotonin and its implication for the management of irritable bowel syndrome. Rev Gastroenterol Disord 2003;3:S25–S34, with permission.)

and acetylcholine. After these interneurons are activated within the ENS, acetylcholine and substance P are released from enteric neurons proximally (orad), which leads to a contractual response in the mucosa. Release of vasoactive intestinal peptide and nitric oxide distally (caudad) result in relaxation of the gut. These actions subsequently result in the peristaltic activity of the intestine (178,179). 5HT$_3$ receptors are located on enteric neurons within the myenteric plexus as well as on vagal and spinal afferents. These receptors are thought to play a role in other intestinal reflexes and modulation of painful and nonpainful (e.g., nausea) sensation, respectively.

Mechanisms exist to regulate how much serotonin is available in the tissue. One of the primary mechanisms that the body has for determining availability of serotonin in the extracellular space is the serotonin reuptake transporter (SERT). SERT is present in both the brain and the gut. The amount of serotonin reuptake that occurs from the extracellular space is genetically determined and is based on the presence of long, short, or heterozygous polymorphisms in the promoter for synthesis of SERT. Presence of the homozygous short variant and presence of the heterozygous variant result in less transcript, less protein expression, and thus less reuptake of serotonin (178). SERT activity is important in influencing serotonin availability to act on serotonin receptors and may influence response to other serotonergic medications such as SSRIs, which are used in the treatment of depression, as well as the novel newer agents for IBS, such as tegaserod and alosetron.

The role of serotonin-related mechanisms in IBS is demonstrated by several studies. The putative role of serotonin in IBS has been supported by higher postprandial serum levels of serotonin in patients with IBS-D compared to healthy controls (180,181). There is also evidence of an increased number of EC cells that contain serotonin in the gut mucosa of patients with PI-IBS (172) and of a decreased number in patients with chronic constipation (182).

In an attempt to determine whether enteric serotonin (5HT) signaling is defective in IBS, mucosal 5HT, tryptophan hydroxylase 1 messenger RNA, serotonin transporter messenger RNA, and serotonin transporter immunoreactivity were measured in patients with IBS, patients with ulcerative colitis (UC), and healthy controls (183). These outcome measures were all significantly reduced in UC, IBS-C, and IBS-D. When 5HT release was investigated under basal and mechanical stimulation conditions, no changes were detected in any of the groups relative to controls. The investigators concluded that IBS and UC are associated with similar molecular changes in serotonergic signaling mechanisms, and that while UC and IBS have distinct pathophysiologic properties, these data suggest that shared defects in 5HT signaling may underlie the altered motility, secretion, and sensation. Although this study is intriguing and demonstrates for the first time significant molecular alterations specific to the gut in patients with IBS, further investigation is needed to more completely understand serotonergic mechanisms in IBS. There is also evidence suggesting that SERT polymorphisms in patients may influence a patient's response to treatment, that is, the 5HT$_3$ antagonist alosetron. A small study of 30 patients (15 women) with IBS-D was conducted in which alosetron at a dose of 1 mg orally twice daily for 6 weeks was given and intestinal transit was measured (184). Only 23 of the subjects (12 women) submitted blood samples for analysis; 8 long homozygote, 4 short homozygote, and 11 heterozygote SERT polymorphisms were identified. When colonic transit was measured, patients with a long homozygous polymorphism (associated with more serotonin reuptake, that is, less serotonin was around to

stimulate the gut and cause peristalsis) had greater slowing of intestinal transit with alosetron than heterozygotes. The importance of SERT and its effect on colonic transit response to alosetron, on its clinical efficacy as well as its relation to adverse events associated with the drug, such as constipation and ischemic colitis (which are potential adverse effects of 5HT$_3$ antagonists), needs to be evaluated.

Genetic Factors

Evidence of heredity in IBS is supported by several studies. There is an increased frequency of IBS in adults with an affected first-degree relative (137,185), which suggests that familial aggregation of IBS occurs, supporting a genetic or intrafamilial environment component, but this may be explained in part by familial aggregation of somatization (185). Levy et al. tried to assess the relative contribution of genetic and environmental (social learning) influences on the development of IBS by comparing concordance rates in monozygotic and dizygotic twins to concordance between mothers and their children (138). Questionnaires soliciting information on the occurrence of more than 80 health problems, including IBS, in self and other family members were sent to both members of 11,986 twin pairs. Concordance for IBS was significantly greater in monozygotic (17.2%) than in dizygotic (8.4%) twins, supporting a genetic contribution to IBS. However, the proportion of dizygotic twins with IBS who have mothers with IBS (15.2%) was significantly greater than the proportion of dizygotic twins with IBS who have co-twins with IBS (6.7%). In addition, having a mother with IBS and a father with IBS were independent predictors of IBS status; both were stronger predictors than having a twin with IBS. This study lends further support that heredity contributes to development of IBS, but social learning (what an individual learns from those in his or her environment) has an equal or greater influence.

Treatment of Irritable Bowel Syndrome

Once the diagnosis of IBS has been made, treatment begins with the establishment of a good physician-patient relationship. Addressing the patients' health concerns about their symptoms and providing reassurance and education about IBS are important (21). While patients need to be informed that this disorder may be associated with increased morbidity (i.e., impact on health-related quality of life), it is not associated with increased mortality and does not lead to more serious disorders like cancer or inflammatory bowel disease.

A dietary history and a 2-week symptom diary may help determine if significant correlations exist between diet, daily activities, emotional factors, and the symptoms of IBS. Certain intolerances to lactose, fructose, and sorbitol may play a role in symptoms, and decreases in these dietary substances may help with diarrhea and bloating. Similarly, patients with constipation may benefit from an increase to 20 to 25 g of fiber per day. Exercise, adequate sleep, and stress reduction may also help to modulate symptoms of IBS.

Traditional Irritable Bowel Syndrome Treatment

Pharmacologic therapy has traditionally been aimed at treating the dominant symptom of diarrhea, constipation, or abdominal pain and bloating. Table 18-5 summarizes the various therapies available for treating the symptoms of IBS. Several excellent systematic reviews evaluating controlled treatment trials for IBS have been performed (186–188). The ACG evaluated many of the available treatments in terms of the evidence available to support their use and their ability to alleviate the symptoms of IBS (188). Therapies were given a grade of A, B, or C depending on the level of evidence available to support their use. Four levels of evidence were identified: (a) level I data was based on high-quality, randomized, placebo-controlled studies (grade A); (b) level II data was based on intermediate quality randomized, controlled trials (grade B); (c) level III data was based on nonrandomized studies (grade C); and (d) level IV data was based on case controls or anecdotal experience (grade C). The therapies based on the highest quality of data were given a grade A recommendation. Unfortunately, the majority of therapies studied, including antispasmodic agents, bulking agents and fiber supplementation, antidiarrheal agents such as loperamide, TCA, and behavioral therapy, were not shown to be more effective than placebo in treating the global symptoms of IBS and therefore were given a grade B recommendation. However, most of these treatment options may relieve individual symptoms of IBS and, therefore, they may be useful in select patients depending on their predominant symptom. Antispasmodic agents are commonly prescribed to treat abdominal pain (187) but may cause side effects such as dry mouth, blurred vision, and urinary retention. Fiber supplementation may help relieve constipation by improving ease of stool passage and stool form but can cause bloating and abdominal cramps. Although antidiarrheal agents may not improve abdominal pain, they help decrease stool frequency and improve stool consistency. Dosing should be adjusted to avoid constipation. TCAs are prescribed for the treatment of chronic-pain disorders. These agents have been shown to be effective when used at low doses for the treatment of abdominal pain via their visceral analgesic effects in patients with FGID. Higher doses are used when treating comorbid affective symptoms, such as depression and anxiety. The efficacy of these agents in IBS are discussed in detail below.

Novel Serotonergic Agents

The discovery of serotonergic molecular targets has led to the development of novel medications and review of older pharmacologic agents that also act on the serotonin system. The goal now is to have therapies that are effective in relieving the global symptoms of IBS, that is, the abdominal pain, bloating, and change in bowel habits. Thus far, two drugs have been given grade A recommendations because they were studied in high-quality, multicenter clinical trials. Each of these therapies targets different serotonergic receptors and therefore different aspects of bowel function.

5HT₃ Receptor Antagonists

The first clinically available 5HT$_3$ antagonists were ondansetron and granisetron, which were approved for the treatment of chemotherapy- and radiotherapy-induced nausea and vomiting. Alosetron is the only medication currently approved in the United States for the treatment of female patients with severe IBS-D. To date there have been 4 clinical trials in almost 2,500 patients comparing the drug

to placebo (113,189–191) and one trial comparing alosetron to a smooth muscle relaxant, mebeverine (192). All studies found that alosetron effectively relieved IBS symptoms. The therapeutic gain has ranged from 12% to 27%. These studies used adequate relief of abdominal pain and discomfort as their primary efficacy endpoint. Alosetron was also demonstrated to improve stool frequency, stool consistency, and urgency in women with nonconstipated IBS. The drug has not been approved for men because at the time of initial approval, men were under-represented in initial phase II trials and, therefore, its true efficacy in men could not be adequately evaluated.

Alosetron is a ligand-gated ion channel receptor, different from all other 5HT receptors, which are G-protein coupled. The 5HT$_3$ receptors act in the gut on postsynaptic 5HT$_3$ receptors (located in the submucosa and myenteric plexus) on myenteric IPANs. Stimulation of the 5HT$_3$ receptors result in fast inward currents that are responsible for mediating a subset of fast excitatory postsynaptic potentials in the ENS. Alosetron is a very potent 5HT$_3$ antagonist that can slow colonic transit, particularly in the left colon (193). It also decreases chloride and water secretion and seems to affect mechanoelastic properties of the colon by increasing colonic compliance (194). Alosetron also appears to have central effects, which probably contribute to its beneficial effects on IBS symptoms. Cerebral blood flow was evaluated using PET in nonconstipated IBS patients randomized to alosetron or placebo (164). This study found that IBS patients taking alosetron (1 to 4 mg twice a day) had a significant reduction of cerebral blood flow to limbic areas such as the amygdala, ventral striatum, and dorsal pons, which significantly correlated with the reduction in IBS symptoms (i.e., abdominal pain). These brain areas are involved in the modulation of emotional, autonomic, peripheral, and neuroendocrine responses to physical and psychological stressors (140). Taken together, these studies suggest that alosetron is effective in relieving IBS symptoms including pain and discomfort and likely improves IBS via its beneficial effects on GI transit, mechanoelastic properties of the colon, and central modulation of painful, emotional, and autonomic responses.

Alosetron is currently prescribed at a dose of 0.5 to 1.0 mg twice a day. The drug is metabolized via the cytochrome P-450 system and has a half-life of 6 to 10 hours. No clinically significant drug interactions are known, but it should be avoided in patients with severe hepatic and renal failure. Unfortunately, after the drug was approved in March 2000, adverse events of severe constipation and serious complications of constipation (ileus, bowel obstruction, toxic megacolon, fecal impaction, and perforation) as well as ischemic colitis occurred. The drug was electively withdrawn by the pharmaceutical company in November 2000. The incidence of serious complications of constipation was approximately 1 in 1,000. Ischemic colitis occurred in 17 of 11,874 patients in clinical trials and 80 of 275,000 (0.02%) patients in postmarketing experience. Seventy-four percent of these cases occurred during the first month of therapy. Fueled by patient and physician protest on the withdrawal of this medication, subsequent discussions were reopened with the FDA that led to the reapproval of the medication in November of 2002 under a restricted use program in which the prescribing physician must be enrolled. The medication is currently

TABLE 18-5 Agents Available to Treat Irritable Bowel Syndrome by Predominant Symptom

DRUG CLASS	GENERIC NAME	TRADE NAME	DOSE
CONSTIPATION			
Fiber[a]	Psyllium	Metamucil, Konsyl, Fiberall	10–20 g qd
	Methycellulose	Citrucel	4 g qd
	Polycarbophil	Fibercon, Equalactin	5–6 mg qd
Laxatives			
Osmotic	Milk of magnesia	MOM	1–2 Tbsp qd to b.i.d
	Magnesium citrate	Citroma	6–12 oz
	Sodium phosphate	Fleet's Phosphosoda	1 tsp in 8 oz fluid
	Lactulose	Cephulac, Kristalose, Enulose	1–2 Tbsp qd to b.i.d
	Polyethelene glycol	Miralax	17 gm in 8 oz fluid
	Sorbitol		1–2 Tbsp qd to b.i.d
Stimulants	Cascara sangrada	Nature's Remedy	325 mg or 1 tsp qhs
	Senna	Perdiem, Senokot	187 mg tabs 1–2 tabs qhs
	Ricinoleic acid	Castor oil	1–2 Tbsp qd
	Diphenylmethane derivatives	Bisacodyl (Ducolax, Correctol)	10 mg 1–2 tabs qhs or 1 suppository qhs
Emollients	Docusates	Colace	100 mg 1–3 tabs qhs
	Mineral oil		1 tsp – 1 Tbsp qhs
5HT$_4$ agonist	Tegaserod	Zelnorm	6 mg b.i.d
Combination 5HT$_4$ agonist and 5HT$_3$ antagonist	Renzapride[b]		1 tab b.i.d
DIARRHEA			
Antidiarrheals	Diphenoxylate	Imodium	1–2 tabs t.i.d
	Loperamide	Lomotil	1 tab q.i.d
Binding agents	Cholestyramine	Questran, Colestid	1 gm b.i.d to q.i.d
5HT$_3$ antagonists	Alosetron[b]	Lotronex	0.5 mg–1 mg qd to b.i.d
	Cilansetron[c]		2 mg t.i.d
TCAs	Amitriptyline	Elavil	10–150 mg qhs
	Doxepin	Sinequan	10–150 mg qhs
	Imipramine	Tofranil	10–150 mg qhs
	Clomipramine	Anafranil	25–100 mg qhs
	Trimipramine	Surmontil	10–150 mg qhs
	Desipramine	Norpramin	10–150 mg qhs
	Nortriptyline	Pamelor	10–150 mg qhs
ABDOMINAL PAIN AND BLOATING			
Antispasmodics	Hyoscamine sulfate	Levsin, Nu-lev, Levbid	0.125 mg sl/po q.i.d prn, 0.375 mg b.i.d (Levbid)
	Dicyclomine	Bentyl	10 mg b.i.d
	Probantheline hydrocholoride	Pro-banthine	15 mg t.i.d a.c and 30 mg qhs
	Clidinium + chlordiazepoxide	Librax	5–10 mg t.i.d to q.i.d
	Hyoscyamine + scopolamine + atropine + phenobarbital	Donnatal	1–2 tabs t.i.d to q.i.d
TCAs	See above	See above	See above
SSRIs	Fluoxetine	Prozac	10–40 mg qd
	Citalopram	Celexa	20 mg qd
	Paroxetine	Paxil	20–50 mg qd
	Sertraline	Zoloft	25–100 mg qd
	Escitalopram	Lexapro	10 mg qd
5 HT$_4$ agonist	Tegaserod	Zelnorm	6 mg b.i.d
Probiotics	Lactobacillus GG	Culturelle	1 tab qd
	VSL no. 3		1 packet b.i.d
	Saccharomyces boulardii	Florastor	250 mg b.i.d

[a] Start with 4 gm/day—gradually increase over 2–3 wk to 20–25 gm/d.
[b] Available through restricted use program.
[c] In phase III trials, not yet commercially available.

indicated for women with severe IBS-D who have chronic IBS symptoms that have been present for at least 6 months, for whom structural and biochemical abnormalities have been ruled out, and who have failed to respond to conventional therapy. IBS is considered severe when there is at least one of the following features: (a) frequent bowel urgency or fecal incontinence, (b) frequent and/or severe pain, or (c) disability or restriction of daily activities due to IBS.

The efficacy of another 5 HT$_3$ antagonist, cilansetron, has been assessed in two large, randomized, placebo-controlled multicenter trials. These trials showed that cilansetron was efficacious in the treatment of both male and female patients with IBS-D (195,196). The dose was 2 mg three times a day. FDA approval of this medication is being planned. Similar to alosetron, the chief side effect of cilansetron was constipation.

5HT$_4$ Receptor Agonists

The prototypical 5HT$_4$ agonist that is currently available in the United States for patients with IBS and constipation is tegaserod. 5HT$_4$ receptors are transmembrane proteins coupled to a G-protein translation that are located on EC cells, enterocytes, smooth muscle cells, and IPANs. They are involved in stimulating the peristaltic reflex (179). Tegaserod works by mimicking serotonin on the luminal surface by stimulating the IPANs via 5HT$_4$ receptors. Therefore, it not only stimulates the peristaltic reflex but also can accelerate oral–cecal transit (197). Tegaserod also increases intestinal chloride secretion, and by this mechanism increases fluid in the stool and improves stool consistency. The effect of tegaserod on visceral sensitivity in human experimental studies is less clear. A recent study found that tegaserod reduced the inhibitory effect of rectal balloon distention on a somatic reflex (RIII) in healthy women (198). This RIII reflex was used as an indirect measure of visceral hypersensitivity because less inhibition of this somatic reflex is suggestive of a reduction in visceral hypersensitivity. However, a recent study compared the effect of tegaserod versus placebo on sensation and mechanoelastic properties of the sigmoid colon to balloon distention in women with IBS-C (199). In these patients, tegaserod at a dose of 6 mg twice daily compared with placebo did increase sigmoid accommodation significantly, although compliance and tone were not altered. The investigators postulated that this change in the mechanoelastic properties of the colon might be a mechanism, in addition to the prokinetic effect on colon transit, by which tegaserod relieves GI symptoms in patients with IBS-C.

Five large multicenter, randomized, double-blind, placebo-controlled phase III clinical trials have evaluated the efficacy of tegaserod in IBS patients with constipation (114–116,200–202). A measure of global symptom relief was the primary efficacy endpoint, and individual GI symptoms, such as abdominal pain, bloating, and stool frequency/consistency were the secondary efficacy endpoints. There were significantly greater responses on all of these outcome measures with tegaserod compared to placebo. The therapeutic gain of the global endpoint ranged from 5% to 19%. Tegaserod has a half-life of 11 ± 5 hours and is taken 30 minutes before breakfast and dinner for the best results. It has no significant drug–drug interactions. Dose adjustment is not needed in the elderly, and it is contraindicated in patients with severe renal or hepatic failure.

Tegaserod is a safe and well-tolerated medication. The two side effects, which occurred more often in patients taking tegaserod compared to placebo, were diarrhea and headache (203). Diarrhea often dissipates with continued use of the drug. There have been no reported associated electrocardiographic effects such as QT prolongation or cardiac arrhythmias with this medication. There is no evidence to suggest an increased incidence of ischemic colitis in patients taking tegaserod compared to the background incidence in the general population or an IBS population (204). Tegaserod has been approved for the treatment of women with IBS and constipation. There have been an insufficient number of male patients enrolled in the clinical trials to assess the efficacy of this agent in this patient population.

Combination 5HT$_4$ Agonist and 5HT$_3$ Antagonist

Renzapride is both a 5HT$_4$ agonist and 5HT$_3$ antagonist, which has shown promise as a treatment for IBS in both men and women. In one study of renzapride in IBS-C patients (205), this medication was shown to increase the frequency of BM and improve stool consistency, but there was no overall significant benefit in terms of relief of abdominal pain and discomfort. In another study, 48 patients with IBS-C who did not have any evidence of pelvic outlet obstruction but did have normal or slow baseline colonic transit were randomized in a double-blind, parallel-group 2-week study to renzapride at a dose of 1, 2, or 4 mg, or placebo (206). Renzapride was associated with acceleration of colonic transit and improvement in bowel function scores. Gastric emptying and small bowel transit were not affected by renzapride. In a clinical trial with patients with IBS-A, renzapride at doses of 1, 2, and 4 mg were given to 168 patients of whom 78% were women (207). Satisfactory relief of overall IBS symptoms for the 2-mg dose was 57% compared with a placebo response of 43%, but this difference failed to reach statistical significance.

Antidepressants

Both TCA and SSRIs have been used in the treatment of IBS. Three observations have led to the use of these agents. First, they may have utility because many IBS patients have associated psychological symptoms such as depression, anxiety, and somatization (208). Secondly, these drugs may have modulating effects either through local gut action or through a centrally mediated action that changes visceral or motor activity or both. Lastly is the fact that both drugs seem to have central modulating effects on pain. Low-dose TCAs (e.g., amitriptyline, desipramine, nortriptyline) are now frequently used in the treatment of IBS, particularly in patients with more severe or refractory symptoms, impaired daily function, and associated depression and anxiety. The temporal effects of TCA on GI function precede those that relate to improvement in mood, which suggests that the therapeutic actions are unrelated to improvement in mental state. A recent systematic review found seven randomized placebo-controlled trials evaluating the effect of TCA in the treatment of IBS. It was found that none of these studies were of high quality due to relatively small sample sizes and that there were poorly defined primary and secondary endpoints (188). However, a recently published study by Drossman et al. (209), which is not included in the systematic review, evaluated the efficacy of the TCA desipramine in treating moderate to severe functional bowel disorders in a large, randomized, 12-week, placebo-controlled trial. Patients taking desipramine were started on a dose of 50 mg per day and then increased in 1 week to 100 mg per day and then to 150 mg per day from week 3 to week 12 as tolerated. Desipramine was shown to have statistically significant benefit over placebo in the per protocol analysis which included only those patients who completed treatment (responder rate 73% vs. 49%) but not in the intention-to-treat analysis. The lack of benefit in the intention-to-treat analysis may have been related to a substantial (28%) drop out primarily due to symptom side effects, thus attesting to the value of carefully monitoring dosage and helping the patient stay on the medication long enough to achieve a treatment response. Desipramine was found to be more effective in the subgroup of patients with less severe symptoms and a history of abuse.

The benefits of SSRIs in the treatment of IBS have not been well studied and their potential central and peripheral effects are less clear. A possible mechanism of SSRIs is through their central effects in reducing the vicious cycle of anxiety and pain. They may also have the peripheral effect of decreasing orocecal transit time, which is presumably the mechanism responsible for the side effect of diarrhea. There is a published study comparing the efficacy of SSRIs (paroxetine) to treatment as usual in reducing abdominal pain, health-related quality of life, and health care costs in a relatively large group of severe IBS patients at 3 months of treatment and 1 year later (210). Between 40% and 48% of the patients had a psychiatric disorder and 12% reported a history of sexual abuse. Paroxetine did not significantly reduce abdominal pain scores although it did decrease days of pain compared to the treatment as usual group. While paroxetine was significantly superior to treatment as usual in improving health-related quality of life, there was no difference between patients with and without a depressive disorder. In a second study that compared the efficacy of a high fiber diet alone and in combination with fluoxetine or placebo in IBS, overall well-being improved more with paroxetine than with placebo (63.3% vs. 26.3%), but abdominal pain, bloating, and social functioning did not (211). These studies provide some preliminary evidence that SSRIs may have some overall efficacy in IBS patients with moderate to severe symptoms. It is still not clear if they are effective in patients with milder symptoms and if they exert their beneficial effect by specifically relieving GI symptoms such as abdominal pain versus decreasing psychological symptoms.

Other Pharmacologic Agents

In a preliminary study, the effects of clonidine, which is an α 2-adrenergic receptor agonist, on GI symptoms, gut transit, and fasting and postprandial gastric volumes were evaluated in patients with IBS-D in a double-blind, randomized, parallel-group, placebo-controlled trial (212). Clonidine, at a dose of 0.1 mg twice a day for 4 weeks, relieved altered bowel habits but not abdominal pain; however, these effects were not associated with significant alterations in transit.

Clonidine did not significantly alter GI transit or gastric volumes. Drowsiness, dizziness, and dry mouth were the most common adverse events with the 0.1-mg dose, but severity of adverse effects subsided after the first week of treatment. Clinical trials with larger sample sizes will be required to more completely assess clonidine's effect in IBS.

Herbal treatments are used throughout the world and have been used by individuals for the treatment of FGIDs such as IBS. However, there are only a few trials that have evaluated herbal remedies in relieving the symptoms of IBS (213,214). In an interesting study, the effect of Chinese herbal medicine (CHM) in the treatment of IBS was assessed in a randomized, double-blind, placebo-controlled trial (213). A total of 116 IBS patients was randomized to 1 of 3 treatment groups: individualized Chinese herbal formulations ($n = 38$), a standard Chinese herbal formulation ($n = 43$), or placebo ($n = 35$). Compared with patients in the placebo group, patients in the active treatment groups (standard and individualized CHM) had significant improvement in bowel symptom scores, global improvement, and reduction in the degree of interference with life caused by IBS symptoms. Chinese herbal formulations individually tailored to the patient proved no more effective than standard CHM treatment. On follow-up 14 weeks after completion of treatment, only the individualized CHM treatment group maintained improvement. In another treatment trial, the efficacy and safety of a commercially available herbal preparation (STW 5) (nine plant extracts) and the research herbal preparation STW 5-II (six plant extracts) were found to be significantly better than placebo in reducing the total abdominal pain score and the IBS symptom score at 4 weeks in 208 patients with IBS (214).

Probiotics are live, microbial food supplements, which are thought to exert beneficial effects by improving intestinal microbial balance. In a 10-week treatment study, the effects of a probiotic formulation, VSL #3 (450 billion lyophilized bacteria per day), on GI transit and symptoms were compared to placebo in 25 IBS-D patients (215). There were no significant differences in mean GI transit measurements, bowel function scores, or satisfactory global symptom relief between the two treatment groups, pre- or posttherapy. However, VSL #3 reduced abdominal bloating compared to placebo. All patients tolerated VSL #3 well.

Behavioral and Psychological Treatment

Psychological treatments used to treat FGIDs include psychotherapy (dynamic- and cognitive-behavioral therapy), relaxation therapy, hypnotherapy, and biofeedback therapy. Psychological treatments can also be combined. Psychological treatments are generally recommended in patients with moderate to severe IBS, when patients fail medical treatment options, or when there is evidence that stress or psychological factors are contributing to symptom onset or exacerbation (21). There are two recent studies that have shown the beneficial effects of psychotherapy (210) and CBT (209) in moderate to severe IBS patients compared to controlled conditions. A review of the psychological treatment studies of IBS supports the superiority of psychological treatment over conventional medical therapy for individual symptoms of IBS (188). Follow-up studies (duration 9 to 40 months) have demonstrated that psychological treatment maintained superiority over placebo, indicating that these methods have lasting value. There are no current studies to support that one type of treatment is superior to the others. The choice of treatment will depend on patient requirements, available resources, and the experience of the therapist.

FUNCTIONAL CONSTIPATION

Definition

Functional constipation comprises a group of functional disorders, which present as persistent, difficult, infrequent, or seemingly incomplete evacuation (22). Surveys have shown that constipation affects up to 28% of the North American population (range 2% to 28%) (216,217) and has been self-reported in 20.8% of women and 8.0% of men (218). A more recent study, which conducted nationwide telephone interview surveys of more than 10,000 individuals, reported the prevalence of constipation in 16% of women and 12% of men (217). The female-to-male ratio was elevated for both the "outlet" type (1.65) and the combined "IBS-outlet" type (2.27) of functional constipation.

Diagnosis

The Rome II criteria view functional constipation as a group of functional disorders in which there is persistent difficult stool, infrequent stool, or a feeling of incomplete defecation. There must be at least 12 weeks of symptoms (not necessarily consecutive) over at least a 12-month period of time that is associated with at least two of the following criteria: (a) straining >25% of the time, (b) hard or lumpy stools >25% of the time, (c) a feeling of incomplete evacuation >25% of the time, (d) a sensation of obstruction or blockage in the anorectal area >25% of the time, (e) manual maneuvers to facilitate a bowel movement >25% of the time, and/or (f) <3 BMs per week. In general, loose BMs should not be present and the patient should have insufficient criteria for IBS (22).

On the basis of the medical history, it is often possible to ascertain the factors that may exacerbate or cause constipation. The chronicity and nature of the symptoms will often dictate the diagnostic studies that are needed. It is helpful to conceptualize chronic constipation as divided into three categories: (a) *extracolonic constipation,* (b) *mechanical constipation,* and (c) *functional constipation.* Table 18-6 lists some of the important considerations in the differential diagnosis of this common condition. *Extracolonic constipation* refers to factors that affect the function of the colon and/or rectum but are not intrinsic to the colon. Included in this category are dietary habits, medications, chronic medical conditions, and neurologic and psychological disorders. Physical abnormalities of the colon or rectum that are either microscopic or macroscopic cause *mechanical constipation,* which include narrowing of the rectum from anal stenosis or colonic narrowing due to diverticular disease, rectal prolapse, or rectocele and Hirschsprung disease. Hirschsprung disease is a congenital disorder due to a loss of ganglia within the ENS in the colon. It usually presents in childhood; however, some individuals may present at a later age due to having only a short

TABLE 18-6	Causes of Chronic Constipation

EXTRACOLONIC
Dietary Habits
  Low fiber intake
  Inadequate fluid intake
  Anorexia
Medications
  Antidepressants (e.g., TCAs)
  Anticholinergics (e.g., hyoscyamine, dicyclomine)
  Antihypertensives (e.g., calcium channel blockers, diuretics)
  Opioid analgesics
  Antiparkinson medications
  Aluminum or calcium based antacids
  Iron supplements
  Anticonvulsants
  Ion exchange resins (e.g., cholestryamine)
  Other psychotropic agents
Metabolic, Endocrine, or Connective Tissue Disorders
  Hypercalcemia
  Hypokalemia
  Renal failure
  Hypopituitarism
  Hyperparathyroidism
  Diabetes mellitus
  Porphyria
  Pregnancy
  Amyloidosis
  Lead poisoning
Neurologic Disorders
  Parkinson disease
  Multiple sclerosis
  Autonomic neuropathy
  Stroke
  Spinal cord injuries
  Chagas disease
  Intracranial tumors
  Von Recklinghausen disease
  Tertiary syphilis
MECHANICAL CONSTIPATION
Narrowing of the Colon, Rectum, or Anus
  Colorectal cancer
  Radiation-induced stricture
  Ischemic colitis with stricture
  Diverticular disease
  Rectal prolapse or rectocele
  Hirschsprung disease
  Familial myopathy
FUNCTIONAL CONSTIPATION
  Slow transit constipation
  Pelvic floor dysfunction (e.g., anismus)
  Irritable bowel syndrome

TCAs, tricyclic antidepressants.

segment of aganglionic distal rectum that fails to relax, producing an obstruction to defecation.

Once extracolonic and mechanical sources for the constipation have been eliminated, chronic constipation is thought to be *functional.* There are three categories of functional constipation: (a) IBS with constipation, (b) slow transit constipation, and (c) defecatory disorders. The medical history may help in determining the etiology of the chronic constipation (219). Presence of constipation symptoms associated with predominant abdominal pain and discomfort supports the diagnosis of IBS-C. Decreased stool frequency (i.e., <3 BMs per week) without an urge or predominant pain is more indicative of slow transit constipation. Excessive straining and use of manual maneuvers in order to have a bowel movement is suggestive of defecatory disorders with pelvic floor or anal sphincter dysfunction. Performing a rectal exam to assess for impacted stool, a rectal mass, anal fissures, external hemorrhoids, rectal prolapse, or abnormal perineal descent during bear down command also helps determine the appropriate diagnostic evaluation. Laboratory tests should include a CBC, TSH, glucose, and serum calcium. Imaging of the GI tract with colonoscopy or barium enema plus flexible sigmoidoscopy to rule out colonic neoplasm is recommended at age 50 or higher for average risk individuals and at age 40 for those individuals with a family history of colon cancer.

In patients without alarm symptoms (e.g., sudden change in bowel habits, weight loss, or signs of gross or occult blood in the stool), it may be reasonable to try a 2-week therapeutic trial of fiber supplementation. Patients who respond to this treatment intervention may not need further diagnostic evaluation. Once medical conditions and medications are sorted out, additional studies may be needed to differentiate patients with chronic constipation due to *slow colonic transit* from those patients with *defecatory disorders*. GI transit time can be measured using radio-opaque markers or scintigraphy. Colon transit assessment using radio-opaque markers is an inexpensive test that may be performed in several ways (220,221). The patient consumes a high fiber diet and takes a capsule with radio-opaque markers daily for 1 to 5 days, depending on the protocol. The number of markers is counted to determine colon transit time (normal <72 hours). A radioisotope marker such as indium[111] bound to microspheres is also used to determine GI transit times (222). The markers can be used to delineate patients with colonic dysfunction where markers are found throughout the colon from patients with anorectal dysfunction where there is retention of markers in the rectosigmoid area (223). The indium[111] test can be used to more clearly delineate transit through the whole large intestine.

Additional studies can be done when defecatory disorders are suspected. These include an anorectal manometry, which assesses anal sphincter pressures at rest and during voluntary squeeze, and the anorectal inhibitory reflex (224). The absence of this reflex in which there is relaxation of the internal anal sphincter during rectal balloon distention is suggestive of Hirschsprung disease or a compliant rectum due to retained stool. In addition, a balloon expulsion test in which a patient must expel a water-filled rectal balloon within 2 minutes can be performed and, if abnormal, would be suggestive of a defecatory disorder such as pelvic floor dyssynergia or anismus (225–227). This diagnosis can be supported by noting a lack of increase in the anorectal angle upon straining during the defecography (228). Defecography, a study where thick barium paste is instilled into the rectum and radiographs are taken, measures anorectal angles and perineal descent and detects intussusception, rectal prolapse, or rectocele with stool retention (229).

Pathophysiology

In slow transit constipation, the time required for the stool to go through the colon is markedly increased. Patients with slow transit constipation have been shown to have abnormalities in myenteric neurons, excitatory and inhibitory neurotransmitters, and a considerable decrease in the number of interstitial cells of Cajal, which are pacemaker cells (224).

Defecatory disorders refer to conditions due to a discoordination in the pelvic floor or anorectal muscles, which results in an impairment in defecation. Patients with pelvic floor dysfunction have either paradoxical contraction of the muscles in this area or failure to relax. This disorder may also be referred to as anismus or puborectalis syndrome. Colonic transit times are usually normal but the patients are not able to defecate normally. The pathophysiology of this disorder is not well understood, but it is not thought to be attributable to any neurologic lesion since at least two thirds of affected patients can learn to relax this musculature with biofeedback training (230). This disorder is believed to be due to maladaptive learned behaviors (231,232).

Treatment

Treatment of chronic constipation depends on the underlying etiology. In general, dietary and lifestyle changes may be helpful, particularly increasing dietary fiber (approximately 20 g per day). Although most clinicians recommend increasing fluids and exercise, these recommendations have actually not been studied, and evidence actually exists that constipated patients have similar fluid intakes and exercise levels when compared to healthy controls (233).

Laxatives are the mainstay of therapy for most forms of constipation. Laxatives can be divided into three groups: emollients (stool softeners), osmotic laxatives, and stimulant laxatives (224,234,235). Emollient laxatives, such as docusate and mineral oil, are anionic detergents that work by softening the stool and allowing more water to enter the stool. Used alone they may help with mild constipation but are most often used in combination with other agents. Mineral oil should be used with care because, if aspirated, it can cause lipoid pneumonia. It also can cause anal seepage.

Osmotic laxatives can be divided into two categories, poorly absorbed ions like magnesium hydroxide or citrate or sodium phosphate and poorly absorbed sugars like lactulose and polyethylene glycol or sorbitol solution (224). They function by increasing stool bulk and by causing an influx of water into the small and large intestine. The poorly absorbed ions are more likely to causes fluxes in electrolytes or volume overload and therefore should be given with care to patients with renal insufficiency or cardiac dysfunction. In contrast, the nonabsorbed sugars are hydrolyzed by the colonic bacteria into various acids. These sugars can be fermented by the colonic bacteria and cause the production of hydrogen gas and carbon dioxide. This in turn can result in more bloating, flatulence, and abdominal cramps. These laxatives often take 1 to 2 days to have a full result. Polyethylene glycol is not hydrolyzed by bacteria and therefore causes less abdominal pain and bloating.

Cascara, senna, castor oil (ricinoleic acid), and diphenylmethane derivatives (e.g., correctol or ducolax) are stimulant laxatives and function by stimulating intestinal contraction by a variety of mechanisms (236). They work within hours and should be used sparingly. Castor oil works primarily in the small intestine and causes significantly more cramps and diarrhea. Tap water enemas work by stimulating the rectum to defecate. They may be helpful in patients with megacolon or disordered defecation.

Until recently, there have been no prokinetic agents that have improved colon transit and symptoms in patients with constipation. Cisapride has been withdrawn from the United States market except under a special program. The 5HT$_4$ agonist, tegaserod, has been shown to increase orocecal transit time (197) and has been shown to be effective in relieving symptoms in patients with chronic constipation (237,238), and is now currently approved for this indication.

If patients with slow colon transit constipation fail to respond to medical management, subtotal colectomy with ileorectal anastomosis may be considered (239). Patients who are considered for this surgical intervention should have normal upper gut and anorectal function and no evidence of significant psychological symptoms. This surgical procedure can be complicated by small bowel obstructions, diarrhea, recurrent constipation, and incontinence (240).

Pelvic floor dyssynergia has been treated with two types of training, anorectal biofeedback and simulated defecation. Biofeedback training uses a sensor in the anal canal to provide feedback to the patient on either striated muscle activity or anal pressures (241). Success rates vary but about 48% to 62% of patients will respond to biofeedback (242,243). In simulated defecation, the patient practices defecating a simulated stool (e.g., a water-filled balloon or a silicon filled condom). Some investigators combine the two techniques (244,245). The exact number of sessions and the timing of these sessions has not been fully studied nor have there been controlled trials comparing it to sham biofeedback or to conventional treatments. However, its overall effectiveness makes this the treatment of choice.

COEXISTENCE OF FIBROMYALGIA AND FUNCTIONAL GASTROINTESTINAL DISORDERS

Many patients with FGID, particularly IBS, report extraintestinal symptoms such as fatigue (12,13), muscle pain (12,13), sleep disturbances (14), and sexual dysfunction (15). IBS patients are twice as likely as comparison groups to be diagnosed with a non-GI chronic-pain disorder (16). One of the more well-studied comorbid conditions seen in IBS patients is FM. IBS and FM are chronic-pain syndromes characterized by visceral and somatic pain and discomfort, respectively. A study of 80 patients demonstrated that 70% of FM patients also had symptoms of IBS, and 65% of IBS patients suffered from FM symptoms (246). Using the diagnostic criteria for both FM (247) and IBS (248), Sperber et al. found that 31.6% of IBS patients met criteria for FM and 32% of FM patients met criteria for IBS (249). These investigators also found that patients with *both* IBS and FM had a significantly poorer health-related quality of life than those with IBS *or* FM (249). These two syndromes have many similar clinical characteristics (19,20): (a) predominant symptom is pain, (b) female predominance,

(c) majority of patients associate stressful life events with initiation or exacerbation of symptoms, (d) increased prevalence of sexual abuse and psychological symptoms, (e) majority of patients complain of disturbed sleep and fatigue, (f) psychotherapy and behavioral therapies are efficacious in treating symptoms, and (g) low-dose TCAs can improve symptoms. However, health-related quality of life is poorer in patients with IBS + FM compared to IBS only. These similarities suggest that these two syndromes may share a common centrally regulated etiology. Studies demonstrate that both IBS and fibromylagia have the following physiologic similarities: (a) are stress-related conditions, (b) are characterized by hyperalgesia, (c) demonstrate evidence of specific hypervigilance and hyperattentiveness, (d) increased activation of the ACC subregion involved in attentional mechanisms, (e) enhanced hypothalamic–pituitary-adrenal axis, (f) autonomic dysregulation, and (g) increased substance P in cerebrospinal fluid (16,20,159,250–252). There is growing evidence in the literature that IBS and FM are both biopsychosocial disorders that can be explained by a neurobiologic model which postulates stress-induced alterations in CNS circuits, resulting in inadequate antinociceptive responses and altered autonomic (e.g., sympathetic nervous system) and hypothalamic–pituitary-adrenal axis responses. Future studies will hopefully elucidate the complex underlying mechanisms responsible for these chronic-pain syndromes and lead to more effective treatment.

SUMMARY POINTS

- FGIDs are commonly diagnosed by primary care physicians and gastroenterologists. These disorders include functional chest pain of presumed esophageal origin, FD, IBS, and chronic constipation.
- These conditions are associated with a considerable health care and economic burden.
- Due to a lack of a diagnostic biologic marker, these FGIDs are diagnosed by symptom-based diagnostic criteria and excluding organic disease.
- A unifying hypothesis to explain FGIDs is that they result from a dysregulation of the brain-gut neuroenteric system, which may result in altered GI motility, visceral perception, autonomic responses, and CNS modulation of visceral sensory information.
- Similar clinical characteristics between IBS and these other syndromes have raised the possibility of a common underlying mechanism.

■ IMPLICATIONS FOR PRACTICE

- The management of FGIDs includes nonpharmacologic (e.g., education and reassurance, psychological treatment) and pharmacologic approaches and should be based on predominant symptoms, symptom severity, and presence of comorbid psychological features.
- Extraintestinal symptoms and psychological symptoms are highly prevalent in IBS patients. The presence of extraintestinal symptoms may be due to comorbidity of other chronic functional disorders, such as FM.

REFERENCES

1. Mitchell CM, Drossman DA. Survey of the AGA membership relating to patients with functional gastrointestinal disorders. *Gastroenterology* 1987;92:1282–1284.
2. Drossman DA, Corazziari E, Talley NJ, et al. Rome II: a multinational consensus document on functional gastrointestinal disorders. *Gut* 1999;45:II1–II81.
3. Thompson WG, Longstreth GF, Drossman DA, et al. C. Functional bowel disorders and D. functional abdominal pain. In: Drossman DA, Corazziari E, Talley NJ et al., eds. *Rome II. The functional gastrointestinal disorders. Diagnosis, pathophysiology and treatment: a multinational consensus*. McLean, VA: Degnon Associates, 2000:351–432.
4. Drossman DA. The functional gastrointestinal disorders and the Rome II process. In: Drossman DA, Corazziari E, Talley NJ et al., eds. *Rome II. The functional gastrointestinal disorders. Diagnosis, pathophysiology, and treatment: a multinational consensus*. McLean, VA: Degnon Associates, 2000: 1–29.
5. Talley NJ, Gabriel SE, Harmsen WS, et al. Medical costs in community subjects with irritable bowel syndrome. *Gastroenterology* 1995;109:1736–1741.
6. Sandler RS, Everhart JE, Donowitz M, et al. The burden of selected digestive diseases in the United States. *Gastroenterology* 2002;122:1500–1511.
7. Aston-Jones G, Rajkowski J, Kubiak P, et al. Role of the locus coeruleus in emotional activation. *Prog Brain Res* 1996; 107:379–402.
8. Longstreth GF, Wilson A, Knight K, et al. Irritable bowel syndrome, health care use, and costs: A U.S. managed care perspective. *Am J Gastroenterol* 2003;98:600–607.
9. Martin BC, Ganguly R, Pannicker S, et al. Utilization patterns and net direct medical cost to Medicaid of irritable bowel syndrome. *Curr Med Res Opin* 2003;19:771–780.
10. Levy RL, Von Korff M, Whitehead WE, et al. Costs of care for irritable bowel syndrome patients in a health maintenance organization. *Am J Gastroenterol* 2001;96:3122–3129.
11. Drossman DA, Li Z, Andruzzi E, et al. U.S. householder survey of functional gastrointestinal disorders. Prevalence, sociodemography and health impact. *Dig Dis Sci* 1993;38: 1569–1580.
12. Whorwell PJ, McCallum M, Creed FH, et al. Non-colonic features of irritable bowel syndrome. *Gut* 1986;27:37–40.
13. Maxton DG, Morris J, Whorwell PJ. More accurate diagnosis of irritable bowel syndrome by the use of 'non-colonic' symptomatology. *Gut* 1991;32:784–786.
14. Fass R, Fullerton S, Tung S, et al. Sleep disturbances in clinic patients with functional bowel disorders. *Am J Gastroenterol* 2000;95:1195–2000.
15. Fass R, Fullerton S, Naliboff B, et al. Sexual dysfunction in patients with irritable bowel syndrome and non-ulcer dyspepsia. *Digestion* 1998;59:79–85.
16. Whitehead WE, Palsson O, Jones KR. Systemic review of the comorbidity of irritable bowel syndrome with other disorders: what are the causes and implications? *Gastroenterology* 2002;122:1140–1156.
17. Whitehead WE, Winget C, Fedoravicius AS, et al. Learned illness behavior in patients with irritable bowel syndrome and peptic ulcer. *Dig Dis Sci* 1982;27:202–208.
18. Whorwell PJ, Lupton EW, Erduran D, et al. Bladder smooth muscle dysfunction in patients with irritable bowel syndrome. *Gut* 1986;27:1014–1017.
19. Chang L. The association of functional gastrointestinal disorders and fibromyalgia. *Eur J Surg* 1998;583:32–36.
20. Chang L. Extraintestinal manifestations and psychiatric illness in IBS: is there a link? In: Holtmann G, Talley NJ, eds. *Gastrointestinal inflammation and disturbed gut function:*
the challenge of new concepts. Dordrecht, The Netherlands: Kluwer Academic Publishers, 2003:10–16.
21. Drossman DA, Camilleri M, Mayer EA, et al. AGA technical review on irritable bowel syndrome. *Gastroenterology* 2002; 123:2108–2131.
22. Drossman DA, Corazziari E, Talley NJ, et al. *Rome II. The functional gastrointestinal disorders. Diagnosis, pathophysiology and treatment: a multinational consensus*. McLean, VA: Degnon Associates, 2000.
23. Kemp HG Jr, Vokonas PS, Cohn PF, et al. The anginal syndrome associated with normal coronary arteriograms. Report of a six year experience. *Am J Med* 1973;54:735–742.
24. Ockene IS, Shay MJ, Alpert JS, et al. Unexplained chest pain in patients with normal coronary arteriograms. A follow-up study of functional status. *N Engl J Med* 1980;303:1249–1252.
25. Richter JE, Bradley LA, Castell DO. Esophageal chest pain: current controversies in pathogenesis, diagnosis and therapy. *Ann Intern Med* 1989;110:66–78.
26. Locke GR III, Talley NJ, Fett SL et al. Prevalence and clinical spectrum of gastroesophageal reflux: a population-based study in Olmsted County, Minnesota. *Gastroenterology* 1997;112:1448–1456.
27. Cormier LE, Katon W, Russo J, et al. Chest pain with negative cardiac diagnostic studies. Relationship to psychiatric illness. *J Nerv Ment Dis* 1988;176:351–358.
28. Tack JF. Chest pain of oesophageal origin. In: Corazziari E, ed. *Approach to the patient with chronic gastrointestinal disorders*. Milan, Italy: Messaggi s.r.l, 1999:153–169.
29. Peters L, Maas L, Petty D, et al. Spontaneous noncardiac chest pain. Evaluation by 24-hour ambulatory esophageal motility and pH monitoring. *Gastroenterology* 1988;94:878–886.
30. Richter JE, Dalton CB, Bradley LA, et al. Oral nifedipine in the treatment of noncardiac chest pain in patients with nutcracker esophagus. *Gastroenterology* 1987;93:21–28.
31. Anderson KO, Dalton CB, Bradley LA, et al. Stress induces alteration of esophageal pressures in healthy volunteers and non-cardiac chest pain patients. *Dig Dis Sci* 1989;34:89–91.
32. Ghillebert G, Janssens J, Vantrappen G, et al. Ambulatory 24 hour intraeosophageal pH and pressure recordings v provocation tests in the diagnosis of chest pain of oesophageal origin. *Gut* 1990;31:738–744.
33. Lynn RB. Mechanisms of esophageal pain. *Am J Med* 1992; 92:11S–19S.
34. Ritchie J. Pain from distension of the pelvic colon by inflating a balloon in the irritable colon syndrome. *Gut* 1973;14: 125–132.
35. Whitehead WE, Holtkotter B, Enck P, et al. Tolerance for rectosigmoid distention in irritable bowel syndrome. *Gastroenterology* 1990;98:1187–1192.
36. Richter JE, Barish CF, Castell DO. Abnormal sensory perception in patients with esophageal chest pain. *Gastroenterology* 1986;91:845–852.
37. Paterson WG, Wang H, Vanner SJ. Increasing pain sensation to repeated esophageal balloon distension in patients with chest pain of undetermined etiology. *Dig Dis Sci* 1995;40: 1325–1331.
38. Clouse RE, Richter JE, Heading RC, et al. A. Functional esophageal disorders. In: Drossman DA, Corazziari E, Talley NJ et al., eds. *Rome II. The functional gastrointestinal disorders. Diagnosis, pathophysiology, and treatment: a multinational consensus*. McLean, VA: Degnon Associates, 2000: 247–298.
39. Fass R, Fennerty MB, Ofman JJ, et al. The clinical and economic value of a short course of omeprazole in patients with noncardiac chest pain. *Gastroenterology* 1998;115:42–49.
40. Kahrilas PJ, Clouse RE, Hogan WJ. American Gastroenterological Association technical review on the clinical use of esophageal manometry. *Gastroenterology* 1994;107: 1865–1884.

41. Hongo M, Traube M, McCallum RW. Comparison of effects of nifedipine, propantheline bromide, and the combination on esophageal motor function in normal volunteers. *Dig Dis Sci* 1984;29:300–304.

42. Bassotti G, Gaburri M, Imbimbo BP, et al. Manometric evaluation of cimetropium bromide activity in patients with the nutcracker esophagus. *Scand J Gastroenterol* 1988;23:1079–1084.

43. Orlando RC, Bozymski EM. Clinical and manometric effects of nitroglycerin in diffuse esophageal spasm. *N Engl J Med* 1973;289:23–25.

44. Kikendall JW, Mellow MH. Effect of sublingual nitroglycerin and long-acting nitrate preparations on esophageal motility. *Gastroenterology* 1980;79:703–706.

45. Mellow MH. Effect of isosorbide and hydralazine in painful primary esophageal motility disorders. *Gastroenterology* 1982;83:364–370.

46. Blackwell JN, Holt S, Heading RC. Effect of nifedipine on oesophageal motility and gastric emptying. *Digestion* 1981; 21:50–56.

47. Cattau EL Jr, Castell DO, Johnson DA, et al. Diltiazem therapy for symptoms associated with nutcracker esophagus. *Am J Gastroenterol* 1991;86:272–276.

48. Richter JE, Dalton CB, Buice RG, et al. Nifedipine: a potent inhibitor of contractions in the body of the human esophagus. Studies in healthy volunteers and patients with the nutcracker esophagus. *Gastroenterology* 1985;89:549–554.

49. Miller LS, Parkman HP, Schiano TD, et al. Treatment of symptomatic nonachalasia esophageal motor disorders with botulinum toxin injection at the lower esophageal sphincter. *Dig Dis Sci* 1996;41:2025–2031.

50. Clouse RE, Lustman PJ, Eckert TC, et al. Low-dose trazodone for symptomatic patients with esophageal contraction abnormalities. A double-blind, placebo-controlled trial. *Gastroenterology* 1987;92:1027–1036.

51. Cannon RO, Quyyumi AA, Mincemoyer R, et al. Imipramine in patients with chest pain despite normal coronary angiograms. *N Engl J Med* 1994;330:1411–1417.

52. Hegel MT, Abel GG, Etscheidt M, et al. Behavioral treatment of angina-like chest pain in patients with hyperventilation syndrome. *J Behav Ther Exp Psychiatry* 1989;20: 31–39.

53. Klimes I, Mayou RA, Pearce MJ, et al. Psychological treatment for atypical non-cardiac chest pain: a controlled evaluation. *Psychol Med* 1990;20:605–611.

54. Quigley EM. Non-erosive reflux disease: part of the spectrum of gastro-oesophageal reflux disease, a component of functional dyspepsia, or both? *Eur J Gastroenterol Hepatol* 2001;13:S13–S18.

55. Talley NJ, Zinsmeister AR, Schleck CD, et al. Dyspepsia and dyspepsia subgroups: a population-based study. *Gastroenterology* 1992;102:1259–1268.

56. Jones RH, Lydeard SE, Hobbs FD, et al. Dyspepsia in England and Scotland. *Gut* 1990;31:401–405.

57. Quadri A, Vakil N. Health-related anxiety and the effect of open-access endoscopy in US patients with dyspepsia. *Aliment Pharmacol Ther* 2003;17:835–840.

58. Talley NJ, Silverstein MD, Agreus L, et al. AGA technical review: evaluation of dyspepsia. *Gastroenterology* 1998;114: 582–595.

59. Muth ER, Koch KL, Stern RM. Significance of autonomic nervous system activity in functional dyspepsia. *Dig Dis Sci* 2000;45:854–863.

60. Kawakami H, Hongo M, Okuno Y, et al. Personality deviation and gastric motility in patients with functional dyspepsia. *J Clin Gastroenterol* 1995;21:S179–S184.

61. Bennett E, Beaurepaire J, Langeluddecke P, et al. Life stress and non-ulcer dyspepsia: a case-control study. *J Psychosom Res* 1991;35:579–590.

62. Talley NJ, Phillips SF, Bruce B, et al. Relation among personality and symptoms in nonulcer dyspepsia and irritable bowel syndrome. *Gastroenterology* 1990;99:327–333.

63. Koch K. Electrogastrography. In: Schuster M, Crowell MD, Koch K, eds. *Schuster atlas of gastrointestinal motility in health and disease.* Hamilton, OH: BC Decker, 2002.

64. Azpiroz F, Malagelada J-R. Gastric tone measured by an electronic barostat in health and postsurgical gastroparesis. *Gastroenterology* 1987;92:934–943.

65. Timmons S, Liston R, Moriarty KJ. Functional dyspepsia: motor abnormalities, sensory dysfunction, and therapeutic options. *Am J Gastroenterol* 2004;99:739–749.

66. Chey W, You C, Lee K, et al. Gastric dysrhythmias: clinical aspects. In: Chey WD, ed. *Functional dyspepsias of the digestive tract.* New York: Raven Press, 1983:175–181.

67. You CH, Lee KY, Chey WY, et al. Electrogastrographic study of patients with unexplained nausea, bloating and vomiting. *Gastroenterology* 1980;79:311–314.

68. Troncon LE, Bennett RJ, Ahluwalia NK, et al. Abnormal intragastric distribution of food during gastric emptying in functional dyspepsia patients. *Gut* 1994;35:327–332.

69. Boeckxstaens GE, Hirsch DP, Kuiken SD, et al. The proximal stomach and postprandial symptoms in functional dyspeptics. *Am J Gastroenterol* 2002;97:40–48.

70. Tack J, Piessevaux H, Caenepeel P, et al. Role of impaired gastric accommodation to a meal in functional dyspepsia. *Gastroenterology* 1998;115:1346–1352.

71. Coffin B, Azpiroz F, Guarnner F, et al. Selective gastric hypersensitivity and reflex hyporeactivity in functional dyspepsia. *Gastroenterology* 1994;107:1345–1351.

72. Mearin F, Cucala M, Azpiroz F, et al. The origin of symptoms on the brain-gut axis in functional dyspepsia. *Gastroenterology* 1991;101:999–1006.

73. Tack J, Caenepeel P, Fischler B, et al. Symptoms associated with hypersensitivity to gastric distension in functional dyspepsia. *Gastroenterology* 2001;121:526–535.

74. Mertz H, Fullerton S, Naliboff B, et al. Symptoms and visceral perception in severe functional and organic dyspepsia. *Gut* 1998;42:814–822.

75. Rhee PL, Kim YH, Son HJ, et al. The etiologic role of gastric hypersensitivity in functional dyspepsia in Korea. *J Clin Gastroenterol* 1999;29:332–335.

76. Holtmann G, Gschossmann J, Neufang-Huber J, et al. Differences in gastric mechanosensory function after repeated ramp distensions in non-consulters with dyspepsia and healthy controls. *Gut* 2000;47:332–336.

77. Saper CB. The central autonomic nervous system: conscious visceral perception and autonomic pattern generation. *Annu Rev Neurosci* 2002;25:433–469.

78. Hobday DI, Aziz Q, Thacker N, et al. A study of the cortical processing of ano-rectal sensation using functional MRI. *Brain* 2001;124:361–368.

79. Aziz Q, Thompson DG, Ng VWK, et al. Cortical processing of human somatic and visceral sensation. *J Neurosci* 2000; 20:2657–2663.

80. Ladabaum U, Minoshima S, Hasler WL, et al. Gastric distention correlates with activation of multiple cortical and subcortical regions. *Gastroenterology* 2000;120:369–376.

81. Thumshirn M, Camilleri M, Choi M-G, et al. Modulation of gastric sensory and motor functions by nitrergic and α_2-adrenergic agents in humans. *Gastroenterology* 1999; 116: 573–585.

82. Trimble KC, Farouk R, Pryde A, et al. Heightened visceral sensation in functional gastrointestinal disease is not site-specific. Evidence for a generalized disorder of gut sensitivity. *Dig Dis Sci* 1995;40:1607–1613.

83. Miwa H, Sato N. Functional dyspepsia and *Helicobacter pylori* infection: a recent consensus up to 1999. *J Gastroenterol Hepatol* 2000;15:D60–D65.

84. Danesh J, Lawrence M, Murphy M, et al. Systematic review of the epidemiological evidence on *Helicobacter pylori* infection and nonulcer or uninvestigated dyspepsia. *Arch Intern Med* 2000;160:1192–1198.

85. Talley NJ, Vakil N, Ballard ED, et al. Absence of benefit of eradicating *Helicobacter pylori* in patients with nonulcer dyspepsia. *N Engl J Med* 1999;341:1106–1111.

86. Blum A, Talley NJ, O'Morain C, et al. (OCAY) Study Group Lack of effect of treating *Helicobactor pylori* infection in patients with nonulcer dyspepsia. Omeprazole plus clarithromycin and amoxicillin effect one year after treatment. *N Engl J Med* 1998;339:1875–1881.

87. McColl K, Murray L, El-Omar E, et al. Symptomatic benefit from eradicating *Helicobacter pylori* infection in patients with nonulcer dyspepsia. *N Engl J Med* 1998;339:1869–1874.

88. Tack J, Coulie B, Wilmer A, et al. Influence of sumatriptan on gastric fundus tone and on the perception of gastric distension in man. *Gut* 2000;46:468–473.

89. Talley NJ, van Zanten SV, Saez LR, et al. A dose-ranging, placebo-controlled, randomized trial of alosetron in patients with functional dyspepsia. *Aliment Pharmacol Ther* 2001;15:525–537.

90. Zerbib F, Bruley des Varannes S, Oriola RC, et al. Alosetron does not affect the visceral perception of gastric distension in healthy subjects. *Aliment Pharmacol Ther* 1994;8:403–407.

91. Tack J, Vos R, Janssens J, et al. Influence of tegaserod on proximal gastric tone and on the perception of gastric distension. *Aliment Pharmacol Ther* 2003;18:1031–1037.

92. Tack J, Delia T, Ligozio G, et al. A phase II placebo controlled randomized trial with tegaserod (T) in functional dyspepsia (FD) patients with normal gastric emptying (NGE). *Gastroenterology* 2002;122:A-20.

93. Tougas G, Chen Y, Luo D, et al. Tegaserod improves gastric emptying in patients with gastroparesis and dyspeptic symptoms. *Gastroenterology* 2003;124:A-54.

94. Finney JS, Kinnersley N, Hughes M, et al. Meta-analysis of antisecretory and gastrokinetic compounds in functional dyspepsia. *J Clin Gastroenterol* 1998;26:312–320.

95. Redstone HA, Barrowman N, Veldhuyzen van Zanten SJ. H2-receptor antagonists in the treatment of functional (nonulcer) dyspepsia: a meta-analysis of randomized controlled clinical trials. *Aliment Pharmacol Ther* 2001;15:1291–1299.

96. Talley NJ, Meineche-Schmidt V, Pare P, et al. Efficacy of omeprazole in functional dyspepsia: double-blind, randomized, placebo-controlled trials (the Bond and Opera studies). *Aliment Pharmacol Ther* 1998;12:1055–1065.

97. Talley NJ, Lauritsen K. The potential role of acid suppression in functional dyspepsia: the BOND, OPERA, PILOT and ENCORE studies. *Gut* 2002;50:iv36–iv41.

98. Peura DA, Kovacs TO, Metz DC, et al. Lansoprazole in the treatment of functional dyspepsia: two double-blind, randomized, placebo-controlled trials. *Am J Med* 2004;116:740–748.

99. Wong WM, Wong BC, Hung WK, et al. Double blind, randomised, placebo controlled study of four weeks of lansoprazole for the treatment of functional dyspepsia in Chinese patients. *Gut* 2002;51:502–506.

100. Moayyedi P, Soo S, Deeks J et al., Dyspepsia Review Group. Systematic review and economic evaluation of *Helicobacter pylori* eradication treatment for non-ulcer dyspepsia. *Br Med J* 2000;321:659–664.

101. Laine L, Schoenfeld P, Fennerty MB. Therapy for *Helicobacter pylori* in patients with nonulcer dyspepsia. A meta-analysis of randomized, controlled trials. *Ann Intern Med* 2001;134:361–369.

102. Talley NJ. Update on the role of drug therapy in non-ulcer dyspepsia. *Rev Gastroenterol Disord* 2003;3:25–30.

103. Malfertheiner P, Megraud F, O'Morain C, et al. Current concepts in the management of Helicobacter pylori infection—the Maastricht 2-2000 Consensus Report. *Aliment Pharmacol Ther* 2002;16:167–180.

104. Mertz H, Fass R, Kodner A, et al. Effect of amitriptyline on symptoms, sleep, and visceral perception in patients with functional dyspepsia. *Am J Gastroenterol* 1998;93:160–165.

105. Tack J, Bisschops R, DeMarchi B. Causes and treatment of functional dyspepsia. *Curr Gastroenterol Rep* 2001;3:503–508.

106. Wu CY, Chou LT, Chen HP, et al. Effect of fluoxetine on symptoms and gastric dysrhythmia in patients with functional dyspepsia. *Hepatogastroenterology* 2003;50:278–283.

107. Soo S, Moayyedi P, Deeks J, et al. Psychological interventions for non-ulcer dyspepsia. *Cochrane Database Syst Rev* 2001;(4):CD002301.

108. Bortolotti M, Coccia G, Grossi G, et al. The treatment of functional dyspepsia with red pepper. *Aliment Pharmacol Ther* 2002;16:1075–1082.

109. May B, Kohler S, Schneider B. Efficacy and tolerability of a fixed combination of peppermint oil and caraway oil in patients suffering from functional dyspepsia. *Aliment Pharmacol Ther* 2000;14:1671–1677.

110. Dundee JW, Yang J, McMillan C. Non-invasive stimulation of the P6 (Neiguan) antiemetic acupuncture point in cancer chemotherapy. *J R Soc Med* 1991;84:210–212.

111. Sandler RS. Epidemiology of irritable bowel syndrome in the United States. *Gastroenterology* 1990;99:409–415.

112. Chang L, Heitkemper MM. Gender differences in irritable bowel syndrome. *Gastroenterology* 2002;123:1686–1701.

113. Camilleri M, Mayer EA, Drossman DA, et al. Improvement in pain and bowel function in female irritable bowel patients with alosetron, a 5-HT$_3$ receptor antagonist. *Aliment Pharmacol Ther* 1999;13:1149–1159.

114. Kellow J, Lee OY, Chang FY, et al. An Asia-Pacific, double blind placebo controlled, randomised study to evaluate the efficacy, safety, and tolerability of tegaserod in patients with irritable bowel syndrome. *Gut* 2003;52:671–676.

115. Müller-Lissner SA, Fumagalli I, Bardhan KD, et al. Tegaserod, a 5-HT(4) receptor partial agonist, relieves symptoms in irritable bowel syndrome patients with abdominal pain, bloating and constipation. *Aliment Pharmacol Ther* 2001; 15:1655–1666.

116. Nyhlin H, Bang C, Elsborg L, et al. A double-blind, placebo-controlled, randomized study to evaluate the efficacy, safety and tolerability of tegaserod in patients with irritable bowel syndrome. *Scand J Gastroenterol* 2004;39:119–126.

117. Naliboff BD, Berman S, Chang L, et al. Sex-related differences in IBS patients: central processing of visceral stimuli. *Gastroenterology* 2003;124:1738–1747.

118. Vanner SJ, Depew WT, Paterson WG, et al. Predictive value of the Rome criteria for diagnosing the irritable bowel syndrome. *Am J Gastroenterol* 1999;94:2912–2917.

119. Svendsen JH, Munck LK, Andersen JR. Irritable bowel syndrome: prognosis and diagnostic safety. A 5-year follow-up study. *Scand J Gastroenterol* 1985;20:415–418.

120. Harvey RF, Mauad EC, Brown AM. Prognosis in the irritable bowel syndrome: a 5-year prospective study. *Lancet* 1987;1:963–965.

121. Owens DM, Nelson DK, Talley NJ. The irritable bowel syndrome: long term prognosis and the physician-patient interaction. *Ann Intern Med* 1995;122:107–112.

122. Cash BD, Schoenfeld P, Chew WD. The utility of diagnostic tests in irritable bowel syndrome patients: a systematic review. *Am J Gastroenterol* 2002;97:2812–2819.

123. American College of Gastroenterology Functional Gastrointestinal Disorders Task Force. Evidence-based position statement on the management of irritable bowel syndrome in North America. *Am J Gastroenterol* 2002;97(Suppl.):S1–S5.

124. Tolliver BA, Jackson MS, Jackson KL, et al. Does lactose maldigestion really play a role in the irritable bowel? *J Clin Gastroenterol* 1996;23:15–17.

125. Newcomer AD, McGill DB, Thomas PJ, et al. Tolerance to lactose among lactase-deficient American Indians. *Gastroenterology* 1978;74:44–46.

126. Suarez FL, Savaiano DA, Levitt MD. A comparison of symptoms after the consumption of milk or lactose-hydrolyzed milk by people with self-reported severe lactose intolerance. *N Engl J Med* 1995;333:1–4.

127. Sanders DS, Carter MJ, Hurlstone DP, et al. Association of adult coeliac disease with irritable bowel syndrome: a case-control study in patients fulfilling ROME II criteria referred to secondary care. *Lancet* 2001;358:1504–1508.

128. Hin H, Bird G, Fisher P, et al. Coeliac disease in primary care: case finding study. *Br Med J* 1999;318:164–167.

129. Holt R, Darnley SE, Kennedy T, et al. Screening for coeliac disease in patients with clinical diagnosis of irritable bowel syndrome. *Gastroenterology* 2001;120:A-757.

130. Sanders DS, Patel D, Stephenson TJ, et al. A primary care cross-sectional study of undiagnosed adult coeliac disease. *Eur J Gastroenterol Hepatol* 2003;15:407–413.

131. Shahbazkhani B, Forootan M, Merat S, et al. Coeliac disease presenting with symptoms of irritable bowel syndrome. *Aliment Pharmacol Ther* 2003;18:231–235.

132. Spiegel BM, DeRosa VP, Gralnek IM, et al. Testing for celiac sprue in irritable bowel syndrome with predominant diarrhea: a cost-effectiveness analysis. *Gastroenterology* 2004;126: 1721–1732.

133. Pimentel M, Chow EJ, Lin HC. Eradication of small intestinal bacterial overgrowth reduces symptoms of irritable bowel syndrome. *Am J Gastroenterol* 2000;95:3503–3506.

134. Pimentel M, Chow EJ, Lin HC. Normalization of lactulose breath testing correlates with symptom improvement in irritable bowel syndrome. A double-blind, randomized, placebo-controlled study. *Am J Gastroenterol* 2003;98:412–419.

135. Pimentel M, Wallace D, Hallegua D, et al. A link between irritable bowel syndrome and fibromyalgia may be related to findings on lactulose breath testing. *Ann Rheum Dis* 2004; 63:450–452.

136. Mayer EA, Raybould HE. Role of visceral afferent mechanisms in functional bowel disorders. *Gastroenterology* 1990; 99:1688–1704.

137. Locke GR III, Zinsmeister AR, Talley NJ, et al. Familial association in adults with functional gastrointestinal disorders. *Mayo Clin Proc* 2000;75:907–912.

138. Levy RL, Jones KR, Whitehead WE, et al. Irritable bowel syndrome in twins: heredity and social learning both contribute to etiology. *Gastroenterology* 2001;121:799–804.

139. Morris-Yates A, Talley NJ, Boyce PM, et al. Evidence of a genetic contribution to functional bowel disorder. *Am J Gastroenterol* 1998;93:1311–1317.

140. Mayer EA, Naliboff BD, Chang L, et al. Stress and the gastrointestinal tract: V. Stress and irritable bowel syndrome. *Am J Physiol Gastrointest Liver Physiol* 2001;280:G519–G524.

141. Dickhaus B, Mayer EA, Firooz N, et al. Irritable bowel syndrome patients show enhanced modulation of visceral perception by auditory stress. *Am J Gastroenterol* 2003;98:135–143.

142. Almy TP. Experimental studies on the irritable bowel syndrome. *Am J Med* 1951;10:60–67.

143. Rogers J, Henry MM, Misiewicz JJ. Increased segmental activity and intraluminal pressures in the sigmoid colon of patients with the irritable bowel syndrome. *Gut* 1989;30:634–641.

144. Sullivan MA, Cohen S, Snape WJ. Colonic myoelectrical activity in irritable-bowel syndrome. Effect of eating and anticholinergics. *N Engl J Med* 1978;298:878–883.

145. Kellow JE, Phillips SF. Altered small bowel motility in irritable bowel syndrome is correlated with symptoms. *Gastroenterology* 1987;92:1885–1893.

146. Camilleri M, Choi M-G. Review article: irritable bowel syndrome. *Aliment Pharmacol Ther* 1997;11:3–15.

147. Chey WY, Jin HO, Lee MH, et al. Colonic motility abnormality in patients with irritable bowel syndrome exhibiting abdominal pain and diarrhea. *Am J Gastroenterol* 2001;96:1499–1506.

148. Clemens CH, Samsom M, Roelofs JM, et al. Association between pain episodes and high amplitude propagated pressure waves in patients with irritable bowel syndrome. *Am J Gastroenterol* 2003;98:1838–1843.

149. Whitehead WE, Engel BT, Schuster MM. Irritable bowel syndrome. Physiological and psychological differences between diarrhea-predominant and constipation-predominant patients. *Dig Dis Sci* 1980;25:404–413.

150. Mertz H, Naliboff B, Munakata J, et al. Altered rectal perception is a biological marker of patients with irritable bowel syndrome. *Gastroenterology* 1995;109:40–52.

151. Naliboff BD, Munakata J, Fullerton S, et al. Evidence for two distinct perceptual alterations in irritable bowel syndrome. *Gut* 1997;41:505–512.

152. Bouin M, Plourde V, Boivin M, et al. Rectal distension testing in patients with irritable bowel syndrome: sensitivity, specificity, and predictive values of pain sensory thresholds. *Gastroenterology* 2002;122:1771–1777.

153. Cook IJ, Van Eeden A, Collins SM. Patients with irritable bowel syndrome have greater pain tolerance than normal subjects. *Gastroenterology* 1987;93:727–733.

154. Chang L, Mayer EA, Johnson T, et al. Differences in somatic perception in female patients with irritable bowel syndrome with and without fibromyalgia. *Pain* 2000;84:297–307.

155. Verne GN, Robinson ME, Price DD. Hypersensitivity to visceral and cutaneous pain in the irritable bowel syndrome. *Pain* 2001;93:7–14.

156. Mayer EA. The neurobiology of stress and gastrointestinal disease. *Gut* 2000;47:861–869.

157. Mertz H, Morgan V, Tanner G, et al. Regional cerebral activation in irritable bowel syndrome and control subjects with painful and nonpainful rectal distension. *Gastroenterology* 2000;118:842–848.

158. Naliboff BD, Derbyshire SWG, Munakata J, et al. Cerebral activation in irritable bowel syndrome patients and control subjects during rectosigmoid stimulation. *Psychosom Med* 2001;63:365–375.

159. Chang L, Berman S, Mayer EA, et al. Brain responses to visceral and somatic stimuli in patients with irritable bowel syndrome with and without fibromyalgia. *Am J Gastroenterol* 2003;98:1354–1361.

160. Berman S, Munakata J, Naliboff B, et al. Gender differences in regional brain response to visceral pressure in IBS patients. *Eur J Pain* 2000;4:157–172.

161. Rainville P, Duncan GH, Price DD, et al. Pain affect encoded in human anterior cingulate but not somatosensory cortex. *Science* 1997;277:968–971.

162. Cremonini F, Delgado-Aros S, Camilleri M. Efficacy of alosetron in irritable bowel syndrome: a meta-analysis of randomized controlled trials. *Neurogastroenterol Motil* 2003;15:79–86.

163. Mayer EA, Berman S, Derbyshire SW, et al. The effect of the 5-HT3 receptor antagonist, alosetron, on brain responses to visceral stimulation in irritable bowel syndrome patients. *Aliment Pharmacol Ther* 2002;16:1357–1366.

164. Berman SM, Chang L, Suyenobu B, et al. Condition-specific deactivation of brain regions by 5-HT$_3$ receptor antagonist alosetron. *Gastroenterology* 2002;123:969–977.

165. Drossman DA, Ringel Y, Vogt BA, et al. Alterations of brain activity associated with resolution of emotional distress and pain in a case of severe irritable bowel syndrome. *Gastroenterology* 2003;124:754–761.

166. Chang L, Drossman DA. Optimizing patient care: the psychological interview in irritable bowel syndrome. *Clin Perspect* 2002;5:336–342.

167. Neal KR, Hebden J, Spiller R. Prevalence of gastrointestinal symptoms six months after bacterial gastroenteritis and risk factors for development of the irritable bowel syndrome: postal survey of patients. *Br Med J* 1997;314:779–782.

168. Spiller RC. Postinfectious irritable bowel syndrome. *Gastroenterology* 2003;124:1662–1671.

169. Chaudhary NA, Truelove SC. The irritable colon syndrome. *QJM* 1962;31:307–322.

170. Marshall JK, Thabane M, James C, et al. Incidence of post-infectious irritable bowel syndrome (PI-IBS) following a food-borne outbreak of acute gastroenteritis attributed to a viral pathogen. *Am J Gastroenterol* 2003;98:S270.

171. Spiller RC, Jenkins D, Thornley JP, et al. Increased rectal mucosal enteroendocrine cells, T-lymphocytes, and increased gut permeability following acute *Campylobacter* enteritis and in post-dysenteric irritable bowel syndrome. *Gut* 2000;47:804–811.

172. Dunlop SP, Jenkins D, Neal KR, et al. Relative importance of enterochromaffin cell hyperplasia, anxiety, and depression in postinfectious IBS. *Gastroenterology* 2003;125:1651–1659.

173. Gwee KA, Collins SM, Read NW, et al. Increased rectal mucosal expression of interleukin 1β in recently acquired post-infectious irritable bowel syndrome. *Gut* 2003;52:523–526.

174. Chadwick VS, Chen W, Shu D, et al. Activation of the mucosal immune system in irritable bowel syndrome. *Gastroenterology* 2002;122:1778–1783.

175. O'Sullivan M, Clayton N, Breslin NP, et al. Increased mast cells in the irritable bowel syndrome. *Neurogastroenterol Motil* 2000;12:449–457.

176. Gershon MD. Review article: roles played by 5-hydroxytryptamine in the physiology of the bowel. *Aliment Pharmacol Ther* 1999;13:15–30.

177. Camilleri M. Serotonergic modulation of visceral sensation: lower gut. *Gut* 2002;51:i81–i86.

178. Gershon MD. Serotonin and its implication for the management of irritable bowel syndrome. *Rev Gastroenterol Disord* 2003;3:S25–S34.

179. Grider JR, Foxx-Orenstein AE, Jin JG. 5-Hydroxytryptamine 4 receptor agonists initiate the peristaltic reflex in human, rat, and guinea pig intestine. *Gastroenterology* 1998;115:370–380.

180. Bearcroft CP, Perrett D, Farthing MJG. Postprandial plasma 5-hydroxytryptamine in diarrhea predominant irritable bowel syndrome. *Gut* 1998;42:42–46.

181. Houghton LA, Atkinson W, Whitaker RP, et al. Increased platelet depleted plasma 5-hydroxytryptamine concentration following meal ingestion in symptomatic female subjects with diarrhoea predominant irritable bowel syndrome. *Gut* 2003;52:663–670.

182. El-Salhy M, Norrgard O, Spinnell S. Abnormal colonic endocrine cells in patients with chronic idiopathic slow-transit constipation. *Scand J Gastroenterol* 1999;34:1007–1011.

183. Coates MD, Mahoney CR, Linden DR, et al. Molecular defects in mucosal serotonin content and decreased serotonin reuptake transporter in ulcerative colitis and irritable bowel syndrome. *Gastroenterology* 2004;126:1657–1664.

184. Camilleri M, Atanasova E, Carlson PJ, et al. Serotonin-transporter polymorphism pharmacogenetics in diarrhea-predominant irritable bowel syndrome. *Gastroenterology* 2002;123:425–432.

185. Kalantar JS, Locke GR III, Zinsmeister AR, et al. Familial aggregation of irritable bowel syndrome: a prospective study. *Gut* 2003;52:1703–1707.

186. Klein KB. Controlled treatment trials in the irritable bowel syndrome: a critique. *Gastroenterology* 1988;95:232–241.

187. Jailwala J, Imperiale TF, Kroenke K. Pharmacologic treatment of the irritable bowel syndrome: a systematic review of randomized, controlled trials. *Ann Intern Med* 2000;133:136–147.

188. Brandt LJ, Bjorkman D, Fennerty MB, et al. Systematic review on the management of irritable bowel syndrome in North America. *Am J Gastroenterol* 2002;97:S7–S26.

189. Camilleri M, Northcutt AR, Kong S, et al. Efficacy and safety of alosetron in women with irritable bowel syndrome: a randomised placebo-controlled trial. *Lancet* 2000;355:1035–1040.

190. Camilleri M, Chey WY, Mayer EA, et al. A randomized controlled clinical trial of the serotonin type 3 receptor antagonist alosetron in women with diarrhea-predominant irritable bowel syndrome. *Arch Intern Med* 2001;161:1733–1740.

191. Lembo T, Wright RA, Bagby B, et al. Alosetron controls bowel urgency and provides global symptom improvement in women with diarrhea-predominant irritable bowel syndrome. *Am J Gastroenterol* 2001;96:2662–2670.

192. Jones RH, Holtmann G, Rodrigo L, et al. Alosetron relieves pain and improves bowel function compared with mebeverine in female nonconstipated irritable bowel syndrome patients. *Aliment Pharmacol Ther* 1999;13:1419–1427.

193. Clemens CH, Samsom M, van Berge Henegouwen GP, et al. Effect of alosetron on left colonic motility in non-constipated patients with irritable bowel syndrome and healthy volunteers. *Aliment Pharmacol Ther* 2002;16:993–1002.

194. Delvaux M, Louvel D, Mamet JP, et al. Effect of alosetron on responses to colonic distension in patients with irritable bowel syndrome. *Aliment Pharmacol Ther* 1998;12:849–855.

195. Bradette M, Moennikes H, Carter F, et al. Cilansetron in irritable bowel syndrome with diarrhea predominance (IBS-D): efficacy and safety in a 6 month global study. *Gastroenterology* 2004;126:A-42.

196. Coremans G, Clouse RE, Carter F, et al. Cilansetron, a novel 5-HT3 antagonist, demonstrated efficacy in males with irritable bowel syndrome with diarrhea-predominance (IBS-D). *Gastroenterology* 2004;126:A-643.

197. Prather CM, Camilleri M, Zinsmeister AR, et al. Tegaserod accelerates orocecal transit in patients with constipation-predominant irritable bowel syndrome. *Gastroenterology* 2000;118:463–468.

198. Coffin B, Farmachidi JP, Rueegg P, et al. Tegaserod, a 5-HT4 receptor partial agonist, decreases sensitivity to rectal distension in healthy subjects. *Aliment Pharmacol Ther* 2003;17:577–585.

199. Naliboff BD, Chang L, Crowell MD, et al. Tegaserod increases sigmoid accommodation in female irritable bowel syndrome (IBS) patients. *Gastroenterology* 2004;126:A-101.

200. Novick J, Miner P, Krause R, et al. A randomized, double-blind, placebo-controlled trial of tegaserod in female patients suffering from irritable bowel syndrome with constipation. *Aliment Pharmacol Ther* 2002;16:1877–1888.

201. Appel-Dingemanse S, Horowitz A, Campestrini J, et al. The pharmacokinetics of the novel promotile drug, tegaserod, are similar in healthy subjects—male and female, elderly and young. *Aliment Pharmacol Ther* 2001;15:937–944.

202. Lefkowitz M, Ruegg P, Dunger-Baldauf C, et al. Validation of a global relief measure in clinical trials of irritable bowel syndrome with tegaserod. *Gastroenterology* 2000;188:A145.

203. Tougas G, Snape WJ Jr, Otten MH, et al. Long-term safety of tegaserod in patients with constipation-predominant irritable bowel syndrome. *Aliment Pharmacol Ther* 2002;16:1701–1708.

204. Cole JA, Cook SF, Sands BE, et al. Occurrence of colon ischemia in relation to irritable bowel syndrome. *Am J Gastroenterol* 2004;99:486–491.

205. Meyers NL, Palmer RMJ, George A. Efficacy and safety of renzapride in patients with constipation-predominant IBS: a phase IIb study in the UK primary healthcare setting. *Gastroenterology* 2004;126:A-640.

206. Camilleri M, McKinzie S, Fox J, et al. Renzapride accelerates colonic transit and improves bowel function in constipation-predominant irritable bowel syndrome (C-IBS). *Gastroenterology* 2004;126:A-642.

207. Henderson JC, Palmer RMJ, Meyers NL, et al. A phase IIb clinical study of renzapride in mixed symptom (alternating) irritable bowel syndrome. *Gastroenterology* 2004;126:A-644.

208. Talley NJ, Boyce PM, Jones M. Predictors of health care seeking for irritable bowel syndrome: a population based study. *Gut* 1997;41:394–398.

209. Drossman DA, Toner BB, Whitehead WE, et al. Cognitive-behavioral therapy versus education and desipramine versus placebo for moderate to severe functional bowel disorders. *Gastroenterology* 2003;125:19–31.

210. Creed F, Fernandes L, Guthrie E, et al. The cost-effectiveness of psychotherapy and paroxetine for severe irritable bowel syndrome. *Gastroenterology* 2003;124:303–317.

211. Tabas G, Beaves M, Wang J, et al. Paroxetine to treat irritable bowel syndrome not responding to high-fiber diet: a double-blind, placebo-controlled trial. *Am J Gastroenterol* 2004;99: 914–920.

212. Camilleri M, Kim DY, McKinzie S, et al. A randomized, controlled exploratory study of clonidine in diarrhea-predominant irritable bowel syndrome. *Clin Gastroenterol Hepatol* 2003;1:111–121.

213. Bensoussan A, Talley NJ, Hing M, et al. Treatment of irritable bowel syndrome with Chinese herbal medicine: a randomized controlled trial. *JAMA* 1998;280:1585–1589.

214. Madisch A, Holtmann G, Plein K, et al. Treatment of irritable bowel syndrome with herbal preparations: results of a double-blind, randomized, placebo-controlled, multi-centre trial. *Aliment Pharmacol Ther* 2004;19:271–279.

215. Kim HJ, Camilleri M, McKinzie S, et al. A randomized controlled trial of a probiotic, VSL#3, on gut transit and symptoms in diarrhoea-predominant irritable bowel syndrome. *Aliment Pharmacol Ther* 2003;17:895–904.

216. Johanson JF, Sonnenberg A, Koch TR. Clinical epidemiology of chronic constipation. *J Clin Gastroenterol* 1989;11: 525–536.

217. Stewart WF, Liberman JN, Sandler RS, et al. Epidemiology of constipation (EPOC) study in the United States: relation of clinical subtypes to sociodemographic features. *Am J Gastroenterol* 1999;94:3530–3540.

218. Everhart JE, Go VLW, Johannes RS, et al. A longitudinal survey of self-reported bowel habits in the United States. *Dig Dis Sci* 1989;34:1153–1162.

219. Mertz H, Naliboff B, Mayer EA. Symptoms and physiology in severe chronic constipation. *Am J Gastroenterol* 1999;94: 131–138.

220. Evans RC, Kamm MA, Hinton JM, et al. The normal range and a simple diagram for recording whole gut transit time. *Int J Colorectal Dis* 1992;7:15–17.

221. Metcalf AM, Phillips SF, Zinsmeister AR, et al. Simplified assessment of segmental colonic transit. *Gastroenterology* 1987;92:40–47.

222. van der Sijp JR, Kamm MA, Nightingale JM, et al. Radioisotope determination of regional colonic transit in severe constipation: comparison with radio opaque markers. *Gut* 1993; 34:402–408.

223. Kuijpers HC. Application of the colorectal laboratory in diagnosis and treatment of functional constipation. *Dis Colon Rectum* 1990;33:35–39.

224. Lembo A, Camilleri M. Chronic constipation. *N Engl J Med* 2003;349:1360–1368.

225. Barnes PR, Lennard-Jones JE. Balloon expulsion from the rectum in constipation of different types. *Gut* 1985;26: 1049–1052.

226. Preston DM, Lennard-Jones JE. Anismus in chronic constipation. *Dig Dis Sci* 1985;30:413–418.

227. Fleshman J, Dreznik Z, Cohen E, et al. Balloon expulsion test facilitates diagnosis of pelvic floor obstruction due to nonrelaxing puborectalis muscle. *Dis Colon Rectum* 1992; 35:1019–1025.

228. Felt-Bersma RJ, Luth WJ, Janssen JJ, et al. Defecography in patients with anorectal disorders. Which findings are clinically relevant? *Dis Colon Rectum* 1990;33:277–284.

229. Wald A, Caruana BJ, Freimanis MG, et al. Contributions of evacuation proctography and anorectal manometry to evaluation of adults with constipation and defecatory difficulty. *Dig Dis Sci* 1990;35:481–487.

230. Enck P. Biofeedback training in disordered defecation: a critical review. *Dig Dis Sci* 1993;38:1953–1960.

231. Wald A. Biofeedback for neurogenic fecal incontinence: rectal sensation is a determinant of outcome. *J Pediatr Gastroenterol Nutr* 1983;2:302–306.

232. Leroi A, Berkelsmans I, Denis P, et al. Anismus as a marker of sexual abuse. Consequences of abuse on rectal motility. *Dig Dis Sci* 1995;40:1411–1416.

233. Klauser AG, Peyeri C, Schindlebeck NE, et al. Nutrition and physical activity in chronic constipation. *Eur J Gastroenterol Hepatol* 1992;4:227–232.

234. Wald A. Slow transit constipation. *Curr Treat Options Gastroenterol* 2002;5:279–283.

235. Borum ML. Constipation: evaluation and management. *Prim Care* 2001;28:577–590.

236. Schiller LR. Review article: the therapy of constipation. *Aliment Pharmacol Ther* 2001;15:749–763.

237. Bardhan K, Schwarz R, Kanty-Okulewicz M, et al. Tegaserod is effective in relieving the multiple symptoms of chronic constipation (CC): pooled data from two phase III studies. *Gastroenterology* 2004;126:A-643.

238. Talley N, Kamm M, Müller-Lissner S, et al. Tegaserod is effective in relieving the multiple symptoms of constipation: results from a 12-week multinational study in patients with chronic constipation. *Am J Gastroenterol* 2003;98:S269–S270.

239. Gasslander T, Larsson J, Wetterfors J. Experience of surgical treatment for chronic ideopathic constipation. *Acta Chir Scand* 1987;153:553–555.

240. Kamm MA, Hawley PR, Lennard-Jones JE. Outcome of colectomy for severe idiopathic constipation. *Gut* 1988;29:969–973.

241. Cox DJ, Sutphen J, Borowitz S, et al. Simple electromyographic biofeedback treatment for chronic pediatric constipation/encopresis: preliminary report. *Biofeedback Self Regul* 1994;19:41–50.

242. Patankar SK, Ferrara A, Levy JR, et al. Biofeedback in colorectal practice: a multicenter, statewide, three-year experience. *Dis Colon Rectum* 1997;40:827–831.

243. Gilliland R, Heymen S, Altomare DF, et al. Outcome and predictors of success of biofeedback for constipation. *Br J Surg* 1997;84:1123–1126.

244. Rao SS, Welcher KD, Pelsang RE. Effects of biofeedback therapy on anorectal function in obstructive defecation. *Dig Dis Sci* 1997;42:2197–2205.

245. Koutsomanis D, Lennard-Jones JE, Roy AJ, et al. Controlled randomised trial of visual biofeedback versus muscle training without a visual display for intractable constipation. *Gut* 1995;37:95–99.

246. Veale D, Kavanagh G, Fielding JF, et al. Primary fibromyalgia and the irritable bowel syndrome: different expressions of a common pathogenetic process. *Br J Rheumatol* 1991;30: 220–222.

247. Wolfe F, Smythe HA, Yunus MB, et al. The American College of Rheumatology 1990 criteria for the classification of fibromyalgia. A report of the Multicenter Criteria Committee. *Arthritis Rheum* 1990;33:160–172.

248. Thompson WG, Dotevall G, Drossman DA, et al. Irritable bowel syndrome: guidelines for the diagnosis. *Gastroenterol Int* 1989;2:92–95.

249. Sperber AD, Atzmon Y, Neumann L, et al. Fibromyalgia in the irritable bowel syndrome: studies of prevalence and clinical implications. *Am J Gastroenterol* 1999;94: 3541–3546.
250. Mayer EA. Emerging disease model for functional gastrointestinal disorders. *Am J Med* 1999;107:12S–19S.
251. Gracely RH, Petzke F, Wolf JM, et al. Functional magnetic resonance imaging evidence of augmented pain processing in fibromyalgia. *Arthritis Rheum* 2002;46:1333–1343.
252. Clauw DJ, Crofford LJ. Chronic widespread pain and fibromyalgia: what we know, and what we need to know. *Best Pract Res Clin Rheumatol* 2003;17:685–701.

19

Genitourinary Associations with Fibromyalgia

Daniel J. Wallace and Swamy Venuturupalli

Depictions of irritable bladder and chronic pelvic pain not attributable to anatomic lesions or infection were briefly mentioned in urologic and gynecologic textbooks and in a handful of articles beginning in the 1960s but not given serious consideration until recently (1). It appears that while these complaints are more prevalent in fibromyalgia (FM) patients, individuals with genitourinary manifestations have a higher frequency of specific psychosocial stressors and issues than others in the syndrome spectrum (see Table 19-1).

IRRITABLE BLADDER OR FEMALE URETHRAL SYNDROME

Characterized by suprapubic pressure or discomfort, frequency of urination, and possibly dysuria, irritable bladder was first reported in women who had symptoms resembling a urinary tract infection but had a normal urinalysis and bacterial culture (2). Although palpation of the bladder by bimanual pelvic exam may be tender and reproduce the symptoms, no other abnormalities are noted. The prevalence of irritable bladder is not known, but it has been estimated that 5% to 20% of urology out-patient referrals relate to the problem, which also accounts for 5 million visits to a gynecologist annually (2,3). Wallace was the first to connect these manifestations with FM, with 6 of 50 patients fulfilling accepted definitions for female urethral syndrome versus none of 50 other rheumatic disease patients ($p<0.05$) (4). These findings were confirmed by Paira, who observed an association in 38 of 212 FM patients (18%) but none of the healthy controls (5). Wolfe queried 256 FM patients and 233 matched rheumatic disease controls about genitourinary symptoms and noted that 59% with FM (versus 41% of controls) complained of nocturia ($p = 0.034$), and 65% (versus 35% of controls) noted urinary urgency ($p<0.01$) (Frederick

Wolfe, personal communication). Chronic pelvic pain (see the next section) is also more common among these patients.

Most patients report frequent urinary tract infections and have had multiple courses of antibiotics (6). Urodynamic studies demonstrate spasticity of the urethral musculature, increased sphincteric tension, and detrusor instability (7,8). One group hypothesized that irritable bladder is a form of female prostatitis (9). Psychological profiles of irritable bladder patients reveal increased tensions and anxieties, childhood sexual abuse, sexual dysfunction, pain levels, and fatigue (10,11). Early efforts to treat the condition with forceful overdilations of the urethra, internal urethral cutting procedures, or surgical excision of periurethral tissue were unsuccessful (8). The best results have been reported with cyclobenzaprine, diazepam, anticholinergic approaches, and hormonal manipulations, as well as biofeedback (12,13).

INTERSTITIAL CYSTITIS

Interstitial cystitis (IC) is a disease of the lining of the bladder and its permeability, which allows certain food substances and beverages to cause significant symptoms of diurnal frequency of urination, urgency, sometimes incontinence, frequent urination at night, and suprapubic discomfort or pain, usually relieved by voiding. IC can be a chronic, progressive, severely debilitating heterogeneous syndrome affecting the urinary bladder. Though known for over a century, its etiology is poorly understood, and universally effective treatments are lacking. IC is nine times more frequent in women than men. The average age for a woman at diagnosis is 40 to 46 years (14). This enigmatic and debilitating bladder syndrome is being diagnosed with increasing frequency and is increasingly recognized by pain clinicians and other physicians. Recent findings also indicate that chronic abacterial prostatitis, prostatodynia in men, and chronic pelvic pain syndrome may be variants of IC (15).

TABLE 19-1	Urogenital Pain Associated with Fibromyalgia

1. Irritable bladder or female urethral syndrome
2. Interstitial cystitis
3. Chronic pelvic pain (excluding infection, scarring, adhesions, myomas)
   a. Vaginal/vulvar: vulvitis, vulvovestibulitis, vaginismus, dyspareunia
   b. Endometriosis (probable)
4. Viscero-somatic symptoms, "chronic pelvic congestion"

PATHOGENESIS

Although the exact cause of IC remains unknown, multiple pathophysiologic mechanisms have been proposed and reported in the scientific literature. Some of the implicated mechanisms for IC include infective agents such as *Escherichia coli* in bladder tissue, mast cell degranulation in damaged urothelium that releases vasoactive and proinflammatory molecules, other angiogenic factors, neuroinflammation from nerve growth factor (NGF), calcitonin gene-related peptide release, extra cellular adenosine triphoshpate (ATP) as a mediator of inflammation, excess substance P urinary excretion, and endocrinologic factors based on the higher prevalence of IC in women (16).

ASSOCIATED CONDITIONS

IC is commonly associated with allergies (to dust, pollen, medications, molds, etc.), sensitive skin, irritable bladder syndrome, and FM (17). Compared with controls, IC patients report increased backache, dizziness, chest pain, joint aches, abdominal cramps, nausea, heart pounding, and headaches (18). FM patients report high rates of bladder symptoms consistent with the female urethral syndrome that includes patients with IC (4,15). There is a significant overlap in symptomatology between FM and IC patients in terms of widespread pain and tender points (TePs), leading to theories that some of the pain in IC may be centrally mediated nociceptive abnormalities rather than strictly peripheral mechanisms involving the bladder (19).

DIAGNOSING INTERSTITIAL CYSTITIS

Currently there is no universally accepted technique for diagnosing IC. In 1988 the National Institutes of Health developed diagnostic criteria for IC for scientific purposes (20). These criteria are strict research criteria; they probably underdiagnose the condition and generally are not recommended for diagnosing IC in the clinical setting. They do, however, highlight the importance of excluding infection, radiation, chemical agents, tuberculosis (TB), and other conditions (21).

The two characteristic symptoms of IC are pain associated with the bladder and urinary urgency. The average IC patient voids 16 times per day with an average voided volume of 106 mL. Patients with IC often have voiding difficulties such as

hesitancy, postvoid fullness, and interruption of the urinary stream. About 85% of patients have pain associated with the bladder. The site of the pain varies and can be suprapubic, perineal, vaginal, in the lower back, or in the medial aspect of the thighs. Constant pain should prompt a look for other causes of pelvic pathology. Patients with IC typically report symptom flares, especially premenstrually and with certain foods such as alcohol, coffee, carbonated drinks, citrus fruits, tomatoes, and chocolate. Voiding diaries, maintained for 3 days, are very valuable in making the diagnosis of IC and in determining the severity of symptoms as well as the ingestion of bladder irritant foods (21).

Physical examination of the abdomen may reveal suprapubic tenderness, which is a sign of IC. The external genitalia should be examined to exclude vulvodynia or vestibulitis, and the vagina should be examined for atrophic vaginitis and infections, especially sexually transmitted diseases (STDs). A characteristic finding of IC is a tender bladder base, which is identified by palpating the anterior vaginal wall during pelvic examination.

Urinalysis and culture are useful to exclude infections because the IC symptoms of urgency, frequency, and suprapubic pain are also classic for urinary infections. A culture for TB, urine cytology, and urethral and cervical cultures to rule out STDs should be performed, if necessary. Urodynamic evaluation shows characteristic findings for IC such as early first sensation of bladder filling (<100 mL), a decreased volume at first desire (<150 mL), and a decreased maximum bladder capacity (<350 mL) (21). Patients with IC have altered epithelial permeability, which can be measured by the potassium permeability test, where 40 mL of potassium chloride solution placed in the bladder produces urgency and pain, while saline does not (22). There is controversy about the application of this test, however (23). In the diagnosis of IC, the main role of cystoscopy is to rule out bladder carcinoma. While performing cystoscopy, Hunner ulcers, which are areas of erythema with small vessels radiating to a central pale scar after bladder filling, are sometimes noted in IC. The bladder is then distended with water and glomerulations and ulcerations are looked for (24). Petechial hemorrhages may be seen. Though widely used to identify IC patients, these tests have been criticized as these lesions are seen in a large proportion of normal women (25,26). Thus, while the findings on cystoscopy help support the diagnosis of IC and rule out other conditions, neither cystoscopy nor biopsy is completely diagnostic for this condition.

MANAGEMENT OF INTERSTITIAL CYSTITIS

The management of IC remains a challenge because no single agent has been proven universally effective. Dimethyl sulfoxide (DMSO) and pentosan polysulfate (PPS) have been evaluated through early placebo controlled trials, and both are Food and Drug Administration (FDA) approved treatments for this condition. Bacillus Calmette-Guerin (BCG) has been studied in two large placebo control trials with contradictory results (27,28). Intravesical hyaluronic acid is currently being evaluated and shows some promise in helping to relieve symptoms (29,30). Gabapentin has shown promising results in clinical trials (31).

Initial therapy should include dietary changes to avoid acidic foods and behavioral therapy. If this fails, oral therapies with PPS, hydroxyzine, amitriptyline, or gabapentin may be tried. Narcotics may be used for refractory pain. Intravesical therapies with DMSO, heparin hydrodistention under anesthesia (which decreases sympathetic nerves fiber density), BCG, and hyaluronic acid may be tried simultaneously. Interventional treatment has been recommended as a last resort for patients who should be very carefully selected (16,32).

CHRONIC PELVIC PAIN

Chronic pelvic pain is an entity encompassing menstrual or nonmenstrual pain of at least 6 months' duration that occurs below the umbilicus and is severe enough to cause functional disability or require treatment. A syndrome and not a disease, epidemiologic surveys suggest that it accounts for 2% of all gynecologic visits annually in the United States. In one study, 65% of women with chronic pelvic pain were never given a specific diagnosis, 31% were given a gynecologic diagnosis, and 4% turned out to have irritable colon, a hernia, or chronic low back musculoskeletal pain. Chronic pelvic pain is self-reported by 15% of women between the ages of 18 and 50; one third of this group seeks medical care for chronic pelvic pain complaints (33,34).

No study has estimated the prevalence of FM in patients with chronic pelvic pain. Further, chronic pelvic pain encompasses a variety of conditions *unrelated* to FM, including pelvic inflammatory disease, adenomyosis, leiomyomata, uterine prolapse, ovarian cysts or masses, cervical stenosis, and pelvic adhesions. The relationship between FM and endometriosis is not clear. Endometriosis is found in 80% with chronic pelvic pain; its relationship to FM is controversial. According to a study conducted at the National Institutes of Health among 3,680 members of the Endometriosis Association, 5.9% had FM, versus 3.4% of the control group ($p<0.0001$) (35).

HISTORY AND CLINICAL COMPLAINTS

Patients with chronic pelvic pain of the types associated with FM have a greatly increased prevalence of mental health issues, including somatoform disorders (as high as 70%), drug-seeking behavior, physical or sexual abuse experiences (voluntarily disclosed in 25%), and depression. A history of physical or sexual abuse may be even higher in women with these types of pelvic pain than that reported with idiopathic FM (36,37). Patients with FM and chronic pelvic pain are often diagnosed with dyspareunia, vulvitis, vaginismus, or vulvovestibulitis. Predisposing factors to fibromyalgia-related chronic pelvic pain include chronic tense pelvic floor holding patterns that develop in childhood as a result of sexual abuse, abnormal bowel patterns, traumatic toilet training, guilt surrounding sexual feelings, dance training, or stress. Also important are repetitive minor trauma or straining at stool; sudden brief severe strains sustained in sports, dance, or gymnastic accidents; referred pain from attaching muscle

groups or viscera; or direct physical trauma from bicycling, childbirth, or instrumentation at pelvic surgery (38).

The history includes identifying the characteristics of the pain (location, magnitude, timing, quality, relationship to activities; a menstrual, contraceptive, sexual, gynecologic, and obstetric history; information about domestic violence, sexual or substance abuse, and a family history of relevant conditions). The physical examination includes a pelvic, abdominal, rectal, and low back musculoskeletal evaluation (38,39).

PATHOPHYSIOLOGY

Chronic pelvic pain conditions such as female urethral syndrome, vulvodynia, vulvar vestibulitis, and IC have many of the underlying features of central sensitization seen in FM and related conditions. Visceral hyperalgesia, a key component of the functional bowel syndrome and its specific parasympathetic interactions, is also an important factor in chronic pelvic pain (40,41). The additive effect of repetitive sensory inputs from tense pelvic floor holding patterns can stimulate the evolution of myofascial trigger points and pelvic floor hypertonus (42). This leads to referred pain in the perineum, low back, or abdomen; urethral pain with urgency and frequency; anal pain; and vaginal discomfort. Entrapment or stretching-induced neuropathies often involve the ilioinguinal, iliohypogastric, genitofemoral, posterior femoral cutaneous, obturator, pudendal, clitoral, or cluneal nerves.

TREATMENT OF CHRONIC PELVIC PAIN

A detailed medical and psychosocial history and evaluation is essential in approaching chronic pelvic pain patients (43). Even in those with anatomic lesions, uncertain outcomes will result unless one's entire environment is assessed. For example, in two pivotal, randomized, prospective studies of lysis of adhesions for chronic pelvic pain at 1 year, there was no difference in pain scores between control and adhesiolysis groups (44,45). Educational programs, biofeedback, acupuncture, transcutaneous electrical nerve stimulation, nerve stimulating devices (including laparoscopic uterosacral nerve ablation and presacral neurectomy), cognitive-behavioral therapy, pelvic relaxation exercises, reassurance, and counseling are mainstays in the management of chronic pelvic pain. Local injections into dermatologic areas sharing innervation with hyperalgesic abdominal, sacral, and vaginal TePs were associated with an 89% success rate in one study. Botox injections may lead to prolonged relief. As with FM, nonsteroidals; tramadol; local anesthetics; tricyclic antidepressants; hormonal interventions with progestins, gonadotropic releasing hormone, or danocrine; anticonvulsants; and specific serotonin reuptake inhibitors are useful adjuncts (43–50). The long-term prognosis of chronic pelvic pain from noninfectious or nonanatomic lesions has never been addressed (51).

SUMMARY POINTS

- Chronic pelvic pain conditions such as female urethral syndrome, vulvodynia, vulvar vestibulitis, and IC are seen more frequently in FM and vice versa.

- These conditions also share many of the same underlying pathophysiologic features as FM and irritable bowel syndrome, such as visceral hyperalgesia and central sensitization.

■ IMPLICATIONS FOR PRACTICE

- Just as with other chronic-pain syndromes, a comprehensive, multidisciplinary approach with medication, specialized exercises, nonaddicting analgesics, local injections, and addressing psychosocial stressors is advised.

ACKNOWLEDGMENT

The authors thank Drs. Jay Stein (Urology) and Paula Bernstein (Gynecology) for reviewing the manuscript for accuracy.

REFERENCES

1. Gallagher GJA, Montgomerie JZ, North JDK. Acute infections of the urinary tract and the urethral syndrome in general practice. *Br Med J* 1965;1:622–662.
2. Karram MM. The painful bladder: urethral syndrome and interstitial cystitis. *Curr Opin Obstet Gynecol* 1990;2:605–611.
3. Hunt J. Irritable bladder syndrome: a void in the research. *Br J Clin Psychol* 1995;34(Pt 3):435–436.
4. Wallace DJ. Genitourinary manifestations of fibrositis: an increased association with the female urethral syndrome. *J Rheumatol* 1990;17(2):238–239.
5. Paira SO. Fibromyalgia associated with female urethral syndrome. *Clin Rheumatol* 1994;13(1):88–89.
6. Zufall R. Ineffectiveness of treatment of urethral syndrome in women. *Urology* 1978;12:337–339.
7. Cukier JM, Cortina-Borja M, Brading AF. A case-control study to examine any association between idiopathic detrusor instability and gastrointestinal tract disorder and between irritable bowel syndrome and urinary tract disorder. *Br J Urol* 1997;79:865–878.
8. Kaplan WE, Firlit CF, Schoenberg HW. The female urethral syndrome: external sphincter spasm as etiology. *J Urol* 1980;124:48–49.
9. Gittes RF, Nakamura RM. Female urethral syndrome. A female prostatitis? *West J Med* 1996;164:435–438.
10. Cardon CC, Osborne D, Segura JW. Psychologic characteristics of patients with female urethral syndrome. *J Clin Psychol* 1979;35:312–313.
11. Romans S, Belaise C, Martin J, et al. Childhood abuse and later medical disorders in women. An epidemiological study. *Psychother Psychosom* 2002;71:141–150.
12. Yoon SM, Jung JK, Lee SB, et al. Treatment of female urethral syndrome refractory to antibiotics. *Yonsei Med J* 2002;43:644–651.
13. Lentz GM, Bevamdam T, Stenchever MA, et al. Hormonal manipulation in women with chronic, cyclic irritable bladder symptoms and pelvic pain. *Am J Obstet Gynecol* 2002;186:1268–1273.
14. Oravisto K. Epidemiology of interstitial cystitis. *Ann Chir Gynaecol Fenn* 1975;64:75–77.
15. Fall M, Aldenborg F, Johansson S, et al. Clinical characteristics support that interstitial cystitis is a heterogeneous syndrome. *Urology* 2001;57(6 Suppl 1):129–130.
16. Oberpenning F, van Ophoven A, Hertle L. Interstitial cystitis: an update. *Curr Opin Urol* 2002;12(4):321–332.
17. Alagiri M, Chottiner S, Ratner V, et al. Interstitial cystitis: unexplained associations with other chronic disease and pain syndromes. *Urology* 1997;49(Suppl. 5A):52–57.
18. Erickson DR, Morgan KC, Ordille S, et al. Nonbladder related symptoms in patients with interstitial cystitis. *J Urol* 2001;166(2):557–561; discussion 561–562.
19. Clauw DJ, Schmidt M, Radulovic D, et al. The relationship between fibromyalgia and interstitial cystitis. *J Psychiatr Res* 1997;31(1):125–131.
20. Gillenwater JY, Wein AJ. Summary of the National Institute of Arthritis, Diabetes, Digestive and Kidney Diseases. Workshop on interstitial cystitis. National Institutes of Health, Bethesda, MD, August 28-29, 1987. *J Urol* 1988; 140(1):203–206.
21. Myers DL, Arya LA. Diagnosing interstitial cystitis in women. *Womens Health Prim Care* 2000;3(12):868–874.
22. Parsons CL, Stein PC, Bidair M, et al. Abnormal sensitivity to intravesical potassium in interstitial cystitis and radiation cystitis. *Neurourol Urodyn* 1994;13(5):515–520.
23. Ratner V. Current controversies that adversely affect interstitial cystitis patients. *Urology* 2001;57(6 Suppl 1):89–94.
24. Rosamilia A, Cann L, Scurry J, et al. Bladder microvasculature and the effects of hydrodistention in interstitial cystitis. *Urology* 2001;57(6 Suppl 1):132.
25. Waxman JA, Sulak PJ, Kuehl TJ. Cystoscopic findings consistent with interstitial cystitis in normal women undergoing tubal ligation. *J Urol* 1998;160(5):1663–1667.
26. Mishra N. To study the effect of hydrodistention on bladder mucosa and submucosa. *Urology* 2001;57(6 Suppl 1):126.
27. Peeker R, Haghsheno MA, Holmang S, et al. Intravesical bacillus Calmette-Guerin and dimethyl sulfoxide for treatment of classic and nonulcer interstitial cystitis: a prospective, randomized double-blind study. *J Urol* 2000;164(6):1912–1915; discussion 1915–1916.
28. Peters KM, Diokno AC, Steinert BW, et al. The efficacy of intravesical bacillus Calmette-Guerin in the treatment of interstitial cystitis: long-term followup. *J Urol* 1998; 159(5):1483–1486; discussion 1486–1487.
29. Morales A, Emerson L, Nickel JC, et al. Intravesical hyaluronic acid in the treatment of refractory interstitial cystitis. *J Urol* 1996;156(1):45–48.
30. Nordling J, Jorgensen S, Kallestrup E. Cystistat for the treatment of interstitial cystitis: a 3-year follow-up study. *Urology* 2001;57(6 Suppl 1):123.
31. Hansen HC. Interstitial cystitis and the potential role of gabapentin. *South Med J* 2000;93(2):238–242.
32. Lukban JC, Whitmore KE, Sant GR. Current management of interstitial cystitis. *Urol Clin North Am* 2002;29(3):649–660.
33. Mathias SD, Kuppermann M, Lieberman RF, et al. Chronic pelvic pain: prevalence, health-related quality of life, and economic correlates. *Obstet Gynecol* 1996;87:321–327.
34. Zondervan KT, Yudkin PK, Vessey MP, et al. Prevalence and incidence of chronic pelvic pain in primary care: evidence from a national general practice database. *Br J Obstet Gynaecol* 1999;106:1149–1159.
35. Sinaii N, Cleary SD, Ballweg ML, et al. High rates of autoimmune and endocrine disorders, fibromyalgia, chronic fatigue syndrome and atopic diseases among women with endometriosis: a survey analysis. *Hum Reprod* 2002;17:2715–2724.
36. Walker E, Katon W, Harrop-Griffiths J, et al. Relationship of chronic pelvic pain to psychiatric diagnoses and childhood sexual abuse. *Am J Psychiatry* 1988;145:75–80.
37. Rapkin AJ, Kames LJ, Darke LL, et al. History of physical and sexual abuse in women with chronic pelvic pain. *Obstet Gynecol* 1990;76:92–96.

38. Prendergast SA, Weiss JM. Screening for musculoskeletal causes of pelvic pain. *Clin Obstet Gynecol* 2003;46:772–782.

39. Scialli AR, Pelvic Pain Expert Working Group. Evaluating chronic pelvic pain, a concensus recommendation. *J Reprod Med* 1999;44:945–952.

40. Hogston P. Irritable bowel syndrome as a cause of chronic pain in women attending a gynaecology clinic. *Br Med J* 1987;294:934–935.

41. Parsons CL, Dell J, Stanford EJ, et al. The prevalence of interstitial cystitis in gynecologic patients with pelvic pain, as detected by intravesical potassium sensitivity. *Am J Obstet Gynecol* 2002;187:1395–1400.

42. Wesselman V, Lai J. Mechanisms of referred visceral pain: uterine inflammation in the adult virgin rat results in neurogenic plasma extravasation in the skin. *Pain* 1997;73:309–317.

43. Gambone JC, Mittman BS, Munro MG, et al. Concensus statement for the management of chronic pelvic pain and endometriosis: proceedings of an expert-panel concensus process. *Fertil Steril* 2002;78:961–972.

44. Peters AA, Trimbos-Kemper GC, Admiraal C, et al. A randomized clinical trial on the benefit of adhesiolysis in patients with intraperitoneal adhesions and chronic pelvic pain. *Br J Obstet Gynecol* 1992;99:59–62.

45. Swank DJ, Swank-Bordewijk SC, Hop WC, et al. Laparoscopic adhesiolysis in patients with chronic abdominal pain: a blinded, randomized, controlled multi-centre trial. *Lancet* 2003;361:1247–1251.

46. Engel CC, Walker EA, Engel AL, et al. A randomized, double-blind crossover trial of sertraline in women with chronic pelvic pain. *J Psychosom Res* 1998;44:203–207.

47. Walker EA, Sullivan MD, Stenchever MA. Use of antidepressants in the management of women with chronic pelvic pain. *Obstet Gynecol Clin North Am* 1993;20:743–751.

48. Sutton C, Pooley AS, Jones KD, et al. A prospective, randomized, double-blind controlled trial of laparoscopic uterine nerve ablation in the treatment of pelvic pain associated with endometriosis. *Gynecol Endosc* 2001;10:217–221.

49. Candiani GB, Fedele L, Vercellini P, et al. Presacral neurectomy for the treatment of pelvic pain associated with endometriosis: a controlled study. *Am J Obstet Gynecol* 1992;167:100–103.

50. Slocumb JC. Operative management of chronic abdominal pelvic pain. *Clin Obstet Gynecol* 1990;33:96–204.

51. Gunter J. Chronic pelvic pain: the myofascial component. *The Female Patient* 2004;29:9–16.

20

Chronic Low Back Pain

Thorsten Giesecke and Michael E. Geisser

EPIDEMIOLOGY

Chronic low back pain (CLBP) is one of the most common and expensive musculoskeletal disorders in all western countries (1,2). Back pain in general affects 70% to 85% of all people at some time in their lives, but 90% of affected individuals recover, typically within 12 weeks (3). Recovery after 12 weeks is slow and uncertain, and this subset of patients with CLBP is responsible for major expenses in the health-care and disability systems (2,4). Patients who develop CLBP account for 70% to 80% of the costs for work-related low back claims (5,6). Annual costs of low back disability in the United States have been estimated to be approximately $50 billion, with the average cost of a single case of work-related back pain exceeding $8,000 (7). Its prevalence also appears to be on the rise, as 31.8% of disability claims in 1990 were due to back pain, compared to 29.2% in 1981 (8).

DIAGNOSTIC EVALUATION

Differential diagnosis of CLBP can be difficult. Although in probably more than 70% of patients complaining about low back pain no exact diagnosis can be given, a number of musculoskeletal or visceral diseases may be causing the pain (see Table 20-1). First intention of the diagnostic evaluation should be to identify or exclude these diseases. In many cases a thorough history and physical examination can answer most questions, and imaging is often unnecessary (9).

MEDICAL HISTORY

Taking a patient's history is an important step toward a trustful relationship between patient and caregiver. The beginning should include a careful definition of the circumstances leading to the onset, character, and precise location of the origin or radiation pattern of the pain. Radicular pain, as in sciatica or pseudoclaudication (leg pain after walking that mimics ischemic claudication) usually suggests neurologic involvement. The leg pain of sciatica or pseudoclaudication is often associated with numbness or paresthesia, and sciatica due to disk herniation typically increases with cough, sneezing, or performance of the Valsalva maneuver. Spinal stenosis due to hypertrophic degenerative processes and degenerative spondylolisthesis is more common in older than in younger adults. The symptoms of spinal stenosis are often diffuse because the disease is usually bilateral and involves several vertebrae (10). Pain, numbness, and tingling may occur in one or both legs. Spinal flexion usually relieves the symptoms, so that patients report less pain when they are sitting or pushing a grocery cart (11). Pain is often increased by extension of the lumbar spine (11). The diagnosis can usually be made on the basis of CT or magnetic resonance imaging (MRI).

Back pain may also be referred, resulting from visceral or spinal disease that shares the same spinal segment distribution as the site where the pain is perceived—for example, pyelonephritis, aortic aneurysm, osteoporosis and compression fractures, and osteomyelitis. Visceral referred pain is not typically affected by motion or relieved by rest; it tends to be more constant and worse at night. However, these findings are not specific for the presence of these conditions. Other clues to underlying systemic disease include the patient's age; a history of cancer, unexplained weight loss, injection-drug use, or chronic infection; the duration of pain; the presence of nighttime pain; and the response to previous therapy.

Prolonged back pain may be associated with the failure of previous treatment, depression, and somatization. Increasing age, female gender, substance abuse, lower levels of formal education, stress, job dissatisfaction, and disability/compensation issues may all play some role in expression of symptoms and in chronicity (2,12–16).

TABLE 20-1	Differential Diagnosis of Chronic Low Back Pain

SPINAL PATHOLOGY	HINTS
Spinal stenosis	Diffuse neurologic deficits, pseudoclaudication; pain is relieved by lumbar flexion and increased by lumbar extension
Herniated disk	Pain increases with cough, Valsalva maneuver
Spondylolisthesis	Age <20
Cauda equina syndrome	Bowel or bladder dysfunction
Tumors	Weight loss, familial history, age >55
Infection	Fever, vertebral tenderness, no relief when lying
Osteoporosis	Female, age >65

VISCERAL DISEASES	
Endometriosis	Other gynecologic symptoms
Prostatitis	Other urologic symptoms
Aortic aneurysm	Age >65, coronary artery disease
Pancreatitis	Other gastrointestinal symptoms
Cholecystitis	Other gastrointestinal symptoms
Gastric/duodenal ulcer	Other gastrointestinal symptoms
Renal diseases	Loin pain with radiation

PHYSICAL EXAMINATION

Low back pain may be associated with tender points (TePs) (i.e., tenderness felt on firm palpation), which may be localized as in myofascial pain syndromes, or widespread as in fibromyalgia syndrome (FMS). Vertebral tenderness has sensitivity for infection but not specificity. Fever suggests the possibility of spinal infection.

Limited spinal motion is not strongly associated with any specific diagnosis, but this finding may help in planning or monitoring physical therapy (9). Chest expansion of <2.5 cm has specificity, but not sensitivity, for ankylosing spondylitis (17).

Among patients with sciatica or pseudoclaudication, a straight-leg-raising test should be performed (1). However, the test is often negative in patients with spinal stenosis. An elevation of <60 degrees is abnormal, suggesting compression or irritation of the nerve roots. A positive test reproduces the symptoms of sciatica, with pain that radiates below the knee, not merely back or hamstring pain. Ipsilateral straight-leg raising has sensitivity but not specificity for a herniated disk, whereas crossed straight-leg raising (with the symptoms of sciatica reproduced when the opposite leg is raised) is insensitive but highly specific (9,18). The remainder of the neurologic examination should focus on ankle and great-toe dorsiflexion strength (the L5 nerve root), plantar flexion strength (S1), ankle and knee reflexes (S1 and L4), and dermatomal sensory loss. The L5 and S1 nerve roots are involved in approximately 95% of lumbar-disk herniations (9,19).

When the neurologic examination is less clear, further physiologic evidence of nerve root dysfunction should be considered before ordering an imaging procedure. Electromyography (EMG), including H-reflex tests, may be useful to identify subtle focal neurologic dysfunction in patients with leg symptoms lasting longer than 3 to 4 weeks (20). Sensory evoked potentials (SEPs) may be added to the assessment if spinal stenosis or spinal cord myelopathy is suspected.

Aortic aneurysm should be suspected among older adults with coronary artery disease or multiple risk factors. Physical examination detects some aneurysms, but ultrasonography, computed tomography (CT), or MRI is often necessary.

ELECTROMYOGRAPHY

EMG records electrophysiological signals from spinal muscles. These signals supposedly consist of motor unit action potentials observed when the muscles are activated. The presumed association between low back pain and muscle fatigue provides the rationale for studying pain with EMG. Nevertheless, an actual association between pain and fatigue has yet to be established. Excessive fatigue due to muscle deconditioning, inhibition of muscle activation secondary to pain, and pain-related action have all been suggested as possible causes of low back pain (21). Needle electromyography (NEMG) and fine-wire electromyography (FWEMG) are the gold standard, but the techniques are invasive and yield limited data (22). Paraspinal mapping using NEMG was developed to assess the extent of denervation of the paraspinal muscles in the low back (23,24). This technique is likewise invasive and painful, which limits its usefulness. Surface electromyography (SEMG) techniques are not invasive and pick up the signal of a greater area. They cannot record single muscle activity. But although two studies found SEMG a useful tool for discriminating between CLBP patients and healthy controls (25,26), the report of the Therapeutics and Technology Assessment Subcommittee of the American Academy of Neurology, a review of more than 2,500 original articles, reviews, and books, considered SEMG unacceptable as a clinical tool in the diagnosis of neuromuscular disease at this time and unacceptable as a clinical tool in the diagnosis of low back pain at this time (22).

IMAGING

Plain radiography provides information about the presence of interosseous pathology, intervertebral disk height, and overall sagittal and coronal plane alignment. Flexion and extension views may dynamically demonstrate increased segmental motion that is not evident on the static films. However, the extent to which such an increase in segmental motion represents instability in the nontraumatic setting is somewhat poorly defined (27). Guidelines recommend plain radiography only for patients with clinical findings suggestive of systemic disease (e.g., fever, unexplained weight loss, a history of cancer, neurologic deficits, and alcohol or injection-drug abuse), an age of more than 50 years, or trauma (28). However, plain radiography is not highly sensitive for early cancer or infection, and therefore systemic diseases should be ruled out only after additional tests like erythrocyte sedimentation rate and a complete blood count (29).

MRI has dramatically increased the ability to assess non-invasively the intervertebral disks and surrounding soft tissue structures. The age-related loss of water content within the disks appears as a loss of bright signal on T2-weighted MRI images and has led to the concept of "dark disk disease." MRI also reveals herniated disks and spinal stenosis, which plain radiography cannot do. In addition, MRI has helped define a number of disk abnormalities, including annular tears (30) and endplate abnormalities (31). But the relationship between disk and other abnormalities and low back pain is controversial, mostly because they are common also among asymptomatic adults (31–33). Degenerated, bulging, and herniated disks are frequently incidental findings and are not predictive for the subsequent development of low back pain (34). Therefore, MRI should be reserved for patients for whom there is a strong clinical suggestion of underlying infection, cancer, or persistent neurologic deficit because it is more sensitive than plain radiography for the detection of early spinal infections and cancers.

A controversial method in the diagnosis of low back pain is that of provocative diskography. The diskography procedure involves the insertion of a needle into the nucleus pulposus, the injection of saline and contrast fluid, measurement of the injection pressure and the subjective pain response to the infusion, and a CT scan to describe the morphologic appearance of the dye within the disk. The purpose of this method is to determine levels for surgical fusion by identifying a "symptomatic disk" when the injection reproduces the patient's back pain symptoms. But although the use of diskography to identify symptomatic disk degeneration is supported in the literature (35), the need for fusion surgery is not, since two-thirds of patients with positive diskography may improve with nonoperative therapy (36).

PATHOGENESIS

SPINAL DEGENERATION

The pathophysiologic causes of CLBP vary but, in general, remain undetermined. Some causes include degenerative changes in the spine, like spinal stenosis and spondylolisthesis. They are usually accompanied by radicular pain and can be detected by MRI. Disk abnormalities, including ruptures, annular tears, and endplate abnormalities, have led to the term "discogenic" low back pain (nonradicular pain in the absence of spinal deformity and instability without neural signs). But despite advances in imaging, in most patients it is impossible to determine whether these identifiable structural or mechanical abnormalities are responsible for the pain (37,38). As mentioned in the imaging section, even when anatomic abnormalities are detected, the significance is unclear, since signs of degeneration like bulging disks or annular tears are found in high percentages of asymptomatic individuals (32,33) and are not predictive for the subsequent development of low back pain (34). However, the vast majority of CLBP patients have no observable underlying organic pathology. White and Gordon indicate that as many as 85% of patients with low back pain have no

identifiable organic pathology (39). These patients usually are given nonspecific diagnoses, such as "lumbar strain or sprain," "chronic intractable benign pain syndrome," (40) and "idiopathic" or "nonspecific low back pain" (41).

PSYCHOSOCIAL FACTORS

This mismatch between anatomic abnormalities and symptoms has led to studies of the psychosocial factors that may contribute to CLBP. These studies show that factors like increasing age, female gender, lower levels of formal education, depression, stress, job dissatisfaction, and disability/compensation issues may play some role in expression of symptoms and in chronicity (12–16).

In a systematic review that included only well-controlled, prospective, longitudinal studies, Linton (42) investigated the association of psychosocial factors on onset and development of CLBP. Using a grading system, he defined level A evidence when at least two studies supported the prospective power of a variable. Level B evidence was defined as support from one study, level C evidence meant inconclusive results, and level D meant no support for prospective power. Chronic distress in daily life, depressive symptoms, and work dissatisfaction were most strongly associated with the onset of back and neck pain. Chronic stress in daily life, work dissatisfaction, depressive symptoms, catastrophizing, fear-avoidance beliefs, and avoidance behavior were clearly linked to the development of chronic pain and disability. Extreme suppressive coping behavior seems to be equally predictive for the development of CLBP. A number of studies have produced at least level B evidence for this association (43,44).

However, all the known demographic and psychosocial factors that might cause CLBP do not explain the symptoms in a significant number of subjects (42,45).

MUSCULOSKELETAL MECHANISMS

In cases where the etiology of CLBP is not readily apparent, traditional medical differential diagnosis would suggest that the cause must then be primarily psychogenic, and this is often inferred (46,47). However, it is unlikely that such a large proportion of CLBP is primarily psychogenic, although this is not to say that psychosocial factors do not influence the experience of CLBP. It is proposed that other potential pathophysiologic factors in chronic pain often tend to go unnoticed or undetected, particularly musculoskeletal causes of pain. Although there are no validated "objective" tests that precisely identify musculoskeletal conditions such as myofascial pain, the neuroanatomical basis for musculoskeletal pain has been described in the literature (48). Lewit reported that over 90% of patients with "nonspecific pain" are affected by myofascial pain syndromes and dysfunctional joints (49). Another study found that 43% of patients evaluated in a 1-year period fulfilled the diagnostic criteria for chronic intractable benign pain (50). Of these patients, all had at least one physical finding suggestive of musculoskeletal dysfunction, such as tender nodules, trigger points, decreased ranges of motion in the back or neck, and rigid musculature. Educating patients about musculoskeletal causes of pain, in addition to providing specific interventions for musculoskeletal dysfunctions, may have important benefits and is discussed further below.

CENTRAL NERVOUS MECHANISMS

Pain in other "idiopathic" chronic-pain conditions, such as irritable bowel syndrome (IBS) and FMS, appears to result from abnormalities in central pain processing rather than from damage or inflammation of peripheral structures. A common finding in these "central" pain syndromes is increased tenderness to pressure, which can be classified as either mechanical hyperalgesia (i.e., increased pain in response to normally painful stimuli) and/or mechanical allodynia (i.e., pain in response to normally nonpainful stimuli) (51,52). These abnormalities are found even in the absence of any identifiable psychological or behavioral factors and thus implicate central mechanisms that exacerbate pain (e.g., "wind-up") or attenuate pathways that begin in the brainstem and normally inhibit the ascending transmission of pain-related activity (53–55).

Clauw et al. were the first to show increased sensitivity to stimulation-evoked pain in a cohort of patients with CLBP (45). In this study they also demonstrated that the measure of pressure-pain sensitivity was the best correlate of pain and functional status, exceeding the predictive value of any other demographic, psychological, or radiographic variables.

Giesecke et al. (56) have recently replicated these findings (see Figure 20-1) and corroborated them by functional brain imaging techniques, which allow visualization of changes in regional cerebral blood flow associated with the application of painful stimuli (see Figures 20-2 and 20-3; Tables 20-2 and 20-3). Functional brain imaging methods infer increased neural activity from highly localized increases in regional cerebral blood flow produced in response to anticipated metabolic demands. These methods can use infusion of radioactive tracers (57,58) or, in the case of functional magnetic resonance imaging (fMRI), use the magnetic character of the level of oxygen in the blood as an indirect, intrinsic tracer (59). Functional imaging studies have consistently shown that painful stimulation produces increased neural activity in structures involved in the processing of sensation, movement, cognition, and emotion (58,60,61).

The experimental pain testing performed in these studies showed that a subset of individuals with idiopathic CLBP has increased pressure-pain sensitivity at a site distant from their region of clinical pain, suggesting central rather than peripheral pain mechanisms. The association of CLBP with a central disturbance in pain processing is congruent with findings in other chronic-pain states. Increased pain sensitivity outside the areas of clinical pain has been reported for other regional pain syndromes, such as tension-type headache (62), temporomandibular disorder (63,64), and localized trapezius myalgia (53). Lowered pain thresholds have also been shown in patients with regional or widespread pain who do not have the 11 TePs required for the diagnosis of FM (65).

The enhanced neural response in pain-related brain regions also contributes to the growing physical evidence of altered physiologic pain processing in CLBP patients. These results are also consistent with other functional imaging studies that have suggested augmented central pain processing in chronic-pain conditions, including FM (66,67), IBS (68), cerebral infarction complicated by allodynia (69), and atypical facial pain (70).

These data suggest that individual pain thresholds of CLBP patients should be evaluated in clinical practice. The finding of a low pressure-pain threshold at neutral sites indicates a central rather than peripheral cause for their pain. This information may guide treatment: Drugs that affect central levels of neuromodulators known to be involved in pain processing, such as tricyclic antidepressants, are more effective for CLBP than alternate classes of compounds that work well for peripheral pain [e.g., nonsteroidal anti-inflammatory drugs (NSAIDs) or opioids] (71,72). Similarly, nonpharmacologic therapies such as aerobic exercise and cognitive-behavioral therapy can be especially useful adjuncts to treating this constellation of symptoms and syndromes (73).

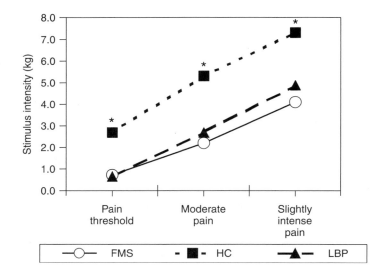

Figure 20-1. Stimulus-response functions for low back pain patients (LBP), fibromyalgia patients (FMS), and healthy controls (HC), obtained by psychophysical pain testing using the multiple random staircase (MRS) paradigm: stimulus intensities for pain thresholds and suprathreshold stimuli sufficient to elicit a rating of moderate pain (7.5/20 units on Gracely pain box scale), and slightly intense pain (13.5/20 units on Gracely pain box scale) in each group. Both patient groups show a significant lowering with almost identical slope (* = $p < .05$).

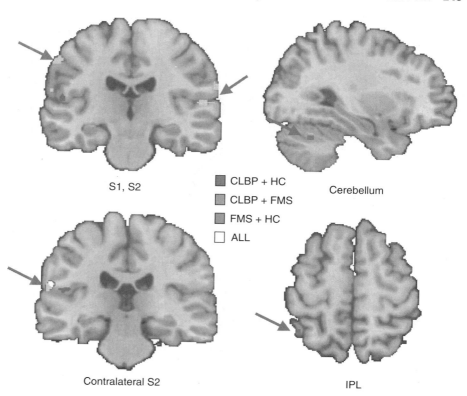

Figure 20-2. Overlapping neuronal activations at equal stimulus condition. Pain-related neuronal activations in chronic low back pain (CLBP), fibromyalgia patients (FMS), and healthy controls (HC) at the equal pressure condition. Significant increases in neuronal activation (*arrows*) are shown in standard space superimposed on a structural T1 weighted magnetic resonance imaging (MRI). Images are shown in radiologic view, with the right brain shown on the left. Overlapping activations appear in shading explained in the legend in the image. Equal pressure intensities result in five overlapping areas of neuronal activation of CLBP and FMS [contralateral primary somatosensory cortex (S1), secondary somatosensory cortex (S2), inferior parietal lobule (IPL), ipsilateral S2, and cerebellum] but only one overlapping area of neuronal activation between HC, CLBP, and FMS (contralateral S2).

TABLE 20-2	Significant Increases in Neuronal Activations for the Equal Pressure (2 kg) Condition					
SIDE	**CORTICAL REGION**	**GROUP**	**X**	**Y**	**Z**	**Z-SCORE**
Contralateral	Primary somatosensory	CLBP	57	−13	43	7.73632
		FMS	59	−15	43	5.15532
	Secondary somatosensory	HC	61	−18	21	4.20553
		CLBP	55	−22	18	7.23976
		FMS	65	−28	16	5.02477
Ipsilateral	Secondary somatosensory	CLBP	−65	−15	12	5.86164
		FMS	−59	−17	10	4.77318
	Inferior parietal	CLBP	46	−144	56	4.45876
		FMS	40	−46	59	4.44034
	Cerebellum	CLBP	−32	−57	−21	3.55417
		FMS	−30	−56	−22	5.27124

CLBP, low back pain; FMS, fibromyalgia; HC, healthy control subjects. X, Y, Z are standard coordinates in mm in the three-dimensional Talairach space. At this stimulus level, only one area (contralateral S2) shows common activation in all three groups, while all other areas show significant activation for CLBP and FMS.

MANAGEMENT

As should be fairly obvious from this chapter so far, in most cases it is impossible to delineate the exact cause of low back pain. Patients suffering from CLBP are most likely not a homogeneous group but a heterogeneous population with a common symptom that is caused by a wide spectrum of conditions. Although the contemporary management of CLBP focuses primarily on conservative treatments, some might profit from a surgical intervention.

CONSERVATIVE TREATMENT

Current conservative treatments for CLBP can be divided into interventions that attempt to "normalize" the physical causes of pain and those that do not necessarily "treat the underlying pathology" but are designed to decrease the experience of pain. Given that many contend that conventional treatments for pain have been unsuccessful (74,75), functional restoration treatments have emerged where the goal of treatment is not to "treat" the etiology of pain or guide treatment by pain reports; rather the focus

TABLE 20-3	Significant Increases in Neuronal Activations for the Equal Pain Condition (Slightly Intense Pain)					
SIDE	**CORTICAL REGION**	**GROUP**	**X**	**Y**	**Z**	**Z-SCORE**
Contralateral	Primary somatosensory	HC	57	−27	46	4.0843
		CLBP	57	−19	42	7.94725
		FMS	57	−13	43	5.39763
	Secondary somatosensory	HC	55	−21	12	4.59193
		CLBP	61	−15	14	7.72307
		FMS	65	−22	18	6.56891
	Inferior parietal lobule	HC	53	−44	50	3.60315
		CLBP	51	−46	48	3.7111
		FMS	42	−40	48	3.70678
	Insula	HC	50	−23	16	4.58386
		CLBP	48	−24	20	5.9398
		FMS	40	2	9	5.06572
	ACC	HC	2	4	46	3.86455
		CLBP	2	12	42	3.94788
		FMS	2	18	40	3.87204
Ipsilateral	Secondary somatosensory	HC	−69	−17	19	6.09707
		CLBP	−63	−17	12	7.51685
		FMS	−67	−17	10	6.88006
	Cerebellum	HC	−36	−65	−22	6.11633
		CLBP	−34	−59	−21	5.44895
		FMS	−34	−61	−22	7.10124

CLBP, low back pain; FMS, fibromyalgia; HC, healthy control subjects; ACC, anterior cingulate cortex. X, Y, Z are standard coordinates in mm in the three-dimensional Talairach space. At this stimulus level, all pain-related cortical areas show common activations in all three groups.

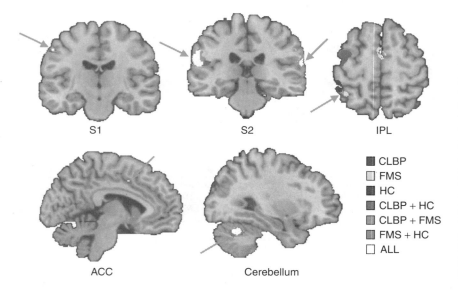

S1 S2 IPL

ACC Cerebellum

■ CLBP
□ FMS
■ HC
■ CLBP + HC
□ CLBP + FMS
■ FMS + HC
□ ALL

Figure 20-3. Overlapping neuronal activations at equal pain condition. Pain-related neuronal activations in chronic low back pain (CLBP), fibromyalgia patients (FMS), and healthy controls (HC) in the equal pain condition. Significant increases in neuronal activations (*arrows*) are shown in standard space superimposed on a structural T1 weighted magnetic resonance imaging (MRI). Images are shown in radiological view, with the right brain shown on the left. Overlapping or adjacent activations appear in shading explained in the legend. Equal subjective pain intensities result in seven overlapping or adjacent areas of neuronal activation in CLBP, HC, and FMS: contralateral S1, S2, IPL, anterior cingulate cortex (ACC), and insula (not shown), ipsilateral S2, and cerebellum.

is on increasing the daily functioning of the patient despite the fact that the patient has pain. Individual treatments, which include medications, injections, electrical stimulation, nontraditional treatments, and cognitive/behavioral therapy, are described below, followed by a discussion of multidisciplinary treatment.

Individual Treatments

Drug Therapy

Drug therapies provide symptomatic relief for pain but do not usually alter pain's underlying physiologic cause (76). Nevertheless, drug therapies are frequently administered to CLBP patients, although there are very few standardized guidelines pertaining to the types of medications that should be administered for specific pain problems. NSAIDs are frequently used to treat CLBP and as a group appear to be superior to placebo and have moderate treatment efficacy (76). However, these medications have been found to have little effect on pain due to sciatica (76). Muscle relaxants also appear to be superior to placebo for treating low back pain (76), but their effectiveness for treating CLBP has rarely been studied. Their mechanism of action is generally unknown. One consideration in prescribing these medications for chronic pain is that nonbenzodiazapine medications [e.g., cyclobenzaprine hydrochloride (Flexeril), methocarbamol (Robaxin), carisoprodol (Soma), and baclofen] may be more appropriate for long-term usage, as these medications have lower potential to produce dependence/tolerance. Cyclobenzaprine hydrochloride is very similar in structure to the tricyclic antidepressants and produces similar side effects. Thus, administering this medication along with a tricyclic antidepressant may produce an undesirable amount of anticholinergic side effects.

Anticonvulsants are frequently used to treat pain of neuropathic origin. It is believed that neuropathic pain is caused at least in part by abnormal firing in central nervous system pain pathways, and anticonvulsants may act to attenuate this abnormal activity, thus relieving pain. Many anticonvulsants have undesirable side effects, such as sedation and bone marrow suppression. Gabapentin has become a popular agent for treating pain, as it appears to have few side effects, and it has good clinical efficacy. A recent study by Serpell (77) found that gabapentin was effective in reducing pain and improving quality of life among persons with a wide range of neuropathic pain syndromes.

Between 2% and 23% of CLBP patients are given antidepressive agents (42). Although depression is common in patients with CLBP, the primary objective in prescribing antidepressants may be to decrease pain rather than to treat depression (42). Within the class of antidepressants, tricyclic compounds are relatively efficacious analgesics, whereas others are not (e.g., highly selective serotonin reuptake inhibitors) (72). The effects of antidepressants may be independent of depression since: (1) antidepressant effects and analgesic effects frequently occur independently of each other in clinical trials and (2) doses of antidepressants necessary to produce analgesia are, in many cases, lower than the dosages required to treat depression (78–82). Several systematic reviews of the efficacy of antidepressants in the treatment of CLBP have reached controversial conclusions: Turner and Denny concluded that there was insufficient evidence to recommend their use (83), and Van Tulder et al. found moderate evidence that they are not effective (84). On the other hand, Salerno (78) found antidepressants to be more effective than placebo, and Staiger et al. (85), by differentiating between different classes of antidepressants, found moderate symptom reduction by tricyclics and tetracyclics but no pain decrease by selective serotonin reuptake inhibitors (SSRIs) and trazodone. The efficacy of various dosages of antidepressants or combinations of antidepressants in chronic-pain patients deserves further study, as a large proportion of patients with chronic pain also suffer from depression (86,87).

The use of opioid medications for the treatment of chronic nonmalignant pain is controversial. There are concerns about the development of addiction, unwanted side effects, and tolerance. Although there is an abundance of literature on the effectiveness of opioids for cancer pain, research examining the efficacy of opioids for treating nonmalignant pain is almost nonexistent. Haythornthwaite et al. (88) reported that 63% of persons with chronic pain treated with opioids had a good treatment response and did not display evidence of impaired cognitive dysfunction. In addition, these patients also displayed significant improvements in mood. A consensus statement published by the American Academy of Pain Management and the American Pain Society (89) proposes that opioids may be of benefit to persons who fail other drug therapies and indicates that many of the commonly held assumptions about opioids, such as the high potential for addiction, need modification.

Transcutaneous Electrical Nerve Stimulation

Transcutaneous electrical nerve stimulation (TENS) is believed to treat or interrupt pain by stimulating large-diameter afferent fibers that modulate pain transmission at spinal or higher levels, thus "closing the gate" on pain transmission (90). Two studies suggest that TENS is superior to placebo in reducing experimental cold induced pain (91) and acute orofacial pain (92). Many types of chronic pain seem to respond to TENS, including peripheral nerve injury, phantom limb pain, shoulder-arm pain, low back pain, and degenerative musculoskeletal disease (90,93). Meyler et al. (93) report that TENS was not as effective in persons with a high degree of psychological and social distress and in persons with pain caused by central and autonomic dysfunction. However, among persons with an initial favorable response, some studies suggest that TENS continues to provide long-term benefits (93,94).

TENS can be varied on several parameters, including the electrode placement, frequency, and intensity of stimulation. There is no apparent consensus in the literature on the optimal parameters for pain control, and, anecdotally, pain control ultimately appears to rely on trial and error giving way to patient preference. Rao et al. found that the location of electrode placement did not appear to influence pain relief (95). High frequency/low intensity TENS is believed to stimulate A-δ fibers and to block pain in the spinal cord, while low-frequency/high-intensity TENS is believed to stimulate β-endorphin production as naloxone blocks the effect of this type of TENS (96). However, some studies have demonstrated that neither type of TENS influences β-endorphin levels in humans (96,97). Some studies have suggested that higher frequency TENS is somewhat superior to lower frequency TENS in terms of reducing both clinical and experimental pain (91,95,98), while other studies report no difference in pain relief produced by high and low-frequency TENS (99). Tulgar et al. found that pain patients preferred frequency modulation and burst stimulation in contrast to conventional continuous stimulation (100). Melzack reports that the duration of pain relief can outlast the period of stimulation by several hours, and on occasion, for days to weeks (90). Thus, TENS may be beneficial even if the stimulation time is limited. Sluka and Walsh (101) report in a recent review on TENS that morphine tolerance reduces the effectiveness of low-frequency TENS in animals; thus high-frequency TENS might be more appropriate among persons taking opioids. In addition, these authors suggest that the effectiveness of TENS might be enhanced if given with certain agonists or antagonists. For example, they indicate that TENS may be more effective in reducing primary hyperalgesia if administered concurrently with morphine or clonidine.

In summary, various studies find TENS to be beneficial in treating several chronic-pain conditions, and it appears to have long-lasting effects in persons who initially respond to the device. A trial period is usually recommended before purchase of the unit. There appears to be a trend for more pronounced benefits produced by higher frequency TENS, and some studies suggest that pain patients prefer burst or frequency modulated stimulation compared to conventional continuous stimulation.

Neural Blockade

Nerve blocks and other types of injections for CLBP have been used both diagnostically and therapeutically for years (102), but have not been extensively investigated in terms of their efficacy in pain diagnosis and treatment (103). Typically, these procedures involve injection of corticosteroids or anesthetic substances, or both. Epidural steroid injections are often used in patients with signs and symptoms of radiculopathy with the belief that steroids will reduce nerve root inflammation, which accompanies the disorder (76). A recent review of studies examining the efficacy of epidural injections indicated that the results of different studies were inconsistent and that the benefits of these injections, if any, seemed to be short-lived (104). Deyo reports that the average clinical effect of epidural steroids is small (10% to 15%) but that even small benefits may be enough to help patients through the acute radicular phase and avoid surgery (76). Small benefits may also help patients progress more quickly in physical therapy or other treatments if employed simultaneously.

Trigger point and tender nodule injections involve infiltration of steroids, anesthetics, or a combination of both into the hypertonic muscle and surrounding tissues. These injections are often used in the diagnosis and treatment of myofascial pain syndrome (103); however, their efficacy has not been demonstrated since less specific techniques (such as needle insertion without injection) have shown results comparable to actual injections (105). Other anesthetic techniques for CLBP include sacroiliac injection and facet blocks (103).

Although these techniques are frequently employed to treat chronic pain, there are few studies examining their efficacy for this (102,103). Most recommend that these procedures be administered within the context of a more comprehensive rehabilitation program to address both the physical and psychosocial aspects of the patient's pain (102). In addition, injections may exacerbate the patient's pain, and substances such as steroids can have undesirable side effects, such as immunosuppression and weight gain (102). Abram and O'Connor (1996) indicate that central nervous system infections may be a complication of repeated epidural injections (106). Further studies appear to be warranted examining the effectiveness of specific types of injections in distinctive subsets of chronic-pain syndromes. Deyo suggests that it

may also be helpful to compare the effectiveness of corticosteroids administered both locally and systemically (76).

Exercise

Exercise is frequently employed in the treatment of CLBP. Exercise may be an important component in the treatment of chronic pain because muscles may become weak and atrophied through disuse (107) and lead to deconditioning, which then may contribute to disability (75). Although it is difficult to tell whether decreased muscle strength among patients with chronic pain is a cause or a consequence of their pain (107), several studies have suggested that decreased strength in the abdominal and spine extensor musculature is associated with the recurrence of persistence of low back pain (108–110). Diminished cardiovascular fitness has also been found to be associated with a higher incidence of back pain disability as well as more frequent episodes of low back pain (109).

In their review of the role of exercise in the treatment of chronic neck and back pain, Rodriquez et al. conclude that nonspecific, general exercise, such as nonspecific strengthening and aerobic conditioning, appears to decrease the intensity of CLBP and protect against recurrence (107). They indicate that little research has been done on the effectiveness of specific types of exercises—for example, whether improvements are related to stretching, strengthening, increased endurance, and/or improved coordination. The optimal frequency and duration of exercise is unknown. In addition, little work has been done to address the issue of compliance with prescribed home exercise programs. Previous studies have demonstrated that compliance with prescribed exercise regimens is poor. Studies indicate that more than 50% of patients in an exercise therapy program will drop out in the first 6 months (111,112).

Clinically, many therapists often prescribe complex regimens that include stretching and strengthening, as well as aerobic exercise. Studies addressing the effectiveness of each of these components, as well as their combination, are warranted, since decreasing the complexity of the regimen may help to increase compliance. Furthermore, it may also be important to examine the effect of general aerobic exercise versus specific adjuvant stretching and strengthening exercises for musculoskeletal dysfunctions.

Education

Although there are little data regarding the effectiveness of educating patients about the physical nature of their pain condition, what data exist suggest that accurate knowledge of the physical etiology of pain, if it can be identified and conveyed to the patient, may be an important determinant of several aspects of the pain experience. Geisser and Roth found that only 32.8% of persons in a chronic-pain sample (predominantly musculoskeletal pain) were able to accurately articulate the cause of their pain, and patients who were unsure of their diagnosis or who disagreed with their actual diagnosis tended to report more dysfunctional pain beliefs, greater psychological distress, higher intensities of chronic pain, and more pain-related disability (113). A path analytic model suggested that lack of knowledge about the etiology of pain was related to greater beliefs that pain is a signal of harm, and that this variable, in addition to affective distress, was significantly related to disability due to pain. Pain intensity was not significantly related to disability. Similar findings have been observed by Lacroix et al. (114) and Roth et al. (115).

Another popular educational intervention for CLBP is back school. Back school is based in part on the work of Nachemson (116), who assessed differences in disk pressure among normals during different functional tasks and found that the highest disk pressures took place while leaning forward or during forward flexion and rotation. Thus, back school in part emphasizes body mechanics during functional tasks that decrease disk pressure. Reviews of the effectiveness of back schools have indicated that many of the studies suffer major methodologic flaws, and outcome results have been mixed (117). In addition, offloading pressure on the spine may place additional stress on other joints and potentially may promote back weakness. Although certainly one should be careful not to overstress the spine, one study found that persons with *acute* low back pain who were prescribed light, normal activity, including bending, actually displayed better outcomes compared to a group of patients who received conservative medical treatment (118).

Manual Therapy

Manual therapy involves the application of specific interventions, such as muscle energy techniques, myofascial release, and thrust techniques to minimize or eliminate musculoskeletal dysfunctions. The mechanism of action is yet unproven, but some authors propose that it involves releasing chronically tight or restricted innervated tissues, thus improving microcirculation, minimizing the corresponding inflammatory response, and decreasing nociception (119). Specific interventions for musculoskeletal conditions have received little empirical attention but include (a) spray and stretch techniques for myofascial pain syndrome (120); (b) various manual therapy techniques, such as joint mobilization and articulartory techniques; (c) muscle energy techniques for specific musculoskeletal dysfunctions, such as hypomobility of spine movement, vertebral malrotation(s), sacroiliac dysfunctions, or innominate dysfunctions (e.g., pelvic asymmetry or torsion) (121); and (d) high-velocity thrust techniques typically employed by chiropractors. In addition to manipulation, Bookhout indicates that instruction on exercises specifically tailored for the patient with chronic musculoskeletal pain and musculoskeletal dysfunction is an important part of treatment (122). These might include specific stretching exercises for shortened muscles, education on proper body mechanics and posture, and self-mobilization exercises. Ideally, the patient can use these techniques as specific pain management tools to improve function and decrease the patient's dependence on ongoing medical care.

Unfortunately, few empirical studies have been conducted on the efficacy of manual therapy and/or specific adjuvant exercises for musculoskeletal dysfunctions. In reviewing the research on manual therapy for chronic pain, Mein (119) indicates that three studies demonstrated positive results (123–125), while one produced negative results (126). Koes et al. (127) identified eight studies examining interventions for subacute and CLBP. Of these, five reported positive results, two reported negative results, and in one

study no conclusion was presented. These authors concluded that the efficacy of manual therapy for CLBP has not been clearly established. A recent study by Hurwitz et al. (128) found that chiropractic care with and without physical modalities and medical care with and without physical therapy produced similar and significant improvements in low back pain. However, the sample was largely comprised of persons with acute low back pain.

Little has been done to examine the combined efficacy of manual therapy and exercise. Recently, Aure et al. (129) examined the impact of manual and exercise therapy in persons with chronic, disabling low back pain. All subjects were prescribed individual home exercises and were encouraged to perform aerobic exercise. Subjects receiving manual therapy underwent sessions twice a week for 8 weeks and were also given exercises specifically designed to treat identified musculoskeletal dysfunctions. The authors found significant improvements in both groups on measures of pain and disability, with the manual therapy group displaying significantly greater gains. However, the study design did not allow for examination of the impact of manual therapy alone, or specific exercise alone, or the combined effect of these interventions. In addition, persons with pain lasting more than 6 months were excluded from the study.

Acupuncture

Acupuncture for pain relief has become increasingly popular in the United States. In terms of providing pain relief, acupuncture is believed to stimulate the production of endogenous opioids. Vincent and Lewith (130) indicate that research regarding the effectiveness of traditional acupuncture for chronic pain, where the needles are placed at classical sites that give rise to a set of sensations referred to as "Teh Chi," is somewhat inconclusive. In fact, acupuncture is somewhat difficult to study empirically, as many control or placebo treatments (e.g., needle insertion at nontraditional sites) may not necessarily be inert (131). Acupuncture also frequently involves electrical stimulation of the needles, thus producing effects similar to TENS. Vincent and Lewith (130) report that in 12 studies comparing classical acupuncture to placebo, 5 demonstrate a significant advantage of acupuncture over placebo and several others show a nonsignificant trend of acupuncture over placebo. In addition, the authors report a slight advantage in terms of response rate of classical acupuncture (60%) over sham acupuncture (40% to 50%) and placebo acupuncture (30%) for chronic pain. Thomas and Lundeberg state that acupuncture with low-frequency electrical stimulation appears to be effective in treating chronic nociceptive musculoskeletal pain (131).

Although there is some evidence that acupuncture may help relieve chronic pain, most studies have employed small samples, and the different parameters of acupuncture that may be particularly effective, such as needle placement and depth of insertion, are not well known. Thomas and Lundeberg suggest that a combination of local and distal needles inserted deeply is optimal (131), but this needs to be investigated further.

Biofeedback and Relaxation Training

These techniques are frequently employed in treating chronic pain. Typically, the goal in biofeedback is to decrease levels of muscle tension in the affected areas. Several studies have suggested that this approach is beneficial in terms of treating back pain (132–135). Flor and Birbaumer (136) found biofeedback to be superior to cognitive-behavioral therapy (CBT) and conservative medical treatment (primarily physical therapy) among patients with musculoskeletal back pain. One study found that patients with the highest electromyographic (EMG) levels responded best to biofeedback (135), while Flor and Birbaumer reported that they obtained the best response in patients with the lowest initial EMG levels (136). Although some studies indicate that biofeedback and relaxation training produce roughly similar outcomes (137), biofeedback may be beneficial among patients with chronic musculoskeletal pain, as these patients have been found to be poor discriminators of levels of muscle tension (138).

Both increased and decreased muscle tension may contribute to chronic pain (139). Studies examining individual subjects suggest that only some patients with chronic pain appear to respond to stress with increased muscle tension (140–142). This suggests that specific recommendations regarding biofeedback may need to be based on an individualized assessment of specific muscle activity patterns.

In addition to examining absolute levels of muscle tension, relative patterns of muscle activity may contribute to CLBP. These include asymmetries in muscle tension or abnormal patterns of muscle activity during dynamic movement. Donaldson et al. report that CLBP patients who underwent single motor unit biofeedback training displayed immediate and sustained decreases in pain, as well as decreased EMG amplitude and asymmetries compared to a relaxation training group and controls (143). Wolf et al. suggest that neuromuscular retraining is an important aspect of treating CLBP (144). On the basis of data from normal subjects, they performed neuromuscular retraining on a back pain patient during trunk movements. The patient reported significantly less pain over time. Thus, biofeedback might be a beneficial adjunct in assisting patients with improving poor body posture, body mechanics, or muscle firing, and ultimately decrease their pain if these are contributing factors.

Relaxation is an important adjunct to biofeedback, as these techniques help generalize the skills learned during biofeedback and help to reduce the effects of stress. Although there is little information about specific relaxation techniques that might be particularly helpful for chronic pain, it is often helpful to teach patients techniques that are practical and can be used while the patient is active, such as deep breathing. Ohrbach and McCall suggest that changes in the muscle stretch receptors may maintain myogenic pain, whereby the contracted muscle state, although painful, actually feels more posturally "normal" to the patient (145). They suggest that contraction-relaxation techniques may be easier for patients with myogenic pain to tolerate, as stretching after the contraction phase is not accompanied by pain.

Cognitive-Behavioral Interventions

The earliest modern psychological interventions and theories of chronic-pain management were primarily based on the work of Fordyce (146), who proposed that environmental contingencies could modify suffering, the behavioral component of pain. Pain treatment programs that followed an operant model were designed to extinguish pain behavior and increase well behavior. Several authors suggest that these interventions are beneficial in treating CLBP (147–149). A study by Roberts et al. found that even a brief, inexpensive outpatient behavioral rehabilitation program was effective in terms of reducing pain and increasing function (150).

In addition to assisting patients in developing more adaptive behavioral responses to pain, modern cognitive/behavioral therapies focus on helping patients to reframe maladaptive thoughts about pain and to employ more adaptive cognitions when faced with pain. Several maladaptive pain beliefs have been identified in the literature, including: (1) the belief that pain is a signal of harm or damage to the body and therefore one should avoid activity or movement; (2) catastrophizing, where patients respond to pain with thoughts that their pain is overwhelming, awful, and horrible; and (3) lack of perceived control over pain, or the belief that nothing one does will change the experience of pain. Research suggests that fear of movement/reinjury significantly contributes to disability and strongly predicts performance during functional tasks (151–154). Catastrophizing has been shown to be related to increased disability, greater pain, and greater emotional distress (155–158). Increasing the patients' perceived control over their pain appears to be related to more favorable chronic-pain adjustment and treatment outcome (152,159,160). Patients can be taught increased control over pain not only through the use of different cognitive/behavioral techniques (e.g., relaxation), but also by remembering to simultaneously use strategies taught by other disciplines, such as the use of icing or stretching encouraged by the physical therapist.

Several studies support the notion that cognitive-behavioral treatment is beneficial in persons with chronic pain. In a recent review of 25 trials of CBT for chronic pain, Morley et al. (161) indicated that the median effect size for these interventions is a standardized mean difference of 0.5, across all outcome domains such as pain, function, and mood. Keefe et al. demonstrated that teaching adaptive pain coping strategies to patients—such as ignoring pain sensations, using coping self-statements, and changing activity patterns—decreased pain and disability (162). Holzman et al. report that distraction may also be an effective coping strategy for patients who tend to focus a great deal on their pain and other bodily sensations (163).

Other studies suggest that additional cognitive/behavioral interventions might be particularly useful for chronic-pain patients whose pain etiology is related to injury or trauma. For example, many authors have reported a high incidence of posttraumatic stress disorder (PTSD) among patients with chronic pain, ranging from 9.5% (164) among patients seen at a multidisciplinary pain clinic to as high as 75% (165) for consecutive patients referred to a psychologist for treatment of headache and other pain resulting from a motor vehicle accident (MVA). Among patients with chronic pain, Geisser et al. found that patients with traumatic pain and high PTSD symptoms displayed the highest levels of disability and pain (166). Turk et al. found that patients with traumatic onset of FM demonstrated greater pain, disability, life interference, and affective distress compared to FM patients whose pain onset was insidious (167). These studies suggest that specific interventions for psychological difficulties that may arise from trauma, such as exposure therapy for PTSD, may be useful adjuncts to treating chronic-pain patients whose pain onset is caused by trauma.

Another important psychological aspect of treating patients with accident-related pain may be the development of feelings of victimization (i.e., one wrongfully suffers because of someone else's mistake or carelessness) and entitlement (i.e., the belief that one is "owed" or should be compensated). DeGood and Kiernan found that chronic-pain patients who blamed their injury on their employer or other source tended to have significantly higher affective distress compared to patients who indicated that no one was at fault for their pain (168). The patients who placed blame also tended to be more refractory to past treatments, were more likely to indicate that their pain would limit their activity, and had higher levels of anticipated pain. Patients who blamed their employer for their pain were also more likely to be unemployed at follow-up.

Multidisciplinary Treatment

It is estimated that there are over 1,000 multidisciplinary pain clinics and pain centers in the United States (40). Given the complexity and multidimensional nature of pain, multidisciplinary treatment is often recommended as the preferred treatment for a number of chronic-pain conditions. Although the specific components of multidisciplinary treatment programs differ, they generally include: (i) ongoing medical care or supervision, (ii) exercise or specific physical therapy intervention, (iii) psychosocial intervention, and (iv) occupational therapy or other services related to daily functioning or vocational rehabilitation, or both. Some programs also offer specialization in pharmacology, dietetics, nursing, and case management. Programs are housed in both inpatient and outpatient settings, although the general trend has been shifting toward providing services through less costly outpatient settings.

A metaanalytic review of multidisciplinary pain treatment for CLBP conducted by Flor et al. concluded that chronic-pain patients treated in multidisciplinary programs were functioning better than 75% of control patients who either received no treatment or patients who were treated by conventional unimodal approaches (169). For example, multidisciplinary treatment was superior to conventional physical therapy alone. Furthermore, these effects appeared to persist over time, and the benefits of multidisciplinary treatment seemed to extend beyond just pain and included increased return to work and decreased use of health care.

A specific type of multidisciplinary approach, labeled functional restoration, has been proposed to be highly effective in treating chronic pain. Given the lack of knowledge regarding "treatable" organic pathology in many chronic-pain patients, functional restoration methods have been proposed as an alternative treatment paradigm. Typically, the focus of the treatment program is to promote function despite the fact that patients experience ongoing pain and other difficulties. Hazard (170) outlines the critical elements of a functional restoration approach, including an interdisciplinary staff, quantification of function to monitor patient status and progress, physical training, and counseling. Two initial studies (171,172) reported that over 80% of patients treated in a functional restoration program were able to return to work

following treatment, and a high percentage were still working at a 1-year follow-up. These studies have been criticized, however, as one of the comparison groups consisted of patients who were not treated due to lack of insurance funding, a group that may differ from the treatment group in terms of other important characteristics (173).

It is unclear what is responsible for the reported success of functional restoration. As many of these programs are intense but brief, it is unlikely that improvement is entirely due to changes in fitness, as some fitness parameters, such as strength, change slowly over time. It is possible that exposure to exercise and activity and decreases in pain-related fear may be in part related to improvement in function in these types of interventions. Exposure to feared activity may have a significant impact on CLBP. Vlaeyen et al. (174) examined six subjects with CLBP who underwent baseline observation and then received either *in vivo* exposure to feared light-normal activity followed by exposure to graded activity (exercise) or graded activity followed by *in vivo* exposure. Among subjects who received *in vivo* exposure first, significant decreases in fear were observed following this exposure and were maintained over time. Subjects who received graded activity demonstrated declines in fear only when *in vivo* exposure was introduced. In addition, *in vivo* exposure also reduced negative thoughts about pain, fear of pain, and self-reported disability. These treatment gains were maintained at a 1-year follow-up. Interestingly, decreases in self-reported pain were also observed, even though pain was not a target of the intervention, and one might expect pain to increase with greater function. The authors propose that declines in pain-related fear may reduce pain vigilance, resulting in declines in reported pain intensity.

Thus, as part of a functional restoration approach, it may be beneficial to identify and target highly feared activities as part of the intervention. This may also be important, as two studies indicate that improvements in function as a result of exposure to feared physical movements do not necessarily generalize to other activities (175,176).

Feuerstein et al. (177) presented a program they termed Multidisciplinary Rehabilitation (MDR), which is a combination of medical management, physical conditioning, pain and stress management, vocational counseling and placement, and education on back safety. The authors indicated that work reentry is the program's primary focus. Among people with chronic back pain, the authors report that 71% of patients who completed the program were working or in vocational rehabilitation at 12-month follow-up, compared to only 44% in corresponding comparison groups.

SURGICAL TREATMENT

Besides the cauda equina syndrome, which is a surgical emergency, the indication for surgical intervention in patients suffering from CLBP is generally given with progressive or severe neurologic deficits, or if they have suffered unremitting pain and functional disability for more than 6 months during which a lengthy and aggressive trial of physical therapy and other conservative treatment options have failed to provide satisfactory relief (178).

According to Kwon et al. the consequences of age-related intervertebral disk degeneration are the leading causative factor in the majority of these cases (178). Such sequelae include the degenerative disks themselves, facet joint arthrosis, and segmental instability. When deciding what pathoanatomy needs to be addressed, one should remember that every diagnostic method has its shortcomings. Patients with both MRI and diskographic abnormalities have been reported to have more reliable outcomes after fusion surgery than those who have normal findings (179,180). Ideally, a patient would display static or dynamic instability on the radiograph, show disk abnormalities in the MRI, have provocative diskography elicit the low back pain symptoms, and have all three investigations pointing at the same segment.

Fusion

Currently, by far the most frequent open surgical management of CLBP is arthrodesis of unstable spine segments by fusion, with additional decompression in cases where symptomatic impingement of nerve roots is apparent (178). The rationale for fusion as a treatment for CLBP stems from other joints in the body, where the elimination of motion by arthrodesis lessens pain. But the complexity of the spinal anatomy and the pathophysiology of CLBP have made it difficult to predict the outcome of surgical procedures (181). However, a large literature review comprising 5,600 patients reported a "satisfactory outcome" in 65% to 87% of the patients after an arthrodesis, with monosegmental fusions having better results than bisegmental or trisegmental fusions (182). And in one of the few prospective, randomized trials of lumbar fusion versus nonsurgical treatment in 294 patients with CLBP of a degenerative nature, excluding patients with a specific radiographic diagnosis such as spondylolisthesis, the investigators found at 2-year follow-up that the surgically treated patients fared significantly better in terms of back pain and functional outcome scores than nonsurgical patients (183). Kwon et al. however, pointed out that the dramatic pain relief in the surgical patients in the first 6 months deteriorated during the subsequent 18 months and raised the question of whether the significant pain relief would be sustained over a longer period of time (178). Furthermore, nearly 15% of patients with operations on the lumbar spine for degenerative causes end up requiring another operation of the lumbar spine (184). Therefore, patients suffering from CLBP seeking a surgical treatment should be approached very cautiously, and every effort should be made to establish an anatomic etiology and to give a realistic estimation of the likelihood that a fusion procedure will lead to improvement of pain. This decision making is probably the most important determinant for successful outcomes after fusion surgery for low back pain (185).

Intradiscal Electrothermal Treatment

Intradiscal electrothermal treatment (IDET) has been proposed for low back pain patients with early nuclear degeneration and minimal-to-no collapse, instability, and arthrosis of the functional spinal unit. A catheter is inserted into the disk identified as causing the pain and heated to 90°C. Nerve endings transmitting the pain become coagulated and the disk is stabilized by a kind of hard-boiling effect. The results, however, are controversial. Spruit and Jacobs conclude that IDET is not effective in reducing pain and improving functional performance in a sample of 20 patients treated for

chronic discogenic low back pain after 6 months follow-up (186). Long-term results are inconsistent, too. At 2-year follow-up, two randomized controlled studies found at least 50% pain relief in 50% (187) and 70% of patients treated (188), respectively. On the other hand, Freedman et al. (189), in a study of active-duty soldiers with chronic discogenic low back pain, concluded that IDET is not a substitute for spinal fusion. Reasonable early results diminished with time, and up to 20% of patients reported worsening of baseline symptoms at final follow-up. Seven of 31 soldiers (23%), all male, went on to spinal surgery within 24 months. In summary, the technique cannot be applied to patients with more advanced nuclear degeneration and a herniated nucleus pulposis, and long-term results are controversial.

Replacement Strategies

Arthrodesis of a joint is generally not considered an optimal solution. Although arthrodesis of a painful motion segment in the lumbar spine has been shown to be an effective treatment (183), perceived disadvantages are that adjacent segment degeneration may occur and excellent long-term results are rarely achieved (190). Hence, a good surgical solution to CLBP is yet to be found. Replacement of the nucleus pulposis or the total disk appears to be an attractive alternative to arthrodesis. Several devices are on the market, but there is only a very small body of literature concerning nuclear or total disk replacement and there are no randomized, controlled studies testing the clinical outcome.

MATCHING PATIENTS TO TREATMENTS

With the numerous available interventions for CLBP, decision making regarding the most appropriate intervention, or course of interventions, can be difficult. Although decisions regarding certain interventions such as surgery are dependent on the pathophysiologic causes of pain, it is generally recognized that psychosocial factors play a significant role in the experience of many types of chronic pain problems. Although more research is needed, several studies suggest that psychosocial factors play a significant role in the outcome of interventions for CLBP, including surgery. Thus, many advocate for the employment of screening procedures prior to interventions such as surgery (191) to attempt to identify persons who possess characteristics related to poor treatment outcome, such as depression (192). Identification of significant risk factors can aid in appropriate intervention prior to the procedure, thus increasing the chances for a successful outcome.

Screening or profiling may also be beneficial for deciding among types of conservative treatments for CLBP, particularly whether a person will benefit most from simpler treatment modalities or is in need of more intensive multidisciplinary care. For example, Turk et al. (193) demonstrated that a multidisciplinary treatment tailored for patients with temporomandibular disorder who had a dysfunctional profile type on the Multidimensional Pain Inventory produced the better outcome compared to physical therapy alone. Haldorson et al. (194) examined treatment outcomes of persons with chronic musculoskeletal pain based on their prognosis score (categorized as good, medium, or bad) and whether they received ordinary care (such as medications and physical therapy), light multidisciplinary treatment, or extensive multidisciplinary treatment. Risk was assessed based on factors such as lifting ability, tenderness, mood, and perceived ability to work. Patients classified as good prognosis patients responded equally well to all interventions. Persons classified as medium prognosis patients benefited most from the two multidisciplinary treatments, while poor risk patients benefited most from extensive multidisciplinary care. Thus, for persons with CLBP with few psychosocial risk factors, simple interventions may prove to be the most cost-effective interventions. However, for persons with moderate or extensive psychosocial risk factors, multidisciplinary treatment may produce the best outcomes.

CONCLUSIONS

The physical causes of CLBP are largely undetermined. Does this mean that CLBP is primarily psychological or does it reflect our lack of knowledge or recognition of certain pathophysiologic causes of CLBP? Although advances still need to be made regarding the various physical and psychosocial factors that influence CLBP, recent research points in two directions. Some studies suggest that musculoskeletal causes of pain tend to go unnoticed or undetected. More recent studies employing sophisticated psychophysical pain testing paradigms and functional MRI provide evidence for central nervous alterations in the pain processing of CLBP patients, similar to changes detected in FM patients. More research in these directions is necessary. Accepted reliable and valid criteria for these disorders need to be developed, and potential interventions for these disorders need to be examined.

Numerous individual interventions appear to have some efficacy in reducing the patient's perception of pain or in decreasing physical contributions to pain. These include medications, TENS, neural blockade, exercise, biofeedback, and CBT. Typically, biofeedback is included as part of a cognitive-behavioral approach to treating CLBP, and some suggest this intervention may change muscle activity patterns that contribute to pain. Tricyclic antidepressant treatment appears to be particularly beneficial among chronic-pain patients. Studies conducted on neural blockade suggest that the efficacy is small and of short duration; however, injections may be beneficial in conjunction with other therapies, as even brief relief may help patients make greater gains, for example, in their exercise program. Acupuncture has some demonstrated efficacy for CLBP; however, its use is somewhat controversial. Manual therapy for CLBP appears to have some initial support; however, its effectiveness in patients with disabling CLBP has not been demonstrated. Exercise appears to have treatment benefits, as well as preventative benefits in terms of reduced risk of recurrence. The issue of compliance with exercise for pain treatment has not been adequately addressed, and empirical studies related to strategies for increasing compliance, such as simplifying prescribed regimens, would be beneficial. The impact of specific exercises and instruction on body mechanics and posture for musculoskeletal dysfunctions as an adjunct to manual therapy has not been examined empirically.

In practice, many of these individual therapies are used as part of multidisciplinary treatment. In general, multidisciplinary treatment appears to be superior to unimodal or no treatment, suggesting that multidimensional treatment should be the preferred method of treatment for CLBP. Given that cost-effectiveness is becoming more of an issue in patient care, studies of multidisciplinary treatment might consider examining the optimal cost-effective parameters of multidisciplinary treatment, such as determining the effective number of sessions or length of treatment, examining which components of treatment are particularly effective, and discovering whether outpatient treatment is more cost-effective than inpatient treatment. In relation to this latter issue, Peters et al. (191) found no differences in the outcomes of inpatient and outpatient chronic-pain patients, while Williams et al. (192) found that inpatients made greater gains and maintained them at 1 year. The authors were able to present the total cost of the programs but not necessarily demonstrate the cost-effectiveness of each individual type of treatment. It would be particularly useful to determine the utility of treatments tailored to empirically determined subgroups of pain patients, as some groups of patients may require more intensive multidisciplinary treatment, although some may respond well to less intensive and less costly interventions.

Another controversial but important issue to address in relation to CLBP treatment is the balance between functional activity and pain. For many patients, complete pain control is not achievable; thus they must work toward managing their pain and increasing their daily functioning despite the fact that they experience chronic pain. Treatments differ to a large degree in their emphasis on pacing or restricting activities to avoid pain versus performing prescribed activities despite increased pain. The progression of increased activity may be critical among patients with musculoskeletal pain, as improving their strength and conditioning may ultimately decrease pain. However, overemphasis on activity pacing to provide pain relief in these patients may actually inhibit rehabilitation. In addition, patients who are fearful of certain activities because they overestimate the amount of pain they will experience may benefit from exposure to these activities, as performing them without experiencing unmanageable pain will likely decrease their fear of movement and increase their functioning. It would be useful to compare the long-term outcomes of different treatment paradigms that emphasize these different approaches to balancing the relationship of pain and functioning. We as pain practitioners do not want to contribute to the disability of patients with CLBP, nor their suffering, yet little is known about how to best balance progression of activity with managing pain.

SUMMARY POINTS

- CLBP patients are most likely a heterogeneous group of patients with a common symptom. An empirical subgrouping is necessary, including anatomical and psychosocial variables and pain sensitivity, with the subsequent development of tailored therapies.
- There is considerable emerging evidence to suggest that many individuals with idiopathic CLBP may have a

regional pain syndrome similar to temporomandibular disorder, tension headache, vulvodynia/vulvar vestibulitis, and so on, with evidence for diffuse hyperalgesia/allodynia, even though the pain is localized.

■ IMPLICATIONS FOR PRACTICE

- Although some patients with CLBP may benefit from surgical therapy or various procedures, many are also made worse by these interventions.
- There are myriad conservative treatment options for CLBP. Current evidence suggests that multimodal therapy with pharmacologic therapies aimed at improving pain and nonpharmacologic therapies aimed at improving function may be superior to unimodal therapy.

REFERENCES

1. Deyo RA, Weinstein JN. Primary care—Low back pain. *N Engl J Med* 2001;344(5):363–370.
2. Andersson GBJ. Epidemiological features of chronic low-back pain. *Lancet* 1999;354(9178):581–585.
3. Shekelle PG, Markovich S, Louie R. An epidemiologic study of episodes of back pain care. *Spine* 1995;20(15):1668–1673.
4. Shekelle PG, Markovich M, Louie R. Comparing the costs between provider types of episodes of back pain care. *Spine* 1995;20(2):221–226.
5. Fast A. Low back disorders: conservative management. *Arch Phys Med Rehabil* 1988;69(10):880–891.
6. Spengler DM, Bigos SJ, Martin NA, et al. Back injuries in industry: a retrospective study. I. Overview and cost analysis. *Spine* 1986;11(3):241–245.
7. Hazard RG, Haugh LD, Reid S, et al. Early prediction of chronic disability after occupational low back injury. *Spine* 1996;21(8):945–951.
8. Deyo RA. Practice variations, treatment fads, rising disability. Do we need a new clinical research paradigm? *Spine* 1993;18(15):2153–2162.
9. Deyo RA, Rainville J, Kent DL. What can the history and physical examination tell us about low back pain? *JAMA* 1992;268(6):760–765.
10. Hall S, Bartleson JD, Onofrio BM, et al. Lumbar spinal stenosis. Clinical features, diagnostic procedures, and results of surgical treatment in 68 patients. *Ann Intern Med* 1985;103(2):271–275.
11. Katz JN, Dalgas M, Stucki G, et al. Degenerative lumbar spinal stenosis. Diagnostic value of the history and physical examination. *Arthritis Rheum* 1995;38(9):1236–1241.
12. Burton AK, Tillotson KM, Main CJ, et al. Psychosocial predictors of outcome in acute and subchronic low back trouble. *Spine* 1995;20(6):722–728.
13. Bigos SJ, Battie MC, Spengler DM, et al. A prospective study of work perceptions and psychosocial factors affecting the report of back injury. *Spine* 1991;16(1):1–6.
14. Croft PR, Papageorgiou AC, Ferry S, et al. Psychologic distress and low back pain. Evidence from a prospective study in the general population. *Spine* 1995;20(24):2731–2737.
15. Frymoyer JW, Rosen JC, Clements J, et al. Psychologic factors in low-back-pain disability. *Clin Orthop* 1985;195:178–184.
16. Greenough CG, Fraser RD. Comparison of eight psychometric instruments in unselected patients with back pain. *Spine* 1991;16(9):1068–1074.
17. Gran JT. An epidemiological survey of the signs and symptoms of ankylosing spondylitis. *Clin Rheumatol* 1985;4(2):161–169.
18. Vroomen PC, de Krom MC, Knottnerus JA. Diagnostic value of history and physical examination in patients suspected of sciatica due to disc herniation: a systematic review. *J Neurol* 1999;246(10):899–906.
19. Deyo RA. Early diagnostic evaluation of low back pain. *J Gen Intern Med* 1986;1(5):328–338.
20. Waddell G. *The back pain revolution.* Edinburgh: Churchill Livingstone, 1998.
21. Roy SH, Oddsson LI. Classification of paraspinal muscle impairments by surface electromyography. *Phys Ther* 1998;78(8):838–851.
22. Pullman SL, Goodin DS, Marquinez AI, et al. Clinical utility of surface EMG: report of the Therapeutics and Technology Assessment Subcommittee of the American Academy of Neurology. *Neurology* 2000;55(2):171–177.
23. Haig AJ. Clinical experience with paraspinal mapping. I: Neurophysiology of the paraspinal muscles in various spinal disorders. *Arch Phys Med Rehabil* 1997;78(11):1177–1184.
24. Haig AJ. Clinical experience with paraspinal mapping. II: A simplified technique that eliminates three-fourths of needle insertions. *Arch Phys Med Rehabil* 1997;78(11):1185–1190.
25. Greenough CG, Oliver CW, Jones AP. Assessment of spinal musculature using surface electromyographic spectral color mapping. *Spine* 1998;23(16):1768–1774.
26. Ambroz C, Scott A, Ambroz A, et al. Chronic low back pain assessment using surface electromyography. *J Occup Environ Med* 2000;42(6):660–669.
27. Nachemson A. Lumbar spine instability. A critical update and symposium summary. *Spine* 1985;10(3):290–291.
28. Bigos S, Bowyer O, Braen G, et al. Acute low back problems in adults. *Clinical practice guideline no. 14.* Rockville, MD: Agency for Health Care Policy and Research, 1994.
29. Deyo RA, Diehl AK. Cancer as a cause of back pain: frequency, clinical presentation, and diagnostic strategies. *J Gen Intern Med* 1988;3(3):230–238.
30. Osti OL, Vernon-Roberts B, Moore R, et al. Annular tears and disc degeneration in the lumbar spine. A post-mortem study of 135 discs. *J Bone Joint Surg Br* 1992;74(5):678–682.
31. Weishaupt D, Zanetti M, Hodler J, et al. MR imaging of the lumbar spine: prevalence of intervertebral disk extrusion and sequestration, nerve root compression, end plate abnormalities, and osteoarthritis of the facet joints in asymptomatic volunteers. *Radiology* 1998;209(3):661–666.
32. Jensen MC, Brant-Zawadzki MN, Obuchowski N, et al. Magnetic resonance imaging of the lumbar spine in people without back pain. *N Engl J Med* 1994;331(2):69–73.
33. Boden SD, McCowin PR, Davis DO, et al. Abnormal magnetic-resonance scans of the cervical spine in asymptomatic subjects. A prospective investigation. *J Bone Joint Surg Am* 1990;72(8):1178–1184.
34. Borenstein DG, O'Mara JW Jr, Boden SD, et al. The value of magnetic resonance imaging of the lumbar spine to predict low-back pain in asymptomatic subjects: a seven-year follow-up study. *J Bone Joint Surg Am* 2001;83-A(9):1306–1311.
35. Guyer RD, Ohnmeiss DD. Lumbar discography. Position statement from the North American Spine Society Diagnostic and Therapeutic Committee. *Spine* 1995;20(18):2048–2059.
36. Smith SE, Darden BV, Rhyne AL, et al. Outcome of unoperated discogram-positive low back pain. *Spine* 1995;20(18):1997–2000.
37. Deyo RA. Diagnostic evaluation of LBP—reaching a specific diagnosis is often impossible. *Arch Intern Med* 2002;162(13):1444–1447.
38. Nachemson A, Vingard E. Assessment of patients with neck and back pain: a best-evidence synthesis. In: Nachemson A, Jonsson E, eds. *Neck and back pain. The scientific evidence of causes, diagnosis and treatment.* Philadelphia, PA: Lippincott Williams & Wilkins, 2000:189–235.

39. White AA III, Gordon SL. Synopsis: workshop on idiopathic low-back pain. *Spine* 1982;7(2):141–149.

40. Crue BL. Multi-disciplinary pain treatment programs: current status. *Clin J Pain* 1986;1:31–38.

41. Coste J, Paolaggi JB, Spira A. Classification of nonspecific low back pain. I. Psychological involvement in low back pain. A clinical, descriptive approach. *Spine* 1992;17(9):1028–1037.

42. Linton SJ. A review of psychological risk factors in back and neck pain. *Spine* 2000;25(9):1148–1156.

43. Hasenbring M, Marienfeld G, Kuhlendahl D, et al. Risk factors of chronicity in lumbar disc patients. A prospective investigation of biologic, psychologic, and social predictors of therapy outcome. *Spine* 1994;19(24):2759–2765.

44. Grebner M, Breme K, Rothoerl R, et al. Coping and convalescence course after lumbar disk operations. *Schmerz* 1999; 13(1):19–30.

45. Clauw DJ, Williams D, Lauerman W, et al. Pain sensitivity as a correlate of clinical status in individuals with chronic low back pain. *Spine* 1999;24(19):2035–2041.

46. Sanders SH. Cross-validation of the back pain classification scale with chronic, intractable pain patients. *Pain* 1985;22(3): 271–277.

47. Weintraub MI. Regional pain is usually hysterical. *Arch Neurol* 1988;45(8):914–915.

48. Mense S. Nociception from skeletal muscle in relation to clinical muscle pain. *Pain* 1993;54(3):241–289.

49. Lewit K. Management of muscular pain associated with articular dysfunction. In: Fricton JR, Awad EA, eds. *Advances in pain research and therapy*, Vol. 17. *Myofascial pain and fibromyalgia*. New York: Raven Press, 1990:315–317.

50. Rosomoff HL, Fishbain DA, Goldberg M, et al. Physical findings in patients with chronic intractable benign pain of the neck and/or back. *Pain* 1989;37(3):279–287.

51. Mense S, Hoheisel U, Reinert A. The possible role of substance P in eliciting and modulating deep somatic pain. *Prog Brain Res* 1996;110:125–135.

52. Granges G, Littlejohn G. Pressure pain threshold in pain-free subjects, in patients with chronic regional pain syndromes, and in patients with fibromyalgia syndrome. *Arthritis Rheum* 1993;36(5):642–646.

53. Leffler AS, Hansson P, Kosek E. Somatosensory perception in a remote pain-free area and function of diffuse noxious inhibitory controls (DNIC) in patients suffering from long-term trapezius myalgia. *Eur J Pain* 2002;6(2):149–159.

54. Staud R, Vierck CJ, Cannon RL, et al. Abnormal sensitization and temporal summation of second pain (wind-up) in patients with fibromyalgia syndrome. *Pain* 2001;91(1-2):165–175.

55. Kosek E, Hansson P. Modulatory influence on somatosensory perception from vibration and heterotopic noxious conditioning stimulation (HNCS) in fibromyalgia patients and healthy subjects. *Pain* 1997;70(1):41–51.

56. Giesecke T, Gracely RH, Grant MAB, et al. Evidence of augmented central pain processing in idiopathic chronic low back pain. *Arthritis Rheum* 2004;50(2):613–623.

57. Casey KL, Minoshima S, Morrow TJ, et al. Comparison of human cerebral activation pattern during cutaneous warmth, heat pain, and deep cold pain. *J Neurophysiol* 1996;76(1): 571–581.

58. Casey KL. Match and mismatch: identifying the neuronal determinants of pain. *Ann Intern Med* 1996;124(11):995–998.

59. Gelnar PA, Krauss BR, Sheehe PR, et al. A comparative fMRI study of cortical representations for thermal painful, vibrotactile, and motor performance tasks. *Neuroimage* 1999; 10(4):460–482.

60. Derbyshire SW. Imaging the brain in pain. *APS Bull* 1999; 9(3):7–8.

61. Peyron R, Garcia-Larrea L, Gregoire MC, et al. Haemodynamic brain responses to acute pain in humans: sensory and attentional networks. *Brain* 1999;122(Pt 9):1765–1780.

62. Teders SJ, Blanchard EB, Andrasik F, et al. Relaxation training for tension headache: comparative efficacy and cost-effectiveness of a minimal therapist contact versus a therapist-delivered procedure. *Behav Ther* 1984;15:59–70.

63. Kashima K, Rahman OI, Sakoda S, et al. Increased pain sensitivity of the upper extremities of TMD patients with myalgia to experimentally-evoked noxious stimulation: possibility of worsened endogenous opioid systems. *Cranio* 1999;17(4): 241–246.

64. Maixner W, Fillingim R, Booker D, et al. Sensitivity of patients with painful temporomandibular disorders to experimentally evoked pain. *Pain* 1995;63(3):341–351.

65. Carli G, Suman AL, Biasi G, et al. Reactivity to superficial and deep stimuli in patients with chronic musculoskeletal pain. *Pain* 2002;100:259–269.

66. Mountz JM, Bradley LA, Modell JG, et al. Fibromyalgia in women. Abnormalities of regional cerebral blood flow in the thalamus and the caudate nucleus are associated with low pain threshold levels. *Arthritis Rheum* 1995;38(7):926–938.

67. Gracely RH, Petzke F, Wolf JM, et al. Functional magnetic resonance imaging evidence of augmented pain processing in fibromyalgia. *Arthritis Rheum* 2002;46(5):1333–1343.

68. Silverman DH, Munakata JA, Ennes H, et al. Regional cerebral activity in normal and pathological perception of visceral pain. *Gastroenterology* 1997;112(1):64–72.

69. Peyron R, Garcia-Larrea L, Gregoire MC, et al. Allodynia after lateral-medullary (Wallenberg) infarct. A PET study. *Brain* 1998;121(Pt 2):345–356.

70. Derbyshire SW, Jones AK, Devani P, et al. Cerebral responses to pain in patients with atypical facial pain measured by positron emission tomography. *J Neurol Neurosurg Psychiatry* 1994;57(10):1166–1172.

71. Clauw DJ, Chrousos GP. Chronic pain and fatigue syndromes: overlapping clinical and neuroendocrine features and potential pathogenic mechanisms. *Neuroimmunomodulation* 1997;4(3): 134–153.

72. Fishbain D. Evidence-based data on pain relief with antidepressants. *Ann Med* 2000;32(5):305–316.

73. Donta ST, Clauw DJ, Engel CC Jr, et al. Cognitive behavioral therapy and aerobic exercise for Gulf War veterans' illnesses: a randomized controlled trial. *JAMA* 2003;289(11): 1396–1404.

74. Loeser JD, Sullivan M. Disability in the chronic low back pain patient may be iatrogenic. *Pain Forum* 1995;4(2): 114–121.

75. Mayer T, Polatin P, Smith B, et al. Spine rehabilitation. Secondary and tertiary nonoperative care. *Spine* 1995;20(18): 2060–2066.

76. Deyo RA. Drug therapy for back pain. Which drugs help which patients? *Spine* 1996;21(24):2840–2849.

77. Serpell MG. Gabapentin in neuropathic pain syndromes: a randomised, double-blind, placebo-controlled trial. *Pain* 2002; 99(3):557–566.

78. Salerno SM, Browning R, Jackson JL. The effect of antidepressant treatment on chronic back pain: a meta-analysis. *Arch Intern Med* 2002;162(1):19–24.

79. Bair MJ, Robinson RL, Katon W, et al. Depression and pain comorbidity: a literature review. *Arch Intern Med* 2003;163(20): 2433–2445.

80. Carter GT, Sullivan MD. Antidepressants in pain management. *Curr Opin Investig Drugs* 2002;3(3):454–458.

81. O'Malley PG, Jackson JL, Santoro J, et al. Antidepressant therapy for unexplained symptoms and symptom syndromes [see Comments]. *J Fam Pract* 1999;48(12):980–990.

82. O'Malley PG, Balden E, Tomkins G, et al. Treatment of fibromyalgia with antidepressants. A meta-analysis. *J Gen Intern Med* 2000;15(9):659–666.

83. Turner JA, Denny MC. Do antidepressant medications relieve chronic low back pain? *J Fam Pract* 1993;37(6):545–553.

84. van Tulder MW, Koes BW, Bouter LM. Conservative treatment of acute and chronic nonspecific low back pain. A systematic review of randomized controlled trials of the most common interventions. *Spine* 1997;22(18):2128–2156.

85. Staiger TO, Gaster B, Sullivan MD, et al. Systematic review of antidepressants in the treatment of chronic low back pain. *Spine* 2003;28(22):2540–2545.

86. Romano JM, Turner JA. Chronic pain and depression: does the evidence support a relationship? *Psychol Bull* 1985; 97(1):18–34.

87. Krishnan KR, France RD, Pelton S, et al. Chronic pain and depression. II. Symptoms of anxiety in chronic low back pain patients and their relationship to subtypes of depression. *Pain* 1985;22(3):289–294.

88. Haythornthwaite JA, Menefee LA, Quatrano-Piacentini AL, et al. Outcome of chronic opioid therapy for non-cancer pain. *J Pain Symptom Manage* 1998;15(3):185–194.

89. Haddox JD, Joranson D, Angarola RT et al, American Academy of Pain Management and the American Pain Society. The use of opioids for the treatment of chronic pain. http://www.ampainsoc.org/advocacy/opioids.htm. 20-8-1996.

90. Melzack R. Prolonged relief of pain by brief, intense transcutaneous somatic stimulation. *Pain* 1975;1(4):357–373.

91. Johnson MI, Ashton CH, Bousfield DR, et al. Analgesic effects of different frequencies of transcutaneous electrical nerve stimulation on cold-induced pain in normal subjects. *Pain* 1989;39(2):231–236.

92. Hansson P, Ekblom A. Transcutaneous electrical nerve stimulation (TENS) as compared to placebo TENS for the relief of acute oro-facial pain. *Pain* 1983;15(2):157–165.

93. Meyler WJ, de Jongste MJ, Rolf CA. Clinical evaluation of pain treatment with electrostimulation: a study on TENS in patients with different pain syndromes. *Clin J Pain* 1994; 10(1):22–27.

94. Fried T, Johnson R, McCracken W. Transcutaneous electrical nerve stimulation: its role in the control of chronic pain. *Arch Phys Med Rehabil* 1984;65(5):228–231.

95. Rao VR, Wolf SL, Gersh MR. Examination of electrode placements and stimulating parameters in treating chronic pain with conventional transcutaneous electrical nerve stimulation (TENS). *Pain* 1981;11(1):37–47.

96. Hughes GS Jr, Lichstein PR, Whitlock D, et al. Response of plasma beta-endorphins to transcutaneous electrical nerve stimulation in healthy subjects. *Phys Ther* 1984; 64(7): 1062–1066.

97. O'Brien WJ, Rutan FM, Sanborn C, et al. Effect of transcutaneous electrical nerve stimulation on human blood beta-endorphin levels. *Phys Ther* 1984;64(9):1367–1374.

98. Tulgar M, McGlone F, Bowsher D, et al. Comparative effectiveness of different stimulation modes in relieving pain. Part I. A pilot study. *Pain* 1991;47(2):151–155.

99. Fox EJ, Melzack R. Transcutaneous electrical stimulation and acupuncture: comparison of treatment for low-back pain. *Pain* 1976;2(2):141–148.

100. Tulgar M, McGlone F, Bowsher D, et al. Comparative effectiveness of different stimulation modes in relieving pain. Part II. A double-blind controlled long-term clinical trial. *Pain* 1991;47(2):157–162.

101. Sluka KA, Walsh D. Transcutaneous electrical nerve stimulation: basic science mechanisms and clinical effectiveness. *J Pain* 2003;4(3):109–121.

102. Gregg RV. Should nerve blocks be used for chronic non-cancer pain? *Am Pain Soc Bull* 1991;1:1–4.

103. Hogan QH, Abram SE. Neural blockade for diagnosis and prognosis. A review. *Anesthesiology* 1997;86(1):216–241.

104. Koes BW, Scholten RJ, Mens JM, et al. Efficacy of epidural steroid injections for low-back pain and sciatica: a systematic review of randomized clinical trials. *Pain* 1995;63(3):279–288.

105. Lewit K. The needle effect in the relief of myofascial pain. *Pain* 1979;6(1):83–90.

106. Abram SE, O'Connor TC. Complications associated with epidural steroid injections. *Reg Anesth* 1996;21(2):149–162.

107. Rodriquez AA, Bilkey WJ, Agre JC. Therapeutic exercise in chronic neck and back pain. *Arch Phys Med Rehabil* 1992; 73(9):870–875.

108. Biering-Sorensen F. Physical measurements as risk indicators for low-back trouble over a one-year period. *Spine* 1984;9(2):106–119.

109. Cady LD, Bischoff DP, O'Connell ER, et al. Strength and fitness and subsequent back injuries in firefighters. *J Occup Med* 1979;21(4):269–272.

110. Troup JD, Martin JW, Lloyd DC. Back pain in industry. A prospective survey. *Spine* 1981;6(1):61–69.

111. Dishman RK, Ickes W. Self-motivation and adherence to therapeutic exercise. *J Behav Med* 1981;4(4):421–438.

112. Martin JE, Dubbert PM. Adherence to exercise. In: Terjung RL, ed. *Exercise and sport sciences reviews*, Vol. 13. New York: Macmillan, 1985:137–167.

113. Geisser ME, Roth RS. Knowledge of and agreement with chronic pain diagnosis: relation to affective distress, pain beliefs and coping, pain intensity, and disability. *J Occup Rehabil* 1998;8(1):73–88.

114. Lacroix JM, Powell J, Lloyd GJ, et al. Low-back pain. Factors of value in predicting outcome. *Spine* 1990;15(6): 495–499.

115. Roth RS, Horowitz K, Bachman JE. Chronic myofascial pain: knowledge of diagnosis and satisfaction with treatment. *Arch Phys Med Rehabil* 1998;79(8):966–970.

116. Nachemson AL. Disc pressure measurements. *Spine* 1981; 6(1):93–97.

117. Turner JA. Educational and behavioral interventions for back pain in primary care. *Spine* 1996;21(24):2851–2857.

118. Indahl A, Velund L, Reikeraas O. Good prognosis for low back pain when left untampered. A randomized clinical trial. *Spine* 1995;20(4):473–477.

119. Mein EA. Low back pain and manual medicine: a look at the literature. *Phys Med Rehabil Clin N Am* 1996;7:715–729.

120. Simons DG. Myofascial pain syndrome due to trigger points. *Int Rehabil Med Assoc Monogr Ser* 1987;1:1–39.

121. Greenman PE. *Principles of manual medicine*. Baltimore, MD: Williams & Wilkins, 1989.

122. Bookhout MR. Exercise and somatic dysfunction. *Phys Med Rehabil Clin N Am* 1996;7:845–862.

123. Evans DP, Burke MS, Lloyd KN, et al. Lumbar spinal manipulation on trial. Part I—clinical assessment. *Rheumatol Rehabil* 1978;17(1):46–53.

124. Ongley MJ, Klein RG, Dorman TA, et al. A new approach to the treatment of chronic low back pain. *Lancet* 1987; 2(8551):143–146.

125. Waagen GN, Haldeman S, Cook G, et al. Short term trial of chiropractic adjustments for the relief of chronic low back pain. *Man Med* 1986;2:63–67.

126. Timm KE. A randomized-control study of active and passive treatments for chronic low back pain following L5 laminectomy. *J Orthop Sports Phys Ther* 1994;20(6):276–286.

127. Koes BW, Assendelft WJ, van der Heijden GJ, et al. Spinal manipulation for low back pain. An updated systematic review of randomized clinical trials. *Spine* 1996;21(24): 2860–2871.

128. Hurwitz EL, Morgenstern H, Harber P, et al. A randomized trial of medical care with and without physical therapy and chiropractic care with and without physical modalities for patients with low back pain: 6-month follow-up outcomes from the UCLA low back pain study. *Spine* 2002;27(20): 2193–2204.

129. Aure OF, Nilsen JH, Vasseljen O. Manual therapy and exercise therapy in patients with chronic low back pain: a randomized,

controlled trial with 1-year follow-up. *Spine* 2003;28(6): 525–531.

130. Vincent C, Lewith G. Placebo controls for acupuncture studies. *J R Soc Med* 1995;88(4):199–202.

131. Thomas M, Lundeberg T. Does acupuncture work? *Pain Clin Updat* 1996;4(3):1–4.

132. Flor H, Haag G, Turk DC, et al. Efficacy of EMG biofeedback, pseudotherapy, and conventional medical treatment for chronic rheumatic back pain. *Pain* 1983;17(1):21–31.

133. Flor H, Haag G, Turk DC. Long-term efficacy of EMG biofeedback for chronic rheumatic back pain. *Pain* 1986; 27(2):195–202.

134. Nigl AJ, Fischer-Williams M. Treatment of low back strain with electromyographic biofeedback and relaxation training. *Psychosomatics* 1980;21(6):495–499.

135. Nouwen A, Solinger JW. The effectiveness of EMG biofeedback training in low back pain. *Biofeedback Self Regul* 1979;4(2):103–111.

136. Flor H, Birbaumer N. Comparison of the efficacy of electromyographic biofeedback, cognitive-behavioral therapy, and conservative medical interventions in the treatment of chronic musculoskeletal pain. *J Consult Clin Psychol* 1993; 61(4):653–658.

137. DeGood DE. What is the role of biofeedback in the treatment of chronic pain patients? *Am Pain Soc Bull* 1993;3(3):1–5.

138. Flor H, Schugens MM, Birbaumer N. Discrimination of muscle tension in chronic pain patients and healthy controls. *Biofeedback Self Regul* 1992;17(3):165–177.

139. Arena JG, Sherman RA, Bruno GM, et al. Electromyographic recordings of 5 types of low back pain subjects and non-pain controls in different positions. *Pain* 1989;37(1): 57–65.

140. Geisser ME, Robinson ME, Richardson C. A time series analysis of the relationship between ambulatory EMG, pain, and stress in chronic low back pain. *Biofeedback Self Regul* 1995;20(4):339–355.

141. Kohler T, Haimerl C. Daily stress as a trigger of migraine attacks: results of thirteen single-subject studies. *J Consult Clin Psychol* 1990;58(6):870–872.

142. Hazlett RL, Haynes SN. Fibromyalgia: a time-series analysis of the stressor-physical symptom association. *J Behav Med* 1992;15(6):541–558.

143. Donaldson S, Romney D, Donaldson M, et al. Randomized study of the application of single motor unit biofeedback training to chronic low back pain. *J Occup Rehabil* 1994; 4:23–37.

144. Wolf SL, Nacht M, Kelly JL. EMG feedback training during dynamic movement for low back pain patients. *Behav Ther* 1982;13:395–406.

145. Ohrbach R, McCall WD. The stress-hyperactivity-pain theory of myogenic pain: proposal for a revised theory. *Pain Forum* 1996;5(1):51–66.

146. Fordyce WE. *Behavioral methods for chronic pain and illness.* St. Louis, MO: Mosby, 1976.

147. Block AR. Mutidisciplinary treatment of chronic low back pain: a review. *Rehabil Psychol* 1982;27:51–63.

148. Keefe FJ, Block AR, Williams RB Jr, et al. Behavioral treatment of chronic low back pain: clinical outcome and individual differences in pain relief. *Pain* 1981;11(2):221–231.

149. Swanson DW, Maruta T, Swenson WM. Results of behavior modification in the treatment of chronic pain. *Psychosom Med* 1979;41(1):55–61.

150. Roberts AH, Sternbach RA, Polich J. Behavioral management of chronic pain and excess disability: long-term follow-up of an outpatient program. *Clin J Pain* 1993;9(1):41–48.

151. Jensen MP, Turner JA, Romano JM. Correlates of improvement in multidisciplinary treatment of chronic pain. *J Consult Clin Psychol* 1994;62(1):172–179.

152. Jensen MP, Turner JA, Romano JM, et al. Relationship of pain-specific beliefs to chronic pain adjustment. *Pain* 1994; 57(3):301–309.

153. Main CJ, Watson PJ. Screening for patients at risk of developing chronic incapacity. *J Occup Rehabil* 1995;5(4): 207–217.

154. McCracken LM, Gross RT, Sorg PJ, et al. Prediction of pain in patients with chronic low back pain: effects of inaccurate prediction and pain-related anxiety. *Behav Res Ther* 1993; 31(7):647–652.

155. Flor H, Turk DC. Chronic back pain and rheumatoid arthritis: predicting pain and disability from cognitive variables. *J Behav Med* 1988;11(3):251–265.

156. Geisser ME, Robinson ME, Keefe FJ, et al. Catastrophizing, depression and the sensory, affective and evaluative aspects of chronic pain. *Pain* 1994;59(1):79–83.

157. Geisser ME, Robinson ME, Henson CD. The coping strategies questionnaire and chronic pain adjustment: a conceptual and empirical reanalysis. *Clin J Pain* 1994;10(2):98–106.

158. Keefe FJ, Brown GK, Wallston KA, et al. Coping with rheumatoid arthritis pain: catastrophizing as a maladaptive strategy. *Pain* 1989;37(1):51–56.

159. Buckelew SP, Parker JC, Keefe FJ, et al. Self-efficacy and pain behavior among subjects with fibromyalgia. *Pain* 1994; 59(3):377–384.

160. Jacob MC, Kerns RD, Rosenberg R, et al. Chronic pain: intrusion and accommodation. *Behav Res Ther* 1993;31(5): 519–527.

161. Morley S, Eccleston C, Williams A. Systematic review and meta-analysis of randomized controlled trials of cognitive behaviour therapy and behaviour therapy for chronic pain in adults, excluding headache. *Pain* 1999;80(1-2):1–13.

162. Keefe FJ, Caldwell DS, Williams DA, et al. Pain coping skills training in the management of osteoarthric knee pain: a comparative study. *Behav Ther* 1990;21:49–62.

163. Holzman AD, Turk DC, Kerns RD. The cognitive-behavioral approach to the management of chronic pain. In: Holzman AD, Turk DC, eds. *Pain management: a handbook of psychological treatment approaches.* New York: Pergamon Press, 1986:31–50.

164. Muse M. Stress-related, posttraumatic chronic pain syndrome: criteria for diagnosis, and preliminary report on prevalence. *Pain* 1985;23(3):295–300.

165. Hickling EJ, Blanchard EB, Silverman DJ, et al. Motor vehicle accidents, headaches and post-traumatic stress disorder: assessment findings in a consecutive series. *Headache* 1992; 32(3):147–151.

166. Geisser ME, Roth RS, Bachman JE, et al. The relationship between symptoms of post-traumatic stress disorder and pain, affective disturbance and disability among patients with accident and non-accident related pain. *Pain* 1996; 66(2-3):207–214.

167. Turk DC, Okifuji A, Starz TW, et al. Effects of type of symptom onset on psychological distress and disability in fibromyalgia syndrome patients. *Pain* 1996;68(2-3):423–430.

168. DeGood DE, Kiernan B. Perception of fault in patients with chronic pain. *Pain* 1996;64(1):153–159.

169. Flor H, Fydrich T, Turk DC. Efficacy of multidisciplinary pain treatment centers: a meta-analytic review. *Pain* 1992; 49(2):221–230.

170. Hazard RG. Spine update. Functional restoration. *Spine* 1995; 20(21):2345–2348.

171. Hazard RG, Fenwick JW, Kalisch SM, et al. Functional restoration with behavioral support. A one-year prospective study of patients with chronic low-back pain. *Spine* 1989; 14(2):157–161.

172. Mayer T, Gatchel RJ, Mayer H, et al. A prospective two-year study of functional restoration in industrial low back injury.

An objective assessment procedure. *J Am Med Assoc* 1987; 258(13):1763–1767.

173. Teasell RW, Harth M. Functional restoration. Returning patients with chronic low back pain to work—revolution or fad? *Spine* 1996;21(7):844–847.

174. Vlaeyen JW, de Jong J, Geilen M, et al. The treatment of fear of movement/(re)injury in chronic low back pain: further evidence on the effectiveness of exposure in vivo. *Clin J Pain* 2002;18(4):251–261.

175. Crombez G, Eccleston C, Vlaeyen JW, et al. Exposure to physical movements in low back pain patients: restricted effects of generalization. *Health Psychol* 2002;21(6): 573–578.

176. Goubert L, Francken G, Crombez G, et al. Exposure to physical movement in chronic back pain patients: no evidence for generalization across different movements. *Behav Res Ther* 2002;40(4):415–429.

177. Feuerstein M, Menz L, Zastowny T, et al. Chronic back pain and work disability: vocational outcomes following multidisciplinary rehabilitation. *J Occup Rehabil* 1994;4(4): 229–251.

178. Kwon BK, Vaccaro AR, Grauer JN, et al. Indications, techniques, and outcomes of posterior surgery for chronic low back pain. *Orthop Clin North Am* 2003;34(2):297–308.

179. Gill K, Blumenthal SL. Functional results after anterior lumbar fusion at L5-S1 in patients with normal and abnormal MRI scans. *Spine* 1992;17(8):940–942.

180. Newman MH, Grinstead GL. Anterior lumbar interbody fusion for internal disc disruption. *Spine* 1992;17(7):831–833.

181. Parker LM, Murrell SE, Boden SD, et al. The outcome of posterolateral fusion in highly selected patients with discogenic low back pain. *Spine* 1996;21(16):1909–1916.

182. Boos N, Webb JK. Pedicle screw fixation in spinal disorders: a European view. *Eur Spine J* 1997;6(1):2–18.

183. Fritzell P, Hagg O, Wessberg P, et al. Volvo award winner in clinical studies: lumbar fusion versus nonsurgical treatment for chronic low back pain: a multicenter randomized controlled trial from the Swedish Lumbar Spine Study Group. *Spine* 2001;26(23):2521–2532.

184. Malter AD, McNeney B, Loeser JD, et al. 5-year reoperation rates after different types of lumbar spine surgery. *Spine* 1998;23(7):814–820.

185. Herkowitz HN, Sidhu KS. Lumbar spine fusion in the treatment of degenerative conditions: current indications and recommendations. *J Am Acad Orthop Surg* 1995;3(3):123–135.

186. Spruit M, Jacobs WC. Pain and function after intradiscal electrothermal treatment (IDET) for symptomatic lumbar disc degeneration. *Eur Spine J* 2002;11(6):589–593.

187. Bogduk N, Karasek M. Two-year follow-up of a controlled trial of intradiscal electrothermal anuloplasty for chronic low back pain resulting from internal disc disruption. *Spine J* 2002;2(5):343–350.

188. Saal JA, Saal JS. Intradiscal electrothermal treatment for chronic discogenic low back pain: prospective outcome study with a minimum 2-year follow-up. *Spine* 2002;27(9): 966–973.

189. Freedman BA, Cohen SP, Kuklo TR, et al. Intradiscal electrothermal therapy (IDET) for chronic low back pain in active-duty soldiers: a 2-year follow-up. *Spine J* 2003;3(6): 502–509.

190. De Kleuver M, Oner FC, Jacobs WC. Total disc replacement for chronic low back pain: background and a systematic review of the literature. *Eur Spine J* 2003;12(2):108–116.

191. Peters J, Large RG, Elkind G. Follow-up results from a randomised controlled trial evaluating in- and outpatient pain management programmes. *Pain* 1992;50(1):41–50.

192. Williams AC, Richardson PH, Nicholas MK, et al. Inpatient vs. outpatient pain management: results of a randomised controlled trial. *Pain* 1996;66(1):13–22.

193. Turk DC, Rudy TE, Kubinski JA, et al. Dysfunctional patients with temporomandibular disorders: evaluating the efficacy of a tailored treatment protocol. *J Consult Clin Psychol* 1996;64(1):139–146.

194. Haldorsen EM, Grasdal AL, Skouen JS, et al. Is there a right treatment for a particular patient group? Comparison of ordinary treatment, light multidisciplinary treatment, and extensive multidisciplinary treatment for long-term sick-listed employees with musculoskeletal pain. *Pain* 2002;95(1-2): 49–63.

21

Reflex Sympathetic Dystrophy Syndrome

Franklin Kozin

BACKGROUND

Silas Weir Mitchell and his colleagues first described reflex sympathetic dystrophy syndrome (RSDS) during the American Civil War when examining gunshot wounds and other injuries in soldiers (1). Some years later Mitchell coined the term "causalgia" for this condition (2). It is thought that "causalgia" is derived from a combination of the words "caustic," in reference to the burning so frequently described by injured soldiers, and "alga," for pain. Leriche later studied this condition during and after World War I; he was the first to use sympathectomy in its treatment. Evans appears to be the first to use the term "reflex sympathetic dystrophy (RSD)" (3,4); however, De Takats used the term "reflex dystrophy" in 1937 (5). Over the ensuing years many investigators introduced different terms to describe the various features of RSD (see Table 21-1).

In 1994 the International Association for the Study of Pain (IASP) introduced the term "complex regional pain syndrome (CRPS)" to describe RSDS, causalgia, and related conditions (6). CRPS type I refers to RSDS, and CRPS type II refers to causalgia. Unfortunately, this change of terminology came about with the introduction of relatively vague criteria (see Table 21-2) (6), leading to greater confusion in the diagnosis and treatment of RSDS/CRPS, in my opinion. A series of recent studies has made significant headway in correcting this problem. Additionally, over the past 10 to 15 years, studies have shown that many painful conditions without features of RSDS/CRPS respond to sympathetic blocks. The change in terminology had the dual goal of eliminating or reducing the frequency of sympathetic blocks in this and related conditions, as well as emphasizing the absence of specificity in the term "RSD."

EPIDEMIOLOGY

The exact prevalence of RSDS/CRPS is not known. It has been estimated to occur in approximately 0.5% of individuals following traumatic injury (7). Studies from Sweden have suggested a prevalence of CRPS of about 10% in upper extremity pain syndromes (1,8). Data has suggested an increased prevalence of RSDS/CRPS, following Colles and other fractures, coronary artery disease, hemiplegia, and possibly cancer, among other conditions (see Table 21-3). In a retrospective review, Allen et al. found that the most common inciting injury was a sprain/strain, accounting for 29% of cases, followed by postsurgical (24%), fractures (16%), contusions/crush injury (8%), spontaneous, other, or unknown (20%) (9). Woman may be 1.6 to 3.1 times more likely to develop RSDS/CRPS than men (9).

CLINICAL FINDINGS

The cardinal features of RSDS/CRPS are listed in Table 21-4. Pain is the primary symptom, although many studies do not find pain in every case. A recent report of five cases of "painless" RSDS/CRPS also supports this finding (10). It is generally accepted that *burning pain* is most characteristic of the syndrome, but a number of other pain descriptors are common. In a prospective study of RSD, it was found that only 25% of patients described burning pain. Pain is usually diffuse in the affected hand/wrist or foot/ankle or other location. When pain is localized to a particular nerve distribution, causalgia/CRPS II should be considered. Whenever pain appears to be disproportionately severe for an injury, RSDS/CRPS should be suspected. Usually the pain syndrome is localized to a distal

TABLE 21-1	Terminology of Reflex Sympathetic Dystrophy Syndrome/Complex Regional Pain Syndrome

Complex regional pain syndrome, type 1
Reflex sympathetic dystrophy syndrome
Reflex dystrophy
Reflex neurovascular dystrophy syndrome
Causalgia
Sudeck atrophy
Acute atrophy of bone
Traumatic angiospasm
Traumatic vasospasm
Shoulder hand syndrome
Shoulder hand finger syndrome
Algodystrophy
Algoneurodystrophy

TABLE 21-3	Primary Conditions Associated with Reflex Sympathetic Dystrophy Syndrome/Complex Regional Pain Syndrome

Major or minor trauma
Fractures, especially of the wrist and ankle
Primary central nervous system disorders
Postoperative
Crush injuries
Hemiplegia
Seizures and/or antiseizure drugs (phenobarbital)
Cervical and or lumbar spondylosis and/or radiculopathy
Ischemic heart disease
Pulmonary tuberculosis and/or medications (isoniazid)
Immobilization in cast or splint

extremity, although bilateral involvement is recognized in up to 20% of cases. In a study of 1,183 patients with RSDS/CRPS, only 10 (0.8%) were found to have symmetrical involvement in the limbs (11). Multiple sites of involvement have also been described (12,13). Less commonly, the knee may also be affected, and others have suggested the presence in the shoulder (adhesive capsulitis) and hip (transient osteopenia of the hip) (14,15). The IASP criteria have allowed for RSDS/CRPS to occur in other locations, including the face, temporomandibular joint, and other sites, but specific criteria for these locations have not yet been developed. Spread of pain proximally is common. Patients will typically develop a myofascial pain syndromelike pain in the neck/upper back when there is upper extremity involvement and in the lower back/gluteal muscles when there is lower extremity involvement. Maleki has reported spread of pain in all 27 subjects with CRPS I; unfortunately, the methods of selection of patients and characteristics of the secondary pain syndrome is not fully explained (16). In this study, 70% of patients experienced spread of pain to a distant, noncontiguous site.

Tenderness of the affected part also is characteristic of RSDS/CRPS. As with the pain, tenderness is usually diffuse in the affected part but tends to be more prominent in the periarticular tissues. Hypersensitivity may occur in the affected part. This may take the form of allodynia (pain with nonnoxious stimuli) or hyperpathia (pain developing with repetitive minimally noxious or nonnoxious stimuli). Allodynia may be produced by joint movement (mechanical allodynia), light touch such as with a tissue (tactile allodynia), vibration (vibratory allodynia), or temperature changes (heat or cold allodynia). The frequency with which these occur in patients with RSD/CRPS is unclear. Price et al. addressed this in a study of mixed patients, which suggested that there may not be correlation among these different forms of hyperalgesia (17).

Dystrophic skin and nail changes occur frequently as well. Skin changes are characterized by shininess, loss of normal wrinkling, fine scaling, and a doughy consistency to the skin and soft tissues. The nails may be brittle and may take on a cloudy/whitish appearance (18).

Vasomotor changes are characterized by changes in skin color and temperature. Typically the affected part will be violaceous or red. Occasionally, the part may be deep blue, and the patient may describe the affected part as being "black." Usually, the affected part is warm within weeks of the initial injury or occurrence of RSDS/CRPS, but later it becomes cool or cold to touch (19). Once again, the color changes and temperature changes should be diffuse in RSDS/CRPS, since localized changes are more likely associated with causalgia/CRPS II or with bone or soft tissue/joint injuries.

Sudomotor changes refer to changes in sweat and hairgrowth patterns. Affected patients typically report increased sweating and increased hair growth and, much less frequently, decreased sweating and decreased hair growth.

TABLE 21-2	International Association for the Study of Pain Criteria for Diagnosis of Reflex Sympathetic Dystrophy Syndrome/Complex Regional Pain Syndrome I

1. A preceding noxious event without (CRPS I) or with (CRPS II) apparent nerve lesion
2. Spontaneous pain or hyperalgesia not limited to a single nerve territory and disproportionate to the inciting event
3. Present or reported edema, skin blood flow (temperature), or sudomotor abnormality in the distal part of the affected limb
4. Exclusion of other diagnoses

From Stanton HM, Baron R, Boas R, et al. Complex regional pain syndromes: guidelines for therapy. *Clin J Pain* 1998;14:155–166, with permission.

TABLE 21-4	Cardinal Clinical Features of Reflex Sympathetic Dystrophy Syndrome/ Complex Regional Pain Syndrome

Pain, characteristically "burning"[a]
Tenderness[a]
Hyperalgesia[a]
Allodynia and hyperpathia[a]
Swelling[a]
Vasomotor changes
   Changes in color or temperature
Sudomotor changes
   Changes in sweat and hair growth
Dystrophic skin and nail changes
   Shiny skin
   Loss of wrinkling in the skin
   Brittle, discolored nails
Motor changes
   Motor neglect
   Joint stiffness
   Problems with coordination
Sensory changes
   Local changes in sensory perception
   Distant changes

[a] These should be diffuse, affecting the entire extremity.

Sensory and motor changes occur. A number of studies have reported tremor or dystonia occurring in patients with RSDS/CRPS (19–21). Others have observed a neglectlike syndrome in these patients and have suggested that this may account for the motor disturbances observed (22). In one study, 84% of 242 patients with RSDS/CRPS were found to have at least one symptom suggesting motor neglect, including akinesia, bradykinesia, deficits in movement amplitude, and reduced frequency of movement. Unusual sensory changes also have been described (23).

Objective measures in the evaluation of patients suspected of having RSDS/CRPS are important, especially in a medical legal setting. These may provide quantitative data to help in assessment of progress during treatment as well. These include measurement of temperature changes, peripheral blood flow, sweat production, heat and or cold allodynia, osteoporosis, scintigraphic changes, and others (see Table 21-5). Temperature measures are usually obtained by thermography or skin temperature measures with temperature tapes or infrared probes, although other techniques are available. Temperature differences of at least 1.5 to 2.0°F and 1.0 to 1.5°C are necessary for a significant difference to be present. These differences should be diffuse and extend beyond a single nerve distribution. Peripheral blood flow may be measured by a number of techniques, including plethysmography, arteriography, magnetic resonance angiogram (MRA), or laser flow analysis (fluometry). It has been suggested that laser cutaneous blood flow may allow for early diagnosis of posttraumatic RSDS/CRPS (8). Quantitative sudomotor axon reflex test (QSART) provides a measure of resting sweat and stimulated sweat production. Quantitative sensory testing (QST) measures sensitivity to heat and cold sensation (as well as vibratory sensation in some instances) and heat and

TABLE 21-5	Objective Measures in Reflex Sympathetic Dystrophy Syndrome/ Complex Regional Pain Syndrome

Swelling	Volumetric measures, ring sizes
Tenderness	Algometers, dolorimeters
Allodynia	Monofilaments, quantitative sensory testing
Temperature	Infrared probe, thermography, others
Sweating	QSART
Vasomotor changes	Three-phase bone scan
Bone changes	Three-phase bone scan
Bone loss	Bone mineral densitometry

cold pain sensitivity (allodynia). QST is useful in identifying small fiber neurologic dysfunction. However, in RSDS/CRPS sensory changes may be seen beyond the area affected (23). The three-phase bone scan has been the most widely studied objective measure of RSDS/ CRPS (24,25). It has been shown to have a relatively high sensitivity and specificity, but false-positive results have been reported.

Sympathetically maintained pain (SMP) is pain that is significantly reduced by sympathetic blockade (26). It is no longer regarded as a useful diagnostic test for RSDS/CRPS. Although a high percentage of patients with RSDS/CRPS will exhibit SMP, response to sympathetic blockade is nonspecific and may occur in a number of conditions not apparently related to RSDS/CRPS. Interpretation of a "positive" sympathetic blockade also is problematic. There appears to be a high rate of placebo response, and since prolonged responses to normal saline for sympathetic blocks (placebo response) may occur, the specificity of the block itself is doubtful (27–29).

CRITERIA FOR DIAGNOSIS OF REFLEX SYMPATHETIC DYSTROPHY SYNDROME/ COMPLEX REGIONAL PAIN SYNDROME

These IASP criteria (Table 21-2) are simple and reasonably straightforward and should alert the observer to the possibility of RSDS/CRPS I. These criteria have not yet been validated empirically. However, in my opinion these criteria lack specificity and may lack objectivity if based primarily on the patients' reports of changes. Much more specific criteria have been offered in the past (30). A study by Galer et al., which found that nearly 40% of patients with diabetic neuropathy met the IASP criteria for CRPS (31), shows a lack of specificity of these criteria. Recently, a multicenter study was performed to further address the criteria that should be used for diagnosis of CRPS (32). These investigators found 123 patients who met the IASP criteria for CRPS. Using an electromyography (EMG)/nerve conduction velocity study in 60 patients, 32% of patients were found to have CRPS type II. Based upon principal components factor analysis to identify statistical groupings of signs and symptoms related to RSDS/CRPS, they suggest that a revision of the previously published diagnostic criteria may be necessary, pending further validation of their findings.

STAGES OF REFLEX SYMPATHETIC DYSTROPHY SYNDROME/COMPLEX REGIONAL PAIN SYNDROME

Clinical stages of RSD syndrome have been proposed over the years. RSDS/CRPS has been staged according to response to sympathetic blockade (sympathetically independent pain vs. SMP), changes in three-phase bone scan (hyperemic vs. vasospastic), and clinical characteristics. The most common clinical stages are those proposed by De Takats (33) and Steinbrocker (34) and their colleagues and by Bonica (35). Many authors have subsequently described these or similar stages (36). I have previously questioned the value of staging RSDS/CRPS in this manner, noting difficulty in distinguishing such stages (25). In addition, prospective studies of patients developing RSDS/CRPS following Colles fracture often demonstrate a limited clinical course without progressing through stages (25). In a recent multicenter study, Bruehl et al. addressed this question in 113 patients meeting IASP criteria for CRPS (37). Using previously published techniques (see 32), and possibly a subgroup of the same patients, a variety of symptoms and signs were statistically analyzed to determine if different stages could be identified. They found that the three CRPS patient subgroups identified from cluster analysis were not significantly different regarding duration of their disorder.

SUBGROUPS OF REFLEX SYMPATHETIC DYSTROPHY SYNDROME/COMPLEX REGIONAL PAIN SYNDROME

The current classification allows for three subgroups, namely, CRPS type I (RSD syndrome), CRPS type II (causalgia), and CRPS undefined. Over the years, a variety of subtypes have been described, including incomplete, partial, limited, abortive, and circumscribed forms of the disorder (25). To address this issue, Bruehl et al. found three statistically distinct subgroups: CRPS subtype 1, which is a limited syndrome with vasomotor signs predominating; subtype 2, which is a limited syndrome with neuropathic pain/sensory abnormalities predominating; and subtype 3, which showed the highest frequency of motor and trophic signs and bone scan abnormalities (37). These findings would appear to correspond to the short duration RSDS/CRPS following such injuries as Colles fracture (subtype 1), CRPS type II or causalgia (subtype 2), and the classical form of RSDS/CRPS type I (subtype 3).

PATHOPHYSIOLOGIC MECHANISMS

A remarkable amount of research has been done in an effort to understand the physiologic processes producing CRPS. A number of questions need to be addressed, including but not limited to the following: What initiates the condition, and does this affect the peripheral or central nervous system, or both? What maintains the condition, and does this affect the peripheral or central nervous system, or both? What role does the sympathetic nervous system play in initiating and maintaining the condition? How do these effects produce the clinical features that we see in CRPS? Are methods available to prevent CRPS from developing or to abort it early in its course?

There are a number of animal models in which partial injury to a peripheral nerve produces behaviors that suggest development of CRPS. Chung et al. used a spinal nerve ligation model of neuropathic pain in rats, tightly ligating one or two segmental spinal nerves that produced partial denervation of a paw (38). The affected paw demonstrated mechanical allodynia, cold allodynia, heat hyperalgesia, and spontaneous pain that may last weeks. Surgical sympathectomy reduced the mechanical allodynia. Data have shown that sympathetic postganglionic fibers sprout into the dorsal root ganglion of the ligated nerves. It is believed that these sympathetic nerves release sympathetic neurotransmitters that may increase the frequency of ectopic discharges from the injured peripheral nerve, thereby increasing pain and allodynia. Additional accumulating experimental evidence has shown that injury-related changes also are observed in noninjured primary afferent fibers following injury to adjacent dorsal roots (39). Studies have shown that injured nerves may up-regulate adrenoreceptors. Sympathetic discharge, therefore, may bind to these receptors, causing increased neural discharge. Sympathetic discharge also has been shown to affect the dorsal root ganglion, also causing increased neural discharge. These latter studies have been recently reviewed (40).

Wasner et al. have investigated RSDS/CRPS in humans (41). They found a number of changes in temperature regulation and sweat production in patients with RSDS/CRPS, which led them to conclude that there was probable central control of these functions. In patients with early RSDS/CRPS, temperatures were almost invariably increased on the affected side, but later in the course of their condition temperatures diminished and the affected side was cooler than the unaffected side. Sweat production was increased early in the course of the disease and diminished later, but sweat production still remained elevated on the affected side. Other studies evaluated the motor function in patients with RSDS/CRPS (42). These demonstrated impairment of motor function that affects target-reaching and grasping, but only minimally affects grip formation, and also suggested central control of these functions.

There is evidence to suggest that immobility alone can lead to many features observed in RSDS/CRPS. Butler has reviewed several of the studies (43). Animal studies, in which the hind limb of rats was immobilized in a plastic splint for 1 week, demonstrated warm hyperalgesia, mechanical allodynia, and cold allodynia (44). In a second study, a contracture was produced by immobilizing a limb in an exaggerated position, causing shortening of certain muscle groups. An increased population of wide-dynamic-range neurons and a diminished population of low-threshold neurons were observed in the dorsal horn. The percentage of dorsal horn cells that responded to passive movement increased from 41% (in controls) to 77% (in treated animals) (45). In separate experiments, the effects of immobilization alone were compared to fracture plus immobilization in rat hind-limbs. Both groups of animals developed hind limb warmth, edema, spontaneous protein extravasation, allodynia, and periarticular osteoporosis similar to what might be observed in RSDS/CRPS. However, in the immobilized animals without fracture the symptoms resolved much faster. Additionally, it was found that a substance P receptor antagonist inhibited these changes, suggesting that substance P contributes to the vascular and nociceptor changes in this model (46). In humans following foot/ankle fracture and immobilization, similar observations were made. In human volunteers, a prospective study of immobilized forearms was undertaken. Clinical examination demonstrated changes that were compatible with RSDS/CRPS and changes in blood flow in the central nervous system. Thus immobilization produces changes suggestive of central sensitization clinically and changes in central nervous system blood flow.

TREATMENT

RSDS/CRPS has remained difficult to treat in spite of advances in our understanding of the pathophysiology of this disorder. For the most part, we still must revert to symptom control until we can identify "mechanism-specific" treatments (47). It is been estimated that only 20% of individuals who are affected may return to normal function (48). If patients can be identified early in the course of their RSDS/CRPS (within 6 to 12 weeks), it is appropriate to start with physical therapy/occupational therapy. Patients should be evaluated frequently to insure progress. For those patients who are not making adequate progress, systemic corticosteroids or a pain management program (see below) should be initiated immediately and physical therapy should be continued. For those patients with longer duration RSDS/CRPS, systemic corticosteroids or a pain management program should be started immediately, followed by physical therapy. Physicians will often provide sympathetic blockade with the goal of enhancing the benefits of physical therapy (49), but I have not found this to be particularly successful.

How effective is physical therapy/occupational therapy in the treatment of RSDS/CRPS? In children these approaches appear to be quite effective, either alone (50) or combined with cognitive-behavioral treatment (51). Other studies have shown mild improvement in adults (52) but may not show significant improvement in impairment when compared to control groups (53).

Other nonpharmacologic treatments also may be successful, including transcutaneous elliptical stimulation, acupuncture (54), and psychological/psychiatric interventions. However, relatively little data support these approaches. A new approach using mirror visual feedback appears promising (55) and is based on the observations of incongruence between motor and sensory output.

Sympathetic blockade, which has long played a major role in the diagnosis and treatment for patients with RSDS/CRPS, has now fallen into disfavor. Systematic reviews of the medical literature have been undertaken and raise serious questions about the value of sympathetic blockade, especially as the primary treatment for RSDS/CRPS (44,45). However,

permanent sympathetic blocks with paralytic agents or thermocoagulation appear to be effective in ischemic pain in patients with advanced peripheral vascular disease, providing up to 50% long-term improved blood flow and decrease in pain (44). Many patients will respond to sympathetic blockade as a therapeutic approach to various pain syndromes; however, the frequency of placebo response appears to be extremely high. In a review of 29 studies, including 1,140 for patients, 29% of the patients had a complete response, 41% of patients had a partial response, and 32% of patients had no response to sympathetic blockade (45). It was not possible to estimate the duration of pain relief in the studies. Clearly, many patients will have transient partial/complete symptomatic relief (70%), but very few subjects will obtain a long-term relief from sympathetic blocks. Occasionally, patients will be treated with weekly blocks to control their pain, but this approach is rarely adequate, and costly. Some patients will have prolonged responses to sympathetic blocks (3 to 6 months), and it may be reasonable to continue sympathetic blockade to control their pain at these intervals. Surgical sympathectomy is still performed occasionally in patients who have excellent responses to sympathetic blocks. Frequently, there is relatively good short-term relief, but long-term (>12 months) benefit is less predictable. This also appears to be true with thermocoagulation of the sympathetic chain. Sympathetic blockade may be achieved by injection of local anesthetics with or without corticosteroids or opiates directly onto the sympathetic chain in the cervical spine or lumbar spine; by epidural injections of local anesthetics or corticosteroids, or both; by infusion of adrenergic agents locally through Bier blocks, such as clonidine (40); or by damage of the sympathetic ganglia/nerve through thermocoagulation, freezing, or chemical ablation (alcohol, phenol).

In a systematic review of the value of sympathectomy for neuropathic pain of both central and peripheral origin, only four studies were judged to be acceptable for analysis. The reviewers concluded that surgical and chemical sympathectomy is based upon poor quality evidence, uncontrolled studies, and personal experience (56), and they suggested that additional studies would be necessary to establish the procedure's overall effectiveness.

Systemic or local steroids have proven beneficial in certain patients with RSDS/CRPS (25), especially those with upper extremity involvement and day "hot" (hyperemic) three-phase bone scan. In such patients, systemic corticosteroids may be curative in 60% to 75% of cases. Although the dose and dosing schedule of corticosteroids has not been studied, I have found that a 28-day tapering course of steroids is effective: 15 mg qid, 10 mg qid, 10 mg tid, 10 mg bid, 15, 10, and then 5 mg qamqaqa for 4 days each. Others have found that infusion of corticosteroids into the affected extremity using the Bier block technique also is effective. In a study of 36 patients, Zyluk found a good response (relief of spontaneous pain, no limitation in finger movement) in 69% and a moderate response in 22% of patients with upper extremity RSDS 1 year after treatment (57).

A medication-based pain management program should be employed in patients who have failed physiotherapy/occupational therapy, systemic corticosteroids, and sympathetic blockade. Generally, antidepressants, anticonvulsants, or opiates are the mainstay of such treatment. In RSDS/CRPS, other drugs may be effective, including α-1 adrenergic receptor blockers, α-2 adrenergic agonists, calcium channel blocking agents, bisphosphonates, N-methyl-D-aspartate (NMDA) agents such as ketamine, and others. Tricyclic antidepressants have been shown to be effective in various neuropathic pain syndromes, including postherpetic neuralgia and diabetic neuropathy (58), as well as in children with RSDS/CRPS (59). Other tricyclic antidepressants have been found to be effective as well, including nortriptyline and desipramine. Anticonvulsants have been used effectively in adults (60) and children (61) with RSDS/CRPS, but a recent review has not found substantial evidence to support their effectiveness in chronic pain (62). Bisphosphonates have been found to be effective as an analgesic drug (63) and in RSDS/CRPS (64). Intrathecal opiates have been used in chronic-pain conditions and may be effective in RSDS/CRPS. Intrathecal baclofen may be helpful for treatment of the dystonia associated with this condition (65).

Implantation of a dorsal column stimulator (spinal stimulator) is a relatively new approach to treatment of RSDS/CRPS, and there is evidence to support the effectiveness of this approach to treatment. The precise mechanism through which spinal cord stimulation reduces pain is uncertain (66). In a randomized, controlled study of spinal stimulation in patients with RSDS/CRPS, Kemler et al. compared the effects of spinal stimulation plus physical therapy with physical therapy alone (67). Twenty-four of the 36 patients assigned to receive a spinal cord stimulator (SCS) improved with a trial period of stimulation and actually received a permanent SCS. These patients were followed for 6 months. Using a number of outcome measures, the authors found significant improvement in pain and health-related quality of life (pain component) but no improvement in function. These changes were present at the 1-month follow-up, and there was no further improvement at the 3- and 6-month follow-ups. Kemler opined that the SCS is a cost-effective approach to treatment in patients with RSDS/CRPS (68). The benefit for pain relief appears to diminish following SCS at 1 and 2 years of follow-up (69). In a recent review of spinal cord stimulation in RSDS/CRPS, Turner et al. concluded that the Kemler study (67) was the only well-designed randomized, controlled trial of appropriate size to address the effectiveness of spinal cord stimulation in RSDS/CRPS. They concluded that the literature on the value of SCS in RSDS/CRPS "remains inadequate to make definitive statements about efficacy in reducing physical disability, work disability, and medication consumption"(70).

REFLEX SYMPATHETIC DYSTROPHY SYNDROME/COMPLEX REGIONAL PAIN SYNDROME AND FIBROMYALGIA

There are a number of similarities between RSDS/CRPS and fibromyalgia. Clinically, both conditions are associated with chronic pain and tenderness, and the pain is often described as "burning" in character. Vasomotor changes and

hyperalgesia, including allodynia, also occur in both conditions. These changes are consistent with central sensitization in both conditions.

Martinez-Lavin has suggested that fibromyalgia is an SMP syndrome due to sensitization of the primary nociceptors, resulting from sympathetic hyperactivity (71). He demonstrated this by showing that norepinephrine-evoked pain was present in 80% of patients with fibromyalgia, compared to 30% of healthy control subjects (72). Therefore, both conditions may share the presence of SMP.

The pathophysiology of fibromyalgia remains poorly understood, and this issue has been addressed recently (73,74). Two studies suggest that fibromyalgia may result from central sensitization. In a very interesting recent study, Sluka et al. injected acidic saline into muscles of experimental animals, which did not produce tissue damage, and produced hyperalgesia and central sensitization. This affect could be blocked by eliminating the acid-sensing ion channels (ASIC-3), but not by blocking ASIC-1 (74). These data suggest a molecular mechanism that may explain the primary features of fibromyalgia and myofascial pain syndromes. Price et al. recently found evidence of central sensitization in studies of patients with fibromyalgia (74). Using repetitive mechanical stimulation of muscle, they showed that the patients exhibited greatly exaggerated temporal summation (wind-up, hyperpathia) compared to normal control subjects. Additionally, temporal summation occurred at a lower frequency of stimulation and at lower forces. Therefore, fibromyalgia appears to share the similar pathophysiologic mechanisms of peripheral sensitization leading to central sensitization.

Finally, fibromyalgia and myofascial pain syndrome will often develop in patients with RSDS/CRPS. I have seen patients with fibromyalgia who were referred for evaluation of their "whole body" RSDS/CRPS. The overlap in symptoms and findings seems to fool some very knowledgeable physicians. Or were they correct?

SUMMARY POINTS

- Complex regional pain syndrome (CRPS) is the currently preferred term for a heterogeneous group of conditions characterized by pain involving extremities, usually accompanied by skin changes and hyperalgesia.
- Although sympathetic overactivity and sympathetically mediated pain are no longer diagnostic criteria for CRPS, they occur very frequently during phases of CRPS.
- There may be a continuum between CRPS and fibromyalgia, with dysautonomia and hyperalgesia being central pathogenic features to both conditions.

■ IMPLICATIONS FOR PRACTICE

- Sympathetic blockade has fallen into disfavor as a definitive treatment for CRPS because of incomplete and short-lived responses and a high placebo rate.
- Many of the same pharmacologic and nonpharmacologic treatments that have been shown to be effective for fibromyalgia may also be of benefit in CRPS.

REFERENCES

1. Mitchell SW, Morehouse GR, Keen WW. *Gunshot wounds and other injuries of nerves.* New York: JB Lippincott Co, 1864.

2. Mitchell SW. *Injuries of nerves and their consequences.* New York: JB Lippincott Co, 1872.

3. Evans JA. Reflex sympathetic dystrophy. *Surg Clin North Am* 1946;26:780–790.

4. Stanton-Hicks M. Reflex sympathetic dystrophy syndrome: a sympathetically mediated pain syndrome or not? *Curr Rev Pain* 2000;4:268–275.

5. De Takats G. Reflex dystrophy of the extremities. *Arch Surg* 1937;34:939.

6. Stanton-Hicks M, Baron R, Boas R, et al. Complex regional pain syndromes: guidelines for therapy. *Clin J Pain* 1998; 14:155–166.

7. Plewes LW. Sudeck's atrophy in the hand. *J Bone Joint Surg* 1956;38:195–203.

8. Schurmann M, Grad LG, Andress HJ, et al. Assessment of peripheral sympathetic nervous system function for diagnosing early post-traumatic CRPS type I. *Pain* 1999;88: 149–159.

9. Allen G, Galer Bs, Schwartz L. Epidemiology of complex regional pain syndrome: a retrospective chart review of 134 patients. *Pain* 1999;80:539–544.

10. Eisenberg E, Melamed E. Can complex regional pain syndrome be painless? *Pain* 2003;106:263–267.

11. Veldman P, Goris RJ. Multiple reflex sympathetic dystrophy: which patients are at risk for developing recurrence of reflex sympathetic dystrophy in the same or another limb? *Pain* 1996;64:463–466.

12. Teasell RW, Potter P, Moulin D. Reflex sympathetic dystrophy involving three limbs: a case study. *Arch Phys Med Rehabil* 1994;75:10008–100010.

13. Lee BH, Scharff L, Sethna NH, et al. Physical therapy and cognitive-behavioral treatment for complex regional pain syndromes. *J Pediatr* 2002;141:135–140.

14. Kozin F. Painful shoulder and reflex sympathetic dystrophy. *Syndrome Arthritis Allied Conditions.*

15. Mailis A, Inman R, Pham D. *J Rheum* 1992;19:758–764.

16. Maleki J, LeBel AA, Bennett GJ, et al. Patterns of spread in complex regional pain syndrome, type I (reflex sympathetic dystrophy). *Pain* 2000;88:259–266.

17. Price DD, Long S, Huitt C. Sensory testing of pathophysiological mechanisms of pain in patients with reflex sympathetic dystrophy. *Pain* 1992;49:163–173.

18. Birklein F, Reidl B, Neundorfer B, et al. Sympathetic vasoconstriction or reflex pattern in patients with complex regional pain syndrome. *Pain* 1998;75:93–100.

19. Jancovic J, van der Linden C. Dystonia and tremor induced by peripheral trauma: predisposing factors. *J Neurol Neurosurg Psychiatry* 1988;51:1512–1519.

20. Schwartzmann RJ, Kerrigan J. The movement disorder of reflex sympathetic dystrophy. *Neurology* 1990;40:57.

21. Deuschl G, Blumberg H, Luckling CH. Tremor and reflex sympathetic dystrophy. *Arch Neurol* 1991;48:1247–1258.

22. Galer BS, Butler S, Jensen MP. Case reports and hypothesis: a neglect-like syndrome may be responsible for the motor disturbance in reflex sympathetic dystrophy (complex regional pain syndrome-one). *J Pain Symptom Manage* 1995; 10:385–391.

23. Thimineur M, Sood S, Kravitz E, et al. Central nervous system abnormalities in complex regional pain syndrome (CRPS): clinical and quantitative evidence of medullary dysfunction. *Clin J Pain* 1998;14:256–267.

24. Kozin F, Genant HK, Bekerman C, et al. The reflex sympathetic dystrophy syndrome. II. Roetenographic and scintigraphic evidence of bilaterality and periarticular accentuation. *Am J Med* 1976;603:32–338.

25. Kozin F. Painful shoulder and the reflex sympathetic dystrophy syndrome. In: Koopman WJ, ed. *In arthritis and allied conditions,* 13th ed. Philadelphia, PA: Williams & Wilkins, 1993.

26. Roberts WJ. A hypothesis on the physiological basis for causalgia and related pains. *Pain* 1986;124:294–311.

27. Price DD, Long SW, Rafii B. A analysis of peak magnitude and duration of analgesia produced by local anesthetics interjected into sympathetic ganglia of complex regional pain syndrome patients. *Clin J Pain* 1998;14:216–226.

28. Verdugo RJ, Ochoa JL. "Sympathetically maintained pain": phentolamine block questions the concept. *Neurology* 1994; 44:1003–1010.

29. Verdugo RJ, Campero M, Ochoa JL. Phentolamine block in painful polyneuropathies. *Neurology* 1994;44: 100010–1001014.

30. Kozin F, Ryan LM, Carerra GF, et al. The reflex sympathetic dystrophy syndrome. III. Scintigraphic studies: further evidence for the therapeutic efficacy of systemic corticosteroids and proposed diagnostic criteria. *Am J Med* 1981;70:23–30.

31. Galer BS, Bruehl S, Harden RN. IASP diagnostic criteria for complex regional pain syndrome: a preliminary empirical validation study. *Clin J Pain* 1998;14:48–54.

32. Hardin RN, Bruehl S, Galer BS, et al. Complex regional pain syndrome: are the IASP diagnostic criteria valid and sufficiently comprehensive? *Pain* 1999;83:211–219.

33. De Takats G, Miller DS. Post traumatic dystrophy of the extremities, a chronic vasodilator mechanism. *Archives of Surgery* 1943; 46:469–479.

34. Steinbrocker O, Argyros TG. The shoulder-hand syndrome: present status as a diagnostic and therapeutic entity. *Med Clin North Am* 1958;42:1533–1553.

35. Bonica JJ. Causalgia and other reflex sympathetic dystrophies. In: Bonica JJ, ed. *Management of pain,* 2nd ed. Philadelphia, PA: Lea & Febiger, 1990:220–243.

36. Schwartzmann RJ, McClellan TL. Reflex sympathetic dystrophy, a review. *Arch Neurol* 1987;44:555–560.

37. Breuhl S, Harden RN, Galer BS, et al. Complex regional pain syndrome: are there distinct subtypes and sequential stages of the syndrome? *Pain* 2002;95:119–124.

38. Chung K, Chung JM. Sympathetic involvement in the spinal nerve ligation model of neuropathic pain in progress in pain research and management. *Prog Pain Res Manage* 2001; 22:19–26.

39. Ringkamp M, Wu G. Role of injured and on the injured afferents in neuropathic pain in progress in pain research and management. *Prog Pain Res Manage* 2001;22:27–37.

40. Habler H-J, Janig W. Neuropathy after spinal nerve injury in rats: a model for sympathetically maintained pain? *Prog Pain Res Manage* 2001;22:39–52.

41. Wasner G, Drummond P, Birklein F, et al. The role of the sympathetic nervous system and autonomic disturbances and "sympathetically maintained pain" and CRPS. *Prog Pain Res Manage* 2001;22:89–118.

42. Schattschneider J, Wenzelburger R, Deuschl G, et al. Kinematic analysis of the upper extremity and CRPS. *Prog Pain Res Manage* 2001;22:119–128.

43. Butler SH. Disuse and CRPS. *Prog Pain Res Manage* 2001; 22:141–150.

44. Boas RA. Sympathetic nerve blocks: in search of a role. *Reg Anesth Pain Med* 1998;23(3):292–305.

45. Cepeda MS, Lau J, Carr DB. Defining the therapeutic role of local anesthetic sympathetic blockade in complex regional pain syndrome: a narrative and systematic review. *Clin J Pain* 2002;18:216–233.

46. Guo T-Z, Offley SC, Boyd EA, et al. Substance P signaling contributes to the vascular and nociceptive abnormalities observed in a tibial fracture were rat model of complex regional pain syndrome type I. *Pain* 2004;108:95–107.

47. Woolf CJ. Pain: moving from symptom control toward mechanism-specific pharmacological management. *Ann Intern Med* 2004;140:441–451.

48. Subbarao J, Stillwell GK. Reflex sympathetic dystrophy syndrome of the upper extremity: analysis of total outcome of management. *Arch Phys Med Rehabil* 1981;62:549–554.

49. Hord ED, Oaklander AL. Complex regional pain syndrome: a review of evidence-supported treatment options. *Curr Pain Headache Rep* 2003;7:188–196.

50. Wesdock KA, Stanton RP, Singsen BH. Reflex sympathetic dystrophy and children. A physical therapy approach. *Arthritis Care Res* 1991;4:32–38.

51. Lee BH, Scharff L, Sethna NH, et al. Physical therapy and cognitive-behavioral treatment for complex regional pain syndromes. *J Pediatr* 2002;141:135–140.

52. Oerlemans HM, Oostendorp RA, de Boo T, et al. Adjuvant physical therapy versus occupational therapy in patients with reflex sympathetic dystrophy/complex regional pain syndrome type I. *Arch Phys Med Rehabil* 2000;81:49–56.

53. Oerlemans HM, Goris JA, de Boo T, et al. Do physical therapy and occupational therapy reduce the impairment percentage in reflex sympathetic dystrophy? *Arch Phys Med Rehabil* 1999;78:533–539.

54. Bar A, Li L, Eichlisberger R, et al. Acupuncture improves peripheral perfusion in patients with reflex sympathetic dystrophy. *J Clin Rheum* 2002;8:6–12.

55. McCabe CS, Haigh RC, Ring EFJ, et al. A controlled pilot study of the utility of mirror visual feedback in the treatment of complex regional pain syndrome (type I). *Rheumatology* 2003;42:97–101.

56. Mailis A, Furlan A. Sympathectomy for neuropathic pain (Cochrane review). *The Cochrane Library* Issue 1, Chichester, UK:2004.

57. Zyluk A. Results of the treatment of post-traumatic reflex sympathetic dystrophy of the upper extremity with regional intravenous blocks of methylprednisolone and lidocaine. *Acta Orthop Belg* 1998;64:452–456.

58. Max M, Culnane M, Muir J, et al. Amitriptyline relieves diabetic neuropathy pain in patients with normal or depressed mood. *Neurology* 1987;37:589–596.

59. Wilder RT, Berde CB, Wolohan M, et al. Reflex sympathetic dystrophy in children: cortical characteristics and follow-up of 70 patients. *J Bone Joint Surg Am* 1992;74:910–919.

60. Mellick GA, Mellicy LB, Mellick LB. Gabapentin in the management of reflex sympathetic dystrophy. *J Pain Symptom Manage* 1995;10:265–266.

61. Wheeler DS, Voux KK, Tam DA. Uses of gabapentin in the treatment of childhood reflex sympathetic dystrophy. *Pediatr Neurol* 2000;22:220–221.

62. Wiffen, P, Collins S, McQuay H, et al. Anticonvulsant drugs for acute and chronic pain (Cochrane review). *The Cochrane Library* Issue 1, Chichester, UK:2004.

63. Lyritis GP, Trovas G. Analgesic effect of calcitonin. *Bone* 2002;30:71S–74S.

64. Kubalek I, Fain O, Paries J, et al. Treatment of reflex sympathetic dystrophy with pamidronate: 2 cases. *Rheumatology* 2001;40:1394–1397.

65. van Hilten BJ, van de Beek W-JT, Hoff JI. Intrathecal baclofen for the treatment of dystonia in patients with reflex sympathetic dystrophy. *N Engl J Med* 2000;343:625–630.

66. Oakley JC, Prager JP. Spinal cord stimulation: mechanisms of action. *Spine* 2002;27:2574–2583.

67. Kemler MA, Barendse AM, van Kleeff M, et al. Spinal cord stimulation in patients with chronic reflex sympathetic dystrophy. *N Engl J Med* 2000;343:618–624.

68. Kemler MA, Furnee CA. Economic evaluation of spinal cord stimulation for chronic reflex sympathetic dystrophy. *Neurology* 2002;59:1203–1209.

69. Forouzanfar T, Kemler MA, Weber WEJ, et al. Spinal cord stimulation in complex regional pain syndrome: cervical and lumbar devices are comparably effective. *Br J Anesth* 2004;92:348–353.

70. Turner JA, Loeser JD, Deyo RA, et al. Spinal cord stimulation for patients with failed back surgery syndrome or complex regional pain syndrome: a systematic review of effectiveness and complications. *Pain* 2004;108:137–147.

71. Martinez-Lavin M. Is fibromyalgia a generalized reflex sympathetic dystrophy? *Clin Exp Rheumatol* 2001;19:1–3.

72. Martinez-Lavin M, Vidal M, Barbosa RE, et al. Norepinephrine-evoked pain in fibromyalgia. A randomized pilot study. *Musculoskelet Disord* 2002;3:2.

73. Arendt-Nielsen L, Graven-Nielsen T. Central sensitization in fibromyalgia and other musculoskeletal disorders. *Curr Pain Headache Rep* 2003;7:355–361.

74. Sluka KA, Price MP, Breese NM, et al. Chronic hyperalgesia induced by repeated acid injections and muscle is abolished by the loss of ASIC 3, but not ASIC1. *Pain* 2003;106:229–239.

22

The Role of Trauma in Chronic Neuromuscular Pain

Samuel A. McLean, Daniel J. Clauw, and David A. Williams

THE ROLE OF TRAUMATIC EVENTS IN PRECIPITATING REGIONAL AND WIDESPREAD PAIN

INTRODUCTION

Can a single traumatic event, such as a motor vehicle collision (MVC), trigger the onset of chronic regional or widespread pain [e.g., "whiplash" syndrome or fibromyalgia (FM)]? Can exposure to particular repetitive movements ("repetitive strain") induce chronic regional or widespread pain? These questions remain unresolved, fascinating, and contentious. In the case of FM, the ability of a traumatic event to trigger the disease is hotly debated. In the case of whiplash syndrome and repetitive strain, a relationship to trauma is accepted but the mechanisms of disease remain ill-defined.

The advancement of scientific knowledge related to these complex issues has been hampered by a paucity of high-quality, prospective data. In addition, the significant financial and social implications of different models of disease, together with the traditional, dichotomous, biomedical model of disease, have encouraged the development of intensely polarized views. Patients may feel vindicated, and their lawyers most remunerated, by conceptions of illness as resulting directly and unavoidably from "the event." In contrast, health care providers and others often believe these illnesses are due to "the individual," describing them either as volitional acts (malingering) or as indicating a character defect or psychiatric disturbances. To even the casual observer the truth may seem more likely to lie between these two extremes. But how then do these diseases develop?

In this chapter we will examine three diseases associated with trauma: whiplash syndrome, FM, and upper extremity repetitive strain injury. The evidence for each association will be reviewed, along with contemporary theories of disease development. In the chapter summary we will consider common themes and practice implications for each disorder.

REGIONAL PAIN AFTER MOTOR VEHICLE COLLISION ("WHIPLASH-ASSOCIATED DISORDERS")

INTRODUCTION/DEFINITION

Whiplash-associated disorders (WADs) are common following MVC and result in patient suffering and tremendous societal costs (1,2). WAD symptoms may include pain in the neck, shoulder, or arm; headache; jaw pain; dizziness; tinnitus; and memory or concentration difficulties (3). The mechanisms that allow a single, often low-speed MVC to trigger this array of chronic symptoms remains unknown. The complexity of defining these disorders, as well as a plethora of associated research challenges, have resulted in relatively few high-quality studies (4). Historically, two relatively polar pathogenic models have characterized the literature: a biomechanical model (5) that attributes chronic pain to the consequences of tissue injury and Ferrari's biopsychosocial model, which attributes chronic pain to largely psychogenic causes (6). In this setting controversy has flourished because the personal and financial consequences of each of these opposing conclusions to the individual and to society (i.e., "blaming the victim" vs. societal costs) have appeared to be profound.

Recent results from an increasing number of high-quality studies suggests that neither of these two extreme models can explain how and why WAD develops. There is increasing evidence that psychosocial factors contribute to disease outcomes (1,7–9), and "state-of-the-art" cognitive-behavioral models of chronic-pain development have been applied to WAD pathogenesis (10). At the same time, central nervous system (CNS) abnormalities have been documented, most notably widespread hyperalgesia (11–14), demonstrating a neurobiological basis for these disorders.

This section reviews contemporary models of WAD development. Candidate neurobiological mechanisms that may be important to disease pathogenesis will be explored, especially the role of the autonomic and hypothalamic-pituitary-adrenal (HPA) systems ("stress response system") in the development of chronic WAD.

MODELS OF PATHOGENESIS: THE BIOMECHANICAL MODEL

The injury or biomechanical model posits that injury to the cervical spine or other tissues sustained at the time of the accident is central to the development of WAD (2). In this model collision biomechanics [e.g., the location of the occupant's head relative to the head restraint (15,16)] and the occupant's anatomy (17) are important factors determining whether sufficient injury is produced to cause chronic symptoms. Proponents of the biomechanical models suggest that one reason that this model is poorly predictive of long-term outcomes is because of methodologic difficulties in accurately measuring injury severity due to the multiplicity of forces acting on the cervical spine during a collision (18).

Continuing injury research has focused particularly on the motion of the head relative to the neck and the resulting shear forces that occur on the zygapophysial joints, especially at C2-3 and C5-6 (19–21). These injuries are often not apparent using conventional imaging techniques, such as CT (22) and magnetic resonance imaging (MRI) (23), and variations in cervical spine characteristics might explain the increased prevalence of WAD observed in women and older patients (17,24). Further, local treatment (radio-frequency ablation) of pain originating in the zygapophysial joint has been found to be effective for chronic neck pain after whiplash injury (25–27). Proponents of this treatment technique have stated that zygapophysial joint pain accounts for approximately half of all cases of whiplash syndrome (25–27). However, it is difficult to generalize with confidence from these radiofrequency ablation treatment studies, which included a relatively small number of patients (due to the time and skill-intensive nature of the intervention) and which included patients with heterogeneous durations and etiologies of pain. Further work is needed to determine the prevalence of zygapophysial injury as a cause of persistent symptoms among more homogenous WAD populations (e.g., patients with persistent neck pain 6 months after an MVC).

Initial injury may also lead to chronic pain via the development of peripheral, spinal, or supraspinal sensitization. Such mechanisms might be set in motion by the initial injury but persist after the initial injury heals, thus explaining continued symptoms in the absence of detectable injury. Mechanisms possibly contributing to the development and maintenance of WAD include the sensitization or activation of peripheral nociceptors and receptors (28,29) and spinal cord sensitization via the destruction of inhibitory interneurons, the development of excitatory connections, and an expansion of dorsal horn receptive fields (30). However, these relatively local mechanisms would be unlikely to explain the widespread hyperalgesia (11,12,14,31) that has been observed in WAD patients soon after MVC (14,31). Other responses to peripheral injury may have more widespread affects, including mechanisms such as glial cell activation (32) and prostaglandin production (33,34).

The biopsychosocial model of whiplash development expands upon the biomechanical model, in that social, cultural, and psychological factors are also believed to contribute to

disease development in many patients. Proponents of the biopsychosocial model point out a number of epidemiologic characteristics of WAD that seem incompatible with a purely biomechanical etiology. First, the population prevalence of chronic pain following MVC is high in some regions, such as North America (1), and very low in other countries, such as Lithuania (35) and Greece (36). Second, decreasing the financial benefit of developing whiplash syndrome has been found to improve WAD outcomes. Cassidy et al. (1) found that the incidence of WAD decreased as much as 40% when the province of Saskatchewan, Canada, changed from a tort-compensation system to a no-fault system. Marked decreases in depressive symptoms and intensity of neck pain were observed, along with improvements in physical function (1). Third, collisions that occur in other settings (e.g., in bumper cars) exert the same biomechanical stress as a low speed MVC (37), yet prolonged WAD after bumper car collisions are rare (38). The physical collision is not even necessary for WAD symptoms, as Castro et al. (8) exposed patients to a "sham" (placebo) rear-end collision and 20% of patients reported whiplash symptoms 3 days after the collision, despite no actual collision. Patients with greater baseline emotional instability were more likely to report symptom development (8). Fourth, there is no "dose effect" between the intensity of the trauma and the likelihood of developing WAD (39–41). In addition, although the severity of initial symptoms is an important predictor of chronic pain (41–43), the assumption that initial symptoms are proportional to initial tissue injury has not been demonstrated.

Proponents of the biopsychosocial model of disease development also point out that it would be unusual for psychological factors (e.g., depressive and/or anxiety symptoms) to have no role in the development of WAD, given the consistent association of such factors with the development of chronic musculoskeletal neck or back pain (44). Symptoms similar to those of WAD can occur as a manifestation of psychological stress: The "sore neck" syndrome, which includes neck pain, headache, tinnitus, and dizziness, is a common manifestation of anxiety disorder among Khmer populations (45). Several prospective studies of WAD patients have found that increased posttraumatic stress disorder (PTSD) symptoms after injury are associated with increased initial pain symptoms (14,46,47) and with an increased risk of chronic WAD (47,46) (discussed in detail below).

The prevailing biopsychosocial model of WAD pathogenesis is that of Ferrari et al. (6,9,36,48,49). According to this theory, an individual involved in a minor MVC who has the expectation of chronic injury [the perceived threat of chronic symptoms (i.e., "whiplash") is high] begins to interpret everyday symptoms as abnormal, severe, and disturbing. This belief in turn leads to illness behaviors, such as changes in posture, activity cessation, and doctor visits. Abnormal postures lead to chronic pain, activity cessation leads to deconditioning, and medications for pain have side effects which lead to further symptoms, illness behavior, and so on. This leads to a progressive worsening of symptoms, which results in chronic WAD.

This model emphasizes that these phenomena play a major role in symptom development and maintenance; the only "biological factors" this model recognizes are common, everyday symptoms unrelated to the accident (48). Chronic symptoms in WAD and other disorders are considered psychogenic, and the possible role of alterations in CNS function in disease pathogenesis is dismissed:

> In light of the failure of research to identify the chronic "damage" or pathology as lying in a muscular, bony, or "connective tissue" site for many chronic pain syndromes like whiplash, fibromyalgia, et cetera, more recent attention has been paid to nervous system structures. We postulate here, however, that the concept of nervous irritation has been prostituted for centuries whenever more concrete structural explanations for chronic pain and other controversial illness have been untenable ... bringing an understanding of this trend will encourage current clinicians and researchers to appreciate the need to abandon this form of speculation...(6).

However, the idea that chronic multisystem illnesses such as WAD and FM are purely "psychogenic" has been refuted by a large body of data demonstrating that CNS abnormalities are indeed present in these disorders (11,31,50–59).

MECHANISMS OF CHRONIC WAD DEVELOPMENT IN THE BIOPSYCHOSOCIAL MODEL

Vlaeyen et al. have proposed a well-known cognitive-behavioral model of chronic musculoskeletal pain pathogenesis (see Figure 22-1) (60,61), and Turk has suggested that this model may also apply to the development of WAD (10). According to this model, patients with musculoskeletal pain who experience negative emotional responses may develop progressive disability:

> Certain cognitive responses (e.g. catastrophizing) in response to painful experience following injury is augmented in people predisposed with high levels of negative affectivity, leading to fear of movement. This fear of movement leads the person to avoid activities that he or she *believes* will aggravate the injury and cause continued pain. Avoidance of activities not only serves to "prevent" further painful experience but also promotes disability and deconditioning due to disuse of muscles. In the short run, this avoidance of activity may lead to a decrease in pain, reinforcing catastrophizing, fear responses, and continued avoidance of movement (10).

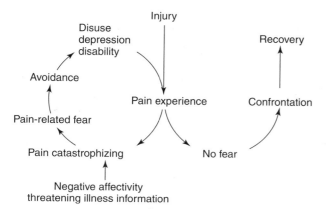

Figure 22-1. Cognitive-behavioral model of chronic-pain pathogenesis. [From Vlaeyen JW, Linton SJ. Fear-avoidance and its consequences in chronic musculoskeletal pain: a state of the art. *Pain* 2000;85:317–332; and Vlaeyen JW, Kole-Snijders AM, Boeren RG, et al. Fear of movement/(re)injury in chronic low back pain and its relation to behavioral performance. *Pain* 1995;62:363–372, with permission.]

Evidence supporting the application of this model to the development of WAD includes the results of several clinical intervention studies (62,63) that have demonstrated the importance of early neck mobilization exercises and avoiding time off work in preventing chronic neck pain after whiplash injury.

Nederhand et al. have applied such cognitive-behavioral models to the examination of the role of musculoskeletal factors in the pathogenesis of WAD (64–66). Using muscle electromyography, they identified cervical muscle hyperactivity in patients with long-standing whiplash syndrome (67) and nonspecific neck pain (65). These data suggested a pain–spasm–pain model of WAD pathogenesis in which sustained muscle hyperactivity plays a role in chronic symptom development. Other studies have also found muscle hyperactivity among WAD patients during the first month after injury (14). However, a subsequent prospective study found no evidence of muscle hyperactivity during the first 6 months after injury in patients developing WAD but a reorganization of muscular activation instead (66). This was hypothesized to be due to cervical muscle "overprotection" from activity avoidance (66). Other studies, with different recruitment strategies and techniques, have shown more sustained activation (68). Such muscular abnormalities may contribute to other symptoms experienced by patients, such as dizziness (69). The precise mechanisms by which musculoskeletal factors interact with other factors to contribute to WAD development remains unknown.

Vlaeyen's model (60) and its application to WAD (66) exemplifies the progress that has been made in the development and testing of conceptual models of candidate psychobehavioral processes involved in the development of WAD. Less progress has been made in identifying candidate neurobiological mechanisms that mediate persistent symptom expression and the development of CNS processing abnormalities, such as widespread hyperalgesia (11,12,14,31). The widespread nature (11,12,14,31) and rapid onset (14,31) of hyperalgesia soon after injury occurrence and the importance of psychosocial factors to WAD outcomes suggest a significant role for supraspinal mechanisms.

EVIDENCE SUGGESTING A ROLE FOR THE STRESS RESPONSE SYSTEM IN WHIPLASH-ASSOCIATED DISORDER PATHOGENESIS

The autonomic and HPA ("stress response") system may be an important central mechanism involved in the development of chronic WAD. Although the role of this system in WAD development has been understudied, many lines of evidence suggest a link: (a) stress response system (HPA and autonomic nervous system) abnormalities have been identified in established psychological sequelae of MVC such as PTSD (70) and in other chronic multisystem pain illnesses such as FM (51,52); (b) WAD, PTSD, and FM have overlapping epidemiologic and clinical features (see below); (c) there is a close association between PTSD symptoms and pain symptoms after MVC, beginning soon after the collision, in those developing WAD (46,47); (d) the stress response system plays a central role in the pathogenesis of PTSD after MVC (71–75); (e) the stress response system is capable of influencing widespread nociception (see below); and (f) the stress response system may contribute to symptom development through multiple mechanisms, including the initial stress response to the MVC, and also through behavior changes that may occur after the collision.

1. *Stress response system abnormalities in PTSD and FM.* The principal components of the human stress response are the HPA axis and locus ceruleus/norepinephrine-sympathetic (LC-NE) system (76,77). Acute stress triggers the release of corticotrophin releasing factor (CRF), which then acts as the "ignition switch" (78) for the human stress response. In addition to activating the HPA and LC-NE systems, CRF also triggers a complex cascade of reactions mediated by many other neurohormonal, neurotransmitter, metabolic, and immunologic mechanisms, including adrenergic, cholinergic, serotonergic, opioid, glutamatergic, gabergic, and cytokine systems (78–80). CRF also initiates its own negative feedback via the stimulation of adrenocorticotropic hormone (ACTH) release from the pituitary (81,82). ACTH stimulates the adrenal glands to release cortisol, which is critical in containing and terminating these stress-related reactions (83).

In patients with PTSD and FM, alterations in neuroendocrine function are believed to be an important feature of the disorder, and abnormalities of both HPA and LC-NE systems have been identified (53–56,78,84–86). Patients with established PTSD often have decreased baseline cortisol levels, increased CRF levels, a hypersensitivity of the hypothalamus and pituitary gland to negative inhibition, and a decreased cortisol response to acute stressors (78,84). Individuals with PTSD exhibit hyperactivity of the LC-NE (autonomic nervous) system (78,84). Although stress response function is acknowledged to be abnormal in FM, the precise nature of the abnormality has been variable among studies (52,87,88). The most consistent finding in FM is hyporesponsiveness of both HPA and autonomic function to standardized stressors (54,88,89). (See Chapters 6,7.)

2. *Overlapping epidemiologic and clinical features of WAD, PTSD, and FM.* WAD, PTSD, and FM have overlapping clinical and epidemiologic characteristics. Female gender (1,41–43,87,90–92), lower socioeconomic status (1,93,94), and preexisting mood disorders (7,8,87,92,95) appear to increase the risk of developing all three disorders. All three disorders are characterized by multisystem complaints (87,96–98), such as headache, axial pain, fatigue, cognitive dysfunction, and sleep disturbances (96,99–101).

Like WAD, PTSD is common after MVC (74,102,103), and PTSD commonly occurs along with chronic-pain conditions, including FM and WAD. Clinically significant PTSD-like symptoms have been found in more than 50% of FM patients (104,105) and in more than 50% of patients receiving treatment for chronic pain after MVC (106,107). At least 15% to 25% of patients with persistent whiplash symptoms meet diagnostic criteria for PTSD (108,109). Patients with chronic pain and PTSD report higher levels of pain and disability relative to patients without PTSD (110,111). In addition, just as PTSD is common in patients with chronic pain, chronic pain is also common in patients with PTSD. Chronic pain is reported by 20% to 30% of outpatients' samples with PTSD (110,112,113) and by 80% of combat veterans with PTSD (110).

FM also appears to occur as a sequela of MVC, although the relationship of MVC to FM has not been well studied.

Between 24% and 47% of FM patients report that injury from MVC was the initiating event for their illnesses (104,114,115). Buskila et al. (116) conducted the only study directly examining the relationship between FM and MVC. This study found that 22% of those with neck pain after MVC developed FM, compared to only 2% of those with leg injury (116). The cumulative direct and indirect evidence for a causal relationship between MVC and FM exceeds that of other rheumatologic conditions for which an environmental trigger has been accepted (117).

3. *Association between PTSD symptoms and WAD symptoms during WAD development.* A limitation of most studies examining the relationship between chronic pain and PTSD is their cross-sectional design. Such studies cannot provide information on disease development—for example, did the diseases develop concurrently or did the presence of chronic pain create a vulnerability for developing PTSD? Studies of WAD indicate that increased PTSD symptoms are associated with increased pain soon after injury (14,46,47), and a longitudinal study that examined PTSD symptoms serially during the development of WAD found that these symptoms continue in patients with persistent moderate or severe WAD symptoms (46). In addition, PTSD symptoms after MVC have been shown to predict the development of chronic WAD. Drottning (47) found that high scores on the Impact of Event Scale (PTSD symptom severity) were found in 70% of patients with significant neck pain 4 weeks after MVC, as opposed to only 26% of those in the low pain group. Sterling et al. (46) found that elevated Impact of Event Scale scores within 1 month of MVC were unique to those with moderate or severe WAD at 6 months.

4. *Stress response system function predicts PTSD development after MVC.* The neurobiological processes involved in chronic-pain development after MVC have not been well studied. However, a number of studies have examined the neurobiology of PTSD development after MVC (71–75). Variations in stress response after MVC have been found to be predictive of PTSD development (71–75) in ways that are consistent with theoretical models that implicate an abnormal stress response in PTSD development (118). As mentioned above, during the response to a stressful event CRF triggers a cascade of reactions, such as the release of catecholamines and cortisol (78). It has been proposed that an exaggerated and/or poorly contained stress response [increased catecholamines and other neuropeptides (119) and/or an insufficient cortisol response (120)] is an important mechanism that contributes to PTSD pathogenesis (119,120). Consistent with this view, both an increased heart rate (74) (increased sympathomimetic response) and decreased cortisol response (71–73) after MVC have been found to predict the later development of PTSD. Shalev et al. found that increased heart rate upon arrival to the emergency department and 1 week after injury (including MVC) predicted PTSD development (74). Several studies have found that a decreased cortisol response in the hours and days after MVC increased the risk of developing PTSD (71–73).

In some prospective studies of PTSD, neurobiological data are better predictors of PTSD development than psychosocial factors (e.g., demographic factors, initial symptoms) (71,118). Preliminary evidence suggests that the secondary prevention of PTSD may be possible using pharmacologic interventions provided in the emergency department to attenuate the stress response (75). In a small pilot study, Pitman et al. found that 40 mg of propranolol given within 6 hours of the traumatic event and continued four times a day was effective in decreasing the subsequent development of PTSD symptoms (75). No studies have examined the importance of the stress response in chronic-pain development after MVC.

In cross-sectional studies, PTSD appears to be particularly common in chronic-pain patients classified as dysfunctional via the Multidimensional Pain Inventory (MPI) (121) and Multiaxial Assessment of Pain (MAP) (122) (i.e., higher pain severity and interference, higher affective distress, and lower levels of self-efficacy). For example, among a sample of patients with work-related chronic pain, 71% of the dysfunctional subgroup, as opposed to 21% of the minimizers/adaptive copers group (i.e., lower pain severity and interference and higher self-efficacy), met criteria for PTSD (123). Another study has reported similar findings (123).

5. *Stress response system is capable of influencing widespread nociception.* In addition to its role in psychological processes, the stress response system is known to influence both opioid and nonopioid descending pain inhibitory pathways (124,125). (See Chapter 5.) The contribution of such mechanisms is suggested by the early onset and widespread nature of the hyperalgesia that develops soon after MVC (14,31) in patients who develop chronic WAD (31). Patients with WAD have been found to have the same widespread hypersensitivity to sensory stimulation as patients with FM (12), and data suggest that descending antinociceptive pathways may be hypoactive in individuals with FM (126–130). Monoamines (e.g., serotonin, norepinephrine) are also involved in the descending modulation of pain (131) and may also contribute to WAD development (12). Specific serotonin genotypes and variants in monoamine metabolism have been linked to increased pain and psychological distress in patients with other chronic multisymptom pain conditions, such as FM, and may help explain variation in patient outcomes (132–134).

6. *HPA system function predicts the development of pain and other symptoms after a standardized experimental stressor.* The above discussion has focused on the MVC event and the hypothesis that an exaggerated and/or poorly contained stress response to an MVC event may contribute to WAD development. However, this is only one of a number of neurobiological mechanisms that may influence alterations in nociceptive processing. First, for some processes stress response measures may only be markers for other neurobiological processes directly involved in nociceptive processing. Second, there are likely to be other potential mechanisms by which the stress response to an MVC event may influence chronic symptom development (78). Third, and perhaps most important, considering this hypothesis in isolation ignores the importance of post-MVC factors on individual outcomes. These post-MVC factors, such as the types of cognitive-behavioral factors proposed in Vlaeyen's model (60), are likely to interact with the initial neurobiological response to the MVC event and may often be more important to chronic symptom development than event-related factors. The mechanisms by which these factors influence alterations in nociception remain poorly understood, but recent studies suggest that some of these cognitive and behavioral responses may cause pain and other symptoms largely via central neurobiological mechanisms. For example, recent studies have identified mechanisms of altered pain processing related to beliefs about pain control (135) and catastrophization (136).

One postevent factor that is known to influence individual outcomes is decreased activity level. Decreased activity after MVC is known to increase the risk of WAD (63), but the mechanisms by which decreased activity may influence nociceptive processing are unknown. Results from a recent study indicate that stress response system function may identify those individuals particularly vulnerable to symptom development resulting from activity decreases (137).

Thus, neurobiological mechanisms involving the stress response system may contribute to cultural variations in WAD prevalence via both MVC-related and/or post-MVC related factors. In countries in which the perceived threat of MVC is high, the MVC event itself may be more likely to result in an exaggerated and/or poorly contained stress response, which in vulnerable individuals may lead to persistent pain or psychological symptoms, or both. In addition, individuals in countries where the perceived threat of MVC is high may also be more likely to decrease their activity level after an MVC (e.g., to "rest up" after the injury), which also may contribute to symptom development in vulnerable individuals via central neurobiological processes. These mechanisms are not mutually exclusive, and in fact may often occur together and be synergistic.

SUMMARY

Recently, Norton and Asmundson (138) proposed an amendment to Vlaeyen's fear-avoidance model of chronic-pain development. Their revised model (see Figure 22-2) places increased emphasis on the importance of physiologic activities in chronic-pain development, which can increase pain (e.g., via increased muscle tension) and augment normal physiologic processes (e.g., cause an increased heart rate), which are then interpreted catastrophically (138). This concept of normal physiologic processes that are interpreted catastrophically is similar to Ferrari's concept of hypervigilance and symptom amplification (48).

Cognitive-behavioral models, such as those of Norton and Asmundson (138), Vlaeyen et al. (60), and Nederhand et al. (66), have focused on the interaction of relatively "peripheral" physiologic processes (such as musculoskeletal factors) in the development of chronic pain. However, increasing data suggest that, for many patients, central neurobiological factors may play a more important role in chronic symptom development than such peripheral factors. Longitudinal studies are needed that examine not only cognitive-behavioral factors but also candidate neurobiological processes, including the stress response system, which appear to contribute to symptom expression in patients with chronic illness. Such studies should also examine the relationship of WAD development to other outcomes after MVC that appear to have overlapping characteristics with WAD, such as PTSD and FM. These studies will allow us to learn more about the rich and complex interactions of the behavioral, cognitive, and physiologic (neurobiological) processes that occur during the transition from acute injury to chronic pain.

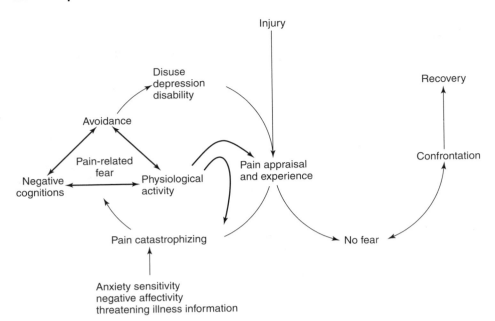

Figure 22-2. Norton and Asmundson's amendment (bold arrows) to Vlaeyen's cognitive-behavioral model.

REGIONAL AND WIDESPREAD PAIN ASSOCIATED WITH OCCUPATIONAL "REPETITIVE STRAIN INJURY"

INTRODUCTION

"Repetitive strain injury" describes chronic-pain conditions of the upper limb that are generally believed to be related to work involving repetitive moment (139). There are many similarities between "whiplash" and "repetitive strain" disorders, beginning with the fact that both disorders carry evocative names suggesting a particular, unproven, solely biomechanical mechanism. Because of this, the term "repetitive strain" has been replaced by other terms such as "work-related upper extremity disorders" (140) and "nonspecific arm pain" (NSAP). The latter term will be used for the purposes of this discussion.

BIOMEDICAL AND PSYCHOSOCIAL RISK FACTORS

As with WAD, both biomechanical and psychosocial risk factors have been identified. Biomechanical factors are important; occupations that involve repetitive movements of the upper extremity are associated with increased risk of disease development (139,141), as are avocations such as wheelchair athletics (139,141) and playing a stringed instrument (139,141). Psychosocial factors are also important (141–143); a recent systematic review found that high perceived job stress and nonwork-related stress were consistently associated with the development of NSAP (142). Macfarlane et al. (141) performed a population-based cohort study of forearm pain development among workers in Manchester, England, during a 2-year follow-up period. Among those who developed the new onset of forearm pain, risk factors included repetitive movements of the arm [relative risk (RR) 4.1], as well

as dissatisfaction with support from colleagues or supervisors (RR 4.7), high levels of psychological distress (RR 2.4), and baseline somatic complaints (RR 1.7) (141).

ASSOCIATION OF NONSPECIFIC ARM PAIN WITH WIDESPREAD PAIN

Evidence suggests that occupation-related NSAP often occurs as part of a more widespread pain condition. In the previously cited study by Macfarlane et al. 45% of those who developed forearm pain also developed chronic widespread pain (141). Two smaller studies also found a high coocurrence of NSAP with widespread pain. Gallinaro et al. found that 59% of those with repetitive strain injury in a Brazilian factory also met diagnostic criteria for FM, as compared to 10% of controls (144). Helfenstein and Feldman found that 71% of workers seeking compensation for repetitive strain injury met diagnostic criteria for FM (145). Further studies are needed to examine the prevalence of widespread pain in those with NSAP, in both population-based and referral samples.

NEUROBIOLOGICAL ABNORMALITIES AND MECHANISMS OF NONSPECIFIC ARM PAIN DEVELOPMENT

The mechanisms of NSAP development and nervous system abnormalities in patients with NSAP have not been well studied. Cohen et al. performed one of the few detailed evaluations of NSAP patients (146,147). They found numerous nociceptive abnormalities in a referral population of patients with refractory NSAP, including hyperalgesia and allodynia in response to both mechanical and electrical stimulation of the affected limb (146,147). They also found abnormalities consistent with sympathetically maintained pain in many patients (147). A recent study by Greening et al. (148) also found abnormalities in sensory function and autonomic response in NSAP patients.

Cohen et al. hypothesized a pathogenesis of NSAP, incorporating ideas first proposed by Livingston in 1943 (149). According to this theory, continuous afferent stimulation from nociceptors and mechanoreceptors in the periphery triggers CNS changes, including alterations in the dorsal horn of the spinal cord. These spinal cord changes result in altered sympathetic and motor efferents, resulting in more pain and a reflexively evoked neuropathic state (147). Cohen et al. suggested that "constrained work postures and movements ... may be sufficient to sensitize WDR (wide dynamic range) neurons so that mechanoreceptive afferent information is processed as nociceptive" (147).

Similarly, other authors have hypothesized that NSAP symptoms result from "multiple levels of nerve compression and muscle imbalance that occur concurrently" in the affected limb (150,151). Several small studies have documented decreased movement of the median nerve in patients with NSAP versus controls (151,152), and such changes have been seen as consistent with a nerve compression pathogenesis (151,152). Further studies of NSAP are needed, including prospective studies that examine the relationship of regional and widespread pain and investigate neurobiological abnormalities during disease development.

FIBROMYALGIA ASSOCIATED WITH MOTOR VEHICLE COLLISION

INTRODUCTION

The ability of physical trauma, such as an MVC, to trigger the development of FM remains the subject of intense debate (153). On the one hand, there are a plethora of case reports and anecdotal accounts of individuals who have developed FM in close temporal association with an MVC (154–157). On the other hand, several authors have raised legitimate arguments regarding the scientific veracity of this linkage and have argued appropriately that prematurely accepting such an association could be more harmful than beneficial—to both individual patients and society (158,159). To date there is only a single case–control study directly examining the relationship between FM and MVC. Buskila et al. found that 22% of patients with neck injury and 2% of patients with leg injury developed FM 1 year after MVC (160).

EVIDENCE FOR A CAUSAL RELATIONSHIP BETWEEN MOTOR VEHICLE COLLISION AND FIBROMYALGIA

To provide explicit criteria for determining the strength of the evidence between an environmental exposure and the development of a rheumatologic disorder, Miller et al. (161) recently proposed a model incorporating the classical principles of establishing causality [originally proposed by Hill (162)]. This model suggested that support for causality be based upon eight elements. The first five of these elements were considered "primary" and included the establishment of (1) a temporal association, (2) a lack of alternative explanations, (3) a biological plausibility, (4) dechallenge (i.e., the result of removing an aspect of the

causal relationship), and (5) rechallenge (i.e., the result of reintroducing a missing aspect of the causal relationship). The remaining three elements were considered "secondary" and included the establishment of (1) analogy (i.e., previous reports of similar cause-and-effect relationships), (2) dose responsiveness (e.g., more of one causal aspect produces more of effect), and (3) specificity (e.g., uniqueness of the cause-and-effect relationship). According to these criteria, at least four out of eight elements must be present (including three primary elements) in order to suspect a causal relationship. The association between MVC and FM will be examined using this methodology.

1. *Temporal association.* There is no disagreement regarding a close temporal association between an MVC and the development of FM. Typically, the progression from acute regional pain to more widespread pain and fatigue predictably occurs within weeks to several months (154,155). If such a pattern is not seen in a given individual, it is unlikely that the MVC had any role in leading to the development of FM.

2. *Lack of likely alternative explanations.* Opponents of the notion that MVC can cause FM cite two possible alternative explanations for symptom development: malingering and psychosocial factors. Although a few people undoubtedly malinger in this setting, even the most ardent opponents of the posttraumatic FM construct concede that this is rare (153,163). In contrast, as noted above, substantial data indicate that psychosocial factors play a significant role in determining who will progress from an acute pain condition to chronic pain (164,165). These psychosocial factors are best understood as a component of a process of chronic symptom development in which biological, psychological, and social factors all play an important role (biopsychosocial model), rather than as an alternative mechanism.

3. *Biological plausibility.* As described above, and in more detail in Chapters 5 and 6, advances in the field of pain research over the past two decades have resulted in new understandings of the mechanisms that are operative in chronic-pain states such as FM. Many of these concepts have also been central to the improved understanding of WAD, and they include an appreciation that (1) CNS changes play a much larger role in chronic pain than "peripheral" factors (e.g., peripheral musculoskeletal injury) (166,167); (2) chronic-pain illnesses are not essentially "psychological" (166–168); (3) chronic-pain syndromes are characterized by abnormalities of CNS pain processing (127,128,169–173); (4) these abnormalities involve the stress response system, and this system is influenced by many factors, including social support and the predictability or avoidability of life stressors (174,175); and (5) the vulnerability of the CNS to developing illnesses such as FM may be influenced by previous life experiences, especially significant stress experienced early in life (175,176), perhaps explaining the association between FM and related conditions and early physical or sexual abuse (177,178).

4. *Dechallenge.* For some environmentally associated rheumatic disorders (e.g., drug-induced lupus) removal of the offending agent leads to resolution of symptoms, strengthening support for a cause-and-effect relationship in this illness. To date little evidence supports a similar relationship in the case of trauma and FM.

5. *Rechallenge.* Patients who experience a second MVC have significant worsening of regional pain (179), and there

is anecdotal evidence that FM symptoms worsen after repeat exposure to trauma.

6. *Analogy; are there previous reports of a similar disorder developing after the exposure in question?* Yes; as previously noted, there are abundant case reports and case series documenting that FM can develop after trauma of various types.

7. *Dose responsiveness.* There is no good evidence of dose responsiveness, if the intensity of trauma, rather than the response to trauma, is considered the "dose." As described above, collisions of a particular magnitude do not appear necessary or sufficient to cause chronic pain after MVC (8,37,39–41,180). In contrast, the emotional distress surrounding the trauma and the personal (7), financial (1), and cultural (181) environments in which the trauma occurs appear to be important factors.

8. *Specificity; are the defining symptoms, signs, and laboratory features of the disorder unique?* FM that occurs after trauma does not have any features that are reliably different from FM that occurs in other settings or under different circumstances. Thus, trauma may be only one of many types of stressors capable of producing symptoms characteristic of FM.

Using these above attribution elements, the association between FM and MVC meets criterion one (temporal association), criterion two (lack of alternative explanations), criterion three (biological plausibility), criterion six (analogy), and possibly criterion five (rechallenge). This meets or exceeds the recommended threshold for suspecting a causal relationship between an exposure and subsequent illness. To put the relationship between FM and trauma in context, there are at least as much data supporting this relationship as there are for many other accepted environmentally associated rheumatic diseases.

SUMMARY

In short, abundant data suggest that it is biologically plausible that physical trauma, acting as a stressor, could lead to the development of chronic widespread pain, as well as a number of other somatic symptoms. Particularly important constructs in this regard are that many different types of stressors are capable of eliciting similar responses, a single exposure to stress can have chronic consequences, and the environment in which the stressor is experienced may largely determine whether or not there is an adverse physiologic effect. These advances in the biology of stress and pain render dualistic arguments of biology versus psychology largely irrelevant. Further case control or other population-based designs are necessary to more firmly establish causation and to better understand the precise mechanisms that are operative. Such research could identify patients at high risk of developing FM after physical trauma and other stressors, identify important biological and psychosocial factors involved in the development of FM, and develop secondary prevention strategies.

CHRONIC NEUROMUSCULAR PAIN AFTER TRAUMA: SUMMARY AND PRACTICE IMPLICATIONS

Several themes emerge from reviewing the relationship between acute or chronic trauma and the development of WAD,

FM, and NSAP. In all three disorders it is clear that biomechanical factors (an MVC or particular repetitive motions) increase one's vulnerability to develop particular types of chronic pain (e.g., whiplash, NSAP). The importance of psychosocial factors in pain pathogenesis has also been demonstrated in the two disorders (whiplash and NSAP) in which risk factors for pain development have been examined.

As noted above, in FM distinct patient subgroups have been identified (59). In some groups psychological factors appear to strongly influence symptom report; in others they do not (59). It is likely that, as other pain disorders related to trauma receive further study, subgroups of patients within these other disorders will also be identified. For example, among whiplash patients, it is likely that at least some individuals have continued occult injury after MVC sufficient to result in chronic neck pain. At the same time, it appears that for many, if not most, patients with these disorders the interplay of psychosocial factors with biomechanical and other factors is necessary for disease development. This interplay of factors may cause the development of chronic pain via more than one mechanism, resulting in patients with varied symptoms within each disorder.

Elucidating the mechanisms by which personal and environmental factors may combine with biomechanical factors to produce disease is complex but achievable. For example, highly developed models of the pathogenesis of occupationally related NSAP have been proposed (182). Although such models of disease development have only begun to be developed and tested, recommendations for patient management need not wait the final conclusions of these studies. Enough information exists on risk factors and probable mechanisms to provide a firm basis for patient care recommendations. For occupationally related NSAP, studies have demonstrated that multimodal interventions are effective in decreasing NSAP, both before and after symptom development (143).

Regarding chronic pain after a traumatic event, such as MVC, evidence suggests that patient outcomes are not determined solely by the event itself. Rather, the postevent environment plays a critical role in disease development, and patient caregivers have an important role in this regard. As far as the CNS effects of stress are concerned, perceived is real, and perceived contingencies need to be recognized as salient stressors along with the trauma itself. Thus, an interpretation of posttrauma symptoms as indicating a significant threat to health appears to increase the risk of chronic symptom development. After clinical evaluation excludes injuries that require immediate intervention (e.g., herniated cervical disc or cervical spine fracture in post-MVC patients) patients should be reassured that their symptoms are common, "normal," and, most important, self-limiting.

In addition, several principles should guide the care, counseling, and advocacy for patients in regards to their interaction with the health system and employers. First, unduly contentious systems, which make patients "prove" that their symptoms are "real," can increase patient distress. Such systems also incentivize symptoms and limitations. This is probably one reason why patients who pursue litigation or compensation are less likely to improve and more likely to end up permanently on disability (183–185). We can and should educate patients about this and tell them that they will rarely reap financial reward or feel as though they have received "justice" in the legal system if they choose this route.

At the other extreme, unduly liberal compensation environments can also incentivize symptoms by providing financial or other motivations for the sick role. Patients should be encouraged to continue usual activities as best they can and to resume full activity as soon as possible. Time off work should be minimized. Among post-MVC patients, for example, immobilization, inactivity, and time off work after MVC have all been shown to increase the risk of developing chronic pain (62,63,186).

There is probably a critical "window of opportunity" in which patients at risk of making the transition to chronic pain can be identified and given more aggressive management. Unfortunately, at present the patient with unresolved acute pain is likely to receive more imaging studies (that frequently detect subtle abnormalities of questionable significance but that reinforce the concept of permanent injury), interventional procedures of unclear efficacy, and/or aggressive physical therapy (which may encourage a passive, helpless approach on the part of the patient). In addition to the above interventions, other more appropriate but rarely utilized interventions include cognitive-behavioral approaches, aggressive activation and exercise programs, pharmacologic therapy aimed at chronic rather than acute pain, and multidisciplinary programs that combine these modalities.

SUMMARY POINTS

- Both biomechanical and psychosocial factors are important in the development of trauma-induced chronic pain. The precise neurobiological mechanisms by which these factors interact to produce chronic symptoms remain poorly understood.
- The stress response system is likely to be an important mechanism mediating the neurobiological changes involved in chronic-pain development after a traumatic event.
- Traumatic events may trigger the development of chronic pain via acting as stressors. In this way many different types of stressors may be capable of eliciting a similar response.
- Patients within each diagnostic group (e.g., whiplash) are unlikely to have identical pathophysiologic mechanisms and symptoms. Important subgroups are likely to exist within each group.
- Relatively few prospective studies examining biopsychosocial mechanisms have been done on any of these disorders. Our understanding of the precise pathologic mechanisms resulting in these diseases is in its infancy.

■ IMPLICATIONS FOR PRACTICE

- After excluding injuries that require immediate intervention, patients with musculoskeletal pain after a traumatic event should be reassured that their symptoms are common, "normal," and, most important, self-limiting.
- After traumatic events, patients should be encouraged to continue usual activities as best they can and to resume full activities as soon as possible. Time off work should be minimized.
- Patients who develop chronic pain after a traumatic event have a neurobiological basis for their symptoms. Malingering is rare.
- Patients should be discouraged from engaging in litigation or compensation claims. Patients are rarely satisfied with the result, and such contention incentivizes symptoms and disability.

REFERENCES

1. Cassidy JD, Carroll LJ, Cote P, et al. Effect of eliminating compensation for pain and suffering on the outcome of insurance claims for whiplash injury. *N Engl J Med* 2000;342:1179–1186.
2. Freeman MD, Croft AC, Rossignol AM, et al. A review and methodologic critique of the literature refuting whiplash syndrome. *Spine* 1999;24:86–96.
3. Spitzer WO, Skovron ML, Salmi LR, et al. Scientific monograph of the Quebec Task Force on whiplash-associated disorders: redefining "whiplash" and its management. *Spine* 1995;20:1S–73S.
4. Cote P, Cassidy JD, Carroll L, et al. A systematic review of the prognosis of acute whiplash and a new conceptual framework to synthesize the literature. *Spine* 2001;26:1.
5. Barnsley L, Lord S, Bogduk N. Whiplash injury. *Pain* 1994;58:283–307.
6. Ferrari R, Shorter E. From railway spine to whiplash—the recycling of nervous irritation. *Med Sci Monit* 2003;9:27–37.
7. Olsson I, Bunketorp O, Carlsson SG, et al. Prediction of outcome in whiplash-associated disorders using West Haven-Yale multidimensional pain inventory. *Clin J Pain* 2002;18:238–244.
8. Castro WH, Meyer SJ, Becke ME, et al. No stress—no whiplash? Prevalence of "whiplash" symptoms following exposure to a placebo rear-end collision. *Int J Legal Med* 2001;114:316–322.
9. Ferrari R, Kwan O, Russell AS, et al. The best approach to the problem of whiplash? One ticket to Lithuania, please. *Clin Exp Rheumatol* 1999;17:321–326.
10. Turk DC. Chronic pain and whiplash associated disorders: rehabilitation and secondary prevention. *Pain Res Manag* 2003;8:40–43.
11. Curatolo M, Petersen-Felix S, Arendt-Nielsen L, et al. Central hypersensitivity in chronic pain after whiplash injury. *Clin J Pain* 2001;17:306–315.
12. Banic B, Petersen-Felix S, Andersen OK, et al. Evidence for spinal cord hypersensitivity in chronic pain after whiplash injury and in fibromyalgia. *Pain* 2004;107:7–15.
13. Sterling M, Jull G, Vicenzino B, et al. Sensory hypersensitivity occurs soon after whiplash injury and is associated with poor recovery. *Pain* 2003;104:509–517.
14. Sterling M, Jull G, Vicenzino B, et al. Characterization of acute whiplash-associated disorders. *Spine* 2004;29:182–188.
15. Svensson MY, Lovsund P, Haland Y, et al. The influence of seat-back and head-restraint properties on the head-neck motion during rear-impact. *Accid Anal Prev* 1996;28:221–227.
16. Lawrence JM, Siegmund GP. Seat back and head restraint response during low-speed rear-end automobile collisions. *Accid Anal Prev* 2000;32:219–232.
17. Stemper BD, Yoganandan N, Pintar FA. Gender dependent cervical spine segmental kinematics during whiplash. *J Biomech* 2003;36:1281–1289.
18. Walz FH, Muser MH. Biomechanical assessment of soft tissue cervical spine disorders and expert opinion in low speed collisions. *Accid Anal Prev* 2000;32:161–165.

19. Bogduk N, Yoganandan N. Biomechanics of the cervical spine. Part 3: minor injuries. *Clin Biomech* 2001;16:267–275.

20. Yoganandan N, Pintar FA, Cusick JF. Biomechanical analyses of whiplash injuries using an experimental model. *Accid Anal Prev* 2002;34:663–671.

21. Yoganandan N, Cusick JF, Pintar FA, et al. Whiplash injury determination with conventional spine imaging and cryomicrotomy. *Spine* 2001;26:2443–2448.

22. Yoganandan N, Cusick JF, Pintar FA, et al. Whiplash injury determination with conventional spine imaging and cryomicrotomy. *Spine* 2001;26:2443−2448.

23. Otte A, Ettlin T, Fierz L, et al. Parieto-occipital hypoperfusion in late whiplash syndrome: first quantitative SPET study using technetium-99m bicisate (ECD). *Eur J Nucl Med* 1996;23:72–74.

24. Yoganandan N, Knowles SA, Maiman DJ, et al. Anatomic study of the morphology of human cervical facet joint. *Spine* 2003;28:2317–2323.

25. Barnsley L, Lord SM, Wallis BJ, et al. The prevalence of chronic cervical zygapophysial joint pain after whiplash. *Spine* 1995;20:20–25.

26. Lord SM, Barnsley L, Wallis BJ, et al. Chronic cervical zygapophysial joint pain after whiplash. A placebo-controlled prevalence study. *Spine* 1996;21:1737–1744; discussion 1744–1745.

27. Lord SM, Barnsley L, Wallis BJ, et al. Percutaneous radiofrequency neurotomy for chronic cervical zygapophysial-joint pain. *N Engl J Med* 1996;335:1721–1726.

28. Treede RD, Meyer RA, Raja SN, et al. Peripheral and central mechanisms of cutaneous hyperalgesia. *Prog Neurobiol* 1992;38:397–421.

29. Schmidt R, Schmelz M, Forster C, et al. Novel classes of responsive and unresponsive C nociceptors in human skin. *J Neurosci* 1995;15:333–341.

30. McMahon SB, Wall PD. Receptive fields of rat lamina 1 projection cells move to incorporate a nearby region of injury. *Pain* 1984;19:235–247.

31. Sterling M, Jull G, Vicenzino B, et al. Sensory hypersensitivity occurs soon after whiplash injury and is associated with poor recovery. *Pain* 2003;104:507–519.

32. Watkins LR, Milligan ED, Maier SF. Glial activation: a driving force for pathological pain. *Trends Neurosci* 2001;24:450–455.

33. Ichitani Y, Shi T, Haeggstrom JZ, et al. Increased levels of cyclooxygenase-2 mRNA in the rat spinal cord after peripheral inflammation: an in situ hybridization study. *Neuroreport* 1997;8:2949–2952.

34. Samad TA, Moore KA, Sapirstein A, et al. Interleukin-1beta-mediated induction of Cox-2 in the CNS contributes to inflammatory pain hypersensitivity [see Comment]. *Nature* 2001;410:471–475.

35. Obelieniene D, Bovim G, Schrader H, et al. Headache after whiplash: a historical cohort study outside the medico-legal context. *Cephalalgia* 1998;18:559–564.

36. Partheni M, Constantoyannis C, Ferrari R, et al. A prospective cohort study of the outcome of acute whiplash injury in Greece. *Clin Exp Rheumatol* 2000;18:67–70.

37. Meyer S, Hugemann RE, Weber M. Zur Belastung der HWS durch Auffahrkollisionen. *Verkehrsunfall Fahrzeugtech* 1994;32:187–199.

38. Castro WH. Correlation between exposure to biomechanical stress and whiplash associated disorders (WAD). *Pain Res Manag* 2003;8:76–78.

39. Kasch H, Stengaard-Pedersen K, Arendt-Nielsen L, et al. Headache, neck pain, and neck mobility after acute whiplash injury: a prospective study. *Spine* 2001;26:1246–1251.

40. Mayou R, Bryant B. Outcome in consecutive emergency department attenders following a road traffic accident. *Br J Psychiatry* 2001;179:528–534.

41. Satoh S, Naito S, Konishi T, et al. An examination of reasons for prolonged treatment in Japanese patients with whiplash injuries. *J Musculoskeletal Pain* 1997;5:71–84.

42. Suissa S, Harder S, Veilleux M. The relation between initial symptoms and signs and the prognosis of whiplash. *Eur Spine J* 2001;10:44–49.

43. Harder S, Veilleux M, Suissa S. The effect of socio-demographic and crash-related factors on the prognosis of whiplash. *J Clin Epidemiol* 1998;51:377–384.

44. Linton SJ. A review of psychological risk factors in back and neck pain. *Spine* 2000;25:1148–1156.

45. Hinton D, Um K, Ba P. A unique panic-disorder presentation among Khmer refugees: the sore-neck syndrome. *Cult Med Psychiatry* 2001;25:297–316.

46. Sterling M, Jull G, Vicenzino B, et al. The development of psychological changes following whiplash injury. *Pain* 2003;106(3):481–489.

47. Drottning M. Acute emotional response to common whiplash predicts subsequent pain complaints: a prospective study of 107 subjects sustaining whiplash injury. *Nord J Psychiatry* 1995;49:293–299.

48. Ferrari R. The biopsychosocial model—a tool for rheumatologists. *Best Pract Res Clin Rheumatol* 2000;14:787–795.

49. Ferrari R, Constantoyannis C, Papadakis N. Laypersons' expectation of the sequelae of whiplash injury: a cross-cultural comparative study between Canada and Greece. *Med Sci Monit* 2003;9:CR120–CR124.

50. Yunus M. Towards a model of pathophysiology of fibromyalgia: aberrant central pain mechanisms with peripheral modulation [Editorial]. *J Rheumatol* 1992;19:846–850.

51. Crofford L, Demitrack M. Evidence that abnormalities of central neurohormonal systems are key to understanding fibromyalgia and chronic fatigue syndrome. *Rheum Dis Clin North Am* 1996;22:267–284.

52. Pillemer S, Bradley L, Crofford L, et al. The neuroscience and endocrinology of fibromyalgia. *Arthritis Rheum* 1997;40:1928–1939.

53. van Denderen JC, Boersma JW, Zeinstra P, et al. Physiological effects of exhaustive physical exercise in primary fibromyalgia syndrome (PFS): is PFS a disorder of neuroendocrine reactivity? *Scand J Rheumatol* 1992;21:35–37.

54. Torpy DJ, Papanicolaou DA, Pillemer SR, et al. Hypersecretory response of adrenocorticotropin to interleukin-6 in patients with fibromyalgia. *Biomedicine* 1997.

55. Qiao ZG, Vaeroy H, Morkrid L. Electrodermal and microcirculatory activity in patients with fibromyalgia during baseline, acoustic stimulation and cold pressor tests. *J Rheumatol* 1991;18:1383–1389.

56. Clauw DJ, Radulovic D, Antonetti D, et al. Tilt table testing in fibromyalgia. *Arthritis Rheum* 1996;39:R20.

57. Clauw DJ, Radulovic D, Heshmat Y, et al. Heart rate variability as a measure of autonomic dysfunction in fibromyalgia and chronic fatigue syndrome. *Arthritis Rheum* 1995;38:R25.

58. Koelbaek Johansen M, Graven-Nielsen T, Schou Olesen A, et al. Generalized muscular hyperalgesia in chronic whiplash syndrome. *Pain* 1999;83:229–234.

59. Giesecke T, Williams DA, Harris RE, et al. Subgrouping of fibromyalgia patients on the basis of pressure-pain thresholds and psychological factors. *Arthritis Rheum* 2003;48:2916–2922.

60. Vlaeyen JW, Linton SJ. Fear-avoidance and its consequences in chronic musculoskeletal pain: a state of the art. *Pain* 2000;85:317–332.

61. Vlaeyen JW, Kole-Snijders AM, Boeren RG, et al. Fear of movement/(re)injury in chronic low back pain and its relation to behavioral performance. *Pain* 1995;62:363–372.

62. Rosenfeld M, Gunnarsson R, Borenstein P. Early intervention in whiplash-associated disorders: a comparison of two treatment protocols. *Spine* 2000;25:1782–1787.

63. Borchgrevink GE, Kaasa A, McDonagh D, et al. Acute treatment of whiplash neck sprain injuries. A randomized trial of treatment during the first 14 days after a car accident. *Spine* 1998;23:25–31.

64. Nederhand MJ, Ijzerman MJ, Hermens HJ, et al. Cervical muscle dysfunction in the chronic whiplash associated disorder grade II (WADII). *Spine* 2000;25:1938–1943.

65. Nederhand MJ, Hermens HJ, Ijzerman MJ, et al. Cervical muscle dysfunction in chronic whiplash-associated disorder grade II: the relevance of the trauma. *Spine* 2002;27: 1056–1061.

66. Nederhand MJ, Hermens HJ, Ijzerman MJ, et al. Chronic neck pain disability due to an acute whiplash injury. *Pain* 2003;102:63–71.

67. Nederhand MJ, Ijzerman MJ, Hermens HJ, et al. Cervical muscle dysfunction in the chronic whiplash associated disorder grade II (WADII). *Spine* 2000;25:1938–1943.

68. Sterling M, Jull G, Vicenzino B, et al. Development of motor system dysfunction following whiplash injury [see Comment]. *Pain* 2003;103:65–73.

69. Treleaven J, Jull G, Sterling M. Dizziness and unsteadiness following whiplash injury: characteristic features and relationship with cervical joint position error. *J Rehabil Med* 2003;35:36–43.

70. Yehuda R. Psychoneuroendocrinology of post-traumatic stress disorder. *Psychiatr Clin North Am* 1998;21:359–379.

71. McFarlane AC, Atchison M, Yehuda R. The acute stress response following motor vehicle accidents and its relation to PTSD. *Ann N Y Acad Sci* 1997;821:437–441.

72. Delahanty DL, Raimonde AJ, Spoonster E, et al. Injury severity, prior trauma history, urinary cortisol levels, and acute PTSD in motor vehicle accident victims. *J Anxiety Disord* 2003;17:149–164.

73. Delahanty DL, Raimonde AJ, Spoonster E. Initial posttraumatic urinary cortisol levels predict subsequent PTSD symptoms in motor vehicle accident victims. *Biol Psychiatry* 2000;48:940–947.

74. Shalev AY, Freedman S, Peri T, et al. Prospective study of posttraumatic stress disorder and depression following trauma. *Am J Psychiatry* 1998;155:630–637.

75. Pitman RK, Sanders KM, Zusman RM, et al. Pilot study of secondary prevention of posttraumatic stress disorder with propranolol. *Biol Psychiatry* 2002;51:189–192.

76. Chrousos G, Gold P. The concepts of stress and stress system disorders. Overview of physical and behavioral homeostasis. *J Am Med Assoc* 1992;267:1244–1252.

77. Gold PW, Goodwin F, Chrousos GP. Clinical and neurobiological manifestations of depression: relationship to the neurobiology of stress (part 1). *N Engl J Med* 1988;319:348–353.

78. Friedman MJ. Future pharmacotherapy for post-traumatic stress disorder: prevention and treatment. *Psychiatr Clin North Am* 2002;25:427–441.

79. Chrousos GP. Stressors, stress, and neuroendocrine integration of the adaptive response. The 1997 Hans Selye Memorial Lecture. *Ann N Y Acad Sci* 1998;851:311–335.

80. McEwen BS. Protective and damaging effects of stress mediators. *N Engl J Med* 1998;338:171–179.

81. Rivier CL, Plotsky PM. Mediation by corticotropin releasing factor (CRF) of adenohypophysial hormone secretion. *Annu Rev Physiol* 1986;48:475–494.

82. Selye H. Thymus and adrenals in the response of the organisms to injuries and intoxications. *Br J Exp Pathol* 1936; 17:234–248.

83. Munck A, Guyre PM, Holbrook NJ. Physiological functions of glucocorticoids in stress and their relation to pharmacological actions. *Endocr Rev* 1984;5:25–44.

84. Yehuda R. Post-traumatic stress disorder. *N Engl J Med* 2002;346:108–114.

85. Crofford LJ, Pillemer SR, Kalogeras KT, et al. Hypothalamic-pituitary-adrenal axis perturbations in patients with fibromyalgia. *Arthritis Rheum* 1994;37:1583–1592.

86. Elam M, Johansson G, Wallin BG. Do patients with primary fibromyalgia have an altered muscle sympathetic nerve activity? *Pain* 1992;48:371–375.

87. Clauw D, Chrousos G. Chronic pain and fatigue syndromes: overlapping clinical and neuroendocrine features and potential pathogenic mechanism. *Neuroimmunomodulation* 1997; 4:134–153.

88. Griep EN, Boersma JW, de Kloet ER. Altered reactivity of the hypothalamic-pituitary-adrenal axis in the primary fibromyalgia syndrome. *J Rheumatol* 1993;20:469–474.

89. Adler GK, Kinsley BT, Hurwitz S, et al. Reduced hypothalamic-pituitary and sympathoadrenal responses to hypoglycemia in women with fibromyalgia syndrome. *Am J Med* 1999; 106:534–543.

90. Versteegen GJ, Kingma J, Meijler WJ, et al. Neck sprain after motor vehicle accidents in drivers and passengers. *Eur Spine J* 2000;9:547–552.

91. Richter M, Otte D, Pohlemann T, et al. Whiplash-type neck distortion in restrained car drivers: frequency, causes and long-term results. *Eur Spine J* 2000;9:109–117.

92. Breslau N, Davis GC. Posttraumatic stress disorder in an urban population of young adults: risk factors for chronicity. *Am J Psychiatry* 1992;149:671–675.

93. Makela M, Heliovaara M. Prevalence of primary fibromyalgia in the Finnish population. *Br Med J* 1991;303: 216–219.

94. Breslau N, Davis GC, Andreski P. Risk factors for PTSD-related traumatic events: a prospective analysis. *Am J Psychiatry* 1995;152:529–535.

95. Linton S. A review of psychological risk factors in back pain and neck pain. *Spine* 2000;25:1148–1156.

96. Berglund A, Alfredsson L, Jensen I, et al. The association between exposure to a rear-end collision and future health complaints. *J Clin Epidemiol* 2001;54:851–856.

97. Andreski P, Chilcoat H, Breslau N. Post-traumatic stress disorder and somatization symptoms: a prospective study. *Psychiatry Res* 1998;79:131–138.

98. Brunello N, Davidson JR, Deahl M, et al. Posttraumatic stress disorder: diagnosis and epidemiology, comorbidity and social consequences, biology and treatment. *Neuropsychobiology* 2001;43:150–162.

99. Kessels RP, Aleman A, Verhagen WI, et al. Cognitive functioning after whiplash injury: a meta-analysis. *J Int Neuropsychol Soc* 2000;6:271–278.

100. Clauw DJ, Chrousos GP. Chronic pain and fatigue syndromes: overlapping clinical and neuroendocrine features and potential pathogenic mechanisms. *Neuroimmunomodulation* 1997;4:134–153.

101. Glass JM, Park DC. Cognitive dysfunction in fibromyalgia. *Curr Rheumatol Rep* 2001;3:123–127.

102. Ehlers A, Mayou R, Bryant B. Psychological predictors of chronic posttraumatic stress disorder after motor vehicle accidents. *J Abnorm Psychol* 1998;107:508–519.

103. Shalev AY, Peri T, Canetti L, et al. Predictors of PTSD in injured trauma survivors: a prospective study. *Am J Psychiatry* 1996;153:219–225.

104. Sherman JJ, Turk DC, Okifuji A. Prevalence and impact of posttraumatic stress disorder-like symptoms on patients with fibromyalgia syndrome. *Clin J Pain* 2000;16:127–134.

105. Cohen H, Neumann L, Haiman Y, et al. Prevalence of post-traumatic stress disorder in fibromyalgia patients: overlapping syndromes or post-traumatic fibromyalgia syndrome? [see Comment]. *Semin Arthritis Rheum* 2002; 32:38–50.

106. Hickling EJ, Blanchard EB. Post-traumatic stress disorder and motor vehicle accidents. *J Anxiety Disord* 1992;6:285–291.

107. Taylor S, Koch WJ. Anxiety disorders due to motor vehicle accidents: nature and treatment. *Clin Psychol Rev* 1995;15: 721–738.

108. Jaspers JP. Whiplash and post-traumatic stress disorder. *Disabil Rehabil* 1998;20:397–404.

109. Mayou R, Bryant B. Psychiatry of whiplash neck injury. *Br J Psychiatry* 2002;180:441–448.

110. Beckham JC, Crawford AL, Feldman ME, et al. Chronic posttraumatic stress disorder and chronic pain in Vietnam combat veterans. *J Psychosom Res* 1997;43:379–389.

111. Geisser ME, Roth RS, Bachman JE, et al. The relationship between symptoms of post-traumatic stress disorder and pain, affective disturbance and disability among patients with accident and non-accident related pain. *Pain* 1996;66: 207–214.

112. Amir M, Kaplan Z, Neumann L, et al. Posttraumatic stress disorder, tenderness and fibromyalgia. *J Psychosom Res* 1997;42:607–613.

113. Hubbard J, Realmuto GM, Northwood AK, et al. Comorbidity of psychiatric diagnoses with posttraumatic stress disorder in survivors of childhood trauma. *J Am Acad Child Adolesc Psychiatry* 1995;34:1167–1173.

114. Greenfield S, Fitzcharles MA, Esdaile JM. Reactive fibromyalgia syndrome. *Arthritis Rheum* 1992;35:678–681.

115. Turk DC, Okifuji A, Starz TW, et al. Effects of type of symptom onset on psychological distress and disability in fibromyalgia syndrome patients. *Pain* 1996;68:423–430.

116. Buskila D, Neumann L, Vaisberg G, et al. Increased rates of fibromyalgia following cervical spine injury. A controlled study of 161 cases of traumatic injury. *Arthritis Rheum* 1997;40:446–452.

117. Clauw DJ, Williams DA. Physical trauma and fibromyalgia. The real question is not whether, but why, and what can we do about it? *Trauma Pers Inj Med Surg* 2002;44:22–34.

118. Yehuda R, McFarlane AC, Shalev AY. Predicting the development of posttraumatic stress disorder from the acute response to a traumatic event. *Biol Psychiatry* 1998;44:1305–1313.

119. Pitman RK. Post-traumatic stress disorder, hormones, and memory. *Biol Psychiatry* 1989;26:221–223.

120. Yehuda R, Harvey H. Relevance of neuroendocrine alterations in PTSD to cognitive impairments of trauma survivors. In: Read D, Lindsay S, eds. *Recollections of trauma: scientific research and clinical practice*. New York: Plenum Press, 1997:221–252.

121. Kerns RD, Turk DC, Rudy TE. The West Haven-Yale Multidimensional Pain Inventory (WHYMPI). *Pain* 1985;23:345–356.

122. Turk DC, Rudy TE. Toward an empirically derived taxonomy of chronic pain patients: integration of psychological assessment data. *J Consult Clin Psychol* 1988;56:233–238.

123. Asmundson GJ, Bonin MF, Frombach IK, et al. Evidence of a disposition toward fearfulness and vulnerability to posttraumatic stress in dysfunctional pain patients. *Behav Res Ther* 2000;38:801–812.

124. Lewis JW, Cannon JT, Liebeskind JC. Opioid and nonopioid mechanisms of stress analgesia. *Science* 1980;208:623–625.

125. Terman GW, Shavit Y, Lewis JW, et al. Intrinsic mechanisms of pain inhibition: activation by stress. *Science* 1984;226: 1270–1277.

126. Kosek E, Hansson P. Modulatory influence on somatosensory perception from vibration and heterotopic noxious conditioning stimulation (HNCS) in fibromyalgia patients and healthy subjects. *Pain* 1997;70:41–51.

127. Kosek E, Ekholm J, Hansson P. Modulation of pressure pain thresholds during and following isometric contraction in patients with fibromyalgia and in healthy controls. *Pain* 1996; 64:415–423.

128. Lautenbacher S, Rollman G. Possible deficiencies of pain modulation in fibromyalgia. *Clin J Pain* 1997;13:189–196.

129. Vaeroy H, Helle R, Forre O, et al. Levels of substance P and high incidence of Raynaud phenomenon in patients with fibromyalgia: new features for diagnosis. *Pain* 1988;32:21–26.

130. Russell IJ, Orr MD, Littman B, et al. Elevated cerebrospinal fluid levels of substance P in patients with the fibromyalgia syndrome. *Arthritis Rheum* 1994;37:1593–1601.

131. Li P, Zhuo M. Cholinergic, noradrenergic, and serotonergic inhibition of fast synaptic transmission in spinal lumbar dorsal horn of rat. *Brain Res Bull* 2001;54:639–647.

132. Bondy B, Spaeth M, Offenbaecher M, et al. The T102C polymorphism of the 5-HT2A-receptor gene in fibromyalgia. *Neurobiol Dis* 1999;6:433–439.

133. Offenbaecher M, Bondy B, de Jonge S, et al. Possible association of fibromyalgia with a polymorphism in the serotonin transporter gene regulatory region. *Arthritis Rheum* 1999;42: 2482–2488.

134. Zubieta JK, Heitzeg MM, Smith YR, et al. COMT val158met genotype affects mu-opioid neurotransmitter responses to a pain stressor. *Science* 2003;299:1240–1243.

135. Farrell M, Van Meter J, Petzke F, et al. Supraspinal activity associated with painful pressure in fibromyalgia is associated with beliefs about locus of pain control. *Arthritis Rheum* 2001;44:S394.

136. Gracely RH, Geisser ME, Giesecke T, et al. Pain catastrophizing and neural responses to pain among persons with fibromyalgia. *Brain* 2004;127:835–843.

137. Glass JM, Lyden AK, Ambrose K, et al. The effect of brief exercise cessation on pain, fatigue, and mood symptom development in healthy, fit individuals. *J Psychosom Res* 2004;57(4):391–398.

138. Norton PJ, Asmundson GJ. Amending the fear-avoidance model of chronic pain: what is the role of physiological arousal? *Behavior Therapy* 2003;34:17–30.

139. McDermott FT. Repetition strain injury: a review of current understanding. *Med J Aust* 1986;144:196–200.

140. Helliwell PS. Diagnostic criteria for work-related upper limb disorders. *Br J Rheumatol* 1996;35:1195–1196.

141. Macfarlane GJ, Hunt IM, Silman AJ. Role of mechanical and psychosocial factors in the onset of forearm pain: prospective population based study. *Br Med J* 2000;321:676–679.

142. Bongers PM, Kremer AM, ter Laak J. Are psychosocial factors risk factors for symptoms and signs of the shoulder, elbow, or hand/wrist? A review of the epidemiological literature. *Am J Ind Med* 2002;41:315–342.

143. Pransky G, Robertson MM, Moon SD. Stress and work-related upper extremity disorders: implications for prevention and management. *Am J Ind Med* 2002;41:443–455.

144. Gallinaro AL, Feldman D, Natour J. An evaluation of the association between fibromyalgia and repetitive strain injuries in metalworkers of an industry in Guarulhos, Brazil. *Joint Bone Spine* 2001;68:59–64.

145. Helfenstein M, Feldman D. The pervasiveness of the illness suffered by workers seeking compensation for disabling arm pain. *J Occup Environ Med* 2000;42:171–175.

146. Arroyo JF, Cohen ML. Unusual responses to electrocutaneous stimulation in refractory cervicobrachial pain: clues to a neuropathic pathogenesis. *Clin Exp Rheumatol* 1992;10: 475–482.

147. Cohen ML, Arroyo JF, Champion GD, et al. In search of the pathogenesis of refractory cervicobrachial pain syndrome. A deconstruction of the RSI phenomenon. *Med J Aust* 1992; 156:432–436.

148. Greening J, Lynn B, Leary R. Sensory and autonomic function in the hands of patients with non-specific arm pain (NSAP) and asymptomatic office workers. *Pain* 2003;104: 275–281.

149. Livingston W. *Pain mechanisms: a physiologic interpretation of causalgia and its related states*. New York: Macmillan, 1943.

150. Novak CB, Mackinnon SE. Nerve injury in repetitive motion disorders. *Clin Orthop* 1998;351:10–20.
151. Greening J, Lynn B, Leary R, et al. Use of ultrasound imaging to demonstrate reduced movement of the median nerve during wrist flexion in patients with non-specific arm pain. *J Hand Surg* 2001;26B:401–406.
152. Greening J, Smart S, Leary R, et al. Reduced movement of median nerve in carpal tunnel during wrist flexion in patients with non-specific arm pain. *Lancet* 1999;354:217–218.
153. Wolfe F. For example is not evidence: fibromyalgia and the law [Editorial; Comment]. *J Rheumatol* 2000;27:1115–1116.
154. Mailis A, Furlong W, Taylor A. Chronic pain in a family of 6 in the context of litigation. *J Rheumatol* 2000;27:1315–1317.
155. Wolfe F. Post-traumatic fibromyalgia: a case report narrated by the patient. *Arthritis Care Res* 1994;7(3):161–165.
156. Jacobsen S, Bredkjaer S. The prevalence of fibromyalgia and widespread chronic musculoskeletal pain in the general population. *Scand J Rheumatolo* 1992;21:261–263.
157. Waylonis G, Perkins RH. Post-traumatic fibromyalgia. A long-term follow-up [see Comments]. *Am J Phys Med Rehabil* 1994;73:403–412.
158. Wolfe F, Aarflot T, Bruusgaard D, et al. Fibromyalgia and disability. Report of the Moss International Working Group on medico-legal aspects of chronic widespread musculoskeletal pain complaints and fibromyalgia. *Scand J Rheumatolo* 1995;24:112–118.
159. Winfield J. Fibromyalgia: what's next? *Arthritis Care Res* 1997;10:219–221.
160. Buskila DNL, Vaisberg G, Alkalay D, et al. Increased rates of fibromyalgia following cervical spine injury. A controlled study of 161 cases of traumatic injury [see Comments]. *Arthritis Rheum.* 1997;40:446–452.
161. Miller F, Hess E, Clauw D, et al. Approaches for identifying and defining environmentally associated rheumatic disorders. *Arthritis Rheum* 2000;43:243–249.
162. Hill A. The environment and disease: association or causation? *Proc R Soc Med* 1965;5:295–300.
163. Gardner G. Fibromyalgia following trauma: psychology or biology? *Curr Rev Pain* 2000;4:295–300.
164. Gatchel R, Polatin P, Mayer T. The dominant role of psychosocial risk factors in the development of chronic low back pain disability. *Spine* 1995;20:2702–2709.
165. Turk D, Okifuji A. Evaluating the role of physical, operant, cognitive, and affective factors in the pain behaviors of chronic pain patients. *Behav Modif* 1997;21:259–280.
166. Clauw D, Williams D, Lauerman W, et al. Pain sensitivity as a correlate of clinical status in individuals with chronic low back pain. *Spine* 1999;24:2035–2041.
167. Hochberg M, Altman R, Brandt K, et al. Guidelines for the medical management of osteoarthritis: Part II. Osteoarthritis of the knee. *Arthritis Rheum* 1995;38:1541–1546.
168. Radanov B, Sturzenegger M, Stefano GD. Long-term outcome after whiplash injury. A 2-year follow-up considering features of injury mechanism and somatic, radiologic, and psychosocial findings. *Medicine (Baltimore)* 1995;74:281–297.
169. Price D, McHaffie J. Effects of heterotopic conditioning stimuli on first and second pain: a psychophysical evaluation in humans. *Pain* 1988;34:245–252.
170. Dirig DM, Yaksh TL. Thermal hyperalgesia in rat evoked by intrathecal substance P at multiple stimulus intensities reflects an increase in the gain of nociceptive processing. *Neurosci Lett* 1996;220:93–96.
171. Park K, Max M, Robinovitz E, et al. Effects of intravenous ketamine, alfentanil, or placebo on pain, pinprick hyperalgesia, and allodynia produced by intradermal capsaicin in human subjects. *Pain* 1995;63:163–172.
172. Derbyshire S. Imaging the brain in pain. *Am Pain Soc* 1999; 9:7–8.
173. Baron R. Brain processing of capsaicin-induced secondary hyperalgesia: a functional MRI study. *Neurology* 1999;53: 548–557.
174. Romero L, Plotsky P, Sapolsky R. Patterns of adrenocorticotropin secretagogue release with hypoglycemia, novelty, and restraint after colchicine blockade of axonal transport. *Endocrinology* 1993;132:199–204.
175. Viau V, Sharma S, Plotsky P, et al. Increased plasma ACTH responses to stress in nonhandled compared with handled rats require basal levels of corticosterone and are associated with increased levels of ACTH secretagogues in the median eminence. *J Neurosci* 1993;13:1097–1105.
176. Sapolsky R. Why stress is bad for your brain. *Science* 1996;273:749–750.
177. Goldberg R, Pachas W, Keith D. Relationship between traumatic events in childhood and chronic pain. *Disabil Rehabil* 1999;21:23–30.
178. Finestone H, Stenn P, Davies F, et al. Chronic pain and health care utilization in women with a history of childhood sexual abuse. *Child Abuse and Neglect* 2000;24:547–556.
179. Khan S, Bannister G, Gargan M, et al. Prognosis following a second whiplash injury. *Injury* 2000;31:249–251.
180. MacFarlane GJ, Croft PR, Schollum J, et al. Widespread pain: is an improved classification possible? *J Rheumatol* 1996;23:1628–1632.
181. Ferrari R, Russell AS. Epidemiology of whiplash: an international dilemma. *Ann Rheum Dis* 1999;58:1–5.
182. Huang G, Feuerstein M, Sauter S. Occupational stress and work-related upper extremity disorders: concepts and models. *Am J Ind Med* 2002;41:298–314.
183. Aaron L, Bradley L, Alarcon G, et al. Perceived physical and emotional trauma as precipitating events in fibromyalgia. Associations with health care seeking and disability status but not pain severity [see Comments]. *Arthritis Rheum* 1997;40: 453–460.
184. Littlejohn G. Medicolegal aspects of fibrositis syndrome. *J Rheumatol Suppl* 1989;19:169–173.
185. Cohen M, Quintner J. Fibromyalgia syndrome and disability: a failed construct fails those in pain. *Med J Aust* 1998;168: 402–404.
186. Radanov B, di Stefano G, Schnidrig A, et al. Role of psychosocial stress in recovery from common whiplash. *Lancet* 1991;338:712–715.

23

Controversial Syndromes and Their Relationship to Fibromyalgia

Swamy Venuturupalli and Daniel J. Wallace

O ver the years, a variety of health professionals have developed terms or phrases to denote seemingly unique clinical combinations of symptoms and signs. Some of these have stood the test of time, whereas most others overlap with syndromes previously described by different specialists. In many instances (e.g., candida hypersensitivity syndrome) these conditions have been proposed by a group of practitioners advocating a "cause" for these symptom complexes. All of these conditions have overlapping features with fibromyalgia (FM) but are not yet recognized as full-blown, legitimate disorders by organized medicine. This chapter will review the current status of research, case definitions, theories of causation, future research needs and trends, and, where appropriate, the therapies for these controversial syndromes that are commonly encountered by clinicians caring for patients with FM.

SECTION I: SYMPTOM BASED CONDITIONS

MULTIPLE CHEMICAL SENSITIVITIES (IDIOPATHIC ENVIRONMENTAL INTOLERANCE)

INTRODUCTION

Multiple chemical sensitivity (MCS) has been referred to as chemical hypersensitivity syndrome, ecologic illness, environmental hypersensitivity disorder, environmental illness, total allergy syndrome, twentieth-century disease, or universal allergic reactivity. It is a term used to describe a disorder characterized by a vast array of somatic, cognitive, and affective symptoms, the cause of which is attributed to exposure to *low*

levels of a variety of chemicals. Typically, patients with MCS do not have any characteristic physical examination findings or laboratory abnormalities (1–4). MCS was first described in 1952 by Randolph, who suggested that exposure to common environmental chemicals could cause a wide variety of symptoms and pathology (5). Substantial controversy exists about various aspects of MCS, including case definitions of MCS, whether MCS is a primary psychiatric disorder or a combination of psychiatric and organic medical syndromes, whether chemical exposure actually causes the symptoms, and the correct treatment of patients who have this syndrome.

DEFINITION

Cullens defined MCS as an acquired disorder characterized by recurrent symptoms referable to multiple organ systems, occurring in response to demonstrable exposure to many chemically unrelated compounds at doses far below those established in the general population to cause harmful effects (6). No single widely accepted test of physiologic function can be shown to correlate with symptoms. This definition has been criticized as being nonspecific (7) and not emphasizing the predictability of exposure-symptom relationships (8). Clinical ecologists are a group of practitioners who define MCS as a chronic multisystem disorder caused by adverse reactions to environmental incitants modified by individual susceptibility and specific adaptation. This definition has been criticized as too broad (9).

Since no relation between exposure and symptoms has thus far been substantiated, the term *idiopathic environmental intolerance* (IEI) has been proposed as a more appropriate description for these phenomena. A working definition of IEI would be that it is an acquired disorder with multiple recurring symptoms associated with various environmental agents which are tolerated well by most people and which cannot be explained by any known somatic, psychiatric, and/or psychosomatic disorder (10).

IS MULTIPLE CHEMICAL SENSITIVITY A PSYCHIATRIC OR PHYSIOLOGIC DISORDER?

Central to the controversy about MCS is whether MCS is a nonpsychiatric organic disorder (11,12) or a psychiatric disorder, such as somatoform disorder, or a combination of both (8,13). Similar debates are currently ongoing in other conditions where there is a dominant psychogenic overlay and a lack of objective physical signs such as in fibromyalgia syndrome (FMS), chronic fatigue syndrome (CFS), and Gulf War syndrome (14). Clinical ecologists are proponents of the physical basis of MCS. Their theories and practices have been severely criticized by mainstream medical organizations (15–19).

CLINICAL FEATURES

The most frequently reported symptoms are headache (55%), fatigue (51%), confusion (31%), depression (30%), shortness of breath (29%), arthralgia (26%), myalgia (25%), nausea (20%), dizziness (18%), memory problems (14%), gastrointestinal (GI) symptoms (14%), and respiratory symptoms (14%) (20). The typical MCS patient is a middle-aged well-educated female, with an average age of presentation between 30 to 50 years (20,21). A majority of the patients work in white-collar professions (20).

ETIOPATHOGENESIS

The exact cause of MCS is unknown at this time. Multiple theories abound regarding the etiopathogenesis of this disorder, which can be broadly grouped as primarily physical theories, primarily psychiatric theories, and a combination of the two. The main etiologic mechanisms that have been proposed for MCS include immunologic dysregulation, limbic kindling, and psychological dysfunction.

1. *Immunologic dysregulation.* Multiple papers have been published stating that individuals with MCS have immunologic abnormalities. However, this entire body of research literature has major flaws. For example, some studies report findings of immunologic abnormalities based on measures of immunoglobulin, lymphocytes, complement levels, or combinations of these. Unfortunately, most of this testing has been done without *a priori* hypotheses, and the fact that multiple parameters have been tested leads to the likelihood of false results. In response, many professional bodies have issued position statements that there is no immunologic basis for the pathogenesis of MCS (15,16,22).

2. *Limbic kindling.* Bell et al. (23) described a model of olfactory limbic kindling for MCS. In this model, permanent increases in limbic neuronal excitability resulted because of repeated stimulation in the olfactory bulb, amygdala, and hippocampus amplified reactivity to low-level chemical exposures. They further hypothesized that the limbic system's role as a central point where the neurologic, endocrine, and immune systems interact, combined with nervous system involvement in all remote organ systems, may explain the wide variety of symptoms seen in MCS patients. There are no experimental data in humans to support or refute the role of limbic kindling in producing MCS (8).

3. *Disturbances in heme synthesis.* A few researchers have noted that MCS may represent mild chronic porphyria because porphyria can be triggered by chemical exposure, and its symptom picture may overlap with that of MCS. However, there is no evidence that laboratory measures of porphyrin excretion or heme synthesis in patients with MCS is altered (24).

4. *Psychological theories to explain the etiology of MCS.* Heightened self-focused attention can result in increased symptom reporting (25). Thus, if actual or perceived toxic exposure activates self-related constructs, ambiguous sensations may be construed in terms of these constructs. Examples of such behavior can be found in injury litigants, who often perceive their preinjury functioning as superior to that of the healthy general population (26). Classic conditioning may play a role in the development of MCS. According to this theory, the initial overexposure is the unconditioned stimulus, and the physical reaction to later exposures is the unconditioned response (27). Other researchers have suggested that MCS may be a variant of atypical depression (28), posttraumatic stress disorder (PTSD), or a panic disorder (29).

RESEARCH LITERATURE ON MULTIPLE CHEMICAL SENSITIVITY

Labarge and McCaffrey (14) conducted an extensive review of research literature in the field of MCS. A few of the key immunologic exposure studies and neuropsychiatric studies are reported in Table 23-1. To summarize, the immunologic studies reviewed showed no consistent evidence to date that supports any immunologic involvement in the etiology and maintenance of MCS (14,17). Similarly, the exposure studies for MCS have significant methodologic flaws, and it cannot be reliably determined whether the symptoms reported by MCS patients are caused by exposure to chemicals. Neuropsychologic studies of MCS patients were unable to demonstrate any consistent differences between patients and controls (14).

Studies investigating psychological factors have been reviewed in detail by Davidoff and Fogarty (30). These studies suggest that a substantial number of individuals with the diagnosis of MCS have a history of physical or psychological problems that existed prior to the inciting exposures that resulted in the MCS. Frequently, these pre-existing problems could account for symptoms that an individual claimed was caused by MCS. However, there appears to be a subset with a diagnosis of MCS whose medical or psychological history does not account for current symptomatology (14). Since criteria for MCS emphasize reproducibility of symptoms on repeat exposure, they may falsely increase the percentage of prior psychiatric illnesses in patients diagnosed with MCS (31).

TREATMENT OF MULTIPLE CHEMICAL SENSITIVITY

Multiple treatment modalities have been proposed for MCS. The clinical ecologists recommend treatments based on

TABLE 23-1	Summary of Studies on Multiple Chemical Sensitivity		
REFERENCE	**STUDY**	**RESULTS**	**COMMENTS**
Studies of Immunologic Dysfunction			
(3)	Complement, lymphocyte, Ig, B-cell, T-cell subsets	All within normal limits	No statistical testing done
(32)	T and B lymphocyte levels vs. controls	MCS patients had statistically lower levels of T8 cells and higher T4/T8 ratios	
(2)	T8 suppressor levels	No significant difference between control and MCS group	Study later criticized for use of lab with unreliable results
(33)	IG and complement components, skin testing for common antigens in 11 patients	No significant or consistent abnormalities	
(34)	IG and complement components in 68 patients with MCS	No consistent changes noted	Initial lab used was same as (3); later the lab was changed
Studies of Exposure to Chemicals			
(35)	50 patients tested with double-blind chemical and placebo challenges	99.4% of challenges produced no reaction	
(36)	20 patients tested with double-blind placebo controlled challenges	Patients not able to reliably identify active agents from clean air controls	Only one chemical per participant was used
Studies of Neuropsychologic Factors			
(37)	23 patients vs. controls were given neuro-psychologic tests	Only one of battery of tests showed any difference	
(2)	41 patients vs. 34 controls were administered tests	No significant differences noted	
Studies of Psychological Factors			
(3)	50 patients with MCS	31/50 patients had features of significant psychological disorders	
(33)	11 patients with MCS	3/11 met criteria for mood disorder; as a group, their MMPI profile was typical of somatoform disorder	
(13)	41 patients vs. 34 controls	No statistically significant difference in prevalence of anxiety and depressive disorders	Prevalence of preexisting somatization disorder higher in MCS group

MCS, multiple chemical sensitivity; MMPI, Minnesota Multiphasic Personality Inventory.

From Labarge X, McCaffrey R. Multiple chemical sensitivity: a review of the theoretical and research literature. *Neuropsychol Rev* 2000;10(4):183–211, with permission.

avoidance strategies. Thus, individuals with MCS may be asked to quit their jobs, move to different parts of the country, use filtering gas masks, avoid certain foods, etc. Clinical ecologists recommend intradermal or sublingual symptom provocation and neutralization as well as the use of vitamin and mineral supplements, antiviral and antifungal drugs, hormones and immunomodulator therapies, etc (38). There are no controlled trials examining the effectiveness of these techniques, and this has prompted many mainstream medical organizations to issue position statements against clinical ecology practices, citing the lack of scientific support for these techniques (15–19). Clinical ecology treatments reinforce misconceptions that individuals with a diagnosis of MCS have regarding their illness and serve to perpetuate negative behavior patterns (39).

Psychogenic and psychiatric therapies are recommended for patients who have no demonstrable underlying medical disorder. The type of therapy depends on the primary psychiatric disorder, that is, whether the patient has depression or an anxiety disorder such as PTSD, panic disorder, or a phobia, and may include cognitive and behavioral techniques such as cognitive restructuring, exposure and response prevention, and appropriate antidepressant or antianxiety medications. It is useful to note that patients with underlying somatization disorder are extremely resistant to these treatments. A few reports of successful treatment of MCS with psychiatric therapies have been published, including the use of cognitive-behavioral therapies and the use of serotonin reuptake inhibitors (40–42).

CONCLUSIONS

There is considerable controversy as to whether MCS is an organic disorder, psychological disorder, or some combination of both. Consistent physical findings and laboratory abnormalities are nonexistent, and there is no compelling evidence that MCS results solely from the exposure to chemicals. At present, there is some evidence to suggest that patients with MCS are a heterogeneous group of individuals with a variety of psychological disorders, though caution must be exercised in classifying MCS as a primary psychiatric illness until further research is performed on elucidating the etiology of MCS. Regardless of etiology, patients with MCS experience considerable suffering and disability, and further research on treatment modalities is sorely needed.

SICK BUILDING SYNDROME

Over the last few decades, a new man-made ecosystem—the controlled indoor environment within the sealed indoor shells of modern office buildings—has developed. More than half the adult work force in North America and Western Europe works in offices or officelike nonindustrial environments. In the past 3 decades, a group of health problems related to the ecosystem of these office settings has emerged (43). Generally, these problems are divided into specific building-related illnesses that have a known etiology and specific physical abnormalities and laboratory findings. Examples of these illnesses are Legionnaire disease, Pontiac fever, and hypersensitivity pneumonitis caused by specific agents found in buildings (44). Sick building syndrome is similar to these disorders in that the symptoms associated with this disorder are caused by building-related factors. However, unlike building-related illnesses, there are no known toxic agents, allergens, or microorganisms (45).

CLINICAL FEATURES

Symptoms are very similar to MCS and include irritation of the skin and mucous membranes of the eyes, nose, and throat, headache, fatigue, and difficulty concentrating. Since there are no characteristic physical findings or laboratory

abnormalities, the symptoms are considered building related even if the only supporting evidence is the worker's reports. The term *nonspecific building-related illnesses* has been proposed as a more appropriate term for sick building syndrome (43).

In cross-sectional surveys, up to 60% of workers reported at least one work-related symptom, and 10% to 25% reported that such symptoms occurred twice weekly or more often (46–48).

The symptoms of this syndrome are associated with a younger age, female sex, and a history of atopy. This may reflect heightened physiologic responses at lower thresholds in these patients, but there is no evidence that there are any psychological differences between symptomatic and asymptomatic office workers (49).

The scientific literature reveals that a number of personal factors appear to be associated with nonspecific building-related illnesses. There is also evidence that symptoms are associated with markers of individual exposure, such as the use of carbonless paper, photocopiers, and video display terminals or the presence of carpets and dust, yet specific factors have not been identified. The importance of building-related factors such as type or presence of mechanical ventilation remains controversial (46–48). The prevalence of symptoms has consistently been shown to be associated with temperature and humidity, but there is no clear relationship between measured chemical and microbial levels.

Nonspecific building-related illnesses can be explained on the basis of three phenomena: a wide range in the threshold of response in any population, a spectrum of response to any given agent, and variability in the exposure within large office buildings (43). These phenomena could explain why large epidemiologic surveys failed to identify relations between environmental factors measured at a limited number of sites and symptoms of all workers within the buildings (50,51).

Thus, nonspecific building-related illnesses are a heterogeneous group of disorders that affect people who may be more susceptible to these illnesses. Although there is no convincing data to implicate specific causative agents, there is indirect evidence to support a number of recommendations, such as maintaining an outdoor air supply of 10 L/sec/person; selecting building materials, furnishings, and equipment least likely to release pollutants such as formaldehyde or volatile organic compounds; and avoiding materials that may act as substrates for the proliferation of microbes and dust mites.

GULF WAR SYNDROME

BACKGROUND

Shortly after the end of the Gulf War in March of 1991, media reports emerged that veterans were experiencing a variety of medically unexplained symptoms including fatigue, headache, aches, pains, and cognitive disturbances. In January 1992, the press reported an outbreak of unexplained symptoms among members of the 123rd Army Reserve Unit in Indiana. Subsequently, more veterans began complaining of similar symptoms, and public concern began growing about a "mystery illness." In 1994, the National Institutes of Health (NIH) convened a Technology Assessment Workshop to determine the adequacy of information on unusual illnesses in Gulf War veterans (52). Since the initial report by the NIH, many controlled epidemiologic studies have been conducted to determine the prevalence of symptoms in Gulf War veterans. The findings of these studies are remarkably consistent, providing evidence of the validity of these results. The most frequently reported symptoms are fatigue, cognitive difficulties, headaches, myalgia, arthralgia, mood disturbances, and sleep problems (53–59). In general, Gulf War veterans are two to three times more likely to experience these symptoms compared to comparison groups.

Several studies have reported relationships between exposures during the Gulf War and subsequent health outcomes. A detailed review of these studies is discussed elsewhere (60). This literature is wrought with methodologic issues and conflicting reports. Independent review committees have been unable to attribute Gulf War symptoms to exposure to any particular stimulus or agent (61–63). Thus, deployment to the Gulf War comprises the only consistently identifiable risk factor for illness among Gulf War veterans.

CASE DEFINITION

In Gulf War illness research, case definition has relied primarily on statistical data driven approaches such as factor analysis (55,64–66). Factor analysis is the statistical technique of developing scales and identifying otherwise latent relationships between multiple variables. These data analytic methods are limited in that they do not address issues of biologic plausibility and are dependent upon initial assessment and inclusion in the analysis of appropriate symptoms and involve subjective interpretation of the factors (60). Reporting of symptoms can vary over time and thus complicate classification (67). Medically unexplained physical symptoms are remarkably prevalent in the community. Although these symptoms are more prevalent among Gulf War veterans than among their nondeployed peers, this pattern of symptoms is not unique to Gulf War service and does not appear to represent unique illness or "Gulf War syndrome." In fact, illnesses similar to Gulf War illness have been noted among veterans of other military deployments dating back to the U.S. Civil War (60,68,69).

RELATIONSHIP OF FIBROMYALGIA TO GULF WAR ILLNESS

Several studies have assessed the prevalence of CFS, FM, and MCS among Gulf War veterans. It is not possible to generalize from the results, but there is a fairly high prevalence of these conditions in Gulf War veterans (55,66,70). Musculoskeletal evaluation of 928 veterans (71) revealed that about 33% had FM, 17% had soft tissue problems, and 9.6% had nonspecific arthralgias. Similar results were reported by others (72,73). Thus, the frequency of rheumatic manifestations of the Gulf War appears to be similar to the symptoms and diagnoses described in previous years, and they are not unique to active-duty soldiers.

TREATMENT OF GULF WAR ILLNESS

Treatment is dictated by the individual patient's predominant symptoms and the presence of concomitant psychiatric or medical diagnoses. In a controlled trial, a program of cognitive-behavioral therapy and exercise appears to effectively improve symptoms in about 20% of patients with Gulf War illness. Exercise, by itself, is effective for several symptoms such as fatigue, distress, cognitive symptoms, and mental functioning, while cognitive-behavioral therapy improves cognitive symptoms and mental functioning (74).

UNDERSTANDING SYMPTOM-BASED CONDITIONS IN THE CONTEXT OF RESEARCH FINDINGS IN FIBROMYALGIA AND CHRONIC FATIGUE SYNDROME

Considerable clinical overlap exists between MCS, FM, and CFS; approximately one half of the individuals who meet criteria for one of these conditions will also meet criteria for one or both of the others (75,76). The term *chronic multisymptom illnesses* (CMI) was coined in a recent Centers for Disease Control and Prevention study (55) to describe this constellation of symptoms and syndromes that includes FM, CFS, MCS, and somatoform disorders.

Symptoms of patients with CFS overlap significantly with FM, and five out of eight criteria for CFS are now pain based (77,78). The demographics of CFS are also similar to FM, with a strong female predominance (79). Similarly, somatoform disorders, which are a group of classified psychiatric disorders defined by the presence of physical symptoms that are not fully explained by a known medical condition, also share many similarities. A less severe form of somatization known as subsyndromal somatization, requiring one or more unexplained symptoms for >6 months, is very common (affecting approximately 4% of the population). Therefore, if the symptoms of FM or CFS are considered *unexplained*, most individuals who meet criteria for one of these illnesses will also meet criteria for a somatoform disorder.

Similar to MCS and CFS, all symptom-based conditions appear as a continuum in the population, with one group of patients who has severe symptoms all the time, another group that has symptoms off and on, and a third group that has very infrequent symptoms (80,81). Other illnesses within this spectrum affect only one organ system or portion of the body, with the seminal features being pain and/or dysfunction in this region (e.g., migraine or tension headaches, irritable bowel syndrome, temporomandibular joint dysfunction, female urethral syndrome, etc.) (77,82).

COMMON ETIOPATHOGENESIS FOR SYMPTOM-BASED CONDITIONS

By synthesizing evidence from studies in the FM and CFS literature, Clauw (31) has described a model to explain the etiology of symptom-based conditions. In this model, a group of individuals may be genetically predisposed to develop this entire spectrum of illnesses. The illness may develop indolently or abruptly after exposure to a stressor or series of stressors, which could be physical, immune, emotional, or chemical, or could act by other mechanisms that disrupt the body's homeostasis. A number of factors, including the environment in which the person is exposed to the stressor, genetic factors, and exposure to prior stressors, may play a role in determining which individuals are most susceptible to develop these illnesses when exposed to stress. Once an individual develops these illnesses, there is typically evidence of one or more of the following: (a) sensory amplification, (b) attenuated hypothalamic-pituitary function, (c) lability of the autonomic nervous system, and (d) psychological and behavioral factors. In this paradigm, changes in the immune system and in the peripheral tissues are de-emphasized because there are data suggesting that these anomalies occur because of these central alterations in the stress system (31).

SECTION II: DISORDERS PROMOTED AS CAUSES FOR UNEXPLAINED SYMPTOM COMPLEXES

CANDIDA HYPERSENSITIVITY SYNDROME

The candida hypersensitivity syndrome is also known as candidiasis hypersensitivity syndrome and yeast hypersensitivity syndrome. This syndrome is based on a theory originally proposed by Truss that certain people develop hypersensitivity to a toxin released from *Candida albicans* (83). The illness consists of multiple symptoms including fatigue, premenstrual tension, GI symptoms, and depression, though there are no characteristic physical findings or laboratory abnormalities (84). Therefore, the illness cannot be distinguished from MCS and other symptom-based conditions. In fact, many patients are diagnosed with a combination of food, chemical, and candida sensitivity. The illness gained popular acceptance with the publication of the book "The Yeast Connection, A Medical Breakthrough" in 1986 (85).

C. albicans is a commensal organism for humans and is found in small quantities in the oral, respiratory, and genital mucosa of most normal individuals. Colonization with *C. albicans* has been described in 4% to 88% of healthy immunocompetent individuals (86). The so-called candida hypersensitivity syndrome should be distinguished from local or systemic candidiasis, which are opportunistic infections facilitated by a breakdown in immune function and which have been well described in the literature.

CLINICAL FEATURES

This syndrome has been applied to patients with numerous subjective symptoms, but it is also held to be the cause or potentiating factor for a number of other diseases such as multiple

sclerosis, psoriasis, schizophrenia, cancer, acquired immunodeficiency syndrome (AIDS), depression, and various behavioral problems (85). There are no characteristic diagnostic physical or laboratory abnormalities. Several factors have been proposed to predispose one to this syndrome, including use of antibiotics, steroids, birth control pills, and diets of yeast-containing foods, sugars, and other carbohydrates (87). A recent systematic review did not find any evidence that nutritional factors, food additives, pollutants, antiovulants, other types of medication, or diabetes mellitus might be predisposing factors for intestinal candidal colonization (86).

Proponents of this syndrome propose an immunologic basis. In support of this, a study describing the isolation of candidotoxin is referenced as are other studies that demonstrate a local immunosuppressive effect of candidal organisms in patients with recurrent vulvovaginitis (88–92). Unfortunately, since there is no accepted definition of this syndrome, it is impossible to verify whether these immune changes are seen more often in patients versus controls. The diagnosis of this syndrome is based entirely on history. Crook provided an entire questionnaire for self-diagnosis that is based on symptoms and prior exposure to presumed risk factors (85). Some physicians supplement the history with a determination of candidal antibodies, but there are no published studies showing any differences between patients and controls.

Treatment includes changes in diet, nutritional supplements, and certain medications. The dietary changes include restriction of sugar, yeast, and other carbohydrates as well as common sense advice such as eating more fruits and vegetables. An elimination diet is recommended to find hidden allergens, and a multitude of nutritional supplements such as magnesium, probiotics, garlic, coenzyme Q10, vitamin B_{12}, etc. are recommended. Antifungals such as nystatin, ketoconazole, and amphotericin B in low doses are also recommended (87). However, there have been no clinical trials evaluating the effectiveness of these regimens to date. A single clinical trial did not demonstrate any difference between nystatin and placebo in relieving symptoms in patients identified with candida hypersensitivity syndrome (84).

In summary, the candida hypersensitivity syndrome is more of a concept that a wide range of subjective symptoms can be caused by immunologic toxicity from the normal reservoir of *C. albicans* than a clinical entity (93). Neither epidemiologic nor therapeutic studies provide evidence for the existence of the so-called "candida syndrome" or "candida hypersensitivity syndrome," and the American Academy of Allergy and Immunology has issued a position statement that the concept is speculative and the treatments potentially dangerous (94). At present, there are no proven treatment indications for antifungal "bowel decontamination" (86).

CHIARI I MALFORMATION

The Chiari I malformation (CM I) is defined as tonsillar herniation of at least 3 to 5 mm below the foramen magnum. Chiari II and III malformations are associated with embryologic defects of the brain and spinal cord and are established as primary neurologic abnormalities. There is increasing clinical and experimental evidence that chronic tonsillar herniation in CM I could be attributable to underdevelopment of the occipital bone and overcrowding of the cerebellum within a too small posterior cranial fossa (PCF). The CM I usually occurs sporadically but can be transmitted genetically in some families. The most constant feature of CM I is a volumetrically small PCF, which predisposes patients to hindbrain overcrowding.

CLINICAL FEATURES

The incidence of Chiari malformation is 0.5% with a 3:2 female-to-male ratio. This syndrome can remain asymptomatic (95). In a prospective study, the mean age of patients was 36 years, and 37% reported histories of lifelong complaints such as headaches and clumsiness. Patients who actually had syringomyelia associated with this syndrome presented at a younger age and were diagnosed earlier. The majority of the patients had a spontaneous onset of symptoms, though 24% cited trauma as a precipitating event. Common misdiagnoses included migraine headaches, FM, and multiple sclerosis. By the time of definitive diagnosis, about 60% had been told by at least one physician that they suffered from a psychogenic disorder (96).

The clinical syndrome of CM I consists of headaches, pseudotumorlike episodes, Ménière diseaselike syndrome, lower cranial nerve signs, and spinal cord disturbances in the absence of syringomyelia. The most common symptom is suboccipital headache reported by 81% of patients and described as a heavy crushing or pressurelike sensation at the back of the head that radiates to the vertex, behind the eyes, and inferiorly to the neck and shoulder. The headaches are pounding when severe but are otherwise nonthrobbing. A distinctive feature of the headaches is their tendency to be accentuated by physical exertion, Valsalva maneuvers, head dependency, and sudden changes in posture. Female patients note worsening of symptoms prior to menses. Ocular disturbances are reported by 78% of patients, and 74% experience otoneurological disturbances (96). Previously, the extent of tonsillar herniation had been reported to correlate with the severity of symptoms (97), though this was not seen in a more recent study (96).

TREATMENT OF CHIARI I MALFORMATION FOR FIBROMYALGIA AND CHRONIC FATIGUE SYNDROME SYMPTOMS

Some patients with FM and CFS have orthostatic intolerance. Some authors have extrapolated this to suggest that CFS and FM represent neurologic problems related to posterior fossa compression. Rosner and Heffez presented abstracts suggesting that posterior fossa decompression improves symptoms in selected patients with FM (98–101). Unfortunately, none of these abstracts has been published in any peer-reviewed publications. These data are also available only in abstract form, and a PubMed search of CM I and CFS or FM done on December 13, 2003 did not yield any publications. A prospective study funded by the National Fibromyalgia Research Association could not confirm that the incidence of cervical stenosis or cerebellar herniation was any greater in the FM patients than in the controlled group (102).

Many reports in the media, especially mainstream television networks, have publicized the relationship between CM Is, FM, and CFS. However, this remains controversial. The American Association of Neurological Surgeons and the CFS/FM website have issued cautionary statements that there is no scientific evidence that CFS is a neurologic disorder or that it requires surgical intervention. Lastly, the hypothesis that some cases of orthostatic intolerance are related to CM I was tested in a retrospective study presented at the 11th International Symposium of Autonomic Nervous System. Magnetic resonance imaging (MRI) scans of the head and the cervical spine were reviewed and these did not show any significant difference between the control groups and the orthostatic group for tonsillar depression (103).

Surgical treatment has been reported to be fairly successful for symptomatic CM I (95). Posterior decompression is the treatment of choice. Cerebrospinal fluid (CSF) diversionary procedures are used when there is increased CSF pressure. The procedures appear to be more successful when there is raised intracranial pressure as opposed to cases where there are symptoms of spinal cord compression and neurologic weakness (104–106). The duration of symptoms has been reported to be inversely related to the success of the procedures (107,108).

Thus, in conclusion, there is some preliminary evidence to support that some patients with CFS, FM, or related syndromes have hindbrain compression with or without CM I and would benefit from decompression surgery (109). However, the literature does not reveal the extent of this association, and it is highly probable that some patients with FM are misdiagnosed as CM I (and vice versa) and that these are unrelated phenomena.

MERCURY AMALGAMS

Dental amalgams have been in use for more than 150 years. They are inexpensive and are thought to be more durable than other types of fillings. The controversy about the deleterious health effects of mercury fillings became heated around 1970, with the discovery that amalgams can release mercury vapors into the oral cavity in concentrations that are higher than those deemed safe by occupational health guidelines. The use of mercury-silver amalgam fillings in dental work has been reported in publications and in the lay media to produce symptoms similar to FM, including chronic fatigue, headaches, cognitive dysfunction, and muscle and joint aches (110). Although subsequent studies have shown the amount of mercury inhaled is small on account of the small size of the oral cavity, inhaled mercury from dental amalgams remains the chief source of exposure to mercury in the general population (111). These fears have been heightened by the recent recommendation by the Environmental Protection Agency (EPA) that the daily recommended intake of mercury be reduced from 0.5 μg/kg/day to 0.1 μg/kg/day (112). The number of amalgam surfaces correlate with blood, brain, and urinary concentrations of mercury, but the level of mercury usually remains far below the toxic level (113,114). Higher urinary concentrations have been reported in persons who chew a great deal (115). Unfortunately, the removal of amalgam fillings can also cause temporary elevations in blood concentrations since the process transiently increases the amount of mercury vapor inhaled (116).

What is the evidence that the exposure to mercury from dental amalgams can cause FM-like symptoms or other diseases? In one uncontrolled study of 20 German patients with FM and dental amalgams, the mean urinary concentrations of mercury were 0.5 μg/L, compared with a mean of 0.9 μg/L in the German general population (117). In several epidemiologic investigations, there is no evidence of a role for amalgam in causing degenerative diseases such as Alzheimer disease, or connective tissue disease, or FM (118,119).

Patients who present to rheumatologists worried about the connection of their symptoms to mercury fillings should be reassured that there is no available evidence to suggest that there is any connection between mercury fillings and their symptoms. Amalgams contain the less toxic ethyl mercury. Furthermore, there is no evidence supporting the removal of amalgams and improvement in FM symptoms. In fact, the removal of amalgams may generate more mercury vapors, causing a rise in serum mercury levels before they subsequently decline (116).

Other sources of mercury exposure in the general population are from the ingestion of fish and from thimerosal preservatives in vaccines. Fish are exposed to methyl mercury from industrial release of mercury into water. The only reported cases of methyl mercury poisoning from fish are from Japan in the 1950s and 1960s. The brain is the targeted tissue in methyl mercury poisoning, with symptoms of paresthesias, visual field constriction, and ataxia. There are speculative reports of correlation between the consumption of methyl mercury and risk of coronary artery disease. This has not consistently been borne out in epidemiologic studies, and prospective studies are needed to confirm this correlation (120). The fetal brain is more susceptible to exposure to mercury, and the Food and Drug Administration has recommended that pregnant women, nursing mothers, and children avoid eating fish with high mercury content (>1 ppm) such as shark, swordfish, tilefish, and king mackerel, or whale meat.

Thimerosal is used as a preservative in many vaccines and effectively kills organisms and prevents the growth of fungi in vaccines. Early toxicologic studies have shown no toxic effects of thimerosal; however, based on studies by Ball et al., who calculated health risks of thimerosal assuming that thimerosal vaccines contain the more toxic methyl mercury rather than ethyl mercury, thimerosal vaccines have been removed from circulation in the United States (121). There is controversy regarding whether the ethyl mercury used in thimerosal vaccines has any chance of accumulating or causing any long-term damage, and the World Health Organization advisory committee concluded that it was safe to continue using thimerosal in vaccines.

In conclusion, all forms of mercury have toxicity at high doses; however, evidence of exposure to low doses of mercury from fish consumption, dental amalgams, and thimerosal in vaccines is open to wide interpretation and is far from being clear.

SILICONOSIS OR SILICONE IMPLANT ASSOCIATED SYNDROME

Since the 1980s, a series of reports have linked silicone breast implants (SBI) to connective tissue disorders such as scleroderma, systemic lupus erythematosus (SLE), and rheumatoid arthritis (RA) (122–125), and later to what has been called "atypical" connective tissue disorders or silicone implant associated syndrome (SIAS) (126). Siliconosis has been proposed as a novel systemic disease with symptoms of chronic fatigue, cognitive dysfunction, sicca syndrome, and arthralgia. The most common symptoms of siliconosis patients are chronic fatigue (77%), cognitive dysfunction (65%), arthralgia (56%), dry mouth (53%), dry eye (50%), alopecia (40%), and dysphagia (35%). The most common findings on physical examination were telangiectasias (60%), erythema of the chest wall (56%), carpal tunnel syndrome (47%), petechiae (46%), lacrimal gland enlargement (26%), thyroid tenderness (22%), thyroid enlargement (21%), and parotid enlargement (18%) (127). Several immunologic changes in response to SBIs have been reported, and the presence of autoantibodies specific to silicone exposure have been reported (127–129).

However, several epidemiologic studies have failed to show any relationship between well-recognized syndromes such as RA, scleroderma, SLE, and SIAS (130–133). These studies have been criticized for not taking into account atypical diseases such as SIAS. There are a number of case reports of SBI patients with SIAS symptoms (126,127,134–138), supporting the existence of a distinct syndrome. However, Wolfe et al. reported that the between 37% and 55% of patients with FM satisfy Bridge's criteria for SIAS and that SIAS does not appear to be a distinct rheumatic disease (139).

There are no prospective studies of patients with SBI to date that describe the occurrence of SIAS or FM after implantation. However, there are several epidemiologic retrospective studies that have attempted to study this question. Several epidemiological retrospective studies (130,140, 141) reported the incidence of various diseases in patients with SBI. They did not find any increase in well-defined rheumatic diseases such as RA, SLE, or scleroderma. Goldman et al. used another approach and looked at patients' various well-defined illnesses and compared the rates of SBI in patients versus controls (131). Again, they did not find any increase in SBI for RA patients versus controls. However, they intriguingly reported that 37 of 43 FM patients with implants had implants before developing FM. Wolfe (139) compared the rates of SBI in FM patients versus control groups and did not find any increase in SBI prior to developing FM (139). Interestingly, they reported that when all implants (before-and after-disease onset of FM) were considered, there was a higher level of SBI in the FM group of patients. They suggested a noncausal association between FM and SBI. Wolfe postulates that the psychosocial features noted in patients with FM and in patients with SBI may be a common denominator, thus suggesting that it is the characteristics of FM that leads to implants rather than implants leading to FM. More recently, Brown et al. surveyed patients with SBI and performed MRIs to diagnose whether there was a rupture of the implants. Using a logistic regression model, they were able to demonstrate a positive correlation between rupture of the silicone implant with extra-capsular silicone and the presence of FM (142), though this could not be confirmed in another study (143). In a small case series, it has been suggested that removal of implants makes symptoms better (144), though in larger studies, even though there was mild improvement in symptoms at 6 months after removal of implants, about 50% of patients decided to have their implants replaced (145).

Thus, there is no evidence that removal of implants definitely improves symptoms, except may be in a small minority of patients who may be allergic to silicone (146).

In conclusion, there is considerable controversy as to whether a separate entity of SIAS exists since a majority of patients with FM may meet criteria for SIAS. There is no evidence that SBIs are linked to well-defined connective tissue diseases. There is some controversy, with contradictory trials, about the association of SBI with FM. SIAS may be related to myofascial pain due to large implants and low self-esteem problems in those getting implants for aesthetic purposes. Prospective studies of SBI patients with monitoring of symptoms pre- and postimplant are sorely needed.

SUMMARY POINTS

- A variety of semantic terms have been used to describe individuals with chronic somatic symptoms.
- Although some of these terms suggest a "cause" for these symptoms and conditions, in general, data do not support the conclusion that these are inherently different from conditions acknowledged to be idiopathic such as FM, CFS, etc.

■ IMPLICATIONS FOR PRACTICE

- Although it is attractive to many patients with chronic somatic symptoms, these individuals may not be well served by the notion that there is a clearly identifiable cause for their symptoms, particularly if this leads them to behaviors or therapies that reinforce chronicity or that have associated morbidity or mortality.

REFERENCES

1. Committee on Environmental Hypersensitivities. *Report of the Ad Hoc Committee on Environmental Hypersensitivity Disorders*. Toronto, Ontario: Government of Ontario Printing Office, 1985.
2. Simon GE, Daniell W, Stockbridge H, et al. Immunologic, psychological, and neuropsychological factors in multiple chemical sensitivity: a controlled study. *Ann Intern Med* 1993; 119(2):97–103.
3. Terr AI. Environmental illness: a clinical review of 50 cases. *Arch Intern Med* 1986;146:145–149.
4. Terr AI. Clinical ecology in the workplace. *J Occup Med* 1989;31:257–261.
5. Randolph T. Sensitivities to petroleum including its derivatives and antecedents. *J Lab Clin Med* 1952;40:921–932.
6. Cullen M. The worker with chemical sensitivities: an overview. *Occup Med* 1987;2:655–661.
7. National Research Council. *Multiple chemical sensitivities: addendum to biologic markers in immunotoxicology*. Washington DC: Academic Press, 1992.
8. Sparks P, Daniell W, Black DW, et al. Multiple chemical sensitivity syndrome: a clinical perspective. 1. Case definition, theories of pathogenesis and research needs. *J Occup Med* 1994;36:718–730.
9. Waddell W. The science of toxicology and its relevance to MCS. *Regul Toxicol Pharmacol* 1993;18:13–22.
10. Lessof M. Report of the Multiple Chemical Sensitivities Workshop, Berlin, Germany, 21-23 February 1996. *Hum Exp Toxicol* 1997;16:233–234.
11. Meggs W. Psychogenic versus biologic basis for chemical sensitivity [Letter]. *J Allergy Clin Immunol* 1997;100:855–856.
12. Meggs W. Neurogenic inflammation and sensitivity to environmental chemicals. *Environ Health Perspect* 1993;103:54–56.
13. Simon G, Deyo RA, Sparks P. Allergic to life: psychological factors in environmental illness. *Am J Psychiatry* 1990;147: 901–906.
14. Labarge X, McCaffrey R. Multiple chemical sensitivity: a review of the theoretical and research literature. *Neuropsychol Rev* 2000;10(4):183–211.
15. American College of Physicians. Clinical ecology. *Ann Intern Med* 1989;111:168–178.
16. American Academy of Allergy and Immunology. Position statement: clinical ecology. *J Allergy Clin Immunol* 1986; 78:269–271.
17. American College of Occupational and Environmental Medicine. ACOEM position statement. Multiple chemical sensitivities: idiopathic environmental intolerance. *J Occup Environ Med* 1999; 41(11):940–942.
18. Council of Scientific Affairs, AMA. Clinical ecology. *JAMA* 1992;268:3465–3467.
19. California Medical Association Scientific Board Task Force on Clinical Ecology. Clinical ecology—a critical appraisal. *West J Med* 1986;144:239–245.
20. Ross G. History and clinical presentation of the chemically sensitive patient. *Toxicol Ind Health* 1992;8:21–28.
21. Cullen M, Pace P, Redlich C. The experience of the Yale occupational and environmental clinics with multiple chemical sensitivities. *Toxicol Ind Health* 1992;8:15–19.
22. Terr AI. Multiple chemical sensitivities. *Ann Intern Med* 1993; 119(2):163–164.
23. Bell I, Rossi J, Gilbert M, et al. Testing the neural sensitization and kindling hypothesis for illness from low levels of environmental chemicals. *Environ Health Perspect* 1997; 105(Suppl. 2):539–547.
24. Daniell W, Stockbridge H, Labbe R, et al. Environmental chemical exposures and disturbances of heme synthesis. *Environ Health Perspect* 1997;105(Suppl. 1):37–53.
25. Williams WC, Lees-Haley PR. Perceived toxic exposure: a review of four cognitive influences on the perception of health. *J Soc Behav Pers* 1993;8:489–506.
26. Lees-Haley P. Manipulation of perception in mass tort litigation. *Nat Resour and Environ* 1997a;4:180–190.
27. Siegel S, Kreutzer R. Pavlovian conditioning and multiple chemical sensitivity. *Environ Health Perspect* 1997;105 (Suppl. 2): 521–526.
28. Schottenfeld R. Workers with multiple chemical sensitivities: a psychiatric approach to diagnosis and treatment. *Occup Med* 1987;2:739–752.
29. Dager S, Holland J, Cowley D, et al. Panic disorder precipitated by exposure to organic solvents in the workplace. *Am J Psychiatry* 1987;144:1056–1058.
30. Davidoff AL, Fogarty L. Psychogenic origins of multiple chemical sensitivities syndrome: a critical review of the research literature. *Arch Environ Health* 1994;49:316–325.
31. Clauw DJ. Potential mechanisms in chemical intolerance and related conditions. *Ann N Y Acad Sci* 2001;933(1):235–253.
32. Rea W, Johnson A, Youdim S, et al. T and B lymphocyte parameters and measures in chemically sensitive patients and controls. *Clinical Ecology* 1986;4:11–14.
33. Fiedler N, Maccia C, Kipen H. Evaluation of chemically sensitive patients. *J Occup Med* 1992;34:529–538.
34. Ziem G, McTamney J. Profile of patients with chemical injury and sensitivity. *Environ Health Perspect* 1997;105(Suppl. 2): 417–436.

35. Rea W, Ross G, Johnson A, et al. Confirmation of chemical sensitivity by means of double blind inhalant challenge of toxic volatile chemicals. *Clin Ecol* 1990;6:113–118.

36. Staudenmayer H, Selner J, Buhr M. Double blind provocation chamber challenges in 20 patients presenting with "multiple chemical sensitivity." *Regul Toxicol Pharmacol* 1993; 18:44–53.

37. Fiedler N, Kipen H, DeLuca J, et al. A controlled comparison of multiple chemical sensitivity and chronic fatigue syndrome. *Psychosom Med* 1996;58:38–49.

38. Levin A, Byers V. Multiple chemical sensitivities: a practicing clinician's point of view. Clinical and immunologic research findings. *Toxicol Ind Health* 1992;8:95–110.

39. Salvagio J, Terr AI. Multiple chemical sensitivity, multiorgan dysthesia, multiple symptom complex, and multiple confusion: problems in diagnosing the patient presenting with multisystemic symptoms. *Crit Rev Toxicol* 1996;26:617–631.

40. Gots R, Hamosh T, Flamm W, et al. Multiple chemical sensitivities: a symposium on the state of the science. *Regul Toxicol Pharmacol* 1993;18:61–78.

41. Haller E. Successful management of patients with "multiple chemical sensitivities" on an inpatient psychiatric unity. *J Clin Pyschiatry* 1993;54:196–199.

42. Andine P, Ronnback L, Jarvholm B. Successful use of a selective serotonin reuptate inhibitor in a patient with multiple chemical sensitivities. *Acta Psychiatr Scand* 1997;96:82–83.

43. Menzies D, Bourbeau J. Building-related illnesses. *N Engl J Med* 1997;337(21):1524–1531.

44. Ryan C, Morrow L. Dysfunctional buildings or dysfunctional people: an examination of sick building syndrome and related disorders. *J Consult Clin Psychol* 1992;60: 220–224.

45. Skov P. The sick building syndrome. In Tucker W, Leaderer B, Molhave L et al., eds. *Sources of indoor air contaminants: characterizing emissions and health impacts.* New York: New York Academy of Sciences, 1992:17–20.

46. Mendell MJ, Fisk WJ, Deddens JA, et al. Elevated symptom prevalence associated with ventilation type in office buildings. *Epidemiology* 1996;7(6):583–589.

47. Mendell MJ, Smith AH. Consistent pattern of elevated symptoms in air-conditioned office buildings: a reanalysis of epidemiologic studies. *Am J Public Health* 1990;80(10): 1193–1199.

48. Bourbeau J, Brisson C, Allaire S. Prevalence of the sick building syndrome symptoms in office workers before and after being exposed to a building with an improved ventilation system. *Occup Environ Med* 1996;53(3):204–210.

49. Bauer RM, Greve KW, Besch EL, et al. The role of psychological factors in the report of building-related symptoms in sick building syndrome. *J Consult Clin Psychol* 1992;60(2): 213–219.

50. Robertson AS, Burge PS, Hedge A, et al. Comparison of health problems related to work and environmental measurements in two office buildings with different ventilation systems. *Br Med J (Clin Res Ed)* 1985;291(6492): 373–376.

51. Skov P, Valbjorn O, Pedersen BV, The Danish Indoor Climate Study Group. Influence of indoor climate on the sick building syndrome in an office environment. *Scand J Work Environ Health* 1990;16(5):363–371.

52. NIH Technology Assessment Workshop Panel. The Persian Gulf experience and health. *JAMA* 1994;272(5): 391–396.

53. Kroenke K, Koslowe P, Roy M. Symptoms in 18,495 Persian Gulf War veterans. Latency of onset and lack of association with self-reported exposures. *J Occup Environ Med* 1998; 40(6):520–528.

54. Murphy FM, Kang H, Dalager NA, et al. The health status of Gulf War veterans: lessons learned from the Department of Veterans Affairs Health Registry. *Mil Med* 1999;164(5): 327–331.

55. Fukuda K, Nisenbaum R, Stewart G, et al. Chronic multisymptom illness affecting Air Force veterans of the Gulf War. *JAMA* 1998;280(11):981–988.

56. Gray GC, Kaiser KS, Hawksworth AW, et al. Increased postwar symptoms and psychological morbidity among U.S. Navy Gulf War veterans. *Am J Trop Med Hyg* 1999;60(5): 758–766.

57. Unwin C, Blatchley N, Coker W, et al. Health of UK servicemen who served in Persian Gulf War. *Lancet* 1999;353(9148): 169–178.

58. Kang HK, Mahan CM, Lee KY, et al. Illnesses among United States veterans of the Gulf War: a population-based survey of 30,000 veterans. *J Occup Environ Med* 2000; 42(5):491–501.

59. Steele L. Prevalence and patterns of Gulf War illness in Kansas veterans: association of symptoms with characteristics of person, place, and time of military service. *Am J Epidemiol* 2000;152(10):992–1002.

60. Barrett DH, Gray GC, Doebbeling BN, et al. Prevalence of symptoms and symptom-based conditions among Gulf War veterans: current status of research findings. *Epidemiol Rev* 2002;24(2):218–227.

61. Presidential Advisory Committee on Gulf War Veterans' Illnesses. *Final report.* Washington, DC: US Government Printing Office, 1996.

62. US Senate Committee on Veterans' Affairs. *Report of the Special Investigation Unit on the Gulf War illnesses.* Washington, DC: US Government Printing Office, 1998.

63. Gunby P. Institute of Medicine calls for coordinated studies of Gulf War veterans' health complaints. *JAMA* 1995; 273(6):444–445.

64. Haley RW, Kurt TL, Hom J. Is there a Gulf War syndrome? Searching for syndromes by factor analysis of symptoms. *JAMA* 1997;277(3):215–222.

65. Ismail K, Everitt B, Blatchley N, et al. Is there a Gulf War syndrome? *Lancet* 1999;353(9148):179–182.

66. The Iowa Persian Gulf Study Group. Self-reported illness and health status among Gulf War veterans. A population-based study. *JAMA* 1997;277(3):238–245.

67. McCauley LA, Joos SK, Lasarev MR, et al. Gulf War unexplained illnesses: persistence and unexplained nature of self-reported symptoms. *Environ Res* 1999;81(3):215–223.

68. Jones E, Hodgins-Vermaas R, McCartney H, et al. Post-combat syndromes from the Boer War to the Gulf War: a cluster analysis of their nature and attribution. *Br Med J* 2002; 324(7333):321–324.

69. Hyams KC, Wignall FS, Roswell R. War syndromes and their evaluation: from the U.S. Civil War to the Persian Gulf War. *Ann Intern Med* 1996;125(5):398–405.

70. Goss Gilroy I. *Health study of Canadian forces personnel involved in the 1991 conflict in the Persian Gulf,* Vol. 1. Ottawa, Ontario, Canada: Department of National Defence, 1998.

71. Escalante A, Fischbach M. Musculoskeletal manifestations, pain, and quality of life in Persian Gulf War veterans referred for rheumatologic evaluation. *J Rheumatol* 1998;25(11): 2228–2235.

72. Grady EP, Carpenter MT, Koenig CD, et al. Rheumatic findings in Gulf War veterans. *Arch Intern Med* 1998;158(4): 367–371.

73. Erickson A, Enzenauer R, Bray V, et al. Musculoskeletal complaints in Persian Gulf veterans. *J Clin Rheumatol* 1998;4:181–185.

74. Donta S, Clauw D, Engel CJ, et al. Cognitive behavioral therapy and aerobic exercise for Gulf War veterans' illnesses: a randomized controlled trial. *JAMA* 2003;289(11): 1396–1404.

75. Goldenberg DL. Fibromyalgia, chronic fatigue syndrome, and myofascial pain syndrome. *Curr Opin Rheumatol* 1991;3(2):247–258.

76. Slotkoff AT, Radulovic DA, Clauw DJ. The relationship between fibromyalgia and the multiple chemical sensitivity syndrome. *Scand J Rheumatol* 1997;26(5):364–367.

77. Clauw DJ. Fibromyalgia: more than just a musculoskeletal disease. *Am Fam Physician* 1995;52(3):843–851, 853–854.

78. McKenzie R, Straus SE. Chronic fatigue syndrome. *Adv Intern Med* 1995;40:119–153.

79. Fukuda K, Straus SE, Hickie I et al., International Chronic Fatigue Syndrome Study Group. The chronic fatigue syndrome: a comprehensive approach to its definition and study. *Ann Intern Med* 1994;121(12):953–959.

80. Wolfe F, Ross K, Anderson J, et al. Aspects of fibromyalgia in the general population: sex, pain threshold, and fibromyalgia symptoms. *J Rheumatol* 1995;22(1):151–156.

81. Wolfe F, Ross K, Anderson J, et al. The prevalence and characteristics of fibromyalgia in the general population. *Arthritis Rheum* 1995;38(1):19–28.

81. Clauw DJ, Chrousos GP. Chronic pain and fatigue syndromes: overlapping clinical and neuroendocrine features and potential pathogenic mechanisms. *Neuroimmunomodulation* 1997;4(3):134–153.

83. Truss C. Tissue injury induced by Candida albicans. *J Orthomol Psychiatr* 1978;7:17.

84. Dismukes W, Wade J, Lee J, et al. A randomized, double-blind trial of nystatin therapy for the candidiasis hypersensitivity syndrome. *N Engl J Med* 1990;323(25):1717–1723.

85. Crook W. *The yeast connection*, 3rd ed. Jackson, TN: Professional Books, 1986.

86. Lacour M, Zunder T, Huber R, et al. The pathogenetic significance of intestinal Candida colonization—a systematic review from an interdisciplinary and environmental medical point of view. *Int J Hyg Environ Health* 2002;205(4):257–268.

87. Crook W. *Chronic fatigue syndrome and the yeast connection*, 2nd ed. Jackson, TN: Professional Books, 1995.

88. Iwata K. Toxins produced by Candida albicans. *Contrib Microbiol Immunol* 1977;4:77–85.

89. Witkin SS, Yu IR, Ledger WJ. Inhibition of Candida albicans induced lymphocyte proliferation by lymphocytes and sera from women with recurrent vaginitis. *Am J Obstet Gynecol* 1983;147(7):809–811.

90. Witkin SS, Hirsch J, Ledger WJ. A macrophage defect in women with recurrent Candida vaginitis and its reversal in vitro by prostaglandin inhibitors. *Am J Obstet Gynecol* 1986; 155(4):790–795.

91. Witkin SS. Immunology of recurrent vaginitis. *Am J Reprod Immunol Microbiol* 1987;15(1):34–37.

92. Witkin SS. Immunologic factors influencing susceptibility to recurrent candidal vaginitis. *Clin Obstet Gynecol* 1991;34(3): 662–668.

93. Bennett JE. Searching for the yeast connection. *N Engl J Med* 1990;323(25):1766–1767.

94. Executive Committee of the American Academy of Allergy and Immunology. Candidiasis hypersensitivity syndrome. *J Allergy Clin Immunol* 1986;78(2):271–273.

95. Cheng JS, Nash J, Meyer GA. Chiari type I malformation revisited: diagnosis and treatment. *Neurolog* 2002;8(6): 357–362.

96. Milhorat TH, Chou MW, Trinidad EM, et al. Chiari I malformation redefined: clinical and radiographic findings for 364 symptomatic patients. *Neurosurgery* 1999;44(5):1005–1017.

97. Stovner LJ, Rinck P. Syringomyelia in Chiari malformation: relation to extent of cerebellar tissue herniation. *Neurosurgery* 1992;31(5):913–917; discussion 917.

98. Rosner M, Guin S, Johnson A. Craniocervical decompression, cerebral blood flow and neuropsychological dysfunction in FMS and CFS [Abstract]. National Fibromyalgia Research Association's Subgroups in Fibromyalgia symposium, September 26–27, 1997. Accessed December 13, 2003. http://www. nfra.net/Subgroups.htm.

99. Rosner M. Decompression of craniovertebral stenosis leads to improvement in FMS and CFIDS symptoms [Abstract]. National Fibromyalgia Research Association's New Dimensions in Fibromyalgia Symposium, September 1997. Accessed Dec 13, 2003. http://www.nfra.net/NewRosner1.htm.

100. Rosner M, D'Amour P, Rowe PC. Neurally mediated hypotension: its surgical evaluation, management and early outcome as part of the fibromyalgia-chronic fatigue syndrome [Abstract]. National Fibromyalgia Research Association's Subgroups in Fibromyalgia Symposium, September 26–29, 1999. Accessed December 13, 2003. http://www.nfra. net/ Subgroups.htm.

101. Heffez D, Clemis J, Elias D. Trivial degrees of tonsillar ectopia may be symptomatic [Abstract]. 75 years of Neurosurgery in Canada 1923-1998 Meeting, Accessed December 13, 2003. http://www.nfra.net/Chiari6.htm.

102. Clauw D, Bennett R, Petzke F, et al. Prevalence of Chiari malformation, and cervical stenosis, in fibromyalgia. *Arthritis Rheum* 2000;43:5173.

103. Anderson J, Garland EM, Black B, et al. Lack of an increase in downward herniation of the cerebellar tonsils (Chiari malformation) in orthostatic intolerance. *Clin Auton Res* 2000; 10:236.

104. Depreitere B, Van Calenbergh F, van Loon J, et al. Posterior fossa decompression in syringomyelia associated with a Chiari malformation: a retrospective analysis of 22 patients. *Clin Neurol Neurosurg* 2000;102(2):91–96.

105. Dyste GN, Menezes AH, VanGilder JC. Symptomatic Chiari malformations. An analysis of presentation, management, and long-term outcome. *J Neurosurg* 1989;71(2):159–168.

106. Paul KS, Lye RH, Strang FA, et al. Arnold-Chiari malformation. Review of 71 cases. *J Neurosurg* 1983;58(2):183–187.

107. Sakamoto H, Nishikawa M, Hakuba A, et al. Expansive suboccipital cranioplasty for the treatment of syringomyelia associated with Chiari malformation. *Acta Neurochir (Wien)* 1999;141(9):949–960; discussion 960–961.

108. Versari PP, D'Aliberti G, Talamonti G, et al. Foraminal syringomyelia: suggestion for a grading system. *Acta Neurochir (Wien)* 1993;125(1-4):97–104.

109. Garland EM, Robertson D. Chiari I malformation as a cause of orthostatic intolerance symptoms: a media myth? *Am J Med* 2001;111(7):546–552.

110. Ahlqwist M, Bengtsson C, Furunes B, et al. Number of amalgam tooth fillings in relation to subjectively experienced symptoms in a study of Swedish women. *Community Dent Oral Epidemiol* 1988;16(4):227–231.

111. *Methylmercury*, Vol 101 of Environmental Health Criteria. Geneva, Switzerland: World Health Organization, 1990.

112. Environmental Protection Agency. *Reference dose for chronic oral exposure to methylmercury*. Greenbelt, MD: Integrated Risk Management System, 2001.

113. Langworth S, Kolbeck KG, Akesson A. Mercury exposure from dental fillings. II. Release and absorption. *Swed Dent J* 1988;12(1-2):71–72.

114. Kingman A, Albertini T, Brown LJ. Mercury concentrations in urine and whole blood associated with amalgam exposure in a US military population. *J Dent Res* 1998;77(3): 461–471.

115. Sallsten G, Barregard L, Schutz A. Clearance half life of mercury in urine after the cessation of long term occupational exposure: influence of a chelating agent (DMPS) on excretion of mercury in urine. *Occup Environ Med* 1994; 51(5):337–342.

116. Molin M, Bergman B, Marklund SL, et al. Mercury, selenium, and glutathione peroxidase before and after amalgam removal in man. *Acta Odontol Scand* 1990;48(3):189–202.

117. Kotter I, Durk H, Saal JG, et al. Mercury exposure from dental amalgam fillings in the etiology of primary fibromyalgia: a pilot study. *J Rheumatol* 1995;22(11):2194–2195.

118. Bjorkman L, Pedersen NL, Lichtenstein P. Physical and mental health related to dental amalgam fillings in Swedish twins. *Community Dent Oral Epidemiol* 1996;24(4):260–267.

119. Ahlqwist M, Bengtsson C, Lapidus L, et al. Serum mercury concentration in relation to survival, symptoms, and diseases: results from the prospective population study of women in Gothenburg, Sweden. *Acta Odontol Scand* 1999; 57(3):168–174.

120. Clarkson T. The three modern faces of mercury. *Environ Health Perspect* 2002;110(Suppl. 1):11–23.

121. Ball LK, Ball R, Pratt RD. An assessment of thimerosal use in childhood vaccines. *Pediatrics* 2001;107(5):1147–1154.

122. Kaiser W, Biesenbach G, Stuby U, et al. Human adjuvant disease: remission of silicone induced autoimmune disease after explanation of breast augmentation. *Ann Rheum Dis* 1990;49(11):937–938.

123. Kumagai Y, Shiokawa Y, Medsger TA Jr, et al. Clinical spectrum of connective tissue disease after cosmetic surgery. Observations on eighteen patients and a review of the Japanese literature. *Arthritis Rheum* 1984;27(1):1–12.

124. Spiera H. Scleroderma after silicone augmentation mammoplasty. *JAMA* 1988;260(2):236–238.

125. Spiera RF, Gibofsky A, Spiera H, et al. Scleroderma in women with silicone breast implants: comment on the article by Sanchez-Guerrero. *Arthritis Rheum* 1995;38(5):719, 721.

126. Bridges AJ. Rheumatic disorders in patients with silicone implants: a critical review. *J Biomater Sci Polym Ed* 1995;7(2): 147–157.

127. Solomon G. A clinical and laboratory profile of symptomatic women with silicone breast implants. *Semin Arthritis Rheum* 1994;24(1 Suppl. 1):29–37.

128. Shanklin DR, Smalley DL. The immunopathology of siliconosis. History, clinical presentation, and relation to silicosis and the chemistry of silicon and silicone. *Immunol Res* 1998;18(3):125–173.

129. Shanklin DR, Smalley DL. Pathogenetic and diagnostic aspects of siliconosis. *Rev Environ Health* 2002;17(2):85–105.

130. Hennekens CH, Lee IM, Cook NR, et al. Self-reported breast implants and connective-tissue diseases in female health professionals. A retrospective cohort study. *JAMA* 1996;275(8): 616–621.

131. Goldman JA, Greenblatt J, Joines R, et al. Breast implants, rheumatoid arthritis, and connective tissue diseases in a clinical practice. *J Clin Epidemiol* 1995;48(4):571–582.

132. Schusterman MA, Kroll SS, Reece GP, et al. Incidence of autoimmune disease in patients after breast reconstruction with silicone gel implants versus autogenous tissue: a preliminary report. *Ann Plast Surg* 1993;31(1):1–6.

133. Hochberg MC, Perlmutter DL, Medsger TA Jr, et al. Lack of association between augmentation mammoplasty and systemic sclerosis (scleroderma). *Arthritis Rheum* 1996;39(7): 1125–1131.

134. Vasey FB, Havice DL, Bocanegra TS, et al. Clinical findings in symptomatic women with silicone breast implants. *Semin Arthritis Rheum* 1994;24(1 Suppl. 1):22–28.

135. Cuellar ML, Gluck O, Molina JF, et al. Silicone breast implant—associated musculoskeletal manifestations. *Clin Rheumatol* 1995;14(6):667–672.

136. Borenstein D. Siliconosis: a spectrum of illness. *Semin Arthritis Rheum* 1994;24(1 Suppl 1):1–7.

137. Kossovsky N, Gornbein JA, Zeidler M, et al. Self-reported signs and symptoms in breast implant patients with novel antibodies to silicone surface associated antigens [anti-SSAA(x)]. *J Appl Biomater* 1995;6(3):153–160.

138. Freundlich B, Altman C, Snadorfi N, et al. A profile of symptomatic patients with silicone breast implants: a Sjogrens-like syndrome. *Semin Arthritis Rheum* 1994;24(1 Suppl. 1):44–53.

139. Wolfe F, Anderson J. Silicone filled breast implants and the risk of fibromyalgia and rheumatoid arthritis. *J Rheumatol* 1999;26(9):2025–2028.

140. Nyren O, Yin L, Josefsson S, et al. Risk of connective tissue disease and related disorders among women with breast implants: a nation-wide retrospective cohort study in Sweden. *Br Med J* 1998;316(7129):417–422.

141. Gabriel SE, O'Fallon WM, Kurland LT, et al. Risk of connective-tissue diseases and other disorders after breast implantation. *N Engl J Med* 1994;330(24):1697–1702.

142. Brown SL, Duggirala HJ, Pennello G. An association of silicone-gel breast implant rupture and fibromyalgia. *Curr Rheumatol Rep* 2002;4(4):293–298.

143. Holmich LR, Kjoller K, Fryzek JP, et al. Self-reported diseases and symptoms by rupture status among unselected Danish women with cosmetic silicone breast implants. *Plast Reconstr Surg* 2003;111(2):723–732; discussion 733–734.

144. Vasey FB, Mills CR, Wells AF. Silicone breast implants and fibromyalgia. *Plast Reconstr Surg* 2001;108(7):2165–2168.

145. Rohrich RJ, Kenkel JM, Adams WP, et al. A prospective analysis of patients undergoing silicone breast implant explantation. *Plast Reconstr Surg* 2000;105(7):2529–2537; discussion 2538–2543.

146. Rohrich RJ. Silicone breast implants and fibromyalgia—reply letter. *Plast Reconstr Surg* 2001;108(7):2165–2168.

24

The Evaluation of Individuals with Chronic Widespread Pain

Daniel J. Clauw

The evaluation of an individual with chronic pain is a complex process. In contrast to most other medical problems, simply arriving at a "diagnosis" is typically insufficient to guide treatment. This is because within any given pain diagnosis, there is tremendous heterogeneity with respect to the underlying causes and contributors to symptoms and the most effective treatments. In particular, individuals with chronic pain can have greater or lesser peripheral nociceptive (i.e., tissue damage, inflammation) and central nonnociceptive (i.e., pain amplification, psychological factors) contributions to their pain. Therefore, the differential diagnosis of chronic pain involves identifying which of these factors are present in which individuals so that the appropriate pharmacologic, procedural, and psychological therapies can be administered.

A careful musculoskeletal history and examination remains the most important diagnostic test for musculoskeletal pain. In other fields of medicine, advances in diagnostic testing have largely rendered a physical examination obsolete. However, in musculoskeletal medicine, technology confuses as much as it helps. For example, a high proportion of the healthy, asymptomatic population has a positive antinuclear antibody, positive rheumatoid factor (RF), or abnormal results of imaging studies (1–3). Worse yet, these diagnostic tests rarely tell us how "severe" the pain is because there is typically a significant discordance between the results of laboratory or imaging studies and the severity of pain and other symptoms that the individual is experiencing (see Chapter 2). Therefore, the musculoskeletal history and examination must allow the clinician to arrive at the diagnosis (or at worst a very narrow differential diagnosis) and then, if necessary, further diagnostic testing should be used to confirm these findings.

Because pain can be a symptom of so many disorders, it is impossible to distill the evaluation of a chronic-pain patient into a single algorithm. Nonetheless, some general principles can be put forth that can guide the evaluation of most individuals.

THE HISTORY

A pain history should elicit information regarding the onset, location, quality, and severity of the pain, as well as aggravating or improving factors, past treatments, and efficacy of these therapies. In clinical practice, it may be useful to use some type of rating scale (e.g., a visual analog scale) to formally rate a patient's pain at the initial and subsequent visits and to track response to therapy. Most physicians and health care providers are quite familiar with this line of inquiry, and the information gained from this evaluation can give important clues to the cause of the pain.

The pain of fibromyalgia and other central pain syndromes frequently waxes and wanes, may be quite migratory, and may be accompanied by dysesthesias or paresthesias following a nondermatomal distribution. In some instances, patients will present with "aching all over," whereas in other instances patients experience several areas of chronic regional pain. In this setting, regional musculoskeletal pain typically involves the axial skeleton, or areas of "tender points (TePs)," and may originally be diagnosed as a local problem (e.g., low back pain, lateral epicondylitis) (see Fig. 24-1). Regional pain involving nonmusculoskeletal regions is also common, including a higher than expected prevalence of both tension and migraine headaches, temporomandibular disorder (TMD) [or temporomandibular joint (TMJ) syndrome], noncardiac chest pain, irritable bowel syndrome, a number of entities characterized by chronic pelvic pain, and plantar or heel pain.

In addition to pain and tenderness, many individuals with fibromyalgia and other nonnociceptive pain syndromes experience fatigue [thus, many also meet criteria for chronic fatigue syndrome (CFS)], memory difficulties, fluctuations in weight, heat and cold intolerance, and the subjective sensation of weakness. They also display a wide array of hypersensitivity symptoms, ranging from adverse reactions to drugs and environmental stimuli to vasomotor rhinitis and hyperacusis.

Symptoms and Syndromes
Commonly Seen in Fibromyalgia

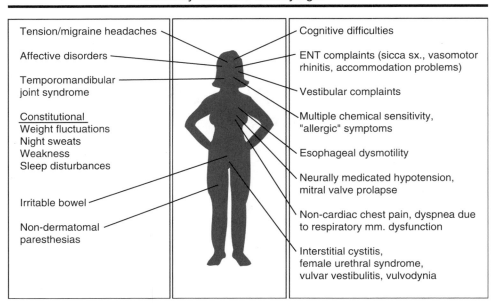

Figure 24-1. Symptoms and syndromes commonly seen in fibromyalgia.

These individuals also suffer from a number of symptoms of "functional" disorders of visceral organs, including a high incidence of recurrent noncardiac chest pain, heartburn, palpitations, mitral valve prolapse, esophageal dysmotility, and irritable bowel symptoms. Neurally mediated hypotension and syncope also occur more frequently in these individuals. Similar syndromes characterized by visceral pain and/or smooth muscle dysmotility are also seen in the pelvis, including dysmenorrhea, urinary frequency, urinary urgency, interstitial cystitis, endometriosis, and vulvar vestibulitis or vulvodynia.

A frequently neglected aspect of the pain history, though, is a thorough evaluation of the psychological, cognitive, social, and behavioral comorbidities that may be present in chronic-pain patients. This evaluation typically takes considerably more time than is allotted to an initial office visit, so it is frequently necessary to gather this type of information via self-report questionnaires or over a period of time as the individual is followed longitudinally. These constructs are covered in detail in Chapter 14, but an overview is given here.

Table 24-1 lists some of the most common psychological comorbidities seen in chronic-pain patients. Most clinicians focus on identifying and treating co-morbid mood disorders. Although this is important, there is increasing evidence that fear (especially of movement), anger, and guilt may be just as important (4–6).

Table 24-2 lists cognitive factors that have been demonstrated to be common in chronic-pain patients and, if present, are predictive of reduced responsiveness to therapies.

Table 24-3 gives examples of sample items from questionnaires that tap into these domains. Table 24-4 lists social factors that negatively impact on chronic pain, and, again, the following table (see Table 24-5) gives examples of questions used to assess these domains. Finally, Table 24-6 lists some of the important behavioral factors that may be present in chronic-pain patients.

THE PHYSICAL EXAMINATION

A thorough musculoskeletal and neuromuscular examination is important to identify any abnormalities that may give a clue to the cause of the pain. In general, in "peripheral" or nociceptive pain syndromes, abnormalities can be identified on physical examination, whereas in "central" pain syndromes, the examination is normal except for the finding of regional or generalized tenderness.

Localizing and characterizing tenderness is arguably the most important aspect of the overall evaluation of the chronic-pain patient. If an individual is only tender in the region in

---

TABLE 24-1 Psychological State

- Heightened emotional reactivity
  - Depression
  - Anxiety
  - Fear
  - Anger
  - Guilt

TABLE 24-2 Cognitions/Beliefs

External locus of control
- Learned belief that personal actions fail to produce desired outcomes

Learned helplessness
- Lack of functioning and depressed affect in the present based upon past failures to effectively control the environment

Catastrophizing
- Wholly negative conceptualization of a condition or situation

Low self-efficacy
- Belief in one's inability to perform a specific behavior

TABLE 24-3	Sample Belief Items

- External locus of control
  - "Whether or not I am in pain depends on what the doctors do for me."
- Catastrophizing
  - "It's awful and I feel that it overwhelms me."
  - "I feel I can't go on."
  - "It's terrible and I think it's never going to get any better."
- Self-Efficacy
  - "How confident are you that you can exercise without making your symptoms worse?" (Not at all/totally confident)

which he or she is experiencing pain, this typically represents a peripheral, nociceptive-pain syndrome. For example, in a regional inflammatory condition such as bursitis, the individual will typically only be tender over the affected bursae. In tendinitis, the tendon may be tender, but more typically the pain can be exacerbated by maneuvers that stretch or use the tendon. Other conditions characterized by local tenderness include arthritis (where it is important to assess for the presence or absence of synovitis, which is an indication of an inflammatory arthritis) and neuropathy.

Any time localized tenderness is identified, the examiner should ascertain whether there is also tenderness in the same location on the opposite side of the body and in other areas of the body such as the forearm or cervical region. These latter areas are good areas to assess an individual's overall pain threshold. Finding bilateral tenderness or tenderness in some of these other regions makes it more likely that the individual has an element of central, nonnociceptive pain, such as fibromyalgia or a related condition. Although a TeP count has classically been recommended for diagnosing fibromyalgia, in reality, individuals with fibromyalgia are tender all over, and the average tenderness in any few regions of the body is highly predictive of overall tenderness (7). It is also important to realize that women are much more tender to digital palpation than men. The requirement for 11/18 TePs is the primary reason that fibromyalgia is an almost exclusively female disease because women are only 1.5 times more likely than men to have chronic widespread pain (8). Thus, the threshold the examiner should use to consider a man "tender" is higher for men than women.

DIAGNOSTIC STUDIES

Considerable clinical judgment is necessary to determine the aggressiveness of the diagnostic evaluation that is necessary for a given individual with chronic pain. For example, individuals with the exact same complaints who present with 6 weeks, 6 months, or 6 years of symptoms would necessitate quite

TABLE 24-4	Social Factors

- Lack of social support
- Family reinforcers of illness
- Medicolegal factors
- Job/role dissatisfaction

TABLE 24-5	Sample Social Support Items

- How would you rate the amount and quality of social support that you currently have from family, friends, and religious activities? (Circle one response in each column.)

(0) None, I don't have anyone I can talk to.	(0) Bad, I don't feel supported.
(1) Some, I have a few people I can talk to.	(1) Fair, I feel somewhat supported.
(2) A lot, I have several people I can talk to.	(2) Good, I feel very supported.

different diagnostic workups. In general, for example, the individual with the most acute or subacute symptoms generally warrants the most aggressive diagnostic evaluation, whereas an individual with chronic waxing and waning of symptoms for many years but a normal physical exam is unlikely to have an unrecognized autoimmune, hormonal, malignant, or infectious disease, and thus the evaluation can be more limited. On the other hand, there are instances when symptoms of short duration require a *less* aggressive workup. For example, individuals who have an acute episode of low back pain generally should have no diagnostic workup unless their symptoms do not resolve in 6 weeks or longer or there are symptoms suggesting severe neurologic compromise (e.g., cauda equina syndrome), malignancy (weight loss), or infection (fever).

DIAGNOSTIC TESTING

A common problem with diagnostic testing in the chronic-pain patient is that of "false-positive" diagnostic tests. This is true for both laboratory testing as well as imaging studies. Antinuclear antibodies (ANA) are a good example of this problem. As many as 30% of the population may have a 1:40 ANA or higher (1), but only 1:2,000 individuals has systemic lupus erythematosus (SLE). Therefore, <1:100 individuals in the population with a positive ANA will have SLE.

For individuals with chronic widespread pain, the differential diagnosis is listed in Table 24-7. A few disorders bear special mention. The two conditions that arguably most closely simulate fibromyalgia are hypothyroidism and polymyalgia rheumatica. For this reason, a thyroid stimulating hormone (TSH) and erythrocyte sedimentation rate (ESR) are suggested in every person in whom the diagnosis of fibromyalgia is being entertained. Because fibromyalgia occurs less frequently in men than women, some have suggested that a further workup may be in order when a man presents with symptoms consistent with fibromyalgia. Examples of entities that simulate fibromyalgia and occur more commonly in men are sleep apnea and hepatitis C infection.

TABLE 24-6	Behavioral Factors

- Decreased activity/isolation
- Decreased function
- Poor sleep
- Disability

TABLE 24-7	Conditions That Simulate Fibromyalgia (see also Chapter 25)

Common
Hypothyroidism
Polymyalgia rheumatica
Hepatitis C
Sleep apnea
Statin-induced myopathy
? Cervical stenosis/Chiari malformation

Less common
Autoimmune disorders (e.g., SLE, RA, etc.)
Endocrine disorders (e.g., Addison disease, Cushing syndrome, hyperparathyroidism)

SLE, systemic lupus erythematosus; RA, rheumatoid arthritis.

SPECIFIC DIAGNOSTIC TESTS

ACUTE PHASE REACTANTS

Nonspecific indicators of the presence of inflammation such as ESR and C-reactive protein (CRP) can be valuable in identifying chronic-pain patients who have an element of systemic inflammatory or autoimmune disorder. The two tests have different utilities, with the ESR being more sensitive and the CRP more specific for inflammation; CRP also rises and falls more rapidly in response to inflammation. In screening a chronic-pain patient, a normal ESR and CRP makes it considerably less likely (but not impossible) that an individual has an active, systemic, inflammatory disease. False-positive ESRs are very common, but false-positive CRPs are less common.

AUTOANTIBODIES

Autoantibodies are qualitatively normal immunoglobulins that are formed by most individuals; higher titers of certain autoantibodies are seen in several autoimmune disorders.

Some autoantibodies are very sensitive for presence of disease (e.g., ANA, which is present in nearly all SLE and scleroderma patients) but not specific, whereas others (e.g., anti-SM and anti-dsDNA antibodies, which are seen in a minority of SLE patients but are rarely found in healthy individuals) are specific but not sensitive.

Because of the high rate of false-positive autoantibodies, these tests should only be ordered in certain clinical settings. For example, ordering ANA for all individuals with myalgia, arthralgias, and fatigue will lead to many more false-positive than true-positive tests (2). However, ANA testing is helpful if the individual has findings on either history or physical examination that are typically seen in autoimmune disorders because negative results of this test ostensibly exclude conditions such as SLE and scleroderma. Table 24-8 gives examples of laboratory testing that are appropriate for differing clinical settings.

The overlap between fibromyalgia and autoimmune disorders deserves special mention. Many individuals early in the course of autoimmune disorders may present with symptoms reminiscent of fibromyalgia, but a larger problem is that many patients with nonspecific symptoms of fibromyalgia have laboratory testing performed that suggests they may have an autoimmune disorder (e.g.,

TABLE 24-8	Appropriate Diagnostic Tests in Chronic Pain Patients

LABORATORY TEST	APPROPRIATE SETTING
ESR, CRP, TSH, routine chemistries, urinalysis	• All chronic-pain patients should have these ordered at least once
Antinuclear antibody	• Abnormal results of above • H + P findings of SLE, scleroderma
Rheumatoid factor	• Synovitis, especially of small joints • Abnormal ESR/CRP
Creatine phosphokinase	• Objective weakness
Lyme titer	• Appropriate rash, arthritis, neurologic findings
More specific autoantibodies (e.g., ENA panels containing RNP, Sm, Ro, La antibodies; ANCA)	• Abnormal ANA • Abnormal ESR/CRP, U/A

ESR, erythrocyte sedimentation rate; CRP, C-reactive protein; TSH, thyroid stimulating hormone; SLE, systemic lupus erythematosus; ANA, antinuclear antibodies.

positive ANA or RF). Symptoms that can be seen in both fibromyalgia and autoimmune disorders include not only arthralgias, myalgias, and fatigue, but also morning stiffness and a history of subjective swelling of the hands and feet. In addition, a Raynaudlike syndrome (characterized by the *entire hand* turning pale or red instead of just the digits), malar flushing (in contrast to a fixed malar rash), and livedo reticularis are all common in fibromyalgia and can mislead the practitioner to suspect an autoimmune disorder.

IMAGING STUDIES

A variety of imaging studies can be useful in arriving at a diagnosis in chronic-pain patients, but again, false-positive test results are a significant problem. For almost any chronic-pain state, there is discordance between the findings seen in peripheral tissues [e.g., joint space narrowing on radiographs, bulging or protruding discs on magnetic resonance imaging (MRI)—see Chapter 2].

Plain radiography is the least expensive and most widely available imaging modality, and it is most helpful when bone or joint pathology is suspected. Computerized tomography (CT) and MRI are more expensive but visualize cartilage, ligaments, and neural tissues, and thus are particularly valuable for imaging the axial skeleton and more complex joints (e.g., the knee). Radionuclide scanning provides insight into physiologic processes, and scintigraphy (e.g., technicium-pyrophosphate targets bone turnover) can be useful to identify pathology. Ultrasonography has increasing utility for identifying regional pain problems such as tendonitis, bursitis, and synovitis.

THE EVALUATION IS OVER. WHAT DOES THE PATIENT HAVE, AND WHAT DO I DO?

Table 24-9 gives an overview of the various elements of the history, physical, and diagnostic workup and how these elements help determine whether the individual has fibromyalgia, some other nonnociceptive pain condition, or has an alternative cause for his or her pain. Again, it is important to emphasize that many individuals have both. Just as it is important that clinicians be vigilant for elements of fibromyalgia in individuals with acknowledged nociceptive pain conditions such as osteoarthritis, the converse is also true. For example, although we consider conditions such as fibromyalgia to be primarily nonnociceptive, if these individuals have comorbid arthritis or other mechanical or inflammatory conditions, these should be identified and treated. This is particularly important because peripheral nociceptive input can lead to phenomena such as windup and central sensitization that lead to hyperalgesia and can worsen the central, nonnociceptive component of that individual's pain.

SUMMARY POINTS

- The history and physical examination give the most important information regarding the correct diagnosis in individuals with chronic pain.
- In addition to chronic pain in multiple regions of the body, individuals with fibromyalgia and other nonnociceptive pain syndromes frequently display other symptoms such as fatigue, insomnia, and difficulty with memory.

TABLE 24-9 Clues to Presence of Nociceptive or Nonnociceptive Pain

	MORE LIKELY TO BE FIBROMYALGIA OR OTHER NONNOCICEPTIVE PAIN SYNDROME	MORE LIKELY TO BE NOCICEPTIVE PAIN
Distribution of pain	More widespread	More focal
Other somatic symptoms such as fatigue, insomnia, headache, memory difficulties	Present	Absent
Tenderness	Regional or none	Widespread or regional
Psychological, behavioral, cognitive comorbidities	More commonly present	Less commonly present but must be identified and addressed
Diagnostic tests	Negative or false positive (e.g., ANA, MRI of axial skeleton)	More likely to be abnormal

ANA, antinuclear antibodies; MRI, magnetic resonance imaging.

- The history should include a careful evaluation of psychological, cognitive, behavioral, and social factors that may be contributing to pain.
- In individuals with fibromyalgia and other similar syndromes, the examination will typically be unremarkable except for the finding of tenderness.
- Diagnostic testing such as serologic assays and imaging studies are frequently abnormal in asymptomatic individuals, making their predictive value poor unless they are obtained in the correct clinical setting.

■ IMPLICATIONS FOR PRACTICE

- Fibromyalgia and other nonnociceptive pain syndromes are the most common cause for chronic widespread pain.
- Even individuals who have a peripheral nociceptive pain syndrome may display elements of fibromyalgia, which must be managed as such.
- The converse is also true. Many individuals with primarily nonnociceptive pain will have elements of local inflammation or damage that lead to nociceptive foci, and these must be addressed and managed or they can worsen the hyperalgesia/allodynia.
- Identification and treatment of psychological, cognitive, behavioral, and social factors that may be contributing

to pain are important in all chronic-pain patients, regardless of the cause.

REFERENCES

1. Tan EM, Feltkamp TE, Smolen JS, et al. Range of antinuclear antibodies in "healthy" individuals. *Arthritis Rheum* 1997;40(9):1601–1611.
2. Pincus T. A pragmatic approach to cost-effective use of laboratory tests and imaging procedures in patients with musculoskeletal symptoms. *Prim Care* 1993;20(4):795–814.
3. Jensen MC, Brant-Zawadzki MN, Obuchowski N, et al. Magnetic resonance imaging of the lumbar spine in people without back pain. *N Engl J Med* 1994;331(2):69–73.
4. Buer N, Linton SJ. Fear-avoidance beliefs and catastrophizing: occurrence and risk factor in back pain and ADL in the general population. *Pain* 2002;99(3):485–491.
5. Turk DC, Okifuji A. Psychological factors in chronic pain: evolution and revolution. *J Consult Clin Psychol* 2002;70(3):678–690.
6. Arntz A, van Eck M, Heijmans M. Predictions of dental pain: the fear of any expected evil, is worse than the evil itself. *Behav Res Ther* 1990;28(1):29–41.
7. Petzke F, Khine A, Williams D, et al. Dolorimetry performed at 3 paired tender points highly predicts overall tenderness. *J Rheumatol* 2001;28(11):2568–2569.
8. Wolfe F, Ross K, Anderson J, et al. The prevalence and characteristics of fibromyalgia in the general population. *Arthritis Rheum* 1995;38(1):19–28.

25

The Differential Diagnosis of Chronic Regional Pain

Kevin P. White

Relatively few disorders mimic the constellation of symptoms that is so pervasive in those with fibromyalgia (FM). Chronic aching all over, a virtual prerequisite for FM, is not generally reported by people with rheumatoid arthritis (RA), osteoarthritis (OA), and other musculoskeletal disorders, except by those who also meet the case definition of FM (1). FM patients often liken this generalized ache to that felt during a severe flu; however, its chronicity distinguishes FM from flu. Similarly, many patients with widely metastatic malignancies or blood dyscrasias (2) may report hurting all over, but such diagnoses usually become apparent relatively quickly and, hence, rarely should be mistaken for FM long term.

Individuals meeting the case definition of chronic fatigue syndrome (CFS) often report such generalized aching, but up to a third of those meeting the case definition for CFS also meet the FM case definition (3,4). There is evidence that those meeting both sets of criteria, for CFS and FM, generally have more symptoms, severer symptoms, and poorer overall function than those meeting the FM case definition alone (5). Epidemics of CFS have also been reported, presumably secondary to viral or other infectious outbreaks (6–9), a phenomenon generally not attributed to FM. Otherwise, however, distinguishing between FM and CFS is rarely useful clinically.

Hence, people who report hurting all over, debilitating fatigue, nonrestorative sleep, and other common FM symptoms, and who also have the generalized body tenderness of FM, almost certainly have FM as the explanation for their symptoms.

What becomes important, however, is that other conditions, including a wide variety of chronic regional pain syndromes, can coexist with FM and may often be missed. This is particularly important when these conditions require treatment that differs from the treatments offered for FM or when these conditions are, in themselves, potentially life or limb threatening.

This chapter initially will address the relatively few conditions that reasonably can be misdiagnosed as FM and for which an accurate diagnosis is essential, such as polymyalgia rheumatica (PMR) and atypical low grade inflammatory polyarthropathies. Then discussion will turn to those conditions that can coexist with FM and potentially be missed and go untreated because of being overlooked. Our discussion cannot possibly be all-inclusive in a single chapter. Our attempt will be to describe those conditions that either are relatively common or for which diagnosis and initiation of appropriate therapy is critical.

DISORDERS THAT REASONABLY MAY BE MISDIAGNOSED AS FIBROMYALGIA

POLYMYALGIA RHEUMATICA

Patients who develop PMR invariably are older—usually 50 or more; in fact, almost all epidemiologic studies of PMR and associated temporal arteritis (TA) have been limited to people 50 or older. Its incidence varies with the population studied, from a low of approximately 130 incident cases per million in Italy (10) to almost 540 cases per million in Olmsted County, Minnesota (11), 1,100 per million in Norway (12), and over 6,000 cases per million in those over age 65 in Cambridge, England (13). The exceedingly high prevalence observed in Cambridge may be secondary to the somewhat older cohort studied since there is evidence that the incidence of PMR follows that of giant cell arteritis, and the latter is known to dramatically increase in incidence with age, from 26 per million in those age 50 to 59 to almost 450 per million in those over 80 (14). Both conditions appear to be more common among Caucasians than other racial groups (14).

Typically, individuals with PMR present complaining of pain and/or stiffness involving the shoulder girdle, pelvic girdle, or both (15). It is often symmetrical, although asymmetrical PMR has been reported (16). Commonly associated features include fevers, weight loss, fatigue, and malaise (17). Headaches, scalp tenderness, amaurosis or other visual changes, and jaw and lingual claudication all are suggestive of comorbid TA (18). The onset of symptoms often is quite sudden: patients often recall the precise day on which their pain and/or stiffness started.

PMR can mimic FM because of the relatively diffuse distribution of pain and stiffness, particularly in the majority of PMR patients who report bilateral pain throughout both the shoulder and pelvic girdles. In this way patients meet the first American College of Rheumatology (ACR) criteria for FM (19) in that they have upper and lower body pain, right and left sided pain, and both axial and peripheral pain. Although pain and stiffness tend to be proximal, approximately half have distal symptoms as well (20). Headaches and jaw pain, very common complaints among FM sufferers, can present in patients with PMR and comorbid TA. Hence, it is not surprising that some patients with PMR may be misdiagnosed with FM. However, every attempt should be made to avoid such a misdiagnosis, for two major reasons. First, both PMR and TA require disease-specific treatment that is highly effective in alleviating symptoms and very different from treatment offered to FM patients; the mainstay of treatment for PMR and/or TA is the prolonged use of systemic corticosteroid (21). Second, failing to diagnose TA may result in failure to prevent severe end-organ damage, to the optic nerve in particular, resulting in usually irreversible vision loss, including total blindness (22).

In essence, any patient over age 50 who presents complaining of shoulder girdle and/or pelvic girdle pain and/or stiffness, particularly of abrupt onset, must be considered to have PMR until proven otherwise. Similarly, anyone over 50 who presents with visual changes, along with amaurosis, new-onset, or altered headaches, scalp tenderness, and/or jaw or lingual claudication, must be considered to have TA until proven otherwise. These diagnoses are not definitively ruled out by obtaining a normal erythrocyte sedimentation rate (ESR), since anywhere from 6% to 22% of individuals with PMR will not have a significant elevation in ESR at presentation (23,24); an elevated C-reactive protein may be more sensitive (25). TA also may be associated with a normal ESR (26). Similarly, although a temporal artery biopsy is indicated when TA is suspected, a normal biopsy does not definitively rule out TA because so-called "skip areas" may result in false-negative biopsies, even in individuals with severe disease culminating in blindness (27,28). PMR and TA essentially are ruled out via an adequate trial of systemic corticosteroid to determine treatment response. Failure to respond to low dose (for PMR) to intermediate dose (for TA) systemic corticosteroid over 3 to 4 weeks generally is considered adequate to rule out either diagnosis (29). The corollary is that a dramatic improvement after 3 to 4 weeks of low to intermediate dose corticosteroid generally is considered confirmatory.

FM and PMR and/or TA may coexist. I have seen several patients who had FM diagnosed only to develop a worsening of their symptoms, heralding the onset of PMR or TA, or both. The key to detecting the onset of the PMR and TA is recognizing either a worsening in pain and/or stiffness, primarily in the neck and shoulder girdle areas, or the onset of other symptoms, such as worsening or changing headaches, low grade fevers, weight loss, and jaw or lingual claudication. As with all patients in whom PMR and/or TA is being considered, a complete history and physical examination, followed by indicated clinical investigations and an adequate trial of low to intermediate dose systemic corticosteroid, is

essential. Responding to corticosteroids resulted in a return to the patient's baseline level of FM symptoms or possibly even to a level of improvement greater than what I had initially perceived to be their baseline.

ATYPICAL RHEUMATOID ARTHRITIS OR OTHER INFLAMMATORY POLYARTHRITIS

Rheumatoid Arthritis and Systemic Lupus Erythematosus

FM truly should not be in the differential as the explanation for one or more visibly or palpably swollen joints. Hence, classically presenting RA, an acute-onset inflammatory polyarthritis, rarely should be mistaken for FM, irrespective of the presence or absence of rheumatoid factor in serum. The same is true of systemic lupus erythematosus (SLE), which also classically presents as an acute onset, chronic inflammatory polyarthritis (30). The potential for confusion lies with patients presenting with oligo- or polyarthralgias in the absence of objective joint swelling with arthralgia rather than obvious arthritis.

Because FM is more common in women and RA is the most common inflammatory arthropathy in women, affecting 0.5% to more than 1% of women in the general population (31–33), RA may cause common confusion. As with FM, the distribution of pain and stiffness in RA typically is diffuse, classically involving all four extremities and frequently the neck as well (34). Even the low back may be involved with RA, although most RA patients with low back pain probably have mechanical rather than inflammatory back pain (35). In one study, 12 of 22 FM patients presenting consecutively to a rheumatology outpatient clinic reported with polyarthralgia as a primary complaint, almost all reporting hand joint pain as well as pain in other joints (36). In a Chinese study of 120 FM clinic patients, 49.2% reported multiple arthralgia (37). Among 100 confirmed FM cases identified in a general population survey, hand pain, especially worsened by exposure to cold, was reported in over 50% (38).

Laboratory and radiographic investigations often are normal or nonspecific early in the course of RA. Detection of rheumatoid factor in serum does not definitively confirm RA, nor does its absence definitively eliminate RA as a diagnostic possibility. As with FM, RA commonly is diagnosed using published classification criteria, one of which is quite subjective (morning stiffness) and others of which are quite observer dependent (e.g., swelling and radiographic erosions) (39).

Early in the course of disease, objective joint swelling likely is the most helpful criterion if considering RA or SLE. If joint swelling is observed, FM cannot be the sole explanation. FM itself is not associated with objective joint swelling. Individuals with FM commonly report swelling, particularly in hands and/or feet, but health practitioners rarely observe it in the absence of synovitis from another cause. Why FM patients so commonly report swelling in the absence of objective evidence has not been scientifically explained, but it likely relates to the neurologic dysfunction associated with this disease. Paresthesias, especially of hands and feet, also are very common in FM (40), and a wide variety of neurohormonal abnormalities are increasingly felt to be central pathophysiologic mechanisms of this disease (41).

In the patient in whom RA or SLE is suspected, despite the absence of joint swelling, a trial of low-dose corticosteroid also may be illuminating. As opposed to patients with active synovitis caused by RA, SLE, or other autoimmune connective tissue diseases, FM patients generally do not respond to low-dose systemic corticosteroid (42). However, comorbid FM is not uncommon in patients with RA (43) and lupus (44,45). A partial response to corticosteroid may add further confusion to any potential placebo response.

The Seronegative Spondyloarthropathies

Whereas most patients with RA present with objective joint swelling, it is not at all uncommon for patients with one of the spondyloarthropathies to present with subtle inflammatory findings, and these patients may have a more equivocal response to corticosteroids than RA and SLE patients. Spondyloarthropathies form a group of conditions that includes ankylosing spondylitis, reactive arthritis, the arthritis associated with psoriasis, the arthritis associated with inflammatory bowel disease (Crohn disease and ulcerative colitis), and a form of juvenile chronic arthritis (46). These conditions involve not only central joints such as the sacroiliac joints, the axial skeleton, and the small joints of the thorax, but also peripheral joints; enthesitis—that is, inflammation of tendon insertion into bone—is common (46,47). Thus, the stage is set in these conditions for patients to experience a type of musculoskeletal pain that can resemble FM. Nocturnal pain, which is typical of spondyloarthritis, may lead to sleep disturbance, another symptom common to the two conditions. Further adding to the possible confusion is the frequent concurrence of FM and irritable bowel syndrome (IBS) (48), which might lead to a mistaken diagnosis of spondyloarthritis due to inflammatory bowel disease in patients with FM and IBS, or vice versa.

Although the prevalence of FM is much higher in association with conditions such as RA and systemic lupus erythematosus than might be expected by chance, the prevalence of FM in spondyloarthritis is unknown. However, pressure pain thresholds appear to be no different from those in healthy controls, at least in patients with ankylosing spondylitis; this is in contrast to patients with RA (49).

It appears that the similarity between certain symptoms of FM and those of spondyloarthritis have led to a number of misdiagnoses. In one Quebec study, 3% of 321 patients referred to a general rheumatology practice over a 1-year period were referred, each with a presumptive diagnosis of FM that the consulting rheumatologist did not confirm; these 11 patients, all women, were considered to have previously unrecognized and clinically subtle spondyloarthropathies (50). It should be noted that patients with FM and with spondyloarthropathy may report equivalent impairment in function (51).

Despite these similarities, overall it should not be difficult to differentiate FM from spondyloarthropathy. The presence of psoriasis, other mucocutaneous reactions, conjunctivitis, uveitis, and urethritis should alert the physician that the patient has spondyloarthritis. The gastrointestinal symptoms of inflammatory bowel disease usually have characteristics that allow differentiation between them and IBS. The onset of ankylosing spondylitis after age 40 is rare (46). The presence

of peripheral joint swelling should raise strong suspicion that the patient has an inflammatory arthritis rather than FM. A family history of spondyloarthritis may be of further help in the differential diagnosis. Finally, x-rays showing sacroiliitis or enthesitis, or both, should be regarded as strong evidence for the presence of spondyloarthritis.

Nonetheless, time and vigilance may be necessary to identify an underlying subtle inflammatory arthropathy in some FM patients. This is a reasonable argument against the practice of some consultants to see any given FM patient only once and to refuse further assessments because "it's just FM."

MULTIPLE SCLEROSIS

A variety of neurologic symptoms are common among individuals with FM. Approximately one-third of adults with FM in a general community sample reported episodic numbness, most commonly in the limbs (40). Other neurologic symptoms include episodic, temporary numbness, shocklike sensations, burning pain, and the sensation of ants crawling on or under the skin. The most likely cause of these symptoms is the disequilibrium and dysfunction that numerous scientific investigators have reported among various neurotransmitters.

Multiple sclerosis (MS) is associated with numerous symptoms classic for FM, including chronic fatigue, sleeplessness, pain, and muscle spasms. All these symptoms may be severely incapacitating.

It is only recently being widely recognized that pain is a common and often severely debilitating symptom of MS. Up to 70% of patients with MS report clinically significant pain (52,53). In one study, 25% of 442 responding members of the King County (Washington) MS Association reported severe pain and/or pain that severely interfered with their activities of daily living (54). Many MS patients report more localized pain, as in trigeminal neuralgia or painful optic neuritis; for others, however, it is more generalized, including diffuse dysesthesias of the limbs (53). As with FM, MS-related pain seems to be difficult to treat (55). As with FM, the underlying causative mechanism of pain often appears to be central rather than peripheral, as evidenced by an incomplete response to intravenous morphine (55).

Chronic fatigue also is being recognized as a frequent, debilitating symptom in MS, and there appears to be a link between fatigue and clinically and electrophysiologically significant sleep disturbance (56,57). Unlike FM, the primary sleep disturbance appears to be in rapid eye movement (REM), rather than in stage IV non-REM, sleep (58). As with FM, fatigue is very difficult to treat in MS, and the mechanism for causation is poorly understood.

Nocturnal muscle spasms, particularly of the lower extremities, are common in MS (59) and FM (60). In both conditions they can be debilitating but also treatable.

As with FM and the inflammatory polyarthritides, FM and MS can coexist. To date, however, there are no published studies on comorbidity of FM and MS. Over the past 14 years, I have identified MS in four patients, all female, whom I had been following for FM. In each case the symptom that triggered further investigation was numbness that persisted. One woman reported numbness along one side of her mouth that started quite abruptly and persisted up through her reporting it to me some 6 months later. In the others, persistent limb numbness was the provocative symptom. I referred each patient for brain magnetic resonance imaging (MRI) and formal neurologic consultation. In every case the consulting neurologist in a university MS clinic considered a diagnosis of MS at least highly likely. To my knowledge, each of these patients has done well and continues to be followed in the MS clinic. My suggestion, therefore, is to consider MS in any FM patient in whom neurologic symptoms become persistent, as opposed to chronic and episodic.

THYROID DYSFUNCTION

A possible association between FM and hypothyroidism has been suspected for a long time. In 1981, Wilke et al. reported eight patients who presented with signs and symptoms of "the fibrositis syndrome" (the name formerly used for FM) and who did not have overt hypothyroid disease but were found to have evidence of hypothyroidism on further investigation; six of these eight patients improved with thyroid treatment (61). Hypothyroidism can give rise to fatigue, myalgias, and arthritis (62). It is obvious that the two conditions could be easily confused. In fact, some have postulated that FM is a form of hormone-resistant hypothyroidism (63). Carette and Lefrancois investigated 100 patients with subclinical or biochemical primary hypothyroidism and found that 19 had symptoms of arthralgia or myalgia; they found, using older criteria for "fibrositis," that only 5% of the whole group had this condition (64). These results suggested that FM is uncommon in patients with primary hypothyroidism.

It is uncertain how often hypothyroidism is missed in patients who are diagnosed as having FM. It has been suggested that it would be wise to order a screening test for hypothyroidism such as a thyroid stimulating hormone (TSH) level in patients who present with symptoms of FM (65), but there are no data to assess this measure's cost-effectiveness. If there were a reasonably high index of suspicion, we would certainly agree that this should be done. Interestingly, there has been little concern about the possibility that thyrotoxic myopathy might present as FM, presumably because muscle weakness and muscle wasting are common clinical manifestations while muscle pain is rare (66).

In summary, the symptoms of FM and hypothyroidism may be difficult to distinguish from each other, but FM seems to be relatively uncommon in patients presenting with hypothyroidism. It is our impression that hypothyroidism also is uncommon in patients presenting with FM, but if there are any suspicious symptoms and signs such as cold intolerance, bradycardia, voice changes, excessive drowsiness, or changes in the tendon jerks, it would be appropriate to order a serum TSH level.

OTHER METABOLIC DISORDERS

A vast array of metabolic diseases can give rise to arthritis/arthralgia or myopathy/myalgia, or both. These include hemochromatosis, Wilson disease, primary oxalosis, McArdle disease, carnitine palmitoyl transferase deficiency, and acute intermittent porphyria, to name only a few. This chapter will address only three endocrine or metabolic abnormalities that could be confused with FM.

Hyperparathyroidism

Hyperparathyroidism can affect bones and joints and give rise to lethargy (67). In one study fatigue and bone pain were the two commonest presenting symptoms (68), while in another smaller study myalgia was reported in 41% of patients (69). It is unknown how often, if at all, hyperparathyroidism is mistaken for FM. Symptoms that should arouse suspicion of hyperparathyroidism in patients with apparent FM would include a history of hematuria or renal stones, fragility fractures, polydypsia, and polyuria.

Vitamin D Deficiency

Vitamin D deficiency seems to be widely prevalent in the population. Common causes include dietary deficiencies, inadequate exposure to ultraviolet light, and malabsorption. Low vitamin D levels can lead to increases in parathyroid hormone concentration. Patients may complain of diffuse bone pain, muscle weakness, paresthesia, fatigue, and malaise (70). Reginato et al. described a series of 26 cases of osteomalacia of whom 23 presented with bone pain; two of the patients had been diagnosed as having FM (71). In a study conducted at a clinic in Minnesota of 150 patients with chronic musculoskeletal pain but without FM, it was found that 93% had low levels of 25-hydroxy vitamin D (72). The implication was that myalgia was due to hypovitaminosis D, but no data are available on whether correction of low vitamin D levels led to improvement of myalgic symptoms. A large percentage of patients with FM are known to have low 25-hydroxy Vitamin D levels (73,74). This might be due to a lack of exposure to ultraviolet light, as these patients tend to be less active and spend less time outdoors. The low levels of vitamin D metabolites seen in these patients do not necessarily imply that they have osteomalacia or that vitamin D would necessarily help their symptoms of FM. Nevertheless, one has to remember, when encountering patients from populations who are at high risk from osteomalacia—for example, those with malabsorption, poor nutrition, lack of exposure to ultraviolet light, and osteodystrophy—that their pain might be due to metabolic bone disease.

Statin-Induced Myopathy

Statins are amongst the most extensively used drugs because of their efficacy in reducing low-density lipoprotein cholesterol levels and reducing the risk of ischemic heart disease. These drugs, however, can also cause myopathy. The mechanisms responsible for this are uncertain and may involve the accumulation of lipids within myocytes and the inhibition of the formation of ubiquinone membrane stabilizer (75). Statin-induced myopathy can result in myositis or even rhabdomyolysis with elevated creatinine kinase (CK) levels and muscle weakness (75). It may also consist of myalgia alone without any objective laboratory findings. Older age, female sex, hypothyroidism, and hepatic dysfunction increase the risk of statin-induced myopathy (75). The concurrent use of a fibrate may also increase the risk of myopathy. Patients with myalgia alone and no elevation of CK levels or other evidence of muscle damage may continue on their medication if their symptoms are tolerable (76). Clearly, statin-induced myopathy might be confused with FM. Important points in the differential diagnosis would include a history of taking a statin prior to the onset of the myalgia, clinical and laboratory evidence of a myopathy, and pain relief by discontinuation of the statin.

DISORDERS THAT MAY COEXIST WITH AND REMAIN UNDIAGNOSED BECAUSE OF FIBROMYALGIA

OSTEOARTHRITIS

Technically, all that an OA patient would require to satisfy the first ACR criterion for FM would be OA causing pain in one finger, a contralateral toe, and the neck or low back. Given that a small percentage of the general population has 11 or more FM tender points (TePs) in the absence of chronic or widespread pain (77), such a patient would satisfy both ACR criteria for FM. Realistically, however, such a patient would almost never be diagnosed with FM in the absence of significant pains elsewhere and/or other significantly troublesome symptoms such as profound fatigue and sleeplessness. In general, OA should not hide FM because OA generally is more localized and asymmetrical than FM. The greater risk is that the presence of FM will delay the diagnosis of OA.

Perhaps the joint for which this is most likely and most clinically relevant is the hip. The primary reason for this is that hip joint swelling can rarely be detected on examination due to the abundance of overlying tissues. On several occasions I have been astounded by the advanced degree of joint space narrowing detected on radiographic imaging of a FM patient's hip, imaging that I had ordered expecting to find no or minimal changes. Knowing when and on whom to order radiographs becomes critical, especially because comorbidity with OA and FM is not at all uncommon (78).

A history of mechanical pain (e.g., pain immediately upon weight-bearing and with minimal stiffness) combined with certain physical findings (e.g., obviously antalgic gait, apparent leg length discrepancy, and pain with log-rolling of the hip) may be sensitive and specific enough to be used as a clinical guide to hip imaging.

DEGENERATIVE ARTHRITIS OF THE CERVICAL AND LUMBAR SPINE

Degenerative changes in the neck and low back are common causes of pain. Although there continues to be some controversy as to the mechanisms of pain in both these regions, there is general agreement that in both the cervical and lumbar spines the facet joints and discs are important sources of pain (79–82). Other possible contributing sites may be the paraspinal muscles and the sacroiliac joints. The pain of degenerative arthritis in either the cervical or the lumbar spine is fairly well localized; in the former, pain will be felt in the neck, shoulders, scapular area, and arms (79), while in the latter it will occur in the low back, buttocks, and thighs. Pain may become more widespread if there is nerve root involvement, as may occur in spinal stenosis, or disc herniation in either of the two spinal regions (79,83). Nevertheless, pain from degenerative changes, with or without neurologic in-

volvement, should be either above or below the waist and therefore easily distinguished from FM, where pain is in both the upper and lower halves of the body. The differential diagnosis between FM and degenerative disease of the spine should therefore be straightforward.

There are some complicating factors. Chronic pain in the neck or back is common. One population study found that 54% of adults had experienced neck pain in the last 6 months, while another study demonstrated a point prevalence of 9% (79). Low back pain is at least as common; several surveys in the United States have shown annual prevalence rates of pain lasting 2 weeks or longer in 10% to 15% of the adult population and a lifetime prevalence in men of 70% (84). This implies that by chance alone there are a large number of patients who have coincidental degenerative arthritis of both the cervical and lumbar spines; in fact, it is likely that the same disease mechanisms partly affect both regions of the spine. In such a case a history of diffuse pain could mislead one to suspect FM. Three points should be made, however. First, the physical examination showing the presence or absence of the requisite number of FM TePs may be useful. Second, the absence of severe debilitating fatigue, nonrestorative sleep, and other FM-associated symptoms makes FM less likely. Third, a definitive diagnosis of FM may not be necessary, since there is no disease-specific therapy usually required for cervical or lumbar spine degenerative arthritis other than surgery for disc resection, which rarely is necessary.

The coincidental occurrence of FM and symptomatic degenerative disease of either or both the cervical and lumbar spines is probably common. A Finnish study of six primary care practices found that patients presenting with neck and shoulder pain frequently also complained of low back pain and pain in many other body sites (85). Similarly, a German regional survey showed that widespread pain was common in patients with low back pain (86). Surprisingly, the prevalence of FM as classified by the ACR criteria was not high. The simultaneous presence of FM and degenerative disease of the cervical and lumbar spines in the same individual may be difficult to diagnose with certainty in the absence of neurologic symptoms. Radiologic investigations are of limited help in determining the presence of symptomatic degenerative arthritis of the spine (80).

One problem with medicolegal implications is that of whiplash-associated disorder (WAD) occurring together with FM. Although the relation of trauma to FM remains controversial (87), evidence suggests that the incidence of FM following cervical spine injury is significantly higher than one would expect by chance (88,89). The diagnoses of WAD and FM can be made independently of each other.

HEADACHE SYNDROMES

Headaches have long been recognized as a common symptom of FM (90,91). In London, Ontario, 82% of 100 confirmed community cases of FM reported frequent headaches, making it the sixth most common symptom, behind pain (100%), fatigue (100%), nonrestorative sleep (92%), weakness (90%), and insomnia (84%). One-third of the cases reported headaches as having been a major problem over the 2 weeks prior to the survey, compared to 12.7% of the general population controls (40). This study made no attempt to categorize different types of headaches.

Migraine headaches may be particularly important to identify in the FM patients for several reasons. First, in most populations studied, migraine headaches traditionally have been characterized as being potentially highly debilitating and highly treatable. There is no evidence that they are any less debilitating or treatable in FM patients. Second, migraines may be particularly common among those with FM; the two conditions may coexist at a greater rate than what would be expected by chance (4), although epidemiologic confirmation of this is lacking. If they do coexist, one scientifically supported explanation is that the two syndromes appear to share a common causative pathway, one that involves disruption involving serotonergic and adrenergic systems (92,93). Third, migraines may exacerbate already the debilitating fatigue that is virtually ubiquitous among FM patients (94).

As stated earlier, no studies suggest that the treatment of migraines in patients with FM is any less effective than in those without. Yet migraines may be ignored in FM patients because of these patients' overall pain. It is important not to do so. Since migraines appear to be highly treatable in almost all patient groups, without scientific evidence that they are untreatable in FM it seems unethical to ignore them in this setting.

Other forms of headaches with treatments that differ from those offered for FM also may be missed in FM patients. I once suspected posterior uveitis in an FM patient who had persistent retro-orbital headaches; this ultimately was confirmed and successfully treated. Headaches due to poor dentition, oral infections, and chronic sinusitis require antibiotics. As stated earlier in this chapter, TA always must be suspected in any patient over 50 who complains of new or different headaches, given the potential for serious complications, including sudden irreversible blindness that can occur if this condition is ignored (22). Temporomandibular joint dysfunction (see below) is a condition that is increasingly being recognized as a cause of chronic headaches (95–98).

TEMPOROMANDIBULAR JOINT DYSFUNCTION

Besides being a potential cause of a variety of headaches, temporomandibular joint (TMJ) dysfunction syndrome and TMJ OA may cause a variety of other complaints, including jaw pain, ear pain, and neck pain, all of which may be confused with pain originating from FM (99,100). A variety of techniques are available and used to diagnose TMJ disease, including computed tomography, MRI, bone scintigraphy, high-resolution ultrasound, and classification criteria (101–104). Practically, referral to a dentist or dental surgeon seems to be a logical first step. For many, a nocturnal bite block (oral splint) to prevent nighttime bruxism is all that is needed to provide significant pain relief (105,106).

BURSITIS AND TENDONITIS

There should be no difficulty in differentiating FM from tendonitis or bursitis since the first is a syndrome of widespread pain and tenderness while the latter two are local conditions. Various monographs lump all three conditions under one chapter or review article heading of "soft tissue rheumatism" for reasons of editorial convenience rather than logic

(107). Bursitis and tendonitis can, of course, occur in patients with FM. Patients with FM self-report a higher incidence of bursitis than normal controls (108). One potential explanation is that hypermobility may be a predisposing factor for FM, tendonitis, and bursitis (109).

The problem arises, again, in missing a diagnosis of bursitis and tendonitis in patients with prediagnosed FM, since the former two conditions may respond to localized treatment that may be ineffective for FM. Such treatments may include localized injections of corticosteroids (110,111).

MYOFASCIAL PAIN SYNDROME

Myofascial pain syndrome is a syndrome of regional muscle pain of soft tissue origin (112,113). The term has also been used to describe a more specific syndrome caused by trigger points (TrPs). TrPs cause regional aching pain when activated and are identified as a localized tender area in "a nodule in a palpable taut band of muscle fibers" (113). Pressure on the TrPs is supposed to evoke a transient twitch of the taut band (113). Needle electromyography is said to give rise to certain motor end plate noise activity. The late Dr. Janet Travell introduced the concept of the myofascial pain syndrome, and she and Dr. David Simons wrote extensively on this subject. Major and minor criteria for the syndrome were proposed; the former include regional pain, pain or altered sensation in the expected distribution of referred pain from a TrP, a palpable taut band, exquisite tenderness at one point along the taut band, and some restricted range of motion; minor criteria include clinical pain, elicitation of a local twitch response, and pain alleviated by stretching the muscle or injecting the TrP (114). The relation between myofascial pain syndrome and FM was at first uncertain, although it was pointed out that many TrPs coincided with the TePs of FM (114). However, Simons et al. then stated that the two conditions should be regarded as separate entities, although the two could, and frequently did, coexist (113). Tunks and Crook reviewed extensively the various concepts of myofascial pain and the evidence for and against it (115). They contrasted two concepts of myofascial pain: one as a name for regional soft tissue pain, the other as the concept that conformed to the criteria outlined above by Simons and which involved TrPs.

The interrater reliability for detecting TrPs is poor, especially in terms of agreeing on palpable bands, or nodular areas (115). On the other hand, there is good interrater reliability for blind dolorimetry and examination by palpation of tender areas in regional pain syndromes (115). It seems that, at best, intensive pretraining must take place before good interrater reliability can occur in TrP detection (116,117). Tunks and Crook also pointed out that there was no satisfactory evidence that there were any proven clinical benefits in distinguishing specific TrP-induced myofascial pain from regional musculoskeletal pain.

Since the ACR classification criteria for FM involved widespread complaints of pain, as well as the finding of at least 11 points on palpation, there should be no confusion between a regional muscular pain syndrome and FM. Confusion, however, could arise if a patient has both conditions, at which time it would be difficult to differentiate one from the other.

Regional pain can be a precursor of FM. A British study found that 10.4% of patients who had regional pain developed chronic widespread pain (defined according to the classification criteria of the ACR, but without necessarily including "TePs") over a period of 7 years, whereas only 2.3% of those without pain developed chronic widespread pain (118). In another British population survey, 19.4% of those with regional pain had 11 or more TePs of FM, as compared to 5.1% of those who had no pain (77). Although regional muscular pain differs, by definition, from FM, evidence suggests it might be a precursor of FM in a substantial percentage of cases.

SUMMARY POINTS

- Although a number of conditions can theoretically simulate FM, practitioners should be comfortable making this diagnosis with minimal trepidation or diagnostic testing in individuals with chronic widespread pain, tenderness, and other somatic symptoms.
- In contrast, there are many conditions that coexist with FM that should be identified and treated.

REFERENCES

1. White KP, Harth M, Speechley M, et al. Testing an instrument to screen for fibromyalgia syndrome in general population studies: the London Fibromyalgia Epidemiology Study Screening Questionnaire (LFESSQ). *J Rheumatol* 1998;26(4): 880–884.
2. Koeller JM. Understanding cancer pain. *Am J Hosp Pharm* 1990;47(8 Suppl):S3–S6.
3. Wysenbeek AJ, Shapira Y. Primary fibromyalgia and the chronic fatigue syndrome. *Rheumatol Int* 1991;10:227–229.
4. Hudson JI, Goldenberg DL, Pope HG Jr, et al. Comorbidity of fibromyalgia with medical and psychiatric disorders. *Am J Med* 1992;92:363–367.
5. White KP, Speechley M, Harth M, et al. Co-existence of chronic fatigue syndrome (CFS) with fibromyalgia syndrome (FMS) in the general population: a controlled study. *Scand J Rheumatol* 2000;29(1):44–51.
6. Daugherty SA, Berch EH, Perterson DL, et al. Chronic fatigue syndrome in Northern Nevada. *Rev Infect Dis* 1991; 13(Suppl. 1):S39–S44.
7. Levine PH, Snow PG, Ranum BA, et al. Epidemic neuromyasthenia and chronic fatigue syndrome in west Otago, New Zealand. A 10-year follow-up. *Arch Intern Med* 1997; 157:750–754.
8. Shefer A, Dobbins JG, Fukuda K, et al. Fatiguing illness among employees in three large state office buildings, California, 1993: was there an outbreak? *J Psychiatr Res* 1997; 31:31–43.
9. Briggs NC, Levine PH. A comparative review of systemic and neurological symptomatology in 12 outbreaks collectively described as chronic fatigue syndrome, epidemic neuromyasthenia, and myalgic encephalomyelitis. *Clin Infect Dis* 1994;18(Suppl. 1):S32–S42.
10. Salvarani C, Macchioni P, Zizzi F, et al. Epidemiologic and immunogenetic aspects of polymyalgia rheumatica and giant cell arteritis in northern Italy. *Arthritis Rheum* 1991;34: 351–356.
11. Salvarani C, Gabriel SE, O'Fallon WM, et al. Epidemiology of polymyalgia rheumatica in Olmsted County, Minnesota, 1970-1991. *Arthritis Rheum* 1995;38(3):369–373.
12. Gran JT, Myklebust G. The incidence of polymyalgia rheumatica and temporal arteritis in the county of Aust Agder, south Norway: a prospective study 1987-94. *J Rheumatol* 1997;24:1739–1743.
13. Kyle V, Silverman B, Silman A, et al. Polymyalgia rheumatica/giant cell arteritis in a Cambridge general practice. *Br Med J (Clin Res Ed)* 1985;291:385–387.
14. Machado EBV, Michet CJ, Ballard DJ, et al. Trends in incidence and clinical presentation of temporal arteritis in Olmsted county, Minnesota, 1950-1985. *Arthritis Rheum* 1988;31(6): 745–749.
15. Kaplan H. Polymyositis, polymyalgia rheumatica, and fibrositis. *Med Times* 1977;105:45–52.
16. Narvaez J, Nolla-Sole JM, Narvaez JA, et al. Musculoskeletal manifestations in polymyalgia rheumatica and temporal arteritis. *Ann Rheum Dis* 2001;60(11):1060–1063.
17. Cohen MD, Ginsburg WW. Polymyalgia rheumatica. *Rheum Dis Clin North Am* 1990;16(2):325–339.
18. Jones JG. Clinical features of giant cell arteritis. *Baillieres Clin Rheumatol* 1991;5(3):413–430.
19. Wolfe F, Smythe HA, Yunus MB, et al. The American College of Rheumatology 1990 criteria for the classification of fibromyalgia. Report of the Multicenter Criteria Committee. *Arthritis Rheum* 1990;33:160–172.
20. Salvarani C, Cantini F, Macchioni P, et al. Distal musculoskeletal manifestations in polymyalgia rheumatica: a prospective followup study. *Arthritis Rheum* 1998;41:1221–1226.
21. Behn AR, Perera T, Myles AB. Polymyalgia rheumatica and corticosteroids: how much for how long? *Ann Rheum Dis* 1983;42:374–378.
22. Gonzalez-Gay MA, Garcia-Porrua C, Llorca J, et al. Visual manifestations of giant cell arteritis. Trends and clinical spectrum in 161 patients. *Medicine (Baltimore)* 2000;79:283–292.
23. Cantini F, Salvarani C, Olivieri I, et al. Erythrocyte sedimentation rate and C-reactive protein in the evaluation of disease activity and severity in polymyalgia rheumatica: a prospective follow-up study. *Semin Arthritis Rheum* 2000;30(1):17–24.
24. Helfgott SM, Kieval RI. Polymyalgia rheumatica in patients with a normal erythrocyte sedimentation rate. *Arthritis Rheum* 1996;39(2):304–307.
25. Cantini F, Salvarani C, Olivieri I, et al. Erythrocyte sedimentation rate and C-reactive protein in the evaluation of disease activity and severity in polymyalgia rheumatica: a prospective follow-up study. *Semin Arthritis Rheum* 2000;30(1):17–24.
26. Wong RL, Korn JH. Temporal arteritis without an elevated erythrocyte sedimentation rate. Case report and review of the literature. *Am J Med* 1986;80(5):959–964.
27. Allsop CJ, Gallagher PJ. Temporal artery biopsy in giant-cell arteritis. A reappraisal. *Am J Surg Pathol* 1981;5(4):317–323.
28. Brownstein S, Nicolle DA, Codere F. Bilateral blindness in temporal arteritis with skip areas. *Arch Ophthalmol* 1983; 101(3):388–391.
29. Weyand CM, Fulbright JW, Evans JM, et al. Corticosteroid requirements in polymyalgia rheumatica. *Arch Intern Med* 1999;159(6):577–584.
30. Tan EM, Cohen AS, Fries JF, et al. The 1982 revised criteria for the classification of systemic lupus erythematosus. *Arthritis Rheum* 1982;25(11):1271–1277.
31. Carmona L, Villaverde V, Hernandez-Garcia C et al., EPISER Study Group. The prevalence of rheumatoid arthritis in the general population of Spain. *Rheumatology (Oxford)* 2002; 41(1):88–95.
32. Cimmino MA, Parisi M, Moggiana G, et al. Prevalence of rheumatoid arthritis in Italy: the Chiavari study. *Ann Rheum Dis* 1998;57(5):315–318.

33. Gabriel SE, Crowson CS, O'Fallon WM. The epidemiology of rheumatoid arthritis in Rochester, Minnesota, 1955–1985. *Arthritis Rheum* 1999;42(3):415–420.

34. Mitchell DM, Fries JF. An analysis of the American Rheumatism Association criteria for rheumatoid arthritis. *Arthritis Rheum* 1982;25(5):481–487.

35. White KP, Harth M. Lumbar planus presenting as cauda equina syndrome in a patient with long-standing rheumatoid arthritis. *J Rheumatol* 2001;28:627–630.

36. Reilly PA, Littlejohn GO. Peripheral arthralgic presentation of fibrositis/fibromyalgia syndrome. *J Rheumatol* 1992;19: 281–283.

37. Xie X, Ye C. Clinical analysis of 120 patients with fibromyalgia. *Hunan Yi Ke Da Xue Xue Bao* 1997;22(2):167–170.

38. White KP, Speechley M, Harth M, et al. The London Fibromyalgia Epidemiology Study (LFES): comparing the demographic and clinical characteristics in 100 random community cases of fibromyalgia syndrome (FMS) versus controls. *J Rheumatol* 1999;26:1577–1585.

39. Arnett FC, Edworthy SM, Bloch DA, et al. The American Rheumatism Association 1987 revised criteria for the classification of rheumatoid arthritis. *Arthritis Rheum* 1988;31(3): 315–324.

40. White KP, Speechley M, Harth M, et al. The London Fibromyalgia Epidemiology Study (LFES): comparing the demographic and clinical characteristics in 100 random community cases of fibromyalgia syndrome (FMS) versus controls. *J Rheumatol* 1999;26:1577–1585.

41. Buskila D, Press J. Neuroendocrine mechanisms in fibromyalgia-chronic fatigue. *Best Pract Res Clin Rheumatol* 2001;15(5): 747–758.

42. Clark S, Tindall E, Bennett RM. A double blind crossover trial of prednisone versus placebo in the treatment of fibrositis. *J Rheumatol* 1985;12(5):980–983.

43. Romano TJ. Incidence of fibromyalgia syndrome (FS) in rheumatoid arthritis (RA) patients in a general rheumatology practice. *Scand J Rheumatol* 1992;94(Suppl):11.

44. Roman TJ. Coexistence of fibromyalgia syndrome (FS) and systemic lupus erythematosus (SLE). *Scand J Rheumatol* 1992;94(Suppl):12.

45. Grafe A, Wollina U, Tebbe B, et al. Fibromyalgia in lupus erythematosus. *Acta Derm Venereol* 1999;79:62–64.

46. Khan MA. Update on spondyloarthropathies. *Ann Intern Med* 2002;136:896–907.

47. Sieper J, Braun J, Rudwaleit M, et al. Ankylosing spondylitis: an overview. *Ann Rheum Dis* 2002;61(Suppl. 3):iii8–iii18.

48. Whitehead WE, Palsson O, Jones KR. Systematic review of the comorbidity of irritable bowel syndrome with other disorders: what are the causes and implications? *Gastroenterology* 2002;122:1140–1156.

49. Incel NA, Erdem HR, Ozgocmen S, et al. Pain pressure threshold values in ankylosing spondylitis. *Rheumatol Int* 2002;22:148–150.

50. Fitzcharles MA, Esdaile JM. The overdiagnosis of fibromyalgia syndrome. *Am J Med* 1997;103:44–50.

51. Hidding A, van Santen M, De Klerk E, et al. Comparison between self-report measures and clinical observations of functional disability in ankylosing spondylitis, rheumatoid arthritis and fibromyalgia. *J Rheumatol* 1994;21:818–823.

52. Solaro C, Lunardi GL, Mancardi GL. Pain and MS. *Int MS J* 2003;10:14–19.

53. Kerns RD, Kassirer M, Otis J. Pain in multiple sclerosis: a biopsychosocial perspective. *J Rehabil Res Dev* 2002;39: 225–232.

54. Ehde DM, Gibbons LE, Chwastiak L, et al. Chronic pain in a large community sample of persons with multiple sclerosis. *Mult Scler* 2003;6:605–611.

55. Kalman S, Osterberg A, Sorensen J, et al. Morphine responsiveness in a group of well-defined multiple sclerosis patients: a study with i.v. morphine. *Eur J Pain* 2002; 6:69–80.

56. Lobentanz IS, Asenbaum S, Vass K, et al. Factors influencing quality of life in multiple sclerosis patients: disability, depressive mood, fatigue and sleep quality. *Acta Neurol Scand* 2004;110:6–13.

57. Attarian HP, Brown KM, Duntley SP, et al. The relationship of sleep disturbances and fatigue in multiple sclerosis. *Arch Neurol* 2004;61:525–528.

58. Plazzi G, Montagna P. Remitting REM sleep behavior disorder as the initial sign of multiple sclerosis. *Sleep Med* 2002; 3(5):437–439.

59. Solaro C, Uccelli MM, Guglieri P, et al. Gabapentin is effective in treating nocturnal painful spasms in multiple sclerosis. *Mult Scler* 2002;6:192–193.

60. Yunus MB, Aldag JC. Restless legs syndrome and leg cramps in fibromyalgia syndrome: a controlled study. *Br Med J* 1996;25;312(7042):1339.

61. Wilke WS, Sheeler LR, Makarowski WS. Hypothyroidism with presenting symptoms of fibrositis. *J Rheumatol* 1981;8: 626–631.

62. McLean RM, Podell DN. Bone and joint manifestations of hypothyroidism. *Semin Arthritis Rheum* 1995;24(4):282–290.

63. Garrison RL, Breeding PC. A metabolic basis for fibromyalgia and its related disorders: the possible role of resistance to thyroid hormone. *Med Hypotheses* 2003;61:182–189.

64. Carette S, Lefrancois L. Fibrositis and primary hypothyroidism. *J Rheumatol* 1988;15:1418–1421.

65. Reilly PA. The differential diagnosis of generalized pain. *Baillieres Best Pract Res Clin Rheumatol* 1999;13:391–401.

66. Segal AM, Sheeler LR, Wilke WS. Myalgia as the primary manifestation of spontaneously resolving hyperthyroidism. *J Rheumatol* 1982;9:459–461.

67. Udelsman R. Primary hyperparathyroidism. *Curr Treat Options Oncol* 2001;2:365–372.

68. Uden P, Chan A, Duh QY, et al. Primary hyperparathyroidism in younger and older patients: symptoms and outcome of surgery. *World J Surg* 1992;16(4):791–797.

69. Helliwell M. Rheumatic symptoms in primary hyperparathyroidism. *Postgrad Med J* 1983;59:236–240.

70. Nellen JF, Smulders YM, Jos Frissen PH, et al. Hypovitaminosis D in immigrant women: slow to be diagnosed. *Br Med J* 1996;312:570–572.

71. Reginato AJ, Falasca GF, Pappu R, et al. Musculoskeletal manifestations of osteomalacia: report of 26 cases and literature review. *Semin Arthritis Rheum* 1999;28:287–304.

72. Plotnikoff GA, Quigley JM. Prevalence of severe hypovitaminosis D in patients with persistent, nonspecific musculoskeletal pain. *Mayo Clin Proc* 2003;78:1463–1470.

73. Huisman AM, White KP, Algra A, et al. Vitamin D levels in women with systemic lupus erythematosus and fibromyalgia. *J Rheumatol* 2001;28:2535–2539.

74. Al-Allaf AW, Mole PA, Paterson CR, et al. Bone health in patients with fibromyalgia. *Rheumatology (Oxford)* 2003;42: 1202–1206.

75. Rosenson RS. Current overview of statin-induced myopathy. *Am J Med* 2004;116:408–416.

76. Thompson PD, Clarkson P, Karas RH. Statin-associated myopathy. *JAMA* 2003;289:1681–1690.

77. Croft P, Schollum J, Silman A. Population study of tender point counts and pain as evidence of fibromyalgia. *Br Med J* 1994;309(6956):696–699.

78. Romano TJ. Presence of fibromyalgia syndrome (FS) in osteoarthritis (OA) patients. *Scand J Rheumatol* 1992; 94(Suppl):11.

79. Rao R. Neck pain, cervical radiculopathy, and cervical myelopathy: pathophysiology, natural history, and clinical evaluation. *Bone Joint Surg Am* 2002;84-A:1872–1881.

80. Bogduk N. Management of chronic low back pain. *Med J Aust* 2004;180:79–83.
81. Borenstein D. Does osteoarthritis of the lumbar spine cause chronic low back pain? *Curr Rheumatol Rep* 2004;6:14–19.
82. Speed C. Low back pain. *Br Med J* 2004;328:1119–1121.
83. Deyo RA, Weinstein JN. Low back pain. *N Engl J Med* 2001;344:363–370.
84. Lawrence RC, Helmick CG, Arnett FC, et al. Estimates of the prevalence of arthritis and selected musculoskeletal disorders in the United States. *Arthritis Rheum* 1998;41:778–799.
85. Rekola KE, Levoska S, Takala J, et al. Patients with neck and shoulder complaints and multisite musculoskeletal symptoms—a prospective study. *J Rheumatol* 1997;24:2424–2428.
86. Hüppe A, Brockow T, Raspe H. Chronische ausgebreitete Schmerzen und tender points bei Rückenschmerzen in der Bevölkerung. *Z Rheumatol* 2004;63:76–83.
87. White KP, Carette S, Harth M, et al. Trauma and fibromyalgia: is there an association and what does it mean? *Semin Arthritis Rheum* 2000;29:200–216.
88. Buskila D, Neumann L, Vaisberg G, et al. Increased rates of fibromyalgia following cervical spine injury. A controlled study of 161 cases of traumatic injury. *Arthritis Rheum* 1997;40:446–452.
89. White KP, Carette S, Harth M, et al. The post-MVC health survey: a controlled epidemiological study to estimate fibromyalgia (FM) incidence post motor vehicle collision [Abstract]. *Arthritis Rheum* 2004;50:S307.
90. Yunus MB, Masi AT, Calabro JJ. Primary fibromyalgia (fibrositis): Clinical study of 50 patients with matched normal controls. *Semin Arthritis Rheum* 1981;11:151–171.
91. Yunus MB. Fibromyalgia syndrome: clinical features and spectrum. *J Musculoskelet Pain* 1994;2:5–21.
92. Nicolodi M, Sicuteri F. Fibromyalgia and migraine, two faces of the same mechanism. Serotonin as the common clue for pathogenesis and therapy. *Adv Exp Med Biol* 1996;398:373–379.
93. Nicolodi M, Volpe AR, Sicuteri F. Fibromyalgia and headache. Failure of serotonergic analgesia and N-methyl-D-aspartate-mediated neuronal plasticity: their common clues. *Cephalgia* 1998;18(Suppl. 21):41–44.
94. Peres MF, Zukerman E, Young WB, et al. Fatigue in chronic migraine patients. *Cephalgia* 2002;22:720–724.
95. Shankland WE. Nociceptive trigeminal inhibition–tension suppression system: a method of preventing migraine and tension headaches. *Compend Contin Educ Dent* 2001;22:1075–1080.
96. Farsi NM. Symptoms and signs of temporomandibular disorders and oral parafunctions among Saudi children. *J Oral Rehabil* 2003;30(12):1200–1208.
97. Vallerand WP, Hall MB. Improvement in myofascial pain and headaches following TMJ surgery. *J Craniomandib Disord* 1991;5:197–204.
98. Quayle AA, Gray RJ, Metcalfe RJ, et al. Soft occlusal splint therapy in the treatment of migraine and other headaches. *J Dent* 1990;18:123–129.
99. Chua EK, Tay DK, Tan BY, et al. A profile of patients with temporomandibular disorders in Singapore—a descriptive study. *Ann Acad Med Singapore* 1989;18:675–680.
100. Campbell CD, Loft GH, Davis H, et al. TMJ symptoms and referred pain patterns. *J Prosthet Dent* 1982;47(4):430–433.
101. Piehslinger E, Schimmerl S, Celar A, et al. Comparison of magnetic resonance tomography with computerized axiography in diagnosis of temporomandibular joint disorders. *Int J Oral Maxillofac Surg* 1995;24(1 Pt 1):13–19.
102. Epstein JB; Rea A, Chahal O. The use of bone scintigraphy in temporomandibular joint disorders. *Oral Dis* 2002;8(1):47–53.
103. Brandlmaier I, Bertram S, Rudisch A, et al. Temporomandibular joint osteoarthrosis diagnosed with high resolution ultrasonography versus magnetic resonance imaging: how reliable is high resolution ultrasonography? *J Oral Rehabil* 2003;30(8):812–817.
104. Rantala MA, Ahlberg J, Suvinen TI, et al. Symptoms, signs, and clinical diagnoses according to the research diagnostic criteria for temporomandibular disorders among Finnish multiprofessional media personnel. *J Orofac Pain* 2003;17:311–316.
105. Radford JR. General practice management of TMDs. *Br Dent J* 2004;197(1):31.
106. Wright E, Anderson G, Schulte J. A randomized clinical trial of intraoral soft splints and palliative treatment for masticatory muscle pain. *J Orofac Pain* 1995;9(2):192–199.
107. Reveille JD. Soft-tissue rheumatism: diagnosis and treatment. *Am J Med* 1997;102(1A):23S–29S.
108. Waylonis GW, Heck W. Fibromyalgia syndrome. New associations. *Am J Phys Med Rehabil* 1992;71:343–348.
109. Hudson N, Fitzcharles MA, Cohen M, et al. The association of soft-tissue rheumatism and hypermobility. *Br J Rheumatol* 1998;37:382–386.
110. Buchbinder R, Green S, Youd JM. Corticosteroid injections for shoulder pain. *Cochrane Database Syst Rev* 2003;(1):CD004016.
111. Huang HH, Qureshi AA, Biundo JJ Jr. Sports and other soft tissue injuries, tendinitis, bursitis, and occupation-related syndromes. *Curr Opin Rheumatol* 2000;12(2):150–154.
112. Simons D. Muscular pain syndromes. *Adv Pain Res Ther* 1990;17:1–41.
113. Simons DG, Travell JG, Simons LS. General overview. In: Simons DG, Travell JG, Simons LS, eds. *Myofascial pain and dysfunction. The trigger point manual*, 2nd ed. Baltimore, MD; Philadelphia, PA: Lippincott Williams & Wilkins, 1998:11–93.
114. Simons D. Muscular pain syndromes. *Adv Pain Res Ther* 1990;17:1–41.
115. Tunks E, Crook J. Regional soft tissue pains: alias myofascial pain? *Baillieres Clin Rheumatol* 1999;13:345–369.
116. Gerwin RD, Shannon S, Hong CZ, et al. Interrater reliability in myofascial trigger point examination. *Pain* 1997;69:65–73.
117. Simons DG, Mense S. Diagnose und therapie myofaszialer triggerpunkte. *Schmerz* 2003;17:419–424.
118. Papageorgiou AC, Silman AJ, Macfarlane GJ. Chronic widespread pain in the population: a seven year follow up study. *Ann Rheum Dis* 2002;61:1071–1074.

26

Assessment Tools and Outcome Measures Used in the Investigation of Fibromyalgia

Stuart L. Silverman and Susan A. Martin

Fibromyalgia (FM) is officially defined by the 1990 American College of Rheumatology (ACR) Operational Criteria as self-report of widespread pain above and below the waist in conjunction with 11 or more of 18 tender points (TePs). However, it is clear that FM is more than widespread pain and for many patients also includes symptom domains of fatigue, sleep, irritable bowel, and cognitive difficulties. These symptoms result in loss of function and health-related quality of life.

In this chapter we will discuss available instruments that measure single domains as well as multidimensional instruments. Use of self-report instruments does not replace history or physical examination. However, it is of interest that there is less variability with self-report instruments than with physical exam parameters and interpretations of diagnostic studies for painful conditions such as low back pain (1). Available instruments may assist clinicians in assessing symptom profiles of an individual patient in order to apply treatment or intervention to the most distressing symptoms and to alleviate the overall burden of FM or to suggest combination therapy. For example, a patient with significant pain may have less pain after treatment for concomitant previously unrecognized anxiety or depression.

CHOOSING AN INSTRUMENT

TYPES OF INSTRUMENT

Patient-reported outcome (PRO) assessments may be either generic or disease specific. Generic PRO assessments are designed for use across most populations, in contrast to disease-specific instruments that are developed to target a particular condition. Generic instruments enable comparisons of the benefit of treatments in varying populations but

may not be adequately sensitive to the impact of a particular disease or treatment.

MEASUREMENT CHARACTERISTICS OF AN INSTRUMENT

The most important characteristics of an instrument are reliability and validity. Reliability refers to whether a measurement is free from random error. Reliability has two major features: reproducibility and consistency. Reproducibility refers to test-retest stability and interobserver or intraobserver reproducibility. Internal consistency refers to the correlation among items in the direction of a change. Validity refers to whether the instrument measures what it purports to measure. There are three main types of validity: content, construct, and criterion validity (2).

Responsiveness refers to the ability to detect change or differences in important outcomes. Adequate responsiveness should include a good signal to noise ratio. Responsiveness may compare baseline and endpoint scale scores, differences in treatment and placebo scores, or changes in scale scores and changes in related measures.

Interpretability is the ability to assign qualitative meaning to quantitative scores. Changes in scores may be compared to scores from defined populations or relationships to clinical factors or life events. Interpretability allows one to evaluate if changes are not just statistically significant but also whether they are clinically significant or meaningful.

The burden of the instruments chosen for a clinical trial or clinical practice should be considered. Burden refers to the respondent burden in terms of time necessary to complete the instrument, energy, or other demands, as well as the administrative burden of training personnel, the financial implications of special scoring equipment or license fees, and so on. An instrument may be responsive but extremely

309

lengthy or difficult to score and therefore difficult to use in a clinical setting.

Instruments may cover several domains or disease features and be multidimensional, or they may focus on only one domain and be a unidimensional assessment. Multidimensional assessment is generally preferred to unidimensional assessment; however, unidimensional assessment may be preferred when there is a desire to focus on one specific domain, such as pain. A multidimensional assessment can also be accomplished by using a battery of instruments that cover several domains, some of which may be multidimensional themselves and some of which may be unidimensional.

Instruments may be self-administered or administered by interview. In most situations self-administered questionnaires are preferred. Although most questionnaires have been administered as hard copy on paper, there is increasing use of computers and handheld device platforms as well as voice recognition systems using telephone-based assessment. Handheld devices also have the capacity to prompt the individual to measure an outcome under study, allowing the opportunity for specification of when assessments are completed as well as documentation of patient compliance in completing the assessment.

Instruments may contain only one item or multiple items. Item response choices can range from numeric rating scales (NRSs) and visual analog scales (VASs) to Likert or verbal response scales. NRSs ask patients to respond on a numerical continuum that usually contains verbal anchors on either end of the scale. A visual analogue scale asks patients to mark a point on a line that is again usually anchored on the ends by either verbal descriptors or numeric values—for example, from 0 to 10. A Likert or verbal response scale asks patients to respond on a multi-level ordinal response scale where each response has a verbal descriptor. Depending on the instrument, the verbal descriptor may also have numbers placed alongside (e.g., 1 = mild pain, 2 = moderate pain, etc.). Any of these may appear horizontally or vertically across the page or computer screen.

POTENTIAL INSTRUMENTS TO QUANTIFY PAIN

Consistent with the 1990 ACR Operational Criteria for fibromyalgia syndrome (FM), pain is usually the primary endpoint of FM clinical studies. Pain is a central nervous system symptom. As defined by the International Association for the Study of Pain, pain is "an unpleasant sensory and emotional experience associated with actual or potential tissue damage or described in terms of such damage." Although pain is often characterized as a sensory experience and quantified by unidimensional means such as a visual analog scale, pain is also multidimensional, including additional emotional or affective attributes as well as cognitive or evaluative attributes. Multidimensional pain instruments may provide a more complete characterization of the pain experience than a unidimensional instrument. Since pain is subjective, all pain instruments are self-reported. Pain instruments may vary in the recall time over which pain is reported.

UNIDIMENSIONAL ASSESSMENTS OF PAIN

NUMERICAL RATING SCALE

A numerical rating scale (NRS) asks a patient to indicate a number, often from 0–10, that bests represents their level of pain. A daily pain diary in the form of an NRS was used in an FM study where 0 was no pain and 10 was worst possible pain. From this NRS question, an endpoint mean pain score, an average of the last seven daily diary entries, was calculated. The endpoint mean pain score was the primary parameter of the study. The study was an 8-week randomized controlled trial (RCT) with 529 patients (3). The endpoint mean pain score was found to be responsive to treatment in that study.

VISUAL ANALOGUE SCALES

VASs have been used in multiple FM studies (4–9) and are often scored either from 0 to 100 mm or 0 to 10 cm. The verbal anchors are generally all some form of no pain (e.g., none, absent, no pain, etc.) at 0 and various descriptors at 10 or 100 to denote very severe pain. In many studies published to date, the actual pain question often is either not explicitly reported or varies from study to study; for instance, some studies may specify a specific recall period, others may ask only about recent pain or present pain, and some specify the pain due to FM while others do not. The nine RCTs of antidepressants reviewed by Arnold et al. (10) used pain VAS items (4–6,11–16). The results of their meta-analysis tended to show moderate effect sizes, with the majority of the nine studies demonstrating effects between 0.40 and 0.50. In addition to these single-item results, the Fibromyalgia Impact Questionnaire (FIQ) (17), discussed further in this chapter, contains several VAS items, one of which relates to pain and is often analyzed individually. The pain item asks the patient over the past week "How bad has your pain been?" from "0 = no pain" to "10 = very severe pain." This was the coprimary outcome (along with the FIQ total score) of a study of fluoxetine for FM (9). The study was a randomized controlled 12-week trial with 60 patients, and the FIQ pain item demonstrated responsiveness in the fluoxetine-treated patients. In a study of duloxetine, which was a randomized controlled 12-week trial with 207 patients (18), the FIQ pain item was also a co-primary and demonstrated numerical improvement but did not achieve statistical significance.

GRACELY PAIN SCALE

The Gracely Pain Scale was developed as a ratio scale of verbal pain descriptors (19). The Gracely Pain Scale contains a horizontal row of boxes containing numbers and verbal descriptors placed at various points along the horizontal row. The scale's measurement properties have been extensively evaluated, and the instrument has demonstrated logarithmic properties in the assessment of pain. The scale also demonstrated responsiveness to treatment in a randomized, controlled, 12-week, trial of milnacipran with 125 patients (20).

LIKERT OR VERBAL RESPONSE PAIN SCALES

Most unidimensional assessments of pain in FM have either been VAS or NRS. Bennett et al. (21) used a verbal response scale to ask about pain relief at the end of their study of tramadol/acetaminophen for the treatment of FM. The 12-week RCT study of 315 patients demonstrated responsiveness for the tramadol/acetaminophen-treated group on the 6-point scale, where "4 = complete pain relief" and "−1 = worse."

MULTIDIMENSIONAL PAIN ASSESSMENTS

McGILL PAIN QUESTIONNAIRE AND SHORT-FORM McGILL PAIN QUESTIONNAIRE

Melzack developed the McGill Pain Questionnaire (MPQ) (22) from a list of 102 adjectives that describe sensory, affective, and evaluative aspects of pain. The MPQ assessment is often considered to be lengthy and to be very dependent on the respondent's language skills. The MPQ was responsive as a secondary outcome in a 6-month study of amitriptyline in 280 patients (23). The MPQ was also included as a secondary outcome and was responsive in a study of fluoxetine treatment (9). A Short-Form McGill Pain Questionnaire (SF-MPQ) has been developed that is brief, has comparable sensitivity, and relies less on language skills. The SF-MPQ (24) consists of 15 descriptors of pain experience on a four-point severity response scale that are summed to create a total score. The SF-MPQ also contains a six-point Present Pain Intensity (PPI) index and a 100 mm pain visual analog scale. The SF-MPQ was used in the pregabalin study (3), with the total score and VAS score improving with treatment and no statistical improvement seen on the PPI. Components of the SF-MPQ also improved with treatment in the milnacipran study (20).

BRIEF PAIN INVENTORY

Cleeland developed the Brief Pain Inventory (BPI) from the Wisconsin Brief Pain Inventory to assess the severity of pain (four items) and the impact of pain on daily functions (seven items) (25). The instrument was originally used in studies of cancer pain but has now been used in many pain models and has undergone extensive measurement evaluation. Each of the questions about pain severity and interference with daily functioning are NRS scales ranging from 0 to 10. The BPI was included as a secondary assessment in a recent study of duloxetine and demonstrated responsiveness to treatment on the average pain and interference from pain items (18).

SPATIOTEMPORAL CHARACTERIZATION OF PAIN

Spatiotemporal characterization of FM pain may be very useful for the clinician. An important part of the pain experience is where the pain is felt and its intensity over time. The spatial characteristics of pain are often represented in a pain drawing as a means of characterizing the location, radiation, and size of the painful areas. The patient is asked to shade in areas that are painful. Total body pain—that is, pain above and below the waist—is characteristic for FM. A pain diagram may be helpful clinically in determining areas of regional barriers in FM that can be addressed with trigger point injection or local therapies. A pain diagram may also be accompanied by a regional verbal rating scale. Regional verbal rating scales have been used clinically but not in research settings. Multiple anatomic regions, such as neck and face, are listed vertically with columns to describe pain intensity (minimal, slight, moderate, severe).

In order to assess the temporal element of pain sensation, patients may complete a day-to-day or hour-by-hour written log or diary of changes in pain intensity and quality as well as influence of external factors such as activity or stress or medication use. Use of a pain diary increases the validity and reliability of average pain estimates (26). Multiple samplings may avoid concerns about regression to mean with a single estimate (27). Use of a handheld Palm© based electronic diary to obtain randomly generated samplings of pain estimates has been validated in a multicenter trial (20).

NONINSTRUMENTAL QUANTIFICATION OF PAIN

Analgesic Consumption

Decreases in patient self-report of analgesic consumption have been used in pain studies as a surrogate measure of analgesic efficacy (28); however, to our knowledge this has not been used in any RCT of FM interventions.

TENDER POINT ASSESSMENT

The TeP count was developed in conjunction with the ACR operational criteria. It measures the presence of subjective tenderness at each of nine pairs of well-defined areas of tenderness bilaterally above and below the waist. Identified control points should not be tender. TeP count does not measure intensity of the self-report of pain and is sometimes included as an outcome measure in clinical studies. Tramadol/acetaminophen-treated patients (21) had fewer TePs at their final visit [13 (±4.9)] in comparison to the placebo group [14 (±4.3)] which was statistically significant. TeP count was also responsive in a study of duloxetine versus placebo (18).

TeP intensity has also been assessed in clinical practice and in clinical studies; however, the method of assessing and recording the intensity has varied. Intensity, sometimes also referred to as a myalgic score, can be assessed through manual pressure applied to TePs or through the use of dolorimetry. The Manual TeP Survey (MTPS) (29) was developed in an effort to standardize the manual assessment of TeP intensity. A clinician applies pressure to the 18 ACR specified TePs and to 3 control points and asks the patient to rate the pain felt, where 0 represents no pain and 10 represents the worst pain imaginable. As manual assessment of TePs attempts to standardize the pressure applied, the responses can be learned, limiting their use in medico-legal evaluations.

A dolorimeter is a semiobjective measure of TeP severity. The dolorimeter uses a gauge with a fixed stopper of 1 cm to apply pressure to TePs and control points. The scale faces away from the patient, who reports when pain is felt, and the observer records the threshold. In medico-legal evaluations, the dolorimeter may be useful in that the absence of symmetry or the absence of lower threshold at TePs or lower threshold at control points may indicate malingering or another illness, such as concomitant depression.

The MTPS was included in a pregabalin study, and, although there was a decrease in the intensity with treatment, the difference did not achieve statistical significance ($p = 0.052$) (3). TeP intensity was calculated in the fluoxetine study (9) by using a Fischer dolorimeter at each of the 18 TePs and then summing the pressure at which the patient first indicated discomfort to arrive at a total myalgic score. An average myalgic score was calculated in the study of tramadol/acetaminophen (21) by using a four-point verbal rating score at each TeP, where "0 = no pain" and "4 = patient" withdraws or flinches." As with the pregabalin study that used the MTPS, the myalgic score also approached, but did not achieve, statistical significance in the study ($p = 0.06$). The assessment of TeP intensity was also evaluated in the meta-analysis of antidepressants by Arnold et al. (10), with results that ranged from high to no responsiveness to treatment and an overall model-estimated effect size of 0.358. This could reflect both a difficulty to treat TeP intensity and that the measurement of intensity was not standardized across these studies, that some of them used manual TeP assessment, and that others employed the use of dolorimetery to obtain an intensity score.

COMPARISON OF PAIN MEASUREMENT TOOLS IN FM

Gendreau et al. (30) compared the responsiveness of unidimensional pain assessment (VAS and Gracely Pain Scale), multidimensional pain measurement (McGill short form), and a multidimensional function instrument (FIQ) in 125 patients in an RCT. Differences between the instruments were observed in terms of differentiating the intervention from placebo. The logarithmic Gracely scale was more sensitive than linear unidimensional instruments such as VAS. Patients who reported improved global assessments were more likely to report improved pain with unidimensional pain assessment.

ANALYSES OF PAIN

Analyses of pain may be categorical—comparing the percent in each group that are defined as "responders" and "nonresponders," for instance—or may be performed on a continuous variable, such as the endpoint mean pain scores between groups.

RESPONDER ANALYSES

Responder analyses are often performed on pain parameters in FM trials. In a responder analysis, the percent of patients reporting at least a fixed percent of pain relief from baseline using a given pain measure is reported. A benchmark of 50% decrease in pain has been used in trials; however, data published from ten pregabalin pain trials suggest that a 30% reduction from baseline corresponds to a clinically important change for individual patients (31). In a study of milnacipran there was a greater proportion of responders defined by at least a 50% reduction in baseline pain in the twice daily group versus placebo (18). The duloxetine study also demonstrated a greater proportion of 50% responders than placebo (20), as did the pregabalin study (3).

POTENTIAL INSTRUMENTS USED TO QUANTIFY PSYCHOLOGICAL DYSFUNCTION

The pain of fibromyalgia may be modulated (increased or decreased) by emotional factors such as anxiety or depression (32,33). Studies of mood disturbance in FM have traditionally been focused on depression, with some studies showing that over half the patients with FM have a lifetime history of depression but that active depression is present in only one-third of FM patients (34–37). Other studies have reported that FM patients have a much lower prevalence of depression than the above estimates (38,39). Increasingly, studies have also focused on the role that anxiety may play in FM.

PATIENT-REPORTED ASSESSMENTS

The Beck Depression Inventory (BDI) is a 21-item questionnaire that was developed as a screening tool for depression (40). The BDI has been widely used to document the prevalence of depressive symptomatology in samples of chronic-pain patients and as an outcome measure in studies of the medical and psychological management of chronic pain. Several BDI items have a somatic focus (sleep, fatigue, etc.) that may be similar to somatic symptoms seen in FM. Therefore the significance of the total BDI score in FM patients is unclear. The use of the total BDI score may give a misleading impression of the nature and degree of the depressive symptoms in patients with FM. A seven-item version that does not include somatic symptoms is available for clinical use. This shorter BDI has not been used in clinical trials. The BDI was used in the milnacipran study but no results were reported. Although numerical improvement was seen with the BDI, there was no statistically significant improvement in one trial with fluoxetine (18) or in the recent study of duloxetine (41). Additionally, depression did not improve as assessed by the BDI in the Goldenberg (4) study of fluoxetine.

The Hospital Anxiety and Depression Scale (HADS) (42) comprises 14 items, each with a four-point categorical response scale. HADS divides into two seven-item subscales that measure the domains of anxiety (HADS-A) and depression (HADS-D scale). Each domain score is the sum of the responses to the seven questions. An estimate of clinically important levels of distress can be made using recommended cutoff scores for each domain. The HADS was used in the pregabalin trial, but neither the anxiety nor depression scale showed statistically significant improvement (3).

The Center for Epidemiological Studies Depression Scale (CES-D) is a 20-item questionnaire that asks patients to rate the frequency of depression symptoms over a 1-week recall period (43). During its development, it was evaluated and found to have positive measurement properties. However, as with the BDI (43,44), it also contains somatic symptom items, causing potential confounding with symptoms seen with FM. The CES-D has not often been used in clinical studies. It was included in a 6-week study of alprazolam, ibuprofen, and placebo (45) but did not show responsiveness in that study. It has been used in some nonpharmacologic studies for the treatment of FM (46–48).

The Arthritis Impact Measurement Scales (AIMS) instrument (49) contains six-item subscales for both depression and anxiety. These subscales were included in a 6-week 42-patient randomized controlled study of fluoxetine (8). Statistically significant differences were not seen in the endpoint intent-to-treat analysis for either anxiety or depression, although depression was statistically improved at 3 weeks as assessed by the AIMS scale.

Single-item visual analogue scales on depression and anxiety are included in the FIQ (17), discussed in more detail below. However, the anxiety item asks "How nervous or anxious have you felt?" and the depression item asks "How depressed or blue have you felt?" In the tramadol/acetaminophen study of FM, the anxiety item showed statistically significant improvement but not the depression item (21). In the fluoxetine trial by Arnold et al. (9), the depression FIQ item, but not the anxiety FIQ item, demonstrated statistically significant improvement over placebo. In the milnacipran study both items improved; however, neither reached statistical significance in the study (20).

CLINICIAN OR INTERVIEW ADMINISTERED ASSESSMENTS

Many assessments [e.g., the Structured Clinical Interview for DSM III-R (SCID) and the Diagnostic Interview Schedule (DIS)] are available that have been developed in the psychiatry field for detailed clinician or interview administered assessment of various mental health conditions. It is recommended that mental health professionals or those who have been specifically trained in the proper administration and scoring of the assessment administer them. For this reason, they are often less used in the clinical trial or physician office setting. The duloxetine (18) and milnacipran trials (20) used a clinician-administered assessment to identify patients with a history of or a present diagnosis of major depressive disorder (MDD) at baseline, but not as a secondary outcome measure. In an 8-week open label study of venlafaxine for FM, Dwight et al. found the SCID and another clinician-rated instrument, the Hamilton Anxiety and Depression scales, to be responsive (50).

MEASUREMENTS OF HEALTH STATUS AND FUNCTIONING

GENERIC

SF-36

The Short Form Health Survey (SF-36) was developed in conjunction with the Medical Outcomes Study (MOS) (51) and is the most commonly used health status measure in the world today. The SF-36 is a 36-item patient-reported outcome measure that results in the following eight domain scores: general health perception, physical role limitations, physical functioning, body pain, vitality, social functioning, emotional role limitations, and mental health. The SF-36 has demonstrated validity and reliability (52,53).

As a generic assessment, the SF-36 is useful in assessing the burden of a given disease state such as fibromyalgia in comparison to other rheumatic illnesses or other medical conditions. Many investigators have demonstrated that patients with FM have a lower health-related quality of life (HRQOL) than patients with other diseases using the SF-36. For instance, Strombeck found HRQOL was lower in fibromyalgia patients than in patients with primary Sjogren or rheumatoid arthritis (54). Other studies have shown that FM patients have lower domain scores in physical function, physical role, bodily pain, and vitality than do systemic lupus erythematosus (SLE) patients (55), that patients with FM have lower scores in the domains of bodily pain and vitality than patients with AIDS, chronic obstructive pulmonary disease (COPD), prostate cancer, urinary incontinence, or hyperlipidemia (56), and that patients with FM can be distinguished by SF-36 scores from other individuals with chronic pain or from normative populations (57).

Despite being a generic health status assessment, the SF-36 has demonstrated responsiveness to both medical and nonmedical interventions. Patients in an RCT of pregabalin showed improvement on the bodily pain, vitality, social functioning, and general health perception domains (3). In an RCT of tramadol/acetaminophen, patients in the treatment group demonstrated improvement on physical functioning and role-physical and bodily pain domains, as well as on the physical component summary score (21). Additionally, nonmedical interventions have demonstrated improvements on various SF-36 domains, such as pool therapy (general health and social functioning) (58) and aerobic fitness (vitality and mental health) (59).

THE NOTTINGHAM HEALTH PROFILE

The Nottingham Health Profile (NHP) (60) consists of two parts. Part one includes 38 items divided into six categories: sleep, physical mobility, energy, pain, emotional reactions, and social isolation. Part two includes seven statements related to the areas of life most affected by health: employment, household activities, social life, home life, sex life, hobbies and interests, and holidays. In the second portion a respondent indicates whether or not a health condition has affected his or her life in these areas. The NHP was found to be responsive to intervention in FM patients receiving moclobemide, amitriptyline, or placebo. Those in the amitriptyline group had statistically significant improvement on the sleep, energy, emotion, and pain categories of the NHP (7).

PHYSICAL FUNCTIONING

Several PROs have focused on assessing physical functioning in patients. The Stanford Health Assessment Questionnaire (HAQ) is one instrument that is used very often in rheumatology (61). The assessment in its totality actually contains four dimensions: discomfort and pain, drug side effects, dollar costs, and disability or functioning. However, the vast majority of studies include only the functioning assessment, which is referred to as the HAQ Disability Index (HAQ-DI). Use of the HAQ-DI in FM has been limited; one study demonstrated that FM patients have a functional impairment similar to patients with RA (62), and another cognitive behavioral therapy study included the HAQ-DI (63). Other versions of the HAQ exist, including the clinical HAQ (CLINHAQ) (8), the modified HAQ (MHAQ) (64), the multidimensional HAQ (MDHAQ) (65), and the childhood HAQ (CHAQ) (66), but few of these have been used in patients with FM. Another version of the HAQ, the Fibromyalgia HAQ (F-HAQ) (67), has been developed based on a Rasch analysis of the HAQ administered to a population with FM and is discussed below.

DISEASE-TARGETED MULTIDIMENSIONAL ASSESSMENTS

FIBROMYALGIA IMPACT QUESTIONNAIRE

The FIQ is a brief ten-item, self-administered instrument that measures physical functioning, work status, depression, anxiety, sleep, pain, stiffness, fatigue, and well-being (17). The FIQ has been translated into many languages and the recall time is 1 week. Statistically significant changes in the FIQ total score were observed in a trial of fluoxetine, amitriptyline, and placebo (4), fluoxetine (2), and tramadol/acetaminophen (21), as well as in nonpharmacologic treatments such as Tai Chi (68), cognitive-behavioral therapy (CBT) (63), education and physical training (69), group treatment (70), and pool exercise and education (71). In one trial of magnetic therapy the FIQ total score was more responsive than TeP number and patient rated pain intensity (72).

FIBROMYALGIA HEALTH ASSESSMENT QUESTIONNAIRE

The F-HAQ has been developed and has undergone psychometric evaluation to assess functioning in patients with FM by Wolfe et al. in the context of the National Databank

rheumatology registry (67). A Rasch analysis was performed of the FIQ, four versions of the HAQ, and the SF-36. The authors found that the FIQ systematically underestimated functional impairment by its handling of activities not usually performed. The authors further concluded that no available functional assessment questionnaire worked well in FM, as they all demonstrated nonunidimensionality and ambiguous items when applied to patients with FM. In addition, scales were found to be nonlinear. In an attempt to address these issues, the 20-item HAQ questionnaire was used as an item bank to develop a new questionnaire more suitable for use in FM, the F-HAQ. This questionnaire fits the Rasch model well, is relevant, linear, and has a long, well-spaced scale, but it has not been tested in clinical trials to assess responsiveness.

PERFORMANCE-BASED ASSESSMENT

Performance-based assessment can compliment patient self-report of functioning, particularly if there is a concern that patients may underestimate or overestimate the degree of functional impairment. Mannerkorpi (58,71) found the 6-minute walk test (6-MWT) responsive in a trial of pool therapy and education with follow-up as well as the FIQ physical functioning items, indicating improvements in both performance and self-report. Two other studies also showed improvement in walking ability; one was an RCT of exercise and education (73), and the other was of group treatment for fibromyalgia (70). Pankoff et al. found that the 6-MWT was not a valid predictor of cardiorespiratory fitness, although it was sensitive to change and was also significantly related to the FIQ total score in patients with FM (74).

POTENTIAL INSTRUMENTS TO MEASURE FATIGUE

Fatigue is an important component of FM; the ACR criteria study found that 81% of FM patients reported fatigue (75). Fatigue is also often considered one of the most difficult symptoms to treat effectively in FM patients.

UNIDIMENSIONAL ASSESSMENT OF FATIGUE

Fatigue is most often been measured using a visual analogue scale (4,6,7,76). Often the VAS is scaled from 0 to 10 with anchors that range from "no fatigue at all" to "extreme fatigue," although the exact wording of the question varied in each of the studies cited above. A study of cyclobenzaprine asked about the actual daily duration of fatigue and analyzed the data as a continuous variable. Scharf et al. (77) assessed fatigue using three numerical rating scales and specified "end of day fatigue," "overall fatigue," and "morning fatigue." Their 24-patient crossover study showed statistical significance with sodium oxybate on all three fatigue NRS items. Milnacipran showed statistically significant improvement in the treatment group on the FIQ fatigue visual analogue scale (20).

Several multidimensional assessment of fatigue measures are available for use in clinical trials or office settings. Many had their origin in cancer research. Belza described six assessments that could be used to assess fatigue in rheumatology patients, depending on the research question: the Multidimensional Assessment of Fatigue (MAF), the Fatigue Scale (FS), the Profile of Mood States (POMS)—fatigue subscale, the Profile of Fatigue-Related Symptoms (PFRS), the Fatigue Severity Scale (FSS), and single-item fatigue questions (78). The PFRS contains 96 items, a length that could make it prohibitive in studies with several other patient-reported outcomes or for use in a clinical setting. The POMS assesses several nonfatigue dimensions that may overlap with other assessments—depression or anxiety, for example. The MAF, the FS, and the FSS are all relatively brief (16, 14, and 9 items respectively), and all have been tested in at least one rheumatology patient population, with the MAF being tested the most extensively in rheumatology, including patients with rheumatoid arthritis, fibromyalgia, and chronic fatigue syndrome (78). The MAF is also the only assessment that has been included in an FM clinical trial (3). It measures four dimensions of fatigue: severity, distress, degree of interference in activities of daily living, and timing. It results in a global fatigue index where 1 represents no fatigue and 50 represents severe fatigue. It showed statistically significant improvement on the global index for two of the three study doses of the pregabalin trial with a small to moderate effect size.

Additionally, the SF-36 Health Survey (see discussion of HRQOL earlier in this chapter) contains a vitality domain that can also be used to assess dimensions of fatigue. The duloxetine (18) and pregabalin trials demonstrated statistically significant improvement on this domain of the SF-36 (3).

POTENTIAL INSTRUMENTS TO MEASURE SLEEP

The ACR criteria study demonstrated that 75% of patients with FM reported nonrestorative sleep (75). Moldofsky et al. have shown that depriving healthy individuals of sleep causes them to have pain symptoms reminiscent of FM (79). Polysomnography studies have demonstrated that FM patients rarely get into the restorative stages 3 and 4 of non-REM sleep (80,81), and nocturnal pain may also interfere with sleep in these patients.

UNIDIMENSIONAL ASSESSMENT OF SLEEP

As with fatigue, clinical studies of FM have most often relied on single-item sleep questions, usually in the form of a VAS (4–8,41,76), although numerical rating scales (3) have also been used. These single items have varied in the question wording—for instance, some ask about sleep quality (3) while others ask about difficulty sleeping (76) or how sleep problems disrupted the patient's life (7). These variations can make it difficult to compare sleep results from study to study or to compare FM values to those of other patient or normative populations. However, they are easy and brief to administer and have demonstrated responsiveness (3,4,6,7,76).

MULTIDIMENSIONAL ASSESSMENT OF SLEEP

Two clinical studies of FM (3,21) have used a multidimensional self-report sleep measure developed as part of the MOS. This 12-item MOS-Sleep Scale (82) yields a sleep problems index and six scale scores: sleep disturbance, snoring, awaken short of breath or with headache, quantity of sleep, sleep adequacy, and somnolence. The subscales and problems index are scored on a 0 to 100 possible range, with higher scores indicating more of the concept being measured; quantity is reported in hours. The scale has been found to have positive psychometric properties in several evaluated populations, including the original MOS chronic patient sample (82), a U.S. general population sample, and U.S. and European samples of patients with neuropathic pain (83,84). The availability of normative values allows demonstration of the high level of disordered sleep seen in these patients and also aids in the interpretation of treatment effects. One of the studies demonstrated statistically significant treatment effects on several of the MOS-Sleep scales, including the overall sleep problems index (3), while the other reported only the sleep problems index results, where numerical improvement but not statistical significance was seen with treatment (21).

The Sleep Assessment Questionnaire (SAQ) is a 17-item, 5-point categorical verbal response questionnaire to evaluate sleep quality. Preliminary information has demonstrated positive measurement properties for the SAQ (85), but to date it has not been used in any RCTs for FM in order to assess responsiveness.

A clinical study of sodium oxybate (77) assessed patients using polysomnography (PSG) and also included five subjective sleep variables. At the end of the 1-month study period, two of the five variables, morning alertness, which was a 5-point categorical verbal response scale, and sleep quality, which was an 11-point numerical rating scale, were statistically significantly improved in the treatment group. The PSG variables of α intrusion, sleep latency, REM sleep, and slow-wave sleep were improved in the treatment group.

POTENTIAL INSTRUMENTS TO MEASURE COGNITION

FM patients often describe difficulties with cognition—the so-called "fibro fog." This may be related to slower speeds of information processing, difficulty doing multitasking, difficulty performing tasks with distraction, and difficulties with short-term memory, nonverbal memory, or executive functioning. Some of these difficulties result in cognitive distress for the individual patient.

Unfortunately, no simple measure of cognitive functioning has been developed for FM patients.

POTENTIAL INSTRUMENTS TO MEASURE IRRITABLE BOWEL SYNDROME

A multidimensional index of irritable bowel severity (the Functional Bowel Severity Index) has been used in one study of patients with FM and Irritable Bowel Syndrome

(IBS) (86). Patients with FM and IBS had greater severity than controls or patients with IBS alone.

GLOBAL ASSESSMENTS

The objective of global assessments is to evaluate all the various aspects of a particular treatment or disease state from either a patient or clinician perspective. For instance, a global evaluation may ask patients to consider all aspects of their experiences since beginning an intervention from efficacy benefits to side effect profile. A global assessment is often a single item and may be a one-time retrospective assessment over the study period, or it can be a prospective evaluation of the patient's overall disease status that is evaluated throughout the study period.

PATIENT GLOBAL ASSESSMENTS

The Patient Global Impression of Change (PGIC) is a seven-item scale in which patients rate their overall change since study start from very much worse to very much improved. The PGIC was used in the pregabalin (3) and milnapracin (20) trials. In the milnapracin trial both qd and bid doses were statistically improved over placebo, and in the pregabalin study two doses of pregabalin were statistically improved over placebo. Earlier studies have also included patient global assessments, many of which did show responsiveness to treatment (4,6,8,10,76,87,88). The increased emphasis on the patient's perspective has resulted in less use of clinical global assessments in favor of patient global assessments.

PHYSICIAN OR CLINICAL GLOBAL ASSESSMENTS

Similar to the PGIC, the Clinical Global Impression of Change (CGIC) asks physicians to rate the overall change in the patient since study start from very much worse to very much improved. The CGIC was used in the pregabalin study and demonstrated statistically significant improvement for two doses (3). As with the patient global assessments, earlier studies often included physician global assessments, several of which demonstrated responsiveness (4,6,45,88).

UTILITY ASSESSMENT

Utility assessment is often used when one wants to perform an economic analysis to compare various treatment options either within a disease area or across disease areas. Utility can be expressed in different ways, but one of the most common is quality-adjusted life years (QALYs). These are computed as the product of the average years of life that remain for the patient and the utility of those years, based on associated quality of life. This utility—a number ranging from 0.0 to 1.0—is determined using various assessment methods, such as the standard gamble, time trade-off, or visual analogue scale. In some cases patient-reported outcome assessments that are more straightforward to administer can be translated into utility scores. Two of the most common PRO assessments for utilities are the Health Utility Index (HUI) (89) and the EuroQoL (EQ-5D) (90). Utilities for patients with FM have been obtained using both rating scales and standard gamble (91), but utility assessment has not been included in an RCT of FM to date.

USE IN CLINICAL PRACTICE

One of the authors (SLS) uses outcome measures routinely in the clinical practice of rheumatology with FM patients. The author gives new patients a packet consisting of (1) a pain diagram, a pain VAS, and a verbal spatiotemporal characterization of pain; (2) a HAQ scale or FIQ to assess functioning, and (3) multidimensional assessment of fatigue and sleep. If difficulty in dealing with anxiety or depression is noted, the Beck Depression or Anxiety Inventory is given to the patient. At routine follow-up the patient will complete at minimum a pain diagram and pain VAS. The Multidimensional Fatigue Assessment may also be administered. Using outcome measures of pain allows one to ascertain if a flare has occurred since the last clinical visit or if a regional barrier has emerged that is acting as a potential pain generator. The author records summary scores in the data section of the chart. In the rehab clinic or with any nonpharmacologic intervention, a PGIC is helpful as an outcome measure combined with a unidimensional measure of pain intensity and a multidimensional measure of pain.

USE IN CLINICAL RESEARCH

Instruments need to be selected based on the intervention studied, the research or clinical objective, and the populations being evaluated.

Assessment of fibromyalgia begins with assessment of the chronic widespread pain. Unidimensional measures of pain intensity such as verbal description, numerical rating, and VAS scores have traditionally been used. However, recently the development of computer technology has increased the use of pain diaries to temporally characterize pain due to the ability to randomly and/or on a regular schedule prompt the patient to enter pain responses. Multidimensional measures like the SF-MPQ help us to define other parts of the pain experience, such as affective response.

Additional suggested outcomes to measure in an interventional trial include a global measure of change, assessment of specific FM domains, such as fatigue and sleep, a measure of functioning, as well as anxiety and depressive symptoms.

SUMMARY POINTS

- Evaluation of patient-reported outcomes in the case of fibromyalgia is an evolving area. The methods for assessment of outcomes continue to be developed, partially in response to the need to evaluate new medications targeted at individuals with FM.
- The multiplicity of instruments available to clinicians and researchers tells us that no single outcome measure has been found for this illness with multiple domains.
- Instruments should be selected based on the setting: clinic, medico-legal, observational trial or RCT, as well as the research or clinical question of interest.

REFERENCES

1. Hoffman RM, Turner JA, Cherkin DC, et al. Therapeutic trials for low back pain. *Spine* 1994;19:2068S–2075S.
2. Staquet MJ, Hays RD, Fayers PM. *Quality of life assessment in clinical trials: methods and practice.* Oxford: Oxford University Press, 1998:7–8.
3. Crofford L, Rowbotham M, Mease P, et al. Pregabalin for the treatment of fibromyalgia syndrome: results of a randomized, double-blind, placebo-controlled trial. *Arthritis & Rheumatism* 2005 (in press).
4. Goldenberg D, Mayskiy M, Mossey C, et al. A randomized double-blind crossover trial of fluoxetine and amitriptyline in the treatment of fibromylagia. *Arthritis Rheum* 1996;39:1852–1859.
5. Bennett RM, Gatter RA, Campbell SM, et al. A comparison of cyclobenzaprine and placebo in the management of fibrositis. A double-blind controlled study. *Arthritis Rheum* 1988;31(12):1535–1542.
6. Carette S, Bell MJ, Reynolds WJ, et al. Comparison of amitriptyline, cyclobenzaprine, and placebo in the treatment of fibromyalgia. A randomized, double-blind clinical trial. *Arthritis Rheum* 1994;37(1):32–40.
7. Hannonen P, Malminiemi K, Yli-Kerttula U, et al. A randomized, double-blind, placebo-controlled study of moclobemide and amitriptyline in the treatment of fibromyalgia in females without psychiatric disorder. *Br J Rheumatol* 1998;37:1279–1286.
8. Wolfe F. Data collection and utilization: a methodology for clinical practice and clinical research. In: Wolfe F, Pincus T, Dekker M, eds. *Rheumatoid arthritis; pathogenesis, assessment, outcome and treatment.* New York: Marcel Dekker, 1994:463–514.
9. Arnold LM, Hess EV, Hudson JI, et al. A randomized, placebo-controlled, double-blind, flexible-dose study of fluoxetine in the treatment of women with fibromyalgia. *Am J Med* 2002;112(3):191–197.
10. Arnold LM, Keck PE Jr, Welge JA. Antidepressant treatment of fibromyalgia. A meta-analysis and review. *Psychosomatics* 2000;41(2):104–113.
11. Carette S, McCain GA, Bell DA, et al. Evaluation of amitriptyline in primary fibrositis: a double-blind, placebo-controlled study. *Arthritis Rheum* 1986;29:655–659.
12. Caruso I, Puttinit PCS, Boccassini L, et al. Double blind study of dothiepin versus placebo in the treatment of primary fibromyalgia syndrome. *J Int Med Res* 1987;15:154–159.
13. Quimby LG, Gratwick GM, Whitney CD, et al. A randomized trial of cyclobenaprine for the treatment of fibromyalgia. *J Rheumatol* 1989;16(Suppl. 19):140–143.
14. Carrette S, Oakson G, Guimont C, et al. Sleep electroencephalography and the clinical response to amitriptyline in patients with fibromyalgia. *Arthritis Rheum* 1995;38:1211–1217.
15. Reynolds WJ, Moldofsy H, Saskin P, et al. The effects of cyclobenzaprine on sleep physiology and symptoms in patients with fibromyalgia. *J Rheumatol* 1991;18:452–454.
16. Bibolotti E, Borghi C, Pasculli E, et al. The management of fibrositis: a double-blind comparison of maprotiline (ludiomil), chlorimipramine, and placebo. *J Clin Trials* 1986;23:269–280.
17. Burckhardt CS, Clark SR, Bennett RM. The fibromyalgia impact questionnaire: development and validation. *J Rheumatol* 1991;18:728–733.
18. Arnold L, Lu Y, Crofford L, et al. A double-blind, multicenter trial comparing duloxetien with placebo in the treatment of fibromyalgia patients with or without major depressive disorder. *Arthritis & Rheumatism* 2004;50:2974–2984.
19. Gracely RH, McGrath P, Dubner R, et al. Validity and sensitivity of ratio scales of sensory and affective verbal pain descriptors. *Pain* 1978;5(1):19–29.
20. Vitton O, Gendreau M, Gendreau J, et al. A double-blind placebo-controlled trial of milnacipran in the treatment of fibromyalgia. *Hum Psychopharmacol Clin Exp* 2004;19:S27–S35.
21. Bennett RM, Kamin M, Karim R, et al. Tramadol and acetaminophen combination tablets in the treatment of fibromyalgia pain: a double-blind, randomized, placebo-controlled study. *Am J Med* 2003;114:537–545.
22. Melzack R. The McGill pain questionnaire: major properties and scoring methods. *Pain* 1975;1(3):277–299.
23. Carrette S, Bell MJ, Reynolds WJ, et al. Comparison of amitriptyline, cyclobenzaprine, and placebo in the treatment of fibormyalgia: a randomized, double-blind clinical trial. *Arthritis Rheum* 1994;37:32–40.
24. Melzack R. The short form McGill pain questionnaire. *Pain* 1987;30:191–197.
25. Cleeland CS. Measurement of pain by subjective report. In: Chapman CR, Loeser JD, eds. *Advances in pain research and therapy, Vol. 12: Issues in pain management.* New York: Raven Press, 1989.
26. Jensen MP, McFarland CA. Increasing the reliability and validity of pain intensity measurement in chronic pain patients. *Pain* 1993;55(2):195–203.
27. Von Korff M. Epidemiology and survey methods: chronic pain assessment. In: Turk DC, Melzack M, eds. *Handbook of pain assessment.* New York: Guilford Press, 1992:391–408.
28. Pun KK, Chan LW. Analgesic effect of intranasal salmon calcitonin in the treatment of osteoporotic vertebral fractures. *Clin Ther* 1989;11:205–209.
29. Okifuji A, Turk DC, Sinclair JD, et al. A standardized manual tender point survey. Development and determination of a threshold point for the identification of positive tender points in fibromyalgia syndrome. *J Rheumatol* 1997;24(2):377–383.
30. Gendreau RM, Williams DA, Clauw DJ. Comparison of several pain measurement tools in fibromyalgia patients. *Arthritis Rheum* 2003b;48(9)suppl:S616–S617.
31. Farrar JT, Young JP, LaMoreaux L, et al. Clinical importance of changes in chronic pain intensity measured on an 11-point numerical pain rating scale. *Pain* 2001;94:149–158.
32. Yunus MB, Ahles TA, Aldag JC, et al. Relationship of clinical features with psychological status in primary fibromyalgia. *Arthritis Rheum* 1991;34(1):15–21.
33. Burckhardt CS, Clark SR, Bennett RM. A comparison of pain perceptions in women with fibromyalgia and rheumatoid arthritis. *Arthritis Care Res* 1992;5(4):216–222.

34. Hudson JI, Pope HG Jr. The relationship between fibromyalgia and major depressive disorder. *Rheum Dis Clin North Am* 1996;22:285–303.

35. Ahles TA, Yunus MB, Riley SD, et al. Psychological factors associated with primary fibromyalgia syndrome. *Arthritis Rheum* 1984;27:1101–1106.

36. Wolfe F, Cathey MA, Kleinheksel SM, et al. Psychological status in primary fibrositis and fibrositis associated with rheumatoid arthritis. *J Rheumatol* 1984;11:500–506.

37. White KP. Chronic widespread pain with or without fibromyalgia: psychological distress in a representative community adult sample. *J Rheumatol* 2002;29:588–594.

38. Walker EA, Keegan D, Gardner G, et al. Psychosocial factors in fibromyalgia and rheumatoid arthritis: I. Psychiatric diagnoses and functional disability. *Psychosom Med* 1997;59: 565–571.

39. Hudson JI, Goldenberg DL, Pope HG Jr, et al. Comorbidity of fibromyalgia with medical and psychiatric disorders. *Am J Med* 1992;92:363–367.

40. Beck AT, Ward CH, Mendelson M, et al. An inventory for measuring depression. *Arch Gen Psychiatry* 1961;4:561–571.

41. Wolfe F, Cathey MA, Hawley DJ. A double-blind placebo controlled trial of fluoxetine in fibromyalgia. *Scand J Rheumatol* 1994;23(5):255–259.

42. Zigmond A, Snaith RP. The hospital anxiety and depression scale. *Acta Psychiatr Scand* 1983;67:361–370.

43. Radloff LS. The CES-D scale: a self-report depression scale for research in the general population. *Appl Psychol Meas* 1977;1:385–401.

44. Weissman MM, Sholomskas D, Pottenger M, et al. Assessing depressive symptoms in five psychiatric populations: a validation study. *Am J Epidemiol* 1987;106:203–214.

45. Russell IJ, Fletcher EM, Michalek JE, et al. Treatment of primary fibrositis/fibromyalgia syndrome with ibuprofen and alprazolam. *Arthritis Rheum* 1991;34:552–560.

46. Turk, Okifuji A, Sinclair JD, et al. Differential response by psychosocial subgroups of fibromyalgia syndrome patients to an interdisciplinary treatment. *Arthritis Care Res* 1998;11: 397–404.

47. Nicassio PM, Radojevic V, Weisman MH, et al. A comparison of behavioral and educational intervention for fibromyalgia. *J Rheumatol* 1997;24:2000–2007.

48. Neilson WR, Walker C, McCain G. Cognitive behavioural treatment of fibromyalgia syndrome: preliminary findings. *J Rheumatol* 1992;19:98–103.

49. Meenan R. The AIMS approach to health status measurement: conceptual background and measurement properties. *J Rheumatol* 1982;9:785–788.

50. Dwight MM, Arnold LM, O'Brien H, et al. An open clinical trial of venlafaxine treatment of fibromyalgia. *Psychosomatics* 1998;39(1):14–17.

51. Ware JE, Sherbourne CD. The MOS 36-item short form health survey (SF-36). *Med Care* 1992;30:473–483.

52. McHorney CA, Ware JEJ, Raczek AE Jr. The MOS 36 item short form health survey (SF-36): II. Psychometric and clinical tests of validity in measuring physical and mental health constructs. *Med Care* 1993;31:247–263.

53. McHorney CA, Ware JE, Sherbourne CD Jr. The MOS 36-item short form health survey (SF-36). Tests of data quality, scaling assumptions, and reliability across diverse patient groups. *Med Care* 1994;32:40–66.

54. Strömbeck B, Ekdahl C, Manthorpe R, et al. Health-related quality of life in primary Sjögren's syndrome, rheumatoid arthritis and fibromyalgia compared to normal population data using SF-36. *Scand J Rheumatol* 2000;29: 20–28.

55. Da Costa D, Dobkin PL, Fitzcharles MA, et al. Determinants of health status in fibromyalgia: a comparative study

with systemic lupus erythematosus. *J Rheumatol* 2000;27: 365–372 .

56. Schlenk EA, Erlen JA, Dunbar-Jacob J, et al. Health-related quality of life in chronic disorders: a comparison across studies using the MOS SF-36. *Qual Life Res* 1998;7:57–65.

57. Neumann L, Berzak A, Buskila D. Measuring health status in Israeli patients with fibromyalgia syndrome and widespread pain and healthy individuals: utility of the short form 36-item health survey (SF-36). *Semin Arthritis Rheum* 2000;29:400–408.

58. Mannerkorpi K, Nyberg B, Ahlmén M, et al. Pool exercise combined with an education program for patients with fibromyalgia syndrome. A prospective, randomized study. *J Rheumatol* 2000;27:2473–2481.

59. Valim V, Oliveira L, Suda A, et al. Aerobic fitness effects in fibromyalgia. [Clinical Trial. Journal Article. Randomized Controlled Trial]. *J Rheumatol.* 2003;30(5):1060–1069.

60. McEwen J. The Nottingham health profile. In: Walker SR, Rosser RM, eds. *Quality of life assessment: key issues for the 90s.* Dordrecht, The Netherlands: Kluwer Academic Publishers, 1992.

61. Fries JF, Spitz P, Kraines G, et al. Measurement of patient outcome in arthritis. *Arthritis Rheum* 1980;23:137–145.

62. Martinez JE, Ferraz MB, Sato EI, et al. Fibromyalgia versus rheumatoid arthritis: a longitudinal comparison of the quality of life. *J Rheumatol* 1995;22:270–274.

63. Singh BB, Berman BM, Hadhazy VA, et al. A pilot study of cognitive behavioral therapy in fibromyalgia. *Altern Ther Health Med* 1998;4:67–70.

64. Pincus T, Summey JA, Soraci SA, et al. Assessment of patient satisfaction in activities of daily living using a modified Stanford health assessment questionnaire. *Arthritis Rheum* 1983; 26(11):1346–1353.

65. Pincus T, Swearingen C, Wolfe F. Toward a multidimensional health assessment questionnaire (MDHAQ): assessment of advanced activities of daily living and psychological status in the patient-friendly health assessment questionnaire format. *Arthritis Rheum* 1999;42:2220–2230.

66. Billings AG, Moos RH, Miller JJ, et al. Psychosocial adaptation in juvenile rheumatic disease: a controlled evaluation. *Health Psychol* 1987;6(4):343–359.

67. Wolfe F, Hawley DJ, Goldenberg DL, et al. The assessment of functional impairment in fibromyalgia (FM): Rasch analyses of 5 functional scales and the development of the FM health assessment questionnaire. *J Rheumatol* 2000;27: 1989–1999.

68. Taggart HM, Arslanian CL, Bae S, et al. Effects of T'ai Chi exercise on fibromyalgia symptoms and health-related quality of life. *Orthop Nurs* 2003;22:353–360.

69. Burckhardt CS, Mannerkorpi K, Hedenberg L, et al. A randomized, controlled clinical trial of education and physical training for women with fibromyalgia. *J Rheumatol* 1994;21: 714–720.

70. Bennett RM, Burckhardt CS, Clark SR, et al. Group treatment of fibromyalgia: a 6 month outpatient program. *J Rheumatol* 1996;23:521–528.

71. Mannerkorpi K, Ahlmén M, Ekdahl C. Six- and 24-month follow-up of pool exercise therapy and education for patients with fibromyalgia. *Scand J Rheumatol* 2002;31:306–310.

72. Dunkl PR, Taylor AG, McConnell GG, et al. Responsiveness of fibromyalgia clinical trial outcome measures. *J Rheumatol* 2000;27:2683–2691.

73. Gowans SE, deHueck A, Voss S, et al. A randomized, controlled trial of exercise and education for individuals with fibromyalgia. *Arthritis Care Res* 1999;12:120–128.

74. Pankoff BA, Overend TJ, Lucy SD, et al. Reliability of the six-minute walk test in people with fibromyalgia. *Arthritis Care Res* 2000;13(5):291–295.

75. Wolfe F, Smythe HA, Yunus MB, et al. The American College of Rheumatology 1990 Criteria for the Classification of Fibromyalgia. Report of the Multicenter Criteria Committee. *Arthritis Rheum* 1990;33(2):160–172.

76. Goldenberg DL, Felson DT, Dinerman H. A randomized, controlled trial of amitriptyline and naproxen in the treatment of patients with fibromyalgia. *Arthritis Rheum* 1986;29(11): 1371–1377.

77. Scharf MB, Baumann M, Berkowitz DV. The effects of sodium oxybate on clinical symptoms and sleep patterns in patients with fibromyalgia. *J Rheumatol* 2003;30:5.

78. Belza B. The impact of fatigue on exercise performance. *Arthritis Care Res* 1994;7(4):176–180.

79. Moldofsky H, Scarisbrick P. Induction of neurasthenic musculoskeletal pain syndrome by selective sleep stage deprivation. *Psychosom Med* 1976;38(1):35–44.

80. Moldofsky H. Sleep and fibrositis syndrome. *Rheum Dis Clin North Am* 1989;15(1):91–103.

81. Drewes AM, Nielsen KD, Taagholt SJ, et al. Sleep intensity in fibromyalgia: focus on the microstructure of the sleep process. *Br J Rheumatol* 1995;34(7):629–635.

82. Hays RD, Stewart AL. Sleep measures. In: Stewart AL, Ware JE, eds. *Measuring functioning and well-being: the medical outcomes study approach.* Durham, NC: Duke University Press, 1992:235–259.

83. Hays R, Martin S, Sesti A, et al. Psychometric properties of the Medical Outcomes Study Sleep measure. *Sleep Medi* 2005;6:41–44.

84. De la Loge C, Viala M, Martin S, et al. Psychometric properties of the MOS-Sleep scale using international clinical trial data. *Qual Life Res* 2003;12:826.

85. Cesta A, Moldofsy H, Sammut C. The sensitivity and specificity of the sleep assessment questionnaire (SAQ) as a measure of non-restorative sleep. *Sleep* 1999;22(Suppl. 1):14.

86. Sperber AD, Carmel S, Atzmon Y, et al. Use of the functional bowel disorder severity index (FBDSI) in a study of patients with the irritable bowel syndrome and fibromyalgia. *Am J Gastroenterol* 2000;95:995–998.

87. Heymann RE, Helfenstein M, Feldman D. A double-blind, randomized, controlled study of amitriptyline, nortriptyline and placebo in patients with fibromyalgia. An analysis of outcome measures. *Clin Exp Rheumatol* 2001;19: 697–702.

88. Simms R, Felson D, Goldenberg D. Development of preliminary criteria for response to treatment in fibromyalgia syndrome. *J Rheumatol* 1991;18:1558–1563.

89. Torrance GW, Furlong W, Feeny D, et al. Multi-attribute preference functions: health utilities index. *Pharmacoeconomics* 1995;7(6):503–520.

90. The EuroQol Group. EuroQol—a new facility for the measurement of health-related quality of life. *Health Policy* 1990; 16(3):199–208.

91. Bakker C, Rutten M, Santen-Hoeufft M, et al. Patient utilities in fibromyalgia and the association with other outcome measures. *J Rheumatol* 1995; 22:1536–1543.

27

Lifestyle and Environmental Interventions in Fibromyalgia and Related Conditions

Stephanie A. Bolling and Thomas M. Susko

Proper self-management of daily activities can play a powerful role in reducing the symptoms of fibromyalgia (FM) and in helping patients break their pain cycle. Guiding patients on how to obtain "wellness" instead of focusing on "the illness" will improve their self-efficacy and allow them to return to a normal lifestyle faster. The self-efficacy principle is based on the theory that if people believe they can accomplish something, they probably can. If people do not believe they can do something, they probably cannot. This chapter's goal will be to review the symptoms of fibromyalgia that are influenced by activities of daily living and the modifications in lifestyles that are needed to control fibromyalgia. The proper approach to sleep, diet, tobacco, climate, fatigue, stress, home modifications, and physical and occupational therapy will be discussed.

ROLE OF SLEEP

Proper sleep is most important in controlling many of the symptoms of fibromyalgia. It is also extremely difficult for most fibromyalgia patients. Sixty to ninety percent of fibromyalgia patients have difficulty sleeping. Besides being unable to fall asleep, many patients suffer from sleep disorders such as nonrestorative sleeping, bruxism, sleep myoclonus, or sleep apnea. The most common sleep disorder is nonrestorative sleep. Patients may sleep enough hours but wake up feeling very fatigued. There are four sleep stages. Normal sleep should consist of about 20% rapid eye movement (REM) stages one and two, containing α and β brain waves. These stages are also known as the dream stages. Eighty percent of normal sleep should be stages three and four, which consist of γ and δ waves. In nonrestorative sleep the deep sleep stages are lacking or interrupted by α waves, which should not be present. Normal sleep is very important

in the production of chemical hormones for the body to function normally. Normal sleep can be defined as the ability to sleep 6 to 8 hours and then wake up fully rested and the ability to fall back to sleep if awakened during the night.

Lack of normal sleep has many consequences besides causing fatigue. It has also been thought to suppress the immune system, causing increased risk of infections as well as decreasing metabolic activity in the thalamus, limbic system, and hypothalamus. The hypothalamus is the master gland that controls many other glands and affects blood pressure, hormonal systems, and temperature regulation (1). For instance, a lack of deep sleep causes a decrease in the production of growth hormone, which can result in decreased energy, decreased exercise capacity, and impaired cognition. The growth hormone is also responsible for creating a substance known as IGF-1 (insulinlike growth factor 1). The body uses IGF-1 for tissue repair. A lack of this hormone may also result in muscles having increased pain levels and increased susceptibility to trauma because muscles are not being repaired while sleeping (2). Proper sleep should be the priority of every fibromyalgia patient because it helps muscles to heal and decreases the pain and fatigue symptoms.

Many things can be done to help promote healthy sleeping besides medication. A proper sleep environment is paramount. Mattresses should be firm with a cushioned top. For patients suffering with neck pain, a cervical pillow may reduce pain. The most commonly recommended cervical pillow is made with polyurethane and two contoured rolls, one to support the neck and the other to elevate the head slightly (e.g., Tempurpedic pillow). Patients with back pain should sleep either on the side with a pillow between the legs or on the back with a pillow under the knees to ease the pressure on the back. Stomach sleeping is not recommended. In the bedroom, light and noise should be reduced and the bed should be used only for reading or sleeping. Plan for 30 minutes to 1 hour of calming activity such as meditation, relaxing television, or reading prior to lights out. Relaxation tapes or soft music can be helpful, and phone calls should be avoided during this time. The sleeping environment needs to always be kept calm and quiet.

Regular bedtime and wake-up times need to be established and adhered to, even on the weekends. Generally, 10 PM to 6 AM or 11 PM to 7 AM is recommended. Try to avoid stressful or busy activities 2 hours before bedtime, including vigorous activity in the late evening. It can be helpful to take a hot bath or a hot shower prior to bedtime. Napping anytime after early afternoon could disrupt sleep. Try not to drink large amounts of fluids in the late evening. Try to cut sugar intake, especially late at night. Eliminate nicotine and decrease alcohol intake or drink only small amounts of alcohol with a meal to avoid disrupting sleep. Alcohol can cause fragmented sleep. Limit caffeine or nonherbal tea to only one cup in the morning or eliminate them completely. If unable to fall asleep within 30 minutes of lights out, try meditation or turn on the lights and continue reading. If still unable to sleep, try using a nonprescription sleep-aid. Getting up is not recommended for difficulty in sleeping or for waking up too early. The most common nonprescription sleep aids are melatonin, Calmes Forte, kava kava, valerian root, Benadryl, Tylenol PM, and Sleep-Eze.

If all the steps to assist in healthy sleep do not restore a normal sleep pattern, it is important to consult a physician regarding proper use of prescription sleep aids or medication.

Since proper sleep is so important for reducing the symptoms of fibromyalgia, use of medication is much less damaging than lack of sleep for a prolonged period of time.

ROLE OF DIET

Searching the Web, patients can find many supplements or diet suggestions to improve fibromyalgia. Research has not yet proven that any specific foods or supplements improve or worsen fibromyalgia. Patients feel better when they eat nutritional, well-balanced meals consisting of proteins, complex carbohydrates (such as vegetables, grains, and fruits), healthy fats, and six to eight glasses of water or noncaffeinated drinks. (See Table 27-1.) One should consume 25 to 40 grams of fiber daily. High-fiber food contains the most vitamins, minerals, and antioxidants with minimal processing. Good nutrition, food with antioxidants, and phytochemicals along with hydration will improve energy level and mental awareness, minimize constant fatigue, and improve sleep.

Since a lack of proper sleep and fatigue are two of the major symptoms of fibromyalgia, some general nutrition guidelines may help. For instance, many patients feel better

TABLE 27-1	Healthy Eating		
PROTEINS			**HEALTHY CARBOHYDRATES**
Nonvegetarian	1/4 **Protein**	1/4 **Healthy Carbohydrates**	1 fist of whole grains or starchy vegetables:
1 palm of Meat Poultry Fish			
Vegetarian 1 cup of dairy 1 oz. low fat cheese 1 egg or 3 whites 2 oz. tofu or soy ¼ cup nuts or 2 tbsp. peanut butter ½ cup beans		1/2 **Fruits and Vegetables**	Whole grain bread Brown rice Whole wheat pasta Baked or boiled potato Whole grain cereal Yam Peas Corn Beans Winter squash

Allow for 5–10 g of added fat and consume 5–10 g of fiber per meal.

FAT (5 G)	FIBER	(G)
1 teaspoon oil/mayo	1 tbsp. wheat bran	(5)
1 pat butter/margarine	½ cup high fiber cereal	(3–13)
1 tbsp. salad dressing	½ cup beans	(5–7)
1 tbsp. sour cream/cream cheese	1 cup cooked vegetables	(2–7)
½ tbsp. nut butter	1 fruit	(1–4)
⅛ avocado	1 slice whole wheat bread	(1–2)
½ oz. cheese	3 rye crackers	(3)
5 large olives		
5 nuts		

From Sarah Mirkin, RD, Cedars-Sinai Medical Network Systems, with permission.

having a slightly larger portion of protein in the morning or at lunch, which may help to improve mental alertness and concentration ability. Consuming alcohol, nicotine, caffeine (in the form of coffee, tea, or chocolate), or sugar late in the day can make it harder for patients to sleep. In addition, consuming a heavy or big meal before bed can increase gastrointestinal symptoms. A slightly smaller portion of protein and more vegetable/carbohydrates for dinner may help patients sleep better because proteins contain amino acids that can block tryptophan from forming serotonin, an important neurochemical needed for proper sleep. A light, low-fat, carbohydrate snack before bed may also to help improve sleep.

Ten percent of fibromyalgia patients may develop food sensitivities. Elimination of the foods or drinks that are most likely causing symptoms is recommended first, followed by reintroducing one food or drink into the diet to determine which is causing the symptoms. Schmidt and associates have been studying the influence of food additives such as monosodium glutamate (MSG) and aspartame on fibromyalgia patients. In their studies a dramatic improvement occurred in some patients when these additives were eliminated from their diet. They concluded that patients with an aggressive form of fibromyalgia or gastrointestinal symptoms could benefit from eradication of dietary additives (3). A nutritionist may be able to guide patients in uncovering foods that are making them feel worse. As patients become healthier, these food sensitivities can diminish.

Vitamins and mineral supplements are recommended especially for patients who are not getting proper nutrition. No particular brand of vitamins has been proven to be more beneficial than another. If patients are taking vitamins, it is generally recommended to take them in the morning or at lunch to avoid interference with sleep. There is currently much discussion on whether liquid vitamins are absorbed more effectively than pills (e.g., Ziquin liquid vitamin products). More research is needed in this area to make a substantial recommendation.

Two minerals should definitely be included in the diet of a fibromyalgia patient. The National Institutes of Health (NIH) recommends 1,200 mg of calcium for women and 1,000 mg for men, in split dosages. For postmenopausal women, the total daily dose is 1,500 mg—again, in split doses (e.g., 500 mg 3 times a day). Calcium is especially needed to avoid osteoporosis, a condition that causes bone loss and increase susceptibility to fractures. Osteoporosis is not unique to fibromyalgia patients, but it is more common in women and most fibromyalgia patients are women.

Magnesium deficiency has been seen in red blood cells of fibromyalgia patients (4). It could be caused by lack of deep sleep resulting in lower amounts of growth hormone. Magnesium is important to many body functions. It is necessary for proper bone function, muscle function, and the activities of hundreds of enzymes that turn food into adenosine triphosphate (ATP), the body's energy source. Taking magnesium and calcium together is recommended because the two minerals work synergistically. Plus, calcium offsets some of magnesium's laxative effects. For fibromyalgia patients, it is generally recommended to take more magnesium than the NIH standards (420 mg for men; 320 mg for women). A 2:1 ratio of calcium to magnesium is most widely recommended (e.g., 1,000 mg calcium, 500 mg magnesium). It is best to spread the dosage throughout the day, and these

TABLE 27-2 Magnesium-rich Foods

FOOD ITEM	SERVING (oz)	MAGNESIUM CONTENT (mg)
Peanuts	$\frac{1}{2}$ cup	131
Tofu	$\frac{1}{2}$ cup	127
Broccoli	2 large stalks	120
Spinach	$\frac{1}{2}$ cup	79
Soybeans	$\frac{1}{2}$ cup	74
Tomato paste	$\frac{1}{2}$ cup	67
White beans	$\frac{1}{2}$ cup	61
Black beans	$\frac{1}{2}$ cup	60
Chili with beans	$\frac{1}{2}$ cup	58
Lima beans	$\frac{1}{2}$ cup	49
Refried beans	$\frac{1}{2}$ cup	49
Pinto beans	$\frac{1}{2}$ cup	47
Blackeyed peas	$\frac{1}{2}$ cup	46
Sweet potato	$\frac{1}{2}$ cup	61
Pumpkin seeds	1 ounce	52
Peanut butter	2 tablespoons	51
Artichoke	1 medium	47
Whole grain cereals, ready-to-eat	1 ounce	47 average (22–134)
Squash, acorn	$\frac{1}{2}$ cup cubes	43
Yogurt	1 cup (8 oz)	37
Milk	1 cup (8 oz)	35 average (28–40)

minerals should be taken with food to avoid stomach upset. For patients who cannot tolerate magnesium supplements, it is suggested to eat magnesium-rich foods, as shown in Table 27-2.

One particular food supplement, malic acid, has been clinically studied. Malic acid is a fruit acid that is extracted from apples and is essential in the function of ATP. Malic acid helps the body make ATP more efficiently. One clinical study combined use of malic acid and magnesium. Fifteen patients ingested 1,200 to 2,400 mg of malic acid and 300 to 600 mg of magnesium for 4 to 8 weeks. The results of the study showed that all patients had significant reduction in pain within 48 hours, and within 4 to 8 weeks all patients had a significant decrease in tender point (TeP) index (5). Jorge Flechas has utilized the combination on over 500 fibromyalgia patients, has found the results to be positive 90% of the time, and highly recommends this combination.

EFFECT OF TOBACCO USE

Nicotine and use of tobacco can aggravate fibromyalgia in several ways. First of all, it can interfere with ability to sleep since it is a strong stimulant. Dr. Yunus at the University of Illinois has demonstrated that there are more sleep problems with smokers than nonsmokers and that smoking causes an increase in pain in patients with fibromyalgia. Furthermore, nicotine causes vascular constriction, which is already a problem in 30% to 40% of fibromyalgia patients (6). Constriction of blood flow results in a decrease in circulation, which can lead to symptoms of numbness, burning, or tingling. Furthermore, smoking has been shown to promote osteoporosis, a condition that results from a loss of calcium in the bones and can cause bones to be more susceptible to fractures. Smoking is also linked to heart disease, emphysema, cancer, stroke, chronic bronchitis, and an increased risk of miscarriage. Giving up smoking should be a high priority for patients with fibromyalgia since smoking will worsen the symptoms of fibromyalgia and is unhealthy for anyone.

EFFECTS OF CLIMATE

Patients with fibromyalgia often report that weather affects their symptoms. It is usually rain or dampness combined with cold or a change in climate from warm to rain that patients complain aggravates their symptoms.

Only a few studies have related pain in fibromyalgia to changes in weather. Fors and Sexton and de Blecourt et al. found no correlation between fibromyalgia pain and weather changes (7,8). Guedj and Weinberger and Strusberg et al. found that high barometric pressure increased fibromyalgia pain (9,10). Strusberg et al. also reported that pain correlated to low temperature. The term of their study was 1 year, compared to most of the other studies, which were 1 month, and possibly explains why a stronger correlation was shown between pain and weather (10). See Table 27-3 for a review of studies relating weather and fibromyalgia pain as adapted by the study done by Donald Quick. In Quick's review, the studies on joint pain and weather found no conclusive scientific evidence between weather changes and pain (11). His interpretation of the literature was that weather-related symptoms may be psychological instead of physiologic.

Raynaud phenomenon is a condition that can occur in patients with autoimmune diseases and causes the fingers or toes to turn red, white, or blue when exposed to cold. This phenomenon is definitely worse in colder weather (12). Occasionally, fibromyalgia patients can have symptoms that mimic this phenomenon. Avoiding cold weather, wearing gloves or socks with warmers, and baths or 10-minute to 15-minute applications of heat on cold days may be helpful in controlling any symptoms of cold sensitivity.

CONTROLLING FATIGUE

Fatigue can be a significant problem for patients with fibromyalgia. For some it is so disabling that they cannot get out of bed. For others, after the fatigue finally remits they feel so behind that they do too much and cause more fatigue. Some patients feel that exercise and medications increase the fatigue, so they do not follow their doctor's recommendations regarding medication and exercise.

Controlling fatigue is extremely challenging for patients with fibromyalgia and cannot be solved by one simple answer. Patients must do many activities to be able to control fatigue:

- Most important is proper sleep. Often fatigue will diminish as sleep improves.
- Proper nutrition is paramount, including well-balanced meals, multivitamins, and minerals containing calcium and magnesium.
- Patients should exercise regularly. Proper exercise will increase endorphins that can help with sleep, increase energy, muscle strength, and flexibility, and help reduce or control weight. Patients should start with the amount of exercise that they can do now and then increase the amount by 10% per week. It is recommended that stretching and exercise be done in the morning to decrease pain and achiness, possibly after a hot shower if the patient is suffering from severe stiffness and pain.
- Schedule the timing of medications with a doctor to avoid taking medications that cause drowsiness during the day.
- Avoid alcohol or illegal drugs.
- Patients need to use their energy wisely.
  - Alternate periods of activity with rest.
  - It is not recommended for patients to stay in bed all day during a flare-up.

TABLE 27-3	Weather Relating to Fibromyalgia Pain (11)			
STUDY DONE BY	Fors, Sexton	de Blucourt et al.	Guedj, Weinberger	Strusburg et al.
REFERENCE No.	7	8	9	10
NUMBER OF SUBJECTS	55	32	11	1,343
TERM	1 month	1 month	1 month	1 year
COUNTRY	Norway	Netherlands	Israel	Argentina
PAIN CORRELATED WITH:				
BAROMETRIC PRESSURE	0	0	High	High
TEMPERATURE	0	0	0	Low
HUMIDITY	0	0	0	0
PRECIPITATION	—	0	0	—

From Quick D. Joint pain and weather. *Minn Med* 1997;80:25–29, with permission.

- Patients need to learn to pace and prioritize by doing the most important responsibility first. Rest, then try the next most important responsibility, and then rest again.
- Patients must plan to perform the tasks requiring the greatest amounts of focus and energy at the time of the day that they function best (generally this is from 10 AM to 2 PM).
- Patients must learn to limit commitments. They must learn to say, "I'll let you know later if I can attend."
- Patients must delegate all responsibilities that have a negative effect on their body or that do not have to be done specifically by them (e.g., heavy lifting).
- Patients need to set realistic goals. When symptoms of fibromyalgia are severe, attempting to accomplish one or two important responsibilities may be the appropriate limit for the day. Patients must be able to let go of doing what is not the most important in the pursuit of controlling fibromyalgia symptoms.
- There must be a balance between activities (work, friends, family, self, environmental maintenance).

CONTROLLING STRESS

All fibromyalgia patients admit that stress can bring on or aggravate their symptoms. Since stress cannot be avoided, it is important for patients to learn how to effectively deal with stress to achieve a happy, productive life. Managing stress includes teaching patients to be mindful and aware of each moment so that they can exert control over the usual unconscious stress reactions. Patients should be able to identify stressors and their usual reactions to stressors. Many patients can be stuck in unhealthy stress reactivity, automatic reactions that usually accompany extreme emotions and compound and exacerbate stress. A healthy stress response can be developed as an alternative to the usual stress reaction (13). Training in effective communication and assertiveness may also help patients who have unhealthy stress reactions to confrontation. Encourage patients not to ignore their symptoms but to listen to their bodies and discuss with a health professional the best ways to overcome their symptoms. Meditation and relaxation training can also be helpful, especially before bed.

EFFECT OF HOME ENVIRONMENT

Disorganization in the home or work environment can increase stress in everyone, not just patients with fibromyalgia. Being organized can add time and energy and significantly increase productivity. Making a house efficient begins by creating a well-thought-out "space organization plan." For instance, all work-related equipment and files should be in one location to avoid excessive getting up and down. Prioritizing the area that needs the most organization or picking the area that is causing the most time and stress is the place to start.

Some patients can afford to hire people to do the space planning and organization for them. If not, it is important to complete one area before starting another area. Consolidate piles of papers by filing those papers that must be kept and creating two simple piles of "to do" and "to read." Have one location where you write down everything, including listening to phone messages and writing down phone numbers.

Consolidate and simplify household chores (e.g., shop for the week, cook two meals at once). Change the body mechanics of chores that are causing pain. For instance, move the dishes or cooking supplies used most frequently to a shelf at waist level. Buy a lightweight or cordless vacuum and step in the direction of the vacuum, moving the entire body, not just the arms. Break up chores with periods of rest. Avoid twisting. The feet should turn in the direction of movement (e.g., loading or unloading a dishwasher). Objects should be directly in front and kept close to the body when lifting or pushing. Generally, pushing objects such as garbage cans is recommended over pulling. When washing windows or dusting, use longer handles or a stepstool. Avoid excessive kneeling or squatting (e.g., gardening). Take frequent breaks or break jobs into small intervals of time over several days. Do low tasks while sitting on a small plastic stool or rolling stool to reduce stress on the knees and back.

Make sure that the house has a proper ergonomic setup to avoid aggravation of pain. For instance, arrange the room so that the television or computer can be faced directly. A work area at home or work should be ergonomic with a chair that supports the lower spine, and the feet should be flat on the floor. The work table should be approximately even with the forearms when they are at a 90-degree angle from the upper arms. The keyboard should also be directly in front of you and at the same 90-degree angle. It can be 5 to 15 degrees higher but not lower. Any angle lower than 90 degrees from your upper arms causes excessive neck flexion and can increase neck pain. Wrist pads can help in reducing wrist pain. Avoid sitting for more than 30 to 45 minutes without walking around for 1 to 5 minutes. Avoid work in bed or reading halfway propped up in bed. For reading in bed, it is recommended to have no more then two pillows under the head and to bend the knees so the reading material can rest on a pillow in your lap.

ROLE OF OCCUPATIONAL AND PHYSICAL THERAPY

The goal of physical therapy is to help restore function, improve mobility and independence, relieve pain, and prevent or limit permanent physical disabilities for patients suffering from musculoskeletal conditions. The goal of occupational therapy is to help people regain, develop, and build skills that are essential for independent functioning, health, and well-being.

Unfortunately, most physical therapists (PTs) and occupational therapists (OTs) have little training in the needs and proper treatment of fibromyalgia. Fibromyalgia patients should definitely seek a therapist who specializes in the treatment of rheumatologic conditions to avoid advice or treatment that could worsen symptoms. For instance, the manual therapy techniques used in physical therapy can be helpful in decreasing pain and muscle spasms. However, a therapist who has not been trained in treatment of fibromyalgia could apply techniques that temporarily cause more pain. Also, a specialized PT will be better at guiding the proper use and progression of exercise. Exercise is extremely important for fibromyalgia patients to do on a regular basis.

Listed below are components of a thorough evaluation and treatment from a therapist and whether an OT or a PT usually performs the procedure. Generally, OTs perform assessments of activities of daily living to see what areas of improvement could be made in energy conservation and joint protection. OTs are experts at designing adaptive equipment such as enlarged handles or specialized braces or tools to decrease joint and muscle strain. PTs focus on the use of manual techniques to reduce muscle spasms and pain and guide patients in movement reeducation and the proper stretching and exercise program to decrease muscle spasms. Both a PT and an OT can guide in the proper ergonomics of a workstation.

An evaluation should include the following (PT or OT):

- Assessment of muscle spasms and most TePs (PT or OT)
- Assessment of muscle flexibility and strength (PT or OT for upper extremity)
- Posture analysis (static and dynamic) (PT or OT)
- Assessment of body mechanics (PT or OT)
- Gait analysis (PT)
- Assessment of functional limitations (PT or OT)
- Aerobic activity assessment (PT)
- Fatigue assessment (PT or OT)
- Sleep hygiene assessment (PT or OT)
- Assessment of stress/anxiety level (PT or OT)
- Discussion of patient's goals (PT or OT)

Treatment should consist of the following:

- Modalities if manual therapy is not tolerated due to hypersensitivity (PT or OT for upper extremity)
- Manual therapy consisting of joint and soft tissue mobilization, manipulation, and/or massage to decrease muscle spasming or TePs (PT or OT for upper extremity)
- Individualized stretching program (PT or OT for upper extremity)
- Proper posture training (PT or OT)
- Body mechanics training (PT or OT)
- Breathing and stress reduction training (PT or OT)
- Proper sleep hygiene training (PT or OT)
- Proper aerobic activity training (PT)
- Safe individualized strengthening training (PT or OT for upper extremity)
- Functional activity training (PT or OT)
- Self-management home treatments to reduce pain during flare-ups (PT or OT)
- Coordination of alternative treatments (PT or OT)
- Communication with doctors regarding patient care (PT or OT)
- Teaching self-trigger point release technique (PT)

ROLE OF A FIBROMYALGIA PROGRAM

Although there is considerable interest in the effectiveness of multidisciplinary rehabilitation programs for patients with fibromyalgia, Karjaiainen et al. screened 1,808 abstracts and found only seven studies that had randomized control trials using a multidisciplinary approach with a physician consultation plus at least one psychological intervention. Although they found a lack of scientific evidence to recommend these programs, they did state that education and physical training showed some positive effects in the long-term follow-up (14).

Sim and Adams reviewed 25 studies using many different interventions, including massage, chiropractic, biofeedback, exercise, education, vibration, electroacupuncture, transcutaneous electrical nerve stimulation, hypnotherapy, pool exercise, and aerobic exercise. Because few of the studies examined used the same modalities or interventions, control groups, or similar outcome measures, the authors found it difficult to form conclusions. Aerobic exercise, education, and relaxation were the interventions most frequently used, and most studies showed a statistically significant difference on at least one outcome measure. However, they also found the statistical power of most studies to be low and the analysis insufficient for meaningful conclusions to be drawn. They found that a multidisciplinary approach showed greater improvements then a single intervention. They concluded that a fibromyalgia program should consist of a multidisciplinary team addressing each patient's specific physical, functional, and psychological needs (15).

SUMMARY POINTS

- A variety of simple and common sense approaches can be helpful to patients with fibromyalgia and related conditions.
- Relatively little research has been performed indicating exactly how this information is best imparted to fibromyalgia patients and which therapies (e.g., exercise, stress management, cognitive-behavioral training, nutrition counseling, body mechanics, and postural training) are necessary in multidisciplinary treatment programs.
- Nonetheless, these programs clearly can be successful and may be especially helpful for individuals who are refractory to previous therapy or who are particularly functionally impaired by their illness.

REFERENCES

1. Teitlebaum J. *From fatigued to fantastic*. Garden City Park: Avery Publishing Group, 2001:27.
2. Wallace D, Brock Wallace J. *All about fibromyalgia*. Oxford: Oxford University Press, 2002:41.
3. Smith JD, Terpening CM, Schmidt SO, et al. Relief of fibromyalgia symptoms following discontinuation of dietary excitotoxins. *Ann Pharmacother* 2001;35:702–706.
4. Eisinger J, Plantamura A, Marie PA, et al. Selenium and magnesium status in fibromyalgia. *Magn Res* 1994;7:285–288.
5. Abraham GE, Flechas JD. Management of fibromyalgia: rationale for the use of magnesium and malic acid. *J Nutr Med* 1992;3:49–59.
6. Wallace D, Brock Wallace J. *All about fibromyalgia*. Oxford: Oxford University Press, 2002:129.
7. Fors EA, Sexton H. Weather and the pain in fibromyalgia: are they related? *Ann Rheum Dis* 2002;61:247–250.
8. de Blecourt ACE, Knipping AA, et al. Weather conditions and complaints in fibromyalgia. *J Rheumatol* 1993;20:1932–1934.

9. Guedj D, Weinberger A. Effect of weather conditions on rheumatic patients. *Ann Rheum Dis* 1990;49:158–159.
10. Strusberg I, Mendelberg R, Serra HA, et al. Influence of weather conditions on rheumatic pain. *J Rheumatol* 2002;29: 335–338.
11. Quick D. Joint pain and weather. *Minn Med* 1997;80:25–29.
12. Wallace D, Weisman M. The role of environmental factors in rheumatic diseases. *Bull Rheum Dis* 2002:51(10).
13. Kabat-Zinn J. *Full catastrophe living*. New York: Dell Bantam Doubleday, 1990:264.

14. Karjaiainen K, Maimivaara A, Van Tulder M, et al. Multidisciplinary rehabilitation for fibromyalgia and musculoskeletal pain in working age adults. *Cochrane Database Syst Rev* 2000; (2):CD001984, updated quarterly.
15. Sim J, Adams N. Systemic review of randomized controlled trials of nonpharmacological interventions for fibromyalgia. *Clin J Pain* 2002;18(5):324–336.

28

The Use of Exercise and Rehabilitation Regimens

Kaisa Mannerkorpi and Maura Daly Iversen

FIBROMYALGIA AND DISABILITY

Fibromyalgia (FM) is a pain disorder that severely impacts quality of life and functional ability. FM is characterized by chronic widespread pain, aching, fatigue, and stiffness, and it is often accompanied by nonrestorative sleep, mood disturbance, irritable bowel syndrome, headache, and paresthesias (1,2). Physical activity, stress, anxiety, tiredness, and poor sleep may aggravate symptoms (3). The currently accepted theory underlying the unpredictable and inconsistent symptomatology is an aberrant central pain-processing mechanism and the complex interaction of multiple biologic, psychological, and sociologic factors. FM commonly occurs during early and middle age and affects women more often than men (4). The prevalence of FM is estimated to be 1% to 3%, and it increases with age (5).

Patients with FM display reduced upper and lower extremity physical performance capacity compared to age-matched and sex-matched healthy controls (6,7). Some studies demonstrate reduced voluntary muscle strength and endurance in patients with FM (8–10), while other studies report no differences between patients and healthy individuals (11,12). Similarly, studies examining aerobic capacity in these patients report conflicting results (6,13,14).

Persons with FM report difficulties in activities in daily life, such as carrying objects and working with the arms in elevated positions (15,16), walking, prolonged sitting, and standing (17). Perceived symptoms and disability can affect all dimensions of life, including social roles, family life, employment, and leisure time. Work-related disability data indicate escalating lost workdays and Social Security payments as well as elevated health care costs (18,19). From a sociological perspective, perception of ill health is not always a consequence of a disorder or a disease but may be associated with personal and environmental factors (20,21). For example, work modifications may enable an individual with FM to remain at work (22). The severity and consequences of FM have been associated with pain, fatigue, helplessness, psychological distress, work status, coping, and level of education (23). However, patients with FM form a heterogeneous population. Some persons with FM appear to manage their symptoms by adapting to their limitations or by struggling to cope with everyday problems, while others perceive themselves helpless and unable to cope with their symptoms and everyday difficulties (24).

CHRONIC WIDESPREAD PAIN

Epidemiologic studies reveal that chronic widespread pain and fatigue are common in the general population (5). Muscle tenderness and positive tender points (TePs) can be found in a variety of pain diagnoses and also in individuals without pain. An increasing number of TePs is associated not only with persistent pain (4,25) but also with other symptoms reflecting ill health, such as depression (4,25), anxiety (4), fatigue (25), and poor sleep (25). Patients with regional and widespread pain can move across pain categories (26), and it is probable that chronic regional pain, chronic widespread pain, and FM represent an overlapping spectrum of illnesses rather than discrete diseases (25,27). However, the concept of FM as a clinical syndrome has provided a framework for evaluating the effects of interventions for patients with severe chronic pain.

TREATMENT

Rehabilitation goals for patients with chronic pain usually focus on maximizing health, function, and independence. The treatment of patients with FM and related syndromes includes explanations of the nature of the syndrome, pharmacotherapy, physical exercise, relaxation, education to promote self-management and prevent inactivity, activities to increase general fitness and physical function, and techniques to reduce pain and develop coping skills (23,28). Most studies of exercise interventions include patients with FM who are treated in outpatient settings (28), while randomized controlled trials of multiprofessional inpatient care are few (29,30). Little is known about the long-term results of therapeutic approaches. One longitudinal study has indicated resolution of symptoms in some patients (31), but this does not appear likely for the majority (18).

In clinical practice the intervention plan is based on the assessment of symptoms and disabilities and a discussion with the patient about goals and preferences (32,33). Physical and occupational therapists commonly use a variety of therapeutic approaches in their treatment of patients with FM to maximize functional ability, general fitness, exercise tolerance, and posture and to provide instruction and education regarding pain management and relaxation (28). Intervention strategies are comprehensive and are designed to address physical and psychosocial factors to improve self-confidence and enhance the patient's ability to manage the disorder.

Interest in evaluating the impact of physical exercise on health outcomes in this population has recently increased. We review randomized controlled studies of physical exercise and exercise plus educational interventions in patients with FM, chronic pain, and chronic fatigue syndrome (CFS). The majority of the studies in this review evaluate the effects of supervised aerobic exercise, including ergometer cycling, aerobic dancing, and outdoor or treadmill walking programs. Some studies have evaluated whole body programs consisting of aerobic, strength, endurance, coordination, balance, and flexibility exercises, and a few studies have focused on whole body exercises in a temperate pool or strength training. We discuss the forms of exercise separately. Since the study designs are not often well described and study samples are small, comparisons between studies are not possible. A summary of the interventions, the between-group results, and follow-up data, when applicable, are presented in tables. Evaluations of exercise as a single modality are presented in Table 28-1, and the evaluations of exercise combined with education are presented in Table 28-2.

AEROBIC EXERCISE BY MEANS OF CYCLING, DANCE, OR WHOLE BODY PROGRAMS

McCain et al. (34) conducted the first trial of aerobic exercise for patients with FM. This study evaluated the effects of moderate-to-high intensity ergometer cycling three times a week for 20 weeks. Patients in the aerobic exercise group improved their aerobic capacity, increased their TeP pain threshold, and reported increases in global well-being compared to the group engaging in flexibility exercise. Only patients who successfully completed a treadmill exercise stress test were included in the study, and this selection criteria is important to remember when translating the results of this clinical trial into clinical practice.

A study conducted by Mengshoel et al. (35) evaluated the effects of supervised aerobic dance performed twice a week over a 20-week period. Aerobic capacity, measured as maximal oxygen uptake, did not improve in the between-group

analysis, but the heart rate during work declined within the exercise group. Improvements were also found in grip strength among the exercisers compared to controls. The researchers identified a decline in lower extremity endurance that may be explained by an increase in anaerobic metabolism in the lower extremity muscles.

Wigers et al. (56) studied the effects of supervised whole body aerobic exercise, performed three times a week at 60% to 70% of the patient's maximum heart rate for 14 weeks. Patients in the aerobic exercise group demonstrated improved aerobic fitness and reductions in TePs and pain distribution, compared to subjects in the relaxation group and usual treatment group. The short-term improvements were, however, not evident at the 4-year follow-up. Verstappen (41) also studied the effects of supervised whole body aerobic and strengthening exercises. However, this trial examined the impact of exercise over 6 months. Participants were taught how to determine and increase the load for aerobic and strengthening exercises. Eighty percent of the patients reported benefits from exercise, including decreased stiffness and increased daily physical activity, although no between-group differences were found when compared to a control group. The majority of patients continued with the exercise program at their own expense after completing the trial. This additional outcome is important to note as continued participation in exercise results in healthier lifestyles. Additional studies of aerobic exercise did not find any between-group differences (39,62).

Martin et al. (38) evaluated the impact of a 6-week program of aerobic walking and muscle strength training performed three times a week. They found slight increases in aerobic fitness among the exercisers compared to subjects in the relaxation group. The number of TePs and TeP score also improved in the exercisers compared to a relaxation group. The short duration of the exercise program and the high drop-out rate may have yielded the small improvements. Isomeri et al. (36) evaluated the effects of 3 weeks of in-hospital treatment, followed by 12 weeks of home therapy. The treatment included aerobic exercises and medication and resulted in decreased pain threshold in the intervention group compared to a group that only received medication.

Two studies compared different intensities and frequencies of aerobic exercise. One study compared low and high intensity of aerobic exercise (62) and another compared the duration of exercise sessions using short and long bouts of aerobic exercise (54). Van Santen et al. (62) found only modest improvements in physical fitness and general well-being with high-intensity training compared to low-intensity training. No significant differences between the two modes were found. Adherence was found to be slightly better in the low-intensity group than in the high-intensity group, and reasons for nonadherence included exercise-induced pain, time constraints, and stress. Schachter et al. (54) enrolled 143 sedentary women with FM and instructed the women allocated to the two exercise groups to exercise three to five times a week beginning with 10 minutes of exercise and progressing to a maximum of 30 minutes over a 16-week period. The target duration for each exercise session was 30 minutes. However, the short bout group performed the exercises in two sessions per day with a 4-hour interval between exercise sessions for a total of 30 minutes. All groups met with a physical therapist or physical therapy student once a month. The two exercise groups trained in their homes

TABLE 28-1		Randomized Controlled Trials of Physical Exercise in Patients with Fibromyalgia (FM) and Related Disorders[a]		
LEAD AUTHOR	**NUMBER OF SUBJECTS WHO COMPLETED THE STUDY**	**TYPE, DURATION, FREQUENCY, AND LENGTH OF EXERCISE**	**RESULTS**	**DROP OUT RATE**
McCain 1988 (34)	38 patients with primary fibromyalgia A. 18 B. 20	A. Supervised cycle ergometry, target heart rate 150–170 bpm, 60 min, 3 ×/wk for 20 wk B. Flexibility	Improved aerobic capacity and pain threshold at TePs in exercise vs. flexibility group. No adverse effects.	A. 14% B. 5%
Mengshoel 1990 (35)	35 female patients A. 18 B. 17	A. Supervised aerobic dance, target heart rate 120–150 bpm, 60 min, 2 ×/wk for 20 wk B. No treatment	Grip strength improved in aerobic dance group compared to control subjects.	A. 39% B. 18%
Isomeri 1993 (36)	45 patients A. 16 B. 15 C. 14	A. Flexibility + amitriptyline for 3 wk inpatient and 12-wk home program B. Strenuous aerobic exercise C. Combined A and B	Pain threshold, measured by means of dolorimeter, improved in the group receiving the combined therapies compared to A or B alone.	
Nichols 1994 (37)	19 patients, 17 women and 2 men	A. Walking at 60%–70% of max heart rate, 20 min, 3 ×/wk for 8 wk B. No treatment	Higher disability score in sickness impact profile physical dimension in A after termination of the program.	A. 17% B. 25%
Martin 1996 (38)	38 patients with FM A. 18 B. 20	A. Aerobic exercise at 60%–80% max heart rate, strength training and flexibility, 60 min session, 3 ×/wk for 6 wk B. 60-min relaxation session, 1 ×/wk for 6 wk	Significant improvements were noted in the exercise group compared to the relaxation group in TePs, total myalgic scores, and aerobic fitness.	A. 40% B. 33%
Norregaard 1997 (39)	23 patients A. 5 B. 11 C. 7	A. Aerobic dance 3 ×/wk for 12 wk B. Steady exercise 2 ×/wk for 12 wk C. Hot packs 2 ×/wk for 12 wk	After 12 wk no improvement in pain, fatigue, general condition, depression, functional status, muscle strength, or aerobic capacity in any group.	A. 66% B. 27% C. 12.5%
Fulcher 1997 (40)	66 patients with CFS; includes a crossover design A. 29 B. 33	A. Supervised graded aerobic exercise up to 30 min for 12 wk plus home program; starting intensity 40% peak O_2 uptake up to 60% peak O_2 uptake B. Flexibility exercises for 12 wk with relaxation	Patients in the graded exercise group (A) rated themselves better (fatigue, physical function) and increased peak O_2 by 13% compared to the flexibility group that increased peak O_2 by 6%. Only 2 patients dropped due to an increase in symptoms.	A. 12% B. 9%
Verstappen 1997 (41)	72 patients A. 45 B. 27	A. Supervised aerobic running and cycling, strengthening, stretching, swimming for 50 min, 2 ×/wk 6 mo + 2 unsupervised sessions B. None	No significant changes between A and B with regard to physical function but programs well received by patients.	A. 22% B. 7%
Wearden 1998 (42)	136 patients with CFS, 34 per group	A. Exercise and 20 mg fluoxetine, B. Exercise and placebo drug C. Appointments and 20 mg fluoxetine D. Appointments and placebo drug All groups enrolled for 26 wk	Fatigue decreased the most and improvements were noted in functional work capacity at 12 and 26 wk in the exercise group. Exercise significantly improved health perceptions and fatigue at 6 mo. Fluoxetine had a significant effect on depression at week 12 only.	29.4% overall drop out rate; drop out rate greater in the exercise group

(Continued)

TABLE 28-1 Continued

LEAD AUTHOR	NUMBER OF SUBJECTS WHO COMPLETED THE STUDY	TYPE, DURATION, FREQUENCY, AND LENGTH OF EXERCISE	RESULTS	DROP OUT RATE
Keel 1998 (43)	27 patients A. 14 B. 13	A. Aerobic stretching, relaxation, and education B. Relaxation Both programs were offered 1 ×/week for 50–60 min for 15 wk	No differences or changes in either group at 15 wk. At 3 mo, pain intensity improved in the exercise group compared to the relaxation group.	
Ramsay 2000 (44)	74 patients, 37 in each group	(A) Graded supervised aerobic exercise, stretching, and relaxation for 60 min, 1 ×/wk for 12 wk (B) One session individualized instruction in aerobic exercise, stretching and relaxation, and written instructions for home-exercise program	Anxiety improved in the group assigned to fitness classes compared to the home-exercise group. At 24 and 48 wk follow-up improvement not sustained.	A. 59% attended 2–3 ×/wk of the sessions B. 5%
Meyer 2000 (45)	21 patients A. 8 B. 8 C. 5	(A) High-intensity walking for 24 wk (B) Low-intensity walking 2–3 ×/wk for 24 wk (C) Control	FIQ improved 8% in high-intensity group and 35% in low-intensity group.	Overall drop out rate 62%; at end of the trial, patients reassigned to treatment group based on exercise log data
Meiworm 2000 (46)	39 patients, 3 men and 36 women A. 27 B. 12	A. Aerobic exercise jogging, cycling, swimming at 50% VO_{2max} for 25 min, 3 ×/wk for 12 wk B. Controls	Increased aerobic capacity, decreased mean number of TePs, mean pain threshold, and percent of painful body surface.	
Saltskår Jentoft 2001 (47)	34 female patients A. 18 B. 16	A. Land aerobic exercise for 60 min, 2 ×/wk for 20 wk (40%–50% of sessions at 60%–80% max. heart rate) B. Pool exercise for 60 min, 2 ×/wk for 20 wk	Grip strength improved more in the land exercise group (A) compared to pool therapy group (B). Within-group improvements were noted for both groups in cardiovascular capacity, walking time, and daytime fatigue. 6-mo follow-up showed within-group improvements for aerobic fitness and walking were maintained.	A. 18% B. 27%
Gowans 2001 (48)	50 patients A. 27 B. 23	A. 30-min progressive exercise (10 min of stretching and 20 min of aerobic exercise) 3 ×/wk for 23 wk; first 6 wk pool-based followed by 1 pool and 2 land-based sessions per wk B. Controls	Significant improvements were noted in 6-min walk test, depression, anxiety, self-efficacy, and mental health in exercisers.	A. 44% B. 69.5%
Häkkinen 2001 (49)	33 patients A. 11 B. 10 C. 12	A. Supervised strength training, starting from 40%–60% and increasing to 60%–80% of 1RM, 2 ×/wk for 21 wk B. None C. Healthy individuals	Muscle strength, EMG-activity, and depression improved in A compared to B.	

(Continued)

| TABLE 28-1 | Continued | | | |

LEAD AUTHOR	NUMBER OF SUBJECTS WHO COMPLETED THE STUDY	TYPE, DURATION, FREQUENCY, AND LENGTH OF EXERCISE	RESULTS	DROP OUT RATE
Jones 2002 (50)	56 female patients A. 28 B. 28	A. Progressive strengthening exercises with 1–3 lb weights and tubing (little eccentric contraction) for 12 wk B. Static flexibility exercises followed by 8–10 min of guided imagery for 12 wk	Significant improvements in strength for both groups but twice the improvement in the group who performed strength training compared to flexibility, no increase in pain.	
Richards 2002 (51)	136 men and women with chronic pain or fibromyalgia from outpatient rheumatology clinic A. 69 B. 67	A. Supervised progressive graded aerobic exercise (walking or cycling) for 60 min, 2 ×/wk for 12 wk B. Relaxation	35% of the exercisers reported improved health compared to 18% in relaxation group. No other improvements noted. Improvements in TeP count still noted at 1 yr in both groups.	18% in each group
Van Santen 2002 (52)	33 female patients A. 18 B. 15	A. Supervised high-intensity aerobic exercise at 70% max heart rate, for 60 min, 3 ×/wk for 20 wk B. Supervised low-intensity aerobic exercise, self-paced for 60 min, 2 ×/wk for 20 wk	AIMS pain score increased in the high-intensity group compared to the low-intensity group. No other differences noted.	
Valim 2003 (53)	76 female patients	A. Aerobic exercise 3 ×/wk for 20 wk B. Stretching 3 ×/wk for 20 wk	Aerobic capacity, function, depression, pain, and mental health improved in A compared to B.	
Schachter 2003 (54)	143 sedentary female patients A. 51 B. 56 C. 36	A. Video led home-based low impact aerobic exercise at 40%–50% HRR progressing to 65%–75% HRR, for 10 min (at start) and progressing to a maximum of 30 min, 3–5 times per wk for 16 wk B. As above, but exercise divided into 2 bouts separated by 4 h C. No exercise All participants also attended monthly group meetings with a physical therapist or physical therapy student	No differences were found in intent-to-treat analysis. 86 patients were included in the efficacy analysis. A improved in disease severity, SE, and well-being compared to C. B improved in disease severity and SE compared to C. Exercise adherence was greater in group A than group B. No differences were found between A and C.	A. 14% B. 38% C. 29%

bpm, beat per minute; FIQ, the fibromyalgia impact questionnaire; ASES, the arthritis self-efficacy scale; QOLS, the quality of life scale; AIMS, the arthritis impact measurement scales; CFS, chronic fatigue syndrome; HRR, heart rate reserve; SE, self-efficacy; TePs, tender points.
[a]Subjects comprise patients with FM only, if no other diagnosis is given.

using exercise videotapes. Both exercise groups improved in self-efficacy and disease severity compared to the control group, but no differences were found between the groups.

A recent meta-analysis (64) found evidence supporting the positive effects of exercise for patients with FM. In this meta-analysis Busch et al. included aerobic exercise programs conducted twice a week for a minimum of 20 minutes and performed at intensity sufficient to achieve 40% to 85% of heart rate reserve or 55% to 90% of predicted maximum heart rate. The results indicated 17% improvement in aerobic performance with aerobic exercise, compared to 0.5% gain in the control group. Subjects who exercised also demonstrated 28% improvement in TeP pain threshold and 11% reduction in pain rating, while the control group slightly worsened on these measurements (64).

TABLE 28-2 Randomized Controlled Trials of Physical Exercise Plus Education in Patients with Fibromyalgia and Related Disorders[a]

LEAD AUTHOR	NUMBER OF SUBJECTS WHO COMPLETED THE STUDY	TYPE, DURATION, FREQUENCY, AND LENGTH OF EXERCISE	RESULTS	DROP OUT RATE
Burckhardt 1994 (55)	86 female patients A. 30 B. 28 C. 28	A. Education only, including planning for outdoor walks, for 1 h, 1 ×/wk for 6 wk B. Education and supervised flexibility, aerobic exercise, and planning for outdoor walks 1.5 h, 3 ×/wk for 6 wk C. No treatment	QOLS and self-efficacy (ASES) for pain, function, and other symptoms was improved in A and B compared to no treatment (C). At 7–11 mo follow-up, FIQ physical function and feeling bad were improved in A, while FIQ physical function, pain, fatigue, stiffness, and distress were improved in B.	
Wigers 1996 (56)	60 patients, 55 female and 5 male (20 patients per group)	A. 45 min of aerobic exercise at 60%–70% max heart rate for 20 min, 3 ×/wk for 14 wk B. Stress management C. Usual treatment	Aerobic capacity, pain distribution, and TeP score improved in exercise group (A) compared to usual treatment (C). TeP score improved in stress management (B) compared to C. Follow-up 4 yr showed a poor compliance. Exercising 3 times a week was perceived stressful.	5% per group
Buckelew 1998 (57)	101 patients A. 26 B. 23 C. 25 D. 27	A. Supervised aerobic walking at 60%–70% of max heart rate, strengthening, and flexibility, 1.5 h, 1 ×/wk for 6 wk + home program for 6 wk B. Supervised exercise and biofeedback C. Biofeedback D. Education	Physical function (AIMS) and self-efficacy (ASES) for function and pain with TeP palpation improved in A and B compared to D. Greatest benefits seen in combination exercise groups (A) even at 2-yr follow-up.	
Gowans 1999 (58)	41 female patients A. 20 B. 21	A. Pool exercise comprising aerobic, endurance, and flexibility exercises for 30 min, 2 ×/wk for 6 wk plus education sessions for 60 min, 2 ×/wk B. No treatment	FIQ fatigue, pain, and aerobic capacity (6-min walk test) improved in the exercise group compared to control. At 3 mo benefits still seen in aerobic capacity and well-being.	
Mannerkorpi 2000 (59)	59 female patients A. 28 B. 29	(A) Low-intensity pool exercise, comprising aerobic, endurance, flexibility, body awareness, and relaxation for 35 min, 1 ×/wk for 6 mo, combined with education at 6 sessions (B) No treatment	FIQ total score, aerobic performance (6-min walk), FIQ physical function and distress, SF36 social role, and grip strength improved in A compared to B. Shoulder endurance deteriorated. At 6 mo, aerobic performance (walk), physical function, pain, fatigue, and distress were maintained in the exercise group. At 2 yr, improvements in pain, fatigue, and social function were maintained.	A. 24% B. 6%
Powell 2001 (60)	127 patients with CFS	A. 2 individualized treatments and 2 follow-up calls supported by educational materials and instruction in progressive home-exercise program B. Control received standardized medical care	No significant between-group differences on main outcomes.	

(Continued)

TABLE 28-2 Continued

LEAD AUTHOR	NUMBER OF SUBJECTS WHO COMPLETED THE STUDY	TYPE, DURATION, FREQUENCY, AND LENGTH OF EXERCISE	RESULTS	DROP OUT RATE
King 2002 (61)	152 patients in intent-to-treat A. 42 B. 41 C. 35 D. 34	A. Aerobic exercise 3 ×/wk for 12 wk B. Education 3 ×/wk for 12 wk C. Aerobic exercise and education 3 ×/wk for 12 wk D. No treatment	Self-efficacy improved in C compared to D and within C. 6-min walk improved in A and C.	A. 28.5% B. 49% C. 28% D. 47%
Van Santen 2002 (62)	118 patients A. 47 B. 43 C. 28	A. Supervised aerobic exercise for 60 min, 2–3 ×/wk for 24 wk B. Biofeedback for 30 min, 2 ×/wk for 8 wk C. Control D. 50% of patients in A and B were randomized to an educational program for 90 min × 6 sessions	No significant differences in any between-group comparisons.	
Thieme 2003 (30)	63 patients in inpatient setting A. 42 B. 21	A. Exercise, education, operant pain treatment, and reduction of medication B. Passive treatments in terms of relaxation, mud bath, light movement therapy in warm water, and antidepressive pharmacologic treatment	Reduction in pain intensity and interference in the multidimensional pain inventory in A compared to B.	A. 5% B. none
Donta 2003 (63)	1,092 Gulf War veterans with 2 or 3 symptoms of 6 mo duration (modified intention-to-treat) A. 266 B. 269 C. 286 D. 271	A. Cognitive-behavioral therapy delivered in small groups (CBT) for 60 min plus supervised aerobic exercise 1 time per week for 60 min and 2–3 times per week independently for 12 wk in addition to usual care B. Supervised progressive low-intensity aerobic exercise (varied forms of exercise) for 60 min once per week and 2–3 times per week independently for 12 wk plus usual care C. CBT delivered in small groups for 60–90 min once per week for 12 wk plus usual care D. Usual care	All groups showed improved function (SF-36). The greatest improvements in function were seen in the CBT alone (18.5%) and CBT plus exercise group (18.4%), compared to exercise alone (11.7%) and usual care group (11.5%). Exercise group improved more in symptom severity than the CBT group. Exercise improvements were also seen in fatigue, distress, cognitive symptoms, and mental health.	Overall drop out rate 8.6% A. 9.4% B. 10.4% C. 8.7% D. 5.9%

bpm, beat per minute; FIQ, the fibromyalgia impact questionnaire; ASES, the arthritis self-efficacy scale; QOLS, the quality of life scale; AIMS, the arthritis impact measurement scales.
[a]Subjects comprise patients with FM only, if no other diagnosis is given.

Aerobic exercise at moderate intensity appears to enhance aerobic capacity and reduce symptoms. However, there is still considerable variability among study results. The discrepancies in findings may be due to differences in exercise intensity, small sample sizes, large drop-out rates, variations in outcome measures, and variations in subject characteristics in terms of function, symptom severity, and psychosocial health.

Individuals with satisfactory baseline cardiovascular fitness (14) may demonstrate little change following participation in an aerobic exercise program, while larger changes are expected in sedentary participants. However, only one study team formally tested baseline function and used it as a criterion for inclusion in their trial (34). A more detailed description of recruitment procedures and patients' characteristics would enable comparisons between programs and aid therapists in interpreting and applying the results of clinical trials into their clinical practice. Few studies have reported detrimental effects following exercise, although it is not unusual for individuals with FM to experience short-term exercise-induced pain. Also, a limited number of studies have reported how many patients followed the prescribed training program. However, van Santen (62) noted that no patient exceeded 130 beats per minute for longer than a few minutes during the exercise sessions, implying that prescribed high-intensity training in fact became low-intensity training. In another study, van Santen (52) discovered that only 50% of the patients managed to fully comply with the training sessions, primarily due to exercise-induced pain.

In sum, patients with FM may improve their aerobic capacity and physical function and diminish their tenderness if they exercise at a moderate intensity at least twice a week. Aerobic exercise prescriptions for patients with chronic pain or FM should be individually tailored to the patient's baseline function, symptom severity, and tolerance for exercise-induced pain. Postexertional pain is a potential adverse effect of exercise and should be closely monitored. Further research is needed to determine the appropriate intensity, dose, and frequency of aerobic exercise for patients exhibiting different levels of symptom severity and function.

WALKING

Walking is a cheap, easily accessible, and safe exercise alternative for sedentary people. Several studies have included walking as a main component of the exercise program. Buckelew et al. (57) studied the effects of 6 weeks of aerobic walking once a week combined with an unspecified home program and found improvements for the ratings of physical function, self-efficacy for function, and TeP assessment. Follow-ups showed that improvements in self-efficacy and symptoms were maintained for 1 year, while the improvements in physical activity and pain were maintained for 2 years.

In a program assessing treadmill walking and cycling, Richards et al. (51) did not find any gains in aerobic capacity or function after 3 months, but 35% of the patients reported feeling better. Exercise was started at a low intensity for a short duration, which then was gradually increased. The number of TePs decreased in the exercise and control group during the 3-month program and during the 1-year follow-up. Meyer and Lemley (45) compared the effects of low- and high-intensity walking. Improvements in function were higher in the patients who walked at low intensity compared to those who walked at high intensity. However, the number of participants was small, and the drop-out rate was high. Subjects had been provided with a description of the walking program, and the unsupervised nature of the program may have contributed to the high drop-out rate.

Burckhardt et al. evaluated the impact of a 6-week education program compared to education plus aerobic and flexibility exercises or delayed treatment (55). The education included planning of outdoor walks and emphasizing the patient's experience of success more than the amount and intensity of exercise. Both intervention groups improved in quality of life and self-efficacy when compared to the control group. At 7-month to 11-month follow-up assessments, the education-only group had improved in their ratings of physical function and well-being, while the combined education and exercise group also improved in pain, fatigue, stiffness, and distress. Based on these findings, the authors concluded that the 6-week program was too short to determine the effects for functioning.

A recently published Brazilian study (53) found that walking was superior to stretching in sedentary women with FM. The exercise group underwent a supervised walking program three times a week of 45 minutes duration for 20 weeks, and the walking speed was determined according to the individual anaerobic threshold during exercise. The walking group improved in maximum oxygen uptake, vital capacity, the Fibromyalgia Impact Questionnaire (FIQ) total score, depression, and mental health when compared to the stretching group. Sixty-six percent of the patients in the exercise group gained at least 15% improvement of their VO_{2max} but so did 33% of the participants in the stretching group, which was not expected. The improvements in the control group were suggested to depend on decrease of pain and an increased effort during the aerobic test.

Adverse effects of walking have been reported in only one study. Nichols and Glen (37) allocated patients to either 20 minutes of aerobic walking three times per week for 8 weeks at 60% to 70% of their predicted maximum heart rate or to a control group. No differences were found for pain, but patients in the aerobic walking group reported impaired functional ability after the trial. To summarize, aerobic walking programs at varying intensities appear to improve function, reduce symptom severity, and enhance overall health in patients with FM.

POOL EXERCISE

Pool exercise is a common therapeutic modality for patients with rheumatic diseases. Exercise programs consist of aerobic, endurance, and flexibility exercises, sometimes supplemented with relaxation and body awareness training. Temperate pool water commonly ranges from 30°C to 34°C, which is supposed to reduce stiffness and to alleviate pain. The viscosity of water provides resistance required in aerobic and endurance exercises, while the buoyancy of water facilitates the performance of movements.

Gowans (58) evaluated the effects of a 6-week pool exercise program, performed twice a week, combined with an educational program. Patients in the exercise group demonstrated improvements in aerobic performance (6-minute walk test) and ratings of fatigue, sleep, and well-being compared to an untreated waiting list control group. At the 6-month follow-up the exercises showed lasting improvements in aerobic performance, symptoms, and well-being. In a subsequent study, Gowans et al. (48) examined the impact of a 23-week aerobic land and water-based exercise program on physical function and mood. Fifty-seven male and female patients diagnosed with FM were enrolled and allocated to either a progressive land and pool-based exercise program or a control group. The exercise program consisted of a 30-minute exercise class, with 10 minutes of stretching and 20 minutes of aerobic exercise, performed three times a week for 23 weeks. During the first 6 weeks, the exercise program was performed in the pool to facilitate compliance and to minimize postexercise pain. Subjects then progressed to two walking classes in a gymnasium and one pool class, where walking was progressed to intermittent jogging. Patients exercised at 60% to 75% of their maximum age-adjusted heart rate. For efficacy calculations, outcomes of 31 patients in training and control groups were included. Twenty subjects were excluded because they changed medication that could potentially affect mood or they did not attend at least 45% of the sessions. The treatment group improved in aerobic performance (6-minute walk test), depression, anxiety, mental health, and self-efficacy compared to the controls. The walk test improved 75 meters in the exercise group. These results were reduced but remained during intention-to-treat analyses.

Mannerkorpi et al. (59) randomized 69 patients either to a 6-month pool exercise program combined with a six-session educational program or to a control group that continued with their usual activities. Seven patients in the treatment group dropped out before the study start or within the first few sessions, and two more dropped out after six sessions. The pool program included aerobic, endurance, flexibility, relaxation, and body awareness exercises, and it was designed to improve overall function and well-being rather than aerobic capacity. During the first weeks the pool exercises focused on teaching patients how to perform the exercises properly and how to modify the exercises to match their threshold of pain and fatigue. Only when a patient was able to perform the movements in a harmonious flow was the patient encouraged to increase the pace and the load of exercises. The treatment group improved in aerobic performance (6-minute walk test), ratings of FM symptoms (the total score of FIQ), physical function, social function, anxiety, and depression when compared to the control group. The 6-month follow-up indicated lasting improvements for aerobic performance, physical function, social function, pain, fatigue, and distress. At 2 years, improvements for aerobic capacity, pain, fatigue, and social function were maintained (65). Most patients reported they had continued exercising after the end of the trial, not only in pools, but walking outdoors. The continued participation in exercise likely sustained the gains from the program.

Saltskår Jentoft et al. (47) compared the impact of 20 weeks of pool-based or land-based aerobic exercise on cardiovascular capacity. Thirty-four women with FM were randomized to one of the two groups. The training intensity and target muscle groups were kept as similar as possible between the two groups. Training intensity was maintained at 60% to 80% of the maximum heart rate in at least half of the training sessions. Between-group differences were found only for grip strength, which improved more in the land group than in the pool group. Within-group improvements were found for aerobic performance (cycle ergometer) and walking (100-meter), both in the pool and land exercise groups. Significant within-group improvements for symptoms were found in both groups. Pain, fatigue, stiffness, and distress improved in the pool group while improvements for fatigue and stiffness were found in the land group, indicating that pool exercise may have some additional effects on symptoms. At 6 months most improvements were maintained.

A Turkish research group recently studied the effects of pool-based exercise and balneotherapy on FM symptoms (66). Fifty patients with FM were randomized either to pool exercise or to balneotherapy—that is, passively relaxing in a temperate mineral water pool. Both groups visited the clinic three times a week for 12 weeks. Within-group improvements were found in both groups for pain, morning stiffness, sleep, TePs, global assessment, and in the FIQ. The exercise group also significantly improved in depression, while the balneotherapy group did not. The 12-week follow-up still showed significant improvements for all the symptoms in the exercise group, and in four of the eight symptom variables in the balneotherapy group. The authors conclude not only that pool-based exercise is a standard treatment, but also that balneotherapy can reduce the severity of symptoms in FM.

To summarize, pool exercise can improve aerobic performance, symptom severity, and distress in patients with FM. Aerobic and strength exercise can be performed at low, moderate, or high intensities. Since movements and exercise load can easily be adjusted to each patient's limitations, this mode of exercise can also be recommended for patients experiencing severe symptoms, exhibiting low function, or who are at risk for exercise-induced pain due to osteoarthritis, tendinitis, or myofascial trigger points.

STRENGTH TRAINING

Strengthening programs enhance muscular strength and contractility, improving patients' ability to perform activities of daily living. Patients with FM are approximately 20% to 30% weaker than their healthy counterparts and are often physically unfit (13,67). Muscle weakness may result from pathologic changes within the tissue, changes in central processing, and/or from sequelae originating from disuse.

Strengthening programs may include static or dynamic exercises, or both. Static exercises generate muscle tension without a change in muscle length or movement through joint range. These exercises are used to prevent muscle atrophy and to prevent exacerbation of symptoms. Dynamic exercises result in a lengthening or shortening of the muscle fibers, allowing the joint to move through a range of motion and generate a force. Patients with FM often complain of pain, muscle fatigue, and exacerbation of symptoms following exercise, creating uncertainty about the intensity and frequency of appropriate exercise prescription and concern about muscle microtrauma and postexertional systemic effects. Unfortunately, there is a paucity of data regarding exercise parameters for strength-training programs.

In one of the few randomized controlled trials of strength training in individuals with FM, Häkkinen (49) enrolled 22 patients with FM and 12 healthy controls in 21 weeks of progressive supervised strength training and assessed the effects of strength training on muscle force production and FM symptoms. Patients with FM were randomly allocated to participate in the exercise program or to continue usual activity. Patients in the intervention group exercised twice a week starting at 40% to 60% of their one-repetition maximum voluntary contraction and gradually increased the intensity to 60% to 80% of their one-repetition maximum. Improvements were seen in muscle strength, mood (as measured by the Beck Depression Scale), and muscle firing patterns in those patients with FM who participated in the strength training program compared to those who were allocated to the usual activity group. In another trial designed to examine the impact of strength training on muscle strength and postexertional symptoms in patients with FM, Jones et al. (50) enrolled 68 women in a 12-week progressive strengthening program. Patients were randomly allocated to the strengthening program or to flexibility exercises and guided imagery. The strengthening exercises were specifically designed to minimize nociceptive input from muscle spindles by limiting eccentric contractions and providing rest between repetitions. Patients in the progressive strengthening program used 1 to 3 lb weights and tubing and were instructed to incorporate a 4-second pause between exercises. Patients in the flexibility program performed static stretching exercises rather than ballistic exercises to minimize the likelihood of side effects from participation. At the 12-week evaluation, women in the strengthening program demonstrated significant improvements in strength on 14 assessments, including knee extensor and flexor strength, total myalgic score, pain, and external and internal shoulder rotation strength. The flexibility group demonstrated significant improvements in seven domains. There were no significant between-group differences at follow-up. Pain did not increase with exercise participation in either group, and program adherence was good. The results of this study indicate that exercises that are performed at low intensity and that are designed to reduce eccentric contractions produce significant improvements in strength without postexertional pain.

In sum, few studies independently examined the impact of strength training, whether static or dynamic, in patients with FM. Among the randomized trials focused on strengthening exercises, data indicate modest improvements in muscle strength, enhanced mood, and, possibly, fatigue reduction. When supervised, low-intensity short-term strengthening programs appear to increase muscle force production. Further research is needed to determine the proper intensity and duration of strength training exercises, the relative contribution of strength training on physical function, muscle force production, and mood state, and whether strength training is safe and effective for patients with various stages of disease severity.

EXERCISE FOR PATIENTS WITH CHRONIC FATIGUE SYNDROME

CFS is defined as severe fatigue lasting more than 6 months that is of unknown etiology. Patients with CFS and those with FM have similar clinical presentations. Both groups of patients report fatigue as a primary symptom. However, it is unclear whether fatigue arises from deficits in muscles or problems with central processing, or whether fatigue is attributed to deconditioning. Most studies in persons with CFS examine the impact of exercise in outpatient settings versus inpatient settings (68).

Bazelmans et al. (69) enrolled 20 patients with CFS and 20 healthy matched controls to compare maximal exercise

performance in each group. The researchers found no significant differences in physical fitness between patients with CFS and healthy controls. To examine the effects of 12 weeks of graded exercise on symptom presentation and fatigue in patients with CFS, Fulcher and White (40) randomized 66 patients who met the Oxford criteria for CFS to either graded aerobic exercise or stretching and relaxing exercises. Patients were excluded if they had a history of psychiatric disorder or appreciable sleep disturbance. Aerobic exercise intensity began at 40% of the peak oxygen consumption and gradually increased to 60%. The duration of exercise also increased over time until the session reached a total of 30 minutes. Fatigue, functional capacity, and fitness were significantly improved in the graded aerobic exercise group compared to the flexibility group. Improvements were maintained at 3 months and at 1 year. The aerobic exercise program was well tolerated. Patients in the flexibility group who agreed to cross over to the graded aerobic exercise program noted improvements following their participation in aerobic exercise. Powell et al. (60) allocated 148 patients with CFS to four groups: standard medical care, telephone intervention, minimal contact intervention, and maximal contact intervention. All intervention groups received two individual treatments and two follow-up calls to educate patients about the benefits of home-based graded exercise. Educational materials supplemented the in-person and telephone contacts. The telephone group received seven telephone calls of 30 minutes duration over 3 months, while the minimal intervention group received two face-to-face sessions of 3 hours duration and the maximal intervention group received an additional seven 1-hour face-to-face sessions. Physical functioning, mood, and fatigue improved in patients in the intervention groups compared to the control subjects. No significant differences were found between the three intervention groups. Marlin et al. (70) evaluated the effects of a multidisciplinary intervention for 51 patients with CFS. The researchers concluded that multimodal interventions including cognitive-behavioral therapy (CBT) and exercise are effective for patients with CFS.

Donta et al. (63) enrolled 1,092 Gulf War Veterans' Illness (GWVI) patients in a study designed to compare the effectiveness of exercise and CBT in GWVI. GWVI is characterized by persistent pain, fatigue, and cognitive symptoms. Men and women were enrolled if they presented with two or three of the following symptoms that had persisted for 6 months: persistent fatigue, musculoskeletal pain involving two or more regions of the body, and cognitive symptoms such as difficulties with memory, concentration, or attention. Researchers used extensive exclusion criteria to reduce the potential for bias and confounding. Study participants were allocated to one of four treatments: (a) CBT delivered in small groups for 60 minutes plus supervised aerobic exercise one time per week for 60 minutes and two to three times per week independently for 12 weeks in addition to usual care, (b) supervised progressive low-intensity aerobic exercise for 60 minutes once per week and two to three times per week independently for 12 weeks plus usual care, (c) CBT delivered in small groups for 60 to 90 minutes once per week for 12 weeks plus usual care, or (d) usual care. A psychologist with previous training in CBT delivered the CBT. The CBT was designed specifically to address physical function and to teach strategies to enhance problem-solving skills. The subjects' physical fitness was assessed using a submaximal bicycle exercise test. The data from the test was also used to establish exercise parameters for the subjects allocated to the exercise interventions. Physical therapists or master's level exercise physiologists supervised the progressive exercise program. They instructed subjects in stretching exercises and activity selection using a perceived exertion scale, target heart rate, and metabolic equivalents (METs). At the end of the trial all groups demonstrated improved function as measured by the SF-36, ranging from 11.5% to 18.5% despite the relatively low adherence rate to exercise sessions (50%). The greatest improvements in function were seen in the CBT alone and CBT plus exercise group, compared to the exercise alone and usual care groups. The exercise group demonstrated significant improvements across all domains of fatigue, as measured by the Multidimensional Fatigue Inventory, and in cognitive symptoms compared to the CBT alone or usual care groups. Participants in the CBT alone and CBT plus exercise group showed improvements only in affective pain as measured by the McGill Pain Questionnaire. Both treatments improved cognitive symptoms and mental health. The modest improvements found in this study may be related to group CBT versus individual CBT sessions, the variability of experience in the psychologists delivering the CBT, and the low compliance rate with sessions.

The data indicate exercise results in improved aerobic performance and function. The inclusion of CBT increases the impact of exercise on function in certain subgroups.

HEALTH EDUCATION IN REHABILITATION INTERVENTIONS

Consequences of illness are influenced by pathophysiologic factors, environmental factors, and by the manner in which individuals conceptualize and respond to their illnesses. Patient education or collaborative reasoning directed at enhancing patients' understanding and management of their disorder and symptoms commonly occurs simultaneously with clinical treatments provided by health care professionals (28,33). Also, standardized educational programs, inspired by psychosocial and cognitive theories about stress and coping (71) and self-efficacy (72), have a long tradition in clinical rheumatology (73–75). These programs are based on the rationale that health can be enhanced through self-management of symptoms and modifications in lifestyle and environment. Teaching practical skills, such as how to alleviate pain, how to apply relaxation techniques, and how to adapt work tasks and exercise to one's own limitations are often incorporated into the exercise intervention (55,59,73–75).

Randomized controlled studies evaluating the impact of physical exercise combined with an educational program demonstrated improvements in self-efficacy (55,58), symptom severity (55,58,59), aerobic performance (58,59), and well-being (55,58,59) in subjects participating in combined programs when compared to control subjects. The combination of exercise and education appears more effective than either treatment alone (61), while a study found no evidence for the hypothesis that education would enhance exercise adherence (62). To conclude, treatment programs combining education and exercise demonstrate improvements in function, symptoms, well-being, and self-efficacy and may be more effective than either one alone.

LOW- OR HIGH-INTENSITY EXERCISE

Early studies of aerobic exercise programs for patients with FM followed established exercise guidelines for healthy people and evaluated programs of vigorous physical exercise at least 20 minutes two to three sessions a week (76). However, patients with FM have variable baseline physical capacity. Some patients with FM can exercise at moderate–high intensity, as shown in an early study of McCain (34), although this is not likely for the majority of patients (62). Van Santen, comparing high- and low-intensity programs, found that the patients felt "broken down" for more than 24 hours after a high-intensity training session (52). Inability to comply with a high-intensity program due to increased postexercise pain was also found in another study attempting to compare the effects of high-intensity and low-intensity exercise (45).

However, the reviewed studies indicate that most patients can engage in low-intensity exercise or in exercise performed at self-selected intensities by adjusting the load and taking pauses during the program. If the patient has been inactive due to disabling pain, fatigue, and distress, it is wise to initiate exercise at a comfortable intensity, at approximately 40% to 50% of the maximum predicted heart rate, and to progress exercise intensity only when the patient feels able to manage it without adverse effects. Walking outdoors or on a treadmill, cycling outdoors or on an ergometer cycle, pool exercise, and flexibility exercises are recommended for all patients. Low-intensity aerobic exercises performed in a group are also recommended, with the caveat that group exercises be performed under the supervision of a trained professional until the patient has learned how to adjust the exercises to his or her limitations.

Whether physical exercise can improve disease-specific symptoms in FM has not been thoroughly studied. The randomized clinical trials produce variable results with regards to pain intensity and fatigue. The decreased number of TePs, which has been found in several trials, is indicative of improvement in patients' health status.

LONG-TERM ADHERENCE

The results of this review indicate that physical exercise is beneficial for patients with FM and related disorders. Physical exercise yields improvements in function, aerobic capacity, symptom severity, and mood. However, motivating patients to continue regular exercise is crucial for maintaining health benefits. In these trials poor adherence to the exercise regimen was due to time limitations, family commitments, employment, the impact of other comorbidities, or postexercise pain due to high-intensity exercise. A patient-provider discussion about exercise should include the rationale for the program and should elicit the patient's preferences, expectations, and perceived barriers to exercise, such as pain, fatigue, and time limitations. It is also important to gather information about previous exercise habits, the patient's self-efficacy for exercise, and perceived social support for exercise, as these factors are known to influence exercise adherence (77). Also, patients who are well-informed about the risks and benefits of exercise and who participate in discussions about alternatives are more likely to adhere to an exercise regimen (78,79). Written instructions also reinforce mutually agreed-upon goals and plans.

Exercise-induced pain may be related to an overload of local musculoskeletal structures, leading to microtrauma or tendinitis or to central sensitization resulting in a "flare" of symptoms. Persistent and severe pain and fatigue are not only disabling and distressing but may be associated with fear of deterioration. To improve adherence, exercise prescriptions should be adjusted to the patient's limitations of pain and fatigue. In general, it is best to initiate exercise at a low intensity and progress the program based on the patient's progress.

Although there are no studies comparing short and long exercise programs, long-term exercise programs are believed to yield better results than short-term ones. As exercise requires a period of adjustment, all exercise programs should be designed on a long-term basis. To enhance long-term motivation, the provider should emphasize exercises that are pleasant and enjoyable. Since patients with chronic pain often associate their body with pain, fatigue, and disabilities, it is important to highlight the body's positive experiences during exercise (80). Exercising in a group may also enhance adherence by providing an opportunity for social interactions and support (80,81). We believe that all successful exercise programs directly and indirectly teach patients how to better manage their symptoms. The goal of an exercise program is to promote regular long-term adherence to an active lifestyle to maximize functioning and well-being.

SUMMARY POINTS

- A variety of different types of exercise regimens have been shown to be helpful for treating FM and related syndromes.
- Individuals who are able to adhere to exercise long-term almost always derive benefit, both with respect to improvements in symptoms as well as improvements in function.
- The largest challenge for research in this area is to develop programs that target adherence and compliance; exercise programs that are combined with cognitive-behavioral approaches can offer promise in this regard.

■ IMPLICATIONS FOR PRACTICE

- Aerobic exercise at adequate intensity can improve aerobic capacity, function, symptoms, and well-being. Pool exercise can have additional effects on mood. Strength training at adequate load improves muscle strength.
- Exercise prescriptions should be individualized, based on the patient's baseline physical function, severity of pain and fatigue, and tolerance to exercise-induced pain.
- Postexercise pain may occur and should be acknowledged by modifying exercise prescriptions accordingly.

The patient may have overloaded sensitive tissues, activated a myofascial TeP, or developed a tendonitis, or the patient may have a "flare" of FM symptoms.
- In the presence of postexertional pain, patients should decrease exercise intensity but continue at the same frequency to prevent further lowered exercise tolerance. Gentle stretching of painful muscles enhances blood circulation and reduces muscle tension.
- Regular exercise also contributes to the prevention of coronary disease, osteoporosis, diabetes mellitus, and other diseases.

REFERENCES

1. Wolfe F. The fibromyalgia syndrome: a consensus report on fibromyalgia and disability. *J Rheumatol* 1996;23:534–539.
2. Wolfe F, Smythe HA, Yunus MB, et al. The American College of Rheumatology 1990 criteria for the classification of fibromyalgia. Report of the Multicenter Criteria Committee. *Arthritis Rheum* 1990;33:160–172.
3. Yunus M, Masi AT, Calabro JJ, et al. Primary fibromyalgia (fibrositis): clinical study of 50 patients with matched normal controls. *Semin Arthritis Rheum* 1981;11:151–171.
4. Wolfe F, Ross K, Anderson J, et al. The prevalence and characteristics of fibromyalgia in the general population. *Arthritis Rheum* 1995;38:19–28.
5. Gran TJ. The epidemiology of chronic generalized musculoskeletal pain. *Best Pract Res Clin Rheumatol* 2003;17: 547–561.
6. Mengshoel AM, Forre O, Komnaes HB. Muscle strength and aerobic capacity in primary fibromyalgia. *Clin Exp Rheumatol* 1990;8:475–479.
7. Mannerkorpi K, Burckhardt CS, Bjelle A. Physical performance characteristics of women with fibromyalgia. *Arthritis Care Res* 1994;7(3):123–129.
8. Jacobsen S, Danneskiold-Samsoe B. Dynamic muscular endurance in primary fibromyalgia compared with chronic myofascial pain syndrome. *Arch Phys Med Rehabil* 1992;73: 170–173.
9. Lindh M, Johansson G, Hedberg M, et al. Muscle fiber characteristics, capillaries and enzymes in patients with fibromyalgia and controls. *Scand J Rheumatol* 1995;24:34–37.
10. Norregaard J, Bulow PM, Lykkegaard JJ, et al. Muscle strength, working capacity and effort in patients with fibromyalgia. *Scand J Rehabil Med* 1997;29:97–102.
11. Elert JE, Rantapää-Dahlqvist SB, Henriksson-Larsén K, et al. Muscle performance, electromyography and fibre type composition in fibromyalgia and work-related myalgia. *Scand J Rheumatol* 1991;21:28–34.
12. Miller TA, Allen GM, Gandevia SC. Muscle force, perceived effort, and voluntary activation of the elbow flexors assessed with sensitive twitch interpolation in fibromyalgia. *J Rheumatol* 1996;23:1621–1627.
13. Bennett RM, Clark SR, Goldenberg L, et al. Aerobic fitness in patients with fibrositis. *Arthritis Rheum* 1989;32:454–460.
14. Nielens H, Boisset V, Masquelier E. Fitness and perceived exertion in patients with fibromyalgia syndrome. *Clin J Pain* 2000;16:209–213.
15. Henriksson C, Gundmark I, Bengtsson A, et al. Living with fibromyalgia. Consequences for everyday life. *Clin J Pain* 1992;8:138–144.
16. Hawley DJ, Wolfe F. Pain, disability and pain/disability relationship in seven rheumatic disorders: a study of 1,522 patients. *J Rheumatol* 1991;18:1552–1557.

17. Waylonis GW, Ronan PG, Gordon C. A profile of fibromyalgia in occupational environments. *Am J Phys Med Rehabil* 1994;73:112–115.

18. Wolfe F, Anderson J, Harkness D, et al. Health status and disease severity in fibromyalgia. *Arthritis Rheum* 1997;40:1571–1579.

19. Robinson RL, Birnbaum HG, Morley MA, et al. Economic cost and epidemiological characteristics of patients with fibromyalgia claims. *J Rheumatol* 2003;30:1318–1325.

20. WHO. *International classification of functioning, disability and health.* Geneva: World Health Organization, 2001.

21. Stucki G, Ewert T, Cieza A. Value and application of the ICF in rehabilitation medicine. *Disabil Rehabil* 2002;24:932–938.

22. Liedberg GM, Henriksson CM. Factors of importance for work disability in women with fibromyalgia: an interview study. *Arthritis Rheum* 2002;47:266–274.

23. Goldenberg DL, Mossey CJ, Schmid CH. A model to assess severity and impact of fibromyalgia. *J Rheumatol* 1995;22:2313–2318.

24. Mannerkorpi K, Kroksmark T, Ekdahl C. How patients with fibromyalgia experience their symptoms in everyday life. *Physiother Res Int* 1999;4:110–122.

25. Croft P, Schollum J, Silman A. Population study of tender point counts and pain as evidence of fibromyalgia. *Br Med J* 1994;309:696–699.

26. Bergman S, Herrstrom P, Jacobsson LT, et al. Chronic widespread pain: a three year follow up of pain distribution and risk factors. *J Rheumatol* 2002;29:818–825.

27. Clauw DJ, Chrousos GP. Chronic pain and fatigue syndromes: overlapping clinical and neuroendocrine features and potential pathogenic mechanisms. *Neuroimmunomodulation* 1997;4:134–153.

28. Sim J, Adams N. Therapeutic approaches for fibromyalgia syndrome in the United Kingdom: a survey of occupational therapists and physical therapists. *Eur J Pain* 2003;7:173–180.

29. Gustafsson M, Ekholm J, Broman L. Effects of a multiprofessional rehabilitation programme for patients with fibromyalgia syndrome. *J Rehabil Med* 2002;34:119–127.

30. Thieme K, Gronica-Ihle E, Flor H. Operant behavioral treatment of fibromyalgia: a controlled study. *Arthritis Care Res* 2003;49:314–320.

31. Granges G, Zilko P, Littlejohn GO. Fibromyalgia syndrome: assessment of the severity of the condition 2 years after diagnosis. *J Rheumatol* 1994;21:523–529.

32. Jones M, Jensen G, Edwards I. Clinical reasoning in physiotherapy. In: Higgs J, Jones M. *Clinical reasoning in health professions*, 2nd ed. Oxford: Butterworth-Heineman, 2002.

33. Higgs J, Jones M. *Clinical reasoning in the health professions*, 2nd ed. Oxford: Butterworth-Heineman, 2002.

34. McCain G, Bell DA, Mai FM, et al. A controlled study of the effects of a supervised cardiovascular fitness training program on the manifestations of primary fibromyalgia. *Arthritis Rheum* 1988;31:1135–1141.

35. Mengshoel AM, Komnaes HB, Forre O. The effects of twenty weeks of physical fitness training in female patients with fibromyalgia. *Clin Exp Rheumatol* 1992;10:345–349.

36. Isomeri R, Mikkelsson M, Latikka P, et al. Effects of amitriptyline and cardiovascular fitness training on pain in patients with primary fibromyalgia. *J Musculoskelet Pain* 1993;3/4:253–260.

37. Nichols DS, Glenn TM. Effects of aerobic exercise on pain perception, affect and level of disability in individuals with fibromyalgia. *Phys Ther* 1994;74:327–332.

38. Martin L, Nutting A, Macintosh BR, et al. An exercise program in the treatment of fibromyalgia. *J Rheumatol* 1996;23:1050–1053.

39. Norregaard J, Lykkegaard JJ, Mehlsen J, et al. Exercise training in treatment of fibromyalgia. *J Musculoskelet Pain* 1997;5:71–79.

40. Fulcher KY, White PD. Randomized controlled trial of graded exercise in patients with the chronic fatigue syndrome. *Br Med J* 1997;314:1647–1652.

41. Verstappen F, van Santen-Hoeuftt H, Bolwijn P, et al. Effects of a group activity program for fibromyalgia patients on physical fitness and well being. *J Musculoskelet Pain* 1997;5:17–28.

42. Wearden AJ, Morris RK, Mullis R, et al. Randomised, double-blind, placebo-controlled treatment trial of fluoxetine and graded exercise for chronic fatigue syndrome. *Br J Psychiatry* 1998;172:491–492.

43. Keel P, Bodoky C, Gerhard U, et al. Comparisons of integrated group therapy and group relaxation training for fibromyalgia. *Clin J Pain* 1998;14:232–238.

44. Ramsay C, Moreland J, Ho M, et al. An observer-blinded comparison of supervised and unsupervised aerobic exercise regimens in fibromyalgia. *Rheumatology* 2000;39:501–505.

45. Meyer BB, Lemley KJ. Utilizing exercise to affect the symptomology of fibromyalgia: a pilot study. *Med Sci Sports Exerc* 2000;10:1691–1697.

46. Meiworm L, Jakob E, Walker UA, et al. Patients with fibromyalgia benefit from aerobic endurance exercise. *Clin Rheumatol* 2000;19:253–257.

47. Saltskår Jentoft E, Grimstvedt Kvalvik A, Mengshoel AM. Effects of pool-based and land-based aerobic exercise on women with fibromyalgia/chronic widespread muscle pain. *Arthritis Care Res* 2001;45:42–47.

48. Gowans SE, deHueck A, Voss S, et al. Effect of a randomized, controlled trial of exercise on mood and physical function in individuals with fibromyalgia. *Arthritis Care Res* 2001;45:519–529.

49. Häkkinen A, Sokka T, Kotaniemi A, et al. Dynamic strength training in patients with early rheumatoid arthritis increases muscle strength but not bone mineral density. *J Rheumatol* 1999;26:1257–1263.

50. Jones KD, Burckhardt CS, Clark SR, et al. A randomized controlled trial of muscle strengthening versus flexibility training in fibromyalgia. *J Rheumatol* 2002;29:1041–1048.

51. Richards S, Scott D. Prescribed exercise in people with fibromyalgia: parallel group randomised controlled trial. *Br Med J* 2002;325:185–189.

52. van Santen M, Bolwijn P, Landewé R, et al. High or low intensity aerobic fitness training in fibromyalgia: does it matter? *J Rheumatol* 2002;29:582–587.

53. Valim V, Oliveira L, Suda A, et al. Aerobic fitness effects in fibromyalgia. *J Rheumatol* 2003;30:1060–1069.

54. Schachter CL, Busch AJ, Peloso PM, et al. Effects of short versus long bouts of aerobic exercise in sedentary women with fibromyalgia: a randomized controlled trial. *Phys Ther* 2003;83:340–358.

55. Burckhardt CS, Mannerkorpi K, Hedenberg L, et al. A randomized, controlled clinical trial of education and physical training for women with fibromyalgia. *J Rheumatol* 1994;21:714–720.

56. Wigers SH, Stiles TC, Vogel PA. Effects of aerobic exercise versus stress management treatment in fibromyalgia. *Scand J Rheumatol* 1996;25:77–86.

57. Buckelew SP, Conway R, Parker J, et al. Biofeedback/relaxation training and exercise interventions for fibromyalgia: a prospective trial. *Arthritis Care Res* 1998;11:196–209.

58. Gowans SE, deHueck A, Voss S, et al. A randomized, controlled trial of exercise and education for individuals with fibromyalgia. *Arthritis Care Res* 1999;12:120–128.

59. Mannerkorpi K, Nyberg B, Ahlmén M, et al. Pool exercise combined with an education program for patients with fibromyalgia syndrome. *J Rheumatol* 2000;27:2473–2481.

60. Powell T, Bentall RP, Nye FJ, et al. Randomised controlled trial of patient education to encourage graded exercise in chronic fatigue syndrome. *Br Med J* 2001;322:387–390.

61. King S, Wessel J, Bhambhani Y, et al. The effects of exercise and education, individually or combined, in women with fibromyalgia. *J Rheumatol* 2002;29:2620–2627.

62. van Santen M, Bolwijn P, Verstappen F, et al. A randomized clinical trial comparing fitness and biofeedback training versus basic treatment in patients with fibromyalgia. *J Rheumatol* 2002;29:575–581.

63. Donta ST, Clauw DJ, Engel CC, et al. Cognitive behavioral therapy and aerobic exercise for Gulf war veterans' illness. *JAMA* 2003;289:1396–1404.

64. Busch A, Schachter C, Peloso P, et al. Exercise for treating fibromyalgia syndrome. In: *The Cochrane library*. Oxford: Update Software, 2002.

65. Mannerkorpi K, Ahlmén M, Ekdahl C. Six and 24-month follow up of pool exercise and education for patients with fibromyalgia. *Scand J Rheumatol* 2002;31:306–310.

66. Altan L, Bingol U, Aykae M, et al. Investigation of the effects of pool-based exercise on fibromyalgia syndrome. *Rheumatol Int* 2003;24(5):272–277.

67. Simms R. Is there muscle pathology in fibromyalgia syndrome? *Rheum Clin North Am* 1996;22:245–265.

68. Lim A, Lubitz L. Chronic fatigue syndrome: successful outcome of an intensive inpatient program. *J Pediatr Child Health* 2002;38:295–299.

69. Bazelmans E, Bleijenberg G, Van Der Meer JWM, et al. Is physical deconditioning a perpetuating factor in chronic fatigue syndrome? A controlled study on maximal exercise performance and relations with fatigue, impairment and physical activity. *J Psychol Med* 2001;31:107–114.

70. Marlin RG, Anchel H, Gibson JC, et al. An evaluation of multidisciplinary intervention for chronic fatigue syndrome with long-term follow-up, and a comparison with untreated controls. *Am J Med* 1998;105:110–114.

71. Lazarus RS, Folkman S. *Stress, appraisal and coping*. New York: Springer, 1984.

72. Bandura A. Self-efficacy: toward a unifying theory of behavioral change. *Psychol Rev* 1977;84:191–215.

73. Lorig K. *Arthritis self-management. Leader's manual*. Palo Alto, CA: Stanford Arthritis Center, 1990.

74. Lorig K. *Common sense patient education*. Victoria, TX: Fraser Publications, 1991.

75. Lorig K, Holmon H. Arthritis self-management studies: a twelve year review. *Health Educ Q* 1993;20:17–28.

76. American College of Sports Medicine. The recommended quantity and quality of exercise for developing and maintaining cardiorespiratory and muscular fitness in healthy adults. *Med Sci Sports Exerc* 1998;30:975–991.

77. Oliver K, Cronan T. Predictors of exercise behaviors among fibromyalgia patients. *Prev Med* 2002;35:383–389.

78. Iversen MD, Fossel AH, Daltroy LH. Rheumatologist-patient communication about exercise and physical therapy in rheumatoid arthritis. *Arthritis Care Res* 1999;12:180–192.

79. Iversen MD, Eaton HM, Daltroy LH. How rheumatologists and patients with rheumatoid arthritis discuss exercise and the influence of discussions on exercise prescriptions. *Arthritis Rheum* 2004;51:63–72.

80. Mannerkorpi K, Gard G. Physiotherapy group treatment for patients with fibromyalgia—an embodied learning process. *Disabil Rehabil* 2003;25:1372–1380.

81. Crook P, Stott R, Rose M, et al. Adherence to group exercise. *Physiotherapy* 1998;84:366–372.

29

Cognitive and Behavioral Approaches to Chronic Pain

David A. Williams

ognitive-behavioral therapy (CBT) is a nonpharmacologic therapy that can be used to manage or treat
medical conditions. Just as there are many types of
medications, there are many types of CBT that can be
matched to specific illnesses. Just as medications induce
biochemical changes associated with healing, CBT alters
biochemical processes associated with thinking and behavior in the service of promoting healing and health. All applications of CBT share common theoretical underpinnings
about how human beings think about, learn about, and respond to illnesses. This chapter provides an overview of
those theoretical underpinnings, gives examples of appropriate therapeutic targets and of specific CBT skills for
managing chronic pain, and provides a review of empirically based support for using CBT in the treatment of fibromyalgia (FM). The chapter concludes with comments
about applying CBT in clinical practice.

BACKGROUND

THE BIOPSYCHOSOCIAL PERSPECTIVE

In order to understand why CBT has become such an important therapeutic tool in the treatment of chronic medical conditions, it helps to understand the perspective of clinicians
who use it. CBT is a therapeutic tool of the biopsychosocial
model of illness. This model attempts to account for the
complex interplay between the individual (e.g., biology,
cognition, and emotion), the environment (e.g., social and
behavioral contingencies), and illness (1). The biopsychosocial model does not draw clear distinctions between biological and psychological factors in the etiology and treatment
of illnesses and does not assume the presence of a psychiatric illness when symptoms elude a biological explanation.
This model assumes that all factors work interdependently
in both the development and resolution of illnesses.

ORIGINS OF COGNITIVE-BEHAVIORAL THERAPY

CBT was originally developed as a therapeutic intervention
for the mental illnesses and has strong empirical support for
the treatment of depression and anxiety disorders (2). In recent years the principles of CBT were applied to more traditional chronic medical conditions such as cardiovascular
disease, cancer, diabetes, asthma, and pain management
(3–5). The goal of any form of CBT is to enhance patients'
expectations for personal control by providing them with
structured learning experiences that offer predictable and effective methods of managing symptoms and concerns. Thus,
CBT is a blending of two forms of therapy: cognitive therapy and behavioral therapy. Although each application of
CBT uses a different set of specific skills, each of the skills
shares a common scientific foundation based on learning
and cognitive principles (6).

Cognitive therapy focuses on the individual's mental environment. The focus of cognitive therapy is to help individuals challenge maladaptive beliefs about their illnesses or
health, eliminate expectations for failure or helplessness,
improve self-efficacy to perform adaptive tasks, and solve
problems that block improvements in health. Cognitive therapy uses personal reflection and draws upon rational thinking to help individuals gain a clearer understanding of their
condition and the options that are available for managing illnesses more successfully (7,8).

Behavioral therapy is a natural compliment to cognitive
therapy because it focuses on the way in which the environment affects how individuals respond to illness through
learning. Knowing the many different avenues by which
learning can occur, a therapist can offer patients structured
opportunities to experience (learn) successful ways to manage their symptoms and problems. These newly learned
skills support the revision of beliefs and expectations regarding the amount of predictability and personal control
one can have over illness. For example, studies show that despite patients' expectations that a pill is the best approach to

treating fibromyalgia syndrome (FMS), exercise and CBT each have equally strong (if not stronger) effects on the symptoms of FMS as medications (9). Most patients, however, will not believe that a "pill-less" intervention will work for them. Thus patients must learn first hand, by trying out various self-management skills, that success is possible with personal effort. Once success is experienced, the patient will find it hard to hold on to the expectation that a pill is the only way to obtain some relief. Getting patients to take that first attempt, however, is one of the most difficult problems clinicians face. Small gradual success is generally best, and good rapport and trust between physician and patient is perhaps the best way to guide patients into treatment options with benefits that are known but that may be inconsistent with initial patient expectations. CBT therapists are also keenly aware that the same forms of learning that promote well-being can also lead to maladaptive experiences. Thus the CBT therapist must be equally facile at facilitating learning as well as interrupting the learned contingencies that maintain maladaptive behavior. Behavior therapy draws upon a number of well-established models of learning, including classical conditioning, operant conditioning, social modeling, and instructional learning.

COGNITIVE-BEHAVIORAL THERAPY IN THE MANAGEMENT OF CHRONIC PAIN

THERAPEUTIC TARGETS OF COGNITIVE-BEHAVIORAL THERAPY FOR CHRONIC PAIN

Historically the most common targets of CBT for pain have been improvements in mood, physical functioning, and pain. The next section reviews how these targets are considered in the context of CBT, where changes in emotions, beliefs, and behavior act as therapeutic agents.

Emotions

Strong evidence supports using CBT with anxiety and depressive disorders, making CBT especially well-suited for treating the common comorbid mood disorders of chronic pain. Depression has 1.6% to 2.9% prevalence in community samples (10) but can range between 30% and 54% in tertiary chronic-pain clinics (11), 14% and 23% for arthritic samples, and 26% and 71% for FM (12). Anxiety disorders also co-occur with chronic-pain conditions. The point prevalence of an anxiety disorder in the general population is 7%, but anxiety disorders such as panic disorder and posttraumatic stress disorder are being increasingly identified as comorbid psychiatric concerns in patients with chronic pain (13).

Changes in mood need not be at pathologic levels (e.g., disordered) for pain perception to be influenced. Evidence from brain imaging data suggests that the afferent central processing of pain is highly dependent upon even subclinical psychological factors to produce the experience of pain (14). Sufficient differences in the clinical presentations of mood disorders and of chronic-pain conditions such as FM have led researchers to conclude that FM and depression are distinct, albeit often co-occurring, entities (15,16). Thus, just as two

medications may be needed to treat two coexisting conditions, it is recommended that when mood disorders are coexpressed with chronic pain both get treated, but as separate entities—which may require separate therapists and separate protocols.

Beliefs

Chronic pain is often considered a major impediment to patients' personal goals. When faced with chronic pain, patients choose between actively overcoming pain-related barriers (e.g., self-corrective actions, compensatory behaviors, altering unsatisfactory life circumstances) and accommodating pain into their lives (e.g., downgrading expectations, positively reappraising failures, revising self-evaluations and personal goals in accordance with perceived deficits) (17). Both approaches can be helpful, and CBT attempts to offer structured "real-life" learning experiences that facilitate these processes. Before patients are open to the idea of trying such learning experiences, however, the CBT therapist must address the common assumption that there is little role for personal effort in the management of illnesses. The basis of this belief typically comes from past failures in this regard, a lack of ideas or skills for self-management, or a lack of guidance and support in adopting more control.

When patients have a history of failures at controlling health, this learned history can support beliefs in helplessness (e.g., learned helplessness) or beliefs that personal effort does not matter in achieving desired outcomes (i.e., external locus of control). Both learned helplessness and an external locus of control are common in patients with chronic pain (18–20) and unfortunately weaken patients' motivation to use self-management strategies. In studies of patients with chronic pain and rheumatologic conditions, a stronger belief in an external locus of control for pain control has been repeatedly associated with greater physical and psychological symptoms and with poorer response to therapy (20–23).

The fostering of an internal locus of control (i.e., believing personal effort affects outcomes) and enhancing beliefs in self-efficacy (i.e., believing in one's ability to perform a specific task) can facilitate improved outcomes. In studies of patients with FM, internal locus of control has been associated with better affect, reduced symptom severity, and less functional disability (20). Beliefs in self-efficacy may or may not reflect actual ability, but perception of self-efficacy influences choices, decisions, and responses to options that can determine the course of an illness (24). In rheumatologic studies, improvements in self-efficacy were highly predictive of improvements in pain, depression, and health status (25). In studies of FM, several studies using both exercise and CBT were helpful in improving this set of beliefs (26,27).

Behaviors

Sometimes patients simply lack the necessary skills for coping with pain and loss of function, such as using exercise to maintain functional status, confiding in others when pain gets intense, or being willing to rely on oneself to reduce tension. Studies of rheumatologic pain suggest that even if coping skills are initially missing, they can be rapidly taught to patients. After such training, osteoarthritis (OA) and rheumatoid arthritis (RA) patients have shown significant improvements in pain and physical disability (28). Improvements in pain and functional status have also been associated with coping skills training in patients with FM (29–31).

When faced with pain, some patients withdraw socially while others become solicitous of help and comfort from others. Temporarily withdrawing to lessen demands from others and regroup mentally may have advantages if this private time facilitates planning for better functioning. Withdrawing long-term, however, may be maladaptive, as longitudinal studies of pain link poor social support with poorer prognoses (32). For many, social support not only offers emotional comfort but also is a source of knowledge for developing additional coping skills and a source of reinforcement for maintaining difficult behavioral programs designed to promote health (e.g., exercise, diet). In general, social support helps pain management, but only if that support is perceived as wanted and of good quality (33).

STRUCTURING A COGNITIVE-BEHAVIORAL THERAPY INTERVENTION FOR CHRONIC PAIN

In application, CBT-based interventions typically include three phases: (1) an educational phase—in which patients learn a model for understanding how and why CBT (a nonpharmacologic intervention) might be helpful, (2) a skills training phase—in which training is provided in a variety of cognitive and behavioral skills aimed at increasing the amount of control the individual can use to predictably and successfully manage problems and symptoms, and (3) an application phase—in which patients learn to apply their skills in progressively more challenging real-life situations. The most common method of delivering CBT is the so-called "smorgasbord" approach where in each session a new and different skill is introduced, tried, and practiced by each patient. An alternative approach capitalizes on the fact that CBT skills are not independent of one another but can be directed toward both a specific therapeutic target and the enhancement of other CBT skills. The following section outlines one approach for structuring a CBT intervention for chronic pain. This approach teaches several basic skills common to all CBT approaches, encourages adoption and practice of several pain-specific skills, and offers a variety of CBT skills that are non-pain-specific but that facilitate the removal of barriers impeding the application of pain management skills in real life or over the long term.

Skill Set A: Education and Cognitive-behavioral Therapy Basics

Given that CBT is very different from taking a pill or relying on a clinician to "fix something," education in CBT helps patients form an important understanding about how and why self-management skills can be helpful in managing pain. Common examples of educational topics include background on what is known about pain and FM, what interventions are useful and why, the gate control theory of pain (34), and an explanation of the biopsychosocial model (1).

Two behavioral skills used by nearly all self-management approaches are behavioral self-monitoring and goal setting. When a medication is given, its presence and actions are often monitored by evaluating lab values. Since this is not possible with behavioral interventions, self-monitoring helps to objectify (i.e., make countable) both symptoms and the use of behavioral strategies over time. Self-monitoring also helps patients identify associations between the use of the interventions and their symptoms. Strong associations between the use of behavioral strategies and decreases in pain reinforce continued use of those strategies. Once monitoring has begun and baseline levels of symptoms are identified, goals can be set for achieving a desired outcome. Goal setting is the process of identifying a desired outcome (e.g., pain level, activity level, number of social encounters) and devising a plan for attaining that outcome. Goals are most often attained when they involve a slight amount of challenge and are specifically defined (e.g., "walk two miles" vs. "get active") and the individual believes that the goal is realistic and attainable. Proper attention to these basic skills early in the therapeutic process (i.e., self-monitoring and goal setting) can help enhance adherence to the more specific skills associated with pain management.

Skill Set B: Pain Management Skills

Some CBT skills appear to have the ability to directly reduce symptoms of pain, whereas others may indirectly affect pain while having a greater impact on pain-related issues such as diminished function. The next four skills are those that appear to have a relatively strong impact specific to pain symptoms.

Relaxation Skills

Patients can learn the relaxation response as a rapid means of reducing pain intensity. The relaxation response is a physiologically based learned response that involves quieting physiologic activity (e.g., muscle tension, heart rate, and breathing) through active and focused mental effort. Although there is no consensus on the best method of teaching the relaxation response (e.g., progressive muscle relaxation, visual imagery, hypnosis, biofeedback), all appear to offer equally useful modalities for learning it. The relaxation response has strong support as a method to manage both pain and insomnia and can lead to improved functioning and concentration (35). The relaxation response is perhaps the single most studied CBT skill for the management of pain.

Aerobic Exercise

Aerobic exercise has been demonstrated to be effective at improving outcomes for a wide range of chronic medical conditions, including FM. The reason for the benefits of exercise in these conditions is likely multifactorial. Aerobic exercise leads to an analgesic effect, probably mediated in part by the release of endogenous opioids (36). Aerobic activity may also increase well-being and control and exert an antidepressant or calming effect (37–39). To reduce the pain associated with exercise, nonimpact exercises such as walking, swimming, or stationary cycling are often recommended. Standard daily or leisure activities such as walking to the mailbox, climbing the stairs at work, and walking from the parking lot to the office can also be considered exercise. Whatever type of activity is chosen, investigators have found a gradual progression in exercise intensity and a focus on adherence to a lifelong program to be most effective (40,41). Although not a behavior learned in traditional CBT, adopting exercise represents a difficult behavioral change. In addition, because exercise must be maintained over time to be effective in improving FM symptoms, it is vulnerable to the same barriers facing any behavioral strategy targeting improved health. Thus self-monitoring and goal setting, as well as many of the CBT skills discussed later in this chapter as facilitating behavioral change, can be applied to help patients maintain exercise over time.

Sleep Hygiene

Sleep disturbances are common in patients with chronic pain. Behavioral strategies that focus on improved sleep (e.g., onset, maintenance, quality), can help individuals get needed restorative sleep with additional benefits in improved mood, better management of pain, less fatigue, and improved mental clarity (42). Sleep hygiene strategies focus on timing strategies (e.g., having regular sleep routines), sleep behaviors (e.g., attempting to sleep only when in need of sleep), and behavioral avoidance of stimulating activities before bed, such as emotionally charged conversations, action movies, and nicotine or caffeine. CBT that targets sleep appears to have a direct impact on pain symptoms and on the interference with goal attainment that has been associated with poor sleep (43,44).

Pleasant Activity Scheduling

Most patients with chronic pain will report that they barely get the essential activities accomplished and that they have very little time for enjoyable activities. This is unfortunate given the benefits of positive mood on pain reduction. Enjoying pleasant activities is a natural way to elevate mood (45). Exposing patients to new pleasurable activities promotes positive affect, new opportunities for social interaction, and confidence in one's body to function at a higher level. This in turn can enhance self-efficacy and a sense of control over pain. With pleasant activity scheduling, patients learn to broaden their range of pleasurable activities by scheduling them into their routine. Scheduling is preferable to spontaneity, given that spontaneity may never occur, or if it does, may occur at a time when the patient is vulnerable to overdoing and risking increased pain.

Skill Set C: Maintenance Strategies

The next set of CBT skills, referred to as maintenance strategies, might directly decrease pain. But when used in conjunction with the pain-specific skills or with one another, they might help eliminate barriers that impede integration of CBT skills into real-life situations or long-term use.

Time–Based Pacing Skills/Graded Activation

Many patients unwittingly worsen pain on "good days" by doing more than personal limitations allow. This overactivity is followed by several "bad days" of symptom flares. An intermittent burst of activity followed by increased pain is a source of frustration for patients, as the ability to plan and predict function becomes limited. Time-based pacing is a method that can improve physical functioning while minimizing the likelihood of pain flare-ups. This approach has been successfully applied to low back populations (46), to rheumatologic populations (47), and to patients having chronic fatigue syndrome (48). The key to this strategy is to limit activities based upon time rather than upon patients' subjective experience of pain or task completion. Active time can be as short as several minutes or as long as several hours depending upon what the patient can initially tolerate without exacerbation. Once a time-based activity program is in place, the therapist and the patient work together to develop a plan that achieves mutually agreed-upon goals for steadily increasing the amount of time spent on specified targeted behaviors (i.e., graded activation). Time-based pacing can be used as a complimentary skill to help insure the long-term application of exercise regimens, work-related activities, and pleasant activities, such as social outings and sports activities.

Problem-solving Strategies and Assertiveness Training

Individuals having chronic pain face interpersonal and functional problems that most healthy individuals never need to consider. Programmatic problem-solving strategies can be taught to patients that help to break large problems down into solvable pieces (49,50). What is taught in therapy is a strategy for solving problems, not solutions to individual problems—thus patients learn a strategy that can be carried into the future as new problems arise. When applied successfully, patients learn to overcome barriers and attain a greater sense of control over the process of adapting to a chronic illness. Since problems of an interpersonal nature are common, assertive communication skills training (51,52) can also be used to help patients obtain the type of assistance or social support they desire in their attempts to improve their condition. Success in problem solving or assertiveness can in turn enhance one's self-efficacy for illness self-management.

Attributional Change

Strong conviction in ones' helplessness, the futility of trying to control illness, and the inability to contribute meaningfully to others are examples of learned automatic thinking patterns that impede the use of CBT skills, evoke negative affect, and exacerbate pain. Cognitive restructuring (7) is one cognitive skill that verbally challenges the rationality of automatic thoughts and seeks to instill thinking that promotes greater function and well-being. This skill is often confused with "positive thinking," which can be perceived as invalid and unrealistic if the suggested thinking patterns are too far outside the perceived reality of the patient with pain. Changes in thinking (or specifically changes in self-efficacy) are best elicited by exposing patients to real-life learning opportunities in which patients can experience success associated with changes in their behavior (53). Thus, contrasting real successful performance with negative automatic thoughts of helplessness begins to lay a foundation for believable revisions in one's beliefs about the manageability of illness.

EVIDENCE SUPPORTING THE USE OF COGNITIVE-BEHAVIORAL THERAPY IN FIBROMYALGIA SYNDROME

DOES COGNITIVE-BEHAVIORAL THERAPY FOR PAIN REALLY WORK?

Numerous studies have successfully explored the utility of CBT with specific forms of pain, including low back pain (54), rheumatologic conditions such as OA and RA (28,55–57), sickle-cell pain (58), headache (59), and burns (60). Summarizing the findings of many of these studies, a review article of CBT trials for chronic pain credited CBT with the ability to produce significant improvements across multiple outcome domains (61). The success of CBT in these other chronic-pain conditions supported the rationale for applying CBT to cases of FM (62), given that the etiology of FM is still largely unknown (63) and the application of pharmacologic agents for symptom palliation continues to help only a minority of cases over the long term (64).

Due to differences in nomenclature, many more studies than those claiming to have used CBT have taught skills to patients with FM using the principles of behavioral and cognitive change. Referring to these skills as "CBT-supported," the next section will review some of the clinical studies fitting this description under three categories: (a) interventions where CBT-supported skills are studied as single modalities, (b) studies in which CBT-supported skills are combined with other nonpharmacologic interventions, and (c) treatment comparison studies.

STUDIES SUPPORTING THE USE OF SINGLE MODALITY COGNITIVE-BEHAVIORAL THERAPY

A few investigations have studied single modalities of CBT, such as studies of relaxation or studies of social support. When studied in isolation, relaxation appears to be best at reducing pain intensity (35), whereas social aspects of CBT appear to affect distress and cognitive factors. Descriptions of several such studies follow.

Biofeedback Assisted Relaxation Training

One of the earliest investigations of a behavioral intervention for FM was the application of electromyography (EMG)-assisted relaxation training (i.e., biofeedback) (65). Six patients were trained in progressive muscle relaxation. The effectiveness of patients' attempts to relax was verified and reinforced through EMG feedback so as to help patients learn how to more effectively produce the relaxation response in their musculature. Six other patients were assigned to a control condition in which false feedback negated any reinforcement that would have contributed to learning the relaxation response. Each group attended their respective biofeedback sessions for 15 twice-weekly sessions. Outcomes for this study included a visual analog scale (VAS) pain rating, tender point (TeP) count, and report of morning stiffness. Analyses between groups were not

reported, but only the accurate biofeedback condition realized pre-posttreatment improvements in VAS pain and morning stiffness. Both groups showed an improvement in TeP counts, suggesting that simple attention (contained in both forms of biofeedback) might help to improve tender points.

Stress Reduction

Two studies from the same working group have suggested that stress-reduction techniques (based largely on relaxation) benefit patients with FM. The first was a single group design that taught CBT-supported stress-reduction techniques in ten weekly 2-hour sessions (66). By using stress-reduction strategies, FM patients gained a 20% improvement in control over pain and substantial reductions in a variety of distress indicators. In a similar study, 42 patients were offered the same stress-management program, 18 were assigned to a wait list control group, and 24 were randomly selected from FM patients showing no interest in the stress-management program. Results indicated that the stress-management program showed significant reduction in pain ratings, whereas the other two groups failed to realize the same benefit in the same time period (67).

Relaxation Alone Versus Mixed Skills Cognitive-behavioral Therapy

In a study that isolated the effects of relaxation from a mixed grouping of skills, relaxation by itself failed to show the benefits across multiple outcomes domains that a mixed skills approach showed. This study combined education, pain-coping skills (including relaxation), social support, and exercise into 15 weekly 2-hour group sessions. The comparison group received only relaxation training in 15 weekly 50-minute sessions. Each group contained 16 patients, and treatment success was determined on the basis of showing improvements in three of six potential outcome measures (i.e., medication use, physical therapy use, sleep improvement, global impression of change, symptoms checklist, or pain rating). Thirty-one percent of the mixed skills therapy group met criteria for success, whereas 0% of the relaxation-only group met the same multidomain criteria (68).

Social Support Versus Mixed Skills Cognitive-behavioral Therapy

One of the few studies to focus on social support compared a mixed set of CBT-supported skills (i.e., education, relaxation, behavioral pacing, social support) to a purely education group that included social support (69). Both interventions were delivered in ten 90-minute group sessions over a 10-week period. Sample sizes for the CBT-supported group and the education/support group were 48 and 38, respectively. At 6-months follow-up, both treatment groups demonstrated improvements in pain behavior, depressive symptoms, myalgic scores, helplessness, and coping. Thus, in this study similar types of improvements were noted whether CBT-supported skills were present or not. This study calls into question the incremental utility of the CBT-supported skills used in this study (i.e., pacing, relaxation) for the outcomes studied while highlighting the potential multidomain impact of social support.

STUDIES SUPPORTING MULTIMODAL AND MULTIDISCIPLINARY USE OF COGNITIVE-BEHAVIORAL THERAPY

Due to its theoretical ties to the biopsychosocial model, CBT as applied to medical conditions tends not to be used as a stand-alone intervention but rather as a companion to other physical modalities. Many of the multimodal and multidisciplinary studies of CBT report benefits when CBT was added to other forms of treatment, given its ability to affect multiple outcome domains of relevance when multiple skills are applied.

Cognitive-behavioral Therapy in an Inpatient Multidisciplinary Pain Program

Several studies have used inpatient pain programs to study CBT. In one study patients with FM attended an inpatient program that included CBT-supported skills in relaxation, coping skills, pacing, and exercise. This single group study found significant improvements in pain, pain behaviors, control over pain, and distress in the 25 individuals receiving this treatment after 3 months (30). In a 30-month follow-up report, the effects of this intervention appeared to be robust, with 22 of the original 25 patients showing maintenance of treatment gains (70). Unfortunately, no control group was included in this study.

A second inpatient study that did include a control group randomly assigned patients with FM to either a standard medical program emphasizing physical therapy ($n = 21$) or to a CBT intervention composed of behavioral medication schedules, increasing activity, and behavioral management of family and social factors ($n = 40$). Both conditions used a group format, and patients met daily over 5 weeks. Sixty-five percent of the CBT group showed clinically significant improvements in targeted areas, whereas 0% of the control condition showed benefit and in fact showed evidence of deterioration (71).

Cognitive-behavioral Therapy in Outpatient Multidisciplinary Pain Programs

Several studies have applied CBT within the context of a large multidisciplinary outpatient pain program. In one, 48 participants were given an intervention consisting of education, physical therapy, occupational therapy, and CBT-supported pain management skills. Delivered in a brief format consisting of three half-day sessions in the first week followed by one half-day session during weeks 2 to 4 (i.e., a total of six half-day sessions), this overall program found significant improvements in pain ratings, distress, and functional disability (29). No control group was used in this study.

A multidisciplinary intervention using CBT that did use a control group offered CBT-supported skills in the context of education, behavioral modification, stress management, instructions in fitness, and social support. The frequency of these sessions was 24 90-minute group sessions. The program had 104 participants, with 70% achieving reductions in TeP counts below 11 and improvements on the Fibromyalgia Impact Questionnaire (FIQ) of at least 25%. Although this was not a randomized trial, a comparison group of FM patients who did not participate in the group failed to show any of the program's benefits. In addition, 33 group participants who were followed for 2 years continued to show benefits from the program, supporting the program's robust effects (72).

Studies of the Effect of Combining Cognitive-behavioral Therapy with Exercise

One of the earliest studies to support the combined use of CBT-supported skills with exercise was a single group design that followed 16 patients through a ten-session intervention. The intervention consisted simply of cognitive problem-solving skills and exercise. Reductions in reported pain were noted immediately posttreatment and at 6 months, as were positive adjustments to lifestyle (73).

A second study in this category compared an exercise/education intervention to a waiting list control condition (74). The exercise consisted of two exercise classes in which patients reached 60% to 75% of their maximal heart rate combined with 12 group sessions covering a variety of educational and CBT-supported skill topics. These educational sessions met twice weekly for 6 weeks. Compared to the waiting list control group, the treated group showed improvements in fatigue, physical movement, and well-being after just 6 weeks. Long-term data were not available for this study.

In a more recent study, 37 patients were offered aquatic-based exercise therapy plus education (75). Pool-based exercise was offered for 35 minutes for 24 weekly sessions. In addition to exercise, all subjects received six 1-hour educational sessions that included CBT-supported skills in coping and lectures on the benefits of activity. The control sample for this study was a group of 32 patients receiving standard medical care for FM. After 6 months significant differences were noted between the groups, with the CBT/exercise group showing improvement on measures of pain, physical functioning, grip strength, walking ability, anxiety and depression, and the total (FIQ). Although the results of this controlled study are quite positive for the patients that remained in the study, it should be noted that, like the other studies involving exercise, adherence was problematic, with 24% of the exercise/education group dropping out of treatment before completing it.

Incremental Utility of Cognitive-behavioral Therapy

It is often difficult to determine the unique contribution of CBT when CBT is delivered concomitantly with other forms of treatment. Several studies have applied study designs that examine the incremental value of adding CBT above and beyond an existing standard of care.

Forty-nine patients with FM were assigned to an education/exercise/cognitive skills group that met for 12 sessions in 6 weeks. This was compared to an education/exercise group that was devoid of the cognitive skills component ($n = 39$). Finally, a third group was a waitlisted control group ($n = 43$). Comparisons between baseline and 12 months follow-up revealed within-group improvements over 12 months for both treatment groups on pain coping and pain control, but no between-group differences for the active treatment groups were noted. The authors concluded that cognitive skills added little to the outcomes but did increase both costs and the therapy burden for staff and patients (76). It should be noted, however, that failure to achieve better results in the cognitive group could have been due to the unusually low educational level of patients used in this study. Additionally, compliance in the group receiving cognitive skills was also low, calling into question whether the active intervention was delivered as intended. This application of CBT was also a bit atypical, as it emphasized cognitive skills while lacking some of the more common behavioral skills used with pain.

In a second study that recruited a particularly challenging sample of patients with FM, an intervention-labeled education that included knowledge about FM and CBT-supported coping skills training such as relaxation was compared to the same education group plus aerobic exercise or to a delayed treatment control group (27). The education/CBT only condition was delivered over 6 weeks in six 90-minute group sessions and the combination education/exercise group added an additional 1 hour per week of exercise. The study sample was particularly challenging as 25% were severely depressed at baseline and 62% were sick-listed. Outcomes that tend to improve in other studies (e.g., pain and function) did not show improvement in this study of extremely disabled patients. What did change, however, was self-efficacy to improve pain and function as well as quality of life. Both groups, the education/CBT plus exercise combination group in particular, appeared to have provided sufficient learning and success experiences to improve self-efficacy, a difficult yet necessary first step in a behavioral program of this nature.

A third study compared standard pharmacologic symptom management in combination with instruction in exercise to the same standard care condition, but to it was added six 1-hour group sessions of CBT that targeted improvements in functional status (31). At 12 months posttreatment, 25% of the patients receiving the additional CBT realized significant improvements in self-reported physical functional status but only 12% of the patients receiving standard care did. The authors concluded that the addition of six brief sessions of CBT to standard care can more than double the number of patients who can receive clinically relevant benefits in functional status. The authors also noted that 75% of the patients receiving CBT failed to gain lasting improvements in functional status, suggesting that the form of CBT used in this study worked extremely well for a subgroup of patients but not for all.

TREATMENT COMPARISON STUDIES

Several studies have sought to test whether CBT is better than other forms of intervention for FM. Rather than assessing the incremental value of adding CBT to an existing standard of care, these studies pit CBT against another form of therapy. The value of such studies may be drawn into question, given that different forms of therapy may interact with the body quite differently, meaning that the relevant outcomes for one form of therapy (e.g., changes in mood) may not be the strength or target of another form of therapy (e.g., improvements in physical capacity). Nevertheless, when CBT is pitted against other forms of therapy (e.g., pharmacologic or physically based modalities), it demonstrates benefits for some patients with FM and at times slightly superior benefits in aggregate (9).

Stress Management versus Aerobic Exercise

One such study compared the benefits of stress management to that of aerobic exercise (41). The aerobic exercise group consisted of 42 45-minute sessions over 14 weeks that had patients achieve 60% to 75% of their maximal heart rate. Twenty subjects were in this condition. Stress management was delivered to 20 patients in 20 90-minute sessions spaced as follows: twice weekly for 6 weeks and then once weekly for 8 weeks. This study also utilized a standard care control condition in which 20 patients participated. Pain report (VAS) and TeP count was improved in both the exercise and stress-management groups compared to the standard care control group. Additionally, exercise was better than stress management in improving measures of fatigue and work capacity, whereas stress management was better than exercise for symptoms of depression.

Education versus Biofeedback versus Exercise versus Combined Exercise/Biofeedback

In a complex study, FM patients were randomly assigned to one of four groups: (a) biofeedback (cognitive and muscular relaxation) delivered to 29 patients in six individual training sessions over 6 weeks, (b) exercise (strength, mobility, endurance) for 30 patients with session frequency matched to biofeedback, (c) a combination of biofeedback and exercise for 30 patients with timing matched to the other two groups, and (d) an educational/attentional control group (with no cognitive problem solving) for 30 patients with timing matched to the other three groups (26). In this study all three active treatment groups produced improvements in self-efficacy to control pain and improve function. TeP counts also improved for all three active groups. The exercise alone and the combination group demonstrated additional benefits in physical functioning. Longer term (e.g., 2 years), the combination group (i.e., exercise/CBT) demonstrated the best maintenance of gains in TeP count, improvements in physical functioning, and improvements in self-efficacy. In contrast, the educational control group not only failed to share in these improvements but also actually deteriorated over time—a finding similar to the inpatient study previously described (71).

SUMMARY AND PRACTICE ISSUES

As was evident from the literature cited, CBT can be composed of many different skills that can be offered alone or in combination with other skills, in group or individual formats, in varying durations of treatment, and with varying outcomes targeted. This lack of standardization can be troublesome for those more familiar with standard drug formulations, but it also reflects the enormous differences between pharmacologic approaches and behavioral interventions. Given that most forms of CBT are delivered face-to-face with a human therapist, it would be impossible to standardize all the interpersonal elements comprising the therapist-patient relationship. Some attempts have been made to standardize the content of therapy through published treatment manuals, but these manuals still fail to address the interpersonal relationship that is likely to be a key ingredient in promoting change and adherence to a behavioral program. Additional considerations that can affect the success of CBT include the degree of therapist training, the presence of comorbid psychiatric considerations, the presence of disability, the degree of adherence to multiple facets of treatment, and how strongly the skills are linked to underlying behavioral theory. Although both group and individual formats can be successful, differing benefits appear to be associated with each format. When CBT is delivered in a group format, greater efficiency at less cost is possible, while individual sessions may be preferable for maximized tailoring of content into patients' lifestyles.

From the existing literature it cannot be stated that CBT cures FM or that all who receive it will benefit significantly. It does, however, appear that in this syndrome, characterized by chronic pain and diminished functioning, there is a subset of individuals who will demonstrate some, or even substantial, improvements if offered CBT in conjunction with pharmacologic management or exercise, or both. To integrate CBT more fully into clinical care, studies are needed to demonstrate generalization of treatment effects to population-based samples, to explore the underlying mechanisms of FM and develop CBT-supported skills that address those mechanisms, to devise better ways of matching skills to patients' capabilities, and to develop improved methods of delivering CBT to a broader group of patients on a less costly, but still effective, basis.

■ IMPLICATIONS FOR PRACTICE

- Clinicians need not wait until their treatments have failed before involving therapists with knowledge of CBT.
- CBT may be more effective if implemented early in the course of a patient's illness.
- When depression and FM co-occur and CBT is being used to treat depression, it is probably best *not* to use the same CBT therapist for both conditions.
- Not all mental health professionals have experience in applying CBT to medical conditions. Postdoctoral fellowships in behavioral medicine help to train clinicians with backgrounds in the principles underlying CBT with application toward medical diseases.
- Specific outcomes must be kept in mind when designing a CBT intervention.
- Individual sessions offer more intense opportunities for learning and tailoring of treatment, but group sessions offer social support and greater efficiency at less cost.
- Monitoring adherence to skills and making sure successful learning of skills is occurring is essential to determining if the therapy is being used as intended.

ACKNOWLEDGMENT

Preparation of this manuscript was supported in part by Department of Army grant DAMD17-00-2-0018.

REFERENCES

1. Engel GL. The need for a new medical model: a challenge for biomedicine. *Science* 1977;196(4286):129–136.
2. Chambless DL, Sanderson WC, Shoham V, et al. An update on empirically validated therapies. *Clin Psychol* 1996;49:5–18.
3. Chambless DL, Baker MJ, Baucom DH, et al. Update on empirically validated therapies, II. *Clin Psychol* 1998;51(1):3–16.
4. Compas BE, Haaga DA, Keefe FJ, et al. Sampling of empirically supported psychological treatments from health psychology: smoking, chronic pain, cancer, and bulimia nervosa. *J Consult Clin Psychol* 1998;66(1):89–112.
5. Emmelkamp PM, van Oppen P. Cognitive interventions in behavioral medicine. *Psychother Psychosom* 1993;59(3-4):116–130.
6. Craighead LW, Craighead WE, Kazdin AE, et al. *Cognitive and behavioral interventions: an empirical approach to mental health problems.* Boston, MA: Allyn and Bacon, 1994.
7. Beck AT, Rush AJ, Shaw BF, et al. *Cognitive therapy and depression.* New York: The Guilford Press, 1979.
8. Lazarus RS, Folkman S. *Stress, appraisal, and coping.* New York: Springer, 1984.
9. Rossy LA, Buckelew SP, Dorr N, et al. A meta-analysis of fibromyalgia treatment interventions. *Ann Behav Med* 1999;21(2):180–191.
10. Blazer DG, Kessler RC, McGonagle KA, et al. The prevalence and distribution of major depression in a national community sample: the National Comorbidity Survey. *Am J Psychiatry* 1994;151(7):979–986.
11. Banks S, Kerns RD. Explaining high rates of depression in chronic pain: a diathesis-stress framework. *Psychol Bull* 1996;119(1):95–110.
12. Bradley LA, Alberts KR. Psychological and behavioral approaches to pain management for patients with rheumatic disease. *Rheum Dis Clin North Am* 1999;25(1):215–232.
13. Eisendrath SJ. Psychiatric aspects of chronic pain. *Neurology* 1995;45(12 Suppl 9):S26–S34.
14. Price DD. Psychological and neural mechanism of the affective dimension of pain. *Science* 2000;288(5472):1769–1772.
15. Okifuji A, Turk DC, Sherman JJ. Evaluation of the relationship between depression and fibromyalgia syndrome: why aren't all patients depressed? *J Rheumatol* 2000;27(1):212–219.
16. Campbell LC, Clauw DJ, Keefe FJ. Persistent pain and depression: a biopsychosocial perspective. *Biol Psychiatry* 2003;54(3):399–409.
17. Schmitz U, Saile H, Nilges P. Coping with chronic pain: flexible goal adjustment as an interactive buffer against pain-related distress. *Pain* 1996;67(1):41–51.
18. Burckhardt CS, Bjelle A. Perceived control: a comparison of women with fibromyalgia, rheumatoid arthritis, and systemic lupus erythematosus using a Swedish version of the rheumatology attitudes index. *Scand J Rheumatol* 1996;25(5):300–306.
19. Gustafsson M, Gaston-Johansson F. Pain intensity and health locus of control: a comparison of patients with fibromyalgia syndrome and rheumatoid arthritis. *Patient Educ Couns* 1996;29(2):179–188.
20. Pastor MA, Salas E, Lopez S, et al. Patients' beliefs about their lack of pain control in primary fibromyalgia syndrome. *Br J Rheumatol* 1993;32(6):484–489.
21. Crisson JE, Keefe FJ. The relationship of locus of control to pain coping strategies and psychological distress in chronic pain patients. *Pain* 1988;35(2):147–154.
22. Jensen MP, Turner JA, Romano JM, et al. Coping with chronic pain: a critical review of the literature. *Pain* 1991;47(3):249–283.
23. Lipchik GL, Milles K, Covington EC. The effects of multidisciplinary pain management treatment on locus of control and pain beliefs in chronic non-terminal pain. *Clin J Pain* 1993;9(1):49–57.

24. Taal E, Rasker JJ, Wiegman O. Patient education and self-management in the rheumatic diseases: a self-efficacy approach. *Arthritis Care Res* 1996;9(3):229–238.

25. Smarr KL, Parker JC, Wright GE, et al. The importance of enhancing self-efficacy in rheumatoid arthritis. *Arthritis Care Res* 1997;10:18–26.

26. Buckelew SP, Conway R, Parker J, et al. Biofeedback/relaxation training and exercise interventions for fibromyalgia: a prospective trial. *Arthritis Care Res* 1998;11(3):196–209.

27. Burckhardt CS, Mannerkorpi K, Hedenberg L, et al. A randomized, controlled clinical trial of education and physical training for women with fibromyalgia. *J Rheumatol* 1994; 21(4):714–720.

28. Keefe FJ, Caldwell DS. Cognitive behavioral control of arthritis pain. *Med Clin North Am* 1997;81(1):277–290.

29. Turk DC, Okifuji A, Sinclair JD, et al. Interdisciplinary treatment for fibromyalgia syndrome: clinical and statistical significance. *Arthritis Care Res* 1998;11(3):186–195.

30. Nielson WR, Walker C, McCain GA. Cognitive behavioral treatment of fibromyalgia syndrome: preliminary findings. *J Rheumatol* 1992;19(1):98–103.

31. Williams DA, Cary MA, Groner KH, et al. Improving physical functional status in patients with fibromyalgia: a brief cognitive behavioral intervention. *J Rheumatol* 2002;29(6):1280–1286.

32. Weinberger M, Tierney WM, Booher P. Social support, stress, and functional status in patients with osteoarthritis. *Soc Sci Med* 1990;30:503–508.

33. Doeglas D, Suurmeijer T, Briancon S. An international study on measuring social support: interactions and satisfaction. *Soc Sci Med* 1996;43:1389–1397.

34. Melzack R, Wall PD. *The challenge of pain*, rev. ed. New York: Penguin Books, 1982.

35. NIH Technology Assessment Panel on Integration of Behavioral and Relaxation Approaches into the Treatment of Chronic Pain and Insomnia. N.I.H. integration of behavioral and relaxation approaches into the treatment of chronic pain and insomnia. *J Am Med Assoc* 1996;276(4):313–318.

36. Janal MN. Pain sensitivity, exercise and stoicism. *J R Soc Med* 1996;89(7):376–381.

37. Sonstroem RJ. Exercise and self-esteem. *Exerc Sport Sci Rev* 1984;12:123–155.

38. McCann IL, Holmes DS. Influence of aerobic exercise on depression. *J Pers Soc Psychol* 1984;46(5):1142–1147.

39. Hammett VB. Psychological changes with physical fitness training. *Can Med Assoc J* 1967;96(12):764–769.

40. Clark SR. Prescribing exercise for fibromyalgia patients. *Arthritis Care Res* 1994;7(4):221–225.

41. Wigers SH, Stiles TC, Vogel PA. Effects of aerobic exercise versus stress management treatment in fibromyalgia. A 4.5 year prospective study. *Scand J Rheumatol* 1996;25(2):77–86.

42. Morin CM, Culbert JP, Schwartz SM. Nonpharmacological interventions for insomnia: a meta-analysis of treatment efficacy. *Am J Psychiatry* 1994;151(8):1172–1180.

43. Affleck G, Tennen H, Urrows S, et al. Fibromyalgia and women's pursuit of personal goals: a daily process analysis. *Health Psychol* 1998;17(1):40–47.

44. Affleck G, Urrows S, Tennen H, et al. Sequential daily relations of sleep, pain intensity, and attention to pain among women with fibromyalgia. *Pain* 1996;68(2-3):363–368.

45. Lewinsohn PM. The behavioral study and treatment of depression. In: Hersen M, Eisler RM, Miller PM, eds. *Progress in behavior modification*. New York: Academic Press, 1975.

46. Lindstrom I, Ohlund C, Eek C, et al. The effect of graded activity on patients with subacute low back pain: a randomized prospective clinical study with an operant-conditioning behavioral approach. *Phys Ther* 1992;72(4):279–290.

47. Gil KM, Ross SL, Keefe FJ. Behavioral treatment of chronic pain: four pain management protocols. In: France RD, Krishnan KRR, eds. *Chronic pain*. New York: American Psychiatric Press, 1988.

48. Deale A, Chalder T, Marks I, et al. Cognitive behavior therapy for chronic fatigue syndrome: a randomized controlled trial. *Am J Psychiatry* 1997;154(3):408–414.

49. D'Zurilla TJ, Goldfried MR. Problem solving and behavior modification. *J Abnorm Psychol* 1971;78(1):107–126.

50. Nezu AM, Nezu CM, Perri MG. *Problem-solving therapy for depression: theory, research and clinical guidelines*. New York: John Wiley and Sons, 1989.

51. Goldfried MR, Davidson G. *Clinical behavioural therapy*. New York: Holt, Rinehart & Winston, 1976.

52. Gombeski WR Jr, Kramer K, Wilson T, et al. Women's Heart Advantage program: motivating rapid and assertive behavior. *J Cardiovasc Manage* 2002;13(5):21–28.

53. Burckhardt CS. Nonpharmacologic management strategies in fibromyalgia. *Rheum Dis Clin North Am* 2002;28(2):291–304.

54. Reid MC, Otis J, Barry LC, et al. Cognitive-behavioral therapy for chronic low back pain in older persons: a preliminary study. *Pain Med* 2003;4(3):223–230.

55. Keefe FJ, Caldwell DS, Williams DA, et al. Pain coping skills training in the management of osteoarthric knee pain—II: follow-up results. *Behav Ther* 1990;21:435–447.

56. Parker JC, Frank RG, Beck NC, et al. Pain management in rheumatoid arthritis patients. A cognitive-behavioral approach. *Arthritis Rheum* 1988;31(5):593–601.

57. Evers AW, Kraaimaat FW, Van Riel PL, et al. Tailored cognitive-behavioral therapy in early rheumatoid arthritis for patients at risk: a randomized controlled trial. *Pain* 2002;100(1-2): 141–153.

58. Thomas V. Cognitive behavioural therapy in pain management for sickle cell disease. *Int J Palliat Nurs* 2000;6(9):434–442.

59. Lake AE III. Behavioral and nonpharmacologic treatments of headache. *Med Clin North Am* 2001;85(4):1055–1075.

60. Haythornthwaite JA, Lawrence JW, Fauerbach JA. Brief cognitive interventions for burn pain. *Ann Behav Med* 2001; 23(1):42–49.

61. Morley S, Eccleston C, Williams A. Systematic review and meta-analysis of randomized controlled trials of cognitive behaviour therapy and behaviour therapy for chronic pain in adults, excluding headache. *Pain* 1999;80(1-2):1–13.

62. Bradley LA. Cognitive-behavioral therapy for primary fibromyalgia. *J Rheumatol—Suppl* 1989;19:131–136.

63. Pillemer SR, Bradley LA, Crofford LJ, et al. The neuroscience and endocrinology of fibromyalgia. *Arthritis Rheum* 1997;40(11):1928–1939.

64. Leventhal LJ. Management of fibromyalgia. *Ann Intern Med* 1999;131(11):850–858.

65. Ferraccioli G, Ghirelli L, Scita F, et al. EMG-biofeedback training in fibromyalgia syndrome. *J Rheumatol* 1987;14(4): 820–825.

66. Kaplan KH, Goldenberg DL, Galvin-Nadeau M. The impact of a meditation-based stress reduction program on fibromyalgia. *Gen Hosp Psychiatry* 1993;15(5):284–289.

67. Goldenberg DL, Kaplan KH, Nadeau MG. A controlled study of stress-reduction, cognitive-behavioral treatment program in fibromyalgia. *J Musculoskelet Pain* 1994;2(2):53–65.

68. Keel PJ, Bodoky C, Gerhard U, et al. Comparison of integrated group therapy and group relaxation training for fibromyalgia. *Clin J Pain* 1998;14(3):232–238.

69. Nicassio PM, Radojevic V, Weisman MH, et al. A comparison of behavioral and educational interventions for fibromyalgia. *J Rheumatol* 1997;24(10):2000–2007.

70. White KP, Nielson WR. Cognitive behavioral treatment of fibromyalgia syndrome: a followup assessment. *J Rheumatol* 1995;22(4):717–721.

71. Thieme K, Gromnica-Ihle E, Flor H. Operant behavioral treatment of fibromyalgia: a controlled study. *Arthritis Rheum* 2003;49(3):314–320.

72. Bennett RM, Burckhardt CS, Clark SR, et al. Group treatment of fibromyalgia: a 6 month outpatient program. *J Rheumatol* 1996;23(3):521–528.

73. Mengshoel AM, Forseth KO, Haugen M, et al. Multidisciplinary approach to fibromyalgia. A pilot study. *Clin Rheumatol* 1995;14(2):165–170.

74. Gowans SE, deHueck A, Voss S, et al. A randomized, controlled trial of exercise and education for individuals with fibromyalgia. *Arthritis Care Res* 1999;12(2):120–128.

75. Mannerkorpi K, Nyberg B, Ahlmen M, et al. Pool exercise combined with an education program for patients with fibromyalgia syndrome. A prospective, randomized study. *J Rheumatol* 2000;27(10):2473–2481.

76. Vlaeyen JW, Teeken-Gruben NJ, Goossens ME, et al. Cognitive-educational treatment of fibromyalgia: a randomized clinical trial. I. Clinical effects. *J Rheumatol* 1996; 23(7):1237–1245.

30

Local Therapy for Fibromyalgia and Nonneuropathic Pain

Lan Chen, Jodi Goldman-Knaub, and Sally Pullman-Mooar

Local therapy for fibromyalgia (FM) and other painful conditions can be an alternative for both patients and their healthcare providers. Local measures can be perceived as going directly to the source of pain, although this is not always the case, but they do generally carry less risk compared to systemic delivery. The "hands on" approach of some these local therapies is also often an important part of a therapeutic relationship. Despite their obvious potential advantages, many patients do not receive local measures. This chapter will review the following local therapy modalities, which can help providers judge for themselves how to use topical drugs, local injections, and various physical measures:

Topical Remedies

Topical nonsteroidal anti-inflammatory drugs

Capsaicin

Local anesthetics

Topical antidepressant

Topical gabapentin (neurontin)

Topical traditional Chinese medicine

Tender Point Injections

Botox

Steroid

Xylocaine

Dry needling

Physical Measures and Other Devices

Massage

Balneotherapy

Heat therapy

Ultrasound

Phonophoresis

Transcutaneous electrical nerve stimulation (TENS)

TOPICAL REMEDIES

An alternative and attractive approach to pain control is to apply drugs locally to the peripheral site of origin of the pain. Topical applications include cream, lotion, gel, oil, aerosol, or patch to somatic sites. These topical remedies allow for a high local concentration of the drug at the site of the pain and lower or negligible systemic drug levels, producing fewer or no adverse drug effects. Other advantages of topical application are the lack of drug interactions and the ease of use.

The general pharmacokinetic principles governing drugs applied to the skin are the same as those involved in other routes of drug administration (1). Major variables that determine pharmacologic response to drugs applied to the skin include the following:

1. Regional variation in the drug penetration. For example, the face, axilla, scrotum, and scalp are far more permeable than the forearm and may require fewer doses for an equivalent.
2. Concentration gradient. Increasing the concentration gradient increases the mass of drug transferred per unit of time.
3. Dosing schedule. Because of the skin's physical properties, the skin acts as a reservoir. For drugs with a short systemic half-life, topical application may be long enough to permit "once-a-day" application.
4. Vehicles and occlusion. An appropriate vehicle maximizes the drug's ability to penetrate the skin's outer layers. Occlusion (application of a plastic wrap to hold the drug and its vehicle in close contact with the skin) is extremely effective in maximizing efficacy.

Topical applications differ from transdermal delivery systems, which are not discussed in detail here. In transdermal delivery systems, the skin is used as an alternative systemic delivery system. For topical application, the target site is immediately adjacent to the site of the delivery, with very limited systemic affects. The actions of topical drugs may decrease production of local inflammatory mediators, block the action of inflammatory mediators or altered impulse generation through actions on up-regulated sodium channels, or attenuate action of the sensory neurons through actions at specific receptors. In chronic-pain states, the effectiveness of a topical approach may depend on the degree of inflammation, the degree of alteration in peripheral sensory processing, and the degree of central sensitization involved. In most chronic-pain conditions, both peripheral and central elements are present. The topical approaches are more likely to be effective where there is a prominent peripheral component (2).

Bioavailability and plasma concentration following topical application are 5% to 15% of those achieved by systemic delivery (3). Adverse effects with topical remedies can be classified as cutaneous and systemic reactions; the local reaction is more commonly compared to systemic reaction. Skin rash and itch at the site of application are accounted for most local reactions (3,4). Systemic adverse effects do occur but much less often compared to systemic delivery (5).

TOPICAL NONSTEROIDAL ANTI-INFLAMMATORY DRUGS

Traditional nonsteroidal anti-inflammatory drugs (NSAIDs) are among the most commonly prescribed drugs worldwide and are responsible for approximately one-fourth of all adverse drug reaction reports. NSAIDs are widely prescribed for patients with rheumatic disease. Topical application of NSAIDs offers the advantage of local, concentrated drug delivery to affected tissues with a reduced incidence of systemic adverse effects, such as peptic ulcer disease and gastrointestinal (GI) hemorrhage.

Steen et al. (6) tested topically applied acetylsalicylic acid (ASA), salicylic acid (SA), and indomethacin in an experimental pain model in humans. In 30 volunteers, sustained burning pain was produced in the palmar forearm through a continuous intradermal pressure infusion of a phosphate-buffered isotonic solution (pH 5.2). In five different, double-blind, randomized crossover studies with six volunteers each, the flow rate of the syringe pump was individually adjusted to result in constant pain ratings of around 20% (50% in study 4) on a visual analog scale (VAS). The painful skin area was then covered with either placebo or the drugs, which had been dissolved in diethylether. In the first study of six volunteers, ASA (60 mg per mL) or lactose (placebo) in diethylether (10 mL) was applied, using both arms at 3-day intervals. Both treatments resulted in sudden and profound pain relief due to the cooling effect of the evaporating ether. With lactose, however, the mean pain rating was restored close to the baseline within 6 to 8 minutes, while with ASA it remained significantly depressed for the rest of the observation period (another 20 minutes). A loss of tactile sensation did not accompany this deep analgesia. The further studies served to show that indomethacin (4.5 mg per mL) and SA (60 mg per mL) were equally as effective as ASA. These antinociceptive effects were felt to be due to local but not systemic actions, since ASA and SA did not reach measurable plasma levels up to 3 hours after topical applications.

Topical application leads to relatively high NSAID concentrations in the dermis. Concentrations achieved in the muscle tissue below the site of application are variable, but they are at least equivalent to that obtained with oral administration (3). NSAIDs applied topically over joints do reach the synovial fluid, but the extent and mechanism (topical penetration vs. distribution via the systemic circulation) remain to be determined. In addition, marked interindividual variability has been noted in all studies; individual skin properties may strongly influence percutaneous absorption. In general, interpretation of clinical studies measuring efficacy of topical NSAIDs in rheumatic disease states is difficult because of a remarkably high placebo response rate, the use of rescue paracetamol (acetaminophen), and a significant variability in percutaneous absorption and response rates between patients. Overall efficacy rates attributable to topical NSAIDs in patients with rheumatic disorders ranged from 18% to 92% of treated patients.

In a clinical context, there have been sufficient studies of soft tissue conditions to demonstrate the superiority of topical NSAIDs over placebo and to suggest equivalent efficacy in comparison to some oral NSAIDs. The effectiveness and tolerability of tolmetin as Tolectin Gel 5% was evaluated in an open, multicentric study (7). Two hundred and five patients suffering from osteoarthritis (OA), spondylarthrosis, soft tissue rheumatism, and posttraumatic pain were treated under conditions similar to practice. The topical preparation was administered alone or when needed, associated with tolmetin 400 mg capsules. Evaluation of symptoms and signs revealed no statistical difference of effectiveness between the two dosage groups. The opinions of the doctors and patients about the clinical course supported this positive result. Dose reduction of oral or other parenteral preparations is often possible by means of concomitant topical treatment. In some types of soft tissue and joint pain, chiefly in mild cases, the local application alone can be sufficient.

Bruhlmann and Michel assessed the efficacy and safety of a diclofenac hydroxyethylpyrrolidine (DHEP) patch in the treatment of symptomatic OA of the knee joint. A double-blind, randomized, placebo-controlled trial was carried out on 103 outpatients for 2 weeks. The main efficacy parameters were spontaneous pain and the Lequesne Index. Secondary endpoints were walking time over a standard distance, global assessment of efficacy and tolerability, and paracetamol consumption. The active treatment group showed a significant improvement in pain, Lequesne Index, and the physician's and patient's global assessment of efficacy. For these parameters the difference between groups was statistically significant in favor of the DHEP patch (8).

NSAIDs administered topically penetrate slowly and in small quantities into the systemic circulation; bioavailability and maximal plasma NSAID concentrations after topical application are generally <5% and 15%, respectively, compared to equivalent oral administration. The adverse event profile of topical agents is reasonable: Minor cutaneous effects occur in up to 2% of patients but tend to be self-limiting (3). GI events appear from the existing literature to be infrequent and minor, although long-term studies are required. Bronchospasm and renal impairment have been reported and may be more frequent in patients who have experienced these effects with oral agents (4), so great caution should be exercised in such patients.

CAPSAICIN

Capsaicin is a natural constituent in pungent red chili peppers. It can selectively activate, desensitize, or exert a neurotoxic effect on sensory neurons, depending on the concentration and the delivery mode (9,10).

Activation of sensory neurons occurs because of interaction with a ligand-gated nonselective cation channel, and receptor occupancy triggers Na^+ and Ca^{2+} ion influx and action potential firing as the burning sensation occurs with spicy food or capsaicin-induced pain (11). Desensitization occurs with repeated administration of capsaicin and is a receptor-mediated process. This process involves Ca^{2+} and calmodulin-dependent phosphorylation of the cation channel. As a consequence of desensitization, secretion of substance P (SP) from both peripheral and central terminals of sensory neurons is inhibited (9). Neurotoxicity is partially osmotic and partially due to Ca^{2+} entry with activation of Ca^{2+}-sensitive protease (10). Repeated application to the skin produces desensitization to this response and thus forms the basis of the therapeutic use of topical capsaicin in chronic-pain conditions (12).

Topical capsaicin preparations of 0.025% and 0.075% are available for human use. It is interesting to know that extracts from red chili peppers have long been used in traditional topical Chinese medication mixes for joint pain. McCarthy and McCarty evaluated topical capsaicin 0.075% for the treatment of the painful joints of rheumatoid arthritis (RA) and OA patients in a 4-week double-blind, placebo-controlled, randomized trial. Twenty-one patients were selected, all of whom had either RA ($n = 7$) or OA ($n = 14$) with painful involvement of the hands. Assessments of pain (VAS), functional capacity, morning stiffness, grip strength, joint swelling, and tenderness (dolorimeter) were performed before randomization. Treatment was applied to each painful hand joint four times daily with reassessment at 1, 2, and 4 weeks after entry. One subject did not complete the study. Capsaicin reduced the tenderness ($p<0.02$) and pain ($p<0.02$) associated with OA but not RA as compared to placebo. A local burning sensation was the only adverse effect noted. These findings suggest that topical capsaicin is a safe and potentially useful drug for the treatment of painful OA of the hands (13).

FM patients commonly have pain in the head and neck. Epstein and Marcoe reviewed an open series of 24 consecutive cases of head and neck pain treated with topical capsaicin. Complete remission of pain was seen in 31.6% of patients; partial remission was achieved in 31.6% of patients. Trigeminal neuralgia with an intraoral trigger was less responsive to topical therapy than neuropathic pain. Further study is needed to clarify the efficacy of topical capsaicin in neuropathic and nonneuropathic pain and the effect of differing dosages and frequency of application (14).

Topical capsaicin is attractive because it is a simple, safe treatment and has been studied in a variety of conditions in uncontrolled and a few controlled trials. However, even though these studies suggest an analgesic effect, it has been impossible to blind even for placebo-controlled trials, due to the burning sensation induced by the capsaicin. A high placebo response rate in the controlled trials is an interesting observation in these studies and may account for the apparent salutary effect reported in the studies lacking a control. A careful scrutiny of the current results of these trials, as well as clinical experience, indicate there is a modest effect with the currently available preparations, although many patients failed to find relief or found the relief insufficient or were unable to tolerate the burning sensation. Occasional patients appear to have very good pain relief, and clinical trials may not reflect these unusual cases. Topical capsaicin is generally not satisfactory as a sole therapy for chronic-painful conditions, although it may serve as an adjuvant to other approaches (15). Topical capsaicin is not associated with any severe systemic adverse effects. However, many patients report stinging and burning, particularly during the first week of therapy (16). Caution must be exercised to avoid touching the eyes. Topical capsaicin merits consideration as a part of multidisciplinary therapy in conditions where the pain can be chronic and difficult to treat.

LOCAL ANESTHETICS (LIDOCAINE PATCHES AND GELS)

Local anesthetics have long been used to abolish pain temporarily by blocking nerve conduction, but local anesthetics, such as lidocaine patch or gel, are now used as an effective treatment for many chronic-pain conditions (17). Local anesthetics block voltage-gated sodium channels (VGSCs), which play a fundamental role in the control of neuronal excitability (2). Alteration in the expression, distribution, and function of VGSCs occurs following chronic inflammation, nerve injury, and other chronic-pain conditions (18).

Systemically administered local anesthetics such as IV lidocaine, oral mexilitine, and oral tocainamide are effective in a number of chronic-pain conditions (17). However, despite this efficacy in different clinical pain conditions, systemic anesthetics are limited by their adverse central nervous system (dizziness, lightheadedness, and somnolence) and cardiac effects. Clinical attention has recently been focused on topical formulations of lidocaine. Topical lidocaine as a 5% gel or patch provides pain relief in several chronic-pain conditions. Galer et al. compared the efficacy of topical lidocaine patches to vehicle (placebo) patches applied directly to the painful skin of subjects with postherpetic neuralgia (PHN) using an "enriched enrollment" study design. All subjects had been successfully treated with topical lidocaine patches on a regular basis for at least 1 month prior to study enrollment. Subjects were enrolled in a randomized, two-treatment period, vehicle-controlled, crossover study. The primary efficacy variable was "time to exit"; subjects were allowed to exit either treatment period if their pain relief score decreased by two or more categories on a six-item pain relief scale for any 2 consecutive days. The median time to exit with the lidocaine patch phase was >14 days, whereas the vehicle patch exit time was 3.8 days ($p<0.001$). At study completion, 25 of 32 (78.1%) subjects preferred the lidocaine patch treatment phase as compared to 3 of 32 (9.4%) who preferred the placebo patch phase ($p<0.001$). No statistical difference was noted between the active and placebo treatments with regard to side effects. Thus, topical lidocaine patches provide significantly more pain relief for PHN than vehicle patches with limited side effects (19).

Topical local anesthetics have shown promise in both un-controlled and controlled studies. Thirty-five subjects with established PHN affecting the torso or extremities completed a four-session, random order, double-blind, vehicle-controlled study of the analgesic effects of topically applied 5% lidocaine in the form of a nonwoven polyethylene adhesive patch (20). All subjects had allodynia on examination. Lidocaine-containing patches were applied in two of the four 12-hour sessions. In one session vehicle patches were applied, and one session was a no-treatment observation session. Lidocaine-containing patches significantly reduced pain intensity at all time points from 30 minutes to 12 hours compared to no-treatment observation and at all time points from 4 to 12 hours compared to vehicle patches. Lidocaine patches were superior to both no-treatment observation and vehicle patches in averaged category pain relief scores. The highest blood lidocaine level measured was 0.1 micrograms/mL, indicating minimal systemic absorption of lidocaine. Patch application was without systemic side effects and was well-tolerated when applied on allodynic skin for 12 hours. This study demonstrates that topical 5% lidocaine in patch form is easy to use and relieves postherpetic neuralgia.

Most published studies of lidocaine gel or patch have focused on PHN. The patch itself provided some pain relief, likely due to the protection afforded to allodynic skin (20).

The question is whether these local anesthetics may also provide pain relief in FM or other nonneuropathic pain conditions. A randomized controlled trial was carried out on patients with chronic muscle pain syndromes. Sixty-one patients (42 with FM and 19 with myofascial pain syndrome [MPS]) completed the trial. Outcome measures included pain intensity, a daily pain diary, headache frequency, sensitivity to pressure using a dolorimeter, anxiety, depression, and sleep quality. Patients were randomized to receive either 4% lidocaine applied over tender points (TePs) or sterile water (placebo) six times over a 3-week period. Both subjects and investigators were blind to treatment allocation. The results showed that 4% lidocaine had no superiority over placebo in any of the outcome measures. Twenty-one subjects (35%) showed a decrease in pain that was >30% of their baseline value. Of these 21 subjects, 10 received lidocaine and 11 received placebo. These data suggest that, in this population, 4% lidocaine is no better than placebo in the treatment of chronic muscle pain (21). This study was done with 4% lidocaine gel rather than the 5% gel or patch used in PHN studies. Further studies are needed to document any efficacy of the lidocaine patch or a higher concentration of lidocaine gel for FM or other more localized nonneuropathic pain conditions.

ANTIDEPRESSANTS

Antidepressants given orally have been used to treat chronic pain for 40 years (22). Tricyclic compounds given systemically have been the most often used agents for treatment of FM (23). Initially, the efficacy of antidepressants was attributed to central action in the spinal cord and at supraspinal levels (24). Recently, peripheral activity also was noted in a visceral pain model (25), a formalin model of tonic pain (26), and a model of neuropathic pain (27). Amitriptyline, a tricyclic antidepressant, can increase local release of adenosine and activation of adenosine A1 receptor (27). These peripheral actions raise the

possibility that topical formulations of antidepressants may be a useful alternative drug delivery system for analgesia. Antidepressants exhibit a number of pharmacologic actions: They block reuptake of noradrenaline and 5-hydroxytryptamine; have direct and indirect actions on opioid receptors; inhibit histamine, cholinergic, 5-hydroxytryptamine, and N-methyl-D-aspartate receptors; inhibit ion channel activity; and block adenosine uptake. But the contribution of these actions to analgesia by antidepressants, locally or systemically, remains to be determined.

Topical doxepin cream has been reported to produce analgesia in one randomized double-blind placebo-controlled study (28). The analgesic efficacy of topical administration of 3.3% doxepin hydrochloride, 0.025% capsaicin, and a combination of 3.3% doxepin and 0.025% capsaicin were assessed in human chronic neuropathic pain. A total of 200 patients were enrolled in this randomized, double-blind, placebo-controlled study. Patients applied placebo, doxepin, capsaicin, or doxepin/capsaicin cream daily for 4 weeks. Patients recorded on a daily basis overall pain, shooting, burning, paraesthesia, and numbness using a 0 to 10 VAS during the week prior to cream application (baseline levels) and for the 4-week study period. Side effects and the desire to continue treatment were also recorded. Overall pain was significantly reduced by all three groups—doxepin, capsaicin, and doxepin/capsaicin—to a similar degree. The analgesia with doxepin/capsaicin was of more rapid onset. Side effects were minor. It was concluded that topical application of 3.3% doxepin, or 0.025% capsaicin, or 3.3% doxepin/0.025% capsaicin produces analgesia of similar magnitude. However, the combination produces more rapid analgesia.

Antidepressants show promise as a useful class of agents to be used as analgesics in chronic-pain conditions. They provide options to both topical applications and systemic delivery.

GABAPENTIN

Gabapentin (GP) is an amino acid that has a mechanism that differs from other anticonvulsant drugs such as phenytoin, carbamazepine, or valproate. Several hypotheses of cellular mechanisms have been proposed to explain the pharmacology of GP:

1. GP crosses several membrane barriers in the body via a specific amino acid transporter (system L) and competes with leucine, isoleucine, valine, and phenylalanine for transport.
2. GP increases the concentration and probably the rate of synthesis of γ-amino-butyric acid (GABA) in the brain, which may enhance nonvesicular GABA release during seizures.
3. GP binds with high affinity to a novel binding site in brain tissues that is associated with an auxiliary subunit of voltage-sensitive Ca^{2+} channels. Recent electrophysiology results suggest that GP may modulate certain types of Ca^{2+} current.
4. GP reduces the release of several monoamine neurotransmitters.
5. Electrophysiology suggests that GP inhibits voltage-activated Na^+ channels, but other results contradict these findings.

6. GP increases serotonin concentrations in human whole blood, which may be relevant to neurobehavioral actions.

7. GP prevents neuronal death in several models, including those designed to mimic amyotrophic lateral sclerosis (ALS). This may occur by the inhibition of glutamate synthesis by branched-chain amino acid aminotransferase (BCAA-t) (29).

Carlton and Zhou (30) reported that local GP has been shown to have antihyperalgesic properties at the site of drug application. Rats received different doses of local GP (intraplantar 20-microl injections of 6, 60, or 600 microg GP). High-dose GP (600 microg) significantly reduced these nociceptive behaviors. The antihyperalgesic effect of GP was not due to a systemic effect, since animals injected with 600 microg GP in one hindpaw and 2% formalin into the contralateral hindpaw developed nociceptive behaviors that were no different from those seen in animals injected with formalin alone. Although the mechanism of action of GP has yet to be elucidated, the results indicated that GP has a peripheral site of action and thus may offer a novel therapeutic agent for topical or local treatment of pain of peripheral origin.

There has been one clinical trial using oral pregabalin in treating FM (31). These preclinical and clinical data support the potential for development of topical formulations of GP.

TOPICAL TRADITIONAL CHINESE MEDICINE

Topical traditional Chinese medicine and other alternative remedies are still widely used, especially in Chinese and other ethnic communities. When all the "modern" preparations have been exhausted, our patients have tried falling back on some "old remedies." Litt (32) has offered a list of 73 alternative topical measures that are often beneficial, mostly for dermatologic disorders. Topical traditional Chinese medicines (TTCMs) have many varieties. A common misconception is that TTCM is a complicated, exotic art. Difficulties in understanding these measures arise because formulations have more than one ingredient, myriad preparations are available, and labels can be confusing, with brands like Tiger Balm, 3-Snake Oil, and Dragon Balm. First and foremost, it must be understood that brand names are just brand names. The names are symbolic. Tiger Balm and 3-Snake Oil do not contain any material from these animals. Indeed, TTCMs are mixtures containing many herbs, ranging from 3 to 20 different types (33). Mixtures are based on the concepts of traditional Chinese medicine. The formulations use different ingredients to balance the body and to balance the opposite properties of different herbs. However, all these many preparations can be grouped into three classes, according to usage. In each class the ingredients revolve around a common theme, with only minor differences. The three classes are: (1) oils, ointments, and pastes for aches and pains; (2) oils, ointments, and pastes for orthopedic injuries; and (3) lotions and ointments for skin diseases. Here, only the first class will be briefly summarized.

The classic example of class 1 TTCMs used for rheumatic pain is Tiger Balm (34). It is oil-based and contains camphor, menthol, and one or more essential oils, such as cinnamon oil, oil of clove, cassia oil, citronella oil, oil of lavender, and cajuput oil. These are mixed in a base oil or petrolatum. The formulation is meant to be soothing, and it is not usually irritating to the skin unless patients are allergic to these ingredients. Other paste preparations are mixtures of various herbs with a petrolatum base. Zingiber officinale rhizoma, polygonum multiflorum radix, peonia lactiflora radix, rhizoma et radix notopterygii, myrrha, and other herbs are commonly used for rheumatic pain, a bi syndrome in Traditional Chinese Medicine (TCM) (34). None of these have been assessed in controlled trials available in English.

TTCMs have been used to soothe pain and still retain some popularity in the modern age. More evidence-based medicine is needed to guide physicians and patients.

PHYSICAL MEASURES AND OTHER DEVICES

Numerous physical measures can be used in the treatment of pain in FM and other nonneuropathic syndromes. Many are drawn from theory, tradition, and belief. However, evidence-based medicine should support the choice of physical interventions in a treatment plan. The efficacy of many physical measures has not been fully established and the physiologic mechanisms for anecdotal improvement in pain, depression, and sleep are being investigated. It is important to realize that FM is a complicated musculoskeletal syndrome that presents with a wide variety of symptoms and considerable overlap with other conditions, such as myofasical pain syndrome and chronic fatigue syndrome. Thus, many different treatment interventions are used to reduce patient symptoms. The remainder of this chapter will discuss some of these interventions, including massage, biofeedback (BFB), heat therapy, balneotherapy, ultrasound, phonophoresis, and TENS.

MASSAGE THERAPY

In the early fifth century B.C., Hippocrates wrote, "The physician must be experienced in many things, but assuredly in rubbing…. For rubbing can bind a joint that is too loose, and loosen a joint that is too rigid." Massage is an ancient treatment for pain relief and is currently being used by 17% to 75% of FM patients (35). The variability in the use of this intervention may be attributed to many factors, including lack of awareness within the medical model, poor insurance reimbursement, and time constraints.

Massage may include both physiologic and psychological components (36). The possible physiologic benefits of massage include stimulation of nonnociceptive nerve endings, which contributes to the release of endorphins and increases serotonin levels (37). The reflex responses can also cause the reduction of blood pressure (38). Massage increases circulation and enhances venous return, which aids in the removal of metabolic waste products, helping to maintain healthy tissues (39). In the "gate theory," the notion is that the pressure receptors stimulated by massage are longer and more myelinated than pain receptors. When pain is experienced and the painful area is rubbed, the pressure message gets to the brain faster than the pain message and the gate is shut, thus blocking the entry of the pain message (40). The "language" of human touch may provide these patients with a feeling of relaxation, warmth, and renewed vitality, which can counteract the stresses and pressures one experiences in everyday life. Massage has been reported to increase mental clarity, reduce anxiety, increase general feelings of well-being, and release unexpressed emotions (39).

Danneskioid-Samsoe et al. (41) studied 26 patients with myofascial pain and found a significant increase in the plasma myoglobin concentration within 2 hours after the first massage. They found a positive correlation between the degree of muscle tension and pain and an increase in plasma myoglobin concentration. After the patients had repeated massage sessions, there was a gradual decline in the increase in plasma myoglobin concentration parallel to a reduction in the muscle tension and pain.

Patients with FM have a significantly elevated concentration of SP in the cerebrospinal fluid compared to normal controls (42,43). SP is a neuropeptide stored in the secretory granules of sensory nerves and released on axonal stimulation (44). The significance of SP continues to be investigated. It has been theorized that it is derived from overactive peripheral nociceptive fibers or from central neurons (44). Field et al. (45) found a significant decrease in SP with massage therapy performed for 30 minutes twice weekly for 5 weeks. This is a promising finding that will require further research.

Ironson et al. (37) demonstrated direct effects of massage on chronic disease outcomes in a group of human immunodeficiency virus (HIV) positive men compared to HIV positive controls. The men who received massage showed a significant increase in the number of natural killer cells, natural killer cytotoxity, soluble CD8, and cytotoxic subset of CD8 cells. Significant decreases in cortisol levels were observed before and after massage. Anxiety and relaxation significantly improved and were correlated with the increased number of natural killer cells (37).

There are many different forms of massage therapy, including classical, cross-fiber friction, connective tissue, myofascial release, soft tissue mobilization, Shiatsu, Swedish, and trigger point. The practitioner's sense of touch is fundamental to the massage technique, as the tactile sensation is the means of communication between the clinician and the patient. Most forms of massage can be used for patients with FM and other nonneuropathic pain syndromes. Pioro-Boisset's (35) interview-based study, however, supports less aggressive forms of massage, reporting greater satisfaction in FM patients when a "more toned down and less rigorous massage was used." This patient population tends to be more sensitive to pressure. Therefore clinicians need to consider patient positioning to promote comfort and to prevent further tension or stress. The therapist may consider beginning the massage in a distal or proximal area of the body to help the patient relax and then slowly work toward the problem areas (39).

Realistic individualized goals should be discussed and established with each patient at the initial evaluation. As treatment advances, the therapist should gradually incorporate active treatment, such as postural and therapeutic exercise. It is recommended that patients strive for independence with an exercise program and the ability to self-manage their

symptoms. It is necessary to establish a network of support because chronic pain can be lifelong.

Numerous studies have suggested the effectiveness of massage in the reduction of pain, stiffness, fatigue, and sleeping difficulties in patients diagnosed with FM (35,45–48).

Brattberg (49) conducted a randomized, controlled trial investigating the effect of 15 sessions of connective tissue massage in a 10-week period in the treatment of 48 FM patients. The findings were positive in a self-reported reduction of pain in 85% of patients and a reduction in analgesic consumption in 30% of subjects. The massage group also showed a reduction in depression and a positive effect on quality of life. However, after a 6-month follow-up, 90% of the pain returned. This study's findings would suggest the need for maintenance massage therapy, as the results did not last long term.

Sunshine et al. (48) found favorable results in 30 FM patients randomly assigned to massage therapy (Swedish massage) or TENS or a no-current TENS group. Thirty treatment sessions were used twice weekly for 4 weeks. All three groups improved on the rheumatologists' assessment of the subject's clinical condition, which suggests that all these forms of tactile stimulation and attention are effective. However, only the massage therapy group improved on both the dolorimeter and the subjects' self reports of pain. The massage group had lower cortisol levels and reported significantly fewer symptoms at the end of the study, including less pain, stiffness, fatigue, and difficulty sleeping. Field et al. (45) supported these results in a similar study when comparing massage therapy to relaxation therapy in 24 FM patients. The authors found that both groups demonstrated a decrease in anxiety and depressed mood. Only the massage group reported an increase in the number of sleep hours and a decrease in their sleep movements, and the patients' physicians assigned lower disease and pain ratings and fewer TeP areas. Field (38) found similar results when investigating massage therapy against a sham TENS control group in patients diagnosed with chronic fatigue syndrome.

Contrary to these studies, Alnigenis et al. (50) completed a randomized, controlled study on the effect of Swedish massage in patients with FM and found no significant benefits in pain reduction, functional status, or psychological distress. High attrition and a small sample limit this study's findings.

Massage is a passive intervention in which the patient is dependent on the practitioner. New research by Field et al. (46) investigated Eutony, a combination treatment of massage and movement therapy. This includes self-administered massage using wooden dowels and tennis balls and stretching movements in lying, seated, and standing positions. Early findings were positive, showing this self-administered treatment effective in decreasing depression, anxiety, and pain. These findings are encouraging because they promote patient independence and may be a progression from passive massage to active therapeutic exercise.

In a recent review of randomized, controlled trials, Holdcraft et al. (51) concluded that there was "moderate" evidence to recommend massage therapy as a therapeutic modality to FM patients. The small sample sizes in most of the studies limit their statistical power and make it difficult to form conclusions on the effectiveness of the massage intervention.

Massage involves considerable one-on-one time, which is problematic in the current healthcare environment. Despite this, massage clearly has some benefit and may be shown to be a cost-effective tool in the treatment of FM and other chronic-pain syndromes.

ELECTROMYOGRAPHIC BIOFEEDBACK

Electromyographic (EMG) BFB is a treatment modality that consists of monitoring a physiologic system (muscle tension) of which the patient is not ordinarily aware, converting it electronically into signals (usually visual or auditory) of which the patient becomes aware and develops strategies for its modification (52). Molina et al. (53) indicated that EMG-BFB training reduced plasma adrenocorticotrophin hormone and β-endorphin levels during treatment of FM patients, signifying an opioid or neuroendocrine basis for some of the observed beneficial effects of EMG BFB.

Ferraccioli et al. (54) conducted an open study administering 20-minute EMG-BFB sessions to 15 FM patients twice weekly for 15 sessions. EMG BFB consisted of patients receiving auditory feedback of ongoing muscle tension in scalp muscles. Clinical improvement (TePs, pain intensity, and morning stiffness) was found in 56% of the subjects at 6 months. Ferraccioli et al. (54) supported these findings in a randomized, controlled study of 12 patients using EMG BFB or sham BFB. Improvement was found in all outcomes in the treatment group, whereas the control had improvement only in TeP count. The authors concluded that EMG BFB in FM appeared reproducible and had long-term effectiveness. Because a small sample size limited their results, further research is needed to confirm them.

Buckelew et al. (55) conducted a randomized, controlled study with 119 FM patients comparing (a) EMG BFB/relaxation, (b) exercise, (c) a combination of EMG BFB/relaxation/exercise, and (d) an educational/attention control program. Subjects received individual training sessions once weekly for 1.5 to 3 hours for 6 weeks. During the maintenance phase of 2 years, the subjects were treated in groups once a month for an hour. Buckelew et al. (55) concluded that all three interventions resulted in improved self-efficacy for physical function and that it was best maintained over a 2-year follow-up by the combination group. As a result, EMG BFB can be an integrated part of a treatment program for chronic-pain patients.

Santen et al. (56) reported contradictory results in a similar study design with a larger sample size. These authors randomized 143 FM patients into a fitness, BFB, or control group. Reliable outcome measures used included the VAS, dolorimetery, the Arthritis Impact Measurement Scales, and the Sickness Impact Profile. After the treatments, the patients did not improve in pain or in any other outcome measure compared to controls. The exercise group did, however, continue with a low impact fitness training at their own expense, which suggests an immeasurable benefit to the this treatment group. The inconsistent results compared to previous studies could be due to high dropout rates, a failure to measure the obvious positive effect of fitness training with fellow sufferers, and the subjectivity of the measurements used for evaluating change in FM (56). In addition, the control group was given treatment, if appropriate, with medication, physical therapy (PT) (excluding exercise or relaxation therapy), and medical counseling.

EMG BFB is a cost-effective treatment modality because it educates patients to have control of their own bodies, whether it be movement control or autonomic, thus giving long-term benefits in both psychological and economic terms. In a recent survey of physical and occupational therapists in their therapeutic approaches to FM, Sim and Adams (57) found limited use of EMG BFB. The authors attribute this to inadequate training in this intervention. Further studies are need to better guide patients and health providers in the beneficial use of EMG BFB.

HEAT THERAPY

The benefits of using hot rocks and thermal baths to reduce joint stiffness and muscle spasm and to promote relaxation have been recognized ever since Hippocrates. The methods of applying heat have progressed since then, but many of the basic principles remain unchanged. Physical and occupational therapists use heating agents to provide pain relief and to prepare stiff joints and tight muscles for stretching and exercise. The physiologic effects of applying heat to the body include increasing blood flow, facilitating tissue healing, decreasing muscle tone, altering viscoelastic properties, altering nerve conduction velocity, and changing muscle spindle firing rates (58). Heating modalities are categorized by the mechanism of action (conduction, convention, and conversion) and the depth of penetration in elevating temperature in the tissues—superficial (1 cm) or deep (3 cm or more). Superficial modalities include hot packs, paraffin, fluidiotherapy, sauna, and hydrotherapy in different forms, such as hot baths, whirlpool, contrast baths, and balneotherapy. Deep heating includes shortwave diathermy and ultrasound.

The Philadelphia Panel (59), using evidence from randomized controlled trials and observational studies, determined that thermal modalities lacked evidence to include or exclude them as therapeutic interventions for chronic low back pain, neck pain, knee pain related to OA, or shoulder pain. Rakel and Barr (60) conducted a literature review and reported weak evidence that thermal modalities have a positive effect on chronic pain and that pain relief was mainly short term. Lin (61) demonstrated that cold packs have a more significant effect in comparison to heating pads in a randomized study comparing the two modalities in testing restriction of knee range of motion. Although cryotherapy is an additional modality used in PT, it is rarely used in FM patients due to their heightened sensitivity. Robinson et al. (62) performed a review of seven randomized, controlled trials on the effect of thermotherapy for treating RA. The authors found no significant effects of ice or heat packs and faradic baths on pain or medication intake; however, there were encouraging results with paraffin wax baths on pain, range of motion, and various functional measures after 4 weeks of treatment.

Superficial heat used in conjunction with an active exercise program may provide greater and longer lasting pain relief (63). The practical benefit of superficial heating is that it can be used at home, it is inexpensive, and there are very few contraindications. Contraindications include infections, acute inflammation, peripheral vascular disease, radiation therapy, malignancy, arterial insufficiency, and impaired circulation, sensation, and cognitive function (64). Treatment plans need to be individualized as FM patients have reported increased pain with heating agents (65). As always, treatment plans need to be individualized and based on goals mutually established by therapist and patient.

BALNEOTHERAPY

Balneotherapy is a treatment modality based on bathing in mineral-containing waters of hot springs or the use of mudpacks. The most popular area for this treatment is the Dead Sea region in Israel, which is the world's lowest and most saline lake (66). The unique climate it offers includes low humidity, high and stable temperatures, and high barometric pressures (the highest in the world) (67). Numerous controlled studies have shown that balneotherapy in this region is effective in the treatment of RA, psoriatic arthritis, and FM (66,68–73).

The mechanism by which these spa treatments work is not fully understood or supported in the literature. There has been no evidence of an actual influence on the disease process. Physiologic changes reported include significant diuresis and natriuresis, hemodilution, and increased cardiac output without significant change in blood pressure (66). The thermal stimuli may produce analgesia on nerve endings by increasing the pain threshold and decreasing muscle spasms (74). Tendon extensibility increases in joints and connective tissue. By causing peripheral vasodilatation, balneotherapy may help to wash out pain mediators (74). There are limited reports of the importance of the trace elements found in the mineral waters and whether they can be absorbed through the skin. This literature review found no adverse side effects of balneotherapy.

Buskila et al. (66) examined the effects of daily 20-minute sulfur baths with water from the Dead Sea in a randomized, controlled trial for 10 days with 48 FM patients. The control included a 10-day stay at the resort without treatment. Blinded assessments revealed that both groups improved on almost all areas measured (FM impact questionnaire, TeP count, tenderness threshold, visual analog scores, functional disability index, fatigue, stiffness, and anxiety). The improvements were significant in the treatment group and lasted for at least 3 months.

Evcik et al. (74) completed a randomized, controlled study with similar design at the natural springs of Afyon, Turkey. The authors compared the effect of balneotherapy in FM with treatments being received 20 minutes daily five times a week for 3 weeks to a control group receiving no treatment except instruction to continue with their daily activities. Their results were very promising for the treatment group, showing statistically significant differences in TePs, visual analog scores, Beck depression index, and FM impact questionnaire scores. After 6 months there was continued improvement in all areas except the depression scores.

Access to these areas of hot springs is limited due to location, expense, and dependability on a therapist. Further randomized controlled studies with longer follow-up periods are needed to strengthen these results.

Flusser et al. (75) performed a prospective, double-blinded, controlled study of 40 patients with knee OA that involved natural mineral-rich mud compresses versus mineral-depleted mud compresses being treated independently in the patient's home. These mud compresses were heated in a microwave or in a pot of hot water and then placed over the painful joints five times a week for 3 weeks. Outcome measures included the Lequesne Index of severity, self-assessments of pain score, and a VAS. Seventy-two percent of the patients in the treatment group had an improvement of more than 20% reduction in self-assessment of knee pain compared to 33% in the control group. Both groups showed significant improvement in pain severity, which was still observed at 3 months after completion of therapy. The authors concluded that efficacy for mud therapy was not clinically dramatic, but was statistically significant. The introduction of a placebo group would have improved the findings, as the local heat in both groups could have played a role in the improvement.

Balneotherapy could be a possible alternative treatment modality in FM and other nonneuropathic pain syndromes (66–74), but this will require continued investigation.

Although the specific mechanism of action of mud pack treatment, sulfur baths, mineral content, and trace elements remains unclear, evidence is mounting to support its use for the treatment of FM and certain chronic-pain syndromes. Balneotherapy may be a safe, practical, and effective physical agent that can be used in a patient's home.

ULTRASOUND

Ultrasound is a physical modality that has achieved recognition for over 40 years as an adjunct in the management of acute and chronic musculoskeletal disorders. It has been used in the treatment of various soft tissue dysfunctions, including scar tissue, tendonitis, bursitis, muscle spasms, joint contracture, OA, and pain. Ultrasound consists of inaudible acoustic waves delivered with a frequency range from 0.75 to 3 MHz and intensity between 0.5 and 3 w per cm^2. The absorption of ultrasound results in molecular oscillatory movements, and this energy transfer is converted into heat proportional to the intensity of the ultrasound (64).

The therapeutic effects include increasing soft tissue extensibility and increasing blood flow. Nonthermal changes occur by mechanical vibration and acoustic streaming, which is performed by using low intensities or a pulsed output of ultrasonic energy (76). The nonthermal properties of ultrasound are less well-defined, but may include altering cellular permeability and metabolism.

Because ultrasound can promote cell proliferation and activity, it is contraindicated over or close to sites of abnormal growth or rapid cell division such as cancer, tuberculosis, or a pregnant uterus. Diagnostic ultrasound, at 2.5 MHz, is used at a significantly lower dose than therapeutic ultrasound ($<0.1\%$ w per cm^2) (64). For similar reasons, it is contraindicated over epiphyseal plates in children, metal implants, cardiac pacemakers, or an area of a thrombus, due to the possibility of dislodgement (64).

Few studies were found on the use of ultrasound with FM or pain syndromes patients. The majority of randomized, controlled trials focused on specific musculoskeletal injuries such as epicondylitis, bursitis, shoulder pain, or tendonitis. Almeida (77) performed a study of 17 patients with FM, comparing the effect of combined therapy, including ultrasound and interferential current, against a sham procedure on pain and sleep. The treatment group underwent 12 sessions in 4 weeks of pulsed ultrasound and interferential current at different painful areas. The results were positive in demonstrating the combined treatment to be a therapeutic option in FM by improving pain manifestations (evaluated by a modified Wisconsin body map, VAS, TeP count, and tenderness threshold) and sleep pattern (assessed by the Brazilian inventory for sleep disorders and polysomnography). The small sample size limits these results.

Baker et al. (76) and Robertson and Baker (78) published reports reviewing randomized, controlled trials on both the biophysical effects and the therapeutic effectiveness of ultrasound. They concluded that there is an absence of evidence for a biologic rationale and provided little clinical evidence for the efficacy of therapeutic ultrasound. Although many clinicians regard ultrasound as a viable treatment, the majority of the literature supporting this application is empirical in nature and comes from studies lacking controls and proper designs (78).

Draper (79) critiqued Roberston and Baker's (76) literature review, pointing out that most of the studies reviewed did not use the generally recommended parameters for ultrasound. For example, the treatment area should be no more than twice the size of the effective radiating area of the crystal, and eight out of ten of the studies did not address this in their treatments. Treatment time was found to be inconsistent throughout the reviewed studies, with two studies with longer treatment times demonstrating ultrasound to be superior to placebo.

It seems that the "jury is still out" on the therapeutic effect of ultrasound (79). Although clinicians widely use ultrasound for localized pain, current reports are conflicting and studies are needed to clarify its efficacy. Ultrasound merits consideration as a treatment modality in conditions in which the pain is localized and difficult to treat.

PHONOPHORESIS

Phonophoresis is a physical modality that uses ultrasound to drive pharmacologic agents (such as hydrocortisone, dexamethasone, salicylates, and lidocaine) transdermally into subcutaneous tissues. Phonophoresis is indicated for musculoskeletal disorders with an inflammatory condition, such as bursitis, plantar fascitis, and epicondylitis. There are theoretical advantages of percutaneous administration of a drug, including: (1) suppression of first hepatic pass effect (2) stable plasma levels, and (3) absence of degradation by the digestive tract (80). The specific physiologic mechanism of phonophoresis remains unclear. Both the thermal and nonthermal properties of ultrasound have been cited as possible mechanisms for the penetration of the medications (81). The mechanisms responsible include increased skin permeability due to increased fluidity of intercellular lipids by heating or mechanical stress and /or by enlarging intercellular space, or by creating permanent or transient holes through corneocytes and keratinocytes as a consequence of cavitation, and/or by driving the drug and the vehicle through the permeabilized skin by convection (80).

The efficacy of phonophoresis has not been established. There have been conflicting results in human-controlled *in vivo* studies demonstrating an absence or mild effects of the technique and effect on skin permeability (80,82). Klaiman (81) discusses five studies that demonstrated drug penetration

as deep as 10 cm, and Bare et al. (83) discussed four studies in addition to their own that failed to demonstrate any transdermal penetration *via* phonophoretic technique.

Early noncontrolled clinical trials showed patients with inflammatory conditions treated with phonophoresis (using 10% hydrocortisone) with decreased pain and improved range of motion (84–86). More recent controlled trials on epicondylitis (hydrocortisone preparations of 1% and 10%) found no significant benefit when comparing phonophoresis to ultrasound alone (87,88).

Klaiman (81) found no significant difference in pain level or pressure tolerance when comparing phonophoresis to ultrasound in the treatment of musculoskeletal disorders. The groups received 8 minutes of continuous ultrasound at 1.5 W per cm^2, three times a week for 3 weeks; the phonophoresis group was treated with a gel containing 0.05% flucocinonide. The results found ultrasound to be effective in decreasing pain, with improved patient tolerance to algometer pressures after 3 weeks of treatment. There was no significant difference with the application of phonophoresis.

There is a paucity of evidence in clinical trials regarding the use of phonophoresis. Lack of standardization exists with preparation, concentration of active ingredients, dosage, treatment prescription, and parameters. Phonophoresis may be a safe alternative or adjuvant treatment to systemic medications. Although further study is recommended, clinicians continue to use this modality for localized musculoskeletal conditions.

TRANSCUTANEOUS ELECTRICAL NERVE STIMULATION

TENS is a noninvasive therapeutic modality widely used in clinical practice for pain relief by electrically stimulating peripheral nerves via skin surface electrodes. Most TENS devices today use an asymmetrical biphasic waveform, with frequency ranges from 1 to 150 Hz, pulse widths from 50 to 300 ms, and amplitudes through 75 mcmp (39). Melzack and Wall (40) attempted to explain the physiologic effect with the "gate theory," by which TENS stimulates the afferent nerve fibers that transmit or inhibit noxious input through the spinal cord to the brain. According to this theory, the analgesic effect is local, taking place in the dermatomes of the spinal segment recruited by the stimulation. The endorphin release phenomenon (89) is a theory in which TENS stimulates the sympathetic nervous system and brain stem nuclei to produce endorphins and possibly inhibit arthritis-related inflammation (63). The main indication for TENS is chronic pain—most commonly low back pain. Contraindications include demand type cardiac pacemaker, epilepsy, loss of sensation, and stimulation over carotid sinus or the eye (64). The major advantage of TENS is the applicability to a home program, which allows the patient to control the treatment independently. Adverse reactions are uncommon, but can include allergic dermatitis from the tape, gel, or electrodes, and, on rare occasions, transient increased pain.

Clinicians need to use the appropriate parameters and electrode placement in order to get the best possible outcome. Motor points, trigger points, and acupuncture points all represent electrically active and identifiable points that enhance the potential flow of current into the target tissue (64).

The bulk of research on TENS focuses on musculoskeletal pain, primarily back pain. FM patients present with multiple TeP areas, which mimic many musculoskeletal conditions. FM patients also typically present with diffuse musculoskeletal pain, while TENS is thought to be effective for localized pain only (65). TENS can be justified for site-specific pain commonly seen at the lateral epicondyle, low back, or upper trapezius area.

Clinical studies demonstrate a wide range of success rates with TENS, varying from 25% to 95% (65). The percentage of patients who benefit from short-term TENS has been reported to range from 50% to 80%, with good long-term benefit for between 6% to 44% (90). In a randomized survey (91) of 2003 chronic-pain patients using TENS for long-term (at least 6 months), the authors found that TENS was associated with a significant reduction in the utilization of pain medication and physical therapy and occupational therapy (PT/OT). Cost simulations of medication and PT/OT indicated that long-term TENS use was associated with a reduction of 55% for medications and up to 69% for PT/OT.

Systematic reviews of TENS in the treatment of chronic pain with placebo and control groups have reported inconclusive results (92–95). Sim and Adams (96) conducted a literature review of randomized controlled trials, finding limited studies showing successful use of TENS in the management of FM. Di Benedetto (97) compared S-adenosyl-L-methionine (SAMe, an antidepressant) to TENS and found that TENS was inferior to SAMe on 3 out of 13 outcomes measures and that there were no significant differences in respect to subjective pain, sleep, or fatigue. Brosseau et al. (98) concluded there was no evidence to support the use or nonuse of TENS in a meta-analysis of TENS in the treatment of low back pain. The Philadelphia Panel (59) evaluated evidence from randomized, controlled trials and observational studies in the use of TENS for chronic low back, knee, shoulder, and neck pain. The panel concluded that TENS was of clinically important benefit for knee OA but not for chronic neck pain. The panel (59) concluded that there was poor evidence to include or exclude TENS alone as an intervention for chronic low back pain.

In contrast, Rushton (99) completed a literature review and reported that TENS was remarkably safe and provided significant analgesia in about half of patients experiencing moderate predictable pain. The author found the implanted devices more effective than TENS used for chronic pain. A randomized survey (100) of 506 chronic-pain patients using TENS for pain management found that 74% were long-time users (more than 6 months) and there was statistically significant change or improvement that paralleled the introduction of TENS use with increased activity level and reduction in pain, drugs, and other therapies. It was suggested that good prognostic factors for the success of TENS in chronic pain include careful training in the use of the device and regular follow-up. Poor prognostic factors included significant depression and a progressive disease state (101).

Clinically, TENS remains a widely used and successful treatment option for some chronic-pain patients despite the conflicting literature. Some research indicated reduced therapy and medication use, increased activities, and improved treatment satisfaction, all contributing to restoring functional ability and an improved quality of life. These improvements, combined with the accompanying cost and complication considerations, are important points that clinicians must weigh when constructing a treatment plan for patients with chronic pain.

SUMMARY POINTS

- Even "central" pain syndromes such as FM depend to some degree on the peripheral activation of primary sensory afferent neurons. Thus, the localized peripheral administration of drugs, such as by topical application, can potentially optimize drug concentrations at the site of origin of the pain while leading to lower systemic levels and fewer adverse systemic effects and fewer drug interactions.
- Primary sensory afferent neurons can be activated by a range of inflammatory mediators, such as prostanoids, bradykinin, adenosine triphosphate (ATP), histamine, and serotonin, and inhibiting their actions represents a strategy for the development of analgesics.
- Peripheral nerve endings also express a variety of inhibitory neuroreceptors, such as opioid, α-adrenergic, cholinergic, adenosine, and cannabinoid receptors, and agonists for these receptors also represent viable targets for drug development.
- At present, topical and other forms of peripheral administration of nonsteroidal anti-inflammatory drugs, opioids, capsaicin, local anesthetics, and alpha-adrenoceptor agonists are being used in a variety of clinical states.
- Given that activation of sensory neurons involves multiple mediators and pathways, combinations of agents targeting different mechanisms and delivery systems may be particularly useful.

REFERENCES

1. Robertson DB, Maibach HI. Topical corticosteroids. *Int J Dermatol* 1982;21(2):59–67.
2. Sawynok J. Topical and peripherally acting analgesics. *Pharmacol Rev* 2003;55(1):1–20.
3. Heyneman CA, Lawless-Liday C, et al. Oral versus topical NSAIDs in rheumatic diseases: a comparison. *Drugs* 2000; 60(3):555–574.
4. Tramer MR, Williams JE, et al. Comparing analgesic efficacy of non-steroidal anti-inflammatory drugs given by different routes in acute and chronic pain: a qualitative systematic review. *Acta Anaesthesiol Scand* 1998;42(1):71–79.
5. Vaile JH, Davis P. Topical NSAIDs for musculoskeletal conditions. A review of the literature. *Drugs* 1998;56(5):783–799.
6. Steen KH, Reeh PW, et al. Topical acetylsalicylic, salicylic acid, and indomethacin suppress pain from experimental tissue acidosis in human skin. *Pain* 1995;62(3):339–347.
7. Fellmann N. Clinical experiences with 5% Tolectin (tolmetin) gel in patients with degenerative joint and spine diseases and soft tissue rheumatism. *Z Rheumatol* 1983;42(5):280–284.
8. Bruhlmann P, Michel BA. Topical diclofenac patch in patients with knee osteoarthritis: a randomized, double-blind, controlled clinical trial. *Clin Exp Rheumatol* 2003;21(2):193–198.
9. Holzer P. Capsaicin: cellular targets, mechanisms of action, and selectivity for thin sensory neurons. *Pharmacol Rev* 1991;43(2):143–201.

10. Winter J, Bevan S, et al. Capsaicin and pain mechanisms. *Br J Anaesth* 1995;75(2):157–168.
11. Caterina MJ, Schumacher MA, et al. The capsaicin receptor: a heat-activated ion channel in the pain pathway. *Nature* 1997;389(6653):816–824.
12. Nolano M, Simone DA, et al. Topical capsaicin in humans: parallel loss of epidermal nerve fibers and pain sensation. *Pain* 1999;81(1-2):135–145.
13. McCarthy GM, McCarty DJ. Effect of topical capsaicin in the therapy of painful osteoarthritis of the hands. *J Rheumatol* 1992;19(4):604–607.
14. Epstein JB, Marcoe JH. Topical application of capsaicin for treatment of oral neuropathic pain and trigeminal neuralgia. *Oral Surg Oral Med Oral Pathol* 1994;77(2):135–140.
15. Watson CP. Topical capsaicin as an adjuvant analgesic. *J Pain Symptom Manage* 1994;9(7):425–433.
16. Rains C, Bryson HM. Topical capsaicin: a review of its pharmacological properties and therapeutic potential in post-herpetic neuralgia, diabetic neuropathy and osteoarthritis. *Drugs Aging* 1995;7(4):317–328.
17. Fields HL. *Excitability blockers: anticonvulsants and low concentration local anesthetics in the treatment of chronic pain.* Berlin: Springer-Verlag, 1997.
18. McCleskey EW, Gold MS. Ion channels of nociception. *Annu Rev Physiol* 1999;61:835–856.
19. Galer BS, Rowbotham MC, et al. Topical lidocaine patch relieves postherpetic neuralgia more effectively than a vehicle topical patch: results of an enriched enrollment study. *Pain* 1999;80(3):533–538.
20. Rowbotham MC, Davies PS, et al. Lidocaine patch: double-blind controlled study of a new treatment method for postherpetic neuralgia. *Pain* 1996;65(1):39–44.
21. Scudds RA, Janzen V, et al. The use of topical 4% lidocaine in spheno-palatine ganglion blocks for the treatment of chronic muscle pain syndromes: a randomized, controlled trial. *Pain* 1995;62(1):69–77.
22. Sindrup SH, Jensen TS. Efficacy of pharmacological treatments of neuropathic pain: an update and effect related to mechanism of drug action. *Pain* 1999;83(3):389–400.
23. Godfrey RG. A guide to the understanding and use of tricyclic antidepressants in the overall management of fibromyalgia and other chronic pain syndromes. *Arch Intern Med* 1996;156(10):1047–1052.
24. Besson A, Privat AM, et al. Dopaminergic and opioidergic mediations of tricyclic antidepressants in the learned helplessness paradigm. *Pharmacol Biochem Behav* 1999;64(3):541–548.
25. Su X, Gebhart GF. Effects of tricyclic antidepressants on mechanosensitive pelvic nerve afferent fibers innervating the rat colon. *Pain* 1998;76(1-2):105–114.
26. Sawynok J, Esser MJ, et al. Antidepressants as analgesics: an overview of central and peripheral mechanisms of action. *J Psychiatry Neurosci* 2001;26(1):21–29.
27. Esser MJ, Sawynok J. Caffeine blockade of the thermal antihyperalgesic effect of acute amitriptyline in a rat model of neuropathic pain. *Eur J Pharmacol* 2000;399(2-3):131–139.
28. McCleane G. Topical application of doxepin hydrochloride, capsaicin, and a combination of both produces analgesia in chronic human neuropathic pain: a randomized, double-blind, placebo-controlled study. *Br J Clin Pharmacol* 2000;49(6):574–579.
29. Taylor CP, Gee NS, et al. A summary of mechanistic hypotheses of gabapentin pharmacology. *Epilepsy Res* 1998; 29(3):233–249.
30. Carlton SM, Zhou S. Attenuation of formalin-induced nociceptive behaviors following local peripheral injection of gabapentin. *Pain* 1998;76(1-2):201–207.
31. Crofford L, Russell IJ, Mease P, et al. Pregabalin improves pain associated with fibromyalgia syndrome in a multicenter randomized, placebo-controlled monotherapy trial. *Arthritis Rheum* 2002;46(9 Suppl):S613.
32. Litt JZ. Alternative topical therapy. *Dermatol Clin* 1989;7(1):43–52.
33. Zizeng Lu, Shude Jiao. *Applied traditional Chinese medicine in rheumatism.* Beijing: Peoples' Health, 1998.
34. Ng SK. Topical traditional Chinese medicine. A report from Singapore. *Arch Dermatol* 1998;134(11):1395–1396.
35. Pioro-Boisset M, Esdaile J, Fitzcharles M. Alternative medicine use in fibromyalgia syndrome. *Arthritis Care Res* 1996; 9(1):13–17.
36. Field T. Massage therapy effects in depression and somatic symptoms in chronic fatigue syndrome. *J Chronic Fatigue Syndr* 1997;3:43–51.
37. Ironson G, Field T, Scafidi F, et al. Massage therapy is associated with enhancement of the immune system's cytotoxic capacity. *Int J Neurosci* 1996;84:205–217.
38. Field T. Massage therapy effects. *Am Psychol* 1998;53(12):1270–1281.
39. Rachlin E, Rachline I. *Myofascial pain and fibromyalgia trigger point management*, 2nd ed. Philadelphia, PA: Mosby, 2002.
40. Melzack R, Wall P. Pain mechanisms: a new theory. *Science* 1965;150:971–979.
41. Danneskiold-Samsoe B, Christiansen E, Anderson RB. Myofascial pain and the role of myoglobin. *Scand J Rheumatol* 1986;15:174–178.
42. Moldofsky H. A chronobiologic theory of fibromyalgia. *J Musculoskelet Pain* 1993;1:49–59.
43. Russell IJ, Orr MD, Littman B, et al. Elevated cerebrospinal fluid levels of substance P in patients with fibromyalgia syndrome. *Arthritis Rheumatol* 1994;37:1593–1601.
44. Clauw D. Fibromyalgia: more than just a musculoskeletal disease. *Disease* 1995;52(3):843–851.
45. Field T, Diego M, Cullen C, et al. Fibromyalgia pain and substance P decrease and sleep improves after massage therapy. *J Clin Rheumatol* 2002;8(2):72–76.
46. Field T, Delage J, Hernandez-Reif M. Movement and massage therapy reduce fibromyalgia pain. *J Bodywork Movement Ther* 2003;7(1):49–52.
47. Gam A, Warming S, Larsen L, et al. Treatment of myofascial trigger-points with ultrasound combined with massage and exercise—a randomised, controlled trial. *Pain* 1998;77:73–79.
48. Sunshine W, Field T, Olga Q, et al. Fibromyalgia benefits from massage therapy and transcutaneous electrical stimulation. *J Clin Rheum* 1996;2(1):18–22.
49. Brattberg G. Connective tissue massage in the treatment of fibromyalgia. *Eur J Pain* 1999;3(3):235–244.
50. Alnigenis MNY, Bradely JD, Wallick J, et al. Massage therapy in the management of fibromyalgia: a pilot study. *J Musculoskelet Pain* 2001;9(2):55–67.
51. Holdcraft LC, Assefi N, Buchwald D, et al. Complementary and alternative medicine in fibromyalgia and related syndromes. *Best Pract Res Clin Rheumatol* 2003;17(4):667–683.
52. Grzesiak R. Psychological considerations in myofascial pain, fibromyalgia, and related musculoskeletal pain. In: Rachlin ES, ed. *Myofascial pain and fibromyalgia trigger point management*, 2nd ed. Philadelphia, PA: Mosby, 2002.
53. Molina A, Cechettin M, Fontana S, et al. Failure of EMG biofeedback (EMG-BF) after sham BFB training in fibromyalgia. *Fed Proc* 1987;46:549.
54. Ferraccioli G, Ghirelli L, Scita F, et al. EMG – biofeedback training in fibromyalgia syndrome. *J Rheumatol* 1987;14:4.
55. Bucklew SP, Conway R, Parker J, et al. Biofeedback/relaxation training and exercise interventions for fibromyalgia: a prospective trial. *Arthritis Care Res* 1998;11:196–209.

56. Van Santen M, Bolwijn P, Verstappen F, et al. Randomized clinical trial comparing fitness and biofeedback training versus basic treatment in patients with fibromyalgia. *J Rheumatol* 2002;29(3):575–581.

57. Sim J, Adams N. Therapeutic approaches to fibromyalgia syndrome in the United Kingdom: a survey of occupational therapists and physical therapists. *Eur J Pain* 2003;7(2):173–180.

58. Michlovitz S. *Thermal agents in rehabilitation*, 3rd ed. Philadelphia, PA: FA Davis Co, 1996.

59. Philadelphia Panel. Philadelphia panel evidence-based clinical practice guidelines on selected rehabilitation for knee pain. *Phys Ther* 2001;81:1675–1700.

60. Rakel B, Barr J. Physical modalities in chronic pain management. *Nurs Clin North Am* 2003;38:477–494.

61. Lin YH. Effects of thermal therapy in improving the passive range of knee motion: comparison of cold and superficial heat applications. *Clin Rehabil* 2003;17:618–623.

62. Robinson V, Brosseau L, Casimiro L, et al. Thermotherapy for treating rheumatoid arthritis (Cochrane Review). *The Cochrane Library*, Issue 4. Chichester, UK: John Wiley and Sons, 2002.

63. Minor MA, Sandord MK. The role of physical therapy and physical modalities in pain management. *Rheumatol Dis Clin North Am* 1999;25:233–248.

64. Behrens B, Michlovitz S. *Physical agents*. Philadelphia, PA: FA Davis Co, 1996.

65. Offenbacher M, Stucki G. Physical therapy in the treatment of fibromyalgia. *Scand J Rheumatol* 2000;29(Suppl. 113):78–85.

66. Buskila D, Mahmoud AS, Neumann L, et al. Balneotherapy for fibromyalgia at the Dead Sea. *Rheumatol Int* 2001;20:105–108.

67. Sukenik S, Baradin R, Codish S, et al. Balneotherapy at the Dead Sea area for patients with psoriatic arthritis and concomitant fibromyalgia. *Isr Med Assoc* 2001;3:147–150.

68. Sukenik S, Buskila D, Neumann L, et al. Sulphur bath and mud pack treatment for rheumatoid arthritis at the Dead Sea area. *Annu Rheumatol Dis* 1990;49:99–102.

69. Sukenik A, Buskila D, Neumann L, et al. Dead Sea bath salts for treatment of rheumatoid arthritis. *Clin Exp Rheumatol* 1990;8:353–357.

70. Sukenik S, Buskila D, Neumann L, et al. Mud pack therapy in rheumatoid arthritis. *Clin Rheumatol* 1992;11:243–247.

71. Sukenik S, Giryes H, Halvey S, et al. Treatment of psoriatic arthritis at the Dead Sea. *J Rheumatol* 1994;21:1305–1309.

72. Sukenik S, Neumann L, Flusser D, et al. Balneotherapy for rheumatoid arthritis at the Dead Sea. *Isr J Med Sci* 1995;31:210–214.

73. Neumann L, Sukenik S, Bolotin A, et al. The effect of balneotherapy at the Dead Sea on the quality of life of patients with fibromyalgia syndrome *Clin Rheumatol* 2001;20:15–19.

74. Evcik D, Kizilay, B, Gokcen, E, The effects of balneotherapy on fibromyalgia patients. *Rheumatol Int* 2002;22:56–59.

75. Flusser D, Abu-Shakra M, Friger M, et al. Therapy with mud compresses for knee osteoarthritis. *J Clin Rheumatol* 2002;8(4):197–203.

76. Baker K, Roberston V, Duck F. A review of therapeutic ultrasound: biophysical effects. *Phys Ther* 2001;81(7):1351–1358.

77. Almeida T, Roizenblatt S, Benedito-Silva AA, et al. The effect of combined therapy (ultrasound and interferential current) on pain and sleep in fibromyalgia. *Pain* 2003;104:665–672.

78. Robertson V, Baker K. 2001) A review of therapeutic ultrasound: effectiveness studies. *Phys Ther* 81(7):1339–1349.

79. Draper DO. Don't disregard ultrasound yet—the jury is still out. *Phys Ther* 2002;82(2):1909–1191.

80. Machet L, Boucaud A. Phonophoresis: efficiency, mechanism and skin tolerance. *Int J Pharm* 2002;242:1–15.

81. Klaiman M. Phonophoresis versus ultrasound in the treatment of common musculoskeletal conditions. *Med Sci Sports Exerc* 1998;30(9):1349–1355.

82. Cagnie B, Vinck E, Rimbaut S, et al. Phonophoresis versus topical application of ketoprofen: comparison between tissue and plasma levels. *Phys Ther* 2003;83(8):707–712.

83. Bare A, McAnaw M, Pritchard A, et al. Phonophoretic delivery of 10% hydrocortisone through the epidermis of humans as determined by serum cortisol concentrations. *Phys Ther* 1996;76(7):738–749.

84. Griffin JE, et al. Patients treated with ultrasonic driven hydrocortisone and with cortisol using phonophoresis. *Phys Ther* 1967;47:595.

85. Kleinkort JA, Wood F. Patients treated with ultrasonic driven hydrocortisone. *Phys Ther* 1975;55:1321.

86. Wing M. Phonophoresis with hydrocortisone in the treatment of temporomandibular joint dysfunction. *Phys Ther* 1982;62:33.

87. Holdsworth LK, Anderson DM. Effectiveness of ultrasound used with a hydrocortisone coupling medium or epicondylitis clasp to treat lateral epicondylitis: pilot study. *Physiotherapy* 1993;79:19.

88. Stratford P, et al. The evaluation of phonophoresis and friction massage as treatments for extensor carpi radialis tendonitis: a randomized, controlled trial. *Physiother Can* 1989;41:93.

89. Kumar VN, Redford JB. Transcutaneous nerve stimulation in rheumatoid arthritis. *Arch Phys Med Rehabil* 1982;63:595–596.

90. Christian L, Kreczi T, Klingler D. Transcutaneous electrical nerve stimulation in the treatment of chronic pain: predictive factors and evaluation of the method. *Clin J Pain* 1998;14(2):134–142.

91. Chabal C, Fishbain DA, Weaver M, et al. Long-term transcutaneous electrical nerve stimulation (TENS) use: impact on medication utilization and physical therapy costs. *Clin J Pain* 1998;14(1):66–73.

92. Carroll D, Moore R, McQuay H, et al. Transcutaneous electrical nerve stimulation (TENS) for chronic pain (Cochrane Review). *The Cochrane Library*, Issue 4. Oxford: Update Software, 2001.

93. Fargas-Babjak, A. Acupuncture, transcutaneous electrical nerve stimulation, and laser therapy in chronic pain. *Clin J Pain* 2001;17:S105–S113.

94. Reeve J, Menon D, Corabian P. Transcutaneous electrical nerve stimulation. *Int J Technol Assess Health Care* 1996;12:299–324.

95. Robinson A. Transcutaneous electrical nerve stimulation for the control of pain in musculoskeletal disorders. *J Orthop Sports Phys Ther* 1996;24:208–226.

96. Sim J, Adams N. Physical and other non-pharmacological interventions for fibromyalgia. *Ballieres Clin Rheumatol* 1999;13(3):507–523.

97. Di Benedetto P, Iona LG, Zidarich V. Clinical evaluation of S-adenosyl-1-methionine versus transcutaneous electrical nerve stimulation in primary fibromyalgia. *Curr Ther Res* 1993;53:222–229.

98. Brosseau L, Milne S, Robinson V, et al. Efficacy of the transcutaneous electrical nerve stimulation for the treatment of chronic low back pain. *Spine* 2002;27(6):596–603.

99. Rushton DN. Electrical stimulation in the treatment of pain. *Disabil Rehabil* 2002;24(8):407–415.

100. Fishbain DA, Chabal C, Abbott A, et al. Transcutaneous electrical nerve stimulation (TENS) treatment outcome in long-term users. *Clin J Pain* 1996;12:201–214.

101. Lampl C, Kreczi T, Klingler D. Transcutaneous electrical nerve stimulation in the treatment of chronic pain: predictive factors and evaluation of the method. *Clin J Pain* 1998;14:134–142.

31

Systemic Therapies for Chronic Pain

Lesley M. Arnold

PHARMACOLOGIC TREATMENT OF FIBROMYALGIA

Although fibromyalgia (FM) affects an estimated 3.4% of women and 0.5% of men in the general U.S. population (1) and is associated with substantial morbidity and disability (2–5), there are few proven effective pharmacologic therapies and, to date, no U.S. Food and Drug Administration (FDA)-approved treatments. Several factors have limited advancements in the pharmacologic treatment of FM. First, the pathophysiology of FM is unknown and treatment studies have been largely empirical. Second, the American College of Rheumatology (ACR) criteria for FM, which include widespread pain of at least 3 months duration and tenderness at 11 or more of 18 specific tender point (TeP) sites on the body (6), do not incorporate other symptoms that commonly occur in patients with FM. Indeed, the clinical presentation of FM is heterogeneous. In the study that established the ACR criteria, 73% to 85% of patients with FM also reported fatigue, sleep disturbance (nonrestorative sleep or insomnia), and morning stiffness. "Pain all over," paresthesias, headache, history of depression, and anxiety were experienced by 45% to 69% of patients, and co-occurring irritable bowel syndrome (IBS), sicca symptoms, and Raynaud phenomenon were less common (<35%) (6). Many patients with FM also report weakness, forgetfulness, concentration difficulties, urinary frequency, dysmenorrhea history, subjective swelling, and restless legs. Although most FM clinical trials have assessed change in the intensity of pain, they have inconsistently evaluated other associated symptoms, which reduces the trials' comparability and clinical applicability. Third, patients with FM frequently have comorbid disorders that may affect their response to treatment. Comorbid mood and anxiety disorders, which are common in patients with FM (7–9), are associated with functional disability (8,10) and persistent FM symptoms (11). Despite evidence of elevated prevalence rates of mood and anxiety disorders in patients with FM and their possible prognostic significance, few clinical trials have systemically evaluated patients for comorbid psychiatric disorders. Patients with FM also have high rates of other chronic-pain disorders, including chronic headache, IBS, and temporomandibular disorder (12). However, most FM trials have not assessed for these conditions or determined the effect of comorbidity on response to treatment. Finally, biomarkers of FM activity remain elusive, and the definition of improvement in trials has relied on clinical impressions. However, there is neither a consensus on clinically important outcome measures nor a definition of clinically meaningful response to treatment in FM trials. It is unclear whether improvement in pain intensity alone should define response to treatment in FM, which is characterized by multiple symptoms in addition to pain. For example, other characteristics of pain might be of particular importance in FM patients, such as the degree to which the pain is widespread and the level of tenderness. It might also be important to include other domains of interest in a measure of response, such as quality of life, physical and emotional function, sleep, fatigue, and cognition.

Despite these limitations, progress has been made in identifying potentially efficacious medications for many of the symptoms of FM. The following is a review of controlled trials of FM, a discussion of the issues that remain to be addressed in further research, and clinical recommendations for the pharmacologic management of FM based on the available evidence. Other chronic nonneuropathic pain disorders that are commonly comorbid with FM will also be addressed. The pharmacologic treatment of FM is a rapidly growing area of research, and it is likely that medication treatment options will continue to expand for patients with FM.

REVIEW OF PHARMACOLOGIC CLINICAL TRIALS

ANTIDEPRESSANT MEDICATION

Most pharmacologic treatment studies in FM have focused on antidepressants. The rationale for studying antidepressants is based on several lines of evidence. First, serotonin and norepinephrine have been implicated in the mediation of endogenous analgesic mechanisms via the descending inhibitory pain pathways in the brain and spinal cord (13–15), and dysfunction of serotonin and norepinephrine-mediated descending pain-inhibitory pathways is a potential mechanism for the pain experienced by patients with FM (16–19). Therefore, antidepressants that enhance serotonin and norepinephrine neurotransmission in the descending inhibitory pain pathways may reduce pain perception in patients with FM (20). Second, antidepressants that increase serotonin and norepinephrine-mediated neurotransmission are effective in the treatment of other chronic-pain conditions (21). Third, antidepressants are effective for the treatment of depressive and anxiety disorders, which are frequently comorbid with FM and possibly share a physiologic abnormality with FM (22). Finally, some antidepressants have other pharmacologic properties, including N-methyl-D-aspartate (NMDA) antagonism and ion-channel blocking activity, which may mediate their antinociceptive effects (23,24).

Tricyclics

The initial impetus for studying tricyclic antidepressants as potential treatments for FM (25,26) was based on the identification of the α-δ non–rapid eye movement (NREM) sleep abnormality in polysomnographic studies of many patients with FM (27). The sleep abnormality consisted of an inappropriate intrusion of α waves [normally seen during wakefulness or rapid eye movement (REM) sleep in sleep electroencephalograms (EEGs)] into deep sleep (characterized by δ waves on sleep EEG) (27). The α-δ NREM sleep abnormality was postulated to be associated with the development of the chronic pain and fatigue characteristic of FM and to be mediated by an abnormality in central serotonergic neurotransmission (28). Thus, tertiary amine tricyclics such as amitriptyline (AMI), with higher ratios of serotonin/norepinephrine reuptake inhibition than secondary amine agents, became the initial candidate antidepressants for the treatment of FM. The antidepressant and antinociceptive effects of the tricyclics may be mediated through reuptake inhibition of serotonin and norepinephrine, which increases the levels of these neurotransmitters. Other properties of the tricyclics, including dopamine reuptake inhibition, NMDA antagonism, and ion-channel blocking activity, might also contribute to their therapeutic effect (23).

Tricyclic agents (TCAs) have been the most common medications studied in randomized, placebo (PB)-controlled FM clinical trials. A recent meta-analysis of PB-controlled trials of tricyclics included nine studies with sufficient statistical data for effect size computations (i.e., means and standard deviations for continuous outcomes, proportions for binary outcomes) (29). The nine studies included two double-blind, PB controlled, parallel-group acute treatment trials of AMI (30) and dothiepin (DTP) (a tricyclic structurally similar to AMI and doxepin) (31), respectively; a parallel-group study comparing AMI, cyclobenzaprine (CBP), and PB for up to 6 months (32); and two parallel-group, double-blind, PB-controlled acute treatment trials of the tricyclic CBP (33,34). Although CBP is classified as a muscle relaxant rather than an antidepressant, it has structural and pharmacologic properties that are very similar to other tricyclics that exert antidepressant effects (35–41). The remaining PB-controlled, double-blind trials included in the

meta-analysis were conducted with crossover designs. These trials included two studies of AMI (42) and CBP (43), respectively; a comparison of clomipramine, maprotiline (MPL), or PB (44); and another multicomparison study of fluoxetine (FLX), AMI, combination AMI and FLX, and PB (only the results of AMI alone were included in the meta-analysis) (45). Seven outcome measures that were most commonly used in the studies were assessed, including the patients' self-ratings of pain, stiffness, fatigue, and sleep, the patient and the physician global (GBL) assessment of improvement, and tenderness as measured by TePs. Table 31-1 summarizes the observed effect sizes for the outcomes in the nine trials. Figure 31-1 presents the observed effects by type of outcome as a box plot. The meta-analysis showed that the overall effect of these agents on FM symptoms was moderate. The largest effect was found in measures of sleep quality, with more modest changes in measures of tenderness and stiffness. Thus the most consistent improvement may be attributed to the sedative properties of these medications (29). Overall, significant clinical response to TCAs was observed in 25% to 37% of patients with FM, and the degree of efficacy was modest in most studies (29).

The results of a meta-analysis of randomized, PB-controlled studies of CBP were consistent with the Arnold et al. (29) meta-analysis, which included CBP as well as other TCAs. For the average patient, CBP treatment resulted in moderate improvement in sleep, modest improvement in pain, and no improvement in fatigue or TePs. Patients were about three times as likely to report improvement in their symptoms compared to those on PB (46).

Another meta-analysis of antidepressants in the treatment of FM included 13 trials that assessed other classes of antidepressants in addition to the tricyclics, including the selective serotonin reuptake inhibitors (SSRIs), FLX (45,47) and citalopram (48); a reversible inhibitor of monoamine oxidase (MAO) A, moclobemide (49); and S-adenosyl-L-methionine (SAMe) (50,51), an over-the counter dietary supplement that is a major methyl donor in the brain and is involved in the pathways for synthesis of norepinephrine, dopamine, and serotonin, as well as hormones, nucleic acids, proteins, and phospholipids (52). However, most of the 13 trials evaluated tricyclic antidepressants, including AMI in eight studies (30,32,42,45,49,53–55), and clomipramine and MPL in one study (44) (CBP was not included in this meta-analysis) (56). Outcome measures for five individual FM symptoms were examined, including the number of TePs, and patients' self-ratings of pain, sleep, fatigue, and overall well-being. The pooled results showed a significant symptomatic benefit of antidepressants that was moderate for sleep, overall well-being, and pain severity, and mild for fatigue and number of TePs. Patients treated with antidepressants were more than four times as likely to improve as those on PB. The magnitude of benefit was similar to that found in the Arnold et al. (29) meta-analysis reviewed above. Furthermore, there was no difference between the efficacy of the SSRIs and the other drug classes, although the small number of SSRI trials precludes firm conclusions about relative efficacy (56).

Two studies of TCAs (42,43) evaluated the effect of the medication on sleep physiology. In the Reynolds et al. (43) study of CBP, the amount of α rhythm occurring during NREM sleep was moderate and unchanged during either PB

TABLE 31-1 The Observed Effect Sizes for Seven Outcomes in Nine Controlled Studies of Tricyclic Medications in the Treatment of Fibromyalgia[a]

STUDY	DESIGN	EFFECTIVE N[b]	DOSAGE (mg/d)	DURATION (wk)	PAIN Pt Gbl	PAIN MD	PAIN Gbl	FATIGUE	SLEEP	TENDERNESS	STIFFNESS
Carette et al. (1986) (30)	AMI vs. PB	59	AMI 50	9	0.58	0.58	0.635	NA	0.70	0.27	0.30
Caruso et al. (1987) (31)	DTP vs. PB	52	DTP 75	8	0.76	1.32	0.45	NA	NA	0.63	NA
Bennett et al. (1988) (33)	CBP vs. PB	63	CBP 10–40	12	NA	0.44	0.42	0.10	0.31	0.59	0.10
Quimby et al. (1989) (34)	CBP vs. PB	40	CBP 10–40	6	0.98	0.98	0.75	0.31	1.19	NA	0.77
Carette et al. (1994) (32)	AMI vs. CBP vs. PB	98 (AMI) /86 (CBP)	AMI 50 CBP 30	26	0.27	0.44	0.45	0.64	0.53	0.03	NA
Carette et al. (1995) (42)	AMI vs. PB	20	AMI 25	8	0.70	0.74	0.80	0.88	0.90	0.25	NA
Reynolds et al. (1991) (43)	CBP vs. PB	9	CBP 20–40	4	NA	NA	0.17	0.55	0.37	−0.34	NA
Bibolotti et al. (1986) (44)	CMI vs. MPL vs. PB	18	CMI 75 MPL 75	3	NA	0.70	NA	NA	NA	0.73	NA
Goldenberg et al. (1996) (45)	AMI + PB vs. AMI + FLX vs. FLX + PB vs. PB + PB	19	AMI 25[c]	6	0.68	0.49	0.68	0.22	0.61	0.14	NA

NA, not assessed; AMI, amitriptyline; PB, placebo; DTP, dothiepin; CBP, cyclobenzaprine; CMI, chlomipramine; MPL, maprotiline; FLX, fluoxetine; GBL, global.
[a]Where repeated measures were taken or multiple treatments were compared, a mean effect size is reported.
[b]Study completers.
[c]Only the results of amitriptyline alone were included in the meta-analysis.
From Arnold LM, Keck PE Jr, Welge JA. Antidepressant treatment of FM. A meta-analysis and review. *Psychosomatics* 2000;41:104–113, with permission.

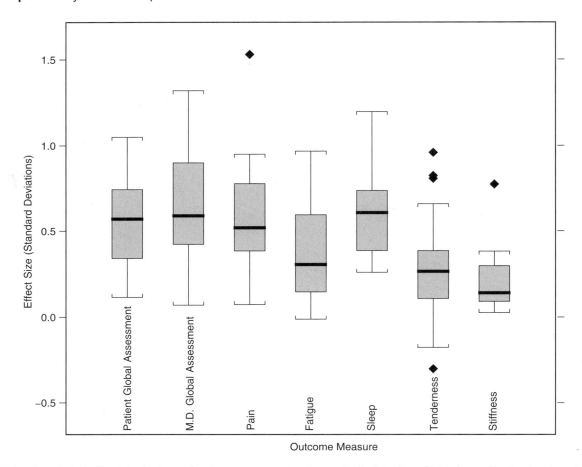

Figure 31-1. Box plot of effect size by type of outcome measure in nine controlled studies of tricyclic medication treatment of fibromyalgia. (The dark line in each box marks the median, the width of the box corresponds to the interquartile range, and the "whiskers" note the 5th and 95th percentiles. Diamond-shaped markers indicate observations lying beyond the 5th and 95th percentiles.) (From Arnold LM, Keck PE Jr, Welge JA. Antidepressant treatment of fibromyalgia. A meta-analysis and review. *Psychosomatics* 2000;41:104–113, with permission.)

or CBP treatment, which was consistent with the lack of change in subjective perception of sleep quality. Similarly, in the Carette et al. (42) study, neither AMI nor PB treatment resulted in any changes in the α ratings during NREM sleep. Therefore, tricyclics agents do not appear to affect the sleep anomaly that was identified as a possible target for treatment by tricyclics (27). Indeed, in the Carette et al. (42) study, only eight patients (36%) exhibited an α NREM sleep anomaly at baseline, leading the authors to conclude that the anomaly is found in a small proportion of patients with FM. Furthermore, the anomaly correlated with more self-reported sleep disturbance but was not associated with other symptoms or signs of FM. Therefore, the role of the sleep disturbance in the pathophysiology of FM remains to be elucidated (42). Tables 31-2 and 31-3 summarize the results of studies of TCAs in FM.

Selective Serotonin Reuptake Inhibitors

SSRIs have a high affinity for the serotonin transporter, although recent evidence suggests that some of the SSRIs increase levels of both serotonin and norepinephrine, particularly at higher therapeutic doses (75,76). SSRIs, although likely to be better tolerated than tricyclics (77), have been

examined in only five double-blind, PB-controlled trials in FM: two with citalopram (48,78) and three with FLX (45,47,79) (see Table 31-4). In the first study of 42 patients with FM who were randomized to citalopram (20–40 mg per day) or PB for 8 weeks, there were no significant differences in efficacy measures between the citalopram and PB groups (48). In the second randomized, double-blind, PB-controlled, 4-month study of 40 women with FM, citalopram (20–40 mg per day) treatment resulted in a significant decrease in depressive symptoms compared to PB. Although there were no significant differences between groups in other symptoms of FM, there was a trend for patients in the citalopram group to report improvement in overall well-being more frequently than those in the PB group (78).

Three randomized, controlled trials have examined FLX in the treatment of FM. The initial FLX trial did not find a significant therapeutic effect over PB (47). However, this trial was limited by a very high (57%) PB dropout rate, small sample size, brief trial duration, and restriction of FLX dose to 20 mg per day. In two other controlled trials, FLX was superior to PB in reducing pain and other symptoms associated with FM (45,79). Goldenberg et al. (45) conducted a double-blind, crossover study in which 19 subjects with FM received four 6-week trials of FLX 20 mg per

TABLE 31-2 Randomized, Double-blind, Placebo-controlled Trials of the Tricyclic Agent (TCA), Amitriptyline (AMI), in Fibromyalgia (FM)

STUDY	FM CRITERIA	N	MEAN AGE	PERCENT WOMEN	DESIGN	DOSAGE, MG/DAY	DURATION WEEKS	OUTCOME MEASURES	TCA SIGNIFICANTLY BETTER THAN PB?
Carette et al. (1986) (30)	Smythe (57)	59	40.9	92	AMI v PB parallel	AMI 50	9	Pain VAS	No
								Dolorimetry	No
								Sleep ordinal scale	Yes
								Duration, AM stiffness	No
								Patient global	Yes
								Physician global	Yes
								≥50% improvement in pain VAS	No
Goldenberg et al. (1986) (58)	Yunus (59)	62	43.8	95	AMI + N v PB + N v AMI +PB v PB + PB parallel	AMI 25 N 1000	6	Pain or stiffness VAS	Yes
								Manual TeP score	Yes
								Sleep VAS	Yes
								Fatigue VAS	Yes
								Patient global	Yes
Scudds et al. (1989) (53)	Smythe (60)	36	39.9	89	AMI v PB crossover	AMI 50	4, with 2-week washout	Physician global	Yes
								McGill Pain Questionnaire (61)	Yes
								Dolorimetry	Yes
								Pain threshold at non-TePs	No
								Pain tolerance at non-TePs	No
Hench et al. (1989) (62)	Yunus (59)	10	NR	NR	AMI v TE v PB crossover	AMI 25 TE 30	2, with 2-week washout	Patient global	Yes
								Pain	No
								Manual TeP number	Yes
								Sleep	No
								Physician global	No

(Continued)

TABLE 31-2 Continued

STUDY	FM CRITERIA	N	MEAN AGE	PERCENT WOMEN	DESIGN	DOSAGE, MG/DAY	DURATION WEEKS	OUTCOME MEASURES	TCA SIGNIFICANTLY BETTER THAN PB?
Jaeschke et al. (1991) (63)	"conventional criteria"	23	55	NR	N-of-1	AMI 5-50	2, with no washout	Symptom questionnaire (energy, tiredness, pain, stiffness, sleep, headaches, bowel problems)	Yes in 7 patients
Carette et al. (1994) (32)	ACR (6)	208	45	94	AMI v CBP v PB parallel	AMI 50 CBP 30	24	Manual TeP count	Yes in 4 patients
								Pain VAS	No
								McGill Pain Questionnaire (61)	No
								Dolorimetry	No
								Sleep VAS	No
								Fatigue VAS	No
								Feeling on awakening VAS	No
								AM stiffness VAS	No
								Patient global	No
								Physician global	No
								SIP (64)	No
								HAQ (65)	No
								AIMS anxiety and depression scales (66)	No
								Simms criteria for improvement (67)	No
Carette et al. (1995) (42)	ACR (6)	22	43.8	96	AMI v PB crossover	AMI 25	8, with no washout	Pain VAS	Yes
Goldenberg et al., (1996) (45)	ACR (6)	31	43.2	90	AMI + PB v AMI + FLX v FLX + PB v PB + PB crossover	AMI 25 FLX 20	4, with 2-week washout	Dolorimetry	No
								Sleep VAS	Yes
								Fatigue VAS	Yes
								Patient global	Yes
								Physician global	Yes
								Pain VAS	Yes
								Manual TeP score	No
								Sleep VAS	Yes
								Fatigue VAS	No

Study	Criteria				Design	Dose	Weeks	Outcome measure	Result
								Feeling on awakening VAS	No
								Patient global	Yes
								Physician global	Yes
								FIQ (68)	Yes
								BDI (69)	No
Ginsberg et al. (1996) (54)	ACR (6)	46	46	83	AMI v PB parallel	AMI 25	8	Pain VAS	
								Manual TeP number	Yes
								Manual TeP score	Yes
								Sleep VAS	Yes
								Fatigue VAS	Yes
								Feeling on awakening VAS	Yes
								Duration of AM stiffness	Yes
								Patient global	Yes
								Physician global	Yes
								Responder: at least 3: 1) ≥50% improvement in patient global; 2) ≥50% improvement in physician global; 3) ≥50% improvement in pain; 4) ≥25% reduction in TeP score	Yes
Hannonen et al. (1998) (49)	ACR (6)	130	49.7	100	AMI v MOCLO v PB parallel	AMI 25-37.5 MOCLO 450-600	12	Primary outcome: physician impression of change	Yes
								Pain VAS	Yes
								Manual TeP number	Yes
								Sleep VAS	Yes
								Fatigue VAS	Yes
								Sheehan disability scale (70)	Yes
								Nottingham Health Profile (71)	Yes (energy, pain, emotion, sleep)
								Physician impression of severity	Yes
Heymann et al. (2001) (72)	ACR (6)	118	53.4	100	AMI v NTP v PB parallel	AMI 25 NTP 25	8	General health VAS	Yes
								Manual TeP number	No
								FIQ total score (68)	No
								Patient global	Yes (AMI) No (NTP)

AMI amitriptyline; PB placebo; VAS visual analog scale; AM morning; N naproxen; NR not reported; TE temazepam; ACR American College of Rheumatology; CBP cyclobenzaprine; SIP Sickness Impact Profile; HAQ Health Assessment Questionnaire; AIMS Arthritis Impact Measurement Scales; FLX fluoxetine; FIQ Fibromyalgia Impact Questionnaire; BDI Beck Depression Inventory; MOCLO moclobemide; NTP nortriptyline; TePs, tender points.

TABLE 31-3 Randomized, Double-blind, Placebo-controlled Trials of Other Tricyclic Agents (TCAs) in Fibromyalgia (FM)

STUDY	FM CRITERIA	N	MEAN AGE	PERCENT WOMEN	DESIGN	DOSAGE (MG/DAY)	DURATION (WEEKS)	OUTCOME MEASURES	TCA SIGNIFICANTLY BETTER THAN PB?
Bibolotti et al. (1986) (44)	Extraarticular pain, variable pain, intensity, and duration, modulated by weather, trigger points, muscle hypertone	37	38.5	100	CMI vs. MPL vs. PB crossover	CMI 75 MPL 75	3, no washout	Hamilton rating scale for depression (73)	Yes (MPL) / No (CMI)
								Number of trigger points	Yes (CMI) / No (MPL)
								Physician global	Yes
								Pain VAS	Yes
Caruso et al. (1987) (31)	Campbell (74)	60	45.2	80	DTP vs. PB parallel	DTP 75	8	Manual TeP index	Yes
								Patient global	Yes
								Physician global	Yes
								Pain VAS	Yes
Bennett et al. (1988) (33)	Chronic, widespread pain, 7/16 TePs, muscle tension, disturbed sleep, AM stiffness, 2 minor criteria	120	49.1	NR	CBP vs. PB parallel	CBP 10–40	12	Manual TeP score	No
								Manual TeP number	No
								Sleep VAS	Yes
								Duration of fatigue	No
								Duration of a.m. stiffness	No
								Physician global	Yes
								Pain (Likert scale)	No
Quimby et al. (1989) (34)	Chronic pain in ≥3 sites, ≥5 TePs by dolorimeter, 3 minor criteria	40	45	100	CBP vs. PB parallel	CBP 10–40	6	Stiffness (Likert scale)	Yes
								Sleep (Likert scale)	Yes
								Fatigue (Likert scale)	No
								Patient global	Yes
								Physician global	Yes
								Pain (Likert scale)	No
Reynolds et al. (1991) (43)	Diffuse aching, fatigue, disturbed sleep, 7/16 TePs	12	43	83	CBP vs. PB crossover	CBP 20–40	4, with 2-wk washout	Manual TeP score	No
								Dolorimetry	No
								Sleep (Likert scale)	No
								Fatigue (Likert scale)	Yes

CMI, clomipramine; MPL, maprotiline; DTP, dothiepin; PB, placebo; VAS, visual analog scale; a.m., morning; CBP, cyclobenzaprine; TePs, tender points.

TABLE 31-4 Randomized, Double-blind, Placebo-controlled Trials of Selective Serotonin Reuptake Inhibitors (SSRIs) in Fibromyalgia (FM)

STUDY	FM CRITERIA	N	MEAN AGE	PERCENT WOMEN	DESIGN	DOSAGE, MG/DAY	DURATION WEEKS	OUTCOME MEASURES	SSRI SIGNIFICANTLY BETTER THAN PB?
Wolfe et al. (1994) (47)	Widespread pain, 7/14 TePs	42	48	100	FLX v PB parallel	FLX 20	6	Pain VAS	No
Goldenberg et al., (1996) (45)	ACR (6)	31	43.2	90	AMI + PB v AMI + FLX v FLX + PB v PB + PB crossover	AMI 25 FLX 20	4, with 2-week washout	Manual TeP count	No
								Manual TeP score	No
								Dolorimetry score	No
								Sleep VAS	No
								Fatigue VAS	No
								Duration of AM stiffness	No
								HAQ (65)	No
								AIMS anxiety (66)	No
								AIMS depression (66)	No
								BDI (69)	No
								Anxiety scale	No
								Global severity	No
								Pain VAS	Yes
Arnold et al. (2002) (79)	ACR (6)	60	46	100	FLX v PB	FLX mean dose 45 ± 25	12	Manual TeP score	No
								Sleep VAS	Yes
								Fatigue VAS	No
								Feeling on awakening VAS	No
								Patient global	Yes
								Physician global	No
								FIQ (68)	Yes
								BDI (69)	No
								FIQ (68) total score	Yes
								FIQ pain score	Yes
								FIQ physical impairment	No
								FIQ days felt good	No
								FIQ fatigue	Yes

(Continued)

TABLE 31-4 Continued

STUDY	FM CRITERIA	N	MEAN AGE	PERCENT WOMEN	DESIGN	DOSAGE, MG/DAY	DURATION WEEKS	OUTCOME MEASURES	SSRI SIGNIFICANTLY BETTER THAN PB?
								FIQ feeling upon awakening	No
								FIQ stiffness	No
								FIQ anxiety	No
								FIQ depression	Yes
								TeP number by dolorimetry	No
								Myalgic score by dolorimetry	No
								McGill Pain Questionnaire (61)	Yes
								≥25% improvement in FIQ total score	No
								≥25% improvement in FIQ pain score	Yes
Nørregaard et al. (1995) (48)	ACR (6)	42	48	NR	CIT v PB parallel	CIT 20-40	8	Pain VAS	No
								Manual TeP count	No
								Fatigue VAS	No
								Sleep VAS	No
								General condition VAS	No
								FIQ (68) physical function score	No
								BDI (69)	No
								Muscle strength	No
								Physician global assessment	No
Anderberg et al. (2000) (78)	ACR (6)	40	48.6	100	CIT v PB	CIT 20-40	16	Pain VAS	No
								FIQ (68)	No
								Depressive symptoms (MADRS) (80)	Yes
								Global assessment of pain	No
								Global assessment of well-being	No

FLX fluoxetine; PB placebo; VAS visual analog scale; AM morning; HAQ Health Assessment Questionnaire; AIMS Arthritis Impact Measurement Scales; BDI Beck Depression Inventory, ACR American College of Rheumatology; AMI amitriptyline; FIQ Fibromyalgia Impact Questionnaire; MADRS Montgomery Asberg Depression Rating Scale; CIT, citalopram; TePs, tender points.

day, AMI 25 mg per day, the combination, or PB. Both FLX and AMI produced significant improvement in pain, global well-being, and function compared to PB. Combination treatment, in turn, produced significantly greater improvement than did either drug alone. Interpretation of the results of this study are limited by the crossover design (potential for carryover effects and unblinding of treatment), low fixed doses of FLX and AMI, and the probable pharmacokinetic interaction between FLX and AMI in the combination treatment group, an interaction that typically elevates tricyclic plasma concentrations (81).

To overcome some of the methodological limitations of earlier trials of FLX, Arnold et al. (79) recently conducted a randomized, PB-controlled, parallel-group, flexible dose, 12-week trial of FLX in FM. Sixty female subjects who did not have any current comorbid psychiatric disorders (including mood and anxiety disorders), a history of substance dependence during the previous 6 months, a history of mania, psychosis, or dementia, or a score of 10 or greater on the 17-item Hamilton Depression Scale (73) were randomized to receive FLX 20 to 80 mg per day or PB and evaluated with the Fibromyalgia Impact Questionnaire (FIQ) (68) total score (score range: 0 to 80, with 0 indicating no impact) and FIQ pain score (score range 0 to 10) as the primary outcome measures. Secondary measures included on the McGill Pain Questionnaire (61), change in the number of TePs by dolorimetry, and total myalgic score (sum of dolorimetry results at the 18 ACR TeP sites). Subjects receiving FLX (mean dose 45 ± 25 mg per day) displayed significantly greater reductions in FIQ total score, and FIQ subscales of pain, fatigue, and depression on the McGill Pain Questionnaire compared to subjects receiving PB. The number of TePs and total myalgic scores improved more in the FLX group than in the PB group, but these differences were not statistically significant. Although threshold severity scores have not been established for the FIQ, a >25% improvement in scores was thought to correspond to clinically meaningful improvement. A >25% improvement in the total FIQ score was observed in 32% of the FLX-treated subjects and 15% of the subjects who received PB ($p = 0.19$), whereas a >25% improvement in the FIQ pain score was observed in 56% of the FLX-treated subjects and 15% of the PB-treated subjects ($p = 0.003$). There was no significant interaction between treatment and either a history of major depressive disorders or by baseline level of depression. Furthermore, the effect of FLX on the FIQ pain score was still significant after adjustment for change in the depression score. Therefore, the effect of FLX on reduction of pain associated with FM appears to be independent of an effect on mood. FLX was well tolerated; there were no significant differences between the two groups in dropouts due to side effects. Applying Cohen's measure of effect size (82), the observed effect sizes in the FLX study were comparable to the treatment effects seen with the tricyclics, with the largest effect of FLX on pain (effect size = 0.95) (83). Given the beneficial effects of higher doses of FLX in this study, some patients who fail to respond to a 20 mg per day dose of FLX may improve with higher doses, if they are tolerated. Several limitations of this study should be considered. Like most studies of antidepressants in FM, this study was limited by small sample size and relatively short

duration of treatment of 12 weeks. Patients with secondary FM and all current and several forms of lifetime psychopathology were excluded, and the results may not generalize to those with certain forms of psychiatric and medical comorbidity. Finally, the results may not generalize to men. However, this is the first randomized, PB-controlled, parallel-group study that showed significant efficacy of an SSRI in FM.

The study of other SSRIs in FM is very limited. Three controlled trials did not use a PB group (84–86). The first trial compared the combination of FLX (20 mg per day) and CBP (10 mg per day) to CBP (10 mg per day) alone in a parallel group, 12-week trial involving 21 women with FM by ACR criteria. Both treatment groups significantly improved in pain, number of TePs, TeP index, and morning stiffness; however, the combination of FLX and CBP was significantly more efficacious than CBP alone (84). As noted above, the efficacy of combined treatment may have been secondary to the pharmacokinetic interaction between FLX and tricyclics that results in elevation of tricyclic plasma levels. In the second study, sertraline (50 to 100 mg per day) was compared to AMI (10 to 25 mg per day) in a parallel group, 12-week trial involving 60 patients with FM by ACR criteria. Both treatment groups experienced significant improvement in pain, fatigue, depressive symptoms, anxiety symptoms, patient and physician global assessment, and total impact of FM as measured by the FIQ. The number of TePs did not significantly improve in either group. There was no difference in the efficacy of AMI compared to sertraline, but sertraline was better tolerated, with significantly fewer dropouts due to side effects (85). In the third study, the SSRI fluvoxamine (mean dose 25 mg per day) was compared to AMI (mean dose 20 mg per day) in a parallel group, 4-week trial involving 68 patients with FM by ACR criteria. A similar percentage of patients on AMI (50%) and fluvoxamine (41%) reported a decrease in pain of at least 50% (86). Although these three controlled studies suggest that SSRIs might be equally as effective as tricyclics in the treatment of FM, it is important to note that none of the trials was powered to detect differences in treatment efficacy. Furthermore, because of the lack of a PB arm, the contribution of a PB effect could not be assessed in any of the trials. Two other trials of SSRIs used single-blind designs (87,88). In the first study, published only as an abstract, 46 patients meeting ACR criteria for FM were treated with sertraline 25 to 200 mg per day for 18 weeks after a 14-day PB run-in period. The investigators' overall assessment of efficacy was good or very good in 63% of patients, and 80% of patients assessed efficacy as good or very good. A significant reduction in TeP score was also observed (87). In the second study, 40 patients with FM by ACR criteria were randomized to receive either paroxetine 20 mg per day or PB for 3 months. Treatment with paroxetine was well tolerated and resulted in significant improvement in the TeP score, pain, morning stiffness, mood, sleep, inclination to work, and capacity to work (88). Lack of adequate blinding limits the conclusions that can be drawn from these studies, and further studies are needed to confirm these preliminary findings and establish the role of sertraline and paroxetine in the management of FM.

Serotonin and Norepinephrine Reuptake Inhibitors

Prior treatment studies with antidepressant medications suggest that inhibition of both the serotonin and norepinephrine reuptake transporters is more effective in treating FM than inhibition of either transporter alone (21). Similarly, there is evidence that medications that combine serotonin and norepinephrine reuptake inhibition are more effective antidepressants than single selective reuptake inhibitors, particularly for severe or refractory depression (89–91). Higher doses of some of the SSRIs, such as paroxetine and FLX, might increase both serotonin and norepinephrine levels and result in better efficacy of these antidepressants. Indeed, FLX at a mean dose of 45 mg per day—higher than the 20 mg per day dose used in a previously negative study of FLX (47)—was efficacious in the treatment of FM, as discussed above (79). Although there are no published randomized, double-blind trials of paroxetine in FM, higher doses of paroxetine (30 to 40 mg per day) were more effective in preventing recurrences of depression and in treating refractory depression than the 20 mg per day dose (92).

Venlafaxine was the first newer-generation antidepressant to be classified as a dual serotonin and norepinephrine reuptake inhibitor. However, recent evidence suggests that venlafaxine is not a dual reuptake inhibitor over its entire dose range. Rather, venlafaxine sequentially engages serotonin uptake inhibition at low doses (75 mg per day) and norepinephrine uptake inhibition at higher doses (375 mg per day), which is consistent with venlafaxine's ascending dose-antidepressant response curve (93). In a preliminary, open-label study of venlafaxine in FM, 15 patients were treated for 8 weeks at a mean dose of 167 (SD±76) and experienced significant improvement in pain, fatigue, sleep quality, feeling upon awakening, morning stiffness, depressive and anxiety symptoms, global assessment, and quality of life. Six (55%) of the 11 study completers had a positive response to venlafaxine, defined as a 50% or greater reduction in both the McGill Pain Questionnaire and the sum of the visual analog scale (VAS) scores for pain, fatigue, sleep quality, feeling upon awakening, morning stiffness, and global assessment. The presence of lifetime, but not current, mood and anxiety disorders predicted response of FM symptoms to venlafaxine (94). By contrast, a 6-week, randomized, PB-controlled, double-blind trial of a fixed, low dose of venlafaxine (75 mg per day) in the treatment of FM (95) found that venlafaxine improved the primary measures of pain [VAS pain today and McGill Pain Questionnaire (60)] but not significantly better than PB. However, the total FIQ and FIQ pain and fatigue subscales improved significantly more in the venlafaxine-treated group than in the PB-treated patients. The short duration of this trial and the low dose of venlafaxine may explain the discrepant results, and more study of higher doses of venlafaxine is needed.

Duloxetine is a new potent serotonin and norepinephrine reuptake inhibitor that lacks the side effect profile of the TCAs that is associated with adrenergic, cholinergic, and histaminergic antagonism. Unlike venlafaxine, the dual reuptake inhibition is active over duloxetine's entire clinically relevant dose range (96). Duloxetine has been shown to be a safe, tolerable, and effective antidepressant at doses of 60 to 120 mg per day (97–99). In a previous trial, duloxetine also significantly reduced the painful physical symptoms, such as headache, back pain, stomach aches, and poorly localized musculoskeletal pain, associated with major depressive disorder (100). Duloxetine has been studied in several animal models of persistent and neuropathic pain and found to be effective in reducing pain-related behaviors at doses that did not cause neuromuscular dysfunction (101–103). Duloxetine was more potent than venlafaxine, AMI, or desipramine and more effective than the SSRI paroxetine and the selective norepinephrine (NE) inhibitor, thionisoxetine, in reducing persistent pain-related behaviors in animals (102). The results from preclinical and clinical studies of duloxetine showing potential efficacy in the treatment of persistent pain symptoms and the painful physical symptoms associated with depression suggest that duloxetine might be efficacious in some chronic-pain disorders such as FM.

In one of the largest clinical trials ever conducted for the treatment of FM, 207 patients meeting ACR criteria for FM with or without current major depressive disorder participated in a randomized, PB-controlled, double-blind, parallel-group multisite study to assess the safety and efficacy of duloxetine, titrated to 60 mg BID (104). After single-blind PB treatment for 1 week, subjects were randomly assigned to receive duloxetine 60 mg bid or PB for 12 weeks. Coprimary outcome measures were the FIQ total score and pain score (68). Secondary outcome measures included mean TeP pain threshold, TeP number, FIQ fatigue, rest, and stiffness scores, Clinical Global Impression of Severity (105), Patient Global Impression of Improvement, Brief Pain Inventory (short form) (106), Medical Outcomes Study Short Form-36 (SF-36) (107), Quality of Life in Depression Scale (108), and Sheehan Disability Scale (70). Duloxetine-treated subjects compared to PB-treated subjects improved significantly more on the FIQ total score but not significantly more on the FIQ pain score. Compared to PB-treated subjects, duloxetine-treated subjects had significantly greater reduction in Brief Pain Inventory average pain severity score and Brief Pain Inventory average interference from pain score, TeP number, and FIQ stiffness score and had significantly greater improvement in mean TeP pain threshold, Clinical Global Impression of Severity, Patient Global Assessment of Improvement, and several quality of life measures. Duloxetine-treated female subjects demonstrated significantly greater improvement on most efficacy measures compared to PB-treated female subjects, while the duloxetine-treated male subjects failed to significantly improve on any efficacy measure. The reasons for the gender differences in response are unclear, but may be related to the small size of the male subgroup [23 (11%) of 207 subjects], reflecting the much higher prevalence of FM in women. Significantly more duloxetine-treated female subjects (30.3%) had a clinically meaningful (>50%) decrease in the FIQ pain score compared to PB-treated female subjects (16.5%). Duloxetine treatment improved FM symptoms and pain severity regardless of baseline major depressive disorder status, and the treatment effect of duloxetine on significant pain reduction in female subjects was independent of the effect on mood or anxiety. Therefore, the effect of duloxetine on the reduction of pain associated with FM appears to be independent of its effect on mood. These results are consistent with prior FLX, AMI, and CBP trials that found no significant relationship between improvement in FM symptoms and change in depression scores, although none of these prior studies evaluated the impact of currently diagnosed major depressive disorder (32,45,79). Duloxetine was well tolerated, and there was no significant difference in the number of patients who discontinued due to adverse events. Duloxetine-treated subjects reported insomnia, dry mouth, and constipation significantly more frequently than PB-treated subjects. Most treatment-emergent adverse events were of mild or moderate severity. Limitations of the duloxetine trial include the relatively short duration of treatment of 12 weeks and the exclusion of individuals with several forms of lifetime psychopathology (e.g., primary anxiety disorders or bipolar disorder), secondary FM, and unstable medical or psychiatric illness. Future studies should assess the long-term efficacy of duloxetine in FM.

Milnacipran is another serotonin and norepinephrine reuptake inhibitor (SNRI) that has been approved for treatment of depression since 1997 in parts of Europe, Asia, and elsewhere but is currently unavailable in the United States. Milnacipran is a dual serotonin and norepinephrine reuptake inhibitor within its therapeutic dose range and also exerts mild NMDA inhibition (23). Like duloxetine, milnacipran lacks the side effect profile of tricyclics associated with adrenergic, cholinergic, and histaminergic antagonism. In a double-blind, PB-controlled, multicenter trial, 125 patients with FM by ACR criteria were randomized to receive PB or milnacipran for 4 weeks of dose escalation to the maximally tolerated dose followed by 8 weeks of stable dose (25 to 200 mg/d). The study evaluated the efficacy and safety of two different dosing regimens of milnacipran (once daily vs. twice daily) for the treatment of FM. The primary outcome measure was based on change in pain recorded in an electronic diary, comparing baseline to endpoint (last 2 weeks of treatment). Secondary outcome measures included the McGill Pain Questionnaire (short form) (109), the FIQ (68), the Beck Depression Inventory (BDI) (69), SF-36 (107), sleep and fatigue assessments, and the Patient Global Impression of Change. The majority of milnacipran-treated patients titrated to the highest daily dose (200 mg), suggesting that milnacipran was well tolerated. The most frequently reported adverse event was nausea, and most adverse events were mild and transient. Patients treated with milnacipran on a twice-daily schedule experienced significant improvement in pain compared to those on PB. Significantly more patients receiving milnacipran twice daily (37%) reported a reduction in the weekly average pain scores by 50% or more, compared to 14% of patients in the PB group. Milnacipran-treated patients on the once daily schedule did not exhibit the same degree of improvement in pain, suggesting that dosing frequency is important in the use of milnacipran for pain associated with FM. Both milnacipran groups (once-daily and twice-daily dosing) had significantly greater improvement on the Patient Global Impression of Change score and the physical function and "feel good" subscales of the FIQ (110). Further study is needed to assess the long-term efficacy of milnacipran in FM.

Other Antidepressants

Three controlled trials of FM treatment have examined medications with putative antidepressant properties (111–113). In an 8-week double-blind, PB-controlled trial, alprazolam (0.5 to 3.0 mg per day), a triazolobenzodiazepine with antide-

pressant effects (114), was compared to ibuprofen (600 mg four times daily), the combination, or PB in 78 patients with FM, diagnosed using criteria by Russell et al. (115). At the conclusion of the study there were no significant differences in improvement in pain, TeP measures, physician global assessment, functional status, depressive, or anxiety symptoms among the four treatment groups (112).

Two controlled trials assessed the efficacy of SAMe (111,113), an over-the counter dietary supplement that is a major methyl donor and involved in the synthesis of norepinephrine, dopamine, and serotonin in the brain (52). In the first study, 17 patients with FM by investigator-derived criteria received SAMe 200 mg per day IM or PB for 21 days in a crossover design, with a 2-week washout (111). SAMe-treated patients experienced significant reductions in the number of trigger points, painful anatomic sites, and depressive symptoms compared to patients receiving PB. In the second, double-blind, parallel-design trial, 44 patients with FM by criteria of Yunus (59) were randomized to SAMe 800 mg per day (orally administered) or PB for 6 weeks. Compared to PB, treatment with SAMe was associated with significant improvement in pain, fatigue, morning stiffness, mood, and physician global assessment of improvement. TeP number did not significantly decrease in the patients treated with SAMe compared to PB-treated patients (113).

The MAO inhibitors (MAOIs) currently available in the United States, phenelzine and tranylcypromine, are associated with risk of potentially life threatening interactions with other medications and foods containing tyramine because of their irreversible and nonspecific effect on the MAO-A and MAO-B enzymes, two types of MAO enzymes that are responsible for the breakdown of monoamines. Newer medications that reversibly inhibit MAO-A, which mainly affects norepinephrine, serotonin, and dopamine, have improved side effect profiles and are effective antidepressants (116). Although not available in the United States, two MAO-A inhibitors, moclobemide and pirlindole, available in parts of Europe, have been studied in FM. In a 12-week, double-blind, PB-controlled study, 130 female patients with FM by ACR criteria, but without current psychiatric comorbidity, were randomized to moclobemide (450 to 600 mg per day), AMI (25 to 37.5 mg per day), or PB for 12 weeks (49). Response to treatment was defined as a rating of minimally improved, much improved, or very much improved on a clinical impression of change scale. Secondary outcomes included changes in the VAS scales for general health, pain, sleep, and fatigue, the manual TeP number, the Sheehan disability scale (70), the Nottingham Health Profile (71), and the physician's clinical impression of severity of FM. Fifty-four percent of patients on moclobemide were judged to be responders, but this did not significantly separate from PB. Similarly, moclobemide treatment improved pain assessed on the pain VAS and the Nottingham Health Profile pain dimension, but this improvement was not significantly better than PB. AMI treatment, on the other hand, led to significant improvement compared to PB on several outcomes (Table 31-2). The treatments were well tolerated, with no differences among the groups in discontinuation rates due to side effects. Another pilot trial of the MAO-A inhibitor, pirlindole, was more promising. In a 4-week, randomized, double-blind,

PB-controlled study of 100 patients with FM by ACR criteria, pirlindole 75 mg twice daily was well tolerated and produced significantly superior improvement in pain, the manual TeP score, and patient and physician global evaluation than PB (117).

LIMITATIONS OF ANTIDEPRESSANT TREATMENT STUDIES AND FUTURE RESEARCH ISSUES

The studies of antidepressants in FM are limited for several reasons (29). First, most studies used low doses of antidepressants and did not examine higher or standard therapeutic doses effective for the treatment of depression. Considering the possible association between depression and FM (118), standard antidepressant doses may be needed to obtain more than moderate improvement in symptoms of FM, and future studies should assess a wider range of antidepressant doses. However, undesirable side effects of the tricyclics from their anticholinergic, antihistaminergic, and α-adrenergic receptor blockade activities reduce tolerability and limit titration. Secondary amine tricyclics (e.g., desipramine, nortriptyline), which have fewer side effects than tertiary amines, have been examined in only one controlled trial in patients with FM. In this study both AMI and nortriptyline, used in low doses, failed to improve symptoms significantly more than PB, except for the patients' assessment of global improvement, which improved significantly more than PB only in the AMI group (72). More trials of the secondary amine tricyclics using higher doses are needed. The studies of higher doses of the SSRI FLX and the SNRIs duloxetine and milnacipran indicate that these doses were well tolerated by most patients and were effective in reducing many of the symptoms of FM (79,104,110). On the basis of these findings, doses of antidepressants at the therapeutic level for the treatment of depression should be attempted if the patient does not respond to, but otherwise tolerates, lower doses.

Second, no tricyclic antidepressant studies obtained plasma concentrations of these agents. The need to monitor tricyclic plasma concentrations is especially relevant to studies that reported greater efficacy for combined tricyclics and FLX (45,84) because the efficacy of combined treatment may have been due, in part, to the pharmacokinetic interaction between FLX and tricyclics that typically elevates tricyclic plasma levels substantially (81).

Third, most of the trials were of short duration, and there is a need for more data on the intermediate and long-term efficacy of antidepressants in the treatment of FM, a disorder that typically has a chronic course. Notably, in the longest study of tricyclics in FM that extended to 6 months (32), neither AMI nor CBP demonstrated significantly greater efficacy than PB after 6 months of treatment.

Fourth, only one controlled tricyclic antidepressant study (49), one controlled study of an SSRI (79), and the two most recent studies of SNRIs (104,110) evaluated patients for a diagnosis of a mood or anxiety disorder, despite evidence of elevated prevalence rates of mood and anxiety disorders in patients with FM and the possible impact of these disorders on response to treatment. An open trial of venlafaxine in FM found that a history of mood or anxiety disorders (not only current disorders) might predict response to antidepressant

treatment of FM, although more study is needed (94). Some of the trials (32,34,44,45,47) administered standardized self-report psychometric instruments to measure depressive or anxiety symptoms, but these measurements are not adequate to establish a psychiatric diagnosis. Only four of the trials that measured depressive symptoms included this assessment in the analysis, and all found no relationship between improvement of FM symptoms and change in depression scores (32,45,79,104). These findings suggest that the antidepressants are having an effect that is independent of improvement in depressive symptoms. However, there has been little assessment of the impact of change in anxiety symptoms on improvement in FM. Future studies should evaluate patients for psychiatric comorbidity using a standardized structured psychiatric interview [e.g., Structured Interview for DSM-IV (119) or Mini International Neuropsychiatric Interview (MINI) (120)] and include an assessment of psychiatric symptoms to determine the impact of the presence of comorbidity and depressive and anxiety symptoms on response to treatment of FM.

Fifth, small sample sizes in many studies and the use of crossover design in several studies limit interpretation of the results. The frequent and noticeable side effects of tertiary amine tricyclics might have affected the blindedness of crossover trials when subjects were switched to or from PB. Two crossover studies (42,44) omitted washout intervals, which may have produced discontinuation symptoms after abrupt cessation of tricyclics, contributing to insomnia and myalgias during PB treatment and decreasing PB response. The crossover trial of AMI and FLX (45) had only a 2-week washout period for FLX, which typically requires a washout interval of 30 days. More double-blind, PB-controlled, parallel-group studies of sufficient sample size and adequate duration are needed.

Sixth, the majority of patients studied in the trials were women, which reflects the much higher prevalence of FM in women (1). The results of the studies may therefore not be generalizable to men with FM. Indeed, gender differences were found in the study of duloxetine in FM. Although the reasons for the gender differences in response to duloxetine are unclear, as discussed above, there may be gender differences in FM that affect treatment response. Studies of FM clinical features have found that women had significantly more TePs than men, as well as more fatigue, sleep disturbance, IBS, and "pain all over" (121). The disparate presentation of FM in women and men suggests that there might be gender differences in the pathophysiology of FM that could affect response to treatment.

Finally, the clinical trials applied different criteria for FM (especially in those studies published before the ACR criteria were established), used dissimilar measures to assess pain and tenderness, and inconsistently evaluated other associated symptoms. For example, none of the studies analyzed by Arnold et al. (29) included all the outcomes that were evaluated in the meta-analysis. Furthermore, the method of evaluating these outcomes varied among studies. For patient-reported outcomes, some studies used 100 mm VASs and others used numerical rating scales or questionnaires. TePs were evaluated using either manual exams or dolorimetry at various TeP sites. Most of the studies did not explore other important outcomes, such as impact on functioning and quality of life. The use of standardized, operationally defined outcome measures of improvement would enhance the comparative value of the treatment trials.

SUMMARY OF ANTIDEPRESSANT TRIALS IN FIBROMYALGIA

Although more research is needed to explore the efficacy of antidepressants in FM, especially in long-term treatment studies, the evidence supports the efficacy of antidepressants in treating pain and other symptoms associated with FM. Therefore, a trial of an antidepressant using adequate doses and duration of treatment should be considered in patients with FM. The TCAs have been the most studied of the antidepressants and are moderately effective in treating the symptoms of FM, although their use is limited by poor tolerability. The SSRIs also have a role to play in treating FM patients, although there have been fewer controlled studies and the results have been mixed. Newer SNRIs that have the dual serotonin and norepinephrine reuptake inhibition activity of tricyclic antidepressants but lack many of the adverse side effects associated with tricyclics show promise in the treatment of FM and may become the first-line choice for antidepressant treatment.

ANTIDEPRESSANTS IN OTHER NONNEUROPATHIC CHRONIC-PAIN DISORDERS

Patients with FM frequently report other chronic-pain disorders, including chronic headache, irritable bowel disorder, and temporomandibular joint disorder. Several recent studies and meta-analyses have demonstrated that these conditions also appear to respond to treatment with antidepressants. Furthermore, major depression, another disorder commonly comorbid with FM, is often associated with painful symptoms (122), which also respond to some antidepressants.

The prevalence of pain symptoms in patients with depression has ranged from 15% to 100% (mean prevalence, 65%) (122). In the general population depression is associated with widespread pain (123), gastrointestinal pain (124), and headache (125). Depressed patients in primary care settings frequently report headache, abdominal pain, joint pain, and chest pain (126). In a large, longitudinal study, depressive symptoms were also found to predict future episodes of low back pain, neck-shoulder pain, and musculoskeletal symptoms (127). The presence and severity of pain symptoms adversely affects depression outcomes. For example, the presence of up to five different pain complaints (abdominal pain, headache, back pain, chest pain, and facial pain) was associated with increased severity of depression (128). In another study increased pain severity at baseline was associated with more severe depression, poor depression outcomes, more pain-related functional limitation, worse self-rated health, more frequent use of opioid analgesics, and more frequent pain-related doctor visits at follow-up (129).

Abnormalities in serotonin and norepinephrine neurotransmission are thought to be involved in the pathophysiology of depression and pain through different but overlapping neuroanatomical pathways, which might account for the high comorbidity of painful symptoms in patients with depression (100). Antidepressants with both serotonin and norepinephrine reuptake inhibition (SNRIs) might therefore be effective in the treatment of painful symptoms that are associated with depression (97–99). The results of three PB-controlled studies of duloxetine, a new SNRI, in depression that included an assessment of pain demonstrated that duloxetine significantly improved painful symptoms in addition to depression. The effects of duloxetine on pain were robust and were significantly different from PB as early as 2 weeks after starting treatment. There was also a low correlation between change in mood and change in pain severity, suggesting that the effect on pain was independent of change in depression (100).

Chronic headache is another common disorder that is frequently reported by patients with FM. A recent meta-analysis of published, randomized, controlled trials in patients with migraine or tension headaches investigated 19 studies of tricyclic antidepressants (most commonly AMI), 18 studies of serotonin-blocking agents (most commonly pizotifen or mianserin), and 7 studies of SSRIs (130). The meta-analysis suggested that antidepressants are effective in reducing chronic headache pain. Patients receiving antidepressants were twice as likely to improve than those on PB. There were similar effects in all three classes of antidepressants (tricyclics, serotonin blockers, and SSRIs), with most consistent benefit from the tricyclic antidepressants and serotonin blockers. Antidepressants also appeared to be equally effective for tension and migraine headaches, which is important, because the clinical differentiation between these two types of chronic headache is sometimes difficult (130). Neither pizotifen nor mianserin is licensed in the United States, although the FDA has approved mirtazapine, a congener of mianserin, for the treatment of depression (130).

Irritable bowel disorder, characterized by abdominal pain with altered bowel habit, is a condition that is commonly comorbid with FM. A meta-analysis of published, randomized, controlled studies identified 11 studies of antidepressant treatment of IBS (9 of the 11 studies) and nonulcer dyspepsia (131). Most of the trials evaluated tricyclic antidepressants (9 of 11) and two trials used the antiserotonin agent mianserin. The results of the meta-analysis suggested that antidepressants might have a clinically important benefit in reducing symptoms of these disorders. There was a large treatment effect on pain associated with these gastrointestinal disorders. There have been very few PB-controlled studies of SSRIs in patients with IBS. A small, 6-week, PB-controlled, crossover trial of 14 patients with IBS evaluated citalopram 20 mg for 3 weeks and 40 mg for the second 3 weeks compared to PB (separated by a 2-week washout). Citalopram was significantly superior to PB in improving abdominal pain, bloating, and global well-being in the treatment of IBS (132). Another small, parallel, double-blind, PB-controlled trial of 40 patients with IBS assessed FLX 20 mg per day versus PB for 6 weeks and found that FLX significantly reduced pain scores, especially in female patients, but not other gastrointestinal symptoms (133). Finally, a study of 257 patients with severe IBS in which patients were randomized to receive eight sessions of individual psychotherapy, paroxetine 20 mg per day, or routine care by a gastroenterologist and general practitioner, found that, after

3 months, the paroxetine group showed a significantly greater reduction in days with pain than the treatment-as-usual group. However, at the 1-year follow-up, both the severity and frequency of pain improved in all three groups, with no significant differences among groups. At 1-year follow-up, the paroxetine and psychotherapy groups showed a significant improvement over usual treatment in improving the physical aspects of health related quality of life (134). The results of these three studies argue for more clinical trials of the efficacy of SSRIs and SNRIs in patients with IBS (134).

Temporomandibular disorders, a group of common chronic orofacial pain disorders, may also respond to antidepressants, although studies are limited. Open-label, low-dose AMI (10 to 30 mg per day) in patients with temporomandibular disorders for up to 1 year resulted in significant reduction in pain and significant improvement in global treatment effectiveness (135). In a small, PB-controlled study, 12 female patients with chronic temporomandibular disorder were randomized to AMI 25 mg per day or PB for 14 days. The amitriptyline-treated patient experienced a significantly greater reduction in pain and discomfort compared to the PB group (136).

ANTIEPILEPTIC MEDICATION

Antiepileptics are frequently used to treat chronic-pain disorders, particularly neuropathic pain disorders and migraine. For example, carbamazepine has long been the treatment of choice for trigeminal neuralgia (137,138), and more recently, divalproex sodium was found to be useful for the prevention of migraine (139). Newer antiepileptics, including gabapentin, lamotrigine, and topiramate, are efficacious in the treatment of several neuropathic conditions and migraine (140). Gabapentin, in particular, has been empirically shown to be beneficial in the treatment of postherpetic neuralgia (141,142), painful diabetic neuropathy (143), and migraine (144) and has an approved indication for postherpetic neuralgia.

Although each antiepileptic's specific mechanism of action may differ, all the antiepileptics generally reduce excitability, decrease ectopic discharge, and reduce neurotransmitter release—effects that may contribute to their antiepileptic and antinociceptive effects (145). Several possible mechanisms of action may account for the antiepileptics' efficacy in chronic-pain disorders; they include sodium channel blockade, calcium channel blockade, enhancement of GABAergic transmission, inhibition of glutamatergic transmission, free radical scavenging, inhibition of nitric oxide formation, and enhancement of serotonergic transmission (140).

There is emerging evidence that FM, like many neuropathic disorders, is associated with aberrant central nervous system processing of pain (146–149). Although the ACR criteria for FM require tenderness in 11 out of 18 discrete regions, patients with FM have increased sensitivity to pain throughout the body. Fibromyalgia patients often develop an increased response to painful stimuli (hyperalgesia) and experience pain from normally nonnoxious stimuli (allodynia) (148). Both hyperalgesia and allodynia reflect an enhanced CNS processing of painful stimuli that

is characteristic of central sensitization (150). The overlap in symptomatology between neuropathic disorders and FM suggests that antiepileptics might also reduce the chronic, allodynic, hyperalgesic pain associated with FM. However, only one randomized, controlled study of an antiepileptic (pregabalin) in the treatment of FM has been completed and presented (151). Pregabalin, like gabapentin, binds to the $\alpha_2\delta$ subunit of voltage-gated calcium channels, resulting in decreased Ca^{2+} influx during depolarization and reduction in the release of several neurotransmitters, including glutamate, norepinephrine, and substance P. Pregabalin was studied in a multicenter, randomized, PB-controlled, 8-week, monotherapy trial of 530 patients with FM, which is the largest FM clinical trial conducted to date. The primary outcome measure was a daily paper pain diary in which patients selected a number on a numerical scale from 0 (no pain) to 10 (worst possible pain) that best described their pain during the past 24 hours. Secondary measures included the Short Form McGill Pain Questionnaire (109), a daily sleep diary (a 0 to 10 numerical scale on the quality of sleep), Multidimensional Assessment of Fatigue (152), Clinical/Patient Global Impression of Change, Medical Outcomes Study Short Form-36 (SF-36) (107), Manual TeP Survey (153), Hospital Anxiety and Depression Scale (154), and the Medical Outcomes Study Sleep Scale (155). Response to treatment was defined as a >50% reduction in the mean of the last seven pain (diary) scores recorded. The outcomes that responded significantly to pregabalin 450 mg/day compared to PB were the mean weekly pain (diary) score, the Short Form McGill Pain Questionnaire total score and Short Form McGill Pain Questionnaire VAS pain score, sleep (diary) score, the Medical Outcomes Study Sleep Scale, Multidimensional Assessment of Fatigue, Clinical/Patient Global Impression of Change, and SF-36 domains of social functioning, bodily pain, vitality, and general health perception. A significantly larger proportion of patients receiving pregabalin 450 mg per day (28.9%) experienced a >50% reduction in the pain (diary) score compared to the PB group (13.2%). Limitations of the trial included the lack of assessment of comorbid psychiatric disorders, the short duration of treatment (8 weeks), and the lack of improvement in TePs. However, the results of the study suggest that pregabalin could have an important role in the management of several symptoms associated with FM. Additional controlled studies of antiepileptics in FM are needed.

SEDATIVE-HYPNOTIC MEDICATION

Although there continues to be debate about the role of sleep disturbance in the pathogenesis of FM, many patients with FM experience disrupted or nonrestorative sleep and benefit from treatment. A few controlled studies have examined sedative hypnotics in the treatment of FM. The short-acting nonbenzodiazepine sedatives zolpidem and zopiclone improved sleep in patients with FM but did not improve pain, limiting their usefulness in FM as monotherapy (156–158). Although the combination of alprazolam and ibuprofen was somewhat beneficial in a pilot trial of FM (112), another study found no significant benefit of another benzodiazepine, bromazepan, over PB in the treatment of FM (159). A recent, preliminary, 4-week, double-blind, PB-controlled crossover trial of 24 women with FM suggested that gammahydroxybutyrate (GHB), a precursor of γ-amino-butyric acid (GABA) with marked sedative properties that is commercially available as sodium oxybate, reduced symptoms of pain and fatigue, decreased the TeP index, and increased slow-wave sleep and decreased α intrusion on polysomnography (160). However, sodium oxybate's abuse potential and its use in cases of date rape (161) will likely limit its usefulness in patients with FM. Safer alternatives for the management of insomnia include TCAs, other sedating antidepressants (e.g., trazodone, which is used clinically to improve sleep, although there is no empirical evidence for its efficacy in FM) and, more recently, antiepileptics, such as gabapentin, that have sedative and well as pain-relieving properties.

ANTI-INFLAMMATORY DRUGS

The corticosteroid, prednisone, was found to be ineffective in FM, and corticosteroids are not recommended in the treatment of FM (162). Patients with FM frequently use nonsteroidal anti-inflammatory drugs (NSAIDs) or acetaminophen, although there is no evidence from clinical trials that they are effective when used alone in the treatment of FM (163), and patients typically report that they offer minimal relief of pain. For example, in one randomized, controlled trial, ibuprofen 600 mg four times daily was not more effective than PB in reducing pain associated with FM (164). The lack of a known significant inflammatory component in the pathophysiology of FM may explain the poor response of FM to NSAID monotherapy. However, studies have documented some benefit of ibuprofen and naproxen when combined with tricyclics (e.g., AMI, CBP) (58,165) or benzodiazepines (112). Furthermore, FM patients with a peripheral pain generator that could be aggravating FM, such as comorbid osteoarthritis or another painful inflammatory condition, would likely benefit from the addition of NSAIDs in the management of their pain.

OPIATES

There is controversy about the use of opiates to manage the pain associated with FM because of the abuse potential of these agents and the limited data supporting their efficacy in FM. However, a survey of academic medical centers in the United States reported that about 14% of FM patients were treated with opiates (166). Interestingly, a small, double-blind, PB-controlled study found that intravenous administration of morphine in nine patients with FM did not result in a reduction of pain intensity (167). A recent 4-year nonrandomized study of opiates in FM discovered that the FM patients taking opiates did not experience significant improvement in pain at the 4-year follow-up compared to

baseline and reported increased depression in the last 2 years of the study (168). These results suggest that opiates may not have a role in the long-term management of FM.

Tramadol is a novel analgesic with weak agonist activity at the mu opiate receptor combined with dual serotonin and norepinephrine reuptake inhibition that may exert antinociceptive effects within both the ascending and descending pain pathways (23). Three controlled studies have evaluated the efficacy of tramadol in FM. The first small study used a double-blind crossover design to compare single-dose intravenous tramadol 100 mg with PB in 12 patients with FM. Patients receiving tramadol experienced a 20.6% reduction in pain compared to an increase of 19.8% of pain in the PB group (169). The second study of tramadol began with a 3-week, open-label phase of tramadol 50 to 400 mg per day followed by a 6-week double-blind phase in which only patients who tolerated tramadol and perceived benefit were enrolled (170). The primary measure of efficacy was the time to exit from the double-blind phase because of inadequate pain relief. One hundred patients with FM were enrolled in the open-label phase; 69% tolerated and perceived benefit from tramadol and were randomized to tramadol or PB. Significantly fewer patients on tramadol discontinued during the double-blind phase because of inadequate pain relief. This study is limited by the possible unblinding of patients in the double-blind phase after open-label treatment with tramadol. Finally, a recent multicenter, double-blind, randomized, PB-controlled, 91-day study examined the efficacy of the combination of tramadol (37.5 mg) and acetaminophen (325 mg) in 315 patients with FM. Patients taking tramadol and acetaminophen (4±1.8 tabs per day) were significantly more likely than PB-treated subjects to continue treatment and experience an improvement in pain and physical function (171). Although tramadol is marketed as an analgesic without scheduling under the Controlled Substances Act, it should be used with caution because of recent reports of classical opioid withdrawal with discontinuation and dose reduction and increasing reports of abuse and dependence (172).

5-HT₃ ANTAGONISTS

5-HT₃ antagonists (e.g., ondansetron and tropisetron) have been found to have analgesic effects (23). A randomized, PB-controlled, double-blind, 10-day trial in 418 patients with FM evaluated the short-term efficacy of tropisetron at doses of 5 mg per day, 10 mg per day, and 15 mg per day. Significant reduction in pain was noted only in those patients taking 5 mg per day and 10 mg per day, while the effects of tropisetron 15 mg per day were no different from PB, suggesting a bell-shaped dose response curve (173). The presence of 5-HT₃ receptors on both the inhibitory dorsal horn interneurons and the primary afferent fibers that relay nociceptive information from peripheral nociceptives to the dorsal horn may explain the pro- and antinociceptive effects of 5-HT₃ receptor blockade. The balance of these opposing effects may be dose-dependent and contribute to unpredictable results with tropisetron (145), but more study of longer-term treatment with 5-HT₃ antagonists is needed.

GROWTH HORMONE

The rationale for studying growth hormone treatment of FM was based on a finding that about a third of patients with FM had low levels of insulinlike growth factor 1 (IGF-1), a surrogate marker for low growth hormone secretion, and experienced many clinical features of growth hormone deficiency, such as low energy, dysphoria, impaired cognition, poor general health, reduced exercise capacity, muscle weakness, and cold intolerance (174,175). A randomized, double-blind, PB-controlled, 9-month study of growth hormone treatment was conducted in 50 women with FM and low IGF-1 levels (175). Subjects gave themselves daily subcutaneous injections of growth hormone or PB; the growth hormone dose was adjusted to achieve an IGF-1 level of about 250 ng per mL. After 9 months, subjects receiving growth hormone showed a significant improvement over the PB group in the total FIQ score, manual TeP count, and patient-reported global improvement. Because 1 month of therapy with growth hormone costs about $1,500, the authors concluded that the cost-benefit ratios would prohibit its use in FM patients with low IGF-1. Furthermore, in another recent study, there were no significant differences in the activity of IGF-1 in premenopausal women with FM compared to that of healthy controls. Notably, increases in age and obesity were both strongly associated with lower activity of the growth hormone-IGF-1 axis, suggesting that these factors should be considered in any study of this axis in FM (176).

N-METHYL-D-ASPARTATE ANTAGONISTS

A possible pathogenic mechanism of the chronic pain associated with FM, central sensitization, is mediated, in part, by the binding of excitatory amino acids (glutamate and aspartate) to the NMDA receptor. NMDA antagonists may inhibit or attenuate central sensitization (177) and potentially reduce pain associated with FM. Two commercially available NMDA antagonists, ketamine and dextromethorphan, have been studied in FM. In a double-blind, PB-controlled study of 11 patients with FM, intravenous ketamine 0.3 mg per kg was found to reduce pain and increase pressure pain thresholds in eight of the patients, four of whom reported decreased pain for up to 5 days after the ketamine infusion. However, ketamine was associated with multiple side effects, including sedation, dizziness, perioral numbness, and dissociative symptoms (167). Another double-blind, PB-controlled study assessed 15 patients with FM who had previously responded to open-label ketamine (0.3 mg per kg) infusion with >50% decrease in pain intensity (178). Before and after ketamine or PB, experimental local and referred pain was induced by musculoskeletal infusion of hypertonic saline into the tibialis anterior muscle. Pain intensity was significantly reduced and pain pressure threshold significantly increased in the patients treated with ketamine compared to the PB group. Although the results of these preliminary studies of ketamine support the possibility that

NMDA receptors are involved in pain mechanism in FM, the long-term clinical use of intravenous ketamine is neither practical nor likely to be tolerated by patients. Only one other clinical study has been published that assesses the effect of NMDA-receptor antagonists in FM. In this study, 48 female patients with FM were treated with an open-label combination of tramadol 200 mg/d and increasing doses of dextromethorphan (50 to 200 mg per day), titrated to therapeutic effect or tolerability. Fifty-eight percent (28 of 48) responded to the addition of dextromethorphan and entered a double-blind phase in which the patients were randomized to dextromethorphan and tramadol or tramadol and PB. A Kaplan-Meier dropout analysis showed that significantly fewer patients on dextromethorphan and tramadol discontinued treatment compared to patients on tramadol alone (179). More study of NMDA-receptor antagonists is needed before clinical recommendations can be made regarding the use of these agents.

SUMMARY AND RECOMMENDATIONS FOR THE PHARMACOLOGIC TREATMENT OF FIBROMYALGIA

Recent large, multicenter pharmacologic trials, particularly the positive results of trials of SNRIs and pregabalin, have shown promise in the treatment of FM. It is, however, important to educate patients about limitations of all the clinical trials and to base recommendations on available evidence from controlled studies, when possible. A treatment algorithm is presented in Figure 31-2. The emphasis in the algorithm is on antidepressants and anticonvulsants because these agents have been shown to be effective in clinical trials and are generally well tolerated by most patients.

Because the clinical presentation of FM is heterogeneous, treatment recommendations must be individualized for each patient. Comorbid medical or psychiatric disorders can affect the outcome of FM treatment and should be identified and treated. There is preliminary evidence that a lifetime history of major depressive disorder and anxiety disorders may predict response of FM to antidepressants, and a trial of these medications using antidepressant therapeutic doses and an adequate duration of treatment (e.g., 6 to 8 weeks at maximally tolerated dose) should be considered in these patients, even if they are not experiencing current episodes. The choice of an antidepressant is based on the evidence for efficacy, as reviewed previously, and tolerability. Since many patients do not tolerate the tricyclics, the SSRIs (e.g., FLX, paroxetine, or sertraline) or SNRIs [e.g., venlafaxine, duloxetine, milnacipran (when available)] may be preferable as first-line antidepressant treatment. In current clinical practice, patients with FM are administered low doses of antidepressants, including the SSRIs and SNRIs, but the evidence from recent studies of FLX and duloxetine suggests that higher doses of antidepressants may be required to achieve a therapeutic response in some patients. Although tertiary amine tricyclics (e.g., AMI) are most commonly used in the treatment of FM, secondary amine agents may be better tolerated, allowing for titration to higher and possibly therapeutic doses. Pregabalin, which has been

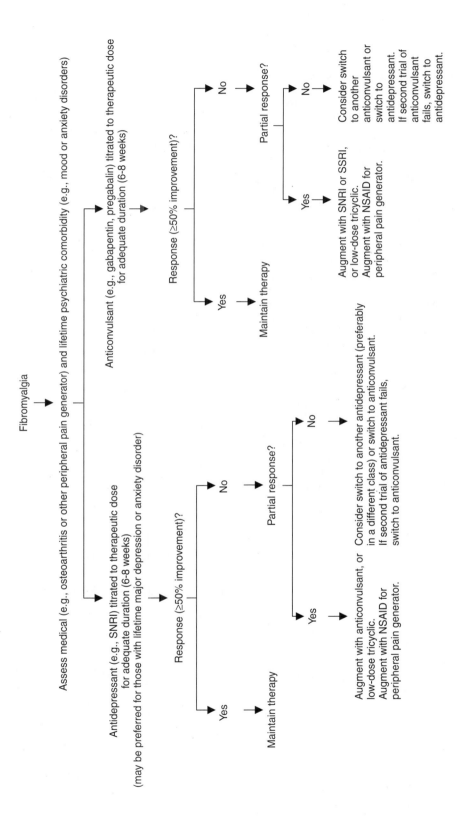

Figure 31-2. Treatment algorithm for fibromyalgia.

found to be effective for FM and generalized anxiety disorder (180,181), is also an option for patients with FM and may be particularly helpful for patients with insomnia or comorbid anxiety because of its sedative properties. Controlled studies of gabapentin, which has a similar mechanism of action as pregabalin, have not yet been published, but gabapentin is commercially available and is another option for patients. Prior studies of gabapentin in other chronic-pain conditions, such as diabetic neuropathy and postherpetic neuralgia, have required doses of 1,800 to 2,400 mg per day to achieve substantial analgesic effects. Therefore, patients with FM who have not responded to gabapentin at lower doses should attempt an increase in dose, if tolerated. Pregabalin and gabapentin, in combination with mood stabilizers, are alternatives to antidepressants in FM patients who have comorbid bipolar disorder in which the use of antidepressants may contribute to increased mood cycling.

Patients with FM are often treated with combinations of medications, and there is some evidence to support this approach (45), although more study of combination treatment is clearly needed. For example, in patients who experience relief of pain, fatigue, and depressed mood with FLX but continue to have insomnia, gabapentin can be added at bedtime, beginning at 300 mg per day and increasing as tolerated by 300 mg per day until there is improvement. Adding a low-dose tricyclic or another sedating antidepressant [e.g., trazodone, at low doses (50 mg)] to an SSRI or SNRI is another option, although it is important to be aware of the pharmacokinetic interaction between tricyclics and SSRIs/SNRIs and the risk of serotonin syndrome when serotonergic agents are combined (182). Adjunctive treatment with the nonbenzodiazepine sedatives zolpidem and zopiclone could also be considered in patients with persistent insomnia, but there is little data on the long-term effects of these medications in FM patients. Although NSAIDs alone have not been found to be very helpful in the treatment of FM, they may be useful in combination with other medications, particularly if there is a comorbid painful condition such as osteoarthritis.

SUMMARY POINTS

- Improved understanding of the pathophysiology of pain and other associated symptoms of FM will lead to more rational approaches to pharmacologic treatment.
- Growing consensus about definitions of clinically important improvement will hopefully pave the way for the establishment of FDA-approved treatments for FM, which will increase therapeutic options for patients.

■ IMPLICATIONS FOR PRACTICE

- Identify and address comorbid medical and psychiatric disorders.
- In general, pharmacologic therapy is most effective for improving the symptoms associated with FM and related conditions, whereas nonpharmacological therapies (e.g., cognitive-behavioral therapy, exercise) are more useful to treat the dysfunction and disability associated with these conditions.

- Consider a trial of antidepressants for patients with a lifetime history of major depressive disorder or anxiety disorders.
- Select antidepressants with effects on both serotonin and norepinephrine [e.g., SNRI or tricyclic (TCA) compounds].
- Titrate to antidepressant therapeutic doses, especially for non-TCA. There is evidence that many SSRIs or SNRIs are more efficacious analgesics at higher doses.
- Anticonvulsants (e.g., gabapentin) can also be used as monotherapy.
- If monotherapy with an antidepressant or anticonvulsant is only partially effective, try combination treatment with these agents.
- For persistent insomnia, consider adding a low-dose tricyclic or an anticonvulsant to the SNRI.

REFERENCES

1. Wolfe F, Ross K, Anderson J, et al. The prevalence and characteristics of fibromyalgia in the general population. *Arthritis Rheum* 1995;38:19–28.
2. Burckhardt CS, Clark SR, Bennett RM. Fibromyalgia and quality of life: a comparative analysis. *J Rheumatol* 1993;20:475–479.
3. Wolfe F, Anderson J, Harkness D, et al. Work and disability status of persons with fibromyalgia. *J Rheumatol* 1997b;24:1171–1178.
4. White KP, Speechley M, Harth M, et al. Comparing self-reported function and work disability in 100 community cases of fibromyalgia syndrome versus controls in London, Ontario. *Arthritis Rheum* 1999;42:76–83.
5. Kaplan RM, Schmidt SM, Cronan TA. Quality of well being in patients with fibromyalgia. *J Rheumatol* 2000;27:785–789.
6. Wolfe F, Smythe HA, Yunus MB, et al. The American College of Rheumatology 1990 criteria for the classification of fibromyalgia. Report of the Multicenter Criteria Committee. *Arthritis Rheum* 1990;33:160–172.
7. Hudson JI, Hudson MS, Pliner LF, et al. Fibromyalgia and major affective disorder: a controlled phenomenology and family history study. *Am J Psychiatry* 1985;142:441–446.
8. Walker EA, Keegan D, Gardner G, et al. Psychosocial factors in fibromyalgia compared with rheumatoid arthritis: I. Psychiatric diagnoses and functional disability. *Psychosom Med* 1997;59:565–571.
9. White KP, Nielson WR, Harth M, et al. Chronic widespread musculoskeletal pain with or without fibromyalgia: psychological distress in a representative community adult sample. *J Rheumatol* 2002;29:588–594.
10. Epstein SA, Kay G, Clauw D, et al. Psychiatric disorders in patients with fibromyalgia. *Psychosomatics* 1999;40:57–63.
11. MacFarlane GJ, Thomas E, Papageorgiou AC, et al. The natural history of chronic pain in the community: a better prognosis than in the clinic? *J Rheumatol* 1996;23:1617–1620.
12. Hudson JI, Goldenberg DL, Pope HG Jr, et al. Comorbidity of fibromyalgia with medical and psychiatric disorders. *Am J Med* 1992;92:363–367.
13. Basbaum AI, Fields HL. Endogenous pain control systems: brainstem spinal pathways and endorphin circuitry. *Annu Rev Neurosci* 1984;7:309–338.
14. Clark FM, Proudfit HK. The projections of noradrenergic neurons in the A5 catecholamine cell group to the spinal cord in the rat: anatomical evidence that A5 neurons modulate nociception. *Brain Res* 1993;616:200–210.

15. Millian MJ. Descending control of pain. *Prog Neurobiol* 2002;66:355–474.
16. Russell IJ, Vaeroy H, Javors M, et al. Cerebrospinal fluid biogenic amine metabolites in fibromyalgia/fibrositis syndrome and rheumatoid arthritis. *Arthritis Rheum* 1992;35:550–556.
17. Russell IJ, Michalek JE, Vipraio GA, et al. Platelet 3H-imipramine uptake receptor density and serum serotonin levels in patients with fibromyalgia/fibrositis syndrome. *J Rheumatol* 1992;19:104–109.
18. Yunus MB, Dailey JW, Aldag JC. Plasma tryptophan and other amino acids in primary fibromyalgia: a controlled study. *J Rheumatol* 1992;19:90–94.
19. Schwarz MJ, Spath M, Muller-Bardorff H. Relationship of substance P, 5-hydroxyindole acetic acid and tryptophan in serum of fibromyalgia patients. *Neurosci Lett* 1999;259:196–198.
20. Millan MJ. Descending control of pain. *Prog Neurobioil* 2002;66:355–474.
21. Fishbain D. Evidence-based data on pain relief with antidepressants. *Ann Med* 2000; 32:305–316.
22. Hudson JI, Pope HG Jr. The relationship between fibromyalgia and major depressive disorder. *Rheum Dis Clin North Am* 1996;22:285–303.
23. Kranzler JD, Gendreau JF, Rao SG. The psychopharmacology of fibromyalgia: a drug development perspective. *Psychopharmacol Bull* 2002;36:165–213.
24. Lawson K. Tricyclic antidepressants and fibromyalgia: what is the mechanism of action? *Expert Opin Investig Drugs* 2002;11:1437–1445.
25. Simms RW. Controlled trials of therapy in fibromyalgia syndrome. *Baillieres Clin Rheumatol* 1994;8:917–934.
26. Goldenberg DL. A review of the role of tricyclic medications in the treatment of fibromyalgia syndrome. *J Rheumatol* 1989;16(Suppl. 19):137–139.
27. Moldofsky H, Scarisbrick P, England R, et al. Musculoskeletal symptoms and non-REM sleep disturbances in patients with "fibrositis syndrome" and healthy subjects. *Psychosom Med* 1975;37:341–345.
28. Moldofsky H, Scarisbrick P. Induction of neuroasthenia musculoskeletal pain syndrome by selective sleep stage deprivation. *Psychosom Med* 1975;38:35–44.
29. Arnold LM, Keck PE, Welge JA Jr. Antidepressant treatment of fibromyalgia. A meta-analysis and review. *Psychosomatics* 2000;41:104–113.
30. Carette S, McCain GA, Bell DA, et al. Evaluation of amitriptyline in primary fibrositis: a double-blind, placebo-controlled study. *Arthritis Rheum* 1986;29:655–659.
31. Caruso I, Puttini PCS, Boccassini L, et al. Double-blind study of dothiepin versus placebo in the treatment of primary fibromyalgia syndrome. *J Int Med Res* 1987;15:154–159.
32. Carette S, Bell MJ, Reynolds WJ, et al. Comparison of amitriptyline, cyclobenzaprine, and placebo in the treatment of fibromyalgia: a randomized, double-blind clinical trial. *Arthritis Rheum* 1994;37:32–40.
33. Bennett RM, Gatter RA, Campbell SM, et al. A comparison of cyclobenzaprine and placebo in the management of fibrositis. *Arthritis Rheum* 1988;31:1535–1542.
34. Quimby LG, Gratwick GM, Whitney CD, et al. A randomized trial of cyclobenzaprine for the treatment of fibromyalgia. *J Rheumatol* 1989;16(Suppl. 19):140–143.
35. Campbell SM, Clark S, Tindall EA, et al. Clinical characteristics of fibrositis. 1. A "blinded" controlled study of symptoms and tender points. *Arthritis Rheum* 1983;26:817–824.
36. Cedarbaum JM, Schleifer LS. Drugs for Parkinson's disease, spasticity, and acute muscle spasms. In: Gilman AG, Rall TW, Nies AM et al., eds. *The pharmacological basis of therapeutics.* Elmsford, NY: Persimmon Press, 1990:463–484.
37. Harsch HH. Mania in two patients following cyclobenzaprine. *Psychosomatics* 1984;25:791–793.
38. Barnes CD, Fung SJ, Gintautus J. Brainstem noradrenergic system depression by cyclobenzaprine. *Neuropharmacol* 1980;19:221–224.
39. Share NN, McFarlane CS. Cyclobenzaprine: a novel centrally acting skeletal muscle relaxant. *Neuropharmacol* 1975;14:675–684.
40. Kobayashi H, Hasegawa Y, One H. Cyclobenzaprine, a centrally acting muscle relaxant, acts on descending serotonergic systems. *Eur J Pharmacol* 1996;311:29–35.
41. Lang IM. Cyclobenzaprine effects on locus coeruleus cells in tissue slice. *Neuropharmacol* 1983;22:249–252.
42. Carette S, Oakson G, Guimont C, et al. Sleep electroencephalography and the clinical response to amitriptyline in patients with fibromyalgia. *Arthritis Rheum* 1995;38:1211–1217.
43. Reynolds WJ, Moldofsky H, Saskin P, et al. The effects of cyclobenzaprine on sleep physiology and symptoms in patients with fibromyalgia. *J Rheumatol* 1991;18:452–454.
44. Bibolotti E, Borghi C, Pasculli E, et al. The management of fibrositis: a double-blind comparison of maprotiline (Ludiomil), chlorimipramine, and placebo. *J Clin Trials* 1986;23:269–280.
45. Goldenberg DL, Mayskiy M, Mossey C, et al. A randomized double-blind crossover trial of fluoxetine and amitriptyline in the treatment of fibromyalgia. *Arthritis Rheum* 1996;39:1852–1859.
46. Tofferi JK, Jackson JL, O'Malley PG. Treatment of fibromyalgia with cyclobenzaprine: a meta-analysis. *Arthritis Rheum* 2004;51:9–13.
47. Wolfe F, Cathey MA, Hawley DJ. A double-blind placebo controlled trial of fluoxetine in fibromyalgia. *Scand J Rheumatol* 1994;23:255–259.
48. Nørregaard J, Volkmann H, Danneskiold-Samsoe B. A randomized controlled trial of citalopram in the treatment of fibromyalgia. *Pain* 1995;61:445–449.
49. Hannonen P, Malminiemi K, Yli-Kerttula U, et al. A randomized, double-blind, placebo-controlled study of moclobemide and amitriptyline in the treatment of fibromyalgia in females without psychiatric disorder. *Br J Rheumatol* 1998;37:1279–1286.
50. Tavoni A, Vitali C, Bombardieri S, et al. Evaluation of S-adenosylmethionine in primary fibromyalgia. *Am J Med* 1987;83(Suppl. 5A):107–110.
51. Jacobsen S, Danneskiold-Samsoe B, Andersen RB, et al. Oral S-adenosylmethionine in primary fibromyalgia. Double-blind clinical evaluation. *Scand J Rheumatol* 1991;20: 294–302.
52. Mischoulon D, Fava M. Role of S-adenosyl-L-methionine in the treatment of depression: a review of the evidence. *Am J Clin Nutr* 2002;76:1158S–1161S.
53. Scudds RA, McCain GA, Rollman GB, et al. Improvements in pain responsiveness in patients with fibrositis after successful treatment with amitriptyline. *J Rheumatol* 1989; 16(Suppl. 19):98–103.
54. Ginsberg F, Mancaux A, Joos E, et al. A randomized placebo-controlled trial of sustained-release amitriptyline in primary fibromyalgia. *J Musculoskelet Pain* 1996;4:37–47.
55. Kempenears CH, Simenon G, Vander Elst M, et al. Effect of an antidiencephalon immune serum on pain and sleep in primary fibromyalgia. *Neuropsychobiology* 1994;30:66–72.
56. O'Malley PG, Balden E, Tomkins G, et al. Treatment of fibromyalgia with antidepressants. A meta-analysis. *J Gen Intern Med* 2000;15:659–666.
57. Smyth HA. Fibrositis and other diffuse musculoskeletal syndromes. In: Kelley WN, Harris ED Jr, Ruddy S et al., eds. *Textbook of rheumatology.* Philadelphia, PA: WB Saunders, 1981:485–493.
58. Goldenberg DL, Felson DT, Dinerman H. A randomized, controlled trial of amitriptyline and naproxen in the treatment of patients with fibromyalgia. *Arthritis Rheum* 1986;29:1371–1377.

59. Yunus M, Masi AT, Calabro JJ, et al. Primary fibromyalgia (fibrositis): clinical study of 50 patients with matched controls. *Semin Arthritis Rheum* 1981;11:151–172.

60. Smythe HA, Moldofsky H. Two contributions to understanding of the "fibrositis" syndrome. *Bull Rheum Dis* 1977;28:928–931.

61. Melzack R. The McGill pain questionnaire: major properties and scoring methods. *Pain* 1975;1:277–299.

62. Hench PK, Cohen R, Mitler MM. Fibromyalgia: effects of temazepam, amitriptyline and placebo on pain and sleep. *Sleep Res* 1989;18:335.

63. Jaeschke R, Adachi J, Guyatt G, et al. Clinical usefulness of amitriptyline in fibromyalgia: the results of 23 N-of-1 randomized controlled trials. *J Rheumatol* 1991;18:447–451.

64. Bergner M, Bobbitt RA, Carter WB, et al. The sickness impact profile: development and final revision of a health status measure. *Med Care* 1981;19:787–805.

65. Fries JF, Spitz PW, Kraines RG, et al. Measurement of patient outcome in arthritis. *Arthritis Rheum* 1980;23:137–145.

66. Meenan RF, Gertman PM, Mason JH. Measuring health status in arthritis: the arthritis impact measurement scales. *Arthritis Rheum* 1980;23:146–152.

67. Simms RW, Felson DT, Goldenberg DL. Criteria for response to treatment in fibromyalgia. *Arthritis Rheum* 1988;31(Suppl. 4):S100.

68. Burckhardt CS, Clark SR, Bennett RM. The fibromyalgia impact questionnaire: development and validation. *J Rheumatol* 1991;18(5):728–733.

69. Beck AT, Steer RA, Ball R, et al. Comparison of Beck depression inventories -IA and -II in psychiatric outpatients. *J Pers Assess* 1996;67(3):588–597.

70. Sheehan DV, Harnett-Sheehan K, Raj BA. The measurement of disability. *Int Clin Psychopharmacol* 1996;11(Suppl. 3):89–95.

71. Hunt SM, McKenna SP, McEwen J, et al. A quantitative approach to perceived health status: a validation study. *J Epidemiol Commun Health* 1980;34:281–286.

72. Heymann RE, Helfenstein M, Feldman D. A double-blind, randomized, controlled study of amitriptyline, nortriptyline and placebo in patients with fibromyalgia. An analysis of outcome measures. *Clin Exp Rheumatol* 2001;19:697–702.

73. Hamilton M. A rating scale for depression. *J Neurol Neurosurg Psychiatry* 1960;23:56–62.

74. Campbell SM, Clark S, Tindall EA, et al. A "blinded" controlled study of symptoms and tender points. *Arthritis Rheum* 1983;26:817–824.

75. Gilmor ML, Owens MJ, Nemeroff CB. Inhibition of norepinephrine uptake in patients with major depression treated with paroxetine. *Am J Psychiatry* 2002;159:1702–1710.

76. Bymaster FP, Zhang W, Carter PA, et al. Fluoxetine, but not other selective serotonin uptake inhibitors, increases norepinephrine and dopamine extracellular levels in prefrontal cortex. *Psychopharmacology* 2002;160:353–361.

77. Versiani M, Ontiveros A, Mazzotti G, et al. Fluoxetine versus amitriptyline in the treatment of major depression with associated anxiety (anxious depression): a double-blind comparison. *Int Clin Psychopharmacol* 1999;14:321–327.

78. Anderberg UM, Marteinsdottir I, von Knorring L. Citalopram in patients with fibromyalgia—a randomized, double-blind, placebo-controlled study. *Eur J Pain* 2000;4:27–35.

79. Arnold LM, Hess EV, Hudson JI, et al. A randomized, placebo-controlled, double-blind, flexible-dose study of fluoxetine in the treatment of women with fibromyalgia. *Am J Med* 2002;112:191–197.

80. Montgomery SA, Asberg M. A new depression scale designed to be sensitive to change. *Br J Psychiatry* 1979;134:382–389.

81. Aranow RB, Hudson JI, Pope HG Jr, et al. Elevated antidepressant plasma levels following addition of fluoxetine. *Am J Psychiatry* 1989;146:911–913.

82. Cohen J. *Statistical power analysis for the behavioral sciences*, 2nd ed. Hillsdale, NJ: Erlbaum, 1988.

83. Arnold LM, Hess EV, Hudson JI, et al. Fluoxetine treatment of fibromyalgia. *Arthritis Rheum* 2001;44:S67.

84. Cantini F, Bellandi F, Niccoli L, et al. Fluoxetine combined with cyclobenzaprine in the treatment of fibromyalgia. *Minerva Med* 1994;85:97–100.

85. Sarzi-Puttini P, Cazzola M, Pettorossi R, et al. Comparative efficacy and tolerability of sertraline vs amitriptyline in patients with fibromyalgia syndrome. *J Funct Syndr* 2001;1(2/3):164–170.

86. Nishikai M, Akiya K. Fluvoxamine therapy for fibromyalgia. *J Rheumatol* 2003;30:1124–1125.

87. Syuertsen JO, Smedsrud T, Lane RM. An open study of sertraline in fibromyalgia syndrome. *Eur Neuropsychopharmacol* 1995;5:315.

88. Giordano N, Geraci S, Santacroce C, et al. Efficacy and tolerability of paroxetine in patients with fibromyalgia syndrome: a single-blind study. *Curr Ther Res* 1999;60:696–702.

89. Nelson JC. Augmentation strategies with serotonergic-noradrenergic combinations. *J Clin Psychiatry* 1998;59:65–68.

90. Thase ME, Entsuah AR, Rudolph RL. Remission rates during treatment with venlafaxine or selective reuptake inhibitors. *Br J Psychiatry* 2001;178:234–241.

91. Nelson JC, Mazure CM, Jatlow PLI, et al. Combining norepinephrine and serotonin reuptake inhibition mechanisms for treatment of depression: a double-blind, randomized study. *Biol Psychiatry* 2004;55:296–300.

92. Franchini L, Gasperini M, Perez J, et al. Dose-response efficacy of paroxetine in preventing depressive recurrences: a randomized, double-blind study. *J Clin Psychiatry* 1998;59:229–232.

93. Harvey AT, Rudolph RL, Preskorn SH. Evidence of the dual mechanisms of action of venlafaxine. *Arch Gen Psychiatry* 2000;57:503–509.

94. Dwight MM, Arnold LM, O'Brien H, et al. An open clinical trial of venlafaxine in fibromyalgia. *Psychosomatics* 1998;39:14–17.

95. Zijlstra TR, Barendregt PJ, van de Laar MAF. Venlafaxine in fibromyalgia: results of a randomized, placebo-controlled, double-blind trial. Presented at the 66th Annual meeting of the American College of Rheumatology, New Orleans, LA, Oct. 25–29, 2002.

96. Bymaster FP, Dreshfield-Ahmad LJ, Threlkeld PG, et al. Comparative affinity of duloxetine for serotonin and norepinephrine transporters in vitro and in vivo, human serotonin receptor subtypes, and other neuronal receptors. *Neuropsychopharmacology* 2001;25:871–880.

97. Goldstein DJ, Mallinckrodt C, Lu Y, et al. Duloxetine in the treatment of major depressive disorder: a double-blind clinical trial. *J Clin Psychiatry* 2002;63:225–231.

98. Detke MJ, Lu Y, Goldstein DJ, et al. Duloxetine 60 mg once daily for major depressive disorder: a randomized double-blind placebo-controlled trial. *J Clin Psychiatry* 2002;63:308–315.

99. Detke MJ, Lu Y, Goldstein DJ, et al. Duloxetine 60 mg once daily dosing versus placebo in the acute treatment of major depression. *J Psychiatr Res* 2002;36:383–390.

100. Goldstein DJ, Lu Y, Detke MJ, et al. Effects of duloxetine on painful physical symptoms associated with depression. *Psychosomatics* 2004;45:17–28.

101. Simmons RM, Li DL, Lee DH, et al. Duloxetine, a potent and balanced dual serotonin and norepinephrine reuptake inhibitor, is efficacious in animal models of persistent pain. Presented at the American Psychiatric Association annual meeting, New Orleans, LA, May 5–10, 2001.

102. Iyengar S, Ahmad L, Simmons RMA. Efficacy of the selective serotonin and norepinephrine reuptake inhibitor, duloxetine, in the formalin model of persistent pain. *Biol Psychiatry* 2002;51(8 Suppl):75S–76S.

103. Jones CK, Peters SC, Iyengar S, et al. Duloxetine, a selective serotonergic and noradrenergic reuptake inhibitor, is efficacious in persistent and inflammatory, but not acute nociceptive, pain states in rodents. Presented at the 10th World Congress on Pain, San Diego, CA, Aug. 17–22, 2002.

104. Arnold LM, Lu Y, Crofford LJ, et al. A double-blind, multicenter trial comparing duloxetine to placebo in the treatment of fibromyalgia patients with or without major depressive disorder. *Arthritis Rheum* 2004;50:2974–2984.

105. Guy W. *ECDEU assessment manual for psychopharmacology*, Revised. US Department of Health, Education, and Welfare publication (ADM). Rockville, MD: National Institute of Mental Health, 1976:76–338.

106. Cleeland CS, Ryan KM. Pain assessment: global use of the Brief Pain Inventory. *Ann Acad Med Singap* 1994;23:129–138.

107. Ware JE, Snow KK, Kosinski M, et al. *SF-36 health survey manual and interpretation guide*. Boston, MA: The Health Institute, New England Medical Center, 1993.

108. Hunt SM, McKenna SP. The QLDS: a scale for the measurement of quality of life in depression. *Health Policy* 1992;22:307–319.

109. Melzack R. The short-form McGill pain questionnaire. *Pain* 1987;30:191–197.

110. Vitton O, Gendreau M, Gendreau J, et al. A double-blind placebo-controlled trial of milnacipran in the treatment of fibromyalgia. *Hum Psychopharmacol Clin Exp* 2004;19:S27–S35.

111. Tavoni A, Vitali C, Bombardieri S, et al. Evaluation of S-adenosylmethionine in primary fibromyalgia. *Am J Med* 1987;83(Suppl. 5A):107–110.

112. Russell IJ, Fletcher EM, Michalek JE, et al. Treatment of primary fibrositis/fibromyalgia syndrome with ibuprofen and alprazolam. *Arthritis Rheum* 1991;34:552–560.

113. Jacobsen S, Danneskiold-Samsoe B, Andersen RB. Oral S-adenosylmethionine in primary fibromyalgia. Double-blind clinical evaluation. *Scand J Rheumatol* 1991;20:294–302.

114. Rickels K, Chung HR, Csanalosi IB, et al. Alprazolam, diazepam, imipramine, and placebo in outpatients with major depression. *Arch Gen Psychiatry* 1987;44:862–866.

115. Russell IJ, Vipraio GA, Morgan WW, et al. Is there a metabolic basis for the fibrositis syndrome? *Am J Med* 1986;81(Suppl. 3A):50–54.

116. Priest RG, Baldwin DS, Bullock T, et al. Recent advances in antidepressant drugs. *S Afr Med J* 1992;6(Suppl):1–4.

117. Ginsberg F, Joos E, Géczy J, et al. A pilot randomized placebo-controlled study of pirlindole in the treatment of primary fibromyalgia. *J Musculoskelet Pain* 1998;6:5–17.

118. Hudson JI, Pope HG Jr. The relationship between fibromyalgia and major depressive disorder. *Rheum Dis Clin North Am* 1996;22:285–303.

119. First MB, Spitzer RL, Gibbon M, et al. *Structured clinical interview for the DSM-IV axis I disorders—patient edition (SCID-I/P)*, version 2.0. New York: Biometrics Research Department, New York State Psychiatric Institute, 1995.

120. Sheehan DV, Lecrubier Y, Sheehan KH, et al. The mini-international neuropsychiatric interview (M.I.N.I.): the development and validation of a structured diagnostic psychiatric interview for DSM-IV and ICD-10. *J Clin Psychiatry* 1998;59(Suppl. 20):22–33.

121. Yunus MB, Inanici F, Aldag JC, et al. Fibromyalgia in men: comparison of clinical features with women. *J Rheumatol* 2000;27:485–490.

122. Bair MJ, Robinson RL, Katon W, et al. Depression and pain comorbidity. A literature review. *Arch Intern Med* 2003;163:2433–2445.

123. Croft P, Rigby AS, Boswell R, et al. The prevalence of chronic widespread pain in the general population. *J Rheumatol* 1993;20:710–713.

124. Walker EA, Katon WJ, Jemelka RP, et al. Comorbidity of gastrointestinal complaints, depression, and anxiety in the Epidemiologic Catchment Area (ECA) study. *Am J Med* 1992;92:26S–30S.

125. Breslau N, Schultz LR, Stewart WF, et al. Headache and major depression: is the association specific to migraine? *Neurology* 2000;54:308–313.

126. Kroenke K, Spitzer RL, Williams JB, et al. Physical symptoms in primary care: predictors of psychiatric disorders and functional impairment. *Arch Fam Med* 1994;3:774–779.

127. Leino P, Magni G. Depressive and distress symptoms as predictors of low back pain, neck-shoulder pain, and other musculoskeletal morbidity: a 10-year follow-up of metal industry employees. *Pain* 1993;53:89–94.

128. Von Korff M, Dworkin SF, Le Resche L, et al. An epidemiologic comparison of pain complaints. *Pain* 1988;32:173–183.

129. Von Korff M, Ormel J, Katon W, et al. Disability and depression among high utilizers of health care: a longitudinal analysis. *Arch Gen Psychiatry* 1992;49:91–100.

130. Tomkins GE, Jackson JL, O'Malley PG, et al. Treatment of chronic headache with antidepressants: a meta-analysis. *Am J Med* 2001;111:54–63.

131. Jackson JL, O'Malley PG, Tomkins G, et al. Treatment of functional gastrointestinal disorders with antidepressant medications: a meta-analysis. *Am J Med* 2000;108:65–72.

132. Broekaert D, Vos R, Gevers AM, et al. A double-blind randomized placebo-controlled crossover trial of citalopram, a selective serotonin reuptake inhibitor, in irritable bowel syndrome. *Gastroenterology* 2001;120:A641.

133. Kuiken SD, Burgres P, Tytgat GNJ. Fluoxetine (Prozac) for the treatment of irritable bowel syndrome: a randomized, controlled clinical trial. *Gastroenterology* 2002;122:A551.

134. Creed F, Fernandes L, Guthrie E, et al. The cost-effectiveness of psychotherapy and paroxetine for severe irritable bowel syndrome. *Gastroenterology* 2003;124:303–317.

135. Plesh O, Curtis D, Levine J, et al. Amitriptyline treatment of chronic pain in patients with temporomandibular disorders. *J Oral Rehabil* 2000;27:834–841.

136. Rizzatti-Barbosa CM, Nogueira MT, de Andrade ED, et al. Clinical evaluation of amitriptyline for the control of chronic pain caused by temporomandibular joint disorders. *Cranio* 2003;21:221–225.

137. Campbell FG, Graham JG, Zilkha KJ. Clinical trial of carbazepine (Tegretol) in trigeminal neuralgia. *J Neurol Neurosurg Psychiatry* 1966;29:265–267.

138. Nicol CF. A four year double-blind study of Tegretol in facial pain. *Headache* 1969;9:54–57.

139. Klapper JA. Divalproex sodium in migraine prophylaxis: a dose-controlled study. *Cephalalgia* 1997;17:103–108.

140. Pappagallo M. Newer antiepileptic drugs: possible uses in the treatment of neuropathic pain and migraine. *Clin Ther* 2003;25:2506–2538.

141. Rowbotham M, Harden N, Stacey B, et al. Gabapentin for the treatment of postherpetic neuralgia. *JAMA* 1998;280:1837–1842.

142. Rice AS, Maton S. Gabapentin in postherpetic neuralgia: a randomized, double-blind, placebo controlled study. *Pain* 2001;94:215–224.

143. Backonja M, Beydoun A, Edwards KR, et al. Gabapentin for the symptomatic treatment of painful neuropathy in patients with diabetes mellitus: a randomized controlled trial. *JAMA* 1998;280:1831–1836.

144. Mathew NT, Rapoport A, Saper J, et al. Efficacy of gabapentin in migraine prophylaxis. *Headache* 2001;41:119–128.

145. Rao SG. The neuropharmacology of centrally-acting analgesic medications in fibromyalgia. *Rheum Dis Clin North Am* 2002;28:235–259.

146. Pillemer SR, Bradley LA, Crofford LJ, et al. The neuroscience and endocrinology of fibromyalgia. *Arthritis Rheum* 1997;40:1928–1939.

147. Lautenbacher S, Rollman GB. Possible deficiencies of pain modulation in fibromyalgia. *Clin J Pain* 1997;13:189–196.

148. Bennett RM. Emerging concepts in the neurobiology of chronic pain: evidence of abnormal sensory processing in fibromyalgia. *Mayo Clin Proc* 1999;74:385–398.

149. Staud R. Evidence of involvement of central neural mechanisms in generating fibromyalgia pain. *Curr Rheumatol Rep* 2002;4:299–305.

150. Baranauskas G, Nistri A. Sensitization of pain pathways in the spinal cord: cellular mechanisms. *Prog Neurobiol* 1998;54:349–365.

151. Crofford L, Russell IJ, Mease P, et al. Pregabalin improves pain associated with fibromyalgia syndrome in a multicenter, randomized, placebo-controlled monotherapy trial. *Arthritis Rheum* 2002;46:S613.

152. Belza BL. Comparison of self-reported fatigue in rheumatoid arthritis and controls. *J Rheumatol* 1995;22:639–643.

153. Okifuji A, Turk DC, Sinclair JD, et al. A standardized manual tender point survey. I. Development and determination of a threshold point for the identification of positive tender points in fibromyalgia syndrome. *J Rheumatol* 1997;24:377–383.

154. Zigmond AS, Smith RP. The hospital anxiety and depression scale. *Acta Psychiatr Scand* 1983;67:361–370.

155. Hays RD, Stewart AL. Sleep measures. In: Stewart AL, Ware JE Jr, eds. *Measuring functioning and well-being.* Durham, NC: Duke University Press, 1992:235–259.

156. Drewes AM, Andreasen A, Jennum P, et al. Zopiclone in the treatment of sleep abnormalities in fibromyalgia. *Scand J Rheumatol* 1991;20:288–293.

157. Grönblad M, Nykänen J, Konttinen Y, et al. Effect of zopiclone on sleep quality, morning stiffness, widespread tenderness and pain and general discomfort in primary fibromyalgia patients. A double-blind randomized trial. *Clin Rheumatol* 1993;12:186–191.

158. Moldofsky H, Lue FA, Mously C, et al. The effect of zolpidem in patients with fibromyalgia: a dose ranging, double-blind, placebo controlled, modified crossover study. *J Rheumatol* 1996;23:529–533.

159. Quijada-Carrera J, Valenzuela-Castano A, Povedano-Gomez J, et al. Comparison of tenoxicam and bromazepan in the treatment of fibromyalgia: a randomized, double-blind, placebo-controlled trial. *Pain* 1996;65:221–225.

160. Scharf MB, Baumann M, Berkokwitz D. The effects of sodium oxybate on clinical symptoms and sleep patterns in patients with fibromyalgia. *J Rheumatol* 2003;30:1070–1074.

161. Nicholson KL, Balster RL. GHB: a new and novel drug of abuse. *Drug Alcohol Depend* 2001;63:1–22.

162. Clark S, Tindall E, Bennett RM. A double blind crossover trial of prednisone versus placebo in the treatment of fibrositis. *J Rheumatol* 1985;12:980–983.

163. Rossy LA, Buckelew SP, Dorr N, et al. A meta-analysis of fibromyalgia treatment interventions. *Ann Behav Med* 1999;21:180–191.

164. Yunus MB, Masi AT, Aldag JC. Short term effects of ibuprofen in primary fibromyalgia syndrome: a double-blind, placebo controlled trial. *J Rheumatol* 1989;16:527–532.

165. Fossaluzza V, De Vita S. Combined therapy with cyclobenzaprine and ibuprofen in primary fibromyalgia syndrome. *Int J Clin Pharmacol Res* 1992;12:99–102.

166. Wolfe F, Anderson J, Harkness D, et al. A prospective, longitudinal, multicenter study of service utilization and costs in fibromyalgia. *Arthritis Rheum* 1997;40:1560–1570.

167. Sorensen J, Bengtsson A, Backman E, et al. Pain analysis in patients with fibromyalgia. Effects of intravenous morphine, lidocaine, and ketamine. *Scand J Rheumatol* 1995;24:360–365.

168. Kemple KL, Smith G, Wong-Ngan J. Opioid therapy in fibromyalgia—a four year prospective evaluation of therapy selection, efficacy, and predictors of outcome. *Arthritis Rheum* 2003;48:S88.

169. Biasi G, Manca S, Manganelli S, et al. Tramadol in the fibromyalgia syndrome: a controlled clinical trial versus placebo. *Int J Clin Pharmacol Res* 1998;18:13–19.

170. Russell IJ, Kamin M, Bennett RM, et al. Efficacy of tramadol in treatment of pain in fibromyalgia. *J Clin Rheumatol* 2000;6:250–257.

171. Bennett RM, Kamin M, Karim R, et al. Tramadol and acetaminophen combination tablets in the treatment of fibromyalgia pain: a double-blind, randomized, placebo-controlled study. *Am J Med* 2003;114:537–545.

172. Senay EC, Adams EH, Geller A, et al. Physical dependence on Ultram® (tramadol hydrochloride): both opioid-like and atypical withdrawal symptoms occur. *Drug Alcohol Depend* 2003;69:233–241.

173. Farber L, Stratz T, Bruckle W, et al. Efficacy and tolerability of tropisetron in primary fibromyalgia—a highly selective and competitive 5-HT3 receptor antagonist. *Scand J Rheumatol Suppl* 2000;113:49–54.

174. Bennett RM, Clark SR, Campbell SM, et al. Low levels of somatomedin C in patients with the fibromyalgia syndrome. A possible link between sleep and muscle pain. *Arthritis Rheum* 1992;35:1113–1116.

175. Bennett RM, Clark SC, Walczyk J. A randomized, double-blind, placebo-controlled study of growth hormone in the treatment of fibromyalgia. *Am J Med* 1998;104:227–231.

176. McCall-Hosenfeld JS, Goldenberg DL, Hurwitz S, et al. Growth hormone and insulin-like growth factor-1 concentrations in women with fibromyalgia. *J Rheumatol* 2003;30:809–814.

177. Henriksson KG, Sörensen J. The promise of N-methyl-D-aspartate receptor antagonists in fibromyalgia. *Rheum Dis Clin North Am* 2002;28:343–351.

178. Graven-Nielsen T, Aspegren Kendall S, Henriksson KG, et al. Ketamine reduces muscle pain, temporal summation, and referred pain in fibromyalgia patients. *Pain* 2000;85:483–491.

179. Clark SR, Bennett RM. Supplemental dextromethorphan in the treatment of fibromyalgia. A double blind, placebo controlled study of efficacy and side effects. *Arthritis Rheum* 2000;43:S333.

180. Feltner DE, Crockatt JG, Dubovsky SJ, et al. A randomized, double-blind, placebo-controlled, fixed-dose, multicenter study of pregabalin in patients with generalized anxiety disorder. *J Clin Psychopharmacol* 2003;23:240–249.

181. Pande AC, Crockatt JG, Feltner DE, et al. Pregabalin in generalized anxiety disorder: a placebo-controlled trial. *Am J Psychiatry* 2004;160:533–540.

182. Keck PE Jr, Arnold LM. The serotonin syndrome. *Psychiatr Annu* 2000;30:333–343.

32

Complementary and Alternative Medicine for Fibromyalgia

Edzard Ernst

Complementary and alternative medicine (CAM) has been defined as "diagnosis, treatment and/or prevention which complements mainstream medicine by contributing to a common whole, by satisfying a demand not met by orthodoxy or by diversifying the conceptual frameworks of medicine" (1), a definition that the Cochrane Collaboration has also adopted. CAM comprises a confusing array of treatments; several hundred different interventions exist. Those most relevant in the context of fibromyalgia (FM) are listed in Table 32-1.

Most chronic conditions are associated with a high level of CAM use (2), and rheumatoid arthritis (RA) is no exception. Thus most patients suffering from FM can be expected to try CAM (3). One survey suggested that 91% of FM patients had used CAM (4). In particular, FM patients frequently try massage, dietary approaches, vitamins and herbal medicines, relaxation, imagery, spiritual healing, acupuncture, and meditation (5). In the majority of cases, CAM is used in addition to, rather than as a substitute for, conventional treatments. Patients' motivations to try CAM can be complex: The wish to take control of their healthcare, the notion that CAM is without risks, and the desire to leave no stone unturned are usually important factors (6).

The high prevalence of CAM use renders it important to critically assess the efficacy and safety of CAM for FM. Recommendations issued in the CAM literature are often uncritically overoptimistic and thus not reliable. Table 32-2 summarizes the CAM treatments recommended in seven CAM books (7). These recommendations are not usually based on evidence; what is more, they also lack consensus among authors.

The aim of this chapter is to summarize and critically evaluate the data from clinical trials or, where possible, systematic reviews of such studies. This is based on electronic searches of the literature and on recent reviews of the subject (8–11). For the purpose of this chapter, treatments such as exercise, biofeedback, physiologic/behavioral therapies, dietary approaches, and low-level lasers are defined as conventional treatments.

ACUPUNCTURE

A systematic review of all randomized clinical trials (RCTs) of acupuncture for FM located only three such studies (12). One of these trials was of good methodologic quality. All studies suggested acupuncture to be effective in alleviating FM symptoms. Thus the collective evidence for acupuncture is positive but small, and further rigorous trials are required before firm recommendations should be provided.

ASCORBIGEN/BROCCOLI

Several American naturopaths tested a food supplement containing 100 mg ascorbigen and 400 mg broccoli powder given daily for 1 month (13). The 12 female FM patients in this study experienced a 20% improvement in their physical impairment, an 18% drop in their total FM impact score, and a trend toward an increase in pain threshold at 18 tender points. After discontinuation of treatment, these effects were reversed. This trial may be encouraging, but the lack of a control group does not allow us to make any conclusions regarding efficacy.

AUTOGENIC TRAINING

This autohypnotic technique was compared to Erickson's relaxation training in an RCT with 53 FM patients (14). The authors found that the latter approach was more suited to FM patients and led to a faster relief of symptoms. This study requires independent replication.

TABLE 32-1 Examples of Complementary and Alternative Medicine (CAM) Used for Fibromyalgia (FM)

NAME	PRINCIPLE	EFFICACY	SAFETY	RISK-BENEFIT BALANCE
Acupuncture	Insertion of needles into the skin for therapeutic preventive purposes	Several studies suggest efficacy	Serious adverse effects are rare; mild ones occur in ~7% of patients	Probably positive
Alexander technique	Training process of ideal body posture and movement; developed by F.M. Alexander	Few clinical trials exist, none in FM	No serious adverse effects	Uncertain
Aromatherapy	Application of essential oils usually through gentle massage techniques; developed by R.M. Gattefossé	Systematic review was inconclusive, no studies in FM	Allergic reactions to oils	Uncertain
Autogenic training	Form of self-hypnosis for relaxation and stress reduction; developed by J. Schultz	One positive study in FM	No serious adverse effects	Positive
Chiropractic	Popular manual therapy based on the assumption that most health problems are due to malalignments of the spine and treatable through spinal manipulation; developed by D.D. Palmer	No sound evidence in FM	Serious adverse effects have been reported, their exact incidence is not known; mild ones occur in ~50% of patients	Negative
Colonic irrigation (or colon therapy)	Cleansing of the colon through water enemas, e.g., to "free the system of toxins"	No sound evidence for effectiveness for any indication	Serious adverse effects reported	Negative
Guided imagery	Mind-body approach creating positive thoughts and images and communicating them with the body	One positive RCT in FM	No serious adverse effects	Positive
Feldenkrais therapy	Technique of body and mind integration based on the assumption that correction of poor habits of movement can improve self-image and health	One positive study in FM	No serious adverse effects	Positive
Homoeopathy	A method using often highly diluted preparations of substances whose effects when administered to healthy subjects correspond to the manifestations of the disorder in the patient	One positive RCT in FM	No serious adverse effects; in ~20% of patients, homoeopaths would expect an initial aggravation of symptoms	Inconclusive

Therapy	Description	Evidence	Adverse effects	Conclusion
Hypnotherapy	Induction of trancelike state to influence the unconscious mind	One positive RCT in FM	Adverse effects probably infrequent	Positive
Magnet therapy	Therapeutic use of magnets or magnetic fields	No sound evidence in FM	No serious adverse effects	Negative
Massage	Various techniques of manual stimulation of cutaneous, subcutaneous, or muscular structures	Some evidence for effectiveness in musculoskeletal and psychological problems	Few serious adverse effects	Positive
Meditation	A technique in which a person empties the mind of extraneous thoughts with the intent of elevating the mind to a different level	No sound evidence in FM	No serious adverse effects	Negative
Osteopathy	Various techniques of spinal mobilization; developed by T. Still	One positive RCT in FM	Adverse effects less than with chiropractic	Inconclusive
Reflexology	Internal organs allegedly correspond to areas on the sole of the feet and can be influenced through massaging these areas	No sound evidence in FM	No serious adverse effects	Inconclusive
Spiritual healing	Umbrella term for techniques of channeling of "healing energy" through a healer into a patient	No sound evidence in FM	No serious adverse effects	Negative
Tai Chi	A system of movements and exercises rooted in ancient Chinese philosophy	No sound evidence in FM	No serious adverse effects	Negative
Yoga	Meditative, postural, and breathing techniques from ancient India	No sound evidence in FM	No serious adverse effects	Negative

RCT, randomized clinical trial.
From Ernst E, Pittler MH, Stevinson C, et al. *The desktop guide to complementary and alternative medicine.* Edinburgh: Mosby, 2001, with permission.

	TABLE 32-2	Complementary and Alternative Medicine (CAM) Modalities Often Recommended for Fibromyalgia

NAME OF THERAPY	NUMBER OF RECOMMENDATIONS IN SEVEN CAM BOOKS	ACTUAL EVIDENCE[a]
Acupuncture	2	Encouraging
Aerobic exercise[b]	1	Good
Homoeopathy	1	Negligible[c]
Hypnotherapy	1	Negligible[c]
Massage	1	Negligible[c]
Mind-body therapy	1	Negligible[c]
Spinal manipulation	1	Encouraging

[a] See also text of this chapter.
[b] Excluded from this chapter.
[c] Only one RCT available.

CHIROPRACTIC

Blunt et al. conducted a randomized, crossover trial with 21 FM patients (15). They were treated with regular spinal manipulation and soft tissue therapy for 4 weeks. The control phases consisted of withholding such treatments. There was a trend for pain and function to improve during chiropractic care. The authors saw their study as preliminary and estimated that a definitive trial should have a sample size of 81.

Hains and Hains later reported another preliminary study with 15 FM patients who received 30 treatments consisting of spinal manipulation and "ischemic compression" (16). Six patients experienced improvements in their pain ratings and were classified as responders. The authors believed that these data "suggest a potential role for chiropractic care in the management of FM." However, without a control group no such conclusion is warranted.

CO-ENZYME Q10/*GINKGO BILOBA*

In a small, uncontrolled study, FM patients were given 200 mg co-enzyme Q10 plus 200 mg *Ginkgo biloba* extract per day for 84 days (17). Quality of life improved progressively during the treatment period. Due to the lack of a control group, no conclusions about the efficacy of this treatment are possible.

GREEN ALGAE (*CHLORELLA PYRENOIDOSA*)

A double-blind, placebo-controlled, crossover RCT tested the efficacy of a green algae supplement for FM (18). Forty-three patients received either 50 tablets of the supplement or placebo for 3 months. Differences at the end of the treatment phases favored the extract over placebo in terms of pain, sleep, and fatigue, all quantified with visual analog scales. These results require independent replication.

GUIDED IMAGERY

Fifty-five women with FM were randomized to receive either guided imagery plus relaxation training, or relaxation training alone, or no such treatments for 4 weeks (19). The results suggested guided imagery to be associated with a more rapid pain relief than that observed in the other two groups. This small but otherwise rigorous trial warrants independent replication.

FELDENKRAIS THERAPY

Twenty FM patients had 3 weekly sessions of Feldenkrais therapy for 15 weeks, while 19 control patients participated in an education plus exercise program for 15 weeks (20). The experimental group showed improvements in balance and lower extremity muscle function. These changes were small and not maintained at 6-month follow-up.

HOMOEOPATHY

Thirty FM patients who were suitable, according to homoeopathic principles, for treatment with homoeopathic dilutions of *Rhus toxicodendrum* 6C were randomized to receiving this intervention or placebos for 1 month following a crossover design (21). The results show superior outcomes for the experimental treatment phases in terms of pain and sleep but not in terms of global assessment. Even though about 15 years old, these encouraging findings have not been replicated.

HYPNOTHERAPY

Forty patients with refractory FM were randomly allocated to regular hypnotherapy or physical therapy for 12 weeks (22).

At the end of the treatment period, the hypnotherapy patients fared better with respect to pain, fatigue, sleep, and global assessment. No intergroup difference was noted in total myalgic score measured by a dolorimeter. This finding deserves to be followed up with further research.

MAGNETS

The effectiveness of static magnets was tested in a placebo-controlled RCT with 119 FM patients (23). They were treated with static magnetic fields or three different sham therapies for 6 months. Pain and number of tender points (TePs) decreased in all four groups. Although there was a trend favoring the magnetic therapy, the differences were not statistically significant.

MASSAGE

In an RCT with three parallel groups, the effectiveness of 10 weeks' regular soft tissue massage was compared to either attention control or no such intervention (24). Compared to the control groups, the experimental group experienced better outcomes in terms of pain, depression, and quality of life. This was a small study ($n = 52$), and its results need to be confirmed by independent replication.

MEDITATION

In an uncontrolled study, 77 FM patients participated in a program of regular meditation for 10 weeks (25). Marked improvements in global well-being, pain, sleep, and fatigue were shown by 51% of these patients. Even though the authors believed that "a meditation-based stress reduction program is effective for patients with FM," no conclusions can be drawn from this study due to lack of a control group.

OSTEOPATHY

Twenty-four female FM patients were randomly assigned to one of four groups: (1) osteopathic manipulation, (2) osteopathic spinal manipulation plus an educational program, (3) local hyperthermia, and (4) no such interventions (26). All patients also received medication. The result showed that the groups receiving spinal manipulations fared best in terms of pain at TePs measured with a dolorimeter as well as pain assessed with several other rating scales. This study requires independent replication.

TAI CHI

Thirty-nine FM patients participated in an uncontrolled study of Tai Chi (27). The program consisted of 1-hour classes twice weekly for 6 weeks. Twenty-one patients completed it. The results showed an improvement in quality of life (SF36) and Fibromyalgia Impact Questionnaire. The authors believe that "Tai Chi is potentially beneficial to patients with FM." Due to the lack of a control group, no such conclusion seems justified.

S-ADENOSYL METHIONINE

The dietary supplement composed of the amino acid methionine and adenosine triphosphate has anti-inflammatory and analgesic properties. In a small but otherwise rigorous RCT, it was shown that oral doses of 800 mg of S-adenosyl methionine given daily to FM patients were superior to placebo in improving disease activity, pain, fatigue, morning stiffness, and mood (28). This finding requires independent replication in a larger trial.

TOPICAL CAPSAICIN

In a placebo-controlled trial involving 45 FM patients, capsaicin (red pepper) plasters were compared to placebo plasters (29). Patients receiving the active therapy experienced less tenderness and a significant increase in grip strength. There were, however, no significant group differences in pain scores.

COMMENT

These data show that some forms of CAM could play a role in the symptomatic treatment of FM: Acupuncture, autogenic training, green algae supplements, guided imagery, Feldenkrais therapy, homoeopathy, hypnotherapy, magnet therapy, massage therapy, and osteopathy have all shown some promising results in controlled clinical trials. Yet the evidence is collectively weak and scarce. Previous reviews of this subject have already pointed out that the methodologic quality of the primary studies is often low (7,9,10). The most frequent and most serious flaws are the small sample size, the lack of a power calculation, the absence of independent replications of promising results, the failure to follow up pilot studies, the use of nonvalidated or FM-irrelevant endpoints, and the drawing of conclusions that the study's results do not support. Moreover, with several interventions it is difficult or even impossible to control for placebo effects. Thus there is uncertainty whether any observed outcomes are due to specific or nonspecific therapeutic effects.

The scarcity of trial data is impressive and, vis-à-vis the popularity of CAM, requires an explanation. Several obvious reasons spring to mind (30). CAM has traditionally not been a research-led area. In fact, many CAM enthusiasts are still not convinced that the rules of science can be applied to their field. Conducting rigorous clinical trials of CAM can be methodologically challenging. For instance, it can be difficult to control for placebo effects of physical interventions such as acupuncture or mind-body approaches such as hypnotherapy. The biggest obstacle to good CAM research, however, is funding. In most countries CAM research funding is overtly out of proportion with the prevalence of CAM use (30).

SUMMARY POINTS

- Although many FM patients try CAM, very few clinical trials in this area are available.
- Some treatments have been associated with encouraging results. These deserve to be followed up with rigorous and well-funded clinical trials.

■ IMPLICATIONS FOR PRACTICE

- Randomized clinical trials of CAM suggest that although many of these treatments are *effective* in clinical practice, they are not *efficacious* when rigorously compared to a placebo or control group.
- When any treatment is effective but has not necessarily been demonstrated to be efficacious, a placebo response may be playing a prominent role.
- As we begin to understand the neurobiological underpinnings and clinical power of the placebo response, we should endeavor to maximize this beneficial effect in clinical practice, using the safest and least expensive techniques possible.
- A safe, inexpensive CAM therapy that leads to clinical improvement in a patient may represent a very useful therapy, even in the absence of "evidence" of efficacy.

REFERENCES

1. Ernst E, Resch KL, Mills S, et al. Complementary medicine—a definition. *Br J Gen Pract* 1995;45:506.
2. Eisenberg D, David RB, Ettner SL, et al. Trends in alternative medicine use in the United States: 1990–1997. *JAMA* 1998; 280:1569–1575.
3. Ernst E. Usage of complementary therapies in rheumatology. A systematic review. *Clin Rheumatol* 1998;17:301–305.
4. Pioro-Boisset M, Esdaile JM, Fitzcharles M-A. Alternative medicine use in fibromyalgia syndrome. *Arthritis Care Res* 1996;9:13–17.
5. Nicassio PM, Schuman C, Kim J, et al. Psychosocial factors associated with complementary treatment use in fibromyalgia. *J Rheumatol* 1997;24:2008–2013.
6. Astin JA. Why patients use alternative medicine: results of a national study. *JAMA* 1998;279:1548–1553.
7. Ernst E, Pittler MH, Stevinson C, et al. *The desktop guide to complementary and alternative medicine.* Edinburgh: Mosby, 2001.
8. Berman BM, Swyers JP. Complementary medicine treatments for fibromyalgia syndrome. *Baillieres Best Pract Res Clin Rheumatol* 1999;13:487–492.
9. Sim J, Adams N. Systematic review of randomised controlled trials of non-pharmacological interventions for fibromyalgia. *Clin J Pain* 2002;18:324–336.
10. Holdcraft LC, Assefi N, Buchwald D. Complementary and alternative medicine in fibromyalgia and related syndromes. *Baillieres Best Pract Res Clin Rheumatol* 2003;17:667–683.
11. White A. Complementary therapies for fibromyalgia. *Focus Altern Complement Med* 2003;8:9–13.
12. Berman B, Ezzo J, Hadhazy V, et al. Is acupuncture effective in the treatment of fibromyalgia? *J Fam Pract* 1999;48:213–218.
13. Bramwell B, Ferguson S, Scarlett N, et al. The use of ascorbigen in the treatment of fibromyalgia patients: a preliminary trial. *Altern Med Rev* 2000;5:455–462.
14. Rucco V, Feruglio C, Genco F, et al. Autogenic training versus Erickson's analogical technique in treatment of fibromyalgia syndrome. *Riv Eur Sci Med Farmacol* 1995;17:41–50.
15. Blunt KL, Rajwani MH, Guerriero RC. The effectiveness of chiropractic management of fibromyalgia patients: a pilot study. *J Manipulative Physiol Ther* 1997;20:389–399.
16. Hains G, Hains F. A combined ischemic compression and spinal manipulation in the treatment of fibromyalgia: a preliminary estimate of dose and efficacy. *J Manipulative Physiol Ther* 2000;23:225–230.
17. Lister RE. An open, pilot study to evaluate the potential benefits of coenzyme Q10 combined with Ginkgo biloba extract in fibromyalgia syndrome. *J Int Med Res* 2002;30:195–199.
18. Merchant RE, Andre CA, Wise CM. Nutritional supplementation with Chlorella pyrenoidosa for fibromyalgia syndrome: a double-blind, placebo-controlled, cross-over study. *J Musculoskelet Pain* 2001;9:37–54.
19. Fors EA, Sexton H, Gotestam KG. The effect of guided imagery and amitriptylene on daily fibromyalgia pain: a prospective, randomized, controlled trial. *J Psychiatr Res* 2002;36:187.
20. Aspegren Kendall S, Ekselius L, Gerdle B. Feldenkrais intervention in fibromyalgia patients: a pilot study. *J Musculoskelet Pain* 2001;9:25–35.
21. Fisher P, Greenwood A, Huskisson EC, et al. Effect of homoeopathic treatment on fibrositis (primary fibromyalgia). *Br Med J* 1989;299:365–366.
22. Haanen HC, Hoenderdos HT, van Romunde LK, et al. Controlled trial of hypnotherapy in the treatment of refractory fibromyalgia. *J Rheumatol* 1991;18:72–75.
23. Alfano AP, Taylor AG, Foresman PA, et al. Static magnetic fields for treatment of fibromyalgia: a randomized controlled trial. *J Altern Complement Med* 2001;7:53–64.
24. Brattberg G. Connective tissue massage in the treatment of fibromyalgia. *Eur J Pain* 1994;3:235–244.
25. Kaplan KH, Goldenberg DL, Galvin-Nadeau M. The impact of a meditation-based stress reduction program on fibromyalgia. *Gen Hosp Psychiatry* 1993;15:284–289.
26. Gamber RG, Shores JH, Russo DP, et al. Osteopathic manipulative treatment in conjunction with medication relieves pain associated with fibromyalgia syndrome: results of a randomized clinical pilot project. *J Am Osteopath Assoc* 2002;102:321–325.
27. Taggart HM, Arslania CL, Bae S, et al. Effects of Tai Chi exercise on fibromyalgia symptoms and health-related quality of life. *Orthop Nurs* 2003;22:353–360.
28. Jacobsen S, Danneskield-Samsoe B, Anderson RB. Oral S-adenosylmethionine in primary fibromyalgia. Double-blind clinical evaluation. *Scand J Rheumatol* 1991;20:294–302.
29. McCarthy DJ, Csuka M, McCarthy G, et al. Treatment of pain due to fibromyalgia with topical capsaicin: a pilot study. *Semin Arthritis Rheum* 1994;23(Suppl. 3):41–47.
30. Ernst E. Obstacles to research in complementary and alternative medicine. *Med J Aust* 2003;179:279.

33

The Economic Impact of Fibromyalgia on Society and Disability Issues

Daniel J. Wallace

The economic burden to society from fibromyalgia-related lost productivity, psychological damage, and disability is significant. How this should be addressed has, unfortunately, been mired in controversy and accusatory discourse. This is further compounded by the failure of compensation systems to adequately deal with subjective complaints, pain, fatigue, and psychological determinants that influence one's ability to work. This chapter will combine an evidence-based approach and practical insights with the goal of formulating a vision of how to deal with this issue.

THE ECONOMIC BURDEN OF FIBROMYALGIA

The cost to society of fibromyalgia (FM) could not be calculated until relatively recently. After the American College of Rheumatology (ACR) approved an ad-hoc committee's proposed criteria for the syndrome in 1990 (1), it took another 5 years for publications to estimate its incidence and prevalence based on these definitions (2). Only at this point could economic impact studies be undertaken. Several clues were available (3): 6 million people in the United States have FM, and they saw an average of four doctors before being correctly diagnosed. The most prominent symptoms of FM are pain and fatigue. Ten million patient visits in the United States annually are for pain; $85 billion is spent annually to diagnose pain, including litigation fees. At any doctor visit in the United States, 15% of patients complain of being tired. Largely because there is no satisfactory drug treatment for FM, the majority of patients use alternative therapies. It has been estimated that $13 billion is spent annually in the United States on these preparations (4). In the mid-1990s, Jon Russell at the University of Texas, San Antonio calculated that the direct and indirect costs of FM were in the $12 to $14 billion range in the United States (J. Russell, *personal communication*). These calculations were never published in

the peer review literature but were used in various presentations, including one to a congressional committee.

The seminal review articles by White et al. note that in terms of pain, quality of life, fatigue, and function, FM patients have as extensive an impact on society as those with systemic lupus and rheumatoid arthritis and a greater impact than those with osteoarthritis (5,6). They critically reviewed papers from Canada suggesting that 700,000 residents have FM leading to $350 million in direct insurance costs and $200 million in private insurance costs. Robinson et al. studied the administrative claims of a Fortune 100 manufacturer where 4,699 individuals had at least one FM health claim submitted to their insurance (7). Compared to a control group, the annual costs for FM claimants was $5,945 versus $2,486 for the typical beneficiary ($p < 0.0001$). For every dollar spent on FM specific claims, an additional $57 to $143 was spent on additional direct and indirect costs. Those with FM and depression had 50% greater health care costs than these without it (7a). FM patients were twice as likely as the control group to become disabled. Another Canadian group derived a 6-month average direct cost of $2,298 (Canadian) for an FM patient. Medication (including complementary remedies) accounted for more than half of this. The presence of disability or a comorbidity increased this burden by 20% (7b).

THE ECONOMIC BURDEN OF FIBROMYALGIA ASSOCIATED FEATURES

Stewart et al. calculated lost productive work time among workers in the United States with depression or pain (8,9). Workers who were depressed had significantly more lost work productivity time (5.6 vs. 1.5 hours per week). Almost half of all lost productivity time was due to depression. Only 30% took antidepressants, and their benefits were slight. An excess of $31 billion per year in lost productivity time compared to peers without depression was estimated. Among a random sampling of 28,902 workers in the United States, 13% lost productive work time in a 2-week period due to a common pain condition. The most common was headache (5.4%), followed by back pain (3.0%), arthritis pain (2.0%), and other musculoskeletal pain (2.0%). This cost totaled $61.2 billion in lost productivity time, of which 76.6% was due to reduced performance while at work rather than work absence. [As a basis for comparison, osteoarthritis leads to $95 billion in lost productivity time out of $149 billion in direct and indirect costs (10).]

In summary, the cost of FM in the United States to society is not known, but by a loose extrapolation, if osteoarthritis accounts for a loss of 3% of our nation's overall productivity, FM accounts for somewhere between 1% and 2%.

THE DISABILITY CONUNDRUM AND FIBROMYALGIA

Many practitioners lose sight of the fact that 90% of Americans with FM who wish to work are working full time (11,12). (Actually, 60% are working and 30% are housewives, househusbands, or retirees). This section will address the following issues: Why are 10% with FM disabled? Why do 30% with FM change jobs or job descriptions to remain employed? The Worker's Compensation system, private disability plans, the Social Security disability system, and private insurance plans are all grossly unfair to both FM patients *and* employers. Why is this so and how can accountability be improved?

WHAT IS DISABILITY?

Much of our understanding of disability has been derived from the World Health Organization, which has published classifications of functioning, disability, and health, and has provided definitions of disability (13–15). Defined as "a limitation of function that compromises the ability to perform an activity within a range considered normal," disability has been explored using enablement-disablement models that fall into the following domains: pathology, impairment, functional limitation, and disability.

Pathology denotes changes at the molecular, cellular, or tissue level secondary to disease, trauma, or congenital conditions. *Impairment* refers to the loss or disruption of physiologic processes at the tissue, organ, or body system level when pathology crosses the clinical threshold. Impairments include pain from work activities (e.g., heavy lifting), emotional stress (e.g., pressure to meet a certain quota), and muscle dysfunction (e.g., polymyositis). A *handicap (or functional limitation)* is a job limitation or something that cannot be done (e.g., blindness, deafness). *Health-related quality of life (HRQOL)* is a subjective, multifactorial measure of wellness that includes physical, functional, emotional, and social domains influenced by disease or medical intervention.

Efforts to manage work disabilities take into account issues such as age, sex, level of education, psychological profiles, past attainments, motivation, retraining prospects, social support systems, self-esteem, stress, fatigue, personal value systems, and availability of financial compensation (16).

CLASSIFICATIONS OF DISABILITY

Persons who can never work again in any capacity are *permanently, totally disabled* and thus are usually eligible for Social Security Disability and Medicare benefits. If one is *permanently, partially disabled,* vocational therapy, occupational therapy, and psychological or ergonomic evaluations can address impairments or handicaps to optimize employment retraining possibilities. *Temporary, partial disability* allows one to work with restrictions (e.g., no heavy lifting, glare-proof screen on computer monitor) while treatment is in progress, while *temporary, total disability* involves a leave of absence from employment while undergoing treatment so that one can return to work.

Disability includes subjective factors (e.g., pain, fatigue) and objective factors (e.g., synovitis, blood pressure readings) and work categories. The latter include light, medium, or heavy work; sedentary work is defined by how much exertion is required over a time interval.

THE EPIDEMIOLOGY OF DISABILITY IN FIBROMYALGIA

Unfortunately, most published studies in the United States come from tertiary centers that inflate the numbers of FM patients on disability. It is this author's belief that over 90% with community FM who wish to work are employed. In a multicentered, university-based survey, 25% of 1,500 patients had received disability payments at some time and 15% were receiving Social Security Disability benefits (17). In the United States, 6% to 15% of employed patients with FM are on some form of disability, whereas in countries with generous benefits, such as Sweden, up to 25% are considered disabled (18). [Early studies were hampered by the lack of a definition of FM, which was not published until 1990, and reported disability rates up to 50% (19).] As a frame of reference, 2% of the nonretirement age adult population in the United States is on some form of disability. In Canada a review of insurance company records found that FM was responsible for 9% of all disability payments, which accounted for an estimated $200 million annually (20). Crook et al. followed 148 Canadian workers with "soft tissue injuries" who had not returned to work after 3 months. Forty percent made no attempt to return to work at 9 months, especially among those who were women and older (21). A bleaker look has been articulated by Hadler and Ehrlich, who start by relating that 5% of the population has chronic widespread pain (22). This group has a lower socioeconomic level of attainment, tends to seek more medical care, and is preoccupied with bodily symptoms. Since one-third will never improve, they posit that the problem should be approached by dealing with psychosocial stressors rather than musculoskeletal symptoms. Ross et al. performed a literature review on the topic of disability and chronic fatigue syndrome (22a). Twenty-two studies related some measure of physical or mental disability between 1988 and 2001 and seven used control subjects. It was found that 13% to 49% with chronic fatigue syndrome were employed versus 71% to 100% percent of controls. Only depression was associated with unemployment. No specific patient characteristics were identified as best predictors of employment outcomes.

HOW IS DISABILITY OR WORK ABILITY "MEASURED"?

Wolfe et al. documented that FM patients perform repetitive tasks well at first but have a decreased rate of performance with time due to musculoskeletal pain and accomplish 59% of the work done by healthy controls (23). Waylonis et al. showed that FM symptoms did not improve after receiving compensation for litigation and were aggravated by computer work or typing (37%), prolonged sitting (27%), stress (21%), and heavy lifting or bending (19%), but not by walking, light sedentary work, teaching, light deskwork, or phone work (24).

How do our current methodologies relating to disability apply to FM (25)? Disability carriers sometimes use measures of pain and fatigue (McGill Pain Questionnaire, West Haven Yale Multidimensional Pain Inventory, Pain Experience Scale), function (Health Assessment Questionnaire, Arthritis Impact Measurement Scales, Fibromyalgia Impact Questionnaire, work simulation tasks, Duke-UNC Health Profile, Quality of Well-being Scale, Activities of Daily Living), limitations (measurements of strength, stamina, and quality), coping strategies [Minnesota Multiphasic Personality Inventory (MMPI), Beck Depression Inventory, Centers for Epidemiologic Studies Depression Scale], and outcomes (Medical Outcomes Study Short Form-36). Most of these instruments have not been validated for FM. For example, the MMPI ignores pain, and measurements of strength do not take into consideration early onset of fatigue in performing repetitive tasks in one who has no decrement in strength. The validity of the handful of published FM-specific instruments is reviewed in Chapter 26, but as of this writing there is no truly accurate combination of instruments to measure disability in an FM patient.

DISPELLING PRECONCEIVED NOTIONS RELEVANT TO FIBROMYALGIA DISABILITY CONSIDERATIONS

Some popular conceptions bias patients, employers, and insurers in approaching disability in an FM patient. First, the prevalence of FM is the same in countries that have a true disability system and those that do not have a compensable disability system, such as Poland and Israel (18). Second, simply because so much of FM is subjective does not mean that it is not real or can be "faked" by a claimant who reads

about the syndrome. Migraine headaches and phantom limb pain are subjective, real, and compensable and in that context are no different from FM. An astute clinician can use control tender points (TePs), forms of distraction during the physical examination, a review of medical records, and a careful interview to assess for malingering. Third, the severity of FM symptoms and signs has little to do with employability. It is well known that many rheumatoid arthritis patients with high sedimentation rates and marked synovitis work full time, while others with normal sedimentation rates and little synovitis sometimes are incapacitated by their symptoms. Last, most functional disability forms filled out by treating physicians and sometimes required by Social Security applicants are misleading in FM. For example, "Can you lift 10 pounds, always, never, or occasionally?" is a common query on disability questionnaires. An FM patient can sometimes lift 10 pounds on 1 day but not on the next, but then for only 10 minutes an hour and on another day 30 minutes an hour.

FACTORS TO BE TAKEN INTO CONSIDERATION RELATING TO DISABILITY

According to Demitrack, the ability to work in FM must take into account certain considerations (26). These include *predisposing factors* such as stressful life events (acute or chronic), psychiatric illnesses (e.g., ergophobia—fear of work), personality (e.g., anxiety, perfectionist tendencies), and constitutional factors (e.g., chronic medical illnesses, allergies); *precipitating factors* such as infection, physical trauma, and emotional stressors; and *perpetuating factors*. These perpetuating factors include not liking work, untreated psychiatric illnesses, unaddressed psychosocial issues, unrecognized illnesses, abnormal illness attributions (e.g., a fixed belief in infection, such as yeast, unsupported by evidence), and disruption in rest activity cycles. Aaron et al. have found a significant correlation ($p = 0.012$) between emotional trauma and functional disability rates in FM (27). White et al. reported that FM patients are four times more likely to be disabled than a control group (28). The risk factors for disability included middle age, previous manual labor, low self-assessment of function, impaired memory or concentration, and complaints of pain, fatigue, or weakness.

In an effort to predict who will become disabled, 1,168 newly hired British workers free of low back pain were evaluated 1 and 2 years later (29). At 1 year, 119 had new onset low back pain and another 81 at 2 years. The predisposing factors for its development were lifting heavy weights, pulling heavy weights, kneeling or squatting for more than 15 minutes, stressful and monotonous work, hot working conditions, and pain at other sites.

PROBLEMS WITH THE SYSTEM AND SOCIAL SECURITY GUIDELINES

Critics of granting FM patients disability should be reminded that Worker's Compensation, private disability benefits, and

Social Security are the only protections a patient has and the patients have to work within a flawed system they did not create. Further, some individuals respond to a rehabilitation program and can resume employment. In 1999 the Social Security Administration issued new guidelines which for the first time stated that FM and chronic fatigue syndrome "are medically determinable conditions" (30,31). An FM or chronic fatigue syndrome patient must have one of the following documented for at least 6 months: swollen or tender lymph nodes; nonexudative pharyngitis; persistent, reproducible muscle tenderness on repeated examinations, including the presence of positive TePs; and fulfilling ACR criteria for FM. Abnormalities in brain imaging, neurally mediated hypotension, abnormal sleep studies, and evidence for exercise intolerance can be used to help establish the impairment. Only a small percentage of individuals who meet this listing will make it over additional hurdles (which are vague) and be granted Medicare insurance and disability benefits. In my experience, most FM patients who are on Medicare qualified by fulfilling psychiatric criteria.

Interviews with patients with FM who cannot work believe that their disability is due to severe pain, poor cognitive function, fatigue, stress, and damp work environments. However, medical and psychiatric evaluations of patients with FM on disability find several common features: low self-esteem, low socioeconomic attainment, hopelessness, severe fatigue, and inability to deal with pain (28,32–35). Although the overwhelming majority of these individuals have Medicare, some achieved total disability on the basis of Worker's Compensation litigation. This is unfortunate. Since almost all the factors related above were evident preexisting, "injury-induced" employment and disability is rarely the fault of the employer who is penalized (by higher insurance rates) for taking a chance on a prospective employee.

CONSEQUENCES OF DISABILITY

In evaluating FM patients for disability, patients have to overcome numerous hurdles that society puts before them. They include the lack of acceptance of the diagnosis, the patient's psychological makeup, self-reported versus observed disability, physician attitudes, compensation as a potential reward, the lack of validated instruments of evaluation, the format of disability evaluations, and the uncertain efficacy of treatment (25). Once disability is granted, patients are almost always worse off. According to Buchwald et al., individuals with FM or chronic fatigue syndrome have significant increased losses in material possessions (e.g., their car), loss of support by friends and family, loss of recreational activities, decreased standard of living, disconnection with intimate partners, and loss of hobbies and socialization (36).

PREVENTING DISABILITY

Since most FM patients are not disabled but differently "abled," how can the system be optimized to best help those who have difficulty working? First, FM patients should seek an agreeable work environment, be up-front and positive with their employers ("This is what I can do"), pace themselves with periods of activity alternating with periods of rest, employ coping strategies, and constructively help themselves. Second, those who are tenuously holding on to a job they cannot optimally perform should seek a change in their job description or workstation or contemplate a career change. Physical therapy, occupational therapy, medication, counseling, vocational training, and ergonomic workstation assessments can make a difference.

SUMMARY POINTS

- FM is responsible for a decrease in U.S. productivity by 1% to 2%, results in direct and indirect expenditures of at least $15 billion, and is inadequately evaluated and managed.
- Even though the overwhelming majority of FM patients who wish to work are employed full time, the syndrome diminishes their quality of life and productivity.
- Improvements need to be made in the compensation system so that nonwork-related psychosocial distress does not penalize employers, ascertainment methodologies for assessing disability are developed and validated, patients are not "stigmatized" and "medicalized" when told they have FM, and rehabilitation, workstation, or ergonomic assistance is made available to those likely to be helped.
- Since placing FM patients on total disability usually harms patients, their families, and society as a whole, a creative approach toward accommodating special needs and optimizing patient skill sets needs to be developed.

REFERENCES

1. Wolfe F, Smythe HA, Yunus MB, et al. The American College of Rheumatology 1990 criteria for the classification of fibromyalgia. Report of the Multicenter Criteria Committee. *Arthritis Rheum* 1990;33:160–172.
2. Wolfe FF, Ross K, Anderson J, et al. The prevalence and characteristics of fibromyalgia in the general population. *Arthritis Rheum* 1995;38:19–28.
3. Wallace DJ, Wallace JB. *All about fibromyalgia.* Oxford: Oxford University Press, 2002.
4. Rao JK, Mihaliak K, Kroenke K, et al. Use of complementary therapies for arthritis among patients of rheumatologists. *Ann Intern Med* 1999;131:409–416.
5. White KP, Harth M, Teasell RW. Work disability evaluation and the fibromyalgia syndrome. *Semin Arthritis Rheum* 1995;24:371–381.
6. White KP, Carette S, Harth M, et al. Trauma and fibromyalgia: is there an association and what does it mean? *Semin Arthritis Rheum* 2000;29:200–216.
7. Robinson RL, Birnbaum HG, Morley MA, et al. Economic cost and epidemiologic characteristics of patients with fibromyalgia claims. *J Rheumatol* 2003;30:1318–1325.
7a. Robinson RL, Birnbaum HG, Morley MA, et al. Depression and fibromyalgia: treatment and cost when diagnosed separately or concurrently. *J Rheumatol* 2004;31:1621–1629.

7b. Penrod JR, Bernatsky S, Adam V, et al. Health services costs and their determinants in woman with fibromyalgia. *J Rheumatol* 2004;31:1391–1398.

8. Stewart WF, Ricci JA, Chee E, et al. Lost productive time and cost due to common pain conditions in the US workforce. *JAMA* 2003;290:2443–2454.

9. Stewart WF, Ricci JA, Hahn SR, et al. Cost of lost productive work time among US workers with depression. *JAMA* 2003;289:3135–3144.

10. Impact of arthritis and other rheumatic diseases on the health care system in the United States. *MMWR* 1999;48:349–353.

11. Aronoff GM, Markovitz A. AADEP position paper: fibromyalgia: impairment and disability issues. *Disability* 1999;8:1–10.

12. Wolfe F, Potter J. Fibromyalgia and work disability: is fibromyalgia a disabling disorder? *Rheum Dis Clin North Am* 1996;22:369–391.

13. Harris-Love MO. Physical activity and disablement in the idiopathic inflammatory myopathies. *Curr Opin Rheumatol* 2003;15:679–690.

14. World Health Organization. *International classification of functioning, disability and health (ICF)*. Geneva: WHO, 2001.

15. World Health Organization. *ICIDH—International classification of impairments, disabilities and handicaps: a manual of classification relating to the consequences of disease.* Geneva: WHO, 1980.

16. Wallace DJ, Wallace JB. *All about fibromyalgia.* New York, London: Oxford University Press, 2001:198–202.

17. Wolfe F, Anderson J, Harkness D, et al. Work and disability status in persons with fibromyalgia. *J Rheumatol* 1997;24:1171–1178.

18. White KP, Harth M, Thorson K, et al. The fibromyalgia problem [Multiple Letters]. *J Rheumatol* 1998;2:1022–1030.

19. Ledingham J, Doherty S, Doherty M. Primary fibromyalgia syndrome—an outcome study. *Br J Rheumatol* 1993;32:139–142.

20. McCain GA, Cameron R, Kennedy JC. The problem of long term disability payments and litigation in primary fibromyalgia: the Canadian perspective. *J Rheumatol* 1989;19(Suppl. 16):174–176.

21. Crook J, Moldofsky H, Shannon H. Determinants of disability after a work related musculoskeletal injury. *J Rheumatol* 1998;25:1570–1577.

22. Hadler NM, Ehrlich GE. Fibromyalgia and the conundrum of disability determination [Editorial]. *J Occup Environ Med* 2003;45:1030–1033.

22a. Ross SD, Estok RP, Frame D, et al. Disability and chronic fatigue syndrome. A focus on function. *Arch Intern Med* 2004;164:1098–1107.

23. Cathey MA, Wolfe F, Kleinheksel SM. Functional ability and work status in patients with fibromyalgia. *Arthritis Care Res* 1988;1:85–98.

24. Waylonis GM, Ronan PG, Gordon C. A profile of fibromyalgia in occupational environments. *Am J Phys Med Rehabil* 1994;73:112–115.

25. Wallace DJ, Hallegua DS. Quality-of-life, legal-financial, and disability issues in fibromyalgia. *Curr Pain Headache Rep* 2001;5:310–319.

26. Demitrack MA. Chronic fatigue syndrome and fibromyalgia. Dilemmas in diagnosis and clinical management. *Psychiatr Clin North Am* 1998;21:671–692.

27. Aaron LA, Bradley LA, Alarcon GS, et al. Perceived physical and emotional trauma as precipitating events in fibromyalgia. Associations with health care seeking and disability status but not pain severity. *Arthritis Rheum* 1997;40: 453–460.

28. White KP, Speechley M, Harth M, et al. Comparing self-reported function and work disability in 100 community cases of fibromyalgia syndrome versus controls in London, Ontario. *Arthritis Rheum* 1999;42:76–83.

29. Harkness EF, Macfarlane GJ, Nahit ES, et al. Risk factors for new-onset low back pain amongst cohorts of newly employed workers. *Rheumatology* 2003;42:959–968.

30. Potter J. Tectonic changes in disability law. *Fibromyalgia Network*, July 1999:14–15.

31. Social Security Administration. Disability evaluation under Social Security, January 2003.

32. Wolfe F. The fibromyalgia syndrome: a consensus report on fibromyalgia and disability. *J Rheumatol* 1996;23:534–538.

33. Henriksson C, Liedberg G. Factors of importance for work disability in women with fibromyalgia. *J Rheumatol* 2000;27:1271–1276.

34. Hallberg LR, Carlsson SG. Anxiety and coping in patients with chronic work-related muscular pain and patients with fibromyalgia. *Eur J Pain* 1998;2:309–319.

35. Bennett RM. Disabling fibromyalgia: appearance versus reality. *J Rheumatol* 1993;20:1821–1823.

36. Assefi N, Coy TV, Uslan D, et al. Financial, occupational, and personal consequences of disability in patients with chronic fatigue syndrome and fibromyalgia compared to other fatiguing conditions. *J Rheumatol* 2003;30:804–808.

34

Prognosis

Arash A. Horizon and Michael H. Weisman

L ittle is known about the natural history and long-term prognosis of fibromyalgia (FM); what is known is based largely on clinical trials and small observational studies. This chapter will review the problems associated with assessing outcomes in FM and will critically review the small number of studies in this area.

BARRIERS AND CONCERNS IN EVALUATING THE PROGNOSIS OF FIBROMYALGIA

FM is a difficult condition to follow for a variety of reasons. First, there is no mortality from it. Second, hospitalizations due to FM are infrequent and rarely listed as such. Next, most FM patients reported in prognosis studies are followed at tertiary centers where disproportionate numbers of patients with psychosocial distress who have failed prior treatment regimens are seen. Further, community FM (see Chapter 3) is not considered in any of the published studies. Since these individuals don't complain of pain or see musculoskeletal specialists, this is an additional confounding factor. Also, since FM is a syndrome and not a disease, secondary factors (e.g., use of corticosteroids, recovery from an infection) are hard to separate from "relief of symptoms." Finally, there is evidence that "early" FM (symptoms for <2 years) is different than "late" FM in that it has a different cytokine profile and is more responsive to therapy (1).

Another area of concern is the lack of surrogates or biomarkers that can be used to assess FM outcomes. There is no accepted or even proposed definition for "remission" of FM. Chapter 26 reviews some of the proposed instruments for evaluating the syndrome for clinical trials, but none has been used for more than 12 months in any patients, let alone prognosis studies. It can be proposed that disability can be an outcome marker for studies, but only 10% of all FM patients are on disability, even though their job descriptions and jobs may have changed as a result of the condition.

Interpretation of these results most certainly needs to take into account how the patients are selected. Almost all clinical trials of pharmacologic agents in FM patients suffer from small sample size and short duration of treatment. Studies are investigator-driven and generally performed at a single site, limiting the number of subjects available for enrollment. Further clouding study outcomes are trial design issues that involve the perception that patients could not tolerate a placebo treatment arm for longer-term studies. Another confounding issue in FM clinical trials is that the most appropriate outcome measures have not yet been clearly defined or identified; tender points (TePs) or pain thresholds may be relatively resistant to treatment, for example.

Another difficult in interpreting clinical trials of patients with FM is the presence of comorbid psychiatric disorders. The degree to which patients in these trials or observational studies possess these confounding conditions will vary from study to study. Many effective pharmacologic and nonpharmacologic treatment approaches act on the psychiatric dimension of FM. It has been hypothesized that similar central nervous system pathways may be affected in patients with FM and patients with anxiety or depression. A major challenge in future clinical trials will be to distinguish between effects of interventions on psychiatric symptoms as separate from altered pain threshold or pain processing. Furthermore, some antidepressant medications may alter pain pathways, which further complicates clinical trial analysis.

CLINICAL STUDIES OF OUTCOMES IN FIBROMYALGIA

Despite the aforementioned study limitations, studies generally indicate that complete remission of FM with complete resolution of chronic pain is rare. Nevertheless, there may be reasons for limited optimism (see Table 34-1).

In the longest follow-up study to date, a 10-year prospective study of 39 clinic patients with FM in Boston, Massachusetts, there are no cases of complete remission, with all

		FEMALE	MEAN AGE (RANGE)	FOLLOW-UP	REMISSIONS[a]
STUDY	N	(%)	IN YEARS	IN YEARS	(%)
Papageorgiou et al. (2)	79	94	48.6 (24–86)	1.5	6.3
Felson and Goldenberg (3)	39	84.6	44.1	2	0
Granges et al. (4)	44	84.1	35.7 (15–61)	2	24.2
Ledingham et al. (5)	72	90.3	52 (18–81)	4	2.8
Baumgartner et al. (6)	45	78.0	50.6	6	0
Bengtsson and Backman (7)	49	—	—	8	"rare"
Kennedy and Felson (8)	29	86.2	43.5	10	0

[a]Remissions are defined as resolution of chronic widespread pain.

subjects reporting some FM symptoms at the study's end (8). In fact, most patients still experienced difficulties by study's end—moderate to extreme fatigue in 59% of subjects, moderate to severe pain or stiffness in 55%, and moderate to severe sleep difficulty in 48%. However at the 10-year follow-up, 66% of the subjects felt they were a little to a lot better than when first diagnosed; 55% felt well or very well, and only 7% felt poor.

The only other long-term FM follow-up study was an 8-year Swedish study of 49 subjects that described remissions as "rare" (7). Furthermore, a larger 4-year British study of 72 patients reported that 97% of patients had continued symptoms for the duration of observation and that 60% were worse, with only 26% improvement noted over baseline (5).

Recently, Baumgartner et al. completed a 6-year prospective study of a cohort of FM patients in a family practice setting. Of the 45 patients that completed the repeat evaluation, 20 (44%) of the patients indicated more pain, 17 (38%) patients did not notice a change in pain, and 8 (18%) reported improvement after 6 years of treatment (6).

A more optimistic clinical picture was presented in a 2-year Australian study of patients with FM not receiving compensation in which almost half the subjects no longer met the case definition for FM at the end of the study (4).

Children may have a more favorable prognosis, as reported by Buskila et al. who found after 30 months that 11 of the 15 children with FM (73%) were no longer fibromyalgic. In addition, none of the children who initially fulfilled the TeP count criteria developed FM (9).

The London, Ontario group presented 18-month-old data on 79 confirmed community FM cases; 16 of 79 (20%) no longer met the full case definition of FM at the termination of the study. In addition, three patients had complete resolution of pain (10).

The London prevalence study also discovered a significant decrease in the prevalence of FM in elderly women compared to younger women (2). This differs from the Wichita study (10), in which the prevalence did not change until the ninth decade. However, this may represent a calculation artifact as the confidence limits were not presented with the Wichita data. FM has generally been considered a noninfectious, chronic, not remitting, noncrippling, nonfatal syndrome (11), and, as such, the prevalence would be expected to rise throughout life. If, in fact, the prevalence of FM does decline after the age of 55, one must ask why.

There are at least three potential explanations for the observed age effect. The first is that of selective mortality. Individuals with FM are more likely to die earlier than age and sex matched individuals in the general population. FM could have a potentially fatal course itself; it could be a confounder through association with other, potentially fatal illnesses; or it could reduce survival in other conditions. As previously mentioned, studies have demonstrated that FM commonly coexists with lupus and rheumatoid arthritis, diseases with a standardized mortality ratio >1.

A second explanation is that FM does remit, particularly in individuals over the age of 55. Although studies show remissions to be rare in FM, many subjects in FM do have mitigation of their symptoms over time. Thus, these patients may no longer report the chronic widespread pain that defines FM, thereby leading to a decrease in the FM prevalence in the elderly.

A third hypothesis is that the differences across age groups reflect different years of birth (a cohort effect) rather than an age effect. Sometime in the past there may have been an epidemic of FM specific to one particular age group. If FM truly is chronic, not remitting, and nonfatal, then this peak of FM prevalence would follow this cohort as it ages. Further study of larger samples would permit a more accurate estimation of age and birth-cohort effect. Allowing for this possibility, the epidemic of FM must then be explained, and the potential for an infectious or other environmental cause must be reexamined.

SUMMARY POINTS

- FM remains a syndrome that is difficult to understand and treat successfully. In general, medical treatments are poorly effective and helpful only for a subset of patients.
- Children, individuals treated in primary care settings, and those with recent onset of symptoms generally have a better prognosis.
- Longer-term studies with larger study populations are needed to define risk factors for prognosis and to determine outcome relative to those risk factors.
- With further understanding of the pathophysiologic abnormalities involved in FM, one would expect to find more effective and possibly longer-lasting medical treatments.

REFERENCES

1. Wallace DJ, Linker-Israeli M, Hallegua D, et al. Cytokines play an aetiopathogenetic role in fibromyalgia: a hypothesis and pilot study. *Rheumatology (Oxford)* 2001;40:743–749.
2. Papageorgiou AC, Croft PR, Ferry S, et al. Estimating the prevalence of low back pain in the general population. Evidence from the South Manchester Back Pain Survey. *Spine* 1995;20:1889–1894.
3. Felson DT, Goldenberg DL. The natural history of fibromyalgia. *Arthritis Rheum* 1986;29:1522–1526.
4. Granges G, Zilko P, Littlejohn GO. Fibromyalgia syndrome: assessment of the severity of the condition two years after diagnosis. *J Rheumatol* 1994;21:523–529.
5. Ledingham J, Doherty S, Doherty M. Primary fibromyalgia syndrome—an outcome study. *Br J Rheumatol* 1993;32: 139–142.
6. Baumgartner E, Finchk A, Cedraschi C, et al. A six year prospective study of a cohort of patients with fibromyalgia. *Ann Rheum Dis* 2002;61:644–645.
7. Bengtsson A, Backman E. Long-term follow-up of fibromyalgia patients. *Scand J Rheum* 1992;21(Suppl. 94): 98.
8. Kennedy M, Felson DT. A prospective long-term study of fibromyalgia syndrome. *Arthritis Rheum* 1996;39:682–685.
9. Buskila D, Neumann L, Hershman E, et al. Fibromyalgia syndrome in children—an outcome study. *J Rheumatol* 1995;22:525–528.
10. White KP, Speechley M, Hart M, et al. The London fibromyalgia epidemiology study: the prevalence of fibromyalgia syndrome in London, Ontario. *J Rheumatol* 1999;26: 1570–1576.
11. Wolfe F, Ross K, Anderson J, et al. The prevalence and characteristics of fibromylagia in the general population. *Arthritis Rheum* 1995;38:19–28.

35

Future Research Directions

Leslie J. Crofford

Fibromyalgia syndrome (FMS) is a chronic multisymptom illness (CMI) characterized by widespread pain and associated with neuropsychological symptoms, including pain, unrefreshing sleep, cognitive dysfunction, anxiety, and depression. Although a discreet cause of FMS has not been identified, it is likely that both genetic factors and environmental triggers contribute to syndrome onset. In fact, many different mechanisms are likely to give rise to a symptom complex that is currently most appropriately diagnosed as FMS but that may be more properly considered as different conditions once specific mechanisms are identified. Understanding specific etiologic factors and pathogenic mechanisms in individual patients will allow clinicians to determine treatments that are most effective for a given patient.

Available evidence implicates the central nervous system (CNS) as a key in maintaining pain and other core symptoms of FMS. Previous research into FMS has taught us a great deal about the confluence of neurobiologic, psychological, and behavioral factors that can maintain central pain. With the availability of increasingly sophisticated methodology for examining the CNS, it is likely that future research will further delineate these relationships. New treatments directed at centrally maintained pain are likely to be developed that will be more effective than the current drugs available for treatment of pain.

The relationship between pain processing alterations and other core FMS symptoms is yet to be fully understood. There is a large void in the understanding of the nonpain symptoms of FMS. Nonpain symptoms such as fatigue predominate in many FMS patients and often precede the development of widespread pain. These neuropsychological symptoms of FMS are shared among many other CMIs that co-occur with FMS, such as chronic fatigue syndrome (CFS), temporomandibular disorder (TMD), irritable bowel syndrome (IBS), and others. These CMIs may or may not exhibit the widespread pain and reduced noxious threshold characteristic of FMS. However, shared mechanisms may be operative between CMI and depression and anxiety, which are present with increased frequency in patients with all these syndromes. Research that seeks to delineate similarities as well as differences in the expression of neuropsychological

symptoms and their underlying mechanisms in FMS and co-occurring syndromes is likely to be fruitful.

With improved understanding of the basic mechanisms underlying these syndromes, there is a tremendous opportunity to develop new pharmacologic and nonpharmacologic therapies. However, it is clear that individual, social, and cultural factors play an important role in the impact of FMS on health. The factors that contribute to refractoriness of symptoms must be identified and methods to improve outcome in all patients must be developed.

DEFINING FIBROMYALGIA SYNDROME

The current American College of Rheumatology (ACR) definition of FMS relies on the presence of chronic widespread pain and the presence of tender points (TePs) (1). There is evidence that measuring altered pain processing using the current TeP criteria captures only a small proportion of those individuals reporting chronic widespread pain. Furthermore, TePs appear to increase selection of women and those with higher levels of neuropsychological symptoms or distress (2,3). A crucial factor in future research of patients with FMS is agreement on whom this syndrome should properly include.

The strength of the current criteria is that they are easily applied and identify a population that has provided insights into the biology of FMS. They have also been useful to identify study populations for clinical trials designed to evaluate response to pharmacologic and nonpharmacologic therapies. Weaknesses include the fact that the TeP criteria impose a dichotomous variable on what is essentially a bell-shaped curve. Do patients with widespread pain and only ten TePs have a different syndrome? Nonpain symptom criteria are not included in the case definition as it is currently formulated. Patients with fewer TePs may complain of neuropsychological symptoms (e.g., fatigue and unrefreshing sleep) in addition to pain, suggesting that they should be considered in the CMI spectrum of illness. Do these patients have a different syndrome? Changing the way

FMS is defined has important implications for biologic and clinical studies in this patient population but should be an important subject for future research (4).

VULNERABILITY AND TRIGGERS

Family studies have suggested an important genetic component contributing to an FMS diagnosis (5,6). It has also been suggested that genetic factors may contribute to shared vulnerability of FMS patients to depression and other CMIs, including CFS, IBS, TMD, and others (7–9). A family study from Arnold et al. compared the prevalence of FMS, tenderness, and depression in first-degree relatives of patients with either FMS or rheumatoid arthritis (RA) (10). They found an odds ratio of 8.5 (95% confidence intervals, 2.8 to 26, $p = 0.0002$) of FMS in the family members of an FMS proband compared to an RA proband. Aggregation was almost entirely among female relatives. There were higher numbers of TePs and myalgic score in relatives of FMS compared to RA patients, which remained true when adjusted for the presence of FMS and mood disorder. There was coaggregation of depression with FMS compared to RA with an odds ratio of 1.8 (95% CI, 1.1 to 2.9, $p = 0.013$). However, the aggregation of FMS in families was independent of mood disorders.

Although not available specifically for FMS, twin studies in CFS also suggest a genetic influence. Buchwald et al. reported that the concordance rate for CFS, as well as non-CFS chronic fatigue, in monozygotic twins was higher than for dizygotic twins. The estimated heritability in liability for CFS was 51% (95% CI, 7 to 96) (11).

Future research should be able to identify specific genes that will segregate into genes that control tenderness and genes that confer shared vulnerability for FMS and depression. There is evidence of possible linkage for genes within the serotonergic system in patients with FMS that have not been confirmed in all studies (12–15). As better understanding of FMS subsets is clarified, phenotyping for genetic studies should proceed more effectively, increasing the ability to understand genetic vulnerability.

Vulnerability may not be genetically determined in all patients but acquired due to events in childhood or perhaps adulthood (16,17). It is clear that factors such as rearing behaviors and stressors such as victimization can permanently affect some of the same CNS pathways identified as altered in patients with FMS and related disorders.

In vulnerable individuals environmental factors are likely to play an important role in the development of FMS. Stressful triggers temporally associated with the development of FMS or other CMIs include physical trauma, certain infections, emotional stress, regional or widespread pain conditions, and autoimmune disorders (8,18–23). The type of stressor and the environment in which it occurs also have an impact on how the stress response is expressed. It has been noted that victims of accidents experience a higher frequency of FMS than those who cause them, which is congruent with animal studies showing that the strongest physiologic responses are triggered by events that are accompanied by a lack of control or support and thus are perceived as inescapable or unavoidable (24,25). In humans, daily "hassles" and personally relevant stressors seem to be more capable of causing symptoms than major catastrophic events that do not personally affect the individual (26–30).

The relationship between FMS and other rheumatic syndromes provides an excellent opportunity. As many as 25% of patients correctly diagnosed with systemic lupus, RA, and ankylosing spondylitis also fulfill criteria for FMS (20). However, the specific risk factors for developing FMS related to these triggers in individual patients has not been determined. Prospective studies to determine the risk factors for developing FMS in those with these and other potential triggers will also help to understand why certain triggers are more potent than others.

Understanding the interactions between genes and environment will continue to be challenging in the study of FMS (see Figure 35-1). Methodology employed by Aaron et al. in patients with CFS may be revealing in determining vulnerability for FMS and other CMIs, as well as dissecting genetic versus environmental determinants of illness (9). These investigators found that an affected twin with fatigue had a markedly increased risk for also having FMS (>70% compared to <10%) and IBS (>50% compared to <5%), suggesting important environmental influences on symptom expression. Regression analysis demonstrated that the burden of illnesses could not be attributed to psychiatric disorders. Studies comparing monozygotic and dizygotic twins, measuring clinical and biologic variables, and recording life experiences in affected versus unaffected twins may shed light on the relative contributions of genes and environment in these groups of illnesses.

DEVELOPMENT AND PERSISTENCE OF CENTRAL PAIN

A key clinical feature of patients with FMS is the presence of evoked pain. Functional magnetic resonance imaging

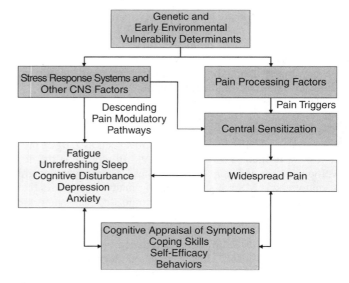

Figure 35-1. Topic areas for future research in the development and persistence of fibromyalgia syndrome.

(fMRI) demonstrations of activation in brain regions associated with noxious stimulation are an objective indication of the veracity of patients' reports of evoked pain (31). A number of observations suggest that FMS is a central pain syndrome—that is, there is no peripheral pain generator that can explain all the patients' pain complaints. Staud et al. demonstrated temporal summation of painful stimuli applied to both skin and muscle (32–34). These data suggest a parallel between pain processing in FMS and the phenomenon of "wind-up" mediated by changes in the dorsal horn (35). Lorenz et al. demonstrated an enhanced evoked response to laser stimulation in FMS patients compared to controls (36). Furthermore, biochemical studies demonstrate altered levels of biochemicals, amino acids, and peptides involved in pain processing (37–43).

It is not known if individuals who develop FMS have pre-existing alterations in pain processing or whether a painful trigger results in changes to pain processing pathways. However, it has been demonstrated that first-degree relatives of FMS patients have increased tenderness (6,10). Similar studies using different methods to assess pain processing will be useful (44). Longitudinal studies of patients at risk for developing FMS may also be useful to assess the relationship between altered pain processing and illness.

In the realm of pain research, specific alterations of dorsal horn neurons and descending modulatory pathways are becoming more clearly understood (45). In addition to changes in neurons, it is becoming clear that glial cells may contribute to persistent pain (46). Milligan et al. demonstrated that when glia become activated, signaling pathways leading to the release of a variety of chemical substances, including proinflammatory cytokines, are enhanced. These pathways contribute to amplification of the pain message (47). Examining hyperalgesia and allodynia in FMS patients compared to individuals with more clearly understood pain syndromes (e.g., inflammatory, neuropathic) will help to clarify FMS pain.

Understanding how to determine the specific alterations of pain processing that are most important in individual patients with FMS may help to understand which treatments may be most effective. This will necessarily involve measurements of pain processing in therapeutic trials.

STRESS AND DISTRESS

Many studies have confirmed the high prevalence of neuropsychological symptoms in FMS (48–53). It is, however, unclear if neuropsychological symptoms or "distress" are a necessary component of FMS. The answer to that question depends, of course, on the definition of FMS.

It is clear that neuropsychological symptoms, such as fatigue, sleep disturbance, cognitive complaints, depression, and anxiety, cluster with multifocal pain in population studies (4). A higher symptom burden is associated with a higher likelihood that an individual will seek health care (54,55). A study by Jones et al. compared patients with FMS to patients who had pain but did not meet criteria for FMS (56). FMS patients were more symptomatic on virtually all measures of psychological distress. Furthermore, individuals with high levels of depression and anxiety had more physical symptoms and had poorer function than those with lower levels. In a simple regression model, the best predictors for both depression and trait anxiety were the total number of symptoms and a physical disability score.

The observation that patients with FMS are at high lifetime risk for other CMIs, depression, and anxiety disorders that are all manifested by similar neuropsychological symptoms has led to a search for shared biological mechanisms. Among these are studies of stress-response systems, including the hypothalamic-pituitary-adrenal (HPA) axis and the sympathetic nervous system (SNS), that are perturbed in FMS and related syndromes (57,58). Stress-response systems may be understood as a set of continuously adaptive physiologic systems that continuously monitor and respond to an individual's physical and psychological state (59). Input to hypothalamic and brainstem regions comes from the periphery (e.g., peripheral nervous system, cytokines, hormones) and higher cortical centers (e.g., limbic and cortical centers). The activity of these systems fluctuates over the day—that is, they exhibit circadian change. These systems respond to a variety of physiologic stressors, including such normal activities as eating and waking, and physical and psychological stressors. The cumulative activity of the stress axes is determined by the set point of the axis as well as the stress load at any given time. Genetic factors, stress, and other physiologic factors such as aging contribute to basal activity levels and the biologic response to stress (60–65).

Patients with FMS and related syndromes have been shown to have altered HPA axis physiology (58,66). Differences in methodology and intersubject variability have made identification of a specific abnormality difficult. Furthermore, it may be that subsets of patients have different types of changes in HPA axis function. Future research will help to clarify these issues.

Also described are specific changes of SNS function (67). Such findings as lack of heart rate variability, particularly during sleep, have been reported (68–71). Alterations of SNS physiology may also define subsets of patients with FMS that will be clarified in future studies. A consensus should be reached on which methods for assessing stress axis physiology should be employed in patients with FMS and other CMIs. Newer methods, including neuroimaging studies that make use of specific receptor ligands, may shed light on central stress system and other brain pathways that may be disturbed in FMS and related syndromes.

It is currently unclear if altered stress system physiology precedes or follows the development of FMS. Studies of patients at risk for developing FMS, including first-degree relatives, will help to clarify this issue. Also unclear is whether previous experiences—sexual or physical abuse, for example—result in changes to stress-response axes that contribute to syndrome onset as has been described for depression and anxiety (17). Studies examining childhood stressors and correlating these experiences with stress axis physiology are needed. Correlation of specific symptoms with specific alterations of stress system physiology should be undertaken. In addition, further studies of these stress-response systems directly comparing FMS to other syndromes should be undertaken.

NONPAIN SYMPTOMS

Among the nonpain symptoms most prominent in FMS are fatigue, unrefreshing sleep, and complaints of cognitive dysfunction. Fatigue is among the most poorly understood symptoms, but studies of chronically fatigued individuals with or without medical or psychiatric comorbidity will help to delineate which tools may be best to study fatigue in FMS. Fatigue may mean different things, and it can be difficult to discern lack of energy from sleepiness or the struggle to overcome inactivity. In the physical domain it may mean weakness, limb heaviness, or postexertional malaise. Fatigue may reflect reduced interest, motivation, or concentration. From a functional standpoint, fatigue may mean difficulty completing daily tasks. Possible etiologies of fatigue in FMS would include sleep disturbances, the fatiguing effect of pain, medications, deconditioning, or abnormal muscle metabolism, or, in a subset of patients, neurally mediated hypotension (69,72,73).

Disturbances in sleep were the first biologic variable described as abnormal in patients with FMS (74). Although three decades have elapsed since Moldofsky described the phenomenon of wakefulness, identified by α activity in slow-wave sleep, little more has been learned. The presence of this normal electroencephalogram (EEG) sign of wakefulness during sleep is linked to complaints of unrefreshing sleep, fatigue, and malaise, which are part of the symptom complex of FMS (75). However, only 40% of overall chronic pain patients exhibit this anomaly, so it cannot be said that this sleep alteration is always the cause of chronic pain (76). Slow-wave sleep is, however, thought to be essential for physiologic restoration, and it has been proposed that the symptoms of FMS could be related. It should be noted that so-called "alpha-delta" sleep is not specific for FMS and there is variable consistency of this anomaly in FMS (76–80). In the most recent study, 70% of FMS patients exhibited phasic or tonic α intrusion, whereas 84% of controls had low α (81). New analytic methods for spectral analyses of polysomnographic data are available that may help to better characterize the sleep alterations of FMS patients and to determine its etiology and clinical associations.

Patients with FMS often complain of difficulty with memory, concentration, and other aspects of cognition, but it has been controversial whether these assessments were accurate. Recent studies have demonstrated that patients with FMS do have significant difficulty with working memory and effortful short-term memory tasks (82,83). Research opportunities exist to determine the reasons for cognitive problems in this group of patients, which may include sleep disturbances, depression, pain, or lack of effort (82,84).

INDIVIDUAL, SOCIAL, AND CULTURAL FACTORS

Individuals can experience pain in markedly different ways. In addition to differences in nociceptive pathways, the cognitive appraisal process contributes to pain perception, emotional response to pain, and pain behaviors (85). Success in dealing effectively with illness is more likely if patients believe that they possess the knowledge and skills to do so, which is called adaptive coping. If a patient lacks these skills, catastrophic thinking and development of anxiety or depression can contribute to ongoing illness. Among the factors that contribute to poor coping skills is lack of, or overly solicitous, social support. In general, social support of good quality facilitates pain management (86). After secondary appraisal shows that coping resources are available, patients determine their ability to take advantage of adaptive resources. Self-efficacy is the perceived ability to perform a specific task in order to achieve a specific outcome (85). In patients with rheumatic diseases, improvements in self-efficacy are highly predictive of improvements in pain, depression, and health status (87). Fear of pain or injury may motivate avoidance of behaviors, such as exercise or work, which may exacerbate symptoms.

Issues related to disability of patients with FMS and other chronic pain conditions have generated significant controversy. Reisine et al. showed that employed women reported significantly less pain, less fatigue, and better functional status than those who were not employed (88), although it is not clear if patients with a higher symptoms burden were simply unable to work. Additionally, the psychological demands of family work were consistently related to all dependent measures of health status, as those with greater psychological demands reported worse health status.

Future research should continue to focus on the therapeutic benefits of increasing adaptive resources and self-efficacy using such interventions as cognitive-behavioral therapy. Furthermore, the factors that predict disability across cultures and how those may be modified should be determined prospectively.

TREATMENT

In order to translate our greater understanding of FMS biology into effective treatment, it is essential to develop appropriate outcome measures. It is desirable that all investigators adopt a similar strategy for measuring FMS activity useful for longitudinal studies as well as for interventional trials. In order to develop outcome measures, general agreement on which domains of FMS are important should be reached. Input from clinicians and patients should be considered. The domains of assessment to date have most commonly included pain, fatigue, depression, function, TePs, health-related quality of life, and global health status. The instruments used to measure these domains have varied from visual analog or numerical rating scales to multidimensional instruments. Measuring function in FMS may include physical function, and also emotional and social function. The Fibromyalgia Impact Questionnaire (FIQ) was developed and validated as an instrument to measure multiple domains in patients with FMS (89). The FIQ total score and elements of the FIQ, such as the pain visual analog scale (VAS), have been used in clinical trials (90). Another strategy would be to use individual measurement instruments and develop an activity or responder index similar to the ACR-20 used in RA. Future research should clarify which outcome measures provide the most meaningful information in FMS.

Surrogate markers or biomarkers that may predict response to therapy will be very useful in this group of patients. Additionally, it will be important to define short-term and long-term outcomes and make recommendations regarding the duration of clinical trials. Ultimately, developing new pharmacologic, nonpharmacologic, and combination therapies to translate improved understanding of FMS biology to the clinic will be the most important research priority.

SUMMARY POINTS

- The definition of FMS affects all forms of research.
- Evidence for a genetic contribution to FMS exists.
- Characteristics of environmental triggers for FMS require further study.
- FMS is a central pain syndrome, and future research should focus on mechanisms underlying the development and persistence of central pain.
- Neuropsychological symptoms of FMS are poorly understood but shared across related syndromes.
- Psychosocial and cultural factors affect health status in FMS patients, and strategies for improving these factors should be studied.
- There is a need to develop and validate outcome measures for FMS that will become the standard for clinical trials.
- Research will guide development of more specific, more effective treatments.

■ IMPLICATIONS FOR PRACTICE

- Strict adherence to the ACR classification criteria in clinical practice is not required for effective management of patients with widespread pain and neuropsychological symptoms.
- Treatments of FMS should be targeted to central pain and neuropsychological symptoms.
- Education of patients on current research in FMS may improve coping and self-efficacy.
- New treatments based on improved understanding of FMS pathophysiology are likely.

REFERENCES

1. Wolfe F, Smythe HA, Yunus MB, et al. The American College of Rheumatology 1990 criteria for the classification of fibromyalgia. Report of the Multicenter Criteria Committee. *Arthritis Rheum* 1990;33:160–172.
2. Petzke F, Gracely RH, Park KM, et al. What do tender points measure? Influence of distress on four measures of tenderness. *J Rheumatol* 2003;30:567–574.
3. Wolfe F. The relation between tender points and fibromyalgia symptom variables: evidence that fibromyalgia is not a discrete disorder in the clinic. *Ann Rheum Dis* 1997;56:268–271.
4. Clauw DJ, Crofford LJ. Chronic widespread pain and fibromyalgia: what we know, and what we need to know. *Best Pract Res Clin Rheumatol* 2003;17:685–701.
5. Buskila D, Neumann L, Hazanov I, et al. Familial aggregation in the fibromyalgia syndrome. *Semin Arthritis Rheum* 1996;26:605–611.
6. Buskila D, Neumann L. Fibromyalgia syndrome (FM) and nonarticular tenderness in relatives of patients with FM. *J Rheumatol* 1997;24:941–944.
7. Hudson JI, Hudson MS, Pliner LF, et al. Fibromyalgia and major affective disorder: a controlled phenomenology and family history study. *Am J Psychiatry* 1985;142:441–446.
8. Hudson JI, Goldenberg DL, Pope HG, et al. Comorbidity of fibromyalgia with medical and psychiatric disorders. *Am J Med* 1992;92:363–367.
9. Aaron LA, Herrell R, Ashton S, et al. Comorbid clinical conditions in chronic fatigue: a co-twin control study. *J Gen Intern Med* 2001;16:24–31.
10. Arnold LM, Hudson JI, Hess EV, et al. Family study of fibromyalgia. *Arthritis Rheum* 2004;50:944–952.
11. Buchwald D, Herrell R, Ashton S, et al. A twin study of chronic fatigue. *Psychosom Med* 2001;63:936–943.
12. Bondy B, Spaeth M, Offenbaecher M, et al. The T102C polymorphism of the 5-HT2A-receptor gene in fibromyalgia. *Neurobiol Dis* 1999;6:433–439.
13. Gursoy S. Absence of association of the serotonin transporter gene polymorphism with the mentally healthy subset of fibromyalgia patients. *Clin Rheumatol* 2002;21:194–197.
14. Offenbaecher M, Bondy B, de Jonge S, et al. Possible association of fibromyalgia with a polymorphism in the serotonin transporter gene regulatory region. *Arthritis Rheum* 1999;42: 2482–2488.
15. Gursoy S, Erdal E, Herken H, et al. Significance of catechol-O-methyltransferase gene polymorphism in fibromyalgia syndrome. *Rheumatol Int* 2003;23:104–107.
16. Weaver IC, La Plante P, Weaver S, et al. Early environmental regulation of hippocampal glucocorticoid receptor gene expression: characterization of intracellular mediators and potential genomic target sites. *Mol Cell Endocrinol* 2001;185: 205–218.
17. Nemeroff CB. Neurobiological consequences of childhood trauma. *J Clin Psychiatry* 2004;65:18–28.
18. Buskila D, Neumann L, Vaisberg G, et al. Increased rates of fibromyalgia following cervical spine injury. *Arthritis Rheum* 1997;40:446–452.
19. Buskila D, Shnaider A, Neumann L, et al. Fibromyalgia in hepatitis C virus infection. Another infectious disease relationship. *Arch Intern Med* 1997;157:2497–2500.
20. Clauw DJ, Katz P. The overlap between fibromyalgia and inflammatory rheumatic diseases: when and why does it occur? *J Clin Rheumatol* 1995;1:335–341.
21. Daoud KF, Barkhuizen A. Rheumatic mimics and selected triggers of fibromyalgia. *Curr Pain Headache Rep* 2002;6: 284–288.
22. Dinerman H, Steere AC. Lyme disease associated with fibromyalgia. *Ann Intern Med* 1992;117:281–285.
23. Drossman DA. Irritable bowel syndrome and sexual/physical abuse history. *Eur J Gastroenterol Hepatol* 1997;9:327–330.
24. Crofford LJ, Demitrack MA. Evidence that abnormalities of central neurohormonal systems are key to understanding fibromyalgia and chronic fatigue syndrome. *Rheum Dis Clin North Am* 1996;22:267–284.
25. Sapolsky RM. Glucocorticoids, stress, and their adverse neurological effects: relevance to aging. *Exp Gerontol* 1999;34: 721–732.
26. Pillow DR, Zautra AJ, Sandler I. Major life events and minor stressors: identifying mediational links in the stress process. *J Pers Soc Psychol* 1996;70:381–394.
27. Van Houdenhove B, Neerinckx E, Onghena P, et al. Daily hassles reported by chronic fatigue syndrome and fibromyalgia patients in tertiary care: a controlled quantitative and qualitative study. *Psychother Psychosom* 2002;71:207–213.
28. Dailey PA, Bishop GD, Russell IJ, et al. Psychological stress and the fibrositis/fibromyalgia syndrome. *J Rheumatol* 1990; 17:1380–1385.

29. Williams DA, Brown SC, Clauw DJ, et al. Self-reported symptoms before and after September 11 in patients with fibromyalgia. *JAMA* 2003;289:1637–1638.

30. Raphael KG, Natelson BH, Janal MN, et al. A community-based survey of fibromyalgia-like pain complaints following the World Trade Center terrorist attacks. *Pain* 2002;100:131–139.

31. Gracely RH, Petzke F, Wolf JM, et al. Functional magnetic resonance imaging evidence of augmented pain processing in fibromyalgia. *Arthritis Rheum* 2002;46:1333–1343.

32. Staud R, Vierck CJ, Cannon RL, et al. Abnormal sensitization and temporal summation of second pain in patients with fibromyalgia syndrome. *Pain* 2001;91:165–175.

33. Staud R, Carl KE, Vierck CJ, et al. Repetitive muscle stimuli result in enhanced wind-up of fibromyalgia patients [Abstract]. *Arthritis Rheum* 2001;44:S395.

34. Staud R, Cannon RC, Mauderli AP, et al. Temporal summation of pain from mechanical stimulation of muscle tissue in normal controls and subjects with fibromyalgia syndrome. *Pain* 2003;102:87–95.

35. Price DD. Psychological and neural mechanisms of the affective dimension of pain. *Science* 2000;288:1769–1772.

36. Lorenz J, Grasedyck K, Bromm B. Middle and long latency somatosensory evoked potentials after painful laser stimulation in patients with fibromyalgia syndrome. *EEG Clin Neurophysiol* 1996;100:165–168.

37. Welin M, Bragee B, Nyberg F, et al. Elevated substance P levels are contrasted by a decrease in met-enkephalin-arg-phe levels in CSF from fibromyalgia patients [Abstract]. *J Musculoskelet Pain* 1995;3:4.

38. Vaeroy H, Helle R, Forre O, et al. Elevated CSF levels of substance P and high incidence of Raynaud's phenomenon in patients with fibromyalgia: new features for diagnosis. *Pain* 1988;32:21–26.

39. Russell IJ, OM D, Lettman B, et al. Elevated cerebrospinal levels of substance P in patients with the fibromyalgia syndrome. *Arthritis Rheum* 1994;37:1593–1601.

40. Russell IJ, Vaeroy H, Javors M, et al. Cerebrospinal fluid biogenic amine metabolites in fibromyalgia/fibrositis syndrome and rheumatoid arthritis. *Arthritis Rheum* 1992;35:550–556.

41. Legangneux E, Mora JJ, Spreux-Varoquaux O, et al. Cerebrospinal fluid biogenic amine metabolites, plasma-rich platelet serotonin and [3H]imipramine reuptake in the primary fibromyalgia syndrome. *Rheumatology* 2001;40:290–296.

42. Larson AA, Giovengo SL, Russell IJ, et al. Changes in the concentrations of amino acids in the cerebrospinal fluid that correlate with pain in patients with fibromyalgia: implications for nitric oxide pathways. *Pain* 2000;87:201–211.

43. Giovengo SL, Russell IJ, Larson AA. Increased concentrations of nerve growth factor in cerebrospinal fluid of patients with fibromyalgia. *J Rheumatol* 1999;26:1564–1569.

44. Gracely RH, Grant MAB, Giesecke T. Evoked pain measures in fibromyalgia. *Best Pract Res Clin Rheumatol* 2003;17:593–609.

45. Dworkin RH, Backonja M, Rowbotham MC, et al. Advances in neuropathic pain: diagnosis, mechanisms, and treatment recommendations. *Arch Neurol* 2003;60:1524–1534.

46. Watkins LR, Milligan ED, Maier SF. Glial proinflammatory cytokines mediate exaggerated pain states: implications for clinical pain. *Adv Exp Med Biol* 2003;521:1–21.

47. Milligan ED, Twining C, Chacur M, et al. Spinal glia and proinflammatory cytokines mediate mirror-image neuropathic pain in rats. *J Neurosci* 2003;23:1026–1040.

48. Yunus MB, Masi AT, Calabro JJ, et al. Primary fibromyalgia (fibrositis): clinical study of 50 patients with matched normal controls. *Semin Arthritis Rheum* 1981;11:151–171.

49. Yunus MB, Ahles TA, Aldag JC, et al. Relationship of clinical features with psychological status in primary fibromyalgia. *Arthritis Rheum* 1991;34:15–21.

50. Hudson JI, Pope HGJ. The relationship between fibromyalgia and major depressive disorder. *Rheum Dis Clin North Am* 1996;22:285–303.

51. White KP, Harth M. To lump or to split. The importance of tender points. *J Rheumatol* 2001;28:2362–2363.

52. Wolfe F, Hawley DJ, Wilson K. The prevalence and meaning of fatigue in rheumatic disease. *J Rheumatol* 1996;23:1407–1417.

53. Wolfe F, Skevington SM. Measuring the epidemiology of distress: the rheumatology distress index. *J Rheumatol* 2000;27:2000–2009.

54. McBeth J, Macfarlane GJ, Hunt IM, et al. Risk factors for persistent chronic widespread pain: a community-based study. *Rheumatology* 2001;40:95–101.

55. White KP, Nielson WR, Harth M. Chronic widespread musculoskeletal pain with or without fibromyalgia: psychological distress in a representative community adult sample. *J Rheumatol* 2002;29:588–594.

56. Jones DA, Rollman GB, White KP, et al. The relationship between cognitive appraisal, affect, and catastrophizing in patients with chronic pain. *J Pain* 2003;4:267–277.

57. Crofford LJ. Neuroendocrine abnormalities in fibromyalgia and related disorders. *Am J Med Sci* 1998;315:359–366.

58. Crofford LJ, Neeck G. Neuroendocrine perturbations in fibromyalgia and chronic fatigue syndrome. *Rheum Dis Clin North Am* 2000;26:989–1002.

59. Chrousos GP, Gold PW. The concepts of stress and stress system disorders: overview of physical and behavioral homeostasis. *JAMA* 1992;267:1244–1252.

60. Rosmond R, Dallman MF, Bjorntorp P. Stress-related cortisol secretion in men: relationships with abdominal obesity and endocrine, metabolic and hemodynamic abnormalities. *J Clin Endocrinol Metab* 1998;83:1853–1859.

61. Pruessner JC, Hellhammer DH, Kirschbaum C. Burnout, perceived stress, and cortisol responses to awakening. *Psychosom Med* 1999;61:197–204.

62. Steptoe A, Cropley M, Griffith J, et al. Job strain and anger expression predict early morning elevations in salivary cortisol. *Psychosom Med* 2000;62:286–292.

63. Wust S, Federenko I, Hellhammer DH, et al. Genetic factors, perceived chronic stress, and the free cortisol response to awakening. *Psychoneuroendocrinology* 2000;25:707–720.

64. Heim C, Newport DJ, Heit S, et al. Pituitary-adrenal and autonomic responses to stress in women after sexual and physical abuse in childhood. *JAMA* 2000;284:592–597.

65. Van Cauter E, LeProult R, Kupfer DJ. Effects of gender and age on the levels and circadian rhythmicity of plasma cortisol. *J Clin Endocrinol Metab* 1996;81:2468–2473.

66. Holsboer F. The rationale for corticotropin-releasing hormone receptor (CRH-R) antagonists to treat depression and anxiety. *J Psychiatr Res* 1999;33:181–214.

67. Petzke F, Clauw DJ. Sympathetic nervous system function in fibromyalgia. *Curr Rheum Rep* 2000;2:116–123.

68. Cohen H, Neumann L, Alhosshle A, et al. Abnormal sympathovagal balance in men with fibromyalgia. *J Rheumatol* 2001;28:581–589.

69. Raj SR, Brouillard D, Simpson CS, et al. Dysautonomia among patients with fibromyalgia: a non-invasive assessment. *J Rheumatol* 2000;27:2660–2665.

70. Cohen H, Neumann L, Shore M, et al. Autonomic dysfunction in patients with fibromyalgia: application of power spectral analysis of heart rate variability. *Semin Arthritis Rheum* 2000;29:217–227.

71. Martinez-Lavin M, Hermosillo AG, Rosas M, et al. Circadian studies of autonomic nervous balance in patients with

fibromyalgia: a heart rate variability analysis. *Arthritis Rheum* 1998;41:1966–1971.

72. Kelemen J, Lang E, Balint G, et al. Orthostatic sympathetic derangement of baroreflex in patients with fibromyalgia. *J Rheumatol* 1998;25:823–825.

73. Rowe PC, Bou-Holaigah I, Kan JS, et al. Is neurally mediated hypotension an unrecognised cause of chronic fatigue? *Lancet* 1995;345:623–624.

74. Moldofsky H, Scarisbrick P, England R, et al. Musculoskeletal symptoms and non-REM sleep disturbance in patients with "fibrositis syndrome" and healthy subjects. *Psychosom Med* 1975;37:341–351.

75. Moldofsky H, Scarisbrick P. Induction of neurasthenic musculoskeletal pain syndrome by selective sleep stage deprivation. *Psychosom Med* 1976;38:35–44.

76. Rains JC, Penzien DB. Sleep and chronic pain: challenges to the alpha-EEG sleep pattern as a pain specific sleep anomaly. *J Psychosom Res* 2003;54:77–83.

77. Horne JA, Shackell BS. Alpha-like EEG activity in non-REM sleep and the fibromyalgia (fibrositis) syndrome. *EEG Clin Neurophysiol* 1991;79:271–276.

78. Jennum P, Drewes AM, Andreasen A, et al. Sleep and other symptoms in primary fibromylagia and in healthy controls. *J Rheumatol* 1993;20:1756–1759.

79. Drewes AM, Gade J, Nielsen KD, et al. Clustering of sleep electroencephalographic patterns in patients with the fibromyalgia syndrome. *Br J Rheumatol* 1995;34:1151–1156.

80. Branco J, Atalaia A, Paiva T. Sleep cycles and alpha-delta sleep in fibromylagia syndrome. *J Rheumatol* 1994;21:1113–1117.

81. Roizenblatt S, Moldofsky H, Benedito-Silva AA, et al. Alpha sleep characteristics in fibromyalgia. *Arthritis Rheum* 2001;44:222–230.

82. Park DC, Glass JM, Minear M, et al. Cognitive function in fibromyalgia patients. *Arthritis Rheum* 2001;44:2125–2133.

83. Grace GM, Nielson WR, Hopkins M, et al. Concentration and memory deficits in patients with fibromyalgia syndrome. *J Clin Exp Neuropsychol* 1999;21:477–487.

84. Suhr JA. Neuropsychological impairment in fibromyalgia. Relation to depression, fatigue, and pain. *J Psychosom Res* 2003;55:321–329.

85. Williams DA. Psychological and behavioural therapies in fibromyalgia and related syndromes. *Best Pract Res Clin Rheumatol* 2003;17:649–665.

86. Doeglas D, Suurmeijer T, Briancon S. An international study on measuring social support: interactions and satisfaction. *Soc Sci Med* 1996;43:1389–1397.

87. Smarr KL, Parker JC, Wright GE, et al. The importance of enhancing self-efficacy in rheumatoid arthritis. *Arthritis Care Res* 1997;10:18–26.

88. Reisine S, Fifield J, Walsh SJ, et al. Do employment and family work affect the health status of women with fibromyalgia? *J Rheumatol* 2003;30:2045–2053.

89. Burckhardt CS, Clark SR, Bennett RM. The fibromyalgia impact questionnaire: development and validation. *J Rheumatol* 1991;18:728–733.

90. Arnold LM, Hess EV, Hudson JI, et al. A randomized, placebo-controlled, double-blind, flexible-dose study of fluoxetine in the treatment of women with fibromyalgia. *Am J Med* 2002;112:191–197.

Appendix
Informational Resources

Compiled by Lynne K. Matallana

Fibromyalgia can be a very confusing syndrome, and a wealth of information and misinformation is available from a variety of web and nonweb-based sources representing different viewpoints, interests, and constituencies. The following list is not intended to be comprehensive, and the editors of this book do not necessarily endorse any of the listings. They are simply provided to the reader as reasonably reliable resources containing repositories of information. Organizations often change their mailing addresses, and checking a current address from a website is advised. The NFA welcomes any additions or corrections to this compilation and feel free to contact us at www.FMaware.org.

ORGANIZATIONS (NONPROFIT)

National Fibromyalgia Association (NFA)
2200 N. Glassell Street, Suite A
Orange, CA 92865
(714) 921-0150
www.FMaware.org

American College of Rheumatology
1800 Century Place, Suite 250
Atlanta, GA 30345-4300
(404) 633-3777
www.rheumatology.org

American Academy of Pain Medicine
13947 Mono Way #A
Sonora, CA 95370
(209) 533-9744
www.painmed.org

American Academy of Physical Medicine
   and Rehabilitation
One IBM Plaza, Suite 2500
Chicago, IL 60611
(312) 464-9700
www.aapmr.org

National Institute of Arthritis and Musculoskeletal
   and Skin Disease
National Institutes of Health
1 AMS Circle
Bethesda, MD 20892-3675
(301) 495-4484 or (877) 22-NIAMS (toll-free)
www.niams.nih.gov

American Pain Society
4700 W. Lake Avenue
Glenview, IL 60025
(847) 375-4715
www.ampainsoc.org

Fibromyalgia Network/American Fibromyalgia
   Syndrome Association
6380 E. Tanque Verde, Suite D
Tucson, AZ 85715
(520) 733-1570
www.afsafund.org

Fibromyalgia Association UK
P.O. Box 206, Stourbridge
DY9 8YL England
www.fibromyalgia-associationuk.org

Oregon Fibromyalgia Foundation
1221 S.W. Yarnhill, Suite 303
Portland, OR 97205
www.myalgia.com

American Pain Foundation
201 N. Charles Street, Suite 710
Baltimore, MD 21201-4111
www.painfoundation.org

International Myopain Society
Barbara Runnels, M.Ed.
IMS Administrative Officer
P.O. Box 690402
San Antonio, TX 78269
(210) 567-4661
www.myopain.org

American Association for Chronic Fatigue Syndrome
27 N. Wacker Drive
Suite 416
Chicago, IL 60606
(847) 258-7248
www.aacfs.org/html/cvs.htm

CFIDS Association
P.O. Box 220398
Charlotte, NC 28222-0398
(704) 365-2343
www.cfids.org

National Family Caregivers Association (NFCA)
10400 Connecticut Avenue, #500
Kensington, MD 20895-3944
(800) 896-3650
www.nfcacares.org

National Headache Foundation
820 N. Orleans, Suite 217
Chicago, IL 60610
(888) NHF-5552
www.headaches.org

National Women's Health Resource Center
157 Broad Street, Suite 315
Red Bank, NJ 07701
(877) 986-9472
www.healthywomen.org

Association for Applied Psychophysiology and Biofeedback
10200 W. 44th Avenue, Suite 304
Wheat Ridge, CO 80033-2840
(303) 422-8436
www.aapb.org

Lupus Foundation of America, Inc.
2000 L Street, N.W., Suite 710
Washington, DC 20036
(202) 349-1155
www.lupus.org

Lupus Research Institute
149 Madison, #205
New York, NY 10016
(212) 685-4118
www.lupusresearchinstitute.org

American Chronic Pain Association
P.O. Box 850
Rocklin, CA 95677
(800) 533-3231
www.theacpa.org

American Lyme Disease Foundation, Inc.
Mill Pond Offices
293 Route 100
Somers, NY 10589
(914) 277-6970
www.aldf.com

American Massage Therapy Association
820 Davis Street
Evanston, IL 60201
(847) 864-0123
www.amtamassage.org

For Grace- RSD
605 W. Olympic Boulevard
Suite 800
Los Angeles, CA 90015
(818) 760-7635
forgrace.org/whatsnew.html

Arthritis Foundation
P.O. Box 7669
Atlanta, GA 30357-0669
(800) 283-7800
www.arthritis.org

AARP
601 E. Street N.W.
Washington, DC 20049
(888) 687-2277
www.aarp.org

National Fibromyalgia Research Association
P.O. Box 500
Salem, OR 97302
www.nfra.net/Reslist.htm

INFORMATIONAL WEBSITES

ImmuneSupport.com
www.immunesupport.com/library/showarticle.cfm/ID/
   3724/e/1/T/CFIDS_FM

Remedy Find
www.remedyfind.com

Teen & Young Adult Guide to FMS
www.angelfire.com/on/teenfms/teenfms.html

Directory of Prescription Drug Patient
   Assistance Programs
www.phrma.org/patients

Healing Well
www.healingwell.com

Co-Cure
www.co-cure.org

Disability—Joshua Potter, Esq.
www2.rpa.net/~lrandall/ssdi_fms.html

Disability—Scott Davis, Esq.
www.disability@scottdavispc.com/articles.html

BioMed Central
www.biomedcentral.com/1523-3774/2?issue=2

Web MD
my.webmd.com/medical_information/
   condition_centersfibromyalgia/default.htm

Web MD
boards.webmd.com/topic.asp?topic_id=92

Medline Plus
www.nlm.nih.gov/medlineplus/fibromyalgia.html

Job Accommodation Network
www.jan.wvu.edu/media/Fibro.html

Co-cure
www.co-cure.org

Government Trials
clinicaltrials.gov/ct/gui/c/w2r/screen/
BrowseAny?recruiting=true&path=%2Fbrowse%2Fby-
condition%2Faz%2FF%2FD005356%2BFibromyalgia&
JServSessionIdzone_ct=yd6zioc151

MedicineNet.com
www.medicinenet.com/script/main/srchcont.asp?SRC=fibr
omyalgia&op=MM

Needy Meds.com
www.needymeds.com

National Sleep Foundation
www.nsaw.org/sleepIQ99i.cfm

U.S. Food & Drug Administration
Food and Drug Interactions
vm.cfsan.fda.gov/~lrd/fdinter.html

Social Security Online
www.ssa.gov/disability

Medline Plus
www.nlm.nih.gov/medlineplus/fibromyalgia.html

Marrtc
www.muhealth.org/~fibro

University of Maryland
www.umm.edu/patiented/articles/what_fibromyalgia_its_sy
mptoms_000076_1.htm

Bibliography of Fibromyalgia Research
www.muhealth.org/~fibro/fmbib.html

Frequently Asked Questions – David Nye, M.D.
www.muhealth.org/~fibro/fm-pt.html

IBS Support
www.ibsgroup.org

Depression.Com
www.depression.com

Restless Legs Syndrome Foundation
www.rls.org

Aquatic Resources Network
www.aquaticnet.com

Arthritis Foundation
www.arthritis.org

BOOKS

Backstrom G with Dr. Bernard Rubin. *When muscle pain won't go away: the relief handbook for fibromyalgia and chronic muscle pain*, 3rd ed. Dallas, TX: Taylor Publishing Company, 1998.

Balch JF, Phyllis A. *Prescription for nutritional healing: a practical A-Z reference to drug-free remedies using vitamins, minerals, herbs & food supplements*. New York: Avery Publishing Group, 2003.

Brown EH. *Healing joint pain naturally*. New York: Broadway Books, 2001.

Bieglow SL. *Fibromyalgia: simple relief through movement*. New York: John Wiley and Sons, 2000.

Dotterer B, Davidson P. *Understanding fibromyalgia, a guide for family and friends*. Stateline, NV: Healthroad Productions, 1996.

Farhi D. *The breathing book*. New York: Henry Holt and Company, 1996.

Fennell PA. *The chronic illness workbook: strategies and solutions for taking back your life*. Oakland, CA: New Harbinger Publications, 2001.

Fransen Jenny RN, Jon Russell I. *The fibromyalgia help book*. St. Paul, MN: Smith House Press, 1996:241.

Goldstein J MD. *Betrayal by the brain: the neurologic basis of chronic fatigue syndrome, fibromyalgia syndrome, and related neural network disorders*. New York: The Haworth Medical Press, 1996.

Goldenberg DL. *Fibromyalgia: understanding and getting relief from pain that won't go away*. London: Piatkus Books, 2002.

Langenfeld C, Douglas L. *Hope and encouragement for people with chronic illness; living better: every patient's guide to living with illness*. Dublin, OH: Patient Press, 2001.

Lasater J. *Relax & renew*. Berkeley, CA: Rodmell Press, 1995.

Matallana LK. *HealthSmart: fibromyalgia personal care organizer*. New York: Penguin Putnam Publishing, 2004.

NFA Book Store. www.fmaware.org/bookstore.htm, 2005

Pellegrino M. *The fibromyalgia survivor*: Columbus, OH: Anadem Publishing, 1995.

Pellegrino M. *Understanding post-traumatic fibromyalgia*. Anadem Publishing, 1996.

Pellegrino M. *The fibromyalgia supporter*. Columbus, OH: Anadem Publishing, 1997.

Pellegrino M. *From whiplash to fibromyalgia*. Columbus, OH: Anadem Publishing, 2003.

Piburn G. *Beyond chaos, one man's journey alongside his chronically Ill wife*. Atlanta, GA: Arthritis Foundation, 1999.

Russell IJ. *The journal of musculoskeletal pain*. TX: The Haworth Medical Press, 2003.

Simmons K. *Natural treatments for fibromyalgia*. Atlanta, GA: Arthritis Foundation, 2003.

Staud R, Christine A. *Fibromyalgia for dummies*. New York: John Wiley and Sons, 2002.

Teitelbaum J. *From fatigued to fantastic*. New York: Avery Publishing Group, 2001.

Wallace DJ, Wallace JB. *All about fibromyalgia: a guide for patients and their families*. New York: Oxford University Press, 2002. (hardcover). (Previous editions were titled "Making sense of fibromyalgia")

Wallace DJ, Wallace JB. *Fibromyalgia: an essential guide for their families and friends*. New York: Oxford University Press, 2003. (paperback)

Williamson ME, Mary AS. *The fibromyalgia relief book: 213 ideas for improving your quality of life*. New York: Walker Publisher, 1998.

MAGAZINES/JOURNALS

Fibromyalgia AWARE Magazine
www.FMaware.org/magazine.html

Digestive Health & Nutrition
www.dhn-online.org

Massage Magazine
www.massagemag.com

Yoga Journal
www.yogajournal.com

Journal of Woman's Health
www.liebertpub.com/jwh/default1.asp

Journal of Chronic Fatigue Syndrome
www.cfs-news.org/jcfs.htm

Journal of Musculoskeletal Pain
www.haworthpress.com/store/Toc/J094v07n01_TOC.pdf

VIDEOS

Exercise
Dr. Sharon Clark
www.myalgia.com

Self Management: A Multi-Disciplined Approach
National Fibromyalgia Association
fmaware.org/store.htm

Associated Symptoms and Diagnostics in FM
National Fibromyalgia Association
fmaware.org/store.htm

Good Moves for Every Body
University of Missouri Arthritis Rehabilitation Research
    and Training Center
www.muhealth.org/~arthritis/gdmvvid.html

INDEX